Contemporary Psychiatric-Mental Health Nursing

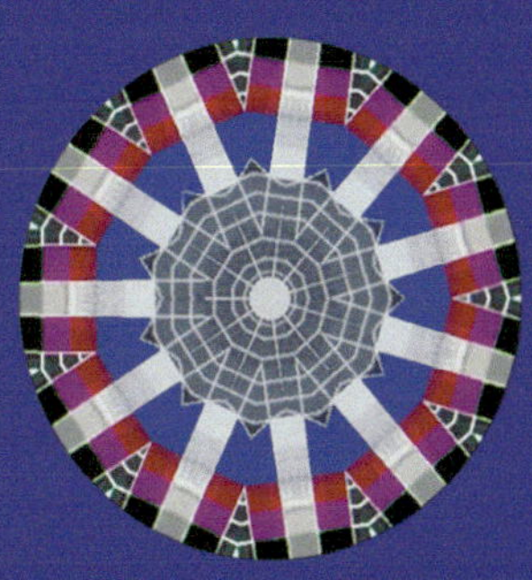
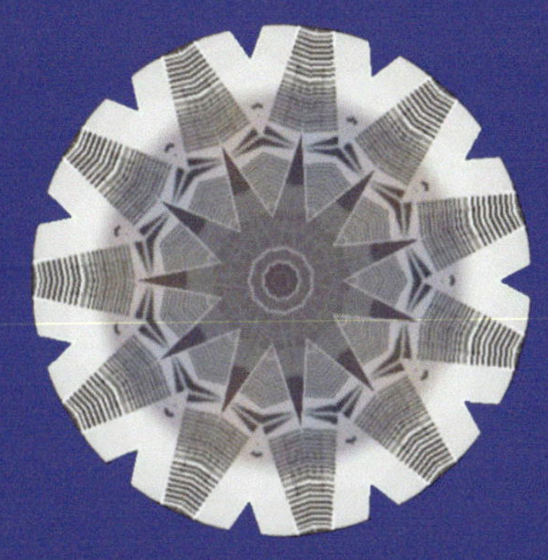

Contemporary Psychiatric-Mental Health Nursing

PARTNERSHIPS IN CARE

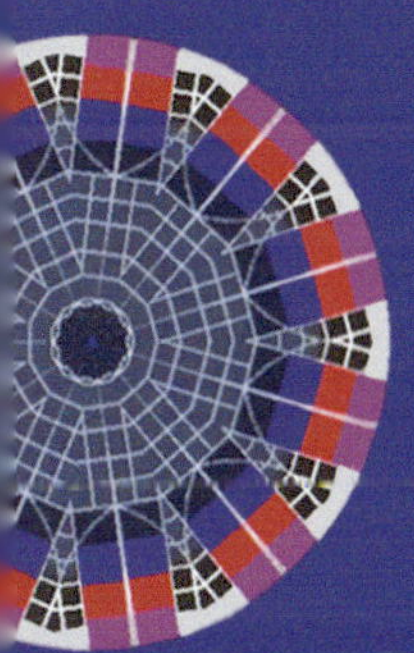
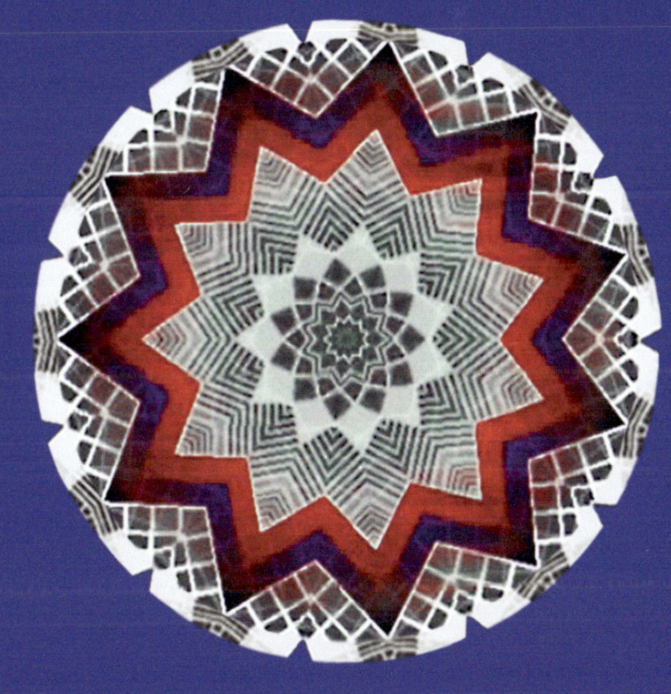
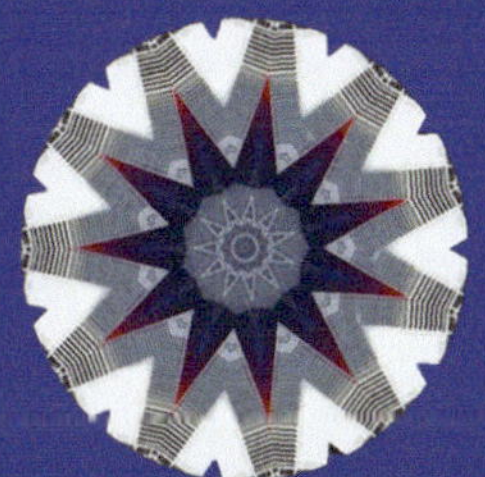
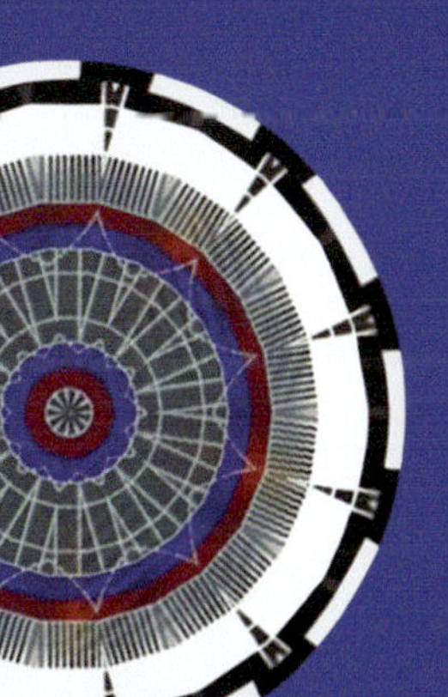

MOXHAM
HAZELTON
MUIR-COCHRANE
HEFFERNAN
KNEISL
TRIGOBOFF

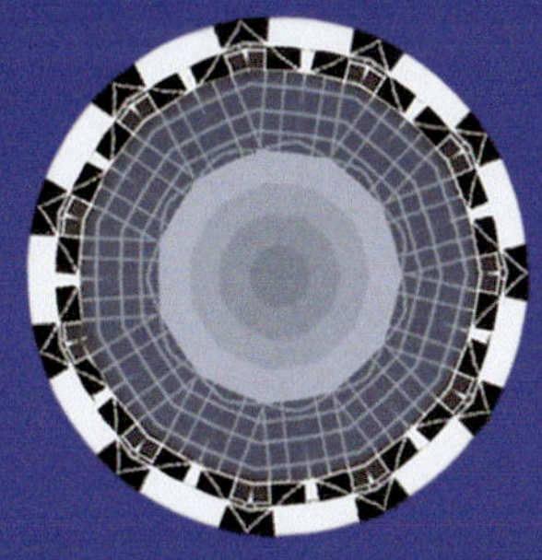

Pearson Australia
707 Collins Street
Melbourne Vic 3008

www.pearson.com.au

Authorised adaptation from the United States edition, entitled CONTEMPORARY PSYCHIATRIC–MENTAL HEALTH NURSING, 3rd Edition, ISBN: 0132557770 by KNEISL, CAROL REN; TRIGOBOFF, EILEEN, published by Pearson Education, Inc, Copyright © 2013.

First adaptation edition published by PEARSON AUSTRALIA GROUP PTY LTD., Copyright 2018.

Senior Portfolio Manager: Mandy Sheppard
Development Editor: Anna Carter
Project Manager: Bronwyn Smith
Editorial and Design Production Manager: Bernadette Chang
Copyright and Pictures Editor: Emma Gaulton
Production Controller: Bradley Smith
Content Developer: Stephen Razos
Lead Editor/Copy Editor: Kate Stone
Proofreader: Maryanne Phillips
Indexer: Graham Clayton
Cover and internal design by Nada Backovic
Typeset by iEnergizer/Aptara®, Ltd.
Printed and bound in Australia by Pegasus Media & Logistics

Cover illustration by Karen Casey. Karen is an Australian interdisciplinary artist who employs a combination of traditional and new media techniques, exploring intersections between the arts, science and society. She has a broad and diverse creative practice spanning printmaking, digital media and public art. She unites her own indigenous perspective of connection to land with a practical and philosophical understanding of the interrelationships between various cultural and spiritual beliefs, along with contemporary Western science.

This publication has been thoroughly checked and reviewed to ensure that procedures, treatments and dosages are as accurate as possible at the time of publication. However, due to ongoing research and changes in regulations, it is advised that the reader verify information described in this book. Neither the authors, contributors nor publisher assume any liability for adverse effects arising from any error in or omission from this publication.

1 2 3 4 5 22 21 20 19 18

National Library of Australia
Cataloguing-in-Publication Data

Creator:	Moxham, Lorna, author.
Title:	Contemporary psychiatric–mental health nursing : partnerships in care / Lorna Moxham [and five] others.
ISBN:	9781486023905 (paperback)
Notes:	Includes index.
Subjects:	Psychiatric nursing—Study and teaching. Mental health services—Australia. Mental health services—New Zealand. Nursing students—Handbooks, manuals, etc.

Pearson Australia Group Pty Ltd ABN 40 004 245 943

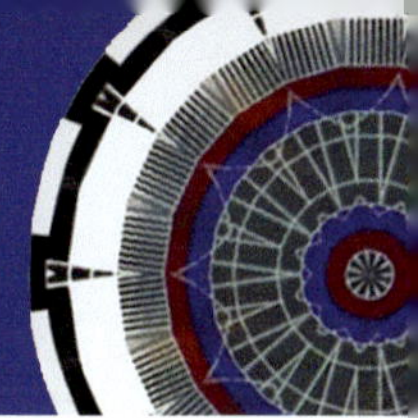

BRIEF CONTENTS

DETAILED CONTENTS

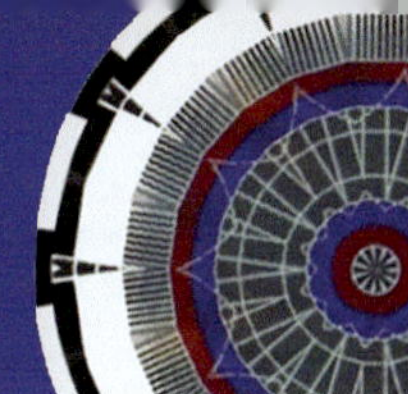

ABOUT THE AUTHORS

LOCAL AUTHORS

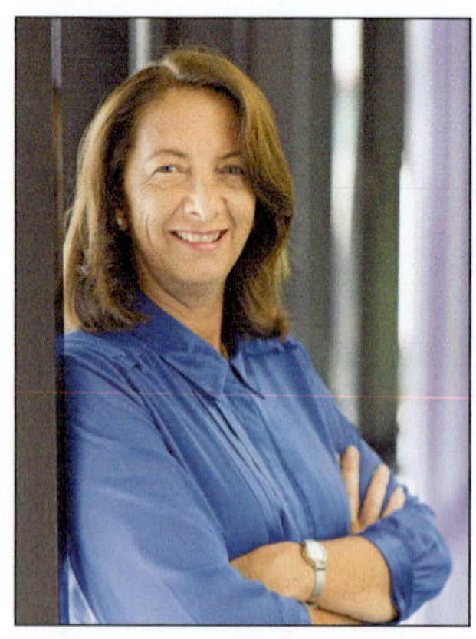

LORNA MOXHAM RN, MHN, PHD, BHSC (UWS), DAS (NSG) (MIHE), MED (UNSW), CERT OH&S (CQU), CERT QUAL MGMT (CQU), CERT IV (TRAINING & ASSESSMENT) (CQIT), FACMHN, FCON

Lorna Moxham is Professor of Mental Health Nursing in the Faculty of Science, Medicine and Health, and the lead for Living Well, Longer in the Global Challenges programme at the University of Wollongong, NSW, Australia. In addition, Lorna is a director of Recovery Camp—http://recoverycamp.com.au. Lorna has been Head of School and Dean of Graduate Research as well as holding numerous other senior governance roles like Chair: Research Committee of Academic Board, and Chair: University Human Research Ethics Committee.

Initially qualified as a registered psychiatric nurse, Lorna continued her passion for lifelong learning, graduating from the University of Western Sydney with a Diploma of Applied Science and Bachelor of Health Science, achieving Golden Key International Honour Society status. She then graduated from the University of New South Wales with a Master's of Education. Lorna also has two Certificates: one in Occupational Health & Safety and one in Quality Management. Additionally she has a PhD.

Lorna has held numerous senior professional and community appointments, including four at ministerial level. These include Chair: Central Queensland Health Community Council, Mental Health Review Tribunal, Regional Planning Advisory Committee and the Queensland Priority Housing Committee. Additionally, Lorna was a board director for Central Queensland Mercy Health and Aged Care, and the Australian College of Mental Health Nurses, and a member of the Executive for the Australian and New Zealand Council of Deans of Nursing and Midwifery. She is a Fellow of the Australian College of Mental Health Nurses and also the Australian College of Nursing.

Passionate about research supervision and the important contributions HDR (higher degree research) students make to research and development, Lorna has twice been awarded a Vice Chancellor's award for Excellence in Research Supervision from two Australian universities. She has supervised numerous students to successful completion, and been invited to examine many doctoral dissertations. Lorna is a prolific author with numerous publications, including 18 books as editor and/or co-author, 16 book chapters, over 80 journal articles and more than 100 conference presentations. Lorna considers this particular book—co-authored with people who have a lived experience—to be particularly rewarding.

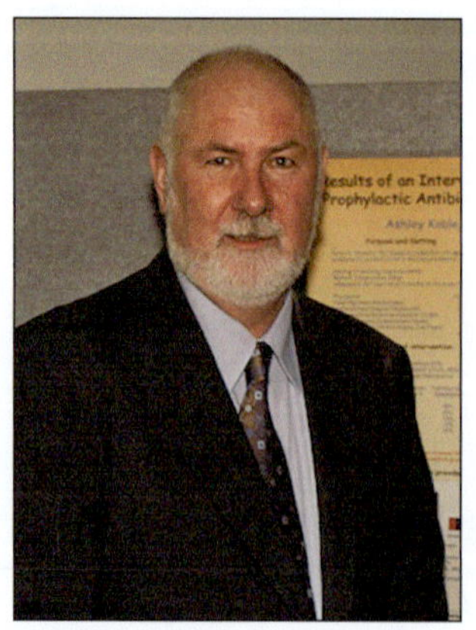

MICHAEL HAZELTON RN BA MA PHD FACMNH (LIFE MEMBER)

Mike Hazelton is Professor of Mental Health Nursing in the School of Nursing and Midwifery, the University of Newcastle, Australia. He is a former Head of Nursing and Midwifery at Newcastle, and also Curtin University and the University of Tasmania, and has been involved in nurse education generally and mental health nurse education specifically for over 30 years. Mike has published over 90 articles, abstracts, books and book chapters on mental health and mental health nursing, and has undertaken consultancies for various governments in Australia. Mike is a former editor of the *International Journal of Mental Health Nursing*, and a current member of the Editorial Advisory Board of the *Australian and New Zealand Journal of Psychiatry*. He has been awarded a number of awards for his research, and is a Life Member of the Australian College of Mental Health Nurses, the highest honour awarded by that professional organisation.

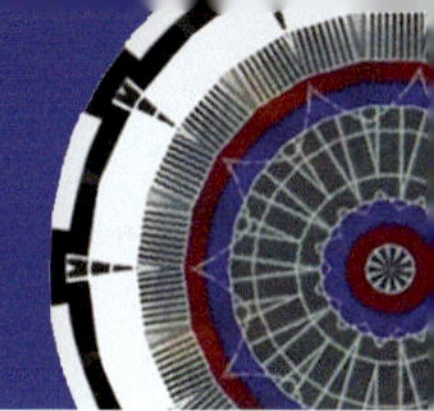

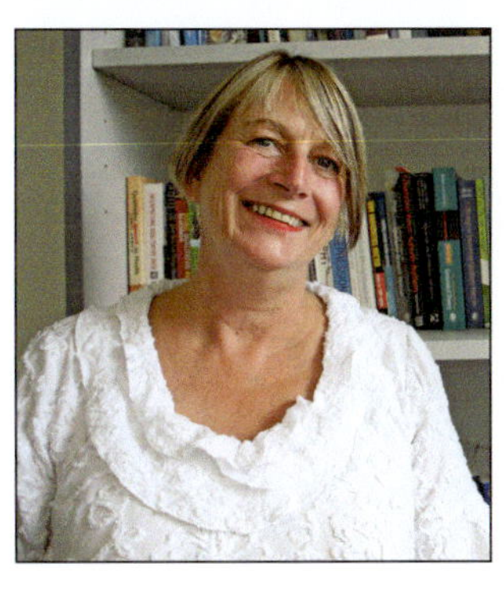

EIMEAR MUIR-COCHRANE BSC (HONS), RN, RMN, GRAD DIP ADULT EDUCATION, MNS, PHD CREDENTIALLED MHN, FELLOW ACMHN

Professor Eimear Muir-Cochrane is Chair of Nursing (Mental Health) and Chair of Senate at Flinders University, Australia, and has been involved in mental health education and research for over 30 years. Eimear has been an architect and course coordinator of mental health courses in undergraduate nursing and postgraduate mental health since 1991. She is also leader of the mental health teaching and research teams at the Faculty of Medicine, Nursing and Health Sciences, Flinders University, a position she has held since 2008. Eimear has provided leadership through Associate Editorship at three national and international journals in Great Britain, Australia and Japan.

Educational research includes the use of new technologies, mental health in education in virtual reality, mental health and culture and communication practices. Eimear has received multiple university awards and grants in Teaching Excellence and has been a awarded a Carrick Citation for Excellence in Australian University Teaching, a Department of Health, South Australia Nurse Excellence Award, and won Best Paper at the National Nurse Education Conference for a paper entitled 'The Book, the MOOC and the App!'

Eimear's outputs include authorship of one book in its third edition, one optimised mobile device, two monographs, over 80 refereed journal articles, multiple keynote invitations to speak and present multiple national and international conference papers. Eimear's research interests focus on the care of the acutely unwell psychiatric patient, and include examination of absconding, restraint and seclusion, with nationally and internationally funded competitive research totalling $2.8 million.

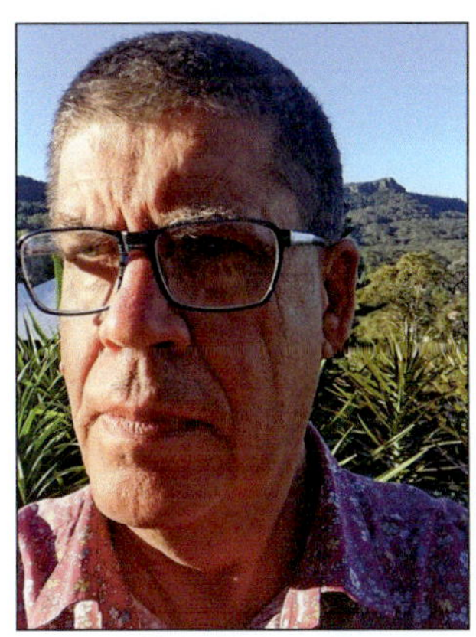

TIM HEFFERNAN

Tim Heffernan is the Mental Health Peer Coordinator for Coordinare, the South East Sydney Primark Health Network, a role to which he brings his lived experience of bipolar 1 disorder and recovery, which began with his first episode of psychosis in 1983. Prior to this position, he worked for almost a decade as a peer support worker with Illawarra Shoalhaven Local Health District. He chaired the NSW Consumer Workers Committee from 2014 to 2017, and is a former member and chair of the Being (NSW Consumer Advisory Group) Board of Trustees. Tim is an executive member of the Illawarra Shoalhaven's Suicide Prevention Collaborative, and has been a member of the NSW Mental Health Commission's Community Advisory Council since its inception in 2014. He is a member of the Agency for Clinical Innovation's Metal Health Network Executive Committee. Tim is also part of the University of Wollongong's Recovery Camp team.

In 2013 Tim participated in Boston University's Centre for Psychiatric Rehabilitation Global Leadership Institute, with a trauma-informed, co-designed, co-delivered alternative to traditional 'aggression management' training called 'Safety for All'. He participated in the National Mental Health Commission/University of Melbourne's Seclusion and Restraint Lived Experience Advisory Group. Tim has been a volunteer rural and regional ambassador and community presenter for the Black Dog Institute since 2007.

An experienced public speaker, Tim has presented papers and led workshops on peer work, consumer-led research and 'mad' poetry at mental health conferences in Sydney, Perth, Canberra, Melbourne and Auckland. He worked for over 20 years as a high-school English teacher, and has published research with the National Schools Network. He has also worked as a disability support worker.

Tim is a poet and he co-edits an online space for 'mad' creative writing—Verity La's 'Clozapine Clinic – The Frater Project'.

US AUTHORS

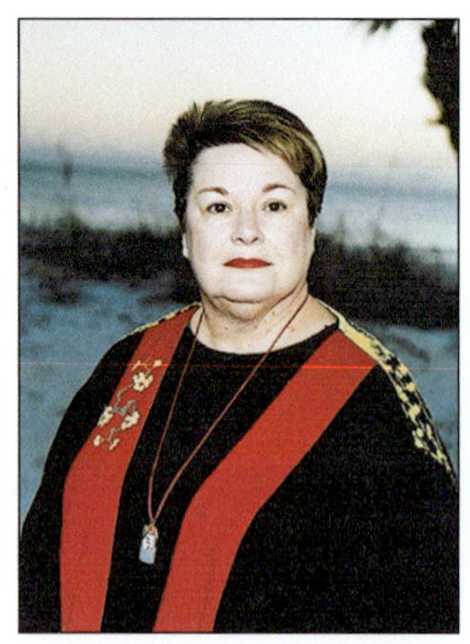

CAROL REN KNEISL RN, MS, APRN, DABFN

Carol Kneisl has had a variety of psychiatric–mental health nursing experiences. She has taught psychiatric–mental health nursing in diploma, baccalaureate and master's programs that prepared clinical specialists in psychiatric–mental health nursing. She has been a staff nurse, a nurse manager, a nursing supervisor and a clinical nurse specialist, and has supervised the group therapy of clinical nurse specialists and psychiatry medical residents. She is currently an adjunct professor of psychiatric–mental health nursing at William Carey University in New Orleans, Louisiana.

Carol is also a nurse entrepreneur. She founded Nursing Transitions, a corporation that provided continuing education for psychiatric–mental health and corrections/forensic nurses. Her company sponsored the first national nursing conference focused on AIDS. She is a national and international speaker, and consults with nurses and mental health and forensic agencies on topics such as group therapy, stress management, self-awareness issues and strategies, implementation of client rights, legal aspects, and creative clinical teaching in psychiatric–mental health nursing.

She has authored or contributed to 28 nursing textbooks and several nursing journals. She has been an associate editor of a psychiatric nursing review journal, and has served on several editorial boards.

Carol was among the first nurses in the country to develop clinical specialist certification, in conjunction with nurses from New York and New Jersey. Their work formed the basis for the national certification granted through the American Nurses Credentialing Center of the American Nurses Association.

She is a graduate of a diploma school, the Millard Fillmore Hospital School of Nursing in Buffalo, New York, from which she received the Alumna of the Century award on the occasion of the school's 100-year anniversary. Carol has a BS in nursing from the University of Buffalo, an MS in nursing as a clinical nurse specialist in adult psychiatric–mental health nursing from the University of California at San Francisco, and has pursued graduate education in community mental health administration and interpersonal communication from the State University of New York at Buffalo.

Carol is the mother of two adult children—a daughter who is a right-brained special-effects artist, and a son who is a left-brained mathematician and the father of her two grandchildren. When she is not commuting to New Orleans, she writes and consults from her home on a Gulf of Mexico beach, in Orange Beach, Alabama.

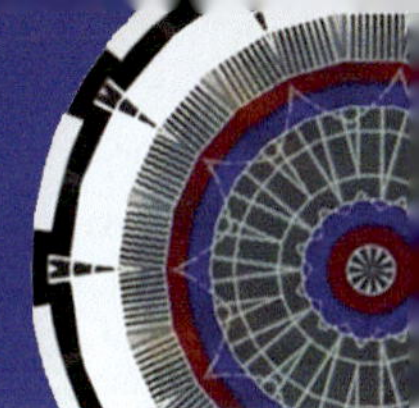

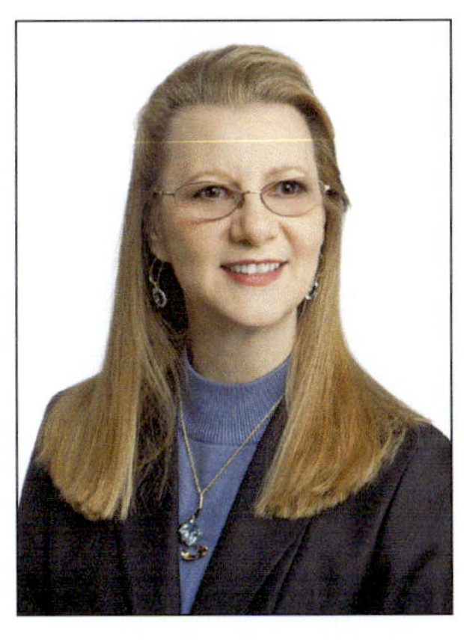

EILEEN TRIGOBOFF RN, PMHCNS-BC, DNS, DABFN, CIP

Eileen Trigoboff is a Clinical Nurse Specialist with a specialty in adult psychiatry/mental health in a private psychotherapy practice in western New York. An important part of her practice is the national and international interdisciplinary supervision of, and consultation with, other mental health and health care professionals. Eileen is the Director of Program Evaluation at the Buffalo Psychiatric Center in Buffalo, New York, and is the Liaison for the Office of Mental Health's Institutional Review Board. She has taught associate degree, Bachelor's degree, and graduate-level nursing students on all aspects of the nursing process, research methodologies, statistics, psychiatric nursing, and pharmacology. Eileen is also the Research Preceptor for the Psychiatric Residency Program at the State University of New York at Buffalo School of Pharmacy Doctoral Residency Program.

Eileen earned her BSN, her MS as a Clinical Nurse Specialist in psychiatric nursing, and her Doctorate in Nursing Science (DNS) in psychiatric nursing from the State University of New York at Buffalo. She received a National Institutes of Mental Health Individual National Research Service Award Pre-Doctoral Research Fellowship for her dissertation research on medication teaching and psychopharmacology. Eileen's research interests include cognitive behavioral nursing interventions with seriously and persistently mentally ill clients, and the safety and efficacy of neuroleptics. She is a Diplomate and Fellow in the American College of Forensic Examiners Board of Forensic Nurse Examiners, and is board certified as an Institutional Review Board Professional (CIP) and in hospital and program accreditation.

Eileen is author, co-author, and contributor to 14 books and numerous journal articles. She presents internationally on a wide variety of clinical, research and professional topics to health care, governmental and corporate organisations. She continues to be an international speaker and consultant on topics including professional issues, assessment, psychopathologies and interventions. She also serves on the editorial boards of several professional journals and is on the editorial panel for a magazine on anxiety and depression. She is active in community service venues, including clinical settings and family support groups. She also serves as a computer systems and statistical consultant, and belongs to numerous professional nursing organisations.

Eileen enjoys her clinical psychologist husband, her Congo African Grey parrot, a large and loving family, good friends, international travel, and reading.

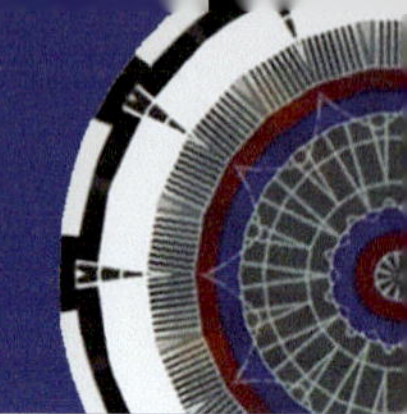

CONTRIBUTING AUTHORS

The lead authors would like to thank the following mental health nursing authors and lived experience authors who have collaborated on each chapter in this text as indicated below. Their contributions reflect the philosophy of this text—to provide a person-centred and recovery-focused resource, with a clearly-heard authentic lived experience voice.

Chapter	Mental health nursing authors	Lived experience authors
Foreword Social and Emotional wellbeing in an Indigenous context	Debra Hocking, University of Wollongong	Debra Hocking, University of Wollongong
Chapter 1 People with lived experience and carers	Mike Hazelton, University of Newcastle	Simon Swinson and Tim Heffernan
Chapter 2 The therapeutic relationship	Mike Hazelton, University of Newcastle	Simon Swinson
Chapter 3 Psychiatric–mental health nurses: who are they and what do they do?	Kim Ryan, ACMHN and Peta Marks, ACMHN	Tim Heffernan
Chapter 4 Self-awareness and the mental health nurse	Lorna Moxham, University of Wollongong, and Paul Robson, Illawarra Shoalhaven Local Health District	Tim Heffernan
Chapter 5 Theories for interdisciplinary care in mental health	Mike Hazelton, University of Newcastle	Simon Swinson
Chapter 6 The biological basis of behavioural and mental disorders	Merrilee Harris, University of Newcastle, and Mike Hazelton, University of Newcastle	Simon Swinson
Chapter 7 The science, practice and experience of psychopharmacology	Mike Hazelton, University of Newcastle	Simon Swinson
Chapter 8 Stress, anxiety and anxiety disorders	Deb O'Kane, Flinders University	Ann Smith
Chapter 9 Therapeutic communication	Deb O'Kane, Flinders University	Ann Smith
Chapter 10 Psychiatric–mental health assessment	Eimear Muir-Cochrane, Flinders University	Franklin D. Bartle
Chapter 11 Ethics, legal issues and the rights of people with a mental illness	Eimear Muir-Cochrane, Flinders University, and Adam Grace, Flinders University	Janne McMahon
Chapter 12 Cognitive disorders	Lorna Moxham, University of Wollongong	Howard James Street
Chapter 13 Substance use disorders	Renee Brighton, University of Wollongong	Kylie Smith

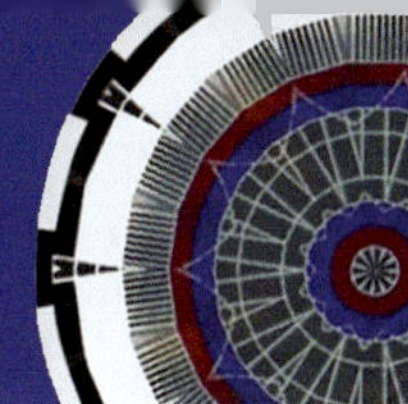

Chapter 14 Working in collaboration with people living with schizophrenia and other psychotic disorders	Mike Hazelton, University of Newcastle	Simon Swinson
Chapter 15 Affective disorders	Christopher Patterson, University of Wollongong	Douglas Holmes
Chapter 16 Dissociative, somatic symptom and factitious disorders	Christopher Patterson, University of Wollongong	Paula Hanlon
Chapter 17 Eating disorders	Renee Brighton, University of Wollongong	Katherine Gill
Chapter 18 Personality disorders	Dr Sue Sumskis, Nan Tien Institute	Erin Howard-Gillis
Chapter 19 People at risk for suicide and self-harming behaviour	Mike Hazelton, University of Newcastle	Carrie Miller
Chapter 20 Family violence	Mike Hazelton, University of Newcastle, and Ellen Sinclair, University of Newcastle	
Chapter 21 The mental health of younger people	Ellen Sinclair, University of Newcastle, and Mike Hazelton, University of Newcastle	Isabella Swinson
Chapter 22 Older people	Bryan McMinn, University of Newcastle	Amtul Shah
Chapter 23 Therapeutic groups	Christine Palmer, Queensland University of Technology	Carolyn Hyde
Chapter 24 Family-focused interventions	Deb O'Kane, Flinders University	Tim Heffernan
Chapter 25 Cognitive and behavioural interventions	Christine Palmer, Queensland University of Technology	Sharon Lawn
Chapter 26 Pathways of care	Christine Palmer, Queensland University of Technology	Matthew Halpin

ACKNOWLEDGEMENTS

The lead authors are aware that there are many people to thank in the construction of such a comprehensive text as this. To those persons who live with a mental illness, your strength, value and resilience and your lived experience expertise are acknowledged. Each author has worked tirelessly to collaboratively construct content that future health professionals will find invaluable. Reviewers have provided the necessary quality assurance and concerned themselves with ensuring practice is evidence-based.

To the Pearson staff who work behind the scenes: you may not have your name in 'lights', but you are all are vital to the development of quality work. We would also like to thank Xanthe Glaw, University of Newcastle, for completing the DSM-5 and ICD-10 Appendix, and finally the editors wish to thank their families who have supported us in our passion to produce a book in collaboration with consumers; a book that has taken countless hours, late nights and sleep deprivation. A heartfelt thank-you to one and all.

REVIEWERS

The authors and publisher are grateful for the expertise provided by nursing faculty and clinicians who gave of their time to review chapters for this book and the material that accompanies it. Thank you for your generosity in sharing your insightful comments with us.

Dr Karen-Ann Clarke
University of the Sunshine Coast

Dr Gayelene Boardman
Victoria University

Dr Jane Clark
University of New England

Sue Willis
University of Western Sydney

Rosemary Saunders
Edith Cowan University

Deb O'Kane
Flinders University

Dr Cheryl Ross
University of Southern QLD

Dr Louise Ward
La Trobe University

Barbara Black
University of Queensland

Ms Rhonda Dawson
University of Southern Queensland

Cheryl Green
University of Adelaide

Dr Terry Froggatt
University of Wollongong

Mr Cameron Peake
Australian Catholic University

Dr Karen Heslop
Curtin University

Mr David Delaney
Victoria University

Ms Rebecca Millar
Victoria University

Mr Hamish Alker-Jones
Charles Sturt University

Ms Pat Mead
University of Adelaide

Mr Keith Skelton
Australian Catholic University

Ms Philippa Harris
Mental Illness Felowship Nth Qld Inc

Mrs Sandra Goetz
Griffith University

Dr Scott Trueman
James Cook University

Ms Patricia Mead
University of Adelaide

Dr Shirley McGough
Curtin University

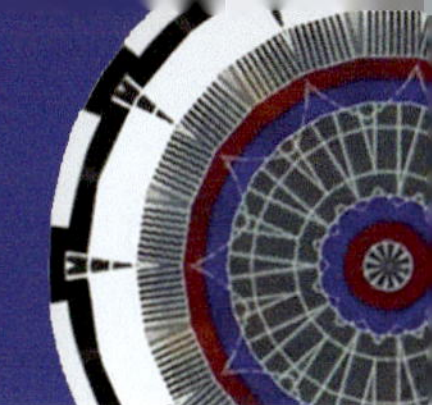

PREFACE

Millions of people around the world face the challenges that living with a mental health issue can bring. In fact, the World Health Organization (WHO) suggests that half of the leading causes of disability in the world today are related to mental health. This is unlikely to change while global mental health resources remain low, and the necessary improvements in early detection and intervention are not addressed by governments locally and nationally.

Adding to the challenges that living with mental health issues brings is the ongoing issue of stigma. The stigma of mental illness is based on a misguided societal perception that mental illness is a blemish of individual character, and is a worldwide problem experienced in all segments of society. Stigma hurts, punishes and diminishes people. Unfortunately, stigma continues to grow around the globe, and is perhaps the main obstacle to better mental health care and quality of life for consumers and their families.

Our goal for this textbook, *Contemporary Psychiatric–Mental Health Nursing: Partnerships in Care*, is to provide the user with a contemporary, evidence-based, culturally competent, authoritative and comprehensive resource. Importantly and most notably, the textbook was co-authored by people with a lived experience of mental illness. Indeed, we set out quite purposefully to ensure a consumer voice was prominent in each chapter of the text. Thus the co-produced resource is designed to enhance your ability to become a therapeutic, non-judgmental, competent and confident psychiatric–mental health nurse. We encourage you to think seriously about what constitutes mental health and mental illness. We would urge you to appreciate the humanity of people who experience mental illness, and to undertake your nursing practice with unconditional positive regard. We think it likely that this will challenge your assumptions about mental illness and those who live their lives with it; we hope it does!

UNDERLYING THEMES

Throughout this book, we value cultural competence in increasingly diverse societies, collaborative-centered care, the relevance of lived experience to shaping recovery and treatment choices, and the need to improve quality and access to mental health care. We believe that mental health nursing must concern itself with the quality of human life, and its relationship to optimal psychobiological health, feelings of self-worth, personal integrity, self-fulfilment, and collaborative care. Thus, we emphasise the importance of empathy and empowerment in the therapeutic relationship.

Understanding people who are searching for personal recovery through interaction in complex times demands the most authoritative and contemporary knowledge and clinical competence. It is through the power of knowledge and clinical competence that psychiatric–mental health nurses work with people as they progress through the journey of personal recovery. Psychiatric–mental health nursing is concerned with sustaining and enhancing the mental health of both the individual and the group, while its practice locale is often found in the community.

In acknowledging the importance and value of lived experience, each chapter offers the voice of the person who lives with a mental health issue. These voices, which are often silent, are vital in knowledge production, and know best how they need to recover. As such, the themes, ideas, knowledge, tools and organisation of this textbook are designed for nursing students who are committed to making a difference in view of contemporary trends. Specifically, this text expects students to recognise the value of lived experience.

Nursing is both a science and an art, and because of advances in neuroscience and the enhancements in the study of the human genome, a solid grounding in psychobiology is threaded throughout the book. Brain imaging and concise yet comprehensive information on the expanding array of psychopharmacological treatment is yet another strong emphasis. *Contemporary Psychiatric–Mental Health Nursing: Partnerships in Care* is explicitly linked to contemporary practices in our field.

ORGANISATION

The book engages with the people you will encounter in your practice and with whom you will work collaboratively. It describes what it means to be a mental health nurse, the professional and personal attributes that enable artful therapeutic practice, and the importance of basing the therapeutic relationship on theoretical understandings, appropriate clinical techniques and the needs and wants of the person who lives with a mental illness.

This text also provides comprehensive coverage of interdisciplinary mental health theories, the biological basis of mental illness, the science of psychopharmacology, the methods by which people attempt to handle stress, and the importance of developing cultural competence. Topics traditionally associated with mental health nursing, such as therapeutic communication, assessment, ethics, advocacy, rights, legal and forensic issues, and therapeutic environments for care are also discussed. Caring for people with a specific DSM mental diagnosis is described by outlining the defining characteristics of each diagnosis, the biopsychosocial theories necessary to understand them, and, importantly, how to apply the nursing process to work with people who live with these illnesses. The authors have also turned their attention to vulnerable populations that require comfort and care from psychiatric–mental health nurses. These populations include people at risk for self-harming behaviour, sexual abuse and family violence, and specific age groups. The textbook provides authoritative coverage of nursing intervention strategies and desired outcomes, including a wide range of modalities from therapeutic groups to family-focused strategies, crisis intervention, and cognitive behavioral interventions; to psychopharmacology, recovery and psychiatric rehabilitation, and complementary, alternative and integrative healing practices; and anger management and violence in psychiatric settings.

AUSTRALIAN EDITION

As lead and chapter authors who have all practised, taught and researched as psychiatric–mental health nurses in the Australian context, we felt it important that Australian nursing students were offered an opportunity to be exposed to contemporary Australian mental health nursing knowledge. Most importantly, though, we felt it important for future health professionals to hear from people with a lived experience. Not only do we believe this is absolutely the right thing to do, it is also the major point of difference about this textbook.

THE TEXTBOOK AS A MAP, A COMPASS AND AN INSPIRATION

Psychiatric–mental health nursing is poised at a crossroads, and every nurse can make a difference. We are challenged to bring complex thinking to a complex world if we are to reduce stigma and actualise our contribution to global mental health—the vision to which this text is dedicated. This book has been crafted to provide you with the best possible evidence generated in research to help you achieve your goal of excellence in practice. It offers a fully integrated perspective, which most importantly includes the voice of people with mental illness. It encourages you to become personally and professionally willing to muster the courage and hope necessary to forge proactive steps in our future, and to make a commitment to work globally in a contemporary landscape and mindscape.

We have the opportunity to forge a new synthesis of professional wisdom in the face of tough mind–body–spirit problems and needs, and the stigmatisation of mental illness. We need to face critical transitions with intelligence, stamina, wit, creativity, skill and moral courage. Global mental health can become a shared, emergent vision constructed in a way that is respectful of the rich diversity of the citizens of our contemporary world. We have created this book to provide you with a map, a compass and an inspiration to succeed in your current work. We hope that it encourages you to become a participant and leader in facing the broader challenges ahead of us.

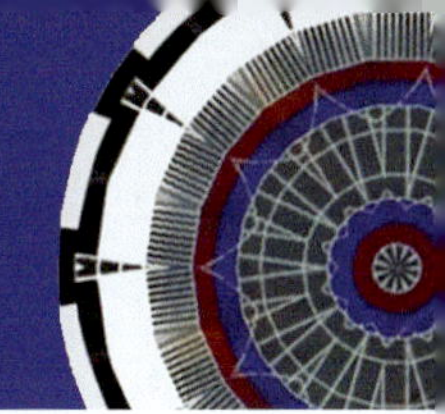

A GUIDE TO *CONTEMPORARY PSYCHIATRIC–MENTAL HEALTH NURSING*

KEY TERMS alert you to the vocabulary used in the chapter. The page numbers indicate where the term is defined.

LEARNING OUTCOMES indicate what important information or skills you will have gained after studying the chapter.

LIVED EXPERIENCE reflects the 'lived-experience' voice of the consumer, which discusses mental health issues that health consumers have encountered.

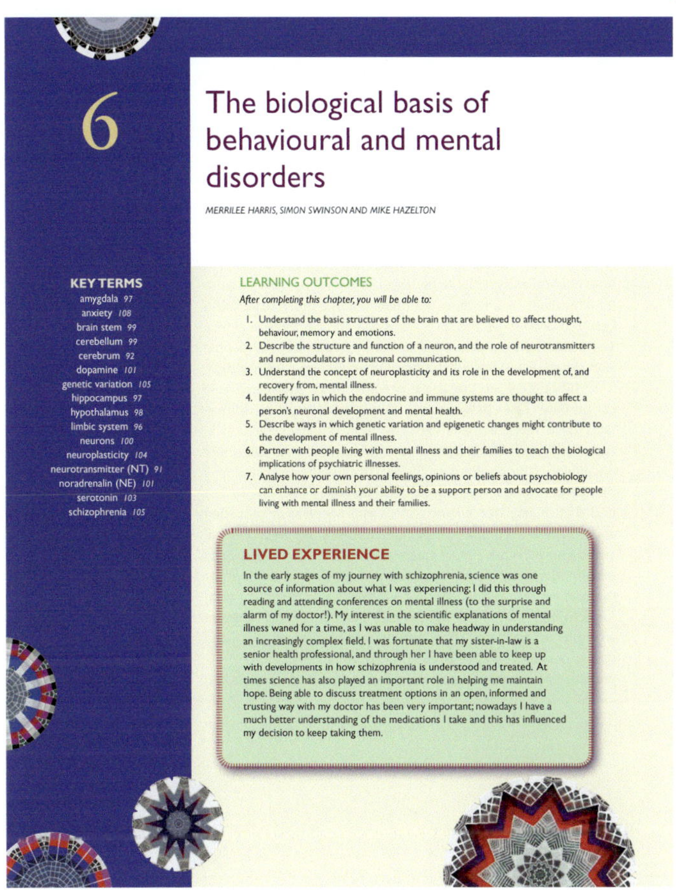

6

The biological basis of behavioural and mental disorders

MERRILEE HARRIS, SIMON SWINSON AND MIKE HAZELTON

KEY TERMS

amygdala *97*
anxiety *108*
brain stem *99*
cerebellum *99*
cerebrum *92*
dopamine *101*
genetic variation *105*
hippocampus *97*
hypothalamus *98*
limbic system *96*
neurons *100*
neuroplasticity *104*
neurotransmitter (NT) *91*
noradrenalin (NE) *101*
serotonin *103*
schizophrenia *105*

LEARNING OUTCOMES

After completing this chapter, you will be able to:

1. Understand the basic structures of the brain that are believed to affect thought, behaviour, memory and emotions.
2. Describe the structure and function of a neuron, and the role of neurotransmitters and neuromodulators in neuronal communication.
3. Understand the concept of neuroplasticity and its role in the development of, and recovery from, mental illness.
4. Identify ways in which the endocrine and immune systems are thought to affect a person's neuronal development and mental health.
5. Describe ways in which genetic variation and epigenetic changes might contribute to the development of mental illness.
6. Partner with people living with mental illness and their families to teach the biological implications of psychiatric illnesses.
7. Analyse how your own personal feelings, opinions or beliefs about psychobiology can enhance or diminish your ability to be a support person and advocate for people living with mental illness and their families.

LIVED EXPERIENCE

In the early stages of my journey with schizophrenia, science was one source of information about what I was experiencing; I did this through reading and attending conferences on mental illness (to the surprise and alarm of my doctor!). My interest in the scientific explanations of mental illness waned for a time, as I was unable to make headway in understanding an increasingly complex field. I was fortunate that my sister-in-law is a senior health professional, and through her I have been able to keep up with developments in how schizophrenia is understood and treated. At times science has also played an important role in helping me maintain hope. Being able to discuss treatment options in an open, informed and trusting way with my doctor has been very important; nowadays I have a much better understanding of the medications I take and this has influenced my decision to keep taking them.

DEVELOPING CULTURAL COMPETENCE boxes are an important link to the cultural forces that influence the experience and expression of mental disorders and pose critical thinking questions.

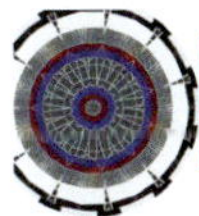

DEVELOPING CULTURAL COMPETENCE

Culture and dementia

Developing cultural competence when working with people who have dementia and their families is important. Cultural factors influence perceptions about what is normal ageing. Look for cultural bias (language, expected response, speed, etc.) in cognitive screening tools, and discuss these biases with colleagues.

Nurses promote effective health practices in the community setting; for example, taking blood pressure, discussing healthy diet, and noticing early symptoms of dementia. Education and outreach to diverse populations can provide support for people with dementia and their families.

CRITICAL THINKING QUESTIONS

1. What are some possible explanations for why different cultures have different attitudes about ageing?
2. Which cultures do you think treat older people with the most respect? Why?

EVIDENCE-BASED PRACTICE boxes show how research evidence shapes the plan of care for a particular client. Critical thinking questions follow each vignette.

EVIDENCE-BASED PRACTICE

Life roles and anorexia nervosa

Suzy, age 45 years, is extremely thin and jogs for several hours every day to maintain her (under) weight. She is 174 centimetres tall, and weighs 55 kilograms. You work with her in an outpatient clinic where she is receiving counselling for marital problems.

Suzy has maintained the same weight since she was 17 years old. Her eating habits have always been tied to her weight. Since she was a teenager, Suzy has added extra distance to her running route, decreased her calorie count, or fasted whenever she was 500 grams over what she considered her ideal weight. The literature reports that adolescence is the peak time for developing eating disorders. Recovery studies will be most helpful to you in understanding and working with Suzy.

As indicated in the following research, many people, through therapy and close relationships, find non-bodily means to express their distress. Events such as committing to a relationship, forming a family, and settling into an identity and occupation all serve to provide a stable platform for overall functioning. Women's drive to be thin tends to decline as they age (conversely, men's drive to be thin tends to increase as they age), but Suzy does not follow that trend. You explore her life roles and what gives her a sense of positive identity (is she a wife, a mother, a daughter, a business executive, a socialite, a student, an athlete, etc.?). Identify the ways in which she expresses a range of negative emotions to determine whether your work with her needs to focus on problematic expression of feelings that may contribute to perpetuating her eating disorder.

You should base action on more than one study, but the following research would be helpful in this situation:

Jenkins, J., & Ogden, J. (2012). Becoming 'whole' again: A qualitative study of women's views of recovering from anorexia nervosa. *European Eating Disorders Review, 20*(1), e23–e31.

CRITICAL THINKING QUESTIONS

1. If Suzy has been maintaining an underweight condition since the age of 17, what are her chances for improvement?
2. What conditions would be necessary for improvement to take place?

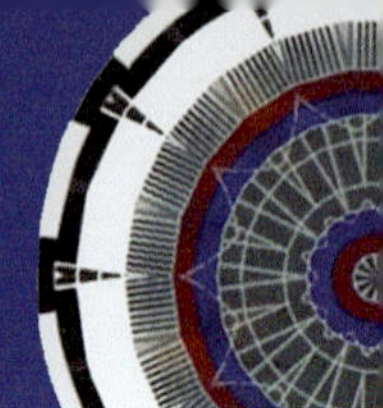

WHAT EVERY NURSE SHOULD KNOW boxes emphasise the importance of recognising mental health problems and applying these practices in all nursing situations.

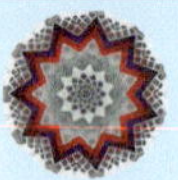

WHAT EVERY NURSE SHOULD KNOW

Suicidal ideation in primary care

Imagine you are a nurse working in a primary care setting, such as a general practice surgery. It is not unusual in primary care settings to see people with suicidal ideation or at high risk for suicide. It is also not unusual for primary care providers to fail to recognise those at high risk for suicide. Suicide risk is increased in both physical and mental illness, especially when both are present. It is important to remember that there is also a strong association between depression, risk for suicide and chronic medical illness. The possibility of suicide risk should be considered in all people with chronic illness, including those with solely physical symptoms.

Although there are more effective medications available to primary care practitioners to treat depression, suicide rates have remained unacceptably high and may be under-reported if unexplained deaths are considered. In instances where uncertainty surrounds a person's death, a psychological autopsy may be performed. A **psychological autopsy** is an assessment tool that reviews the circumstances and events that preceded an individual's completed suicide. Reviews of psychological autopsies and other similar methods have revealed that a high percentage of suicide victims have a comorbid mental disorder (such as mood disorders and/or substance use disorders) and, furthermore, that they were under-treated, despite contact with mental health or other health care services. Recognising this association, screening for it, and providing treatment is a primary care imperative and may prevent unnecessary tragedies.

COLLARBORATIVE CARE boxes emphasise the value of including the family in psychiatric–mental health care. This feature provides key topics to discuss with families, allowing them to understand the characteristics of the disorder.

COLLABORATIVE CARE

Teaching about a low-tyramine diet

MAOIs combined with certain foods and medications may produce a significant increase in blood pressure, which can be a health hazard. In general, foods that cause this reaction are those that have been ***pickled, fermented, smoked or aged***. The list below includes the main foods, fluids and medications that should be avoided while taking a MAOI and for at least two weeks after discontinuation of a MAOI. It should be noted that preservatives in foodstuffs and beverages can change over time, and thus dietary restrictions should be updated regularly.

Foods and beverages to avoid completely

Meats and fish: Pickled herring, dried fish, aged/dried/cured meats, unrefrigerated fermented fish, liver, caviar, fermented sausage (salami, pepperoni), fermented oyster sauces used in Asian dishes, jerky, meat extracts, miso, soy sauce, teriyaki sauce.
Vegetables: English broad beans, Chinese pea pods, fava beans, banana peels, Italian or broad green beans, fermented cabbage, lentils, lima beans, sauerkraut, overly ripe fruits, peanuts, spinach.
Dairy products: Yoghurt, many types of cheese (e.g. English Stilton, mozzarella, Parmesan).
Beverages: Chianti, aged wines, imported beers, aged beers.
Combination foods: Breads made with aged cheeses, and meats, or yeast extracts; homemade or high-yeast breads; pizza; lasagna; macaroni and cheese; quiche; liver pâté; Caesar salad; all yeast products (e.g. brewer's yeast, yeast extracts such as Vegemite and Marmite).
MSG: MSG is frequently used in Asian dishes as a meat tenderiser and flavour enhancer; many prepared and processed foods also use MSG (e.g. canned soups, packaged noodle meals, frozen prepared meals, salad dressings).
Medications: Cough and cold medications, nasal decongestants (tablets, drops, sprays), hayfever and allergy medications, weight-reduction preparations, anti-appetite medications, asthma inhalants.

Foods and beverages that can be taken in small amounts

Dairy products: Most processed cheeses bought in a supermarket.
Fruits: Raisins, prunes, bananas, avocados, plums, canned figs.
Caffeine sources: Coffee, chocolate, colas.
Beverages: Domestic red wines; domestic beers, ales, stouts; sherry. (Note: alcohol is a CNS-depressant, and so should be avoided by individuals in treatment for depression.)

Allowed foods

Beverages: White wines. (Note: alcohol is a CNS-depressant, and so should be avoided by individuals in treatment for depression.)
Baked goods: Raised with yeast, but not high in yeast.
Dairy products: Cottage cheese, cream cheese, milk, cream, ice cream.

Additional information

St John's wort: This naturally occurring MAOI, less potent than pharmaceutical grade; is not regulated and may cause inconsistent access to the active ingredient. It has the same dietary and medication restrictions as pharmaceutical-grade MAOIs.

PRACTICE EXAMPLE features provide real-life scenarios that students may encounter, and point out the challenges involved.

Practice example

A young man who was hospitalised at a mental health assessment unit complained to other consumers and staff members that he had been 'odenated', and he became increasingly frustrated and anxious when it became apparent that he wasn't being understood. Rather than simply writing him off as confused, his primary nurse recognised that 'odenated' most likely had a private meaning. With some help, he was able to explain that he was upset about having been moved to a different room. The room was, he said, so dark and dingy that it looked like a cave. Animals live in caves that are called 'dens'. In his view he had been o-den-ated—put into a cave.

MENTAL HEALTH IN THE MEDIA features depict how mental illness in the media affects our attitudes and behaviour. They also highlight the successes and difficulties faced by those in the media.

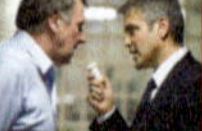

MENTAL HEALTH IN THE MEDIA

Michael Clayton

Michael Clayton is a movie about an attorney, Michael Clayton (played by George Clooney), who fixes problems in law firms caused by the idiosyncratic behaviours of various attorneys. Crimes, sexual misconduct and ethics issues, along with behaviours related to mental disorders, are his usual assignments. One of the attorneys he is asked to extract from an embarrassing situation is a brilliant man who happens to have bipolar disorder. Arthur Edens (played by Tom Wilkinson) has had a bizarre outburst in the middle of a deposition in a class action lawsuit against a conglomerate. Michael arrives to fix the situation for his good friend and colleague. He convinces the authorities to let Arthur out of jail, and brings him back to their hotel where he is successfully sedated. However, Arthur escapes from the hotel in the middle of the night.

The lawyers for the conglomerate obtain Arthur's briefcase and discover that Arthur has documentation detailing the conglomerate's decision to manufacture a chemical they know to be carcinogenic. Public knowledge of this decision would severely disrupt the finances of the conglomerate. In addition, the lawyers know about Arthur's bipolar disorder, his failure to take his medications and his outbursts. They follow Arthur, tap his phone and bug his apartment. The conglomerate's lawyers have Arthur assassinated in a manner designed to resemble suicide, a common occurrence with people who are bipolar and unmedicated.

Michael, saddened by the death of his friend and colleague, is suspicious about the circumstances. He cannot reconcile his friend's beliefs and energies with suicidal intent. Because he searches for and finds Arthur's evidence and plans to publicise it, he is also targeted for assassination. However, the attempt is botched. The movie resolves with Michael recording the admission of murder and attempted murder.

Photo courtesy of CAP/FB Supplied by Capital Pictures/Newscom.

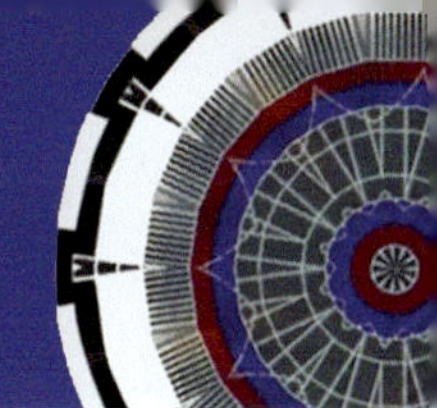

HOW I WILL USE MY MENTAL HEALTH SKILLS IN PRACTICE *AND* WHY I CHOSE TO WORK IN MENTAL HEALTH present the personal stories of those who work in mental health nursing.

HOW I WILL USE MY MENTAL-HEALTH SKILLS IN PRACTICE

Madison's story

I was 17 years old when I began working as a nurse's aide in a small long-term care facility. I was just starting university to become a nurse, and wanted experience working in the field. There were not very many people being cared for in the facility, because it was a private enterprise with the goal of making it as homelike as possible. I became close to all of the residents while learning to take care of them.

One woman, Louise, was extra special. She was only 50 years old, but had such debilitating and deforming arthritis that she could not care for herself and was no longer able to work as a psychiatric–mental health nurse. She was bright and personable, and I admired her strength of character in dealing with a chronic illness. Louise's roommate, Ida, was a bitter and negative woman, who rarely said anything neutral about her world or the people in it. A positive statement from Ida was unheard of. Ida's granddaughter came in to visit her, and she was so excited to show off her boyfriend's gift—a pretty pearl ring in a gold band. Ida's only comment was: 'Pearls mean sorrow.' Ida's granddaughter was devastated and left in tears. Ida's response to her roommate was: 'See? Pearls do mean sorrow.' Louise then reassured Ida that, even though her granddaughter was becoming close to her boyfriend, no one could take Ida's place. Ida, Louise told her, would always be Grandmother, and nothing could change that.

When I asked Louise later, in private, what was the connection between Ida being mean-spirited and Louise reassuring Ida, Louise's reply opened my eyes to the value of psychological sophistication. Louise said, 'When people feel threatened about being hurt by someone, they will put the energy into hurting that person first. Ida wasn't being mean, she was being hurt.' Being able to help someone cope with feelings, with what I now know are psychiatric–mental health nursing interactions, helped me choose the area for my nursing career.

WHY I CHOSE TO WORK IN MENTAL HEALTH

Kim Ryan

I first began my nursing career as a general registered nurse, and then under took psychiatric nurse training. Back then it wasn't uncommon for nurses to hold double or triple certificates—in general, midwifery and psychiatry.

During my general nurse training, I didn't really learn about mental health—as a result, when I first started psychiatric nursing I had little understanding of mental illness or the way in which people exhibited mental illness. What I discovered was that it's not that easy to divide a person into 'the mind' or 'the body'—so much that happens in the mind affects the body and vice versa.

Deinstitutionalisation had also just started: the big psychiatric hospitals were being opened up, and people who had lived in institutions, in some cases for many years, were being transferred back into the community. I quickly realised that most of society didn't understand mental illness. I was humbled by the very difficult lives that many of the people I encountered had experienced. They were misunderstood, they were stigmatised, they were removed from their family, and the medications they were taking could have debilitating side-effects. However, they were (and still are) some of the most resilient people I have ever had the privilege to meet. I guess that is why I stayed in mental health, rather than moving on to another nursing specialty.

Mental health nursing is a wonderful career, you meet some great characters, you laugh and you cry, but, best of all, you can make a difference to people's lives.

Are there any aspects of Kim' story that you relate to? What is important to you about the work that you do? When you are at the other end of your nursing career and you look back, what would you like to have achieved, what would you like to have stood for?

SELF-AWARENESS boxes engage the reader in a process of introspection and self-questioning that is essential to the therapeutic use of self.

SELF-AWARENESS
Reflecting on feedback from consumers and carers

Input—both positive and negative—from consumers, carers, classmates, tutors, staff, family and friends can help you to become aware of your 'blind spots', the characteristics about yourself that you ignore, deny or defend. Protecting oneself through self-deception interferes with both relating and communicating. To become more self-aware, do the following:

- think about a recent interaction with a consumer and how they responded to you
- identify the positive/negative elements in the interaction
- try to determine what the consumer was telling you about yourself in this interaction (i.e. What characteristic(s) do you have that enables people to openly express their thoughts and feelings? What characteristic(s) do you have that prevents people from openly expressing their thoughts and feelings?)
- discuss the interaction and your interpretation of it with a supervisor
- ask for feedback on your behaviour from others—family members, classmates, staff, friends.

DIAGNOSTIC FEATURES provide diagnostic criteria for mental health disorders, followed by descriptive text.

DIAGNOSTIC FEATURES
Cognitive disorders

Delirium: Delirium is a disturbance of consciousness with a reduced ability to focus, sustain or shift attention. There is a change in cognition, and the disturbance develops over hours to days, and tends to fluctuate during the day. Medical conditions can also contribute to these difficulties.

Dementia of the Alzheimer's type (DAT): DAT involves multiple cognitive deficits, with memory impairment and aphasia, apraxia, agnosia and/or a disturbance in organising. This causes impairment and decreased functioning in important areas. It starts gradually and is progressive, and problems are not due to other sources.

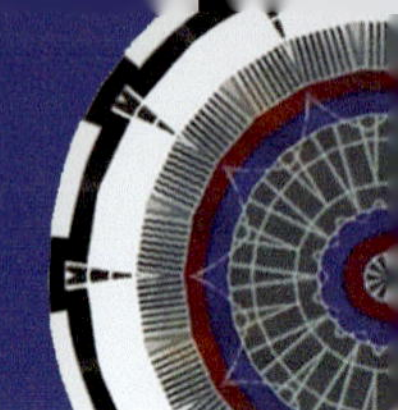

COMMUNICATION boxes offer sample dialogues between nurses and clients. In addition, they provide the rationale for at least two different but helpful alternatives. This feature is designed to provide students with a beginning repertoire of useful communication interventions when interacting with mental health clients.

COMMUNICATION

A person with clang associations

PERSON: 'The dining room lining trying to eat forever.'

NURSE RESPONSE 1: 'Jack, are you having a problem getting your food?'	NURSE RESPONSE 2: 'Come with me and let's get you set up.'
RATIONALE: A direct question allows the person experiencing clang associations to answer with a 'yes' or 'no' response, models how the communication can be stated, and labels the situation as a problem.	*RATIONALE:* This response reinforces the appropriateness of the person coming to the nurse with a problem and concretely shows the person how to resolve the problem.

NURSING CARE PLANS are included in the chapters dealing with specific disorders. They represent a different way to view care for clients diagnosed with specific mental disorders according to the DSM-5.

NURSING CARE PLAN: AN ADULT SURVIVOR OF CHILDHOOD SEXUAL ABUSE

Identifying information

Jill is 35 years old and, with her husband John, co-owns and operates a local newsagent business. The couple have been married for 15 years, and have three children aged 14, 12 and 7.

Jill was sexually abused by her grandfather from a very young age until she was about 11 or 12. She states that she told her mother about the abuse when she was 9 or 10, but that her mother just ignored it. Her mother now denies that Jill told her about the abuse when it was occurring. Jill has tried to ignore her abuse history, until several months ago when she saw a television program about incest. She has periods when she is filled with rage at her parents and grandfather.

History

No prior psychiatric history.

Jill is the third child of five in an intact family. She describes her mother as 'strict . . . she would threaten by saying "wait until your dad comes home".' When asked about her father, Jill states, 'He wasn't around . . . he was working . . . he was always distant.' She describes the family communication as 'dysfunctional; only certain people talked to certain other people. For example, none of us kids could talk directly to Dad. We always had to go through Mum.'

Jill describes herself as a 'homebody'; she works in the newsagency several days a week while the children are at school, and says 'the shop is my chance to get out of the house each week.' In the past, she went out with her husband regularly, but says she never really enjoyed doing so. Since having children, Jill's life has increasingly involved parenting, home duties and the newsagency. She states that she has never had close friends and her only friend is her husband, but she also feels intimidated by him. She has a very close relationship with her children.

Jill has no current or past medical problems. She states that she is in good health except for feeling 'down a lot of the time'.

Current mental status

Jill is oriented to person, place and time. Her affect appears dysphoric, irritable and constricted in range. At times she is filled with rage, saying, 'I am mad . . . Mad at the world in general, and at having to deal with all of this.' She states that during her entire life she has spent much of her energy in 'not thinking', 'not imagining' and 'not remembering' the abuse. She has attempted to keep a sense of distance from her inner emotional life. After viewing the television program on incest, she now experiences 'painful, bitter, brooding thoughts about the abuse'. Jill is an anxious and angry woman with extremely low self-esteem and intense feelings of inadequacy. She views herself as unable to function in an autonomous, self-directed and self-reliant fashion, and sees the world as untrustworthy, betraying and often cruel.

Unable to rely on her own resources or depend on the support of others, Jill feels a sense of bitter futility and resignation.

YOUR INTERVENTION STRATEGIES
Reducing and modifying the occurrence of burnout

- Address staff–consumer ratios. Giving more attention to each person enables time to focus on the positive, non-problematic aspects of the person's life.
- Recognise that no one is perfect. The people to whom you provide care deserve the best you can provide; it may not always be perfect care, and it isn't 24-hours-a-day, 7-days-a-week care.
- Take sanctioned breaks rather than guilt-provoking escapes from the work situation.
- Talk over your problems to get advice and support when you need it. Clinical supervision is important for mental health nurses.
- Express, analyse and share your feelings about burning out. This lets you get things off your chest, and gives you the chance to get constructive feedback from others and perhaps a new perspective as well.
- Understand your own motivations in pursuing a mental health nursing career, and recognise your own expectations for working with consumers. Deal with the issues of the people you are caring for, not your own.
- Listen to and then attend to your own internal stress signals.
- Pursue happiness and satisfaction in your personal life, through things you enjoy and being around positive people.
- Work with a peer support worker to get a different recovery perspective.

YOUR ASSESSMENT APPROACH *AND* YOUR INTERVENTION STRATEGIES present clinically-relevant strategies in a succinct, user-friendly format. Your Assessment Approach contains lists of assessment points. Your Intervention Strategies list specific nursing intervention strategies along with their rationales.

YOUR ASSESSMENT APPROACH **Signs of a working relationship**

The following criteria may be useful in determining whether a one-to-one relationship is moving into the working, or middle, phase.

For nurse

- Sense of making contact with the person
- Sense that the person is responding well to the relationship
- Sense that the nurse can facilitate growth in the person regardless of the severity of dysfunction
- Sense of commitment to addressing the person's problems

For consumer

- Non-verbal and verbal evidence of liking the nurse
- Sense of relaxation with the nurse
- Sense of confidence in the nurse
- Non-superficial (in nature and depth) problems addressed

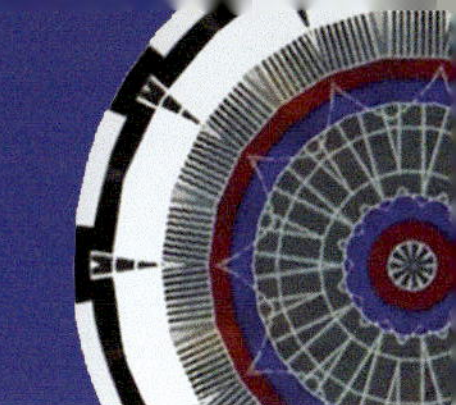

EDUCATOR RESOURCES

A suite of resources is provided to assist with delivery of the text, as well as to support teaching and learning.

SOLUTIONS MANUAL

The Solutions Manual provides educators with detailed, accuracy-verified solutions to all of the in-chapter and end-of-chapter problems in the book.

TEST BANK

The Test Bank provides a wealth of accuracy-verified testing material. Updated for the new edition, each chapter offers a wide variety of true/false, short answer and multiple-choice questions, arranged by learning objective and tagged by NMBA standards.
Questions can be integrated into Blackboard or Moodle.

POWERPOINT LECTURE SLIDES

A comprehensive set of PowerPoint slides can be used by educators for class presentations or by students for lecture preview or review. They include key figures and tables, as well as a summary of key concepts and examples from the text.

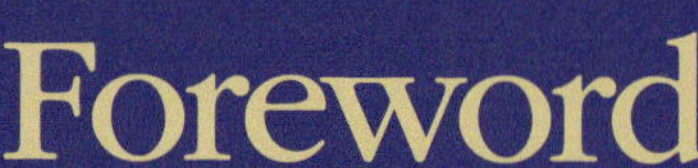

Foreword

Social and emotional wellbeing in an Indigenous context

DEBRA HOCKING

Debra is a lecturer with the University of Wollongong, coordinating Postgraduate Indigenous Health subjects. She is a Palawa (Tasmanian Aboriginal) person who descends from the Mouheneenner people from south-east Tasmania. She is a Stolen Generations survivor who has lived the journey of trauma and distress as many Aboriginal Australians have done. She has worked in Aboriginal Affairs/Health for almost two decades, and undertakes continual research into the effects of trauma on Aboriginal individuals, families and communities. She is the recipient of two United Nations awards for humanitarian activities in Australia.

The cultures of Aboriginal Australians are the oldest living cultural history in the world, dating back at least 60 000 years. How we have survived may be attributed to the ability to adapt and adjust our worldviews over time, and also the affinity with our environment may elucidate why and how we have endured for so many millennia.

'Aboriginal' refers to individuals of Aboriginal descent and who are recognised by the community in which they live, or who identify as Aboriginal.

This contribution to the book is not designed to invoke guilt, but to tell a story based on fact and lived experiences. Readers may find it challenging, and even feel a sense of responsibility; but where the responsibility lays in contemporary terms is to provoke empathy and understanding from a historical misguidance of people ignorant of the severe negative impacts that the actions that governments and individuals took would have on Aboriginal people, with devastating effects. To appreciate fully the need for trauma-informed practice today, there must be an understanding of the history of contact and invasion, and the attitudes of the colonisers to the First Nations people then and now.

SOCIAL AND EMOTIONAL WELLBEING (SEWB)

In 2004, the Social Health Reference Group (SHRG) for the National Aboriginal and Torres Strait Islander Health Council and National Mental Health Working Group—which were responsible for developing the *National strategic framework for Aboriginal and Torres Strait Islander peoples' mental health and social and emotional well being 2004–2009*—articulated a distinction between the concepts of *social and emotional wellbeing* (SEWB) used in Aboriginal settings, and the term *mental health* used in non-Aboriginal settings:

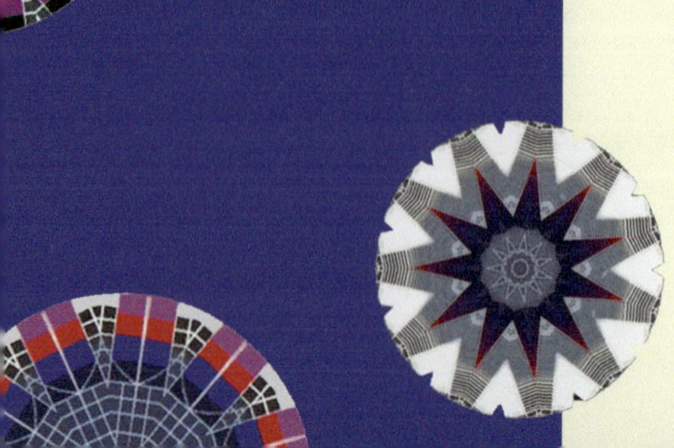

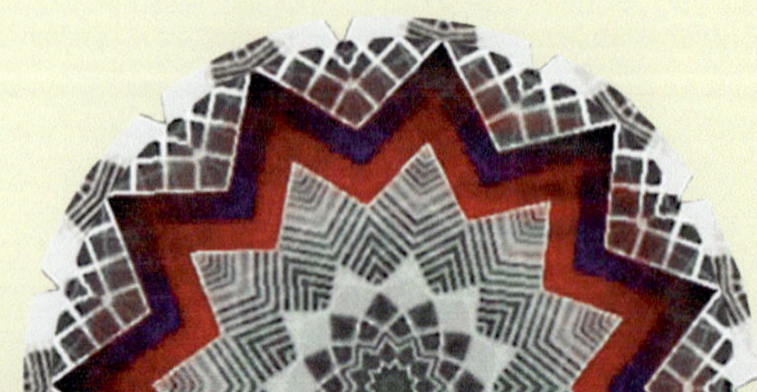

The concept of mental health comes more from an illness or clinical perspective and its focus is more on the individual and their level of functioning in their environment.

The social and emotional wellbeing concept is broader than this and recognises the importance of connection to land, culture, spirituality, ancestry, family and community, and how these affect the individual. (SHRG, 2004)

The concept of SEWB attempts to encompass our extended formation of the self, which involves a pattern of vital interconnections with others and the environment. It also recognises that achieving optimum conditions for health and wellbeing requires a holistic and whole-of-life insight of health that comprises the social, emotional, spiritual and cultural wellbeing of the whole community.

Health is a multi-faceted concept that has been defined and shaped most strongly by a non-Indigenous Western biomedical discourse of health. It is a model of health that frames it with a reference to disease or how a person presents according to their symptomology. The focus is also based on a curative framework rather than on attending to the whole person (Van Loon, 2011).

COLONISATION/COLONIALISM OF AUSTRALIA

The basis in (European) international law for the progressive takeover of the continent was the doctrine of '*terra nullius*'—land belonging to no one (Hollinsworth, 2006, pp. 68–69). This meant that Aboriginal lands were Crown lands in the eyes of the (British) law. There is often confusion when discussing the concepts of colonisation and colonialism. *Colonisation* is a fundamental process by which species spread. The settlement of the British was not peaceful, and is increasingly accepted as being a countrywide invasion. As the colonies spread across the continent, traditional lands were taken over and Aboriginal peoples became trespassers on their own lands. All over Australia there was Aboriginal resistance, but this was written out of history (Hollinsworth, 2006, pp. 70–79). Colonisation is the essential factor in human expansion, and is generally the product of a growing population and finite resources, whereas colonialism is the power exercised through occupation and subsequently majority settlement (as in North and South America, Australia and New Zealand) (Hampton & Toombs, 2013, p. 31). To simplify this, one is an extension into a new territory using a natural process; the other is the result of enforced settlement in a subservient setting.

Colonialism experienced by Aboriginal Australians reflects a history of loss of culture, identity, spirituality and dispossession. The other factor of colonialism in Australia saw the introduction and expansion of Christianity.

ADAPTING ABORIGINAL WORLDVIEWS

Aboriginal Australians now had to deal with elements of life that were not a part of their original worldviews. The challenge was to adjust (quickly) to new people who looked different, had no connection to the land, and could not be fitted into existing structures of kinship. There were now new commodities, such as flour, sugar, tea, metal, blankets, cotton and alcohol. There was also the arrival of animals such as sheep, cattle, rabbits, horses and foxes. Guns were introduced. The foundations of Aboriginal spirituality were shaken, in much the same way that Christianity was shaken by scientific discoveries about how the world was created (Hocking, 2014).

ASSIMILATION POLICY

The policy of assimilation was developed to absorb us into the colonist society. In 1937, the Commonwealth Government convened a conference with the states, where it was agreed that the aim for those Indigenous people not of 'full blood' should be their ultimate absorption in the wider population, with some form of protection for the 'semi-civilised' people of the north and centre of Australia. Two recommendations were tabled at the conference.

1. The destiny of the native of Aboriginal origin but not the full-blood lies in their ultimate absorption by the people of the Commonwealth, and . . . all efforts should be directed to that end.
2. Efforts by all state authorities should be directed towards the education of children of mixed blood at white standards, and their subsequent employment under the same conditions as whites with a view to taking their place in the white community on an equal footing with whites. (Bell, 1959)

In 1951, this policy was extended to all Aboriginal people. The aim of assimilation policies was that the 'Aboriginal problem' would ultimately disappear—the people would lose their identity within the wider community. It stated that all Aborigines should attain the same manner of living as other Australians, enjoying the same rights and privileges, accepting the same responsibilities, observing the same customs and being influenced by the same beliefs, hopes and loyalties (Lippman, 1981).

THE CHILD-REMOVAL POLICY — THE STOLEN GENERATIONS

The term *Stolen Generations* generated from the *Bringing them home* report (BTH). The fact that 'Generations' is in the plural reflects that this misguided government policy was not just relative to a particular period of Australia's history, but has had a continuing effect on the lives of undoubtedly most, if not all, Indigenous people of Australia. The overwhelming evidence is that the impact does not stop with the children removed; their children and families inherit it. The effects on family and structure have been documented in the context of war-related trauma, or even family terrorism. The effects of trauma for Indigenous Australians have therefore been widespread and enduring, recurring across generations (Bessarab & Crawford, 2013).

This was perhaps the most brutal of policies to be bestowed on our people. As a Stolen Generations survivor, I experienced first-hand the implications of this process. Born in Tasmania in 1959 to an Aboriginal mother, father unknown, it became government practice to remove what the authorities considered to be half-castes. I was removed in 1961, aged

18 months, and was not going to see my mum again until the age of 20. I was sent to various foster homes, as according to my government file I was 'fretful' and difficult to manage. What child would not be fretful being taken like that? Although at the time I was not aware of this, due to my age; it was not until I retrieved my Welfare file that I read of my history. All I knew is that the family I was to spend the next 16 years with was not mine. I was told when old enough that my mother did not want me, and that this family could show me a better life. I remained in this foster home, and from the age of five endured abuse in every sense on a daily basis.

This story is very similar to what happened around the country due to the assimilation policy. It gave authorities the right to arrive without any notice and take your children. Parents were powerless, and in many cases the police were used to doing this. Many of the Stolen children have never met—and more than likely will never meet—their parents or families.

SUBSTANCE MISUSE

In studies of non-Indigenous communities, the extent of such traumatic separation, loss, abuse, dislocation and dehumanisation can only be found in populations subjected to systemic torture, genocide, concentration camps or urban or family violence. It is interesting to note that there is a belief that drugs and alcohol were introduced by Europeans upon settlement. Substance use and abuse among Aboriginal Australian communities is at high levels, and includes tobacco, alcohol, prescription medicines, solvents and, of course, illicit drugs. Much of this appears to stem from issues arising from the impacts of colonisation, dispossession and segregation (Hampton & Toombs, 2013, pp. 169–70).

Few Aboriginal Australians have escaped from this anguish, or the self-destructive behaviour that has been particularly associated with the harmful use of alcohol and other psychoactive substances. Until the collective and essential determinants of good social and emotional wellbeing are addressed, the comorbidity of substance misuse and mental distress among Aboriginal Australians will remain.

LIVED EXPERIENCE

Aunty Dianne

Background

There are increasing concerns that the assessment tools used to evaluate mental distress for Aboriginal Australians do not provide a true diagnosis of the extent of trauma that individuals, families and communities experience. The lack of understanding of Australian Aboriginal culture and worldview, the potential cultural bias and monoculturalism, the trans-generational effects of government policy, and the differing contexts of mental health make it difficult to find easy solutions.

Aunty Dianne's story

We were sitting in the local park drinking when the police came to us and said we were not allowed to be drinking in the park. They asked to see our identification, but we didn't have any. They said we must have some form of identification and did not believe us.

The coppers grabbed my bag and tried to steal it off me, and of course I resisted. I was taken by police car down to the local police station and they put handcuffs on me. I didn't like them handcuffs, so I tried to kick one of the police, and was thrown to the ground and he put his boot into my back and held me there. Next thing I know there is an ambulance and they threw me inside and I didn't know where they were taking me. They had me strapped down so I couldn't move. When the ambulance finally stopped I had no idea where I was, but I kept screaming at them to let me go.

I was taken into a big building and some people in white coats took hold of me and the police left. They shoved me into a room which only had a bed in it. They laid me on the bed and rubbed some smelly stuff on my arm and came towards me with a big needle. Even then I was still resisting, but they jabbed it in my arm and I couldn't stay awake, just fell right to sleep. Next thing I remember was waking up in a strange room with other people. They had taken most of the ties off me so I could sit up on the bed. I felt so giddy, it was like the whole world was spinning and I couldn't see much. I tried to stand, but my legs wouldn't work, they just felt like they weren't mine. I was kept in that room for a long time, and as much as I could I resisted them. Each time I did that they would jab a big needle into me again.

After the last big needle I woke up in this place. I don't really know where I am, but I asked why I can't go home. They said that I could only go home if family came to get me, and although they had been contacted, no one had come. I wait every day for them to come to take me away from here, I'm sure they will come soon and I can go home.

I felt so sad for Aunty, and didn't understand why the family had not come to get her. She finished painting her flag, and I thanked her for sharing her story, but I had just one more question: 'How long have you been here, Aunty?' One of the staff heard

Aunty Dianne's story (*continued*)

me ask the question, and she leaned forward and whispered, 'Thirty years.'

Amazing, sad, but true.

As I left the hospital in complete dismay, I wanted to learn more of this situation, so when I returned to the university I sat down with my lecturer, who explained how this situation happened. She explained that when you are apprehended by police, if you resist you are taken to the psychiatric hospital, where you receive a tranquiliser to calm you down. The tranquiliser lasts for a long time, and it is the hope that you will stop resisting and then the police come and interview you. The police will not do this until the hospital is satisfied that you will no longer resist. This was/is the law in Western Australia; no one can fight against it. I then asked why the family would not come to see Aunty, and it was explained that once you have medicine like that you may be possessed by the devil, so families are scared of you. There is a real stigma with these kinds of facilities, and the fear of going there under any circumstances is very real. Aunty Dianne was not the only one who was not collected by her family, and most of the other patients had been there for many years.

Graylands Psychiatric Hospital is listed as one of the most antiquated psychiatric hospitals in Australia. Many attempts to close it down have for various reasons failed, and the hospital continues to be a talking point between health authorities and media.

FAMILY VIOLENCE

Domestic or family violence occurs at a higher rate in Indigenous communities compared to non-Indigenous communities. Domestic violence is carried out by partners, spouses or parents. A major trigger is often alcohol or drug use. This is exacerbated by poverty, overcrowding, lack of education or parenting skills, and unemployment (Hampton & Toombs, 2013, p. 231).

The issue of family violence and sexual abuse in Aboriginal Australian communities, more specifically the Northern Territory, has been subjected to stringent reporting from the media over the past several years. This issue is not new. There have been constant inquiries and reports over the past decade that have documented the high occurrence of violence in Aboriginal Australian communities. However, many of these documents and, in particular, their recommendations have been ignored. This may be due to funding restraints, the seeming difficulty of implementing them, or, in some cases, the need for federal or state reform.

LATERAL VIOLENCE

The term *lateral violence* is being used to describe the kind of violence Aboriginal Australians inflict on each other. Lateral violence comes from being colonised and invaded. It comes from being told you are worthless and being treated as worthless for a long period of time. Naturally you don't want to be at the bottom of the pecking order, so you turn on your own. Lateral violence is not just an individual's behaviour; it often occurs when a group of people work together to attack or undermine another individual or group. It can also be a sustained attack on individuals, families or groups (Frankland, 2011).

Lateral violence may have stemmed from the practice of removing Aboriginal Australians of different tribes from their land and forcing them to live on missions, which meant there was more than likely a clash of cultures as individuals/groups found it difficult to maintain cultural practices. I can relate to this explanation, as over the years I have served as a committee and board member to a variety of community groups. I have witnessed this behaviour often, and was even targeted on occasion, which was extremely stressful, traumatic and debilitating. It was not until this behaviour was named, and a definition given to it, that any of us understand what was taking place. Lateral violence does not discriminate; it can occur anywhere, anytime. In my experience, the sad thing is that many Aboriginal Australians have become numb to the occurrence of day-to-day violence. It has just become a way of life.

IMPACT OF TRAUMA

The traumatic experiences of introduced diseases, physical violence, rape, starvation, torture and death are not those of individuals alone. Rather, these traumas were both individual and collective. Furthermore, any one of these disasters as a traumatic event could be passed through the adult and child survivors to their children and grandchildren. The multiple layers have compounded the trauma. Today, the trauma remains in the hearts, minds and souls of Aboriginal families whose ancestors survived these times (Atkinson, 2002).

I remember some years ago having a conversation with Elders from my community, and they explained many things that disturbed me. They spoke of the deaths of my ancestors at the hands of the colonisers, and of many other atrocities. It was only when retrieving my Welfare file from the authorities some years ago that I realised the devastation my mother had had to endure. Explaining it to my children at an appropriate age, I saw in their reactions the same things that I had felt in learning of our history. The hardest thing was that I could not explain why these things had happened, but I cautioned them about prolonged blame, which is easy to do. Transference of trauma can occur so easily, but I had to make sure the cycle stopped with me. Although my children had to learn the truth of our family history, I stressed for them not to be angry. Anger, I explained, can make you sick, and I reminded them of so many people they knew who had these characteristics. This is my philosophy even today.

According to the Healing Forum Working Group (2009) there are four types of unresolved trauma impacting on the lives of Aboriginal and Torres Strait Islander people which stem from the process of colonisation and the repercussions of government policy. These are:

1. *situational trauma*—where specific situations, such as death or forcible removal, produce traumatic responses
2. *ecological trauma*—where chaotic environments contribute to trauma
3. *cumulative trauma*—where traumas such as daily racism, daily abuse or violence or poverty are repeated
4. *inter-generational trauma*—where trauma left unresolved in one generation is often unwittingly handed down to the next generation through fear, shame, violence or abusive behaviour, for example.

TRAUMA-INFORMED PRACTICE—WHAT DOES THIS MEAN?

According to the Aboriginal and Torres Strait Islander Healing Foundation Development Team (2009):

> . . . many of the problems prevalent in Aboriginal and Torres Strait Islander communities today—alcohol abuse, mental illness and family violence . . . have their roots in [the] failure of Australian governments and society to acknowledge and address the legacy of unresolved trauma still inherent in Aboriginal and Torres Strait Islander communities.

One example where trauma-informed practice is imperative is the misuse of alcohol. The devastation alcohol causes in some Aboriginal families is well documented, albeit from a biomedical perspective. Just dealing with the symptoms is not enough, and investigating causative factors is imperative. Alcohol may be used as self-medication to block trauma and the associated thoughts. It may also be used as a slow method of suicide. To assess a person with such a condition, it is imperative to encourage them to disclose their traumas in a safe, nonjudgmental environment, without fear of prejudice. Understanding trauma for Aboriginal Australians due to colonisation is imperative for any health care worker. There may be multiple traumas present, caused through loss of connection to land, family or community. This is not an easy process, as some traumas are entrenched very deep, so dealing with them one at a time is suggested. Of course this means that the process will take time, but it will provide meaningful care with hopefully positive outcomes (Hocking, 2014).

THE CONCEPT OF HEALING

Healing means different thought processes for different people, which may depend on historical factors, spiritual/religious and cultural beliefs. According to Atkinson (2012):

> Aboriginal peoples, as individuals and within their families and communities, have been profoundly hurt across generations by layered historic, social and cultural (complex) trauma. 'Closing the Gap' on Aboriginal 'disadvantage' must acknowledge that where there is hurting, there has to be a healing. In healing, people's Trauma Stories become the centrepiece for social healing action, where the storyteller is the teacher and the listener is the student or learner.

As stated by the Aboriginal and Torres Strait Islander Healing Foundation Development Team (2009):

> Healing is about bringing feelings of despair out into the open, having your pain recognized and, in turn, recognizing the pain of others. It is a therapeutic dialogue with people who are listening. It is about following your own personal journey but also seeing how it fits into the collective story of Aboriginal and Torres Strait Islander trauma.

This foreword has presented lived experience and information, supplemented by activities designed to deepen the understanding of:

- social and emotional wellbeing in an Aboriginal context
- worldviews—understanding your own, and how the worldviews of Aboriginal Australians have had to accept the non-Aboriginal domain and adjust under forced circumstances
- how an important part of understanding mental distress for Aboriginal Australians is to appreciate the trauma which has been experienced from the losses incurred by colonisation
- the impact on assessment of Aboriginal Australians in a mental health context using trauma-informed practice
- the healing process for Aboriginal Australians is at different stages—it is an individual process.

REFERENCES

Aboriginal and Torres Strait Islander Healing Foundation Development Team. (2009). *Voices from the campfires: Establishing the Aboriginal and Torres Strait Islander Healing Foundation.* Canberra, Australia: Commonwealth of Australia, pp. 4–6, 11.

Atkinson, J. (2002). Trauma trails, recreating song lines: The transgenerational effects of trauma in Indigenous Australia. North Melbourne, Australia: Spinifex Press.

Atkinson, J. (2012). An educaring approach to healing generational trauma in Aboriginal Australia. Retrieved 21 April 2015 from http://aifs.gov.au/institute/seminars/2012/atkinson/index.php

Bell, J. (1959). Official policies toward the Aborigines of NSW. *Mankind, 5*(8), 345–355.

Besserarb, D., & Crawford, F. R. (2013). Trauma, grief and loss: The vulnerability of Aboriginal families in the child protection system. In B. Bennet, S. Green, S. Gilbert, & D. Bessarab (Eds.), *Our voices: Aboriginal and Torres Strait Islander social work.* Melbourne, Australia: Palgrave Macmillan.

Frankland, R. (2011). Bullying and lateral violence. *Creative Spirits.* Retrieved from https://www.creativespirits.info/aboriginalculture/people/bullying-lateral-violence (Accessed 2015, March.)

Hampton, R., & Toombs, M. (Eds). (2013). *Indigenous Australians and health: The wombat in the room.* South Melbourne, Australia: Oxford University Press.

Healing Forum Working Group. (2009). A Healing Foundation discussion paper. Retrieved from http://aboriginalhealth.flinders.edu.au/Newsletters/2009%20Team%20Discussion%Paper.pdf (Accessed 2015, April 20.)

Hocking, D. (2014). The social and emotional well-being of Australian Aboriginals and the collaborative consumer narrative. In N. Procter, H. P. Hamer, D. McGarry, R. L. Wilson, & T. Froggatt (Eds.), *Mental health: A person-centred approach.* Melbourne, Australia: Cambridge University Press.

Hollinsworth, D. (2006). *Race and racism in Australia*. South Melbourne, Australia: Thompson Social Science Press.

Lippmann, L. (1981). *Generations of resistance: The Aboriginal struggle for justice*. Melbourne, Australia: Longman Cheshire.

Social Health Reference Group. (2004) *National strategic framework for Aboriginal and Torres Strait Islander peoples' mental health and social and emotional well being 2004–2009.* Canberra, Australia: National Aboriginal and Torres Strait Islander Health Council and National Mental Health Working Group.

Van Loon, A. (2011). Contexts of community nursing. In D. Kralik & A. Van Loon (Eds.), *Community nursing in Australia* (2nd ed.) (pp. 46–84). Milton, Australia: John Wiley & Sons.

1

People with lived experience and carers

SIMON SWINSON, MIKE HAZELTON AND TIM HEFFERNAN

LEARNING OUTCOMES

After completing this chapter, you will be able to:

1. Analyse why the term *deviant behaviour* lacks a definition that covers all situations.
2. Define and explain *mental illness*.
3. Compare and contrast the essential characteristics of mental health with mental illness.
4. Identify five types of mental illness that rank among the top 10 causes of disability worldwide.
5. Explain how societal attitudes, philosophical viewpoints and definitions of *mental illness* have changed over time.
6. Explore the lived experiences of people with mental illness and of their families and friends.
7. Explore the meaning and impact of stigma for people living with mental illness, their families and friends, mental health service providers and the wider community.

KEY TERMS

consumer 4
comorbidity 7
deviance 3
disability 5
distress 5
epidemiology 6
hardiness 4
interpersonal 4
intrapersonal 4
mental disorder 4
mental health 4
mental illness 4
nervous breakdown 17
psychopathology 5
resilience 4
stigma 15

LIVED EXPERIENCE

Simon Swinson

One does not grow up intending to become a mental health consumer. It is something that life thrusts upon you, and society labels you with in the course of developing specific kinds of (mental) health problems. You start off with a blank sheet of possibilities, only to find that life is severely limited by the labels and experiences that surround mental illness. Fortunately, society is starting to find ways of being more responsive to, and supportive of, the real needs of people who live with mental illness. Slowly but surely, consumers are having a greater say in the services they receive as part of the constant project of personal recovery.

Increasingly, the consumer voice is being sought out in ways that it never was previously—by governments, health service managers, health professional practitioners and university academics. Nonetheless, many consumers still lack access to the resources that would enable them to be heard. Such problems are especially likely to occur: in rural and remote areas; in places of high socioeconomic disadvantage; among people of uncertain citizenship status, such as refugees and asylum seekers living in immigration detention centres.

Unfortunately, not all health professionals are as yet open to the consumer voice; for many consumers, exposure to mental health services, which invariably occurs under distressing circumstances, can be profoundly unsatisfactory. As the next generation of health professionals, you are encouraged to take on board the concepts of 'consumer voice' and 'recovery-oriented practice', and put these at the heart of your studies in mental health.

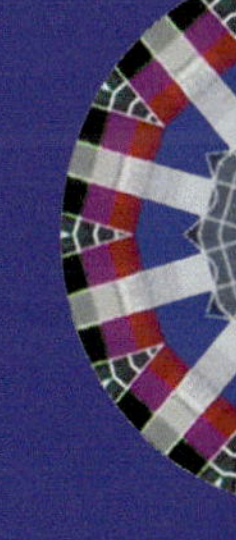

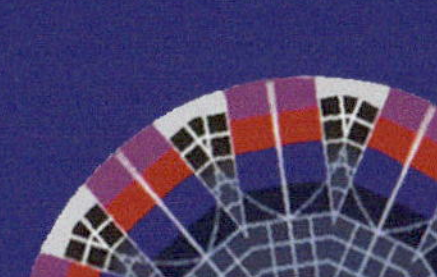

INTRODUCTION

The World Health Organization (WHO; 2014b) asserts that mental health is integral to all health, and that there is no health without mental health. The WHO (2007) also considers nurses to be an essential human resource for mental health care globally, and in low- to middle-income countries may be the only formal providers of care to people living with mental illness. Strategically, nurses are in a prime position to contribute to mental health and overall health outcomes; to provide comfort and support to people experiencing trauma and distress. While doing this work well requires rigorous formal education, another important source of learning is from people with a lived experience of mental illness and from those family members and friends who care for them.

Much of the work undertaken by nurses in the mental health field is different to that found in other areas of nursing. In particular, psychiatric–mental health nursing is about making interpersonal connections and using relationships as the basis to providing help. There are occasions when the work is unpredictable. Facing the unknown in a mental health setting can produce anxiety in students, new graduates and even more experienced nurses. It is not unusual for students and new graduates to ask:

- What kinds of people will I meet in a mental health setting?
- Will these people be hard to talk to?
- What do I have in common with them?
- What if I do something or say something wrong?
- How do I make a connection with them?
- Will I know what to do if a person becomes angry or upset?

This chapter discusses some of these questions. Other common concerns of nursing students and new graduate nurses are more fully addressed in Chapters 2 and 9 (see especially the Self-awareness feature in Chapter 2 on page 22).

What do you have in common with people who use mental health services? How can you ever hope to understand them? There are many approaches to understanding people—history, sociology, anthropology, philosophy, anatomy, physiology and psychology, among others. Each is like a searchlight, illuminating some facts while leaving others in shadow. One of the challenges you will face in your clinical experiences, in your classroom lectures, tutorials and discussions, and in reading this textbook, is how to judiciously and appropriately blend knowledge from these diverse sources. Learning from people with lived experience will almost certainly change the way you think about mental health issues. We have no doubt that had this chapter and other chapters in this textbook been written by nursing authors only, it would have been less relevant personally, professionally and educationally.

LIVED EXPERIENCE

Tim Heffernan

Mental health consumers are people just like you. In fact, if you look around your lecture theatre or workplace, at least 20 per cent of you and your colleagues are mental health consumers. Over your lifetime—say at your 50th high-school reunion—probably 50 per cent of your classmates will have experienced mental illness.

The thing is, they are still your workmates and classmates, and you are probably unaware of their struggles, their 'illness'. We, the people you will work with if you choose to become a mental health nurse, are mostly not much different than your friends and colleagues. Despite our illness, we all hope to be able to attend our 50th-year reunion, and we hope to reclaim or gain our place in the workforce and in the community.

When I talk to student nurses, I often say that yours is the most wonderful job in the world. How good is it to be able to help people heal and begin their journey of recovery? How good is it to find out later that that hopeless person now has a job and family? How good is it to make a difference most days at work?

We are all recovering, and most consumers understand that their illness is a normal human reaction to extraordinary life experiences. For many, this means adverse childhood experiences or trauma; for others, it can be bullying or a lack of love during those crucial teenage years. We mostly reject the medical or biological model of mental illness—we mostly don't believe that we have a brain disease.

The idea of disease was a good one initially. If it is a disease, we can cure it. But we now know that it is much more complex than this. We think that the best way nurses can assist us on our recovery journey is to be with us, share bits of yourself with us, be our confidant, listen to us, laugh with us, cry with us. Mental health nursing is so special because you are sometimes nursing our soul, our most vulnerable being.

Mostly, we see nurses who are task-driven—checking off the clipboard or on the computer writing things we never own. Some seem scared of us, and like to spend most of the shift behind the 'fishbowl' looking out over us. Some, the ones I remember, stayed with us on the floor, asked about our lives, took an interest and then the best shared something of themselves. They said: 'You are a person, I am a person—let's share.'

As for mental illness being a global problem, we have to recognise that our global, national and local problems cause mental illness. We are not a problem: if you get to know us, you will discover that we hold many solutions. We need to be strong together.

Most people with mental illness do not seek treatment. We get the blame. The reality is that historically the treatment has alienated us, traumatised us and made us wary of the mental health system.

You can make this history.

The strategies in this book are designed to help you become a therapeutic, confident and safe psychiatric–mental health nurse. This chapter discusses what it means to live with mental illness, sometimes also referred to as 'mental disorder'. We review the attitudes and philosophical viewpoints that have influenced the understandings and approaches to mental health care throughout history, and the stigma connected with mental illness. We also identify the burden of mental illness, both nationally and globally. Our goals in this text are to encourage you to think seriously about what constitutes mental health and mental illness, to appreciate the humanity of people who live with mental illness, and to approach your mental health professional practice in a confident, open-minded and respectful manner.

It is possible that your studies in mental health and associated clinical placements may lead to anxiety, or self-doubt. We encourage you to approach psychiatric–mental health nursing with energetic enthusiasm, and an eagerness to understand and develop your skills in this critically important field. In doing so, you will find the humanity, creativity, caring and joy inherent in the people with whom you are working.

THE CONCEPTS OF DEVIANCE, MENTAL HEALTH AND MENTAL ILLNESS

Defining what is 'normal' *and* what is 'abnormal' is not as simple as it might seem. Whatever else they imply, concepts such as *deviance, mental health* and *mental disorder* are social constructions which derive their meaning from how society defines certain behaviours by certain people. Accordingly, we advocate taking a critical look at the social conditions (Hewitt & Shulman, 2011) under which someone is called 'mentally ill'.

Deviance

You will undoubtedly hear about, and see, 'deviant' behaviour. We use a sociological definition in approaching **deviance**—behaviour outside or away from the social norm of a specific group—in this text. Within its social context, *deviant* does not mean 'bad' or abnormal (Cockerham, 2011). Behaviour that is considered bizarre or unreasonable in one cultural context or in one particular time span may be considered acceptable in another. For example, 20 or 30 years ago, tattoos and body piercings (see Figure 1.1 ■) would have been thought to be extremely deviant. Today, such forms of body adornment are not unique. Not only are they commonplace, they are also considered fashion statements in some social contexts.

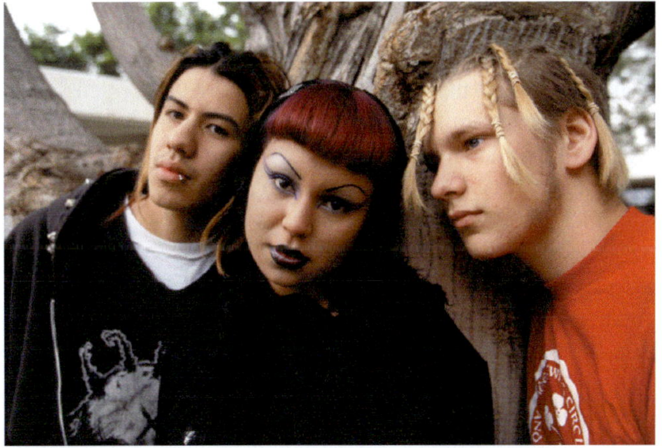

FIGURE 1.1 ■ Nonconforming behaviour or appearance that flouts social norms is an example of social deviance—not evidence of psychopathology or abnormal behaviour.
Photo courtesy of Michael Newman/PhotoEdit.

Further, your ideas about deviant behaviour are likely to be influenced by your upbringing, what you have seen and heard in your own communities and neighbourhoods (as illustrated in the Practice Example on the next page), what you have read about in newspapers or magazines, or what you have seen and read about on the internet and in social media. All of these experiences influence your attitudes towards, and beliefs about, deviance, mental health and mental illness.

You will also find that people living with mental illness are everyday, ordinary people. They are your neighbours, your friends, your family members; your teacher, your doctor; or even yourself. It is highly likely that you know someone who has been diagnosed with a mental illness or has sought mental health counselling to deal with problems in living.

Practice example

A mental health nurse, recalling her childhood experiences with what were then considered community deviants, described how she and her friends taunted 'Crazy Helen', causing her to shout incoherently at them.

Peter, a student in the Bachelor of Nursing, recalled that one of his close schoolfriends had an older brother who was said to be very smart but 'odd'; in his early teenage years he used to feel both apprehensive and intrigued when visiting his friend—wondering whether the older brother would answer the door. Peter admitted to similar feelings of anxiety and fascination as he prepared to undertake his first mental health clinical placement.

People, not patients

As you work through the chapters in this text, you will notice the terms *person, individual* or **consumer**, not client or patient, being used to refer to persons who seek or receive mental health services. We prefer the terms *person, individual* and *consumer* over patient because of their association with empowerment and self-responsibility, respect and an optimistic belief that people are capable of recovery. The term *patient* is associated with the traditional sick role, in which people relinquish responsibility to health care experts who have decision-making authority. We believe that in the traditional sick role, people are vulnerable and disempowered.

More people than ever before engage in partnerships with their health care providers and act on their own behalf (or, an advocate does, if the person is unable). Not all people are capable of participating in their own health care all of the time—for example, in some emergency situations, when comatose, or when a mental or physical condition prevents it. However, they are more likely to do so when they are informed consumers of mental health care and know that options exist, and when they are encouraged, and even expected, to do so. The term 'partnership' is a reminder—to all of us—that, among other things, recovery involves collaboration with others.

In health care today, the power balance has shifted. The same principles apply to the use of the terms *adherence* and *compliance.* These days, people are supported to adhere to a treatment protocol rather than to 'comply' with it; that is, people should be active participants in the treatment regimen.

Mental health

There is no one overall accepted definition of **mental health**. In general, a person is considered to be mentally healthy when what that person does (the person's behaviour), how that person relates to others (the person's **interpersonal** relationships between oneself and others), and how that person relates to him- or herself (the person's **intrapersonal** relationships within the mind or the self) give evidence of psychological, emotional and social health. It is a lifelong process of growing towards one's potential. Just as physical health is more than the absence of disease, mental health is more than the absence of mental illness.

Mentally healthy people are independent and autonomous. They think well of themselves and others, but are also realistic about their own and others' abilities and shortcomings. They can accept the ups and downs of life, and often come out even stronger than before. They have a wide range of behaviours, emotions and values that are usually consistent with one another. These and other characteristics of mentally healthy people are discussed in Box 1.1.

Mental illness

Mental illness and mental health, we believe, are outgrowths of both intrapersonal and interpersonal processes. Determining that someone has a mental illness is often a matter of judgment. The appropriateness of behaviour depends on whether it is judged plausible or not (e.g. deviant) according to a set of social, ethical and legal rules that define the limits of appropriate behaviour and reality within particular social, cultural and historical contexts. For example, if a man on a street corner says he is the King of England, people will not believe him and will consider him deviant and his statement symptomatic or disturbed. If a man at a fancy-dress party says he is the King of England, people reach a different conclusion, because in that social setting his behaviour and dress fit the norm. We would not label deviant political, religious or sexual behaviour, or conflicts primarily between an individual and society, as a **mental disorder** unless the deviance or conflict is a symptom of dysfunction in the individual.

With the preceding as philosophical background, we understand the concept of **mental illness** as a group of

Box 1.1 Characteristics of people considered to be mentally healthy

People who are considered mentally healthy:

- ***function independently and autonomously***—mentally healthy individuals respect and seek out the opinions of others, but assume responsibility for solving their own problems; they can plan ahead and formulate realistic goals
- ***hold a positive attitude toward themselves***—their self-esteem is combined with a realistic estimate of their abilities and their limitations
- ***take life's disappointments in stride***—mentally healthy people have a variety of coping mechanisms that help them to deal with the ups and downs of everyday life
- ***remain healthy even under high levels of stress or in the face of loss or trauma***—this characteristic is called **hardiness**
- ***adapt successfully to even very difficult experiences***—this characteristic of being able to bounce back to normal functioning or an even higher level of functioning is called **resilience**
- ***integrate their emotions, behaviours and values into a coherent whole***—their emotions, behaviours and values are consistent and fit together
- ***experience a wide range of emotions***—the emotions that mentally healthy people experience run the gamut—sadness, hopefulness, anger, joy, anxiety, disgust, fear, surprise, elation and happiness, among others
- ***master their environment***—mastering the environment includes being able to capably deal with what goes on around them, thus achieving a sense of connectedness, harmony and balance among themselves, their families, their friends and the community
- ***perceive reality clearly***—the mentally healthy person can distinguish between fact and fantasy and lives in the real world.

symptoms, such as a pattern or a syndrome, in which the individual experiences significant **distress** (the person suffers psychologically) and **disability** (impairment in one or more important areas of functioning in daily life), or causes them to harm themselves or others.

The signs and symptoms of mental illness are known as **psychopathology** (literally, 'pathology of the mind'). Mental health professionals refer to mental illnesses as psychopathological conditions. Mental illnesses are identified, standardised and categorised in two diagnostic classification systems: the *Diagnostic and statistical manual of mental disorders* (DSM-5) of the American Psychiatric Association, the 5th edition of which became available in late 2013; and the International Classification of Diseases (ICD-10) of the World Health Organization, a new 11th edition of which is expected to be released in 2018. Later in this textbook, you will learn about major types of mental illness, some of which are as follows:

- *disorders of mood*, such as depression and bipolar disorder, which can significantly interfere with a person's thoughts, behaviour, mood, activity and physical health
- *schizophrenia*, a disorder of thinking characterised by social withdrawal, distortions of thinking and perception, and bizarre behaviour, that first develops in the later teenage and early adult years
- *anxiety disorders*, with the common theme of excessive, irrational fear and dread
- *personality disorders*—persistent and rigid behaviour patterns that can significantly affect the person's ability to reasonably function in society
- *cognitive disorders* or disorders of thinking, which usually develop in the later adult years
- *substance-related disorders* that include addictions to alcohol, drugs, tobacco and other substances
- *dissociative disorders*, complex disorders in which a cluster of events is beyond the person's ability to recall
- *somatic symptom disorders* in which symptoms suggest physical disorders for which there is no evidence, and factitious disorders in which a person intentionally produces or feigns physical or psychological symptoms
- *eating disorders* in which disturbed eating patterns develop as a way of coping with stress
- *disorders specific to children*.

Given the right circumstances, anyone can develop a mental health problem, ranging from a mild, temporary increase in anxiety to the most severe types of mental illness. Fame, status and money do not ensure mental health or happiness, at least not according to the celebrities we hear about—actors, sports stars, authors, musicians, singers, movie directors and scientists. Many celebrities are speaking out about their experiences with mental illness, such as those in the following list:

- Paula Abdul has spoken about her experience with the eating disorder, bulimia.
- Jessica Rowe and Brooke Shields have spoken about their post-natal depression.
- Drew Carey has spoken about bouts of depression and suicide attempts.
- Catherine Zeta-Jones, Mel Gibson and Carrie Fisher have spoken about living with bipolar disorder.
- Matthew Mitcham and Ruby Rose have spoken about having depression, and Garry McDonald has spoken about having both anxiety and depression.

People, especially those who are public figures who openly discuss their mental health problems or write books about their experiences, help increase public awareness. They contribute to making it easier for others to reveal their own struggles and seek help. The Mental Health in the Media feature, below, highlights Carrie Fisher's success in coping with problems with drugs and alcohol, addiction to prescription medications, and bipolar disorder.

Like many concepts in the human sciences, the concept of mental illness lacks a definition that covers all situations. In addition, definitions of mental illness have shifted throughout history. The historical shifts in attitude and philosophical viewpoints from preliterate cultures to the present day are reviewed later in this chapter. The history of mental health nursing is reviewed in Chapter 3, and the history of psychiatric treatment in Chapter 5.

MENTAL ILLNESS AS A GLOBAL PROBLEM

How many people worldwide have a diagnosable mental illness? Answers to this important question, most of which are derived from epidemiological studies, contribute to the planning and implementation of mental health services.

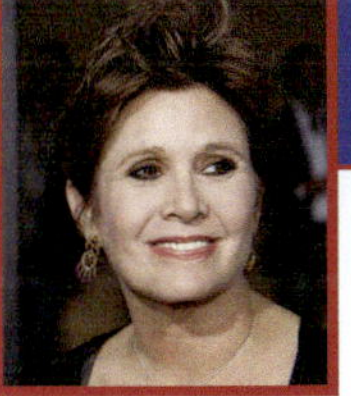

MENTAL HEALTH IN THE MEDIA
Carrie Fisher

As the daughter of Debbie Reynolds and Eddie Fisher, Carrie Fisher was a real-life Hollywood princess before she became Princess Leia of the Star Wars movie trilogy in the 1970s. As an author, Fisher wrote *Postcards from the Edge (1987)*, a semi-autobiographical novel that discussed her addiction to cocaine and other drugs. *Postcards from the Edge* became a movie, for which she also wrote the screenplay. She became a Hollywood script 'doctor', working on and refining the screenplays of other authors, writing other novels and screenplays, and acting in movies, television and stage plays. Her memoir *Wishful Drinking* was published in 2008. She recently returned to the role of Princess Leia in *Star Wars: The Force Awakens*.

Carrie Fisher publicly discussed her problems with drugs and alcohol, addiction to prescription medications, and bipolar disorder. A highly productive person, Carrie Fisher's successes provided hope to others in coping with and recovering from mental illness. Carrie Fisher passed away in December 2016.

Photo courtesy © Allstar Picture Library/Alamy.

Psychiatric **epidemiology** is the study of the distribution and determinants of mental illness in human populations, and is used to do the following:

- determine causative factors for specific types of illness
- identify groups of people at high risk of developing specific types of illness
- recognise changes in health problems, especially the emergence of new problems
- plan for current health needs and predict future needs
- evaluate preventive and therapeutic measures.

Psychiatric epidemiology can assist psychiatric mental health nurses to better understand the prevalence of mental illness and the organisation of mental health services. Information about mental health in Australia can be obtained from the Australian Institute of Health and Welfare (AIHW).

Australian epidemiological data is collected in a number of data sets: Admitted Patient Mental Health Care Data Set; Mental Health Establishment Data Set; Community Mental Health Care Data Set; and the Residential Mental Health Care Data Set. In addition, the National Minimum Data Sets Mental Health Care are gathered by state and territory governments annually. All data element definitions have been agreed by the National Health Information Standards and Statistics Committee to ensure alignment with national standards. These are available at www.aihw.gov/mental-health-information-sources/.

In addition to these Australian data sets, international mental health data can be obtained from the World Health Organization (see www.who.int/mental_health/en/).

Mental illness in Australia

Mental illness affects a large number of Australians every year; for adults, this is estimated to be up to 20 per cent of the population, and for children and adolescents up to 25 per cent. Up to 45 per cent of Australians aged 16–85 will experience a mental illness at some point in their lifetime. Anxiety disorders affect about 14 per cent and depression about 6 per cent of adults annually. The remainder are affected by substance use disorders, psychotic illness such as schizophrenia, personality disorders and other conditions. While mental illness is common, a large number of those affected do not seek any form of help for their problems—far fewer than for physical health problems. For depression this is about 25 per cent; for other common forms of mental illness it is higher, about 60 per cent for people living with anxiety disorders and over 75 per cent for those living with substance use disorders (Australian Bureau of Statistics [ABS], 2007).

For some people, the extent of disability caused by mental illness is so great that participation in society is severely compromised. Schizophrenia can be a particularly disabling condition that affects about 1 per cent of Australians at some stage in their lives. In severe forms of mental illness such as schizophrenia, mental health professionals typically give priority to managing the symptoms. However, for people living with mental illness the priorities can be different. When asked about the challenges they expected to face in the coming year, participants in the Survey of High Impact Psychosis (SHIP) ranked financial concerns, loneliness/social isolation, lack of employment and poor physical health above uncontrolled symptoms of mental illness (Carr, Whiteford, Groves, McGorry & Shepherd, 2012). It has been estimated that up to 75 per cent of homeless people have a mental illness (Mental Health Council of Australia, 2009).

Most people living with mental illness receive their care from a primary care practitioner, a general (medical) practitioner or a mental health nurse working in a community mental health team, or in schemes such as the Mental Health Nurse Incentive Program (MHNIP). However, Australia is a large continent, and the majority of mental health services are located in highly urbanised locations, such as capital cities or regional centres. Access to mental health care is much more difficult in rural and remote areas.

It is estimated that mental illness is responsible for almost 13 per cent of the total burden of disease in Australia, placing it third as a disease group after cancer and cardiovascular disease (Australian Institute of Health and Welfare [AIHW], 2016). Thus, the principles of psychiatric mental health nursing that you will learn in this textbook have major implications for your work in nursing, regardless of your future area of specialisation.

Comorbidity of mental disorders

Many people living with mental illness have two or more psychiatric disorders—particularly depression, anxiety, and alcohol and other substance abuse—at any one given time or during their lifetime. People living with mental illness are also much more likely to experience poor physical health when compared to the general population, with life expectancy

LIVED EXPERIENCE

Simon Swinson

With the commencement of my National Disability Insurance Scheme (NDIS) Plan, I have been able to participate in regular gym sessions as part of an exercise plan developed in collaboration with my service provider. This involvement has been made possible by a recent Commonwealth Government initiative and community donations (of equipment), and has enabled me to address long-term concerns regarding my cardiovascular health. Weight has been a constant issue associated with the use of prescribed antipsychotic medication and an illness-related sedentary lifestyle. Such opportunities have been rare up until now, and I believe represent changes in the way society thinks of and responds to people living with mental illness. I now feel that my life is valuable.

being reduced by as much as 30 years (Ehrlich, Kenall, Frey & Compton, 2014). In the past few decades, metabolic syndrome has emerged as a problem, especially for people living with psychotic disorders such as schizophrenia (Morgan et al., 2012). Living with more than one form of illness is referred to as **comorbidity**. Issues related to comorbidity are receiving significant attention in mental health research.

Over a decade ago, Kessler and colleagues (2005) replicated an earlier North American comorbidity study to examine what changes, if any, had occurred in the prevalence of mental disorders in the years since the original study. The comorbidity replication study is one of the most extensive studies of psychiatric disorders to date. It was found that the prevalence of mental disorders had not changed during the decade in question. The main findings of this study are summarised below, and were consistent with previous research:

- Women had higher rates of affective and anxiety disorders.
- Men had higher rates of substance abuse disorders and antisocial personality disorder.
- Most disorders declined with age and with higher socioeconomic status.
- Fewer than 40 per cent of those with a lifetime disorder had ever received professional treatment.

A most striking finding is that mental illnesses are more highly concentrated than previously recognised in approximately 14 per cent of the population who have had a history of three or more comorbid disorders. When severity is considered, this group also includes the great majority of those with severe disorders. Less than 50 per cent of this highly comorbid group ever obtained specialty mental health treatment, despite the number and severity of their disorders. These North American findings are consistent with the Australian data (ABS, 2007), and point to the need for community-based preventive programs aimed at more outreach. There is also a need for more research on barriers, including cultural barriers, to accessing mental health services.

Help-seeking patterns in mental health care

The research on help-seeking patterns may be summarised as follows:

- Most people with mental disorders do not seek professional treatment.
- Comorbidity increases the likelihood that a person will seek treatment. Still less than half of the highly comorbid group identified by Kessler and colleagues (2005) ever obtained specialty mental health treatment, despite the number and severity of their disorders.
- When seeking treatment, most people living with mental illness seek treatment from primary care practitioners such as general practitioners, who prescribe the majority of medications. Yet there is a lack of general practitioners with mental health expertise, especially in rural and remote areas.
- Individuals with chronic mental illness comprise the majority of those who seek treatment.

Awareness of these help-seeking patterns is essential in order to address the problems of nonuse or misuse of mental health services. Pivotal issues are the availability, accessibility, cost and quality of mental health services, especially because prognosis is affected by the duration of any mental disorder.

Severely under-served groups in relation to mental health services include the following:

- people with substance use disorders
- people from culturally and linguistically diverse backgrounds
- people living with severe socioeconomic disadvantage
- people who are homeless.

Unfortunately, mental health funding in Australia has tended to go to services that are reactive rather than proactive, situational rather than long-term and strategic, and rehabilitative rather than preventive. In addressing these problems, the Commonwealth Government recently announced a major reallocation of funding from mental health services in hospitals to community mental health and primary care services.

Adequacy of mental health services

Australia has a number of government and non-government organisations that provide advice and support to people living with mental illness, their families and health professionals. The contact details of some of these are provided in Table 1.1 ■.

Mental illness around the globe

A classic and still relevant major study by the WHO has shown an underestimation of the incidence of mental illness worldwide. The Global Burden of Disease study, which collects and compares health data from across the globe, indicates that mental illnesses such as depression are among the leading causes of disability worldwide (WHO, 2014a). Globally, about 400 million people of all ages live with depression, with more women affected than men, 60 million people live with bipolar disorder, and schizophrenia affects about 21 million people worldwide (WHO, 2014a).

The WHO's Mental Health Action Plan 2013–2020 recognises the essential role of mental health in achieving health for all people. The Action Plan includes the following objectives:

- more effective leadership and governance for mental health
- provision of comprehensive, integrated mental health and social care services in community-based settings
- implementation of strategies for promotion and prevention
- strengthened information systems, evidence and research.

More information on the Action Plan can be obtained at www.who.int/mental_health/publications/action_plan/en/.

Researchers suggest that the personal, social and economic costs associated with mental illness are very high, and are likely to be underestimated. Under-reporting due to stigma and a lack

TABLE 1.1 ■ Mental health support organisations

Organisation	Purpose	Contact details
SANE	To help Australians affected by mental illness lead a better life. SANE pursues its mission through three key areas of activity to promote a better life for all Australians affected by mental illness: support, training and education.	https://www.sane.org/
Beyond Blue	Beyond Blue was established in 2000 as a national initiative to create a community response to depression. The aim was to move the focus on depression away from a mental health service issue and towards one which is understood, acknowledged and addressed by the wider community.	http://www.beyondblue.org.au Tel: 1300 22 4636
Headspace	Headspace was established in 2006 and is the National Youth Mental Health Foundation. Headspace helps young people who are going through a tough time. People aged 12–25 years can get health advice, support and information about general health, mental health and counselling, education, employment and other services, and alcohol and other drug services	http://www.headspace.org.au
The Black Dog Institute	The Black Dog Institute is dedicated to improving the lives of people affected by mood disorders through high-quality translational research, clinical expertise and national education programs.	http://www.blackdoginstitute.org.au Bipolar Disorders Clinic Tel: (02) 9382 2991 Depression Clinic Tel: (02) 9382 2991 Psychology Clinic Tel: (02) 9382 2991
Kids Helpline	Kids Helpline is Australia's only national 24/7 telephone and online counselling and support service for young people aged between 5 and 25 years.	http://www.kidshelp.com.au Tel: 1800 55 1800
Lifeline	Lifeline is a national charity providing all Australians experiencing a personal crisis with access to 24-hour crisis support and suicide prevention services.	https://www.lifeline.org.au Tel: 13 11 14
Mental Health Carers ARAFMI Australia	Mental Health Carers ARAFMI is a collective of organisations whose members are mental health carers. ARAFMI represents the views and perspectives of carers, and has advocated for changes and services to improve the lives and wellbeing of people affected by mental illness, including carers and family members. Members include: Mental Health Carers ARAFMI Qld; Mind Australia, ARAFMI Tasmania; Mental Health Carers ARAFMI NSW; Mental Health Carers ARAFMI WA; and Mental Illness Fellowship of Australia (NT).	http://www.arafmiaustralia.asn.au Tel: (03) 8640 5683
Mental Illness Fellowship Australia (MIFA)	A national network of community-based organisations that provide a range of services to people living with mental illness, their carers and the community	www.mifa.org.au

of awareness of the connection between mental disorders and other health conditions are likely contributing factors. Mental illnesses may interact to increase risk for communicable diseases (e.g. alcohol and other drugs for HIV/AIDS), non-communicable diseases (e.g. depression and coronary heart disease), and intentional and unintentional injuries (e.g. alcohol as a risk factor in traffic accidents). Conversely, many health conditions may increase the risk of mental illness (e.g. depression subsequent to debilitating chronic illness).

The prediction of the WHO is that the burden of mental disorders will increase even more by the year 2020, because global mental health resources remain low, and improvements in the past few decades have been minimal. Moreover, the impacts of rapid technological development, widespread civil disturbance, terrorism and climate change will likely contribute to an increasing risk of mental illness. It is also possible to identify groups of people whose life circumstances make them especially vulnerable to developing mental illness. In many cases this vulnerability stems from sociocultural dislocation, disadvantage or exposure to violence. Some of these groups are included in Table 1.2 ■. Clearly, mental illness is one of global health's greatest challenges (Patel & Prince, 2011), which is unlikely to be adequately addressed unless nurses play a leading role.

Throughout this text, we will continue to remind you of these serious concerns. We will remind you of the humanity

Table 1.2 ■ Sociocultural dislocation, violence and mental illness
People exposed to bullying Bullying is associated with youth violence, but can occur with adults, too. Bullying is defined as unwanted repeated aggressive behaviour towards others, involving power imbalance, and can be physical, verbal or relational in nature. Cyber-bullying is bullying through information communication technology. Bullying is a major, modifiable risk factor for mental illness, and can contribute to depression, anxiety, sleep disturbance and poor school adjustment (Kozlowska & Durheim, 2013). **See:** www.cdc.gov/violenceprevention
People subjected to intimate partner violence Intimate partner violence refers to behaviour within an intimate relationship that causes physical, psychological or sexual harm to those in the relationship. Such physical violence, psychological abuse and controlling behaviour is often associated with harmful levels of alcohol consumption, and is most often perpetrated by men. Exposure to intimate partner violence significantly increases the risk of depression, anxiety, suicide and drug and alcohol abuse. Public policy responses include awareness-raising campaigns, reporting of cases, and advocacy to protect survivors and bring perpetrators to justice. **See:** www.who.int/violence_injury_prevention/violence/world_report/factsheets/ft_intimate.pdf
People living with disability Disability is the interaction between individuals with a health condition and personal and environmental factors. Worldwide, a billion people have some form of disability, many with mental illness. There is high unmet need for health care among people living with disability, especially among people living with mental illness: in developed countries, 35–50 per cent of those affected do not receive any form of help; in developing countries, this can be as high as 76–85 per cent. Policy responses include: awareness-raising campaigns; accurate data collection and dissemination; capacity building within health and social care services; and strategies to ensure that people living with disabilities are knowledgeable about their health conditions. **See**: http://www.who.int/mediacentre/factsheets/fs352/en/
Child maltreatment Up to a quarter of adults report having been physically abused when they were children, with females (1 in 5) being at higher risk than males (1 in 13). Child maltreatment includes: physical and/or emotional ill-treatment, sexual abuse, neglect and commercial exploitation. The consequences of child maltreatment include severe physical and mental health problems that may persist for life. Approaches to prevention include supporting parents and teaching parenting skills through home visits to provide support and education, and group-based effective parenting courses. In many countries, child protection checks and reporting of actual or suspected cases are mandatory for health and social care professionals and students. **See:** www.who.int/mediacentre/factsheets/fs150/en/
The mental health of indigenous people Worldwide, there are about 370 million indigenous peoples living in more than 70 countries. They represent a rich diversity of cultures, religions, languages and traditions; however, many are socially and politically marginalised, and as a population group have much poorer health than their non-indigenous counterparts. Human rights and social justice concerns often underpin poor health, and this is especially so for indigenous peoples: they are at higher risk of poor living conditions, alcohol and substance misuse and suicide. Interventions include: improved health data collection and dissemination; improved access to housing, social services, education and employment; and the development of culturally appropriate health services. **See:** www.who.int/mediacentre/factsheets/fs326/en/
The mental health of people during and after emergencies People can develop a wide range of mental health problems during and long after being involved in emergency situations. The likelihood of recovery is improved if people feel safe and remain connected, calm and hopeful. With access to social, physical and emotional support, many will find ways to help themselves. Intervention involves the provision of basic services through to services that are highly specialised, to help match community needs to required levels of expertise. Despite their adverse effects on mental health, humanitarian crises and emergency situations are also opportunities to build better mental health systems; as individuals, communities and countries recover, resilience increases. **See:** www.int/mediacentre/factsheets/fs/383/en/
Refugees and asylum seekers Cultural factors may influence the presentation, assessment and treatment of mental illness. Escape from conflict zones, the experience of long and often dangerous journeys, and the uncertainty and distress of potentially long-term (onshore and offshore) immigration detention contribute to the high rates of mental illness among refugees seeking to enter Australia. Psychiatric–mental health nurses and other practitioners must be aware of how individual refugees and family groups understand and respond to mental illness, and how such understandings are likely to influence the expression of distress, patterns of (non-) help-seeking and (non-) adherence to treatment. Working with refugees and asylum seekers involves: understanding how cultural beliefs may present as psychiatric symptoms; communicating effectively using (telephone and face-to-face) interpreters; establishing rapport with people distrustful of government officials and services; managing the possibility that symptoms might be feigned to gain support to stay in Australia from treating staff; recognising and responding to the psychological and emotional impact of prolonged immigration detention. Galletly and colleagues (2016, pp. 451–452) have outlined cultural considerations in the treatment of psychoses in refugee and asylum-seeker populations. Box 1.2 outlines questions that may be used on assessing people from refugee and immigrant backgrounds.

Box 1.2 Questions for assessing people from refugee and immigrant backgrounds

- Can you tell me about what brought you here? What do you call_____? [Use the person's words for their problem]
- When do you think it started, and why did it start then?
- What are the main problems it is causing you?
- What have you done to try to stop/manage ______ to make it go away or make it better?
- How would you usually manage _______ in your own culture, or make it go away or make it better?
- How have you been coping so far with ______?
- In your culture, is your _______ considered 'severe'? What is the worst problem ______ could cause you?
- What type of help would you be seeking from me/our service?
- Are there people in your community who are aware that you have this condition?
- What do they think or believe caused _______? Are they doing anything to help you?

Source: Galletly et al. (2016, 451, citing Procter [2007]).

of people living with mental illness—of the family and friends we love, the neighbours we know, and celebrities we hear about. We will also continue to remind you that the lived experience of mental illness not only has distressing effects on the lives of those affected, but also can encourage extraordinary clarity, insight and creative potential.

FAMILIES, FRIENDS AND CARERS OF PEOPLE LIVING WITH MENTAL ILLNESS

Your work as a nurse is also likely to bring you into contact with members of another very important group of stakeholders—the carers of people living with mental illness. The number of informal carers in Australia is estimated to be 2.7 million (12 per cent of the population). Of these, just under one-third are primary carers, providing the majority of help and support for the person being cared for. More than two-thirds of primary carers are women caring for a close relative, such as a partner, parent or child (Hughes, 2007; Pirkis et al., 2010; ABS, 2016).

Carers are essential to the effective working of mental health care in Australia, and the replacement value of informal caregiving is likely to be in the tens of billions of dollars. Carers provide a range of emotional and practical supports to close relatives living with mental illness, including help in crisis situations, supervision with medications, financial support, and support to attend medical appointments. It is important to recognise the considerable burdens that may accompany caregiving—worry, anxiety, depression and the pressure of caring-associated financial costs (Pirkis et al., 2010). Caregiving is itself a risk factor for mental illness.

Carers are important stakeholders in the mental health system. It is important that mental health nurses and other health professionals acknowledge and value the very important role they play in supporting people living with mental illness. Carers Australia (www.carersaustralia.com.au) and ARAFMI Mental Health Carers of Australia (www.arafmi.australia.asn.au) are two national organisations that provide advocacy on behalf of carers.

HISTORICAL PERSPECTIVES

People who have been called 'mentally ill' have been with us throughout history—to be feared, marvelled at, ignored, banished, laughed at, pitied or tortured. A historical review of mental illness and the people who have lived with these experiences shows that societies have 'understood' and reacted to the phenomenon differently over time:

- Dominant social attitudes as well as religious and philosophical viewpoints have influenced the understanding of, approach to, and treatment of mental illness throughout recorded history, and probably before.
- Ideas that may be considered contemporary at one time often have roots in earlier centuries.
- The modern medical concept of 'madness' as an illness is open to the same scrutiny as interpretations of the past, such as beliefs about witchcraft or mysticism.

The timeline in Figure 1.2 ■ illustrates the shifting approaches to mental disorder throughout history.

IMPORTANT DATES IN THE SHIFTING APPROACHES TO MENTAL DISORDER

Era of magico–religious explanations

It is thought that in preliterate cultures the causes of mental and physical suffering were not differentiated. Both were attributed to forces acting outside the body. Consequently, no distinctions were made between magic, medicine and religion. Primitive healers quite logically dealt with the 'spirits of torment' with appeal, reverence, prayer, bribery, intimidation, appeasement, confession, punishment, exorcism, magical ritual and incantation. In some cultures, beliefs and practices similar to these continue today, and are directed towards 'banishing' the mental illness.

Behaviour considered to be a mental illness by modern Western cultures was attributed in preliterate cultures to the violation of taboos, the neglect of ritual obligations, the loss of a vital substance from the body (such as the soul), the introduction of a foreign and harmful substance into the body (such as evil spirits), or witchcraft.

Era of organic explanations

In the 4th century BCE, Hippocrates proposed a medical concept to explain mental suffering. He rejected demonology, and proposed that mental illnesses were caused mainly by imbalances in body humours: blood, black bile, yellow bile and phlegm. For example, an excess of black bile was thought to cause melancholy (Wallace & Gach, 2011).

One important consequence of these beliefs was that emotional suffering came within the realm of medical practice, to include words (interpretation of dreams and talking) and medical treatments (purging, bloodletting and ritual purification).

Era of alienation

At the height of their civilisation, the citizens of ancient Greece found their inner security in knowledge and reason. The Romans adopted the intellectual heritage of Greece, but placed greater reliance on their social institutions and the rational organisation of society, supported by law and military might. When these institutions disintegrated and the Roman Empire went into a decline, fear tore apart the fabric of society.

The collapse of Rome signalled a general return to the magic, mysticism and demonology from which people had retreated during the age of Greek rationality. During the Middle Ages, the period between approximately 400CE and the Renaissance (1300–1600CE), madness was seen as a dramatic encounter with secret powers. Troubled minds were thought to be influenced by the moon (see Figure 1.3 ■). *Lunacy* literally means a disorder caused by the moon.

In the Arab world, people who were insane were believed to be divinely inspired and not victims of demons. An asylum for people with mental illness was built in Fez, Morocco, early in the 8th century. Other asylums were soon established in Baghdad, Cairo and Damascus. The care in these asylums was usually benevolent and kindly. Contrary to the pejorative meanings often associated with 'mental asylum', the term 'asylum' literally means 'a place of safety'.

The first European hospital devoted entirely to people with mental illness was built in 1409 in Valencia, Spain. The problems of the mind, however, remained the domain of theologians. A book called *Malleus maleficarum* (translated as *The witches' hammer;* Institoris, H. & Sprenger, J. [1970; original ed. 1498]) became the basis for witch hunts. The *Malleus* details the destruction of dissenters, heretics and the 'mentally ill', most of whom were women, and all of whom were labelled *witches*. Theological rationalisations and magical explanations were used to justify burning witches at the stake.

People considered to be the 'violent insane' were shackled in prisons. In Europe, the belief developed that people who had mental illness could be sent on voyages of symbolic importance to find their reason (sanity). While the existence of actual boatloads of 'ships of fools' is now disputed, the idea persisted for centuries and possibly contributed to the social abandonment of people with mental illness.

Era of confinement

Unlike the Middle Ages, when people with mental illness were generally driven out of, or excluded from, community life, during the Renaissance they were confined. Tamed, retained and maintained, 'madness' was reduced to silence through a system of mutual obligation between the afflicted and society. People with mental illness—known as 'mad' persons—had the right to be fed, but were morally constrained and physically confined.

Seventeenth-century society created enormous houses of confinement. In these establishments, society incarcerated the mad, the poor and people who were considered deviants. A landmark date is 1656, when by decree the Hôpital Général in Paris was founded. It was not a medical establishment, but rather a threatening institution, complete with stakes, irons and dungeons. The 'insane' were completely under the jurisdiction of the institution, and had no recourse to appeal their incarceration. The Hôpital Général and other, similar institutions were primarily established to maintain social order. In London, the hospital of St Mary of Bethlehem became famous as *Bedlam*, illustrated in Figure 1.4 ■, where, for the entertainment of onlookers on a Sunday afternoon outing, mad persons were publicly beaten and tortured.

Those chained to cell walls were no longer considered people who had lost their reason or sick persons, but rather beasts seized by frenzy. During this period, it was believed that madness could be overcome only by discipline and brutality.

Era of moral treatment

The 18th and early 19th centuries were an era characterised by internal contradictions. Although people with mental illness were unchained, the medical treatment they received consisted of what amounted to torture with special paraphernalia. To grasp the incredible inhumanity with which people with mental illness were treated in what became known as 'the era of enlightenment', consider the following:

- The nature of mental illness could not be explained by any of the prevailing concepts—black humours could not be seen, demons or animal spirits could not be observed, and knowledge of anatomy could not be applied to the workings of the mind.
- Because mental illness could not be satisfactorily explained, the deeply felt dread of the insane could not be dispelled.
- Mental illness was believed to be incurable and mad persons were thought to be dangerous.

Even the most sensitive physicians did not try to understand the sources of mental suffering. Because they had no way to explain or understand mental illness, they developed and focused on elaborate and detailed systems of classification (see Chapter 5).

During this period, a general spirit of reform and humanitarianism swept Western Europe and the United States. Social reform and moral enrichment saw people released from their chains, systematised brutality with chains and whips was abolished, nourishing foods were provided, and the importance of treating people with kindness was acknowledged. This movement was first led by Philippe Pinel (1745–1826) (see Figure 1.5 ■) in France, and the Quakers in England under William Tuke (1732–1822).

Moral treatment in the United States—associated with Benjamin Franklin, Benjamin Rush (called 'the father of American psychiatry', 1745–1813), and others—was an alternative to mere confinement. Despite his association with humanitarianism and moral treatment, Rush was a major follower of the ideas of Scotland's William Cullen (1710–1790). Cullen believed that mental illness was due to decay, either of the intellect or of the involuntary nervous system; that is, a matter of disordered physiology. Rush advocated bloodletting, the restraining chair illustrated in Figure 1.6 ■, the gyrating chair and other devices that we now consider inhumane.

Important dates in the shifting approaches to mental disorder

Preliterate times

Era of magico-religious explanations

- Mental and physical suffering not differentiated.
- 'Spirits of torment' acting outside the body are responsible for ills.
- No distinctions made between medicine, magic and religion.
- Primitive healers address spirits by appeal, prayer, bribery, intimidation, appeasement, punishment.
- Healing methods include exorcism, magical ritual, incantation.

Early civilisation

Era of organic explanations

- Hippocrates (460–370) rejects demonology and proposes that psychiatric illnesses are caused by imbalances in 'body humours': blood, black bile, yellow bile, and phlegm.
- Psychiatric suffering comes within the realm of medical practice.
- Imbalances in body humors often corrected by bloodletting.

The medieval period

Era of alienation

- Return to the magic, mysticism and demonology of preliterate times.
- Madness viewed as dramatic encounter with secret powers and influenced by the moon (lunacy).

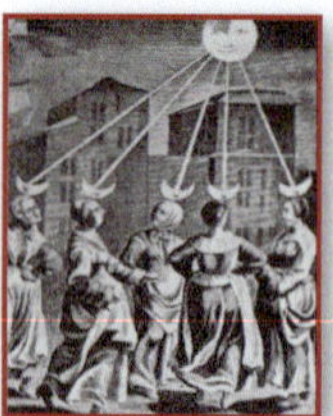

- *Malleus Maleficarum* (The Witches' Hammer) by Dominican monks Johann Sprenger and Heinrich Kraemer, published in 1487, rationalised mental illness in terms of magical explanation.
- Violent insane shackled in prisons or sent to sea 'in search of reason'.

Early 20th century

Era of psychoanalysis

- Emil Kraepelin (1856–1926) creates system of distinct disease entities and differentiates biopolar disorder from schizophrenia.
- Sigmund Freud (1856–1939) explains human behaviour in psychological terms and demonstrates that behaviour can be changed through psychoanalysis.

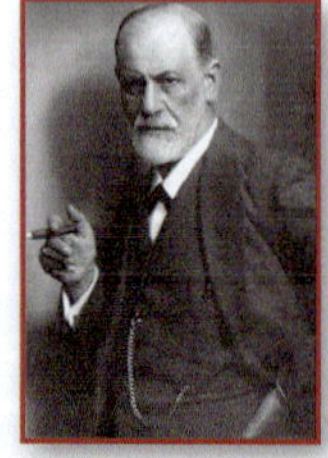

- Pavlov's discovery of the conditioned response forms the basis for modern-day cognitive behavioural therapy.

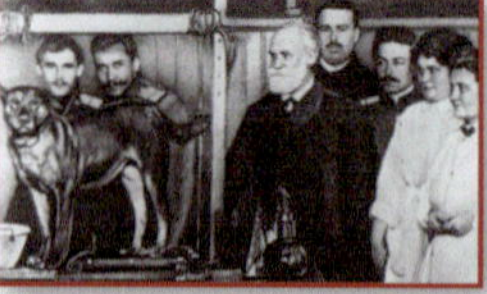

Mid 20th century

Era of ideological expansion

- From the mid-1940s to mid-1950s, a strong rift between biological orientation and dynamic orientation develops.
- By the early 1950s, several drugs for the treatment of mental disorder were in common use.
- Harry Stack Sullivan developed the interpersonal theory of psychiatry, Erik Erikson formulated his psychosocial theory of development, and Abraham Maslow proposed an order, or hierarchy, of basic human needs leading to self-actualisation.
- Group therapy, family therapy and short-term therapy recognised as options to costly long-term therapy.
- Milieu therapy developed by Maxwell Jones in England.

Late 20th century

Deinstitutionalisation and the community mental health movement

- By the early 1960s, a shift from institutional to community-based care and toward preventive services, consumer participation and the development of community mental health centres began.
- Between 1955 and 1975, the number of people resident in state mental hospitals decreased substantially as the community mental health movement gained in influence.
- By the 1960s, family therapy had become both a diagnostic tool and a mode of treatment.
- Politicians and the public become more aware of the difficulties the mentally ill face.

FIGURE 1.2 ■ *Photo source top to bottom by column:* SZ Photo/Scheri/Alamy; Photo Researchers, Inc.; Maslow, Abraham H./Frager, Robert D./Fadiman, James, *Motivation and Personality*, 3rd Ed., ©1987. Reprinted and electronically reproduced by permission of Pearson Education, Inc., Upper Saddle River, New Jersey; Philosophical Library; Photo Researchers, Inc.; Photo Researchers, Inc.; Philosophical Library; Philosophical Library; ajt/Shutterstock.

The renaissance

Era of confinement

- In 1656, Hôpital Général in Paris founded to confine the mad, poor and various deviants.
- The 'insane' have no recourse to appeal.
- Madness not linked to medicine; could only be mastered by discipline and brutality.
- Radical physicians like Johann Weyer (1515–1588) believed that 'those illnesses whose origins are attributed to witches come from natural causes'.

The 18th and early 19th centuries

Era of moral treatment

- Physicians classify symptoms of mental disorders without understanding the sources of mental suffering.
- In 1794, Philippe Pinel (1745–1826) treated inmates in the French institutions Bicêtre and Salpêtrière with humanity and was thus considered mad.

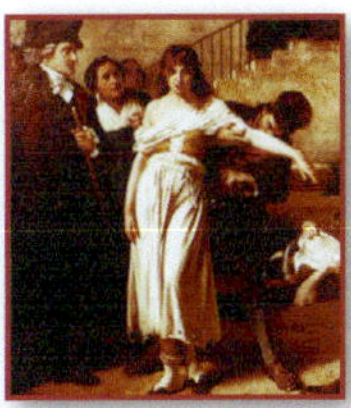

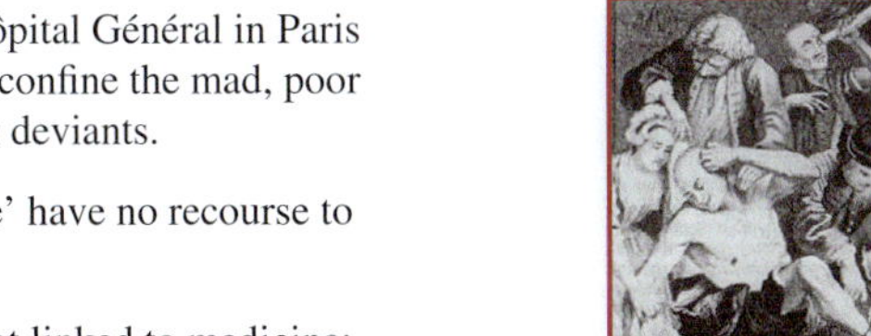

- In England, William Tuke (1732–1822) focused on 'moral treatment' in a humane milieu called the York Retreat, to counter conditions in settings such as 'Bedlam.'
- In America, Benjamin Rush (1746–1813) focused on moral treatment and humanitarianism at the Pennsylvania Hospital.

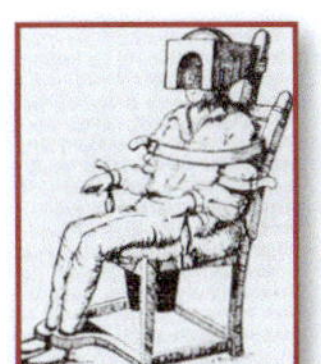

Late 19th and early 20th centuries

Era of public mental hospitals

- Dorothea L. Dix (1802–1887) founds or enlarges over 30 mental hospitals.
- Moral treatment replaced by custodial care.
- Clifford Beers (1876–1943) published his book describing his own intense suffering and mental anguish, leading to the development of preventive psychiatry and the formation of child guidance clinics.

The 1990s

The decade of the brain

- The primary innovation of the 1990s is the 'biological revolution': collaboration of science and technology to expand concepts of mental disorder proposed by psychological, behavioural and psychoanalytic theories.
- The gains made in research-based knowledge about the epidemiology, diagnosis, treatment and prevention of major mental illnesses constitute substantial progress in understanding of the brain.

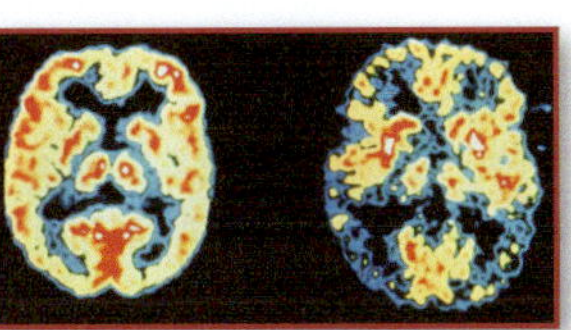

- Consumer advocacy groups welcome psychiatry's shift toward psychosocial rehabilitation for consumer self-care.

The new millennium

Era of health care reform

- Reform of psychiatric care has decreased length of stay and increased consumer acuity.
- Developments in neuroscience have reshaped our conception of the bases of mental disorders.
- Innovations in technology have informed diagnostic practices such as brain imaging.

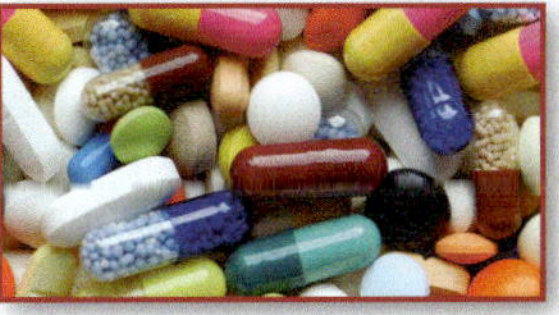

- The range of available psychopharmacological treatments continues to expand.
- Populations of people with mental illnesses include growing numbers of older people, more people with co-existing substance use disorders, more comorbidities with chronic illnesses and expanding cultural diversity.
- The study of genomes and the biology of the brain touch ethical, moral and political nerves.

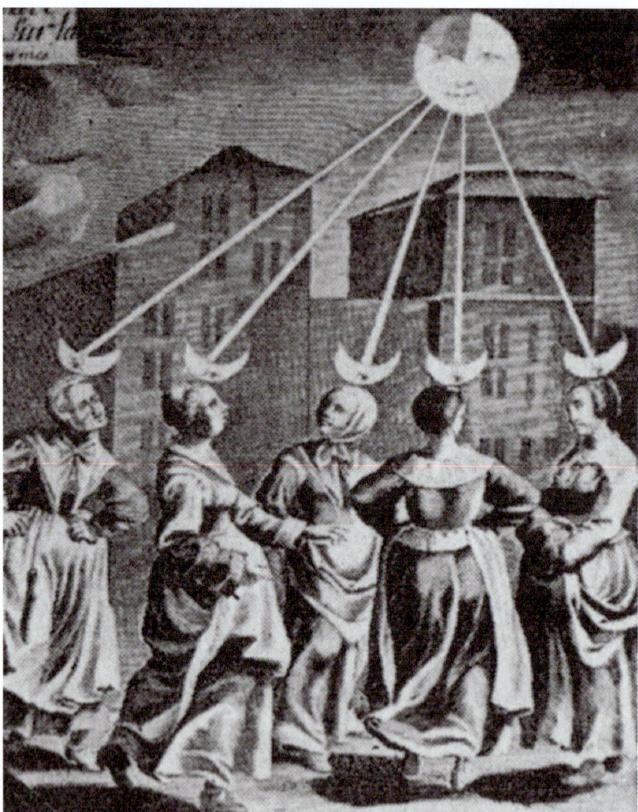

FIGURE 1.3 ■ Moonstruck women dancing in a 17th-century square. This activity is the source for the word 'lunatic'.
Photo courtesy of Philosophical Library.

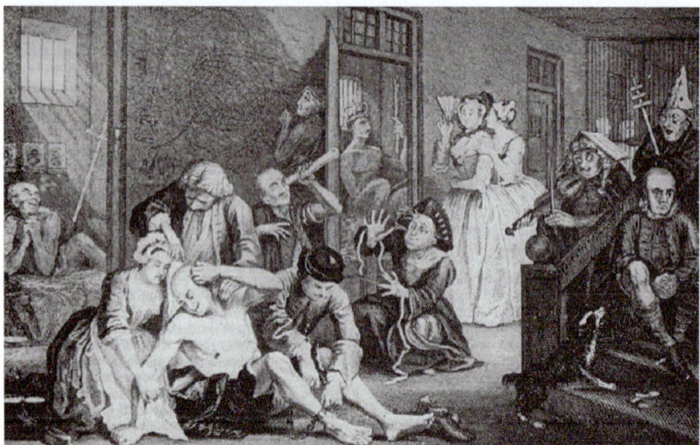

FIGURE 1.4 ■ A ward in Bethlehem Hospital, about 1745. A patient is being chained in the foreground, and in the background are two Sunday visitors on an entertainment outing.
Photo courtesy of Philosophical Library.

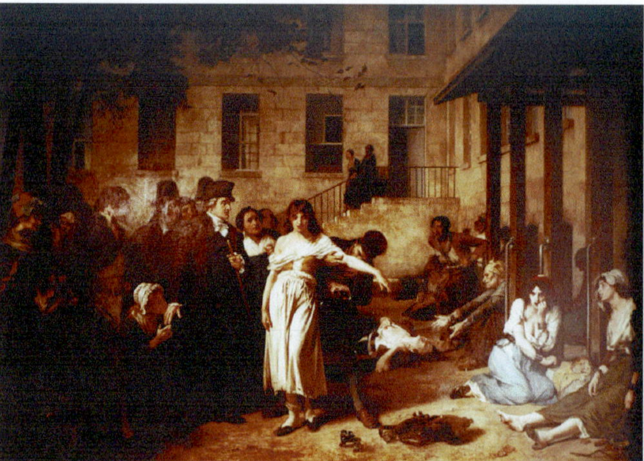

FIGURE 1.5 ■ A landmark event—Philippe Pinel unchaining the insane in the Bicêtre Hospital in Paris.
Photo courtesy of Charles Ciccione/Photo Researchers, Inc.

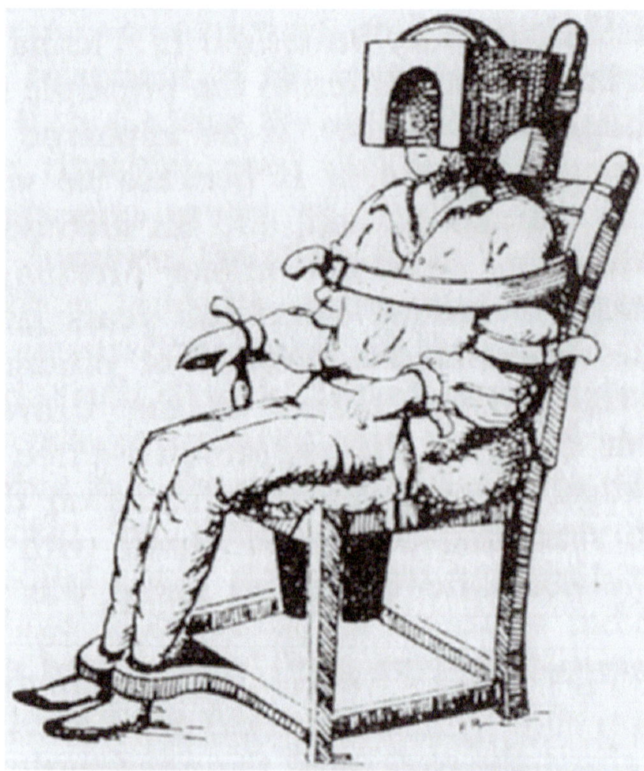

FIGURE 1.6 ■ Benjamin Rush, the 'father of American psychiatry' and an idealist and humanitarian, nevertheless favoured physical theories such as 'excitement of the brain' to explain mental illness. He was preoccupied with somatic treatments, such as bleeding and purging, and developed the tranquilising chair to quieten the insane.
Photo courtesy of Philosophical Library.

Era of psychoanalysis

During the late 19th and early 20th centuries, the number of mental hospitals, both private and government-run, grew. Beliefs about mental illness began to change again. Mental illness was linked to faulty life habits, and treated with new forms of physical or somatic therapies. Some clinicians were inclined towards an organic, neurophysiological explanation of mental illness. The emphasis on the classification of distinct disease entities continued.

These developments formed the background for the work of one of the most influential figures in the history of psychiatry, Sigmund Freud (1856–1939). He succeeded in explaining human behaviour in psychological terms. Freud's contributions to psychiatry are discussed in greater detail in Chapter 5.

Contemporary developments

By the mid-20th century, psychiatric thinking was expanding and moving towards an emphasis on the importance of the social dimension. Dissatisfaction with psychoanalytic explanations for mental illness became more common, and pharmacological treatments for mental illness were being developed in the early 1950s. Research into chemotherapy and the aetiology of mental illness increased.

The primary innovation of the 1990s—known as The Decade of the Brain—was the so-called biological revolution: the collaboration of science and technology to expand concepts of mental illness proposed by psychological and behavioural theories. During this period, considerable progress was made in understanding the brain. For example, research on brain function resulted in a major reconceptualisation of the diagnosis and treatment of several mental disorders. Researchers discovered a variety of disturbances of brain functions, including ventricular enlargement, cerebral atrophy and disturbances in neurotransmitters (discussed in Chapter 6).

This medical approach is reflected in contemporary psychiatric mental health nursing literature, including this text. Research in the 21st century is focused on such areas as:

- the bases of mental illness
- the continuing development of newer generations of medications with fewer side-effects
- the effects of various medications on the neurotransmitters in the brains of people living with mental illness
- the role of nutrients in brain function
- the influence on mood and behaviour of disruptions of biological rhythms
- the role of viruses in mental illness
- the influence of the endocrine system on the brain and behaviour
- the role of the brain in producing physical illnesses
- the identification of biological markers that might signify the onset of mental illness
- the interrelationship between genetics and mental illness
- the prevention of mental illness
- the lived experience of mental illness, learning directly from people who have a mental health condition.

We can expect that, as the result of contemporary research, health professional and societal conceptualisations of mental illness will continue to shift.

THE STIGMA OF MENTAL ILLNESS

One of the negative consequences of being diagnosed with a mental illness is stigmatisation. The **stigma** of mental illness is based on a societal perception that mental illness is a blemish of individual character (Cockerham, 2011). Stigmatisation of mental illness is a worldwide problem experienced in all segments of society, but is especially prevalent in deprived, marginalised and minority communities (Lamb, Bower, Rogers, Dowrick & Gask, 2011). In North America, the actor Glenn Close, whose sister is living with bipolar disorder, established a national anti-stigma campaign called Bring Change 2 Mind. SANE Australia also has an anti-stigma campaign called Say No to Stigma (www.sane.org/stigmawatch).

Stigma is about disrespect. It:

- hurts, punishes and diminishes people
- harms and undermines interpersonal relationships
- appears in behaviour, language, attitude and tone of voice
- causes others to keep their distance from someone who has an illness, and results in social isolation for the stigmatised person.

Stigma is an attitude that leads to prejudice and discrimination. It affects the judgments of family, friends, co-workers, health care providers, and others about the person who has a mental illness. SANE Australia has produced a detailed report on stigma entitled *A life without stigma*, which can be obtained from https://www.sane.org/images/stories/media/ALifeWithoutStigma_A_SANE_Report.pdf. Examples of inaccurate beliefs about mental illness that lead to or perpetuate stigma and discrimination against people living with mental illness are given in Box 1.3.

Box 1.3 Stigmatising beliefs about mental illness

- ***MYTH: People with a mental illness are dangerous and violent.*** *FACT: People with mental illness are not more violent than other people. They are more frequently the survivors of violence than the perpetrators.*
- ***MYTH: People with a mental illness have a low IQ.*** *FACT: People with mental illness have the same range of intelligence as the 'normal' population. They may have temporary difficulty performing at a 'normal' level. People with an intellectual disability may also have a mental illness.*
- ***MYTH: People with a mental illness cannot hold down a job.*** *FACT: People who live with a diagnosis of a mental illness not only hold down jobs but may excel at work. They often face discrimination when applying for jobs.*
- ***MYTH: People with a mental illness have nothing to contribute to society.*** *FACT: People with mental illness are contributing members of society. They are scientists, musicians, astronauts, sports stars, singers, actors and contribute to society in a wide range of areas.*
- ***MYTH: People with mental illness lack willpower.*** *FACT: People with mental illness can, and do, exert willpower and control in their daily lives. Most difficulties are due to the impacts of medication, discrimination and stigma, and not to a lack of willpower.*
- ***MYTH: People with mental illness come from low-income families.*** *FACT. People with mental illness come from any income bracket, race, religion, age and educational background. Mental illness is an equal-opportunity disorder.*
- ***MYTH: People with mental illness are lazy.*** *FACT: People with mental illness are not lazy. Their symptoms and the medications they take can sometimes make it hard to be active.*
- ***MYTH: People with mental illness cause their own problems.*** *FACT: People with mental illness have often experienced trauma, discrimination and stigma, which create disruptions in their thinking, feeling, mood, daily functioning, and an ability to relate to others.*
- ***MYTH: People with mental illness should just 'shape up'.*** *FACT: People with mental illness can shape up if they can choose the mental health 'gymnasiums' they know work.*
- ***MYTH: Mental illness does not exist.*** *FACT: This one is in dispute. Many people believe that what they are experiencing is a normal human reaction to extraordinary experience. The dominant medical model believes that people with mental illness have an actual illness that is every bit as factual as a physical illness.*

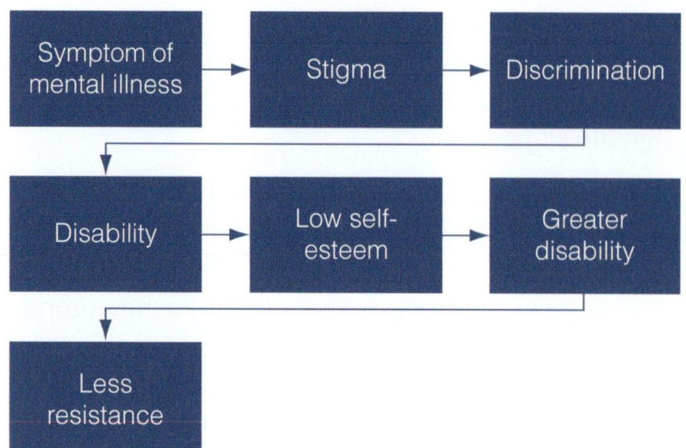

FIGURE 1.7 ■ The effect of stigma on recovery from mental illness. The person's symptom is the marker that leads to stigmatisation by society. Eventually, the effects of stigmatisation negatively influence the person's ability to recover from mental illness.

In his early classic work on stigma, the sociologist Erving Goffman (1963) equated stigma with having a *spoiled identity*. The person incorporates societal perceptions of not being normal, or right, or worthwhile, and comes to believe that they do indeed fall short of what they should be. This internalisation, or self-stigma, leads to feeling unworthy, having low self-esteem and losing hope—all characteristics that work against coping with, or recovering from, mental illness. This process is illustrated in Figure 1.7 ■.

Despite advances, stigma continues to grow around the globe, and is one of the main obstacles to better mental health care and quality of life for people living with mental illness, their families, communities and staff members who deal with mental health disorders.

According to the Programme against Stigma and Discrimination of the World Psychiatric Association (WPA), stigma extends to not only people living with mental illness and their families, but also to the medications used for treatment, the agencies that provide mental health treatment, staff members in those agencies (Sartorius et al., 2010), and even the sites on which they are located. Stigma affects everyone in the global mental health community.

Practice example

In Australia, job-seekers who tell a prospective employer about their mental illness risk not being hired. On the other hand, if they do not tell or have a relapse, they risk being fired despite the anti-discrimination laws. In India, people are reluctant to tell their neighbours about a mental illness, because it might hurt a child's or sibling's chances of being married. In Japan, people with mental illness are kept at home to do domestic chores, and out of the public eye. In China, mental illness is seen as a family problem that is hidden, and the responsibility for managing it is kept within the family. In all of these countries, stigmatisation is a significant motivating force.

LIVED EXPERIENCE

Simon Swinson

In my experience, internalising stigma is a very painful and almost unavoidable consequence of mental illness. Even before diagnosis, people turn away from you; people who have been close don't want to know you—schoolfriends, close friends, family members. However, I was fortunate in that my immediate family stood by me, including my sister-in-law. Things started to improve once I was well-established on medication. Self-confidence returned with time, some old friends reconnected and I have made new friends, many from within the mental health consumer movement.

Language matters

Although aberrant behaviour is a source of stigma, labels also reinforce stigma (Theurer, Jen-Paul, Cheyney, Koro-Ljungberg & Stevens, 2015). It would be nice if the old saying 'Sticks

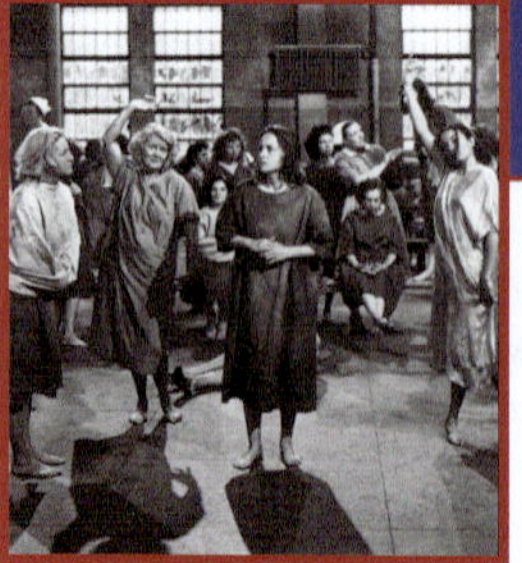

MENTAL HEALTH IN THE MEDIA

The Snake Pit

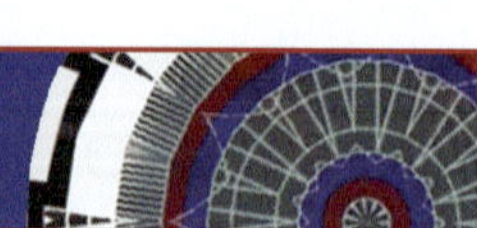

In this 1948 classic film and exposé of the dire conditions at many state hospitals in the United States, Virginia Cunningham, played by Olivia de Havilland, is an inpatient in a state insane asylum (as mental health facilities were known then). *The Snake Pit* was an adaptation of a best-selling novel by Mary Jane Ward, who had been an inpatient in a mental hospital for more than eight months. Many of the characters were composites of the nurses, doctors and patients she met during her hospitalisation.

Prior to *The Snake Pit*, mental illness in the movies was either the butt of jokes in comedies or romanticised as a byproduct of tragic love. The film authentically portrayed the dehumanising conditions that existed at the time in large mental institutions—a fearful and insensitive staff focused on regimentation to control and manage the asylum's inmates, overcrowding, facilities designed like prisons, and typical treatments such as cold water hydrotherapy. Even so, the portrayals of psychoanalysis, hypnosis and the reasons behind the main character's mental illness were too simplistic to do justice to the complexities involved in living with a mental illness.

Nonetheless, the film had a significant impact on the conditions in psychiatric facilities in the United States. By 1949, journalists were keeping track of the number of states to institute reforms, and 20th Century Fox claimed that 26 of the 48 states had enacted reform legislation as a result of *The Snake Pit*.

Photo courtesy of Everett Collection.

and stones can break my bones, but words can never hurt me' was true. As it relates to stigma in mental health, words are powerful. Stigmatising language builds barriers to the understanding and treatment of persons with mental disorders.

Many terms have been used to describe aberrant behaviour or mental illness. You may have used some or all of these terms yourself, and you may hear them used in mental health settings and in the community at large. As you learn more about mental illness and the effects of stigma, you will gain a greater appreciation of the humanity of people living with mental illness, and find that you have edited demeaning, denigrating and stigmatising labels from your vocabulary.

In the earlier Practice Example on page 4, young people amused themselves by taunting 'Crazy Helen'. When used by people who do not identify as having a lived experience of mental illness, crazy is an informal, denigrating and stigmatising term that carries with it unfounded and negative implications. People probably described 'Crazy Helen' as having had a **nervous breakdown**—a general, non-specific term for an incapacitating but otherwise unspecified type of mental illness. Other stigmatising and denigrating terms are 'wacko', 'looney', 'psycho', 'lunatic', 'maniac', 'bananas', 'cuckoo', 'head case' and 'nuts'.

Many of the terms that society uses to describe aberrant behaviour have a convoluted history and have travelled over time and between languages, as shown in the historical perspectives section of this chapter. It is important that you not only educate those who use stigmatising language, and advocate for others to treat people living with mental illness respectfully and ethically, but also that you serve as a role model. The Nursing and Midwifery Board of Australia in its Code of Ethics for Nurses (2008), Code of Professional Conduct for Nurses in Australia (2008) and Registered Nurse Standards of Practice (2016) identifies respect for persons as a core principal integral to professional nursing. Respectful language is discussed in the Self-awareness feature. We also discuss the ethics of stigmatising labels in Chapter 11.

LIVED EXPERIENCE

Tim Heffernan

Driving to work today, a Tasmanian senator, who shall remain nameless, commented that people who believe that renewable energy can make a difference to climate change 'are deluded and should be locked up'. Politicians and the media use language about mental illness very carelessly, and in ways that reinforce and entrench stigma and marginalisation. It is essential that those who care for consumers when we are in distress and vulnerable use language for the opposite effect: to destigmatise, humanise, include and educate.

Language is most important within the therapeutic relationship, where two people are travelling together on a recovery journey. It is not just the words that are chosen that are important, but the tone and the context of delivery. Adult consumers experiencing psychological distress are not children, yet we frequently feel we are patronised when in inpatient care. Similarly, many of us have heard the language of 'deficits', where 'we can't do this, can't do that'. I am reminded of the lyrics of 'School' by Supertramp, a formative band of my youth, in which attempts to make the singer a good boy, by telling him what to do or not do, ends with the response 'do they know where it's at?'

Your language should be uplifting, positive and strengths-based. Really, you will only have partial knowledge of where a consumer is 'at', but you can choose, through your choice of words, the way you say them and when you say them, to either facilitate or undermine a consumer's journey to recovery.

The most difficult thing you will do, but you will have to do it, is to challenge inappropriate language in the workplace. How will you react when at handover you hear the language that seeks to dehumanise and oppress us? I don't need to write down examples, because unfortunately you will already have heard plenty.

It is an ethical issue for you; a human rights issue for us.

SELF-AWARENESS

Respectful language to combat stigma

You can help to combat stigma by using respectful language when you refer to mental illness or to people living with mental illness. This requires that you become aware of the language you use, and modify it, if necessary. The suggestions below are designed for your use. However, they can also be implemented in a psychoeducation teaching plan for people living with mental illness, family members, mental health staff and others in the community. Guidelines for recovery-oriented language in mental health can be obtained for the Mental Health Coordinating Council (MHCC) (mob.mhcc.org.au/media/5902/mhcc-recovery-oriented-language-guide-final-web.pdf). Following the MHCC Guideline, you can:

- Say *mental disorder, mental illness* or *psychiatric disability* (terms that show respect). Avoid saying *crazy, cuckoo, wacko, nuts, psycho, lunatic, bananas* or *head case* (terms that disrespect and stigmatise).
- Say *person with bipolar disorder, person who has schizophrenia, person who has cognitive difficulties* (terms that put people first, not their disabilities). Avoid saying *manic, bipolar, schizophrenic* or *demented* (terms that emphasise limitations and depersonalise).
- Say *person coping with, managing* or *recovering from depression* (terms that focus on positive abilities). Avoid saying *afflicted with, suffering from, victim of* (terms that sensationalise a disability).

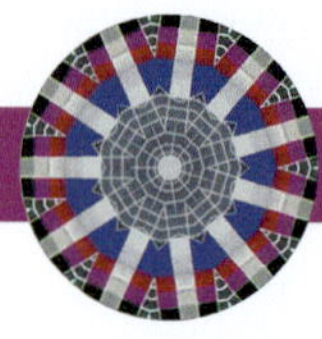

REFERENCES

Australian Bureau of Statistics (ABS). (2007). *National Survey of Mental Health and Wellbeing: Summary of results*. (Document 4326.0.) Canberra, Australia: ABS.

Australian Bureau of Statistics (ABS). (2016). *Disability, ageing and carers, Australia: Summary of findings, 2015*. (Document 4430.0.) Canberra, Australia: ABS.

Australian Institute of Health and Welfare (AIHW). (2016). *Mental health services in Australia: Prevalence, impact and burden*. Canberra, Australia: AIHW. Retrieved from https://mhsa.aihw.gov.au/background/prevalence/ (Accessed 2016, February 5.)

Carr, V., Whiteford, H., Groves, A., McGorry, P., & Shepherd, A. (2012). Policy and service development implications of the second Australian National Survey of High Impact Psychosis (SHIP). *Australian and New Zealand Journal of Psychiatry, 46*(8), 708–718.

Cockerham, W. C. (2011). *Sociology of mental disorder* (8th ed.). Upper Saddle River, NJ: Prentice Hall.

Ehrlich, C., Kenall, E., Frey, N., & Compton, D. (2014). Improving the physical health of people with severe mental illness: Boundaries of care provision. *International Journal of Mental Health Nursing, 23*(3), 243–251.

Galletly, C., Castel, D., Dark, F., Humberstone, V., Jablensky, A., Killackey, E., . . . Tran, N. (2016). Royal Australian and New Zealand College of Psychiatrists clinical practice guidelines for the management of schizophrenia and related disorders. *Australian and New Zealand Journal of Psychiatry, 50*(5), 410–472.

Goffman, E. (1963). *Stigma: Notes on the management of spoiled identity*. Englewood Cliffs, NJ: Prentice Hall.

Hewitt, J. P., & Shulman, D. (2011). *Self and society: A symbolic interactionist social psychology* (11th ed.). Upper Saddle River, NJ: Prentice Hall.

Hughes, J. (2007). 'Caring for carers': The financial strain of caring. *Family Matters, 76*, 32–33.

Institoris, H., & Sprenger, J. (1970; original ed.1498). *Malleus Maleficarum*. New York: B Blom.

Kessler, R. C., Demler, O., Frank, R. G., Olfson, M., Pincus, H. A., Walters, E. E., & Zaslavsky, A. M. (2005). Prevalence and treatment of mental disorders, 1990 to 2003. *New England Journal of Medicine, 352*(24), 2515–2523.

Kozlowska, K., & Durheim, E. (2013). Is bullying in children and adolescents a modifiable risk factor for mental illness? *Australian and New Zealand Journal of Psychiatry, 48*(3), 288–289.

Lamb, J. D., Bower, P., Rogers, A., Dowrick, C., & Gask, L. (2012). Access to mental health in primary care: A qualitative meta-synthesis of evidence from the experience of people from 'hard to reach groups'. *Health, 16(1)*, 76–104.

Mental Health Council of Australia. (2009). Home truths: Mental health, housing and homelessness in Australia. Deakin, Australia: Mental Health Council of Australia.

Morgan, V., Waterreus, A., Jablensky, A., Mackinnon, A., McGrath, J., Carr, V., . . . Saw, S. (2012). People living with psychotic illness in 2010: The second Australian national survey of psychosis, *Australian and New Zealand Journal of Psychiatry, 46*(8), 735–752.

National Institute of Mental Health. *Leading categories of diseases/disorders*. Retrieved from http://www.nimh.gov.

Nursing and Midwifery Board of Australia. (2008). *Code of professional conduct for nurses in Australia*. Melbourne, Australia: Nursing and Midwifery Board of Australia: wwwnursingmidwiferyboard.gov.au (retrieved 9 February 2017).

Nursing and Midwifery Board of Australia. (2008). *Code of ethics for nurses*. Melbourne, Australia: Nursing and Midwifery Board of Australia: wwwnursingmidwiferyboard.gov.au (Accessed 2017, February 9.)

Nursing and Midwifery Board of Australia. (2016). *Registered nurse standards of practice*. Melbourne, Australia: Nursing and Midwifery Board of Australia: wwwnursingmidwiferyboard.gov.au (Accessed 2017, February 9.)

Patel, V., & Prince, M. (2011). Global mental health. *Journal of the American Medical Association, 303*(19), 1976–1977.

Pirkis, J., Burgess, P., Hardy, J., Harris, M., Slade, T., & Johnstone, A. (2010). Who cares? A profile of people who care for relatives with a mental disorder. *Australian and New Zealand Journal of Psychiatry 44*(10), 929–937.

Procter, N. (2007). Mental health emergencies. In K. Curtis, C. Ramsden, & J. Friendship (Eds.), *Emergency and trauma nursing* (pp. 625–642). New York: Elsevier Press.

Sartorius, N., Gaebel, W., Cleveland, H. R., Stuart, H., Akiyama, T., Arboleda-Flórez, J., . . . Tasman, A. (2010). WPA guidance on how to combat stigma of psychiatry and psychiatrists. *World Psychiatry, 9*(3), 131–144.

Stein, M. B., Roy-Byrne, P. P., Craske, M. G., Campbell-Sills, L., Lang, A. J., Golinelli, D., . . . Sherbourne, C. D. (2011). Quality of and patient satisfaction with primary health care for anxiety disorders. *Journal of Clinical Psychiatry, 72(7), 970–976.*

Theurer, J. M., Jen-Paul, N., Cheyney, L., Koro-Ljungberg, M., & Stevens, B. R. (2015). Wearing the label of mental illness: Community-based participatory action research of mental health stigma. *The Qualitative Report, 20*(1), 42–58.

Wallace, E. R., & Gach, I. (2011). *History of psychiatry and medical psychology*. New York, NY: Springer-Verlag.

World Health Organization (WHO). (2007). *Nurses in mental health* 2007. Geneva, Switzerland: WHO.

World Health Organization (WHO). (2014a). *10 facts on the State of Global Health*. Geneva, Switzerland: WHO. Retrieved from http://www.who.int/features/factfiles/global_burden/facts/en/ (Accessed 2016, February 5.)

World Health Organization (WHO). (2014b). *Mental health: Strengthening our response*. Fact Sheet No. 220 (August 2014). Geneva, Switzerland: WHO.

The therapeutic relationship

2

MIKE HAZELTON AND SIMON SWINSON

LEARNING OUTCOMES

After completing this chapter, you will be able to:

1. Understand that people living with mental illness expect to engage in a therapeutic relationship that is equal and reciprocal.
2. Encourage the systematic use of abilities and behaviours most often associated with growth-producing outcomes.
3. Analyse how phenomena such as resistance, transference, countertransference, critical distance, gift giving, the use of touch, and personal values affect the therapeutic relationship.
4. Incorporate an understanding of the three phases of the therapeutic relationship, and the main objectives and therapeutic tasks of each phase, into one-to-one work.
5. Apply the nursing process to the three phases of the therapeutic relationship.
6. Establish and maintain one-to-one relationships within the context of a person's cultural background.
7. Understand and appreciate the experience of living with mental illness.

KEY TERMS

LIVED EXPERIENCE

I can recall once having a case manager who refused to deal with me; not because she didn't like me, but I suspect because she felt pressured in her work. On a number of occasions she mentioned that of course I wouldn't want to talk about my experience of psychosis. I am not sure why she thought that; perhaps it was considered a taboo topic, or she felt I didn't need to talk about it. However, at that stage I desperately needed to talk about it; I was busting to talk about it. I had just been diagnosed with schizophrenia, and she didn't want me to talk about it! I did find people to discuss my concerns with through my involvement in Clubhouse—an NGO-based psychosocial rehabilitation service. For the most part, those I spoke to had experienced mental illness or were carers. Several years later, I was taken on by a very good therapist in the public mental health service; he was always available by phone; listened with great empathy; and was about my age. Towards the end of my time with him, he told me that for some time he had looked forward to having a coffee with me every second Monday. Looking back on it now, I feel he really helped me to develop my resilience.

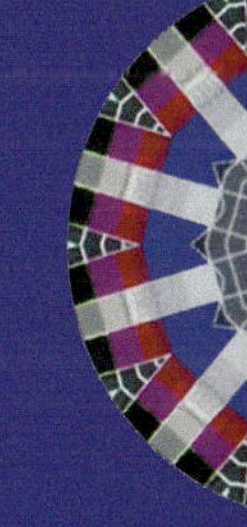

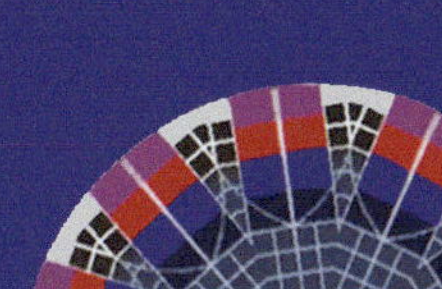

INTRODUCTION

In the 21st century, psychiatric–mental health nursing continues to cautiously expand its neuropsychiatric focus. There have been advances in knowledge concerning the possible neurobiological basis of mental illness, in diagnostic technology and in the discovery of newer psychopharmacologic approaches (see Chapters 6 and 7) that suggest a neuropsychiatric paradigm of care. At the same time that people touched by issues with mental illness (hereafter referred to as 'people living with mental illness' or 'consumers') may have their needs for safety, structure and medication addressed, they also expect to be directly involved in decisions concerning their treatment. The challenge is to integrate both biological and psychosocial concepts while maintaining a collaborative focus on caring. The therapeutic relationship provides the opportunity to meet this challenge.

The **therapeutic relationship**, also called the *nurse–client relationship* or *one-to-one relationship*, is one which uses theoretical understandings, personal attributes and appropriate clinical techniques such as those in Figure 2.1 ■ to provide the opportunity for a sustaining and positive emotional experience for people receiving treatment from mental health services. The therapeutic relationship has evolved as the cornerstone of psychiatric–mental health nursing theory and practice. Initially based on Hildegard Peplau's work on interpersonal relations in nursing (Peplau, 1952; 1997), the theory and practice of one-to-one work in nursing has been further developed by commentators such as Barker (1999). Current understandings of the importance of the therapeutic relationship in nursing must now take account of changing public and professional expectations of how mental health services ought to be organised and delivered; models of care are increasingly collaborative, and reflect the growing influence of the mental health consumer movement (Shattell, Starr & Thomas, 2007).

We are challenged to creatively adapt the well-established principles of Peplau's work under changing conditions, such as briefer psychiatric hospitalisations and the increase in outpatient and community treatment. The current health care economic climate and the emergence of health consumerism have changed the face of the traditional therapeutic relationship advocated by Peplau and others. Nevertheless, the same key principles are incorporated in the everyday work of nurses—brief encounters, as well as consistent long-term relationships.

It is also important to consider the increasing impact of information-communication technology (ICT) on human communication and social interaction broadly, and the therapeutic relationship more specifically. Some decades ago, McLuhan (1964) noted the ways in which the form of communication may influence the meaning and importance of what is being transmitted. Nowadays, almost all human communication is mediated by electronic devices (Schultz, 2001). However, the implications of ICT-mediated human communication for the

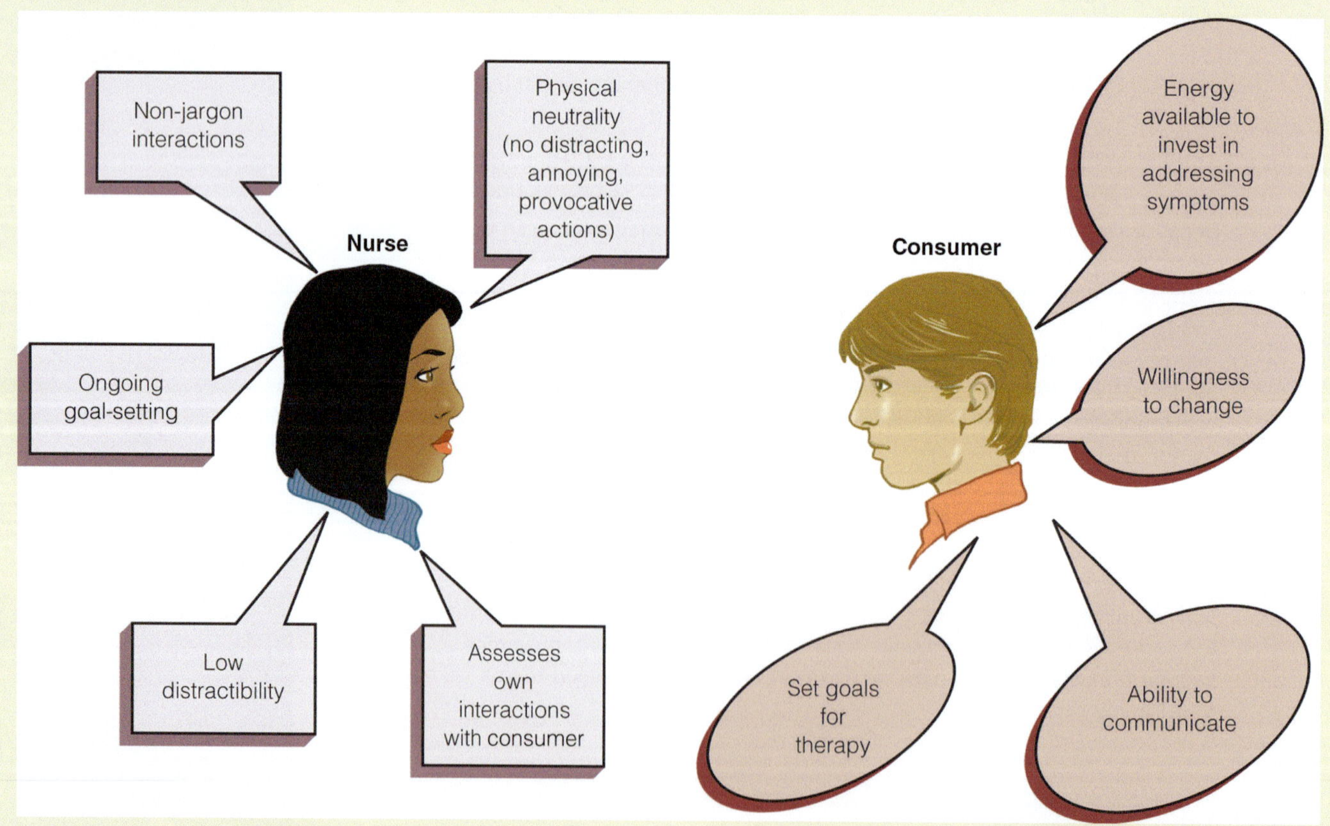

FIGURE 2.1 ■ Nurse and consumer characteristics that enhance the one-to-one therapeutic relationship.

therapeutic relationship are poorly understood. Increasingly, the written and spoken word is being modified to fit the transmission modes of electronic devices; the internet and mobile phones are increasingly relocating interpersonal communication to cyberspace, and are doing so in ways that (re)shape how we think and express ourselves (Hazelton & Morrall, 2011).

The increasing use of what has been referred to as *e-mental health*—'mental health services and information delivered or enhanced through the internet and related technologies' (Jorm, Morgan & Malhi, 2013)—imply transformations in the nature and processes of therapeutic work. Traditionally, discussions of the therapeutic relationship have assumed a face-to-face interaction, involving a nurse (or other health care provider) and the person/s receiving mental health care. The rapid development of e-mental health is changing the nature of service delivery, so that, for instance, comprehensive mental health assessment and consultation can now be provided using audio-visual technology (Saurman, Perkins, Lyle, Patfiled & Roberts 2011), and a range of psychological interventions can be delivered online (Christensen & Petrie, 2013). Such modes of service delivery imply a 'therapeutic relationship' that need not be conducted face-to-face or in real time. If such initiatives have the potential to increase access to mental health treatments, they also raise questions regarding the potential for 'technological developments to overshadow the fundamental need of people with mental health problems for human care' (Jorm et al., 2013, p. 106).

This chapter demystifies the characteristics, processes, phases and problems of one-to-one relationships, so that students and beginning mental health nurses can approach them with increased awareness of their own interpersonal effectiveness. Practical guidelines on how to facilitate interpersonal effectiveness within one-to-one work are included. The principles, processes and phases discussed in this chapter also apply to family, group and community interventions or therapies. One of the authors of this chapter is a senior nursing academic with expertise in mental health nursing. The other author has 30 years of lived experience of mental health issues, and currently leads a Hearing Voices Movement support group and works as a volunteer for Schizophrenia Fellowship (NSW). The intention is to approach the therapeutic relationship as a collaboration that is meaningful and beneficial to both participants.

THE ONE-TO-ONE RELATIONSHIP

The one-to-one relationship between a psychiatric–mental health nurse and a person living with mental illness is a mutually defined, collaborative and goal-oriented professional relationship. It may be viewed as a series of sequential interactions with the following additional elements:

- the interactions occur over a designated period of time (daily, weekly, monthly)
- the interactions take place in a unique structure, characterised by specific phases, processes and problems
- the interactions occur in a designated setting (home, private practice office, community mental health centre, inpatient psychiatric unit, medical ward, emergency department).

In addition, a one-to-one relationship has three distinct phases, as follows:

1. the *orientation (beginning) phase*, characterised by the establishment of contact between the health care practitioner and the person with whom they are working
2. the *working (middle) phase*, characterised by the maintenance and analysis of contact
3. the *termination (end) phase*, characterised by the termination of contact.

Each phase of a one-to-one relationship is distinguished by important goals and therapeutic tasks. These phases are discussed in detail later in the nursing process section of this chapter.

The time required for each phase ideally depends on the severity of dysfunction experienced by the person, the number and types of problems experienced, and the type of therapeutic contract. Although these phases are presented in this chapter in their entirety in order to develop a comprehensive theoretical framework, nurses rarely experience them in such detail and sequence. You are more likely to experience the development of several short-term goals, and to experiment with several subsequent interventions in any phase of relationship work. Nevertheless, an exploration of each phase will increase your familiarity with the flow—that is, 'what comes next'—and may also provide a framework in which you can see the participants' actions as partial expressions of a specific phase.

The amount of time available to establish a one-to-one relationship can be contingent on a variety of circumstances. Despite policy initiatives designed to improve access to mental health care, it remains the case that a person's financial circumstances and level of health insurance coverage may restrict access to mental health services. This is especially so for services provided by psychiatrists, psychologists or nurses in private practice. In addition, practitioners working in public sector mental health services often carry heavy caseloads, resulting in long waiting times for outpatient appointments, and a lack of follow-up after discharge from inpatient care. In rural and remote locations, it may not be possible to easily access specialist mental health care.

Therapeutic alliance

The one-to-one relationship begins with the creation of a **therapeutic alliance**, a conscious, growth-facilitating relationship between a helping person (the psychiatric–mental health nurse) and a consumer. This is fundamental to the process of making adaptive change (Horvath, Del Re, Fluckiger & Symonds, 2011). Students and new graduate nurses may have concerns about the process of creating a therapeutic alliance. The questions and answers in the following Self-awareness: Common Concerns of Nursing Students and New Graduate Nurses address those concerns.

SELF-AWARENESS

Common concerns of nursing students and new graduate nurses

Many of the interactions you have with people with mental illness will be straightforward on a person-to-person basis. However, there will be times when you are concerned. Review these common concerns, and the suggestions that relate to them, before your mental health clinical placement experience.

- ***The person I am caring for won't talk to me.*** It is true that at times people living with mental illness may not want to talk, or their symptoms may make it difficult for them to interact with you. You can offer to remain with the person (if that is acceptable to them) without an expectation that they talk to you. Demonstrate your genuine interest in the person by offering to return at another time and by giving them the opportunity to seek you out or let you know when they wish to talk.
- ***The person I am caring for tells me to go away or seems angry when I approach them.*** Refrain from imposing your goals on the person, and indicate that you respect their wishes. Let them know that you will try again at another time. Recognise that the rejection or anger is not likely to have anything to do with you, but is probably a reflection of the person's emotional distress.
- ***I am afraid of hurting the person I am caring for by saying the wrong thing.*** There is no one wrong thing that will make things worse for the person. If you show genuine interest, respect the person's dignity, and truly care, these qualities will be apparent in your non-verbal behaviour. If you say something that you think is wrong or came out in a way you did not intend, let the person know. You can always say something like: 'That didn't sound right. What I really meant to say is . . .'
- ***I am scared that people with mental illness can be dangerous.*** If this is your first experience in a psychiatric setting, much of what you think you know about people with mental illness comes from the movies and television. Actually, few people with mental illness are dangerous to others. Of course, you must keep safety factors in mind—note which people the staff say are aggressive, be with these people in an open area rather than a closed room, provide space between yourself and the person, and seek the assistance or presence of your clinical facilitator or a registered nurse.
- ***I feel sorry for people I am caring for who do not have money for personal use.*** Giving money or doing personal favours is a form of gift giving (see the section on gift giving in the Nursing Process section), and may impair the therapeutic relationship.
- ***What do I do if I am asked to give personal information—my home address, telephone number—or if I am being asked to see the person I am caring for socially outside of the psychiatric setting?*** Realise that some people with mental illness have difficulty recognising interpersonal boundaries. Explain the difference between a social relationship and a professional relationship, and tell the person that yours is a professional relationship. Giving personal information or agreeing to meet socially would be a professional boundary violation.
- ***The person I am caring for is sexually inappropriate.*** Recognise that sexually inappropriate behaviour is a boundary violation on the part of the other person. You can use the same strategies described earlier. Make it known that the behaviour is inappropriate, but do so in a way that protects the person's dignity.
- ***What do I do if I see someone I know being treated in the mental health facility?*** Take your cue from the person concerned—they may not wish to acknowledge your previous relationship. Discuss this situation with your clinical facilitator to determine the best course of action. If you are assigned to work elsewhere, respect the person's privacy and do not read their record.
- ***What do I do if I run into a person I have cared for at a restaurant, grocery store or some other public place?*** Again, take your cue from the person concerned. They may not wish others to know that they receive, or have received, mental health treatment. Do not acknowledge the person unless they acknowledge you first. Monitor what you say in order to keep the person's confidentiality.
- ***I am scared of admitting that I am anxious about the clinical experience.*** Many students and new graduate nurses are anxious about the clinical experience connected with mental health services, and your lecturers and clinical facilitators recognise that. Your clinical facilitator can be a source of help to you to overcome or reduce your anxiety, but not if you do not share these concerns in the spirit of learning and growing.

LIVED EXPERIENCE

Anxiety is a human experience; in all likelihood the person or persons you will be dealing with will be considerably more anxious than you are. I think it is important to come across as confident even if you don't feel that way, because anxiety can be contagious, and this can easily be communicated to the person experiencing mental illness.

The goal in the therapeutic alliance is to facilitate personal growth by collaboratively addressing problems and concerns in order to handle unresolved problems constructively. More specifically, the nurse works with the person to identify and understand patterns of behaviour, abilities and strengths, using therapeutic communication skills (discussed in Chapter 9). These assets can then be used in working through unresolved problems constructively.

Establishing a therapeutic alliance is essential in one-to-one relationships. Such a binding alliance allows the one-to-one relationship to continue, especially when a person experiences increased anxiety and resistance to change. Investing time, persistence and patience in the therapeutic relationship promotes

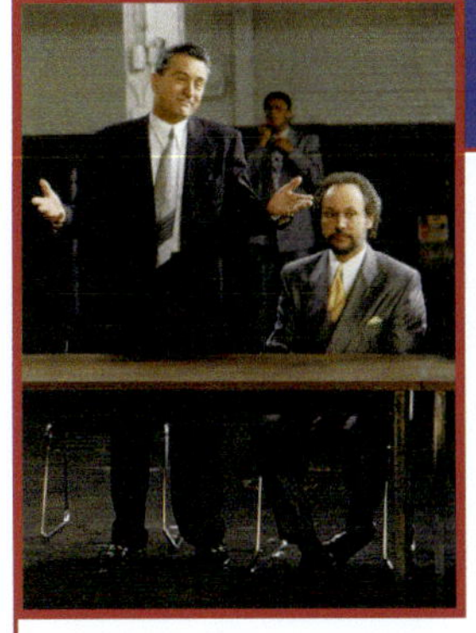

MENTAL HEALTH IN THE MEDIA

Analyze This

Analyze This is the story of a calm, cool and collected psychiatrist (Dr Ben Sobel, played by Billy Crystal) and his new patient, the most powerful crime boss in New York City (Paul Vitti, played by Robert DeNiro), an emotionally vulnerable man who has begun to experience incapacitating panic attacks. The odd-couple chemistry between the two men is engaging, as the psychiatrist is forced to help the gangster get in touch with his feelings. The sessions between psychiatrist and patient are witty—as Dr. Ben Sobel puts it, 'What is my goal here? To make you a happy, well-adjusted gangster?' Later in the movie, Vitti tries out some of what he has learned in therapy, attempting to talk about his feelings to a rival crime boss with whom he is angry.

The movie is not all slapstick comedy, though. It treats Vitti's emotional problems seriously. We come to understand the crime boss's feelings of stress, anxiety and depression, as well as the psychiatrist's complicated family situation that brings him stresses of his own. In *Analyze That*, the sequel to the film, Sobel and Vitti continue to deal with the nuances of their therapeutic relationship in a variety of unusual situations.

Photo courtesy of Alamy A.F. Archive.

the long-term goal of helping to bring about change in established response patterns. Forming a strong therapeutic alliance may enhance recovery and rehabilitation among persons with major mental illnesses (Priebe, Richardson, Cooney, Adedejo & McCabe, 2011). One version of forming a therapeutic alliance is critiqued in Mental Health in the Media.

Characteristics of therapeutic relationships

In addition to having three distinct phases, the therapeutic relationship has several specific, inherent characteristics.

Professional

One-to-one relationships reflect a professional, rather than a social, relationship. We use our personalities, interpersonal skills and techniques, and theoretical knowledge of psychiatric–mental health nursing practice in a purposeful, goal-directed manner to facilitate a useful change in the life of a person. This professional relationship differs from a social relationship in several significant ways that are summarised in Table 2.1 ■.

A professional one-to-one relationship can be either informal or formal. Spontaneous, informal relationships are at one end of the continuum, and formal, individual counselling or psychotherapy (by advanced-practice mental health nurses) is at the other end.

Informal relationships Informal relationships may be prearranged and planned, but more often they occur spontaneously—between a nurse and a person with leukaemia, between a nurse and an offender in prison, between a nurse and a high-risk pregnant woman, between a community nurse and a person with emphysema, or between a nurse and a person living with mental illness. An example of an informal one-to-one relationship is described in What Every Nurse Should Know on the next page.

These relationships consist of a set of interactions limited in time. There is minimum structure and a sense of immediacy. They occur in numerous clinical and non-clinical settings, and are particularly common in psychiatric inpatient units and community mental health settings.

Formal relationships The more formal one-to-one relationship is used in crisis intervention, counselling or individual psychotherapy. It requires more planning, structure, consistency, professional expertise and time. The formal one-to-one relationship occurs in various mental health settings, including psychiatric inpatient units, community mental health centres and private practice.

High levels of symptoms can compromise a person's level of functioning, and thus the ability to establish a formal

TABLE 2.1 ■ Differences between professional and social relationships

Characteristic	Professional relationship	Social relationship
Purpose	Systematic working-through of troublesome thoughts, feelings, and behaviours Planned evaluation (through stages)	Companionship, pleasure, sharing of interests Evolves spontaneously
Role delineation	Specific roles for the nurse and the person, with explicit use of psychiatric nursing skills and interventions	Generally not present, except for broad social norms governing the particular type of relationship (friend versus lover)
Satisfaction of needs	The person is encouraged to identify, develop and assess ways to meet their own needs more effectively Does not address the personal needs of the nurse	Mutual sharing and satisfaction of personal and interpersonal needs
Timeframe	Usually time-limited interactions with an expected termination	Usually not time-limited, in either duration or frequency of contact No planned termination

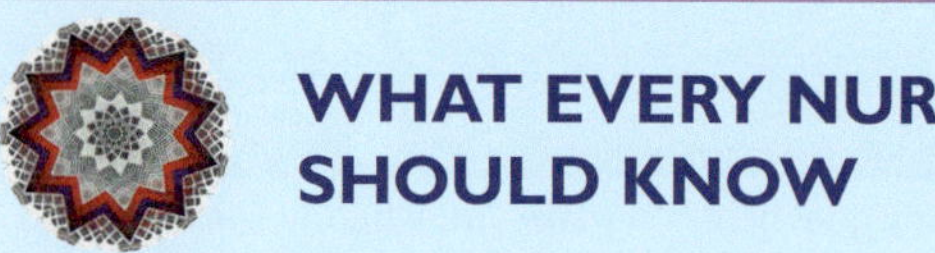

WHAT EVERY NURSE SHOULD KNOW

The therapeutic relationship with parents of a premature infant

Imagine that you are working in neonatal intensive care. When an infant has been born prematurely or has physical problems upon birth (such as low birth weight), the infant may be placed in a neonatal intensive care unit (NICU). Emotions can run high in the NICU as the infant's health fluctuates.

Your ability to act as a liaison between the other health professionals and the parents throughout the infant's stay in the NICU may take place within a one-to-one relationship. You will incorporate a number of one-to-one strategies when you work with parents: recognising and respecting the boundaries of the therapeutic relationship, acknowledging how the parents' anxiety affects communication with their infant as well as the NICU staff, adjusting the speed and volume of your information-sharing so as not to overwhelm the stressed adults, and discussing the emotional tone the parents have while interacting with their infant.

You can use the information in this chapter, specifically information about the therapeutic alliance, cultural context and goal-directed behaviours, to shape how you proceed in situations such as this.

LIVED EXPERIENCE

In my experience, once a diagnosis of schizophrenia has been confirmed, many health professionals, especially those working outside of mental health services, tend to treat you with what I might call 'excessive professionalism'. In other words, they read the 'rules' to you all the time, are typically hyper-vigilant, establish and maintain a high degree of 'professional distance', and seem to want to get you off their books as soon as possible.

relationship. If a one-to-one relationship already exists when symptoms worsen, your therapeutic interactions must be skilled and flexible enough to change your pace and expectations. When the goal of the therapeutic relationship is to promote major changes in emotional states, the person must be able to participate in a focused and abstract effort (Smith & Greenberg, 2007). The nurse must be a skilled partner in achieving that goal.

Table 2.2 ■ highlights the similarities and differences of informal and formal relationship work. The differences are also discussed throughout this chapter.

Mutually defined

A one-to-one relationship is mutually defined by the two participants. That is, both you and the person voluntarily enter the relationship and specify the conditions under which it is to evolve (Spiers & Wood, 2010). For example, immediate relief from symptoms may be sought rather than long-term individual psychotherapy. Decisions regarding where and when to meet, and the conditions of participation, are jointly agreed. This is a part of the contract that is explored further in the discussion of the beginning (orientation) phase of therapy, later in the chapter. Once the one-to-one relationship is established, maintaining it depends on the commitment of both participants.

TABLE 2.2 ■ Similarities and differences in informal and formal one-to-one relationships

Characteristic	Informal relationship	Formal relationship
Setting	Varied	Generally, clinical settings
Frequency and duration of contact	Flexible, depending on individual need or tolerance; example: short, frequent intervals, daily	Structured; example: once weekly, with possible crisis sessions; duration usually set at 30 minutes or 1 hour
Duration of relationship	May or may not involve time commitment Generally a few days to a few weeks	Involves time commitment: weeks to months, for short-term work; months to years, for long-term work
Type of dysfunction	In general, more effective with severe dysfunction	In severe dysfunction, may be useful after stabilisation on medication has been achieved
Use of therapeutic contract	May involve a simple therapeutic contract	Utilises a therapeutic contract; the more specific, the better
Fees	Usually not relevant	May be relevant; may be part of therapeutic contract
Degree of skill required	Nursing student or psychiatric–mental health nurse	Postgraduate qualification in mental health nursing beneficial but not essential
Degree of supervision	Some degree and type of supervision always necessary	Consistent supervision or consultation usually necessary
Degree of effectiveness	Depends on individual level of functioning, the skills of the psychiatric–mental health nurse, and time allotment	Depends on individual level of functioning, the skills of the psychiatric–mental health nurse, and time allotment

Collaborative

Both you and the person enter a relationship in which goals, strategies and outcomes evolve within the context of the therapeutic work together. Mutual collaboration implies that each of you brings personal abilities, capabilities and power to the relationship. You have an impact on each other. However, it is important to not assume responsibility for the behaviours of the other person, but to actively work with them to assess the self-defeating and growth-promoting aspects of specific behaviours. Recognising, supporting and emphasising the person's capacity to have control over their own health and life (Hudson, St. Cyr-Tribble, Bravo & Poitras, 2011) is a growth-producing opportunity.

The person is responsible for change following a joint assessment of problematic behaviours and emotional states (Hudson et al., 2011). Working in concert with a nursing professional in a therapeutic alliance has the added effect of supporting psychological wellbeing by crafting healthy interdependence (Steelman, 2007). Mutual collaboration also means that we assess and are accountable for our own behaviour in therapeutic relationships. Ongoing clinical supervision often helps us to meet these particular goals.

Goal-directed

A therapeutic relationship is always goal-directed. The person is expected to identify and achieve specific physical, emotional and social goals within the context of the relationship. These goals vary widely in type and depth. For example, in informal relationship work, a goal may be to initiate one peer relationship within an inpatient psychiatric unit. Other examples include resolution of a divorce involving children and shared personal possessions, or coming to terms with impending death. Often, the initial goal is to solve an immediate problem, and this serves as a basis for establishing more extensive psychosocial goals.

The psychiatric–mental health nurse and the person collaborate in formulating therapeutic goals to enhance the growth-producing elements of the relationship. People in inpatient services with serious symptomatology may have difficulty in connecting behaviours and modifying them in the time allotted. Goals that can be worked on in the future and in various settings are more likely to be achieved.

Open

The one-to-one relationship may be viewed as an experience in *shared dignity*. The psychiatric–mental health nurse adapts to allow the person to reveal their humanness freely and openly. Each aspect of your verbal and non-verbal behaviour either encourages or inhibits the other person from being open themselves. Evidence-based Practice, below, shows how one nurse demonstrated openness using several interventions to encourage discussion of a difficult topic.

Negotiated

In the one-to-one relationship, the person is an active decision-maker and is personally accountable for the work. The atmosphere of give-and-take within the relationship emphasises mutuality, reciprocity and interpersonal fairness. Establishing a clearly defined, mutually agreed-upon therapeutic contract represents a prime example of negotiation in one-to-one work. (The therapeutic contract is covered later in the chapter.)

EVIDENCE-BASED PRACTICE

Pregnancy and antidepressants

Sharon is a 25-year-old with a history of depression. She is currently pregnant, and is wondering if she should continue taking anti-depressant medications during her pregnancy, or stop and risk having her symptoms return. Sharon has been discussing her concerns with you and the rest of the team during her prenatal care appointments. She has not discussed them with anyone other than her health care providers, because she is afraid of what they might say.

During your one-to-one interactions with Sharon, you state your concern for her welfare, and assure her that her concerns will be discussed on a regular basis. You tell her that the two of you will work on a solution together as you have in the past with other problems.

The one-to-one relationship maintained in this situation has a positive effect on Sharon's ability to discuss a difficult topic. You remain available, without withdrawing, despite Sharon's distress, fears or silence. You promote trust by stating your concern for Sharon's welfare and offering to discuss the issue together. Your intervention should be based on more than one study, but the following research would be helpful in this case.

Gawley, L., Einarson, A., & Bowen, A. (2011). Stigma and attitudes toward antenatal depression and antidepressant use during pregnancy in healthcare students. *Advances in Health Science Education, Theory, and Practice*, *16*(5), 669–679.

Gentile, S. (2011). Drug treatment for mood disorders in pregnancy. *Current Opinion in Psychiatry*, *24*(1), 34–40.

Mahli, G. S., Bassett, D., Boyce, P., Bryant, R., Fitzgerald, P. B., Fritz, K., . . . Singh, R. B. (2015). Royal Australian and New Zealand College of Psychiatrists clinical practice guidelines for mood disorders. *Australian New Zealand Journal of Psychiatry*, *49*(12), 1165–1166.

Petersen, I., Gilbert, R. E., Evans, S. K., Man, S. L., & Nazareth, I. (2011). Pregnancy as a major determinant for discontinuance of anti-depressants: An analysis of data from The Health Improvement Network. *Journal of Clinical Psychiatry*. *72*(7), 979–985.

See, also, the Australian Categorisation of Risk of Medication Use in Pregnancy: <http://www.tga.gov.au/medicines-pregnancy.htm>

CRITICAL THINKING QUESTIONS

1. If antidepressants have even an unlikely potential to affect the baby, should Sharon stop taking them?
2. Should women who take psychotropic medications avoid pregnancy?
3. Why is it important that Sharon's symptoms of depression do not return?

Committed

Commitment is based on the therapeutic contract between the nurse and the person. The contract establishes the limits of the relationship, as well as the time and energy allotted to it. At some point in the relationship, you will be confronted by the reality of the distress experienced by the person with whom you are working. Because of personal discomfort, some beginning nurses may respond by actively colluding to deny or ignore the dysfunction, and remain on a superficial, social level of communication. This collusion protects the nurse from having to address the person's helplessness, desperation, hostility or raw grief. Not allowing expression of these feelings signals that you are not sufficiently committed to the other person.

The opposite may also be non-therapeutic. Assuming an omnipotent or rescuer role to provide a 'cure' signals over-commitment. This role robs the other person of active decision-making power and accountability.

Be aware that your commitment may be tested in some phase of the relationship. Both participants in the therapeutic relationship need to deal with this test explicitly on verbal and non-verbal levels. A sense of positive connectedness with the other person strengthens the sense of commitment.

Culturally sensitive

Because cultural context influences nursing care, a sensitive and systematic consideration of a person's cultural and ethnic background is an essential part of the psychiatric–mental health nursing process in one-to-one relationship work. Cultural forces shape the expression of distress and the formation of symptoms. Culture also influences the expectations of the therapeutic relationship, and interpretations of the events that take place within it. It is important to consistently evaluate the influence of culture within the one-to-one relationship, as well as the effects of the therapeutic relationship on the person's values and life experiences. A sensitive and systematic consideration of cultural and ethnic background is important at each phase of the one-to-one relationship. How to keep culture in mind is interwoven throughout this and other chapters, and is further discussed in the Foreword: Social and Emotional Wellbeing in the Indigenous Context.

PHENOMENA OCCURRING IN ONE-TO-ONE RELATIONSHIPS

Sometimes you may initially feel a sense of unease or confusion about what is happening in the therapeutic relationship. This uneasiness may be difficult to identify, describe and explore. Remember to keep the following phenomena in mind when you are attempting to 'make sense' of a one-to-one relationship.

Resistance

Resistance refers to all of the phenomena that interfere with and disrupt the smooth flow of feelings, memories and thoughts. It inevitably surfaces in the course of any informal or formal psychotherapeutic work, and most often occurs as the person begins to address self-defeating thoughts, feelings and behaviours.

Resistance is often mistakenly seen as being directed against the nurse. Instead, the person is struggling against the anxiety associated with change, against self-awareness, and against responsibility for actions (Smith & Greenberg, 2007). Thus, resistance in therapeutic one-to-one relationships is best understood as a person's struggle against change. These behaviour patterns may have self-defeating aspects, but at the same time they have also provided some satisfaction or prevented some discomfort. In other words, they have 'worked' in the past.

Evaluating behaviour as resistive

In general, you may suspect resistance when the person's behaviour appears to block the progress of the relationship. However, caution should be exercised in evaluating behaviour as resistive. There may be other explanations for the emotional atmosphere in the one-to-one interaction. For example, a silence may indicate pensiveness, a pause before emotive expression, or a sense of completion. Habitual lateness may indicate real difficulties in adjusting a full personal schedule to accommodate the sessions. The person who resists discussing specific topics or concerns may not be ready for investigative work. Likewise, resistance to giving up a defence mechanism such as rationalisation or projection (see Chapter 8) may indicate a desperate need to keep anxiety about unbearable thoughts and impulses, or anxiety about a present situation, at manageable levels.

Remember that people have the right to resist any aspect, or the entirety, of the therapeutic process as a matter of choice. However, resistive behaviour should be openly discussed, rather than ignored.

General intervention strategies with resistance

Several consecutive approaches are used as intervention strategies for resistance. They begin with awareness of the resistance. Helpful intervention strategies include the following:

- Label the resistant behaviour with the person. You may allow the resistance to occur several times to demonstrate its presence. It is as if you are holding up a mirror, reflecting and clarifying the specific resistant behaviour.
- Explore the accompanying emotion, and the history of its development.
- Explore what function the resistance may serve, especially any self-defeating aspects.
- Facilitate working through the resistance by fully understanding and appreciating its implications in the person's life.

This sequence may occur repeatedly before a resistant behaviour is resolved.

Acting out as resistance

Acting out is a particularly challenging form of resistance, in which the emotional conflicts are put into action (that is, are 'acted out'). It is important to recognise that this is the externalisation of an inner conflict to people in the immediate environment. Rather than verbalising conflicts or feelings, the person displays inappropriate behaviours. Some examples of acting out include forcefully slamming a door, dressing provocatively, or slapping someone.

In acting out, a person acts towards a partner, friend, relative or other person those feelings and attitudes that they do not express towards the nurse. An example of acting out is developing third-person relationships to absorb the emotions and fantasies that belong in the therapeutic relationship. Exaggerated feelings of intense hostility towards the nurse may lead to violence or physical harm to themselves, the nurse or a third person. Intense feelings of affection for the nurse or therapist may precipitate a desire for emotional involvement with the nurse or a third person.

Intervention strategies with acting out Acting out contains a vital seed for change. That is, it can form the basis for an understanding of, and eventual giving up of, destructive and inappropriate behaviours. The one-to-one therapeutic relationship can transform acting out (for example, rageful behaviours) into adaptive emotions and behaviours by facilitating change (Smith & Greenberg, 2007). Acting out is difficult to deal with, because the person does not talk about the feelings that precipitate the behaviour, and later tends to conceal or rationalise the behaviour. Acting out can abruptly disrupt the relationship or psychiatric treatment, unless it is identified and dealt with explicitly.

Specific interventions relating to acting out include the following:

- bring the acting-out behaviour to the attention of the person concerned
- encourage *talking about* impulses rather than acting them out
- encourage identification of feelings *before* putting them into action
- increase the frequency of contact
- look for evidence of transference phenomena towards the nurse (discussed in the next section).

LIVED EXPERIENCE

I suspect that for many practitioners acting out involves physically aggressive if not violent behaviours. My experience of it has been different. My experience of dealing with those I considered authority figures, such as the nurse who was my case manager following a really severe psychotic episode, was more passive and fearful behaviour. I now consider that to have been acting-out behaviour, and I think, among other things, that it might have made it too easy for the nurses and doctors to dismiss me and not listen to what I wanted to say at a time when I desperately needed to discuss my psychosis with someone.

With repeated dangerous acting-out behaviours, consider withdrawing from the relationship unless the limits can be set on these behaviours.

Transference

Transference is a normal phenomenon that may surface and inhibit effectiveness in any phase of one-to-one relationship work, and in any setting, including non-mental health settings. **Transference** is a set of feelings and thoughts about significant others in a person's past and current life that is transferred to the caregiver. It can be considered a lens through which an individual sees their relationships. Transference typically happens quickly, and generally unconsciously, in the therapeutic relationship (Schaeffer, 2007). Therapeutic effectiveness requires working with transference issues within a person's cultural framework, and developing options for expressing emotions and behaving adaptively in interpersonal relationships.

A study of early transference reactions (Beretta et al., 2007) noted that people tend to have a limited number of types of relationship patterns (parents, romantic, family, friendship, colleague and impersonal). It is possible that people will repeat their particular patterns with you and re-enact the patterns they use outside the therapeutic relationship. The following Practice Example illustrates how transference may surface in a clinical setting.

Practice example

Nick, hospitalised for depression, was assigned to a case manager, a male psychiatric–mental health nurse. Over the course of several meetings with his case manager, Nick assumed a cowering, ingratiating manner. He seemed to resemble a little boy awaiting punishment from an intimidating, punitive father. This interpersonal orientation was observed by other male staff members in their informal interactions with Nick. Nick was eventually able to discuss his views of older men based on his relationship with a stern, demanding father.

The recognition of transference signals that it is time to explore this interaction in order to reduce interpersonal problems in the one-to-one relationship (Ryum, Stile, Svartberg & McCullough, 2010). Expect that transference issues are likely to arise in a therapeutic relationship. Work collaboratively, using the transference as a therapeutic tool, to foster adaptive and positive changes in the people with whom you are working.

Explore the meaning of individual words, gestures, events and situations in the current one-to-one relationship to determine how these reflect or replay distortions in other past or current relationships. The therapeutic task is to separate feelings, thoughts and behaviours that belong to the current one-to-one relationship from those that represent unresolved conflicts in other relationships.

Increasing awareness of the transference process often frees a person to work through conflicts and explore the more creative, self-actualising aspects of personal identity as they evolve. It is important that you do not take on the role of parent or any other transference figure. Rather, help the person bring an unconscious event into consciousness, to examine its cause and meaning. Remember to seek supervision from your clinical facilitator or other experienced nursing staff member when you suspect a transference reaction.

Positive transference

Transference may be positive or negative. *Positive transference*—that is, positive feelings for the therapist—occurs when a person generally has had satisfying past relationships with significant others during childhood. The therapeutic relationship is usually able to progress in this instance.

Negative transference

In *negative transference*, a person shows a number of reactions based on forms of hate (hostility, loathing, bitterness, contempt, annoyance). Although there are both positive and negative aspects to every transference, a predominantly negative transference is uncomfortable for both you and the person with whom you are working. They do not like to be aware of and express this hate, and you will not like being the target of it. When negative transference appears unresolvable, seek clinical supervision with a knowledgeable and trusted colleague. It may be advisable to terminate the relationship rather than run the risk of further dysfunction in the person concerned.

Countertransference

While transference involves a person's reactions to the psychiatric–mental health nurse, **countertransference** involves the nurse's reactions to a person. You may develop powerful counterproductive fantasies, feelings and attitudes in response to transference phenomena or type of personality. Countertransference is thought by some to be almost inevitable in psychotherapeutic situations (Ellis, 2001).

Countertransference is suspected when the nurse repeatedly assigns meaning to the therapeutic relationship that belongs to the nurse's other relationships. In countertransference, the psychiatric–mental health nurse's ability to assess interactions with a person becomes confused or thwarted by unresolved conflicts. This conflict may be expressed in acts of omission or commission that may be covert or overt. That is, you may unconsciously use behaviours (as parent, sibling, lover or friend) that attempt to replay some conflict with significant others. Some examples are as follows:

- placing hands on the hips or pointing a finger while setting limits on behaviour (parental)
- patting on the shoulder and offering reassurance (parental)
- dressing suggestively (erotic)
- blushing and giggling when a sexual remark is made (sexual)
- being sarcastic in response to an expression of concern (hostile).

Parental or caretaker behaviours that express the need to nurture are the most common among beginning psychiatric–mental health nurses. These behaviours may discount a person's ability to ensure their own wellbeing and encourage acting out. Be alert for actions that are out of line with standard expectations for professional psychiatric–mental health nursing care. Look for cues to the presence of countertransference, such as those discussed in Self-awareness: Countertransference.

SELF-AWARENESS
Countertransference

Look for the following cues in your own behaviour that signal the presence of countertransference:

- overfamiliarity towards the person
- excessive concern about the person
- reacting with annoyance or irrational hostility towards the person
- feeling uneasy during or after meeting with the person
- dreaming or fantasising about the person
- being preoccupied with thoughts of the person during leisure time
- any actions that are out of line with standard expectations for professional and therapeutic behaviours.

Countertransference is a normal occurrence, requiring clinical supervision or consultation to prevent degeneration of the one-to-one relationship. Clinical supervision may enable you to separate feelings, thoughts and behaviours that belong to the current relationship from those that represent unfinished conflicts in other relationships. It is reassuring that most countertransference problems can be resolved by self-assessment with professional supervision. Once the countertransference process is identified, you can consciously develop therapeutic, goal-directed responses. Avoid self-disclosure of countertransference to people with whom you are working. Sharing these feelings may overwhelm and burden them in a destructive way (Beretta et al., 2007). In the rare instance that controlling these disturbed attitudes and emotions requires extended work, making a referral to another nurse or mental health professional is appropriate.

Conflict between caretaker and therapist roles

A one-to-one relationship requires that you work collaboratively with a person to actively explore the meaning underlying their pain, distress or discomfort. Avoid the caretaker role in which you alleviate pain. Rather, encourage people to develop ways to do so for themselves. Similarly, the caretaker role requires nurses to make decisions for people; it does not encourage recovery.

Assuming the caretaker role also undermines your therapeutic effectiveness. The caretaker role tends to involve sympathy rather than empathy. The difference between these two responses (discussed in Chapter 9) is significant to therapeutic outcomes. How effective you are when you interact with a person in a one-to-one relationship is based on your intentions and emotions. The path of the relationship depends on your self-knowledge of these factors discussed in Chapter 4.

Critical distance

It is important to observe how the person with whom you are working uses physical space. Individual preferences, as well as culture, will dictate the specific distance between individuals, depending on the relationship between them. Allow physical distance, especially early in a relationship. This distance promotes verbal communication and minimises any existing anxiety and hostility the person may have. Moving rapidly towards closeness, especially in establishing the therapeutic relationship, may lead to feelings of being overwhelmed and increased anxiety.

Physical distance can be indicative of other therapeutic processes. For example, a person may sit in a chair at a great distance from you during initial meetings, but move closer and closer as the working relationship is established. Assess the possible interpersonal implications of proximity (nearness) for each person. As the relationship progresses, assess whether physical distance or proximity reduces anxiety. The need for critical distance during the therapeutic process usually increases as panic or near-panic levels of anxiety are experienced. See Chapter 9 and Figure 9.3.

Gift giving

The giving of gifts may be a special concern in therapeutic relationships (Forrester, 2010). Gift giving may take various forms: a fleeting social amenity (the purchase of a cup of coffee), a gesture (the loan of a favourite book), or the presentation of a valued object (the giving of an original painting). Like self-disclosure (discussed later in this chapter), gift giving in any instance must be met with ongoing assessment and evaluation to determine its form, intent, appropriateness and meaning in the context of the therapeutic relationship. Nurses from specialty areas other than psychiatry may have more leeway in this regard (Weeks, Cowell, Scullion, & Tanton, 2007). However, professional ethics and therapeutic integrity bar any but the most token of gifts (Nursing and Midwifery Board of Australia, 2008a, 2008b). No rule covers all instances of gift giving. Guidelines to help evaluate particular situations are discussed in each phase of the one-to-one relationship in the nursing process section of this chapter.

Use of touch

Physical contact is used cautiously in therapeutic work. It is best to avoid unplanned physical contact without therapeutic rationale. Some people with poor ego boundaries may become intensely threatened and feel overwhelmed by physical contact. For example, a person may lose the ability to distinguish self from the nurse during simple hand contact. Such contact may be perceived as a hostile or sexual gesture, although you do not intend it that way. In contrast, a person who is acutely grief-stricken, too distraught to focus on words, might receive needed support from being held. When considering any use of touch, ask yourself:

1. Does touch meet the therapeutic goals for this person, or does it meet my needs?
2. Does touch foster a more productive therapeutic relationship?
3. Will touch respect the personal space for this person?
4. How does touch fit with the cultural background of this person?

Evaluate the use of touch, like self-disclosure, in the context of the therapeutic relationship, paying attention to its timing, appropriateness and type. For example, a person is thrilled to achieve an on-the-job goal that has taken much personal time and effort. You determine that a firm handshake and a statement of congratulations are facilitative in this instance and at this working phase of the relationship. If you are unsure of the effect of such a gesture, a frank inquiry may be in order: 'How did you feel when I shook your hand a few moments ago?' Again, the person's reaction and subsequent exploration can be a gauge for measuring how they perceive and respond to the use of touch.

Self-disclosure

Self-disclosure means being open to personal feelings and experiences, being 'real' as opposed to hiding behind a façade. This is an expectation we have of the people with whom we work; we encourage them to be real, to self-disclose as a necessary step in their move towards mental health. But what about self-disclosure on our part? While being 'real' is a quality of authenticity (see Chapter 4), it is important to also recognise that self-disclosure is a complex phenomenon.

How much should you share? Under what circumstances is it appropriate? The wisdom of disclosing personal information has been the subject of much debate. Some argue that self-disclosure impedes therapeutic work, and undermines the relationship because it violates boundaries between professional and social roles (Pope & Keith-Spiegel, 2008). Others argue just the opposite—that self-disclosure can facilitate therapeutic work depending on the circumstances—in cognitive behavioural therapy, with children, with persons with diminished capacity, in social skills training, and in psychopharmacological and supportive treatments (Psychopathology Committee of the Group for the Advancement of Psychiatry, 2001). A review of the literature on self-disclosure found divergent results from one study to the next, indicating that the implications of self-disclosure on the mental health professional's part are unclear (Henretty & Levitt, 2010). How much to share, and under what circumstances, remains an area for further research. Nursing students should be cautious about personal self-disclosure, and should always discuss self-disclosure with a clinical facilitator first.

Pay attention to the timing, appropriateness and degree of self-disclosure. For example, use self-disclosure cautiously when working with people who are severely distressed, or with people with poor ego boundaries. In circumstances such as these, a person may struggle to separate thoughts and feelings that belong to the self from those that belong to you. They might misinterpret your self-disclosure, or might not be able to make sense of the disclosure. There may also be fear of engulfment; that is, your feelings might be perceived as threatening or overwhelming. Self-disclosure should foster the development of the therapeutic relationship rather than threaten its continuance. The right time and reason for self-disclosure become clearer after answering the questions in Self-awareness: Self-disclosure.

SELF-AWARENESS
Self-disclosure

Determining whether or not to self-disclose will be made clearer by answering the following questions:

- What is the purpose of the revelation? Who is this self-disclosure for?
- Does this self-disclosure meet the therapeutic goals for the person with whom I am working, or does it meet my needs?
- Will this self-disclosure take the focus away from the person with whom I am working?
- Does this self-disclosure foster the development of a more productive therapeutic relationship?
  1. Will it encourage the person with whom I am working to disclose what they have withheld or suppressed?
  2. Will it encourage the person with whom I am working to cooperate?
  3. Will it help the person with whom I am working to consider another point of view?
  4. Will it support the person's positive movement in addressing life problems?
  5. Will it encourage empathic understanding?

Personal self-disclosures require evaluation. Students should seek consultation from a lecturer or a clinical facilitator. Practising nurses should seek consultation through peer review (Jain & Roberts 2009) or clinical supervision (Hazelton, Rossiter & Sinclair, 2010).

Culture, values and beliefs

Values and beliefs that may interfere with adaptive functioning will need to be addressed. Some examples of people who hold values and beliefs that may interfere with constructive change are:

- the person who believes that their partner should be subservient, and, conversely, the partner who defers personal needs to preserve the relationship
- the parent who believes that to 'spare the rod' is to 'spoil the child'
- the child raised with the family injunction that family problems should not be discussed outside the home, and may view your actions as an invasion of privacy
- the woman who believes that because God takes care of His people there is no need to solve personal problems
- the man who believes that divorce and homosexuality are sins that will never be forgiven.

Initially, you should become aware of the specific values and beliefs that influence the immediate relationship work. It is often useful to label the value or belief with the person, exploring its history, importance, cultural context and impact. Nonjudgmental, alternative values may be discussed if the other person initiates such an exploration. The humanistic nurse respects values, beliefs and choices regarding personal value systems (Todres, Galvin & Holloway, 2009). Your earnest interest in how a person is coping with emotional stressors provides the encouragement and support that facilitates health-related behaviour change (Weiss & Lewis, 2007).

LIVED EXPERIENCE

About 15 years ago when I was entering a mental health service, I was asked about my sexual orientation by a female nurse who disclosed that she was a lesbian. While I did not feel compromised or obliged to give her an answer, I did feel that the question and her disclosure were inappropriate. It wasn't so much that she asked the question, it was the timing; this was my first interaction with her.

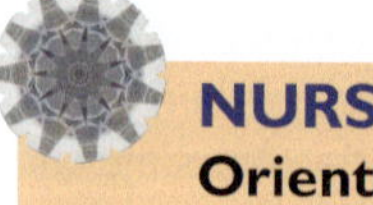

NURSING PROCESS
Orientation (beginning) phase

The primary goal of the orientation phase is to establish contact and begin developing a working relationship with the person. Establishing contact includes the initial encounters, how the two participants approach and interact with each other, both verbally and non-verbally. An example of early dialogue in the orientation phase can be found in the Communication feature.

COMMUNICATION
The initial contract

CONSUMER: 'What, exactly, are we supposed to be doing together?

NURSE RESPONSE 1: 'I'd like to meet with you every day while you're here. This will give you an opportunity to talk about yourself and the things that are of concern to you.'

RATIONALE: In addition to providing structure about the sessions, the nurse lays the groundwork for the focus on the person with whom they will be working.

NURSE RESPONSE 2: 'That's something that you and I can decide together tomorrow morning when we meet here at 9.30.'

RATIONALE: The nurse reminds the person of the time for their meeting, and sets the stage for mutual collaboration and negotiation.

In informal relationships, contact usually begins when the nurse seeks out the person they will be working with. Establishing contact may involve making your presence known and working to establish verbal communicate with the person. In formal relationships, contact may begin when a person enquires about services or when the psychiatric–mental health nurse follows up a referral. In both formal and informal relationships, the sense of working together in a therapeutic alliance enables the person to endure anxiety and deal with resistance to change, which inevitably surface during the course of one-to-one relationships.

This phase of the therapeutic relationship concludes with mutual agreement on a therapeutic contract, which may be verbal and quite simple. The contract spells out the goals for treatment and the nurse's professional responsibilities.

Assessment

Assessment begins at the first moment of contact and continues throughout the therapeutic relationship, but is particularly important during the orientation phase. Remember that shortcuts taken in assessment procedures almost always jeopardise the ultimate quality of care, because crucial areas of concern may go unaddressed or be treated superficially.

An important part of assessment is to determine what is likely to be accomplished in the time allotted. Consider the extent of the person's responsiveness to you during this early stage of relating, the severity of their symptoms, the level of resistance, and the priorities for the care provided. Emphasise the treatment needed to reach the most important and obtainable goals. Together, you and the person take this opportunity to shape the nature of the care within the limits of the current health care environment.

Subjective data

Observation, a process long regarded as essential to clinical nursing practice, is of particular importance in one-to-one relationship work. Note any elements in the interaction that are missing, distorted or imbalanced. What is avoided in discussion is often more crucial than what is shared.

An effective one-to-one relationship requires observation of the behaviour and facial expressions, the content of communication, and other cues about involvement in the process. Keep in mind that you will also be sending the message that you understand, care about and respect the person. Being aware of and using the cues you observe helps you adjust your interventions as necessary during the session. Your goal is to promote the therapeutic relationship and allow the therapeutic process to continue.

An awareness of changes in non-verbal behaviour—such as crossing the arms across the chest, leaning back in the chair, and appearing to withdraw from the interaction with you—is an important component of maintaining a one-to-one relationship. In this instance, an appropriate therapeutic response is 'I'm noticing as we're talking that you've crossed your arms and leaned back in the chair away from me. I wonder how you're feeling right now.' This therapeutic response acknowledges the **here-and-now**, that is, the processes and dynamics at that very moment in the interaction. The importance of tuning in to process is emphasised later in this chapter.

Objective data

Objective data collection ideally includes the following: mental status examination, complete physical examination, history-taking, and psychological testing, as needed. Which examinations are done, and by whom, are generally determined by the service in which the psychiatric–mental health nurse works, and by the psychiatric–mental health nurse's expertise in these specific areas.

The initial interview

Interviewing is a process that serves several purposes in the orientation phase of one-to-one relationships. Although a psychiatric–mental health nurse may use a structured initial interview in formal one-to-one work, it is rarely used in informal relationships. In informal relationships, consider using the applicable principles and concepts during your initial meeting.

The initial interview has the following purposes:

- to initiate trust building
- to establish rapport with the person
- to obtain pertinent data
- to initiate assessment
- to make practical arrangements for treatment.

The initial interview is crucial because it sets the stage for subsequent therapeutic contact. As you begin to work together to identify the issues the person intends to work on, you further the development of the one-to-one relationship. You are more likely to intervene effectively if you understand how a therapeutic relationship will fit into the person's life and consider the direction they wish to take (Gary, 2007).

Structure Structure the initial interview to establish rapport, decrease anxiety and convey willingness to address personal distress. Begin by introducing yourself, inviting the person to be seated, and making a statement about the information thus far known about their contact with services. An open-ended question such as 'How is it that you are here today?' or 'What brought you to the hospital?' provides an opportunity for the person to talk about their concerns. Indicate that the purpose of the initial interview is to obtain an overview of the person's current situation and then determine the availability of appropriate services.

Essential data One primary purpose of structuring the initial interview is to collect essential data (see Chapter 10). Address resistance if it surfaces during the initial interview. This resistance may occur when the person has initiated services at someone else's request or insistence, has fears and misconceptions about therapy, or has had an unsatisfactory therapeutic experience in the past. Explore resistance before collecting further data.

A person who is anxious may be confused about or misinterpret the information you give during the initial interview. You may need to repeat information several times or in subsequent meetings. You will also need to determine whether confusion or misinterpretation could be a manifestation of resistance instead of anxiety, as in the Practice Example that follows.

Practice example

One of the doctors in the medical practice where you work has asked you to see Rowena. On checking her medical record, you note that Rowena is a 35-year-old woman who has had several appointments for minor medical problems. You note from the record a pattern of repeat prescriptions for anti-anxiety medication. You also note that she was referred for mental health care on two other occasions, but failed to keep those appointments.

In thinking about the information Rowena presented in the first session, you review her comments on having not followed through on the other two referrals. There are many possible reasons a person may miss appointments, some having to do with insufficient motivation for treatment, some having to do with psychiatric symptoms, and others attributable to unavoidable life circumstances. Rowena's explanations indicate no external interfering life stressors or difficulties with transportation.

During that first session, Rowena was upset and apologetic for not following through on the referrals, which she attributed to her anxiety symptoms. Specifically, she has been experiencing increasing difficulty leaving her home. The farther she gets from home, the more anxious she becomes. She cannot leave her home, even to run important errands, without taking anti-anxiety medications. Rowena cannot really specify the reason for her anxiety other than a sense of impending catastrophe. Rowena's behaviour, self-reports and history are all consistent with what would be expected in an anxiety disorder. You note the lack of defensiveness in her presentation, and you conclude that, at this point, there is no avoidance or resistance that would undermine the initiation of a one-to-one relationship.

LIVED EXPERIENCE

I am aware of friends who live with mental illness for whom anxiety can sometimes be so overwhelming that it interferes with the capacity to engage in the normal activities of life. Situations such as this indicate the extent to which it is important to think through very carefully the reasons why a person may or may not engage with treatment. For some people there can be practical concerns—such as childcare responsibilities or fear of running into certain people—that can hinder even leaving the house. This is the case with several people with whom I am friendly.

Knowing about a person's typical emotions and defences is valuable, because it provides direction for making an appropriate formulation related to both behaviour and affect, identifying appropriate outcomes, setting individualised goals, and implementing appropriate interventions.

Diagnosis

Organise all of the data collected during the assessment phase, and make a preliminary formulation. The word *preliminary* is used to imply the ongoing potential for revision as the person's behaviours unfold during the course of the therapeutic relationship.

The goal in organising the data is to understand the data as they reflect the person's unique, private world. Look for dominant themes or central issues in the person's responses. The dominant themes and central issues will be unique to each individual.

Outcome identification

The major outcomes of the orientation phase are establishing contact and beginning to form a working relationship between the participants. The working relationship in this initial phase is the framework within which behavioural change is constructed, a challenging task, in the next phase. Your Assessment Approach, below, highlights the common signs of a working relationship. Look for these signs to determine whether the one-to-one relationship is moving into the working phase. Other individual outcomes will be determined by the person's specific dominant themes and central issues.

Planning and intervention

The following interventions are common elements during the orientation phase. The development of additional interventions is based on assessment and formulations for each individual person with whom you work.

Developing the therapeutic contract

A plan for action actually forms the *therapeutic contract* negotiated in a one-to-one relationship. The therapeutic contract is a concrete, detailed and mutually negotiated acknowledgment of a person's personal goals for treatment, plus the nurse's professional responsibilities. Essentially, this involves a discussion of how the two of you will work together. Be certain to discuss the timeframe for your work together during this phase, and reinforce it during the other phases,

YOUR ASSESSMENT APPROACH Signs of a working relationship

The following criteria may be useful in determining whether a one-to-one relationship is moving into the working, or middle, phase.

For nurse

- Sense of making contact with the person
- Sense that the person is responding well to the relationship
- Sense that the nurse can facilitate growth in the person regardless of the severity of dysfunction
- Sense of commitment to addressing the person's problems

For consumer

- Non-verbal and verbal evidence of liking the nurse
- Sense of relaxation with the nurse
- Sense of confidence in the nurse
- Non-superficial (in nature and depth) problems addressed

so that it does not come as a surprise when it is time to terminate the relationship.

The contract may be modified over time, but always serves as a tool for evaluating the benefit to the person and the effectiveness of the nurse. In an informal therapeutic relationship, the therapeutic contract may differ from the usual care plan often developed in outpatient and inpatient settings. For example, an initial contract may begin as a very simple agreement concerning the time and place of subsequent meetings together.

Personal goals for treatment may be long-term or short-term goals, but they always specify detailed, observable outcomes, as in the following Practice Example.

Practice example

Nicole is a 30-year-old woman admitted to an inpatient psychiatric unit following an overdose of risperidone (Risperdal). During past hospitalisations, Nicole has been emotionally labile, has had trouble following her treatment schedule, was frustrated by the limits and compromises of living in the hospital, demanded medication, and threatened suicide. The clinical nurse specialist has proposed that she and Nicole work together to identify goals and behaviours for improved personal and interpersonal functioning. Nicole identified problems of feeling empty, having poor relationships with others, and being angry; she chose to focus on the overall goal of improved social skills. Nicole agreed to the following expectations:

- I will participate in a one-to-one relationship with the clinical nurse specialist and express my feelings verbally.
- I will identify uncomfortable situations involving other people, and discuss the interactions with the clinical nurse specialist at appointed times.
- I will continue my routine treatment activities until the appropriate time to meet with the clinical nurse specialist.

LIVED EXPERIENCE

I have often found the non-verbal to be much more important than the verbal. I have long recognised that my body will sometimes react to situations I don't like or people I don't feel drawn to before I respond emotionally. In some instances, I have not been aware of my feelings about a particular person or topic, and my body has provided guidance by reacting physically. Mental illness can interfere with your capacity to feel, and the body reacts as a kind of early warning system.

Therapeutic goals most often contribute to the establishment of a working relationship when they are specific, address intrapersonal or interpersonal behaviour patterns, and specifically delineate the degree of change necessary for the person to feel satisfied. Strive for the most concise, detailed and accurate description of therapeutic goals in the beginning phase. Clearly stated goals facilitate subsequent mutual evaluation during the middle and end phases of one-to-one work. Goals may focus on the following:

- decreasing or eliminating troublesome behaviours
- increasing socialisation
- increasing living skills
- engaging in education
- securing employment.

At times, such goals may be long-term or even unrealistic. In this situation, help can be offered to define initial steps towards the long-term goal. For example, a person readmitted with mental illness may pinpoint discharge as an important goal. You may then work together to identify the steps needed to achieve this goal. One step may be to maintain self-care in the area of bathing/hygiene. When severe dysfunction limits a person's input into planning, the nursing staff may supplement goals that are determined to be beneficial to that person.

In a formal therapeutic relationship, as in individual psychotherapy, the therapeutic contract is more detailed and generally includes three practical matters:

1. determining the place, duration and time of the meetings
2. establishing capacity to meet the costs associated with treatment
3. considering optional referral sources, should the person be unable to meet the costs of treatment

The therapeutic contract does not always reflect a person's problems and strengths in their entirety. For example, it may not be acknowledged that an area is, in fact, a problem. Thus, the therapeutic contract reflects the *person's* definition of personal goals at one moment in time. In this instance, remain aware of other probable problem areas, and engage with the person in reassessing these areas and modifying or deleting goals in subsequent phases.

Regardless of the form that goal identification takes, the therapeutic contract serves the following purposes:

- facilitating humanistic involvement with the person as an individual
- involving the person as a full partner in the therapeutic process
- serving as a basis for communication in the therapeutic process
- providing continuity for the person and everyone involved with them.

Establishing trust

Concerns about trust surface in this first phase of the relationship. Trust evolves over time as the person tests the emotional climate of your interactions together, risks self-disclosure, and observes that you are responsible and do what you say you are going to do. You can promote trust by responding to all of the person's feeling states without being judgmental or attempting to control their expression of emotions. The process recording in Table 2.3 ■ demonstrates how one nurse began to promote trust early in the orientation phase. Note that she was self-assured enough to encourage the sharing of concerns about trust. It is important

Table 2.3 ■ Process recording of an orientation phase session

Verbatim interaction	Nursing intervention	Rationale
Consumer: 'It's so difficult for me to talk . . . to let you know about me.' (30-second pause)	None.	Allows person to proceed at own pace; if silence is uncomfortably long in the first few contacts, you may use reflection, e.g., 'I sense how difficult talking is for you.'
Consumer: 'Every time I start to tell anybody about myself, they usually end up laughing at me.'		
Nurse: 'Give me an example.'	Encourage elaboration.	Explores meaning of this statement to the person.
Consumer: 'Well, just last week I started talking to my neighbour. I told him that I was laid off from work again. Next thing you know, he's laughing, slapping my back, and saying, "Hey, hard times, eh?" '(Shifts in chair, avoids eye contact.)		
Nurse: 'What was this like for you?'	Explore the person's reaction, especially accompanying feelings.	Further explores meaning of this specific incident as perceived by the person.
Consumer: 'Awful . . . lousy . . . that's all.' (Pause.)		
Nurse: 'I wonder if you're concerned that the same might happen here—that you'll be laughed at?'	Connect the person's concern regarding this emotionally difficult interaction to the here-and-now, i.e., the one-to-one therapeutic relationship.	Issues concerning the person's immediate life situations often reflect parallel issues in the therapeutic relationship.
Consumer: 'Well, maybe . . . I don't know you, so how do I know what you might do? You don't look like the type, but then again, how do I know?'		
Nurse: 'It sounds like you're wondering if it's safe to trust me.'	Identify what appears to be the underlying central concern or theme.	Reflection of what appears to be the central concern (theme) encourages assessment by the person through validation or correction of your statement.
Consumer: 'Yeah . . . No offence, though.'		
Nurse: 'Let's talk about how safe you feel today and as we continue to work together.'	Focus on trust as an issue for further exploration; acknowledge that there is stress in evolving a working relationship.	Avoid premature reassurances so that trust can evolve and be assessed periodically.

to be consistent and to be self-aware of the part your feelings play in the interactions.

In addition to being consistent and self-aware of the part your feelings play in such interactions, the following positive and helpful behaviours may encourage initial trust and help the person to feel safe while disclosing uncomfortable, even forbidden feelings, wishes or behaviours:

- listening attentively to the person's feelings
- responding to the person's feelings
- exhibiting consistency
- viewing situations from the person's perspective.

These behaviours constitute positive, helpful influences in encouraging trust. It is also important to avoid giving premature reassurances about trust, which may inhibit exploration of this vital therapeutic issue and create distance.

Keeping confidentiality

Concerns about the level of confidentiality also surface in this first phase of the therapeutic relationship. Maintaining confidentiality is a legal and ethical responsibility (see pages 213 and 223–224 in Chapter 11). However, circumstances do exist (for example, intent to kill oneself, intent to harm others) in which it is necessary to disclose a person's information. Be sure to provide information about the limits of confidentiality. Doing so actively demonstrates caring behaviour by protecting the dignity and respecting the autonomy of the person with whom you are working (Fisher & Oransky, 2008).

Be aware of your responsibilities in relation to confidentiality. Explicitly address the issue of confidentiality when even a vague reference is made to it. Explicitly state which people will have access to personal information (clinical facilitator, case manager, consultant treating doctor, nursing colleagues on the treatment team), and explore how the person feels in response to this situation.

Tuning in to process

The nursing student or new graduate nurse often attends carefully to the *content* of such sessions—what the person says—and only after considerable experience becomes actively attuned to *process*, the dynamics of the here-and-now situation. Avoid focusing solely on your technique. This produces mechanical, unfeeling responses and interferes with

> **LIVED EXPERIENCE**
>
> What the person will very likely want out of an initial meeting is a sense of going forward positively; you don't want things to be entirely focused on the past—all those things that have gone wrong; you want things to be forward-looking. For me, there is nothing more dispiriting than spending an hour rehashing my past to someone who is taking detailed notes. Focusing too much on the past is unhelpful, and I am sick of retelling my history to professionals who often feel to me as if they don't care.

your ability to be aware of process. *Process* as used here (and discussed in Chapter 9) does not mean nursing process. Processing is a complex communication skill that enables the nurse to focus on several aspects of the one-to-one relationship at the same time. Process involves attending to all non-verbal and verbal behaviours. It involves responding to personal themes, such as anger, hopelessness and powerlessness.

The experienced nurse is simultaneously aware of both content and process, interweaving both for maximum therapeutic effectiveness. The challenge is to develop sufficient know-how to learn what to ignore and be sensitive enough to know what to emphasise (Guy & Brady, 2001).

Addressing suffering

Directly address the person's experience within the context of their cultural and ethnic background. This intervention allows people to share how they perceive, experience and manifest the problem. The accompanying Practice Example illustrates how a nurse encouraged a person with depression to 'move outside himself'.

> **Practice example**
>
> **Person:** 'This depression is like a tonne of bricks weighing me down.'
>
> **Nurse:** 'How would I know that you are suffering in this way? What would I see and hear?'
>
> **Person:** 'Well . . . I sigh a lot . . . I don't move a lot, only when I have to . . . I wouldn't look at you, or bother talking to you. I guess when I feel like this, I shut people out. Yeah, I shut everyone out, even my wife.'
>
> **Nurse:** 'So when you suffer in this way, you shut people out. And what is this like for you?'
>
> **Person:** 'I'm alone and lonely. There is no one who cares for me.'

Addressing suffering is never easy. Avoid the temptation to offer reassurance or sympathy, or change the topic, in the hope that you will ease the person's burden. Doing so will only demonstrate that it is not safe to talk about painful topics.

Clarifying purpose, roles and responsibilities

An additional therapeutic task in this beginning phase is to intervene directly in clarifying the purpose of the relationship work, the role of the nurse, and the responsibilities of the person with whom you are working. When this preliminary exploration of purpose, roles and responsibilities is explicit and detailed, each participant better understands how to move within the relationship. It also decreases anxiety and the chance that the relationship may be used to obtain special privileges. From the first meeting, you have the opportunity to reinforce effective coping skills and increase the person's self-esteem. Your Intervention Strategies, below, summarises the goals, tasks and subsequent nursing interventions of the orientation phase of one-to-one relationships.

YOUR INTERVENTION STRATEGIES Goals, tasks and interventions of the orientation phase

Goal: Establish contact and begin to form a working relationship with the consumer

Therapeutic tasks	Nursing interventions
Clarify the purpose of relationship work, and the roles and responsibilities involved.	Provide information regarding the purpose, roles and responsibilities in relationship work, to alleviate the person's initial anxiety. Immediately and explicitly address any misconceptions, fantasies and fears regarding relationship work and/or the nurse.
Address suffering directly, offering to work with the person towards its alleviation.	Use therapeutic communication techniques, especially empathic understanding, discussed in Chapter 9. Avoid premature reassurance (allow trust to evolve).
Address issues of confidentiality.	Be explicit about the degree of confidentiality, and who has access to information about the person.
Negotiate a therapeutic contract (the person's definition of personal goals for treatment and the nurse's professional responsibilities).	Whenever possible, encourage delineation of goals that are specific, address intrapersonal and interpersonal behavioural patterns, and designate the degree of change necessary for the person to feel satisfied that progress is being made.

Gift giving during the orientation phase

During the orientation phase of a therapeutic relationship, you may be offered or asked for a gift. This gesture may be as incidental as offering you a cigarette or asking you for one. Examine this overture, keeping in mind several possible motivations:

- the person may seek to bribe or manipulate you, thereby seeking to control the direction of the therapeutic relationship (Chapter 18 deals with manipulation)
- the person may seek to 'buy' your time and attention
- the person may ask for small gifts to reinforce a helpless, 'take-care-of-me' interpersonal stance
- the person may have no covert intent, and may simply want something they think you can provide.

In the orientation phase, it may be helpful not to accept or give any gift you feel uncomfortable about, or that may signal a boundary violation (Forrester, 2010). Explore the person's intent. Often, this mutual exploration not only clarifies the intent, but also helps define the parameters of the evolving relationship and models the exploratory process.

Evaluation

In the orientation phase, evaluation includes your initial comprehensive evaluation of the person's behaviours, any initial steps towards the development of self-evaluation, and your ongoing self-evaluation. The more specific and goal-oriented the therapeutic contract, the easier it is for both participants to evaluate the effectiveness of the therapeutic relationship.

In addition to evaluating the effectiveness of each therapeutic task, you must evaluate the important goal of the orientation phase: has a working relationship developed between yourself and the person with whom you are working, and, if so, to what degree? Review the Your Assessment Approach: Signs of a Working Relationship, on page 32, to assess readiness to move into the working phase.

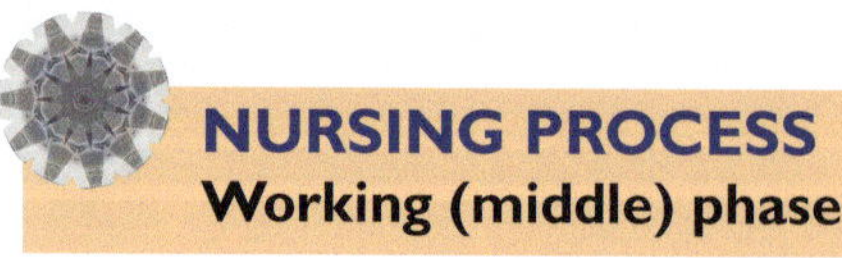

NURSING PROCESS
Working (middle) phase

Once contact is established, attention turns to maintenance and analysis of contact in the working phase. *Analysis of contact* refers to an in-depth exploration of how the person relates to others as manifested in the therapeutic relationship. In this working phase, developmental and situational problems may be addressed, as well as interpersonal problems. It is called the *working phase*, because during this phase both participants actively and systematically identify, explore, link, modify and evaluate specific behaviours, especially those determined to be dysfunctional for the person.

The person's clearly stated goals in the therapeutic contract are now explored. This involves the following two therapeutic goals:

- *Behavioural analysis.* Mutually determine the dynamics of the person's response patterns, especially those considered to be dysfunctional. Such analysis also addresses dysfunctional thought and emotive patterns, because these inevitably alter behaviour.
- *Constructive change in behaviour.* This applies particularly to dysfunctional response patterns.

Thus, both participants work together to analyse behaviour and institute behavioural change.

Assessment

Assessment is continued, detailed and expanded upon. Your observations of non-verbal, verbal and environmental responses continue to have vital importance as the person begins to address personal response patterns. In addition, you continue to assess emotive, cognitive, cultural and behavioural aspects.

By filling in gaps of information not obtained in the orientation phase, you may now acquire a detailed assessment about a subject the person was unable to share or had ignored earlier. The following Practice Example illustrates that what is not said (that is, what is avoided, blocked, rejected) may have more significance than what is shared.

Practice example

During initial appointments, 18-year-old Maureen avoided any inquiries about her parents, other than to say that she lived alone. After several meetings, the nurse again asked about the parents. Maureen replied softly, with tears welling in her eyes, 'They're dead. They died in a car crash two years ago.' She slowly related how, since their deaths, she had spent so much energy trying to survive that she barely felt much of anything. Subsequent meetings dealt with her apparent delayed grief reaction.

The new data caused the nurse to revise and update the tentative formulation, and initiate a marked change in the direction of the meetings. Such shifting is not uncommon in one-to-one relationships. When a change in direction occurs, assess if the sudden change indicates either the need to avoid a certain topic or a move toward a deeper level of emotive expression.

In the working phase, you facilitate many aspects of assessment with the person. First, collaborate in identifying important behavioural trends and patterns. Knowing the issues that promote or inhibit therapeutic progress is essential to success (Balkin, Leicht, Sartos & Powell, 2011). Once you identify a pattern, explore it in elaborate detail to determine its origin, causes, operation and effects on the person and those in their world. Environmental factors (familial, political, economic or cultural) are separated from any intrapersonal factors (depression or anxiety) contributing to the pattern. The person figuratively holds the pattern to the light to examine and make sense of its every aspect. The elements of one pattern will inevitably link with others, so that the major life patterns gradually unfold. The first part of Your Intervention Strategies summarises the therapeutic tasks undertaken to achieve the objective of behavioural analysis, and offers specific approaches to providing help.

YOUR INTERVENTION STRATEGIES Goals, tasks and interventions of the working phase

Goal: Behavioural analysis (mutual determination of dynamics of response patterns identified by the consumer, especially those considered dysfunctional)

Therapeutic tasks	Nursing interventions
Identify and explore important response patterns in detail.	Explore the origin, causes, operation and effect of response patterns (intrapersonally and interpersonally). Separate environmental factors (familial, political, economic, cultural) from intrapersonal factors. Link elements of one response pattern to other patterns, as appropriate, for a gradual unfolding of central life patterns.
Jointly analyse the mode of conflict resolution to be used.	Encourage detailed exploration of how the person reacts to reduce anxiety associated with conflict. Increase awareness of the defences employed to ward off anxiety awakened by such exploration.
Facilitate self-assessment of growth-producing and growth-inhibiting response patterns.	Encourage evaluation of each response pattern to determine which are self-defeating and/or thwart the gratification of basic needs.

Goal: Constructive change in behaviour, especially in dysfunctional response patterns identified by the consumer

Therapeutic tasks	Nursing interventions
Address the forces that inhibit desired change (troublesome thoughts, feelings and behaviours).	Help the person challenge personal resistance to change. Use problem-solving strategies, active decision-making and personal accountability. Help the person learn and apply problem-solving strategies. Encourage the person to assert their own needs when external environmental conditions (group, agency, institution) are an inhibiting force.
Create an atmosphere offering permission for active experimentation to test and assess the effectiveness of new behaviours.	Allow freedom to make and assess mistakes and blunders. Avoid parental judgment of any behavioural experimentation; encourage self-assessment instead.
Facilitate development of coping skills to deal with anxiety associated with constructive changes in behaviour.	Address, rather than avoid, anxiety and its manifestations. Strengthen existing growth-promoting coping skills, especially regarding unalterable conditions (terminal illness, physical deformity, loss of significant other by death). Encourage development of new coping skills and their application to actual life experiences.

There are two noteworthy considerations regarding the therapeutic tasks of the first goal, behavioural analysis:

1. As people begin to describe and re-experience conflict, they consciously or unconsciously use defences to ward off the anxiety this awakens. The development of a good working relationship enables increased anxiety to be tolerated in the working phase.
2. As people become familiar with self-assessment, they may modify original personal goals, or develop additional goals, in keeping with what they have learned.

It is important during the working phase to encourage the person's self-assessment of growth-facilitating and growth-inhibiting behaviours. After assessing one specific response, the person is often able to transfer this skill to begin assessing other aspects of life as well. A realistic self-assessment process is perhaps the most valuable skill that can be 'taken home'. It is often exciting to experience a person 'taking over' and further applying realistic assessment skills developed in one-to-one work.

Diagnosis

In the working phase, earlier formulations may be revised, expanded or deleted to more accurately reflect a central pattern of concern in the evolving one-to-one relationship. As the working phase proceeds, priorities may change—for example, when the person is able to implement positive change in some areas. Actions considered risky, or to pose a risk, may move up or down on the priority list, depending on what interventions, if any, have been effective. An area of concern may decrease in priority after preventive health education, if there is mutual agreement that this intervention is beneficial.

Outcome identification

The initial goal of behavioural analysis of the person's response patterns continues throughout the working phase. The major identified outcomes are as follows:

- develops an awareness of current behavioural patterns
- understands how and when those patterns manifest themselves

LIVED EXPERIENCE

I find that in working with me the therapist should adopt a strategy of cautious intervention; by this I mean you let me talk, and you show that you are listening. I respond to interest being shown in me, and appreciate it when the therapist gives indications of having listened and can replay that back to me. Feeling that I have been fully involved in decision-making regarding myself is absolutely crucial to me. I have had the experience of being discussed by two professionals—a case manager and a psychiatrist—as if I wasn't there, and found this to be an especially humiliating experience.

- may gain insight into the potential causes of those patterns
- assesses which behavioural patterns are ineffective and self-defeating
- attempts to change ineffective behavioural patterns and develop new, more effective behaviours.

Be aware that the quality of the therapeutic relationship predicts outcomes—the better the relationship, the better the outcomes (Priebe et al., 2011).

Planning and implementation

In the working phase, planning is ideally done collaboratively. When planning has been systematic and thorough, there is hardly a moment to worry about 'what to do'. The short-term and long-term treatment goals in the form of the therapeutic contract comprise a map indicating the direction, the momentum and the steps that are needed to reach a designated point.

There is, however, a potential danger in the implementation of the planning component: moving too quickly and incompletely through an exploration of feelings and thoughts in an attempt to reach a designated goal. *Slowness* and *thoroughness* are all-important here. Change needs to take place in the person's feelings, thoughts and behaviours. If change does not occur in all aspects, then it is destined to be short-lived and ineffectual in the long run, and may cause discouragement.

When working on an issue that is unresolved at the end of a meeting, it is often helpful to summarise the unfinished work for the next meeting. This technique may help the person anticipate, plan or prepare to tackle this area of concern again. Personal experiments, such as trying out new behaviours in real situations, may be encouraged between sessions. Some people may be able to continue working through a problem on their own between meetings. Indeed, as engagement with treatment strengthens, this is to be encouraged.

Active intervention is especially important to achieve the second goal of the working phase, constructive changes in behaviour, particularly in self-defeating, growth-inhibiting behaviour patterns. Behavioural change flows from the first goal of behavioural analysis. The objectives are interrelated and essential for successful therapeutic work. Understanding and insight need to be complemented by behavioural implementation. Failure to make adaptive behavioural changes stymies progress and sabotages the therapeutic experience (Martin & Pear, 2007). A person may consistently generate and thrive on sophisticated insights while continuing to assume a powerless stance about implementing constructive change in their condition. Your Intervention Strategies on page 37 highlights therapeutic tasks and specific nursing interventions for both goals of the working phase—behavioural analysis and constructive change in behaviour.

Testing the effect of new behaviours

Active experimentation can also be used to test the effect of new behaviours. The introverted male who resolved to feel more comfortable in initiating conversations with other people may try out various approaches with both male and female nurses to determine which seem to work best. Permission to 'try on' or role-play new behaviours must also include the freedom to make mistakes. Errors and blunders are rich sources of additional learning and occasional fun. Those who can see humour in errors have acquired a new skill. Encourage the use of such techniques, and any other coping skills learned in relationship work, in dealing with normal maturational and situational challenges encountered throughout life.

In inpatient settings, communicate with other staff members to make the whole team aware when a person is trying out new behaviours that may be exaggerated at first. For example, a person who is depressed may be encouraged to verbalise anger and begin by shouting. If there is no staff collaboration they may receive negative feedback, such as room restrictions or a loss of certain privileges, for testing out new coping skills.

Implementing problem-solving strategies

Problem-solving strategies, as a mode of intervention, are particularly important in the working phase. Problem-solving strategies are essential after important behavioural patterns have been identified, explored and assessed. Encourage the sequential problem-solving strategies discussed in Your Intervention Strategies, on the next page. Reminding a person to be patient is supportive and reassuring. Problem-solving abilities improve with time and experience.

Challenging resistance to change

Challenging resistance to change is an appropriate intervention in the working phase. There are two major categories of forces that inhibit desired change, as follows:

1. *intrapersonal forces*, which may arise from troublesome thoughts, feelings or behaviours; thoughts that hamper sense of worth, inability to control and express emotion appropriately, or the inability to relate to others in a meaningful manner
2. personal *resistance to change*, which is the greatest inhibiting force—in fact, the person's challenge to this resistance constitutes the major work in one-to-one relationships.

YOUR INTERVENTION STRATEGIES Problem-solving strategies

- ***Observation.*** Observation as a problem-solving strategy involves gathering and analysing facts about a potential problem area. It eliminates opinions and impressions, and emphasises facts. Observation as an aspect of assessment is discussed in the section on subjective assessment.
- ***Definition.*** Definition is perhaps the most significant and far-reaching problem-solving strategy. It involves an initial specification of a problem, followed by a question. Starting a problem-solving exploration with the word 'How' ('How is it?' 'How does it manifest itself?' 'How has this come about?') puts the focus on the process of a specific problem. It is generally more useful than asking 'Why?', which emphasises rationale. Questioning as a communication technique is explored in Chapter 9.
- ***Preparation.*** Preparation involves collecting additional pertinent data related to the basic problem that may prove useful in later stages of problem-solving strategies. This enables the nurse and the person to anticipate which data might be most useful.
- ***Analysis.*** As a problem-solving strategy, analysis involves breaking down the relevant material into sub-problems, so that each sub-problem may be assessed separately.
- ***Ideation.*** Ideation involves accumulating alternative ideas on how to resolve the basic problem.
- ***Incubation.*** Incubation involves setting aside the problem-solving process or one aspect of it for a period of time to allow for illumination.
- ***Synthesis.*** Synthesis involves putting together all elements of the basic problem, sub-problems, and possible alternatives.
- ***Evaluation.*** Evaluation consists of making judgments about the ideas that result.
- ***Development.*** As a final problem-solving strategy, development involves planning the implementation of these ideas.

LIVED EXPERIENCE

These strategies sound very good, providing problem-solving involves a truly collaborative enterprise. For me, and I am sure it is true for many others, if I am excluded from the process I will become resentful and unhappy; and these are not sound pre-conditions for good outcomes. It is much better to participate in the decision-making than to have it done for you.

Problems of resistance and general intervention strategies were discussed earlier in the chapter. Of equal significance is the previous discussion of transference and countertransference phenomena, since these may require careful, planned interventions. Sometimes transference and countertransference are so intense that they become a problem for the new graduate nurse.

Gift giving during the working phase

During the working phase, particularly after a person has shown positive growth, they may offer a gift in the form of a craft or skill. As in the orientation phase, the intent of the gift needs to be made explicit. Most ethics and professional conduct boards set overall limits on the monetary value of gifts, and agree that professionals must consider the symbolic meaning of the gift (Nursing and Midwifery Board of Australia, 2008a; 2008b). Encourage this exploration by asking questions such as 'How is it that you are sharing this gift with me?' or 'What feelings might you want to share with this gift?' Be careful to establish and maintain professional boundaries in relation to gifts (Forrester, 2010).

A person might wish to give a gift during the working phase for several reasons. For example, the gift may:

- acknowledge the mutual work that has taken place
- show appreciation for being allowed to share concerns with another person
- act as a smoke-screen to block further exploration of a major dynamic
- outwardly cover up anger or frustration felt inwardly
- indicate the perception that the therapeutic work is finished.

In every instance, assess the intent of the gift, as well as its timing and appropriateness, in the context of the therapeutic relationship. Nursing students and new graduate nurses should always discuss gifts with their clinical facilitator or another senior member of the nursing staff.

Evaluation

Several levels of evaluation occur simultaneously in the working phase. First, do an ongoing evaluation of the person's various levels of intrapersonal and interpersonal functioning. Feedback from family, community agencies or an employer may enhance any current comprehensive evaluation. For example, does the person seem to be facing an impending crisis? If so, you may choose to switch from intrapersonal exploration to a crisis intervention strategy. Second, encourage self-evaluation, as explored in the previous discussion. Finally, constantly reflect on and evaluate your own practice in terms of developing skill and experience. Reflection and self-evaluation is done by informal discussions with staff and other mental health care personnel, and by formal clinical supervision.

On-the-spot evaluations of relevant short-term and long-term goals can occur during any meeting with the person with whom you are working. For example, as the person with whom you are working talks about increasing their socialisation skills, you may reflect: 'Let's look at our contract together. You originally wanted to go out with a woman of your choice for two hours during an evening without having to leave. How do you think this compares with what you're now saying has happened?' Support any effort at self-evaluation, and explore what else needs to happen to achieve the short-term goal. An additional area of evaluation involves 'trying on' alternative behaviours to determine whether these new behaviours may work.

There should be mutual evaluation of the appropriateness of goals in any one of the following areas in light of the person's current functioning:

- degree of success in achieving specific goals
- growth-producing and growth-inhibiting behaviour patterns
- unfinished business that must be resolved to achieve a desired goal

The working phase may also involve ongoing evaluations of the status, characteristics and depth of the therapeutic relationship. You may be viewed in different ways (parent, sibling, friend) at various times. It is only when these views are made explicit that you may intervene to clarify roles and responsibilities in a facilitative manner.

The first two phases of the therapeutic relationship have been worked through when the following occurs:

- a working relationship has been established
- the dynamics of behavioural patterns have been mutually analysed
- behavioural changes consistent with the therapeutic contract have been effectively instituted.

In informal relationship work, you may touch on only one or two aspects of the working phase. Even the advanced psychiatric–mental health nurse rarely addresses all therapeutic tasks in this phase of relationship work.

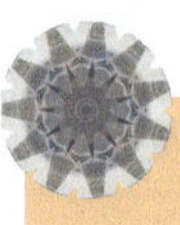

NURSING PROCESS
Termination (end) phase

During the termination or resolution phase of one-to-one relationships, the psychiatric–mental health nurse works towards discontinuing contact. This phase is as important as the previous two phases, although both the nurse and the person frequently avoid it because of past difficulties with separation.

The goal of the end phase is termination of the one-to-one relationship in a mutually planned, satisfying manner. Remind the person that termination was first addressed in the orientation phase, when the duration of the relationship was discussed. Also emphasise the extent of personal growth and the positive aspects of the relationship, rather than focusing exclusively on separation.

A smooth and complete termination sometimes occurs in actual practice. In informal relationship work in inpatient settings, termination more often occurs with an abrupt departure or planned discharge from hospital. Even in formal relationship work in community settings, contact often ceases without explanation after a series of missed appointments, or with a phone call in which the decision to terminate is voiced, or with a person abruptly leaving a session and failing to resume subsequent contact. If this happens, you can call or write and suggest an additional session either to deal with the therapeutic goodbye or to continue the relationship work. Termination requires careful preparation, adequate time for the person to work through the feelings about ending the relationship, and an opportunity for you to explore your personal reactions with a clinical facilitator, mentor, colleague or supervisor.

Assessment

Assessment as a component of the nursing process in the resolution phase deals primarily with determining when the person may be ready to terminate, how they deal with termination, and how the nurse deals with termination. Criteria that indicate readiness for termination are presented in Your Assessment Approach, below.

Many factors influence how a person reacts to termination. These factors include the following:

- *Degree of involvement.* The greater the degree of involvement by the person, the more intense the reaction to termination.
- *Length of treatment.* In general, the longer the therapeutic relationship lasts, the more time should be spent in exploring all aspects of termination.

YOUR ASSESSMENT APPROACH
Termination readiness

The following criteria may be useful to determine whether a person is ready to terminate:

- ***The person has experienced relief from the presenting problem.*** Symptoms no longer interfere with personal comfort, or can be managed more effectively.
- ***The treatment goals have been achieved.*** These ideally are planned goals included in the therapeutic contract.
- ***Social functioning has improved.*** The person experiences increased satisfaction in interpersonal relationships.
- ***Adaptive coping strategies have been acquired.*** Ideally, these strategies include the use of effective problem-solving strategies on a daily basis.
- ***More effective defence mechanisms.*** A person who cannot achieve adaptive coping strategies should develop more effective defence mechanisms to ensure stabilisation.
- ***There is increased self-dependence.*** The person experiences self-satisfaction, and no longer needs to depend on the nurse for a sense of wellbeing.
- ***There has been a major impasse in the one-to-one relationship.*** Stubborn resistances may surface and persist on the part of the person. Uncontrollable countertransference may develop on the nurse's part.

LIVED EXPERIENCE

I have had both good and not-so-good experiences of termination. A good experience was being invited out for cake and coffee by my therapist immediately after our last session together. I was very much touched by that experience; it made me feel like a full person at a time when I had been struggling with severe depression and intense feelings of guilt associated with my psychosis. A not-so-good example was being misdiagnosed with a suggestion that I might contact another service. At the time this felt very much like I was being dumped; the news that I was being discharged from the service was conveyed in a way that made me feel uncared for.

- *Past history of significant losses.* A person who has lost significant others may re-experience past conflicts and emotional responses.
- *Ability to separate from others.* The reaction to termination is influenced by how well the early separation–individuation phase of development has been mastered (see Erikson's eight developmental stages in Chapter 5).
- *Degree of success achieved.* Reaction to termination depends on how successful and satisfying the relationship has been for the person.
- *Degree of transference in the relationship.* The greater the transference in the therapeutic relationship, the more intense the reaction to termination.

Be alert to a range of possible responses during termination. Any number of responses—repression, regression, anger, denial, sadness, withdrawal, avoidance, acceptance, joy—may surface, and it is not unusual for several to surface at once. With repression, there may be no emotional response. Regression is an extremely common response to termination. Regressive behaviour may range from statements of abandonment and hopelessness to an inability to tend to personal hygiene. The central message conveyed is: 'See? I can't make it without you!'

Nurse's self-awareness

Finally, assessment involves how you personally manage separation in the one-to-one relationship. You can also have any number of responses. Some common responses are as follows:

- regret that more was not achieved
- being dependent on, and hesitant to give up, the relationship
- colluding to prolong sessions to avoid the inevitability of separation.

Diagnosis

The focus during termination should be on the termination behaviours that emerge. There are a range of possibilities here, including those that stem from regression, such as deficits in self-care, hopelessness, powerlessness and ineffective coping. It may be necessary to modify earlier formulations as the person moves through the termination experience.

Outcome identification

The ideal outcome occurs when the therapeutic relationship terminates after achieving all of the identified and measurable personal behavioural changes. Such resolution seldom occurs in acute-care inpatient settings, especially since brief hospital stays are now the rule rather than the exception. Often, more limited behavioural changes are achieved, and there is agreement to return for future work or referral as necessary. At other times, only symptom relief is achieved.

Outcomes are compromised when a person is unable to make progress due to lack of insight or mental capacity. Chronic catastrophic life circumstances (such as severe medical illness, life-threatening poverty, prison, and so on) may interfere with growth-producing behaviours. On rare occasions, a person's condition deteriorates and they are unable to benefit from the therapeutic relationship.

Planning and implementation

Planning involves preparing for the final goodbye, and for where and under what circumstances the person may seek future help if the need arises.

Intervening in specific consumer termination behaviours

Intervention strategies vary according to the behaviours that are presented. You may respond to the person who is repressing the reality of termination by repeatedly observing that they are not addressing the issue of the impending separation. You may then attempt to jointly explore this avoidance with the person.

Useful interventions for people who are regressing in response to termination include the following:

- addressing the possible underlying fears of abandonment
- emphasising the growth achieved
- continuing to focus on the realities of separation.

The person who acts out may protest termination in numerous ways before the termination date, such as attempting suicide, requiring psychiatric hospitalisation, quitting a job, or rejecting the nurse.

In general, underlying feelings, fears and fantasies need ventilation, exploration and working through, as do reactions of anger, depression and grief. An exception to this general guideline is the person who uses distraction manoeuvres to prevent termination, such as introducing explosive new material in final sessions. In this situation, you may use limit-setting rather than exploration because of time constraints. In other words, there may be 'unfinished business' despite appropriate planning and effort.

Providing for an explicit and therapeutic goodbye

You have the final task of participating in an *explicit and therapeutic goodbye* with the person. Nursing responsibilities in this final phase include anticipating your own personal

YOUR INTERVENTION STRATEGIES **Goals, tasks and interventions of the termination phase**

Goal: Terminate contact in a mutually planned, satisfying manner

Therapeutic tasks	Nursing interventions
Help the person evaluate the therapeutic contract, and the therapeutic experience in general.	Encourage realistic appraisal of personal therapeutic goals (motivation, effort, progress, outcome) as these evolved in treatment. Provide appropriate feedback regarding the appraisal of goals. Review the person's assets and therapeutic gains. Review areas for further therapeutic work.
Encourage the transference of dependence to other support systems.	Encourage the person to develop reliance on others in their immediate environment (spouse, relative, employer, neighbour, friend) for empathic, emotional support.
Participate in an explicit, therapeutic goodbye with the person.	Be alert to the surfacing of any behaviour arising on termination (repression, regression, acting out, anger, withdrawal, acceptance). Help the person work through any feelings associated with these behaviours. Anticipate your own reaction to separation, and share in a manner that does not burden the person. Allow time and space for termination; the longer the duration of the one-to-one relationship, the more time is needed for the termination phase.

reaction to separation and, optionally, expressing this reaction in a manner that does not burden the person. In addition, you may share a special wish, based on their particular assets within the therapeutic relationship.

A therapeutic goodbye gives a sense of freedom to move on to other relationships. The end phase may take from one meeting to several months of meetings, depending on the duration of the one-to-one relationship. In general, the longer the duration of the relationship, the longer the time needed to deal explicitly with the termination of contact. Your Intervention Strategies, above, summarises the goal, therapeutic tasks and specific interventions of the termination phase.

Ideally, feelings regarding separation can be completely worked through so that there is no unfinished business between the participants in the therapeutic relationship. The therapeutic relationship has given the opportunity to depend on another in a realistic and mature manner. The direct, explicit goodbye is sometimes the first such experience for a person with mental illness. It is usually a moment of unique humanness for both of the people involved.

Gift giving during the termination phase

Gifts are most often given during the termination phase of one-to-one relationships. In this phase, a gift may have several overt and covert meanings. It may:

- be given as a token of appreciation for the positive personal growth that has taken place
- express a desire to change the therapeutic relationship into a social one
- represent a wish to prolong the sessions to avoid the final goodbye.

Some nurses accept a small gift from a person with whom they have been working at the time of termination if feelings regarding the gift have been explored and clarified. (The gift may be an appropriate remembrance of a mutual and positive growth experience.) In so doing, it is important to follow the guidelines set down for the acceptance of small tokens of appreciation in codes of professional conduct (Nursing and Midwifery Board of Australia, 2008a; 2008b). Exploring the significance of a termination gift will ensure the maximum therapeutic benefit for the person offering the gift. A nurse's refusal to accept a gift of any type may hinder the opportunity to learn the important skill of being able to accept gifts from others (Duffin, 2007). The nurse, as role model, has an opportunity to model appropriate gift giving and gift receiving. You may find receiving a gift at times awkward and insincere. Yet such a situation gives the opportunity to facilitate the further development of self-expression and self-knowledge.

Referring for follow-up

When a referral is made to another psychiatric–mental health nurse or therapist, a community nurse, a self-help group, or a non-government organisation, it is often wise to arrange for an initial contact with the referred person or organisation before the therapeutic relationship terminates. This is a way to identify and deal with any initial misconceptions about what will take place after discharge, and to ensure follow-up. The shift to dependence on other support systems (family, friends, health care providers) is a therapeutic task that should be jointly managed, at least initially, by the nurse and other members of the therapeutic team.

Evaluation

Evaluation is a vital component of the nursing process during the termination phase. The task is to work jointly to evaluate the therapeutic contract. The criteria for evaluation are the goals formulated in the orientation and working phases of the one-to-one relationship. Each goal is evaluated in terms of measurable, observable behaviour. Were the goals appropriate, practical and specific to the individual? What are the therapeutic gains? What are the areas for possible further therapeutic work? How does the person evaluate motivation, effort, progress and outcome? Have most feelings about separation from the nurse been worked through?

It will also be important to evaluate the therapeutic experience in general, which may set the stage for future psychotherapeutic work. Would the person seek a similar experience in the future if deemed necessary? Having the opportunity to discuss the work and the outcome can be an empowering exercise for people who use mental health services.

The nurse's own personal, ongoing self-evaluation also warrants emphasis here. It is essential to continuously evaluate which of your own behaviours consciously or unconsciously promote, inhibit or actively block the growth-producing abilities of people seeking your help. For experienced psychiatric–mental health nurses, clinical supervision can be considered for this purpose. For more junior nurses and students, mentorship from more senior and experienced colleagues can be considered.

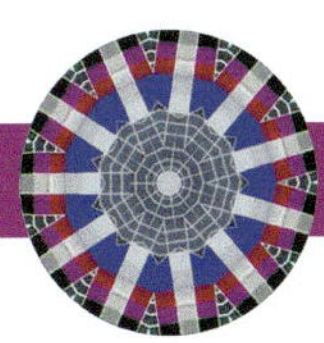

REFERENCES

Balkin, R. S., Leicht, D. J., Sartos, T., & Powell, J. (2011). Assessing the relationship between therapeutic goal attainment and psychosocial characteristics for adolescents in crisis residence. *Journal of Mental Health, 20*(1), 32–42.

Barker, P. (1999). *The philosophy of psychiatric nursing*. Edinburgh, Scotland: Churchill Livingstone.

Beretta, V., Despland, J. N., Drapeau, M., Michel, L., Kramer, U., Stigler, M., & de Roten, Y. (2007). Are relationship patterns with significant others reenacted with the therapist? A study of early transference reactions. *Journal of Nervous and Mental Disease, 195*(5), 443–450.

Christensen, H., & Petrie, K. (2013). State of the e-mental health field in Australia: Where are we now? *Australian and New Zealand Journal of Psychiatry, 47*(2), 117–120.

Duffin, C. (2007). NMC proposal to ban gifts 'could harm staff–patient relationships'. *Nursing Standard, 21*(32), 10.

Ellis, A. (2001). Rational and irrational aspects of countertransference. *Journal of Clinical Psychology, 57*(8), 999–1004.

Fisher, C. B., & Oransky, M. (2008). Informed consent to psychotherapy: Protecting the dignity and respecting the autonomy of patients. *Journal of Clinical Psychology, 64*(5), 576–588.

Forrester, K. (2010). What you see may not be what you get: Beware of patients bearing gifts. *Journal of Law and Medicine, 18*(2), 268–274.

Gary, J. M. (2007). Counseling adult learners: Individual interventions, group interventions, and campus resources. In J. A. Lippincott & R. B. Lippincott (Eds.), *Special populations in college counseling: A handbook for mental health professionals* (pp. 99–113). Alexandria, VA: American Counseling Association.

Gawley, L., Einarson, A., & Bowen, A. (2011). Stigma and attitudes toward antenatal depression and antidepressant use during pregnancy in healthcare students. *Advances in Health Science Education, Theory, and Practice. 16*(5), 669–679.

Gentile, S. (2011). Drug treatment for mood disorders in pregnancy. *Current Opinion in Psychiatry, 24*(1), 34–40.

Guy, J. D., & Brady, J. L. (2001). Identifying the faces in the mirror: Untangling transference and countertransference in self psychology. *Journal of Clinical Psychology, 57*(8), 993–997.

Hazelton, M., & Morrall, P. (2011). Nursing, information technology and the humanization of health care. In A. Cashion & R. Cook (Eds.), *Evidence-based practice in nursing informatics: Concepts and applications* (pp. 135–149). Hershey, PA: Medical Information Science Reference.

Hazelton, M., Rossiter, R., & Sinclair, E. (2010). Lost in transition: Bridging the gap and supporting newly qualified practitioners. In T. Warne and S. McAndrew (Eds.), *Creative approaches to health and social care education* (pp. 213–229). Houndmills, Basingstoke, England: Palgrave MacMillan.

Henretty, J. R., & Levitt, H. M. (2010). The role of therapist self-disclosure in psychotherapy: A qualitative review. *Clinical Psychology Review, 30*(1), 63–77.

Horvath, A. O., Del Re, A. C., Fluckiger, C., & Symonds, D. (2011). Alliance in individual psychotherapy. *Psychotherapy, 48*(1), 9–16.

Hudson, C., St. Cyr-Tribble, D., Bravo, G., & Poitras, M. E. (2011). Enablement in health care context: A concept analysis. *Journal of Evaluation in Clinical Practice, 17*(1), 143–149.

Jain, S., & Roberts, L. W. (2009). Ethics in psychotherapy: A focus on professional boundaries and confidentiality practices. *Psychiatric Clinics of North America, 32*(2), 299–314.

Jorm, A. F., Morgan, A. J., & Malhi, G. S. (2013). The future of e-mental health. *Australian and New Zealand Journal of Psychiatry, 47*(2), 104–106.

McLuhan, M. (1964). *Understanding media: The extensions of man*. New York, NY: McGraw-Hill.

Martin, G., & Pear, J. (2007). *Behavioral modification: What it is and how to do it* (8th ed.). Upper Saddle River, NJ: Pearson Education.

Nursing and Midwifery Board of Australia. (2008a). *Code of professional conduct for midwives in Australia*. Melbourne, Australia: Nursing and Midwifery Board of Australia. Retrieved from wwwnursingmidwiferyboard.gov.au (Accessed 2014, January 24.)

Nursing and Midwifery Board of Australia. (2008b). *Code of professional conduct for nurses in Australia*. Melbourne, Australia: Nursing and Midwifery Board of Australia. Retrieved from wwwnursingmidwiferyboard.gov.au (Accessed 2014, January 24.)

Peplau, H. E. (1952). *Interpersonal relations in nursing*. New York, NY: Putnam.

Peplau, H. E. (1997). Peplau's theory of interpersonal relations. *Nursing Science Quarterly, 10*(4), 162–167.

Petersen, I., Gilbert, R. E., Evans, S. K., Man, S. L., & Nazareth, I. (2011). Pregnancy as a major determinant for discontinuance of antidepressants: An analysis of data from The Health Improvement Network. *Journal of Clinical Psychiatry, 72(7)*, 979–985

Pope, K. S., & Keith-Spiegel, P. (2008). A practical approach to boundaries in psychotherapy: Making decisions, bypassing blunders, and mending fences. *Journal of Clinical Psychology, 64*(5), 638–652.

Priebe, S., Richardson, M., Cooney, M., Adedejo, O., & McCabe, R. (2011). Does the therapeutic relationship predict outcomes of psychiatric treatment in patients with psychosis? A systematic review. *Psychotherapy and Psychosomatics, 80*(2), 70–77.

Psychopathology Committee of the Group for the Advancement of Psychiatry. (2001). Reexamination of therapist self-disclosure. *Psychiatric Services, 52*(11), 1489–1493.

Ryum, T., Stile, T. C., Svartberg, M., & McCullough, L. (2010). The role of transference work, the therapeutic alliance, and their interaction in reducing interpersonal problems among psychotherapy patients with Cluster C personality disorders. *Psychotherapy*, *47*(4), 442–453.

Saurman, E., Perkins, D., Lyle, D., Patfiled, M., & Roberts, R. (2011). Case study: Mental health emergency care rural access project: Assessing rural and remote emergency mental health in Western New South Wales Australia by videoconference technology. In A. Cashion & R. Cook (Eds.), *Evidence-based practice in nursing informatics: Concepts and applications* (pp. 191–203). Hershey, PA: Medical Information Science Reference.

Schaeffer, J. A. (2007). *Transference and countertransference in non-analytic therapy: Double-edged swords*. Lanham, MD: University Press of America.

Schultz, T. (2001). Distance communication. *Soziologie*, *30*(2), 85–102.

Shattell, M., Starr, S., & Thomas, S. (2007). 'Take my hand, help me out': Mental health service recipients' experience of the therapeutic relationship. *International Journal of Mental Health Nursing*, *16*(4), 274–284.

Smith, K. W., & Greenberg, L. S. (2007). Internal multiplicity in emotion-focused psychotherapy. *Journal of Clinical Psychology*, *63*(2), 175–186.

Spiers, J. A., & Wood, A. (2010). Building a therapeutic alliance in brief therapy: The experience of community mental health nurses. *Archives of Psychiatric Nursing*, *24*(6), 373–386.

Steelman, J. R. (2007). Relationship dynamics: Understanding married women's mental health. *Advances in Nursing Science. Women and Aging*, *30*(2), 151–158.

Todres, L., Galvin, K., & Holloway, I. (2009). The humanization of healthcare: A value framework for qualitative research. *International Journal of Qualitative Studies in Health and Well-being*, *4*, 68–77.

Weeks, S., Cowell, R., Scullion, J., & Tanton, E. (2007). Readers panel. Refusing gifts. *Nursing Standard*, *21*(39), 26–27.

Weiss, M. A., & Lewis, L. (2007). Respect for the patient. *American Journal of Nursing*, *107* (Supp.), 12.

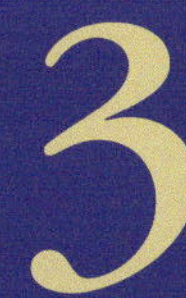

Psychiatric–mental health nurses: who are they and what do they do?

3

KIM RYAN, PETA MARKS AND TIM HEFFERNAN

LEARNING OUTCOMES

After completing this chapter, you will be able to:

1. Apply knowledge of current practice and professional performance standards to the delivery of contemporary psychiatric–mental health nursing.
2. Compare and contrast the differences and similarities among the roles of the psychiatric–mental health nurse and other members of the team.
3. Analyse the factors that influence the success with which the mental health team achieves collaboration among its members, and with people who have mental illness and their support networks.
4. Describe how the role of the psychiatric–mental health nurse has changed over the years from that of custodian to a multi-faceted role.
5. Discuss the nursing theory concepts and principles that have particularly shaped psychiatric–mental health nursing.
6. Explain why you should be capable of functioning in all theories of care.

KEY TERMS

credentialling *52*
credentialled mental health nurse (CMHN) *52*
mental health nurse practitioner (MHNP) *51*
mental health nursing *46*

LIVED EXPERIENCE

For many of us, the onset of a major mental health issue can be devastating. It can seem like the world we once knew is falling away the more we try to hold onto it. It can seem like our identity is stripped away by the illness, the system and the medication. We lose our sense of self and stumble to find our own way forward. The cornerstone of recovery is the time when we begin to regain our identity and move to a place where the illness is just one small part of the whole person. During our vulnerability, when the self is fogged and frightened, we need authentic, therapeutic relationships with those who are entrusted with our care.

Self-awareness is an essential state of being for the mental health nurse. The development and nurturing of the therapeutic relationship is most ideal when people are able to share something of themselves, and to have the strength to empathise with those who might be vulnerable, distressed and confused. It is difficult to walk in the shoes of another person, if you are not first comfortable in your own. A therapeutic relationship is a helping relationship that is based on mutual trust and respect, the nurturing of faith and hope, being sensitive to self and others, and assisting the consumer to fulfil their physical, emotional and spiritual needs. For many of us, the therapeutic relationship is more important than the therapy.

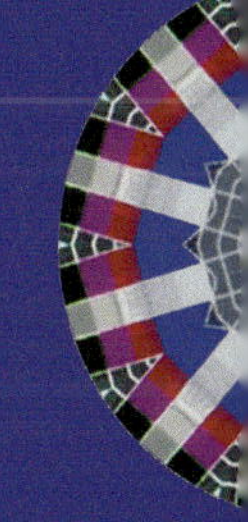

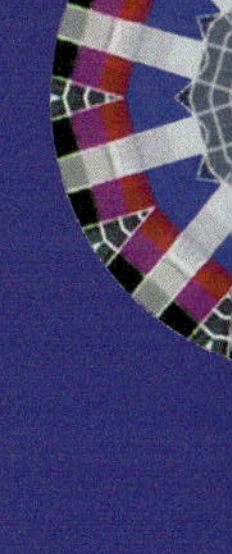

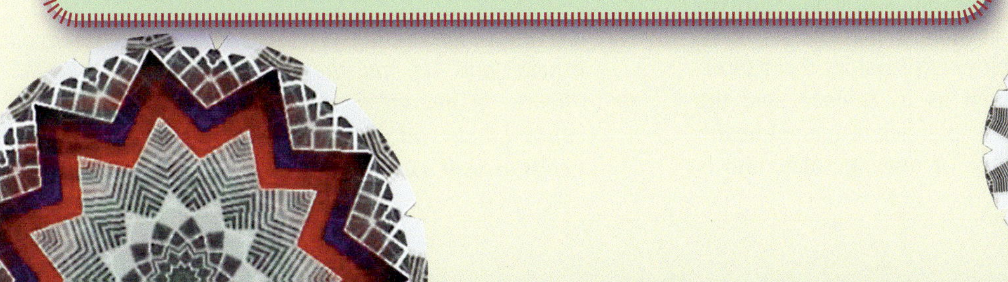

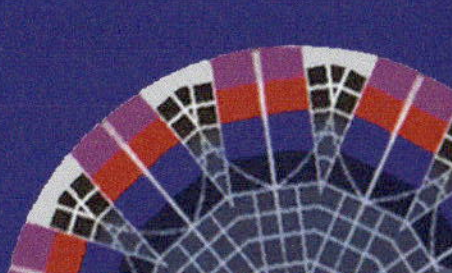

INTRODUCTION

This chapter describes development of the psychiatric–mental health nursing profession, from our early beginnings as attendants, through the numerous ideological and social changes of the 20th century. It describes the way mental health nurses have reacted and adapted in the face of paradigm shifts, sector reform, theoretical and policy developments, right up to contemporary approaches and ways of thinking.

While the chapter grounds us in where we have been and how we have arrived at this point in our history, one thing that it highlights is the enormous capacity that psychiatric–mental health nurses have to adapt to change, and to modify practice to meet the demands of the time. The challenge moving forward is for the profession (both at an individual and a collective level) to take more of a leadership role in setting the agenda, rather than simply responding to the agenda set by others. We have a unique perspective and insights to offer, and we are well positioned to collaborate with consumers and carers, and, of course, with other professions, towards a radical transformation of the way mental health services are provided.

Now, more than ever, psychiatric–mental health nurses are challenged to step up to the opportunities that are available to them—across primary care, private practice, throughout the health care sector and beyond. Envision a future for yourself, identify the type of practitioner you want to be, and how you want to engage and connect with the community around you. Ensure you have solid educational and clinical preparation, then step into that reality. Psychiatric–mental health nursing is a dynamic profession with an ever-expanding scope of practice. Jump on board!

WHAT IS MENTAL HEALTH NURSING?

What does it mean to be a mental health nurse? According to the Australian College of Mental Health Nurses (ACMHN) Standards of Practice for Australian Mental Health Nurses 2010: *'A mental health nurse is a Registered Nurse who holds a recognised specialist qualification in mental health [nursing]. Taking a holistic approach, guided by evidence, the mental health nurse works in collaboration with people who have mental health issues, their family and community, towards recovery as defined by the individual'* (ACMHN, 2010, p. 5).

Mental health nurses make a distinct contribution, in that there is purposeful and time-intensive contact with the person accessing mental health services. Mental health nurses engage with the person's everyday lived experience, and can recognise and understand how that experience is complicit in their health and wellbeing. Mental health nurses negotiate interventions and execute them based on acquired experience, knowledge and evidence (Santangelo, 2015).

Contemporary **mental health nursing** is person-centered and recovery-focused. It provides recovery-oriented and trauma-informed care to people from all cultures, across all age groups and across diverse settings, including primary care, community health, outpatient and inpatient services. Mental health nurses work with people across the health and mental health spectrum—undertaking promotion/prevention, early intervention, collaborative treatment and nursing care. The practice of mental health nursing is nested within a holistic theoretical and clinical framework. It aims to encompass all aspects of the person and the community—including biological, cognitive, cultural, educational, emotional, environmental, functional, mental, occupational, physical, psychological, relational, sexual, social and spiritual elements. This specialised area of nursing practice is a core mental health discipline that employs explanatory theories of, and research on, human behaviour as its science, and the purposeful use of self as its art. The practice of mental health nursing encompasses a wide range of nursing roles, and is characterised by engagement and relationship-building, partnership and collaboration, and personal and professional reflection (ACMHN, 2013).

The Australian College of Mental Health Nurses identifies the Standards of Practice for Australian Mental Health Nurses (2013), which will be discussed later in this chapter. First, though, because the purposeful use of 'self' is at the heart of mental health nursing practice and, because mental health nursing requires practitioners to achieve a level of competence not only in professional knowledge, skills and behaviours, but also in a personal context, it is important to consider the *personal* qualities and experiences which shape the work of mental health nurses.

The capacity for reflective practice is vital—particularly around one's own values, attitudes and beliefs, and how these impact on the relationships we develop with the people we work with and their families. Our own personal awareness and insights, our culture, our background life experiences and interests all combine with our professional and practice development experiences to enhance our expertise. Our own personal nursing philosophy, and the theories and strategies we use in our practice, are important in shaping our work.

Contemporary mental health nursing care has strong theoretical foundations. It is evidence-based and evidence-informed, and is underpinned by values which ensure that care and treatment is therapeutic. While some core values are not unique to mental health nursing, they underpin the learning outcomes and the principles of learning and teaching required for mental health nursing. This distinct way of relating and interrelating with consumers distinguishes mental health nurses in their practice, and contributes to the development of a conceptual framework for practice (ACMHN, 2016):

1. *The nature of nursing is influenced by its 'service to others' and its 'on the ground' interaction with clients. In mental health this facilitates a client-centred focus that is intimately in tune with their life needs as well as health needs (Bulletins 9 & 10);*

2. *Mental health nursing practice is determined by the nature of the nursing world view and delivers broad, flexible, time intensive care that goes beyond health and professional paradigms to individual commitment to client generated care (Bulletins 11 & 12);*
3. *Outcomes of mental health nursing care are facilitated by acknowledging and responding to client needs that is generated by a special collaboration with clients and others and result in mutual benefits (Bulletins 13 & 14);*
4. *The distinctive contribution by mental health nursing is characterised by care that is collaborative, co-constructed with the client and as a consequence, committed to a recovery approach that results from the special way in which nurses view, relate and respond to individual client needs (Bulletins 15 & 16).*

(Santangelo, 2015; Bulletins 13–17 in ACMHN, 2016)

EMERGENCE OF THE DISCIPLINE

Although nursing functions have existed since ancient times, the profession of nursing, particularly mental health nursing, is a product of the late 19th and 20th centuries. Awareness of the history can provide a basis for focusing on the developments that have shaped the knowledge and practice of mental health nursing as a specialty and profession.

Like the history of mental health care more broadly, the mental health nursing history in Australia is for the most part inglorious (ACMHN, 1999, p. 1). It is also relatively difficult to research; there is a lack of documentation (original texts, narratives, case notes) that describes the historical development of the profession (Sands, 2009), and mental health nursing and education is often completely overlooked in general nursing history texts (Henderson & Martyr, 2013).

Prior to the establishment of asylums, people with mental illness were incarcerated in gaols, under harsh and difficult conditions, and were supervised by 'keepers' and 'wardens' (Sands, 2009). In Western Australia, convicts provided 'care' to people with mental illness until 1903, when they were replaced by 'attendants'. Perhaps as a result of this early history, the 'attendants' who worked in asylums were more gaoler than nurse—the role was custodial, mechanistic and always directed by psychiatrists. Attendants were mostly males, selected for their strength and fighting ability rather than their interpersonal skills (ACMHN, 1999). The focus was on the physical needs of the person and on the physical environment of the institution; however, coercion and punishment by attendants was commonplace, and being an attendant was a poorly paid and undesirable job (Sands, 2009).

The first large-scale state-run 'mental asylum' in Australia was built at Castle Hill, NSW, in 1811. Asylums were often grand edifices that corralled not only those who were considered 'mentally unstable', but people branded as 'idiots', 'imbeciles' or 'mentally retarded' (e.g. those with acquired brain injury or who had epilepsy), paupers, 'derelicts' and itinerant workers who had nowhere else to go. They also included wards of the state, women with neurotic disorders, and people with 'diseases' that are no longer recognised as mental illnesses. On the whole, people with mental illness were considered to be 'hopelessly incurable', and lifelong internment was considered likely.

In developing psychiatry and psychiatric care, Australia followed Great Britain and America, and tended to reflect the views of medical superintendents who migrated to the colonies to oversee asylums (Happell, 2007). Around 1800 in Great Britain, literature on the occupation of the 'keeper' appeared, which noted the occupation as an essential service and advocated for a register to be established (Spearitt, 1980). This was also the time of the emergence of the 'moral treatment' movement, which considered that mental illness could best be managed with humanity and kindness, and through useful work (Sands, 2009). This was underpinned by the view that mental illness *may* be treatable and had a psychological dimension, and signalled the idea of upgrading care. The term 'psychotherapy' appeared, and 'nurse', 'attendant' and 'superintendent' were used interchangeably. Legislation was introduced to provide for people with mental illness and confirm the role of the institution, while psychiatry was becoming more respectable, and control of the care and who delivered the care was in the hands of the medical practitioners (Nolan, 1993).

WHY I CHOSE TO WORK IN MENTAL HEALTH

Kim Ryan

I first began my nursing career as a general registered nurse, and then under took psychiatric nurse training. Back then it wasn't uncommon for nurses to hold double or triple certificates—in general, midwifery and psychiatry.

During my general nurse training, I didn't really learn about mental health—as a result, when I first started psychiatric nursing I had little understanding of mental illness or the way in which people exhibited mental illness. What I discovered was that it's not that easy to divide a person into 'the mind' or 'the body'—so much that happens in the mind affects the body and vice versa.

Deinstitutionalisation had also just started: the big psychiatric hospitals were being opened up, and people who had lived in institutions, in some cases for many years, were being transferred back into the community. I quickly realised that most of society didn't understand mental illness. I was humbled by the very difficult lives that many of the people I encountered had experienced. They were misunderstood, they were stigmatised, they were removed from their family, and the medications they were taking could have debilitating side-effects. However, they were (and still are) some of the most resilient people I have ever had the privilege to meet. I guess that is why I stayed in mental health, rather than moving on to another nursing specialty.

Mental health nursing is a wonderful career, you meet some great characters, you laugh and you cry, but, best of all, you can make a difference to people's lives.

Are there any aspects of Kim' story that you relate to? What is important to you about the work that you do? When you are at the other end of your nursing career and you look back, what would you like to have achieved, what would you like to have stood for?

Attempts to improve the calibre of attendants in Australia began from the mid-1850s. Policy documents, such as the Victorian Lunacy Department's Regulations, described the duties of asylum employees; lectures on nursing were established for attendants; trained general nurses were appointed; and examinations for attendants were conducted towards the end of the 1800s (Sands, 2009; Finnane, 2008). There were also a number of investigations and Royal Commissions conducted across the colonies, revealing poor management and practice within institutions, which didn't improve despite recommended reforms (Schultz, 1991).

In the early part of the 20th century, hospital-based training programs, which led to a Certificate of Mental Nursing/Psychiatric Nursing, were established. However, jurisdictional differences were significant (e.g. 1912 in Queensland, 1917 in Western Australia, 1935 in Tasmania, and not until the late 1950s in Victoria), and there was little consistency in training between hospitals (Henderson & Martyr, 2013; Finnane, 2008; ACMHN, 1999). Over this period, policy developments and changes in terminology (e.g. 'hospitals for the insane' became known as 'mental hospitals'; 'lunatics' as 'mental patients'; 'lunatic attendants' as 'mental nurses') reflect conceptual changes, and represent a significant step in the professional development of mental health nursing (Happell, 2007).

Although psychiatric nurse training was determined by each hospital, generally, the course was three years long; the theoretical component was provided by doctors. A *handbook for the instruction of attendants of the insane* was commissioned in 1894 in England, to assist attendants in understanding the work that they were to undertake (Nolan, 1993; Henderson & Martyr, 2013). This became the basis for studies in parts of the new Australian federation, and it was transformed in the 1920s into the *Handbook for mental nurses*, commonly known as the 'Red Book'. Shorter, 18-month programs were developed for general trained nurses wanting to do a psychiatric nursing certificate.

During the period of educational preparation, students were also employees of the hospital, and undertook training across a range of clinical settings. Hospital-based training, following the Nightingale system, was seen to improve the quality of nursing services more broadly, and so remained substantially unchanged in Australia for some 100 years. However, it also provided a cheap, heavily-disciplined hospital workforce, where the needs of the hospital took precedence over the education of nurses, and the theoretical component of the course was seen to be less important than the clinical component. Learning by doing, and by trial and error, were a feature of nursing courses of the day (Russell, 1990).

Mental health nursing in the 1900s

The development of the mental health nursing profession is also subject to the reforms and underpinning principles in mental health care, and new technologies for better treatment of people with mental illness. The opening decades of the 19th century brought new ideas for 'cure', such as those based on Pinel's 'moral treatment' and the establishment of the asylums.

Despite the increase in training, the psychiatric nurse role was still largely custodial and focused on the physical. Between the World Wars, people with mental illness were exposed to somatic treatments, such as inducing fever with malaria for psychosis, insulin therapy for schizophrenia, lobotomy, cardiac stimulation and electroconvulsive therapy (ECT) (Sands, 2009; Maude, 2001).

Nurses were involved with procedures, including the application of cold dressings and poultices, fomentations and enemas, administering early medications (such as chloral hydrate and paraldehyde), supervising the use of 'therapies' (such as hydrotherapy, psychosurgery, ECT), monitoring those in isolation rooms and using various forms of restraint, and overseeing the nutrition and physical care of patients (Boling, 2003). Commonly, nurses also undertook or oversaw the housekeeping tasks, general maintenance and operation of the facility, although these roles were curtailed as the 'nursing' functions of the role became more pronounced (Finnane, 2008).

The 1940s and 1950s

From the 1940s, psychiatric theory expanded to encompass the interpersonal and emotional dimensions of mental illness. Sigmund Freud published his works on psychoanalysis, Adolph Meyer's *commonsense psychiatry* had a great impact in the United States and Great Britain, and Harry Stack Sullivan introduced the concept of *milieu therapy* as a new approach to treating people in psychiatric hospitals. While the role of the psychiatric nurse was slowly evolving, these ideological changes in psychiatry, and the changes that were occurring across nursing more broadly (e.g. the 1943 Kelly Report, which made recommendations around the professional development of nursing and nurse education), did not have a noticeable influence on psychiatric nursing care or education at that time. Until the early 1950s, psychiatric nurses formulated only vague concepts about how nurses might participate in one-to-one relationships with the people in their care.

Ambiguity about professional psychiatric nursing roles characterised this period. Most psychiatric patients were still cared for in large state mental hospitals, where relatively small numbers of staff were expected to manage large numbers living in crowded conditions. Somatic treatments were more practical in these settings than talk therapies (or psychotherapy), which were often reserved for the private clients of psychiatrists.

The 1950s and 1960s

The post-war 1950s and 1960s were a period of immense change in mental health (and in nursing), in Australia and overseas. Philosophical debates around mental health and mental illness informed policy objectives and changed the focus of service delivery and organisation. For example, the idea of the 'assimilation' of previously separated groups back into society gained prominence. That, coupled with the chronic overcrowding of mental hospitals, resulted in mental health service design focusing on community-based rather than institutionally-based services. At the same time, there was concern around attempting to increase community understanding of psychiatric concepts—what we now call 'mental health literacy' (Robson, 2008; Hickie et al., 2014). The World Federation of Mental Health was established in 1948 by the World Health Organization, and its focus was on mental 'health', rather than on mental 'illness'. This broader public health perspective, and the idea of *prevention* of mental health problems, were reflected in Australian health policy of that period.

Significantly, a range of inquiries into psychiatric hospitals were also conducted in Australia over the 1950s and 1960s, and these identified appalling conditions and brutality. Overcrowding and understaffing remained key issues impacting on both patients and nurses, with some nurses becoming disillusioned by the archaic nature of psychiatric hospitals, and others using understaffing as an excuse for inaction (Nolan & Hopper, 2000). Not surprisingly, the 'anti-psychiatry' movement also emerged during this period.

From a biological and treatment perspective, the 1950s saw new psychopharmacological agents being developed, the safer application of ECT, the use of group therapy and other psychotherapies, the provision of day treatment, and the development of rehabilitation services (Austin & Boyd, 2010), all of which had an impact on the nurse's role. An influx of post-war immigrants joined the mental health workforce, which went some way towards redressing the chronically understaffed wards and, as such, the working conditions for psychiatric nurses improved marginally.

Interestingly, some consider that the 1960s was a period of professional disintegration rather than growth, because, while the structure of the institutions offered security to nurses, who had a strong sense of safety and their place within them, within this context nurses didn't need to define their role, or identify underpinning values or knowledge bases; nor could they grow and evolve their sense of professional identity, because there was no room for independent thinking (Nolan & Hopper, 2000).

Overseas impacts on psychiatric nursing in the 1950s and 1960s included the work of three key figures: Hildegard Peplau, Gwen Tudor and Frances Sleeper.

Hildegard Peplau Hildegard Peplau's *Interpersonal relations in nursing* was published in 1952. It was the first systematic theoretical framework in psychiatric nursing, and a milestone in the development of psychiatric nursing theory and practice. Peplau identified skills, activities and roles for psychiatric nurses, and emphasised the interpersonal nature of nursing, and the need for nurses to understand and use psychodynamic concepts and counselling techniques in their practice. Under Peplau's leadership, the first graduate degree in psychiatric–mental health nursing was awarded by Rutgers University in the United States in 1954. Peplau's theoretical contributions are discussed in greater detail later in this chapter.

Gwen Tudor When Gwen Tudor published an article in the journal *Psychiatry* in 1952, this was a major feat, because this journal for psychiatrists had never before published an article by a nurse (and no psychiatric nursing journals existed at the time). Tudor used socio-psychiatric theory to explain a mutual pattern of avoidance that emerged among the nursing staff, physicians and one particular female client (Tudor, 1952), and designed and tested a nursing intervention to disrupt the pattern of avoidance. Tudor's unique contribution demonstrated that:

- psychiatric nurses can have a profoundly positive or a profoundly negative effect on the person they are caring for
- the social milieu of the psychiatric ward can maintain deviant patterns of behaviour
- the psychotherapeutic nursing role can be taught to others
- nurses can carry out scholarly research.

Hers is the classic scholarly psychiatric nursing research study, significant for its dramatic impact on nursing and its contribution to an understanding of the effects of the milieu.

Frances Sleeper Finally, Frances Sleeper, in an address to the American Psychiatric Association, advocated the use of psychiatric nurses as psychotherapists. Her advocacy ushered in a heated, 10-year controversy over 'caretaker versus psychotherapist' roles for psychiatric nurses in the United States, a discussion that would be replicated in Australia.

The 1970s and 1980s

In the 1970s and 1980s, the process of 'deinstitutionalisation' began in earnest. Therapeutic environments were created, community care increased, and mental health nurses were established in the community. The introduction of mainstreaming mental health services within the broader health care system also began, and the consumer-driven Recovery movement was born (NSW Consumer Advisory Group—Mental Health & Mental Health Coordinating Council, 2009). In Australia, these changes had implications for the future education and practice of mental health nurses, and it was during this milieu of change that a national organisation of Australian mental health nurses appeared. The First National Mental Health Nurses Congress was held in 1975, and in 1977 the Australian Congress of Mental Health Nurses was formalised into a non-industrial, non-sectarian and non-politically-aligned organisation.

The 1990s

By 1991, the Australian Congress of Mental Health Nurses had established itself as a college, and in 1994 New Zealand mental health nurses were invited to join the college as a branch. The Australian and New Zealand College of Mental Health Nursing (ANZCMHN) operated until in late 2004 New Zealand formed its own college, Te Ao Māramatanga/New Zealand College of Mental Health Nurses, and the college's name reverted to the Australian College of Mental Health Nurses (ACMHN). The first Standards of Practice for Mental Health Nurses in Australia were published by the college in 1983 and revised in 1995. Those important documents, which were used to help define and guide the practice of mental health nursing in the various settings it is practised, provided a beacon for the profession's aspirations, goals and objectives, until the Standards were again revised in 2010 after a research, consultation and review process lasting two and a half years. (See the Standards, outlined below.)

During the 1990s, psychiatry underwent a paradigm shift to include the neurobiological domains. Research studies that focused on psychobiology provided new biological strategies for assessments and interventions. Mental health nursing leaders urged the inclusion of biological therapies along with the use of more traditional psychotherapy, psychosocial therapies and combination therapies—and for mental health nurses to become fundamentally re-associated with care and caring (McBride, 1990). Peplau (1989) made additional recommendations to:

- promote political savvy in advocating psychiatric–mental health care resources
- continue developing out-of-hospital services, including those offered on a private practice basis
- pursue evaluation and outcome clinical studies
- inform the public and others of the work that mental health nurses do
- keep emphasising the human aspects of mental health work, even as psychiatry moves in the direction of psychobiological practice.

Despite all of the advances, an Australian Human Rights and Equal Opportunity Commission inquiry into the human rights of people with a mental illness (producing the Burdekin Report [Burdekin, 1993]) found: widespread, systematic discrimination against people with mental illness; the consistent denial of rights and services to which people were entitled; a lack of crisis teams to help with emergency situations; oversight of, or actual abuse of, human rights in inpatient services; and the observation that the money saved by deinstitutionalisation of mental health services had not followed people into the community.

The resulting National Mental Health Strategy, along with ongoing five-year plans to improve consistent delivery of mental health services nationally, the routine use of consumer- and clinician-rated outcome measures and, more recently, the shift in focus to primary mental health care, have contributed to the widening of the context in which mental health nurses practise, the development of mental health nursing roles, and the expansion of knowledge and skills.

The new millennium

The new millennium has seen the knowledge explosion in psychobiology continuing, characterised by a broader understanding of the biology of the mind, and the biological foundations of behaviour and temperament. Significant knowledge about the genetic basis of inherited mental disorders has resulted from genetic research, and our understanding of neuroplasticity and neurogenesis—the capacity of the brain to adapt to major changes and challenges by remodelling and refining its existing connections—is rapidly expanding. The brain, once considered to be a fixed and stable organ, is now viewed as dynamic, flexible and adaptive (Kays, Hurley & Taber, 2012).

This expanding knowledge has informed contemporary mental health nursing practice in a variety of ways. For example, a trauma-informed approach, which recognises the impact of trauma on the developing brain, requires a fundamental shift in philosophy, culture and practice. It promotes the understanding that recovery is not possible until a person is physically and emotionally safe from violence and abuse, and that therapeutic services need to be well-integrated to reflect the centrality of trauma in the person's life and lived experience (Bateman & Henderson, 2013).

Other transformative processes, early in this new millennium, have sparked significant changes in the delivery of mental health services and the practice of mental health nursing:

- The inclusion of and collaboration with service users and carers in the planning, development, delivery and evaluation of mental health services across the sector, including:
  - a recovery orientation being adopted as an overarching philosophy to guide mental health practice, and embedded into policy and standards nationally
  - a focus on reducing restrictive practices with the aim of ending seclusion and restraint practices within mental health services
  - the emergence of the consumer- and carer-identified workforce and their involvement in the education of mental health professionals.
  - Concern with the significant physical health problems of people with mental illness and their reduced life expectancy. In particular, the relationship between mental illness and modifiable risk factors (e.g. smoking, obesity, poor nutrition culminating in metabolic syndrome), as well as high levels of diabetes, cardiovascular, respiratory disease and cancer, which account for 80 per cent of deaths of people with mental illness (http://www.bmj.com/press-releases/2013/05/21/life-expectancy-gap-widens-between-those-mental-illness-and-general-popula).
  - It is widely recognised that working with people with co-existing disorders is core business of both drug and alcohol and mental health services, and this should be the expectation rather than the exception (National Mental Health Commission, 2013, the 'Report Card'). A 'no wrong door' approach underpins Australian health policy for services supporting those with co-existing problems.
  - The shift to primary care as a point of entry for mental health care (Jackson, Passamonti & Kroenke, 2007; Kroenke, Spitzer, Williams, Monahan & Lowe, 2007) and the emergence of effective primary care models, such as the Mental Health Nurse Incentive Program (MHNIP), where credentialled mental health nurses are engaged in primary care, working in collaboration with GPs or psychiatrists, to provide mental health nursing care to people with complex and enduring mental illness.
  - The emergence of psychological therapies aimed at working with people whose symptoms were

previously considered untreatable; for example, 'open dialogue' or using the Maastricht Approach (see: http://www.dirkcorstens.com/maastrichtapproach/) for accepting and working with voices and dialogical behavioural therapy (DBT) for people who struggle with overwhelming emotions and deliberately self-harm; and of therapies that can be used across the mental health, wellbeing and illness spectrum; for example, mindfulness practices.

- The introduction of **mental health nurse practitioner** roles within Australian health care services to complement and improve access to services and health care outcomes for consumers. MHNPs have progressed and acquired both an advanced level of formal education and considerable experience and expertise within a particular clinical specialty or setting; they are clinical experts making complex decisions about what care is required. Authorisation as a nurse practitioner in Australia enables nurses to prescribe and administer certain medications germane to their specialty area, based on an agreed formulary, and to initiate focused diagnostic investigations, such as pathology tests and medical imaging. Authorisation also formalises the right to refer to specialists (Wand & White, 2007).

THE EDUCATION OF MENTAL HEALTH NURSES

In the 1960s, issues such as recruitment and retention, and high attrition rates of nurses, were becoming problematic. An enrolled nursing tier of nurses was established as one of the solutions. While there was a lot of disagreement as to how the problems of nursing should be addressed, there was considerable agreement that change was essential and that nursing education should be a target of change. Discussions among nursing leaders addressed the venue for nurse education, the service priorities of the apprenticeship system, the entry standard and what should be taught in the nursing curricula. A range of alternatives were piloted (e.g. pre-registration nursing programs within Colleges of Advanced Education, combined nursing/arts/science degrees) (Russell, 2005). The NSW College of Nursing and the College of Nursing Australia (Vic) were established, and began devising and delivering postgraduate nursing courses.

Internationally, nursing leaders had already begun to question the wisdom of single-focus schools of psychiatric nursing. In the United States, a 1948 report entitled *Nursing for the future* (Brown, 1948) recommended their elimination. The needs of nursing could best be served, the report indicated, if the psychiatric hospitals conducting schools of nursing made their facilities widely available to students in basic schools of nursing. Shortly thereafter, in 1955, the provision of a clinical experience in psychiatric nursing was made a requirement for the accreditation of nursing schools. Requiring both coursework and hands-on clinical experience further cemented the mainstreaming of psychiatric nursing in the United States.

In Australia, it wasn't until 1974 that the first tertiary-based nursing program was established in Victoria, but these graduates could only register as general nurses and couldn't work in mental health.

In 1983, the NSW government announced the transfer of all basic nursing education into the higher-education sector by 1985: at a comprehensive undergraduate level, preparing nurses for practices in all major areas—general medical/surgical, psychiatric and developmental disability nursing (Russell, 2005). In 1984, the Australian government announced in-principle support for the complete transfer of nursing education into the tertiary sector—again, at comprehensive level. The last intakes into general hospital-based programs were to happen in 1990, with the full transfer to be completed by 1993. In 1992, the decision was made that comprehensive undergraduate pre-registration programs for nurses Australia-wide would be in the form of a Bachelor of Nursing (Russell, 2005).

In the decade after the transition to 'comprehensive' nurse education, a number of Australian studies (Clinton, 1997, 2001; Clinton & Hazelton, 2000) identified that Australian universities had not been successful in preparing undergraduate students for the role of beginning practitioner in mental health nursing. Issues around the quality and quantity of the mental health content, and the access to and quality of mental health clinical placements, were highlighted as deficient. These deficiencies were reiterated by a 2002 National Review of Nursing Education (Commonwealth of Australia), a 2002 Senate Inquiry Report (Senate Community Affairs References Committee), and again in the 2008 report by the Mental Health Nurse Education Taskforce (MHNET; MHNET, 2008)—a subcommittee of the Australian Health Ministers' Advisory Council's (AHMAC) Mental Health Workforce Advisory Committee (MHWAC). The MHNET proposed a framework for mental health in preregistration nursing, and provided technical advice and recommendations on the development of national policy and strategic directions for mental health nurse education (MHNET, 2008).

The establishment of postgraduate mental health nursing education following the transfer of nurse education to the higher-education sector was slow to start. Psychiatric nurse education began the transition to the tertiary sector in 1989 in Victoria, where mental health-focused Diploma then Bachelor programs were provided until 1993, when these direct-entry programs ceased in favour of comprehensive undergraduate programs. Elsewhere, direct-entry and post-basic programs continued to be provided in psychiatric hospital settings until October 1991, when Queensland's Wolston Park Hospital commenced the last hospital-based direct-entry three-year pre-registration mental health nursing program in Australia.

A review of postgraduate mental health nursing programs in the late 1990s identified a limited number of courses and students; then, a 2011 scan of postgraduate mental health nursing programs conducted by the ACMHN identified a range of problems, including a very limited focus on profession-based standards of practice, inconsistent interpretation of the words 'specialist' and 'advanced' in relation to mental health nursing practice, and inconsistencies in relation to the amount, level and appropriateness of content across various programs. In response, the ACMHN has recently completed the development of a National Framework for Postgraduate

Mental Health Nursing Education in Australia (ACMHN, 2016), which will provide a benchmark for the education of mental health nurses into the future.

TRANSITION TO A NATIONAL REGISTER AND CREDENTIALLING FOR MENTAL HEALTH NURSES

Until a National Registration and Accreditation Scheme (2011–2014) was devised by the Australian Health Practitioner Regulation Agency (APHRA), states and territories passed their own nursing registration Acts. Psychiatric nursing registration was recorded on a separate register to general nursing, and was established in different jurisdictions at different times (e.g. 1926 in Tasmania, 1944 in Western Australia, and 1952 in Victoria) (ACMHN, 1999).

As mental health nursing courses were phased out in the 1990s, and in response to the changes that had occurred to nursing education and regulation policy in Australia, the Australian College of Mental Health Nurses proactively increased its self-governance role, developed practice standards and undertook to develop a mental health nurse credentialling program—the Credential for Practice Program (CPP).

Currently in Australia, there are three categories of nurse authorised under law to practice nursing: enrolled nurses, registered nurses and nurse practitioners—'mental health nurse' and 'psychiatric nurse' are not protected titles under the national law. During transition to the national register, any identification as a mental health nurse by title or endorsement through statutory regulation was ceased. Mental health nurses were registered nurses, and some mental health nurses were endorsed as nurse practitioners.

Credentialling is a core component of clinical/professional governance or self-regulation where members of a profession set standards for practice and establish a minimum requirement for entry, continuing professional development, endorsement and recognition. The ACMHN CPP recognises the skills, expertise and experience of nurses who are practising as specialist mental health nurses, and is the only nationally consistent recognition for specialist mental health nurses in Australia. A valid and reliable credential program confirms to consumers, employers and regulators that a nurse has been prepared to a level that will enable the delivery of contemporary mental health nursing care.

In 2005, credentialling by the ACMHN was identified as the standard for mental health nurses to participate in certain Commonwealth Government-funded primary care programs provided for people with mental illness. Credentialled mental health nurses met eligibility criteria for allied health professionals providing Medicare services as 'mental health workers'. Being a **credentialled mental health nurse™** is also a requirement for nurses working under the Mental Health Nurse Incentive Program (MHNIP), which was implemented by the Australian government in 2007. By the end of 2010, nurses practising in other mental health settings started to enquire about credentialling, particularly when specialist endorsements or specialist registration of mental health nurses under statutory regulation ceased. Implementation of the ACMHN CPP has progressed over the past 10 years, with some minor, but no major, modifications to the program, and since its inception over 3000 mental health nurses have received a Credential in Mental Health Nursing.

STANDARDS OF PRACTICE FOR AUSTRALIAN MENTAL HEALTH NURSES

Standards of Practice provide practical benchmarks to guide and measure how care is provided. They are concerned with the performance of mental health nurses across a range of clinical environments, and include professional knowledge, skills and attitudes (attributes).

The ACMHN Standards of Practice for Australian Mental Health Nurses 2010 specify the minimum level of performance required for a registered nurse practising in any mental health setting. The ACMHN Standards of Practice are underpinned by the following core values:

- working in partnership with the individual affected by mental health issues and significant others, such as family, carers, support agencies and other health care providers
- acknowledging the personal experience and expertise of the individual, supporting their potential for recovery and assisting them to achieve optimal quality of life
- recognising the human rights of people affected by mental health issues, as proclaimed by the United Nations Principle on the Protection of People with a Mental Illness and the Australian Health Ministers' Mental Health Statement of Rights and Responsibilities, utilising an evidence base for practice and quality improvement processes, to provide the highest attainable standard of care
- enabling cultural safety, taking into account the age, gender, spirituality, ethnicity and health values of the people affected by mental health issues.

Standard 1

The mental health nurse acknowledges diversity in culture, values and belief systems and ensures his/her practice is non-discriminatory, and promotes dignity and self-determination.

Rationale

Recognising the cultural context in which mental health issues occur is critical to providing culturally competent services. Understanding cultural diversity is essential to working therapeutically with people whose experiences differ from those of the nurse.

Practice outcomes

This standard is being met when:

1. people with mental health issues report that they feel respected and safe in terms of their cultural background
2. cultural considerations affecting assessment and intervention processes are documented and acted upon
3. culturally appropriate support agencies have been accessed where appropriate.

Standard 2

The mental health nurse establishes collaborative partnerships that facilitate and support people with mental health issues to participate in all aspects of their care.

Rationale

Understanding the value of partnership(s) in promoting optimum practice outcomes is essential in the context of a holistic care framework.

Practice outcomes

This standard is being met when:

1. people with mental health issues confirm they have been involved in key aspects of their care and express satisfaction with the process and outcomes of the partnership
2. the health care/treatment plan identifies the outcomes of collaborative assessment and consultation
3. collaborative partnerships with consumers, families, community, government and non-government organisations are established across all aspects of the person's care and recovery.

Standard 3

The mental health nurse develops a therapeutic relationship that is respectful of the individual's choices, experiences and circumstances. This involves building on strengths, holding hope and enhancing resilience to promote recovery.

Rationale

The recovery journey is a subjective experience, defined by the individual.

Practice outcomes

This standard is being met when:

1. people with mental health issues confirm that their skills and experience have been valued and utilised, and that they feel supported in their individual recovery journey
2. the mental health nurse interprets and contributes to the health care/treatment plan with respect to the principles of recovery.

Standard 4

The mental health nurse collaboratively plans and provides ethically based care consistent with the mental, physical, spiritual, emotional, social and cultural needs of the individual.

Rationale

This standard recognises the mental, physical, spiritual, emotional, social and cultural needs of people affected by mental health issues, and supports best-practice outcomes.

Practice outcomes

This standard is being met when:

1. people with mental health issues identify that their mental, physical, spiritual, emotional, social and cultural needs have been consistently considered
2. where ethical dilemmas exist, the mental health nurse uses ethical practice principles to ensure the consumer's mental, physical, spiritual, emotional, social and cultural needs are best met
3. where they exist, breaches in ethical practice are appropriately documented and investigated.

Standard 5

The mental health nurse values the contributions of other agencies and stakeholders in the collaborative provision of holistic, evidence-based care and in ensuring comprehensive service provision for people with mental health issues.

Rationale

Promoting and facilitating the contribution of others promotes the best practice outcome for people affected by mental health issues.

Practice outcomes

This standard is being met when:

1. people with mental health issues identify that the mental health nurse utilised the skills and knowledge of other individuals, organisations and groups wherever necessary
2. the contributions of other agencies and stakeholders are valued and identified in documentation.

Standard 6

The mental health nurse actively pursues opportunities to reduce stigma and promotes social inclusion and community participation for all people with mental health issues.

Rationale

The recognition of, and taking action to address, the stigma that surrounds and influences the lives of people affected by mental health issues is an important contributor to improving practice outcomes.

Practice outcomes

This standard is being met when:

1. people identify that they experience an improved sense of community integration and reduced experiences involving stigma
2. the mental health nurse demonstrates active participation in health-promoting, stigma-reducing activities
3. the mental health nurse engages in opportunities to review and/or develop strategies and policies that promote community integration and reduce stigma.

Standard 7

The mental health nurse demonstrates evidence-based practice and actively promotes practice innovation through lifelong education, research, professional development, clinical supervision and reflective practice.

Rationale

Understanding the value of and utilising evidence-based practice is essential to promote best-practice outcomes for persons affected by mental health issues. Ongoing professional development, education, clinical supervision and reflection provide the basis for the consistent evolution of practice required to enhance recovery for people with mental health issues.

Practice outcomes

This standard is being met when the mental health nurse:

1. consistently engages in activities to use and develop an evidence base for practice, and utilises practice innovation where evidence is lacking or a novel approach is required
2. demonstrates regular engagement in activities of research, education and professional development, clinical supervision and reflective practice
3. engages in activities which support others in activities of research, education and professional development, clinical supervision and reflective practice.

Standard 8

The mental health nurse's practice incorporates and reflects common law requirements, relevant statutes and the nursing profession's code of conduct and ethics. The mental health nurse integrates international, national, local and state policies and guidelines with professional Standards and competencies.

Rationale

Legal requirements and professional codes of practice are incorporated into clinical practice to safeguard the rights of people with mental health issues.

Practice outcomes

This standard is being met when:

1. people affected by mental health issues and/or relevant others identify that the mental health nurse's practice is consistent with common law requirements, relevant statutes, policies, standards, competencies, guidelines and the nursing codes of conduct and ethics
2. the mental health nurse utilises legislation, relevant statutes, policies, standards, competencies, guidelines and the nursing codes of conduct and ethics in their practice
3. the mental health nurse acts to safeguard the rights of people with mental health issues, the family, carers and the community.

Standard 9

The mental health nurse holds specialist qualifications and demonstrates advanced specialist knowledge, skills and practice, integrating all the Standards competently and modelling leadership in the practice setting.

Rationale

Recognising the value of standards for clinical practice promotes optimal care for people with mental health issues, and establishes the role of specialist mental health nurses as leaders in the promotion and provision of optimal care.

Practice outcomes

This standard is being met when:

1. the mental health nurse is acknowledged by peers as expertly integrating all of the standards with advanced specialist knowledge, skills and practice.

PARTNERSHIP AND COLLABORATION

Mental health nursing is a collaborative endeavour:

- with consumers, their families and support networks
- with nurses from other specialties, as well as other members of the health and mental health team
- with social services and community organisations
- with government and non-government agencies.

Wherever mental health nurses practise, they plan and share with others to deliver effective, evidence-informed, individualised mental health services to individuals and their families. The purpose of partnering and collaborating with others is to make the best use of the different abilities of mental health team members, so that the person and their family receive the most effective and relevant service available.

The mental health team

Mental health services are provided by a variety of professionals—mental health nurses, psychiatrists, clinical psychologists, social workers, marriage and family therapists, occupational therapists, recreational therapists, and creative arts therapists—who have received many forms of specialised training. These professions require formal academic instruction, often at postgraduate level, and extensive clinical experience. Peer workers, who are people with a lived experience of mental illness, also provide mental health services and support to people with mental illness, and may have formal or on-the-job training.

In general, the number of professionals who supply mental health services has expanded dramatically since the 1990s. Role definitions that were traditionally assigned to specific disciplines have become increasingly blurred. Many functions are now shared across disciplines when the team member has been appropriately educated for the task, and when laws and regulations permit the sharing of functions. Roles are less specifically defined, and in many community settings mental health professionals take on whichever functions they do best. However, these roles involve more than the transfer of skills—they also involve a reconfiguration of power relationships from one professional group to another (Rana, Bradley & Nolan, 2009). While it is undeniable that many roles can be shared among the professions, it is also important that each discipline maintains that which is unique about its practice.

Collaboration with colleagues

Contemporary mental health nursing practice is all about collaboration. Working together in cooperation ensures movement towards the common goal; goals which should be determined by the person, who is at the centre of care.

Effective collaboration is based on respect for the position from which another participant acts. Our values and attitudes, as well as our cultural backgrounds, influence our beliefs and the climate in which we operate. Knowing this, we can become aware of the values and culture of others and, in turn, respect them.

Clinical supervision and peer support creates an atmosphere in which nurses are free to share their knowledge, skills and evolving ideas. Such support increases creativity, depth and perspective in nursing. Self-exploration and self-assessment, through reading and dialogue with other nurses and mental health team members, can help nurses embrace a spirit of cooperation.

Collaboration with individuals and their families

Family members, friends and members of the mental health team are a central influence in each individual's life. Wherever possible, the person and their significant others are partners in the collaborative process of the mental health team. The notion of self-determination is focused on the way in which a person acquires new health behaviours and maintains them over time—with services that afford people autonomy and support their confidence to self-regulate and sustain behaviours that are conducive to their health and wellbeing, considered more likely to enhance adherence to treatment and improve health outcomes (Taylor et al., 2016). People are more likely to adopt values and behaviours promoted by those to whom they feel connected and in whom they trust (Ryan, Patrick, Deci & Williams, 2008).

Unfortunately, the process of socialisation into a profession may make it difficult for a person to respect, accept and trust the position of another. As students become committed to a profession through the process of socialisation, they tend to view members of other disciplines with suspicion. Review the strategies for collaboration in the following Your Intervention Strategies, which identify some of the aspects of successful collaboration that are particularly important.

It is important that individuals and their family members are able to participate in team discussions, which often have an important place in the functioning of mental health services and may have a number of purposes. Remember, it may feel overwhelming for a person to participate in team meetings, particularly where the discussion involves collaboration among several agencies or several mental health care workers who are moving towards similar goals, so supporting the person to attend, helping them to prepare for the discussions and to identify what they want, is the role of the mental health nurse.

Discuss with the person the information to be shared with family members and the other members of the mental health team. When the boundaries of confidentiality are not clear, discuss this with a colleague or a clinical supervisor to determine what is appropriate to be shared. Decisions around confidentiality should always take safety into consideration, as well as what agreement exists with regard to sharing information, and how the person or agency receiving the information will use that information in the person's best interest. Refer to Chapter 11 for a thorough discussion of rights and responsibilities as they relate to confidentiality.

YOUR INTERVENTION STRATEGIES
Lessons on collaboration

1. First, know your own reality. Determine your values, attitudes, biases and goals.
2. Value diversity, and turn differences into assets.
3. Acknowledge that conflict is natural and develop constructive conflict resolution skills.
4. Recognise your own power base, and share it with others (colleagues, consumers and their families).
5. Master interpersonal communication skills and processing skills.
6. Approach collaboration as lifelong learning. The more you collaborate with others, the better you get at it.
7. Place yourself in interdisciplinary situations whenever possible—be present, both physically and mentally, at team forums.
8. Appreciate that collaboration is often spontaneous, and that you must be ready to seize the moment.
9. Balance unity with autonomy. That is, work neither exclusively as a member of a team (collaboration is not required for all decisions) nor in isolation.

NURSING'S THEORETICAL HERITAGE

Mental health nursing is based in theories that help us to organise assessment data, identify problems or areas for development, plan interventions, generate goals and nursing actions, and determine and evaluate outcomes.

A few of the best-known nursing theorists, and the concepts and principles of their theories or models most relevant to mental health nursing, are examined in this section. Each of the early nursing theorists has revisited her original formulation to move closer to mental health nursing values of humanism, interactionism, cultural competence, the relevance of meaning, and the importance of empathy and empowerment in the nurse–client relationship. Hildegard Peplau, Joyce Travelbee, Josephine Paterson, Loretta Zderad, Jean Watson and Patricia Benner are theorists whose existential and interactional origins and subsequent conceptualisations are particularly congruent with the philosophy of mental health nursing advocated in this text.

Peplau

Hildegard Peplau (see Figure 3.1 ■) has had a greater impact on mental health nursing than any other nursing theorist to date. Peplau published her groundbreaking nursing theory in the classic book *Interpersonal relations in nursing* (1952), where she defined nursing as a significant therapeutic interpersonal process. Peplau was strongly influenced by the psychiatrist Harry Stack Sullivan and other theorists of the interpersonal school.

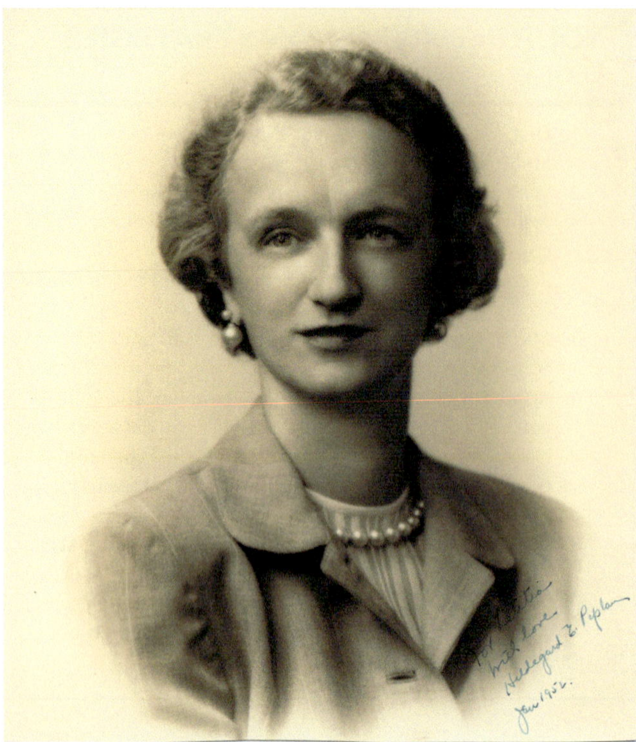

FIGURE 3.1 ■ Hildegard Peplau. Peplau's theory continues to guide the heart of psychiatric–mental health nursing practice.
Photo courtesy of Letitia Anne Peplau.

Peplau conceptualised the one-to-one nurse–client relationship as the situation in which consumers can accomplish tasks such as learning to trust or learning to collaborate, and practise healthy communication and behaviours. The core concepts of Peplau's theory of interpersonal relations (1997) were the three phases of what she identified as the nurse–client relationship, as follows:

1. *orientation phase:* mutually defining the problem/issues
2. *working phase:* assisting the person to identify problem-solving alternatives
3. *termination phase:* dissolving the links between the nurse and the person.

There are several similarities between Peplau's stages and the nursing process. Some say that Peplau's stages are the ancestor of the phases of the nursing process.

One of Peplau's many major contributions was the demonstration of how nurses could implement the nursing roles she wrote about (1978) that were central in the creation of a therapeutic relationship. The roles are:

- *teacher:* imparting knowledge that sheds light on a need or interest
- *resource:* providing specific information that aids in understanding a problem or a new situation
- *counsellor:* using specific skills and attitudes to help another to identify, cope with and resolve problems that interfere with wellbeing
- *leader:* carrying out and maintaining the therapeutic relationship through interacting with the person in specific phases
- *technical expert:* using clinical skills in giving physical care
- *surrogate:* taking the role of another, as in providing a corrective emotional experience; see Chapter 2.

Memorial tributes to Peplau by nurses from around the world, upon her death in 1999, recognised her as the 'mother of psychiatric nursing' (Barker, 1999; Haber, 1999). She developed the first Master's level clinical specialist program in psychiatric–mental health nursing, at Rutgers University in 1954, and also practised what she preached in a private practice in psychiatric nursing, with the World Health Organization and the National Institute of Mental Health (NIMH), the Nurse Corps, and in other schools of nursing in North America and abroad. Mental health nurses continue to use Peplau's teachings to understand and guide decisions in the one-to-one therapeutic relationship. Chapter 2 details the one-to-one therapeutic relationship between consumer and nurse.

Travelbee

Joyce Travelbee is another nurse theorist who focuses on the meaning in nurse–client interactions. Travelbee (1966) explained in detail the concepts of sympathy, rapport and suffering, and emphasised the importance of communication and stages in nurse–client relationships. She emphasised the importance of being motivated by compassion—of 'walking the walk with you' (George, 2011). Her view of humanity, uniqueness, existential encounters and nursing is highly congruent with values in mental health nursing.

Paterson and Zderad

Josephine Paterson and Loretta Zderad's 1976 book, *Humanistic nursing,* republished in 1988, and again in 2008, reflected the contemporary nature of their original ideas. They were a decade ahead of their time in rejecting a mechanistic cause-and-effect view of nursing science, and urged instead that observations of the experience of nurses in practice should be the basis of any useful nursing theory.

Their theory portrays nursing as a live dialogue in which both the nurse and the person they are caring for are present in the experience in an existential way that includes mutuality and intimacy. Their theory relies heavily on existential philosophers and emphasises humanism—the freedom of human choice and responsibility for one's actions (George, 2011). It is a highly abstract theory, with a major focus on the process of interaction (or dialogue) between nurse and individual.

Watson

Jean Watson's theory of human caring was influenced by Jungian psychology, feminist theory and Maslow's concept of self-actualisation (Watson, 1988). She credits much of her thinking on therapeutic relationships and communication to the work of Carl Rogers, identifying congruency, empathy and warmth as foundational to a caring relationship that conveys authenticity and genuineness, and facilitates the expression of emotions.

Caring–healing within Watson's framework is based on values such as kindness, concern, love of self and others, and the ecology of the Earth, and involves what she originally called *carative* factors: a humanistic–altruistic value system, faith–hope, and sensitivity of self and others (Watson, 1999). Watson now uses the term *clinical caritas processes*; *caritas* meaning 'to cherish, to give special and/or loving attention'. This shift in terminology demonstrates Watson's emphasis on the spiritual dimensions of the human experience. In fact, she likens caring science to sacred science. Watson's 10 clinical caritas concepts are described in Box 3.1.

Box 3.1 Watson's clinical caritas processes

1. Embrace altruistic values and practise loving kindness with others.
2. Instil faith and hope and honour others.
3. Be sensitive to self and others by nurturing individual beliefs and practices.
4. Develop helping–trusting–caring relationships.
5. Promote and accept positive and negative feelings as you authentically listen to another's story.
6. Use creative scientific problem-solving methods for caring decision-making.
7. Share teaching and learning that addresses the individual needs and comprehension styles.
8. Create a healing environment for the physical and spiritual self that respects human dignity.
9. Assist with basic physical, emotional and spiritual human needs.
10. Open to mystery and allow miracles to enter.

Source: Dr Jean Watson's human caring theory: Ten caritas processes. Retrieved from http://watsoncaringscience.org/caring_science/10caritas.html

Her theory emphasises sensitivity to self, and values clarification regarding personal and cultural beliefs that might pose barriers to transpersonal caring. Establishing a helping–trusting human care relationship is pivotal to Watson's theory.

Watson (2008) also develops the notion of spiritual environment and the interconnectedness of all things, including the connection between natural healing approaches, self-knowledge, self-control, self-caring, self-healing potential, and caring, healing relationships with the self and others. Watson's theory is philosophically congruent with contemporary global approaches to health and health promotion (Pilkington, 2007), and with the philosophical approach of this textbook.

Benner

Patricia Benner (1983, 1996, 1999), part philosopher, part theorist, has added to nursing's understanding of the language of caring. Her ideas have been generated by observing and interviewing expert nurses engaged in clinical practice. Her goal has been to disclose the nature of clinical wisdom, particularly around caring and comforting practices. She argues for the importance of forming nurse–client relationships, teaching and coaching, and bearing witness to the illness experience.

Implications for mental health nursing practice

The interpersonal theory of mental health nursing originated by Hildegard Peplau remains the nursing theory that has shaped mental health nursing most directly. More contemporary nurse theorists, however, have also laid the foundation for concepts that are central to mental health nursing practice. The nursing theorists discussed here have had the following effects on psychiatric–mental health nursing:

- differentiated nursing from medicine, with emphases on caring rather than curing
- placed the importance of interpreting meaning at the centre of their theories
- focused on interaction between the nurse and the person in their care
- advocated humanistic and existential values of dignity, freedom and responsibility, authenticity and caring as crucial to quality of care.

LIVED EXPERIENCE

Self-awareness allows us to understand our humanity—our personal humanity and our social humanity. It allows us to communicate effectively, take risks, make errors and achieve success. It allows us to understand that much mental 'illness' is about what's happened to people, not what's wrong with people. The majority of people treated by public mental health and substance abuse services have trauma histories. Trauma-informed care is the new 'recovery', so we need to be careful that it is not co-opted into inflexible systems. In Australia, Adults Surviving Child Abuse (ASCA) has published *'The last frontier': Practice guidelines for treatment of complex trauma and trauma informed care and service delivery*.

The core principles of trauma-informed care are safety, trustworthiness, choice, collaboration and empowerment. Individuals who have experienced trauma 'need access to systems of care, protection and justice that are knowledgeable, understanding, accepting and validating, and which can offer interventions that become part of the solution rather than part of the problem' (Kezelman & Stavropoulos, 2012).

Historically, many consumers have been traumatised by their experiences of coercive, involuntary mental health services, and so we hope that trauma-informed care will be a powerful force for change.

Dr Cathy Kezelman & Dr Pam Stavropoulos. (2012). 'The last frontier': Practice guidelines for treatment of complex trauma and trauma informed care and service delivery, Kiribilli, Australia: Adults Surviving Child Abuse.

These theories provide the beginnings for directing practice, focusing nursing research, and developing a framework of concepts integral to the preparation of professional nurses.

Approaches associated with two or more different nursing theories or the psychiatric theories discussed in Chapter 5 are often used in combination. For example, self-destructive behaviour may be ameliorated by the judicious use of medication, so that the person is more available for a caring, healing relationship with a mental health nurse. Such a combined or eclectic approach demands that mental health nurses are capable of functioning according to all theories of care, depending on which is best for the individual and best fits the resources and limitations of the situation. If you give adequate consideration to the theoretical framework of the way you practise mental health nursing, you will foster practice-oriented research and clinical judgments that you can articulate and share with others. Research is a tool for developing mental health nursing theory that synthesises the most useful elements of these theories.

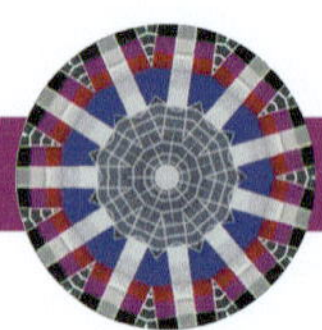

REFERENCES

Austin, W., & Boyd, M. A. (2010) *Psychiatric and mental health nursing for Canadian practice*. Philadelphia, PA: Lippincott Williams & Wilkins.

Australian College of Mental Health Nurses (ACMHN). (1999). *Setting the standard: A history of the Australian and New Zealand College of Mental Health Nurses Inc.* Canberra, Australia: ACMHN.

Australian College of Mental Health Nurses Inc (ACMHN). (2010). Standards of practice for Australian Mental Health Nurses 2010. Canberra, Australia: ACMHN.

Australian College of Mental Health Nurses (ACMHN). (2013). *Scope of practice of mental health nurses in Australia 2013.* Canberra, Australia: ACMHN.

Australian College of Mental Health Nurses (ACMHN). (2016) *National framework for postgraduate mental health nursing education.* Canberra, Australia: ACMHN.

Barker, P. (1999). Hildegard E. Peplau: The mother of psychiatric nursing. *Journal of Psychiatric and Mental Health Nursing, 6*(3), 175–176.

Bateman, J., & Henderson, C. (2013). Trauma-informed care and practice: Towards a cultural shift in policy reform across mental health and human services in Australia—a national strategic direction. Retrieved from http://www.mhcc.org.au/media/44467/nticp_strategic_direction_journal_article__vf4_-_jan_2014_.pdf

Benner, P. (1983). Uncovering the knowledge embedded in clinical practice. *Image: Journal of Nursing Scholarship, 15*(2), 36–41.

Benner, P. (1996). *Expertise in nursing practice: Caring, clinical judgment and ethics.* New York, NY: Springer.

Benner, P. (1999). *Clinical wisdom and interventions in critical care: A thinking-in-action approach.* Philadelphia, PA: Saunders.

Boling, A. (2003). The professionalization of psychiatric nursing from doctors' handmaidens to empowered professionals. *Journal of Psychosocial Nursing and Mental Health Services, 41*, 10–26.

Brown, E. L. (1948). *Nursing for the future.* New York, NY: Russell Sage Foundation.

Burdekin, B. (1993). *Human rights and mental illness: Report of the National inquiry concerning the human rights of people with mental illness* (Vols 1 and 2). Canberra, Australia: Australian Human Rights Commission. Retrieved from: http://apo.org.au/node/29708

Byrd, S., & Marshall, M. (1963). *Clinical approaches to psychiatric nursing.* New York, NY: Macmillan.

Clinton, M. (1997). National review of specialist nurse education. *Australian and New Zealand Journal of Mental Health Nursing, 6*(3), 91–92.

Clinton, M. (2001). *Scoping study of the Australian mental health nursing workforce 1999.* Canberra, Australia: Commonwealth Department of Health and Aged Care.

Clinton M., & Hazelton, M. (2000). Scoping mental health nursing education. *Australian and New Zealand Journal of Mental Health Nursing, 9*(1), 2–10.

Finnane, M. (2008). Wolston Park Hospital, 1865–2001: a retrospect. *Queensland Review, 15*(2), 39–58.

George, G. B. (2011). *Nursing theories: The base for professional nursing practice* (6th ed.). Upper Saddle River, NJ: Pearson.

Greehan, M. 'Nursing', in *The Encyclopedia of Women and Leadership in Twentieth-Century Australia.* Melbourne, Australia: Australia Women's Archives Project 2014. Retrieved from http://www.womenaustralia.info/leaders/biogs/WLE0337b.htm

Haber, J. (1999). Hildegard Peplau: The mother of psychiatric nursing. *Nursing and Health Care Perspectives, 20*(4), 228.

Happell, B. (2007). Appreciating the importance of history: A brief historical overview of mental health, mental health nursing and education in Australia. *International Journal of Psychiatric Nursing Research, 12*(2), 1439–1445.

Happell, B. M., Cowin, L., Roper, C., Lakeman, R., & Cox, L. (2013). *Introducing mental health nursing: A service user-oriented approach.* (2nd ed.) Sydney, Australia: Allen & Unwin.

Henderson, A. R., & Martyr, P. (2013). Too little, too late: Mental health nursing education in Western Australia, 1958–1994. *International Journal of Mental Health Nursing, 22*(3), 221–230. doi: 10.1111/j.1447-0349.2012.00861.x

Hickie, I. B. McGorry, P. D., Davenport, T. A., Rosenberg, S. P., Mendoza, J. A., Burns, J. M., . . . Christensen, H. (2014) Getting mental health reform back on track: A leadership challenge for the new Australian Government. *Medical Journal of Australia, 200*(8), 445–448.

Jackson, J. L., Passamonti, M., & Kroenke, K. (2007). Outcome and impact of mental disorders in primary care at 5 years. *Psychosomatic Medicine, 69*(2), 217–229.

Kays, J. L., Hurley, R. A., & Taber, K. H. (2012). The dynamic brain: Neuroplasticity and mental health. *Journal of Neuropsychiatry and Clinical Neurosciences, 24*(2), 118–124.

Kezelman, C., & Stavropoulos, P. (2012). 'The last frontier': Practice guidelines for treatment of complex trauma and trauma informed care and service delivery. Kiribilli, Australia: Adults Surviving Child Abuse. Retrieved from http://www.recoveryonpurpose.com/upload/ASCA_Practice%20Guidelines%20for%20the%20Treatment%20of%20Complex%20Trauma.pdf

Kroenke, K., Spitzer, R. L., Williams, J. B., Monahan, P. O., & Lowe, B. (2007). Anxiety disorders in primary care: Prevalence, impairment, comorbidity, and detection. *Annals of Internal Medicine, 146*(5), 317.

Maude, P. (2001). From lunatic to client: A history/nursing oral history of the treatment of Western Australians who experienced a mental illness. (Unpublished doctoral thesis, University of Melbourne, Melbourne). Retrieved from http://dtl.unimelb.edu.au/view/action/singleViewer.do?dvs=1334291362766~462&locale=en_AU&VIEWER_URL=/view/action/singleViewer.do?&DELIVERY_RULE_ID=7&search_terms=SYS%20=%20000029896&adjacency=N&application=DIGITOOL-3&frameId=1&usePid1=true&usePid2=true

McBride, A. B. (1990). Psychiatric nursing in the 1990s. *Archives of Psychiatric Nursing, 4*(1), 21–27.

Mental Health Nurse Education Taskforce. (2008). Final report: Mental health in pre-registration nursing courses. Melbourne, Australia: Mental Health Nurse Education Taskforce.

National Mental Health Commission (NMHC). (2013). *A contributing life: The 2013 national report card on mental health and suicide prevention.* Sydney, Australia: NMHC.

Nolan, P. (1993). *A history of mental health nursing.* London, England: Chapman and Hall.

Nolan, P., & Hopper, B. (2000). Revisiting mental health nursing in the 1960s. *Journal of Mental Health, 9*(6), 563–573. doi:10.1080/jmh.9.6.563.573

NSW Consumer Advisory Group—Mental Health (NSW CAG), & Mental Health Coordinating Council (MHCC). (2009). *Developing a recovery oriented service provider resource for community mental health organisations: Literature review on Recovery.* Sydney, Australia: NSW CAG & MHCC. Retrieved from: http://mhcc.org.au/media/2498/nsw-cag-mhcc-project-recovery-literature-review.pdf

Paterson, J. G., & Zderad, L. T. (2008). *Humanistic nursing*. Retrieved from http://www.paterson-zderad-humanistic-nursing.com. Previously published 1988 (Publication No. 41–2218). New York, NY: National League for Nursing.

Peplau, H. E. (1952). *Interpersonal relations in nursing.* New York, NY: Putnam.

Peplau, H. E. (1978). Psychiatric nursing: Role of nurses and psychiatric nurses. *International Nursing Review, 25*(2) 41–47.

Peplau, H. E. (1989). Future directions in psychiatric nursing from the perspective of history. *Journal of Psychosocial Nursing, 27*(2), 18–27.

Peplau, H. E. (1997). Peplau's theory of interpersonal relations. *Nursing Science Quarterly, 10*(4), 162–167.

Pilkington, F. B. (2007). Envisioning nursing in 2050 through the eyes of nurse theorists: Leininger and Watson. *Nursing Science Quarterly, 20*(1), 8.

Rana, T., Bradley, E., & Nolan, P. (2009). Survey of psychiatrists' views of nurse prescribing. *Journal of Psychiatric and Mental Health Nursing, 16*(3), 257–262.

Robson, B. (2008) From mental hygiene to community mental health: Psychiatrists and Victorian public administration from the 1940s to 1990s. *Provenance: The Journal of Public Record Office Victoria*, Issue 7. Retrieved from http://prov.vic.gov.au/publications/provenance/provenance2008/from-mental-hygiene-to-community-mental-health

Russell, R. L. (1990). *From Nightingale to now: Nurse education in Australia.* Sydney, Australia: Harcourt, Brace and Jovanovich.

Russell, R. L. (2005). *From hospital to university—the transfer of nurse education.* Council of Deans of Nursing and Midwifery, Australia and NewZealand. Retrieved from: http://www.cdnm.edu.au/wp-content/uploads/2011/09/HistoryNursingEducation.pdf

Ryan, R. M., Patrick, H., Deci, E. L., & Williams, G. C. (2008). Facilitating health behaviour change and its maintenance: Interventions based on self-determination theory. *European Health Psychologist, 10*(1), 2–5. http://openhealthpsychology.com/ehp/index.php/contents/article/viewFile/ehp.v10.i1.p2/32

Sands, N. (2009) Round the bend: A brief history of mental health nursing in Victoria, Australia 1848–1950s. *Issues in Mental Health Nursing, 30*, 364–371. doi: 10.1080/01612840802422631

Santangelo, P. (2015). What's special about mental health nursing? Being in the here and now, side by side, co-constructing care: A substantive grounded theory of recovery-focused mental health nursing. (Unpublished doctoral thesis. Faculty of Health School of Health Sciences, Nursing and Midwifery, University of Tasmania, Hobart.)

Shultz, B. (1991). *A tapestry of service: The evolution of nursing in Australia. Volume 1: Foundation to Federation 1788–1899.* Melbourne, Australia: Churchill Livingstone.

Spearitt, D. (1980). A role model for the psychiatric nurse in state institutions and some implications for methodology and training. *Journal of the Australian Congress of Mental Health Nurses, 1*(1), 7–11.

Taylor, E., Perlman, D., Moxham, L., Pegg, S., Patterson, C., Brighton, R., . . . Heffernan, T. (2016). Recovery Camp: Assisting consumers toward enhanced self-determination. *International Journal of Mental Health Nursing*, May 27, 1447-0349.

Travelbee, J. (1966). *Interpersonal aspects of nursing.* Philadelphia, PA: Davis.

Tudor, G. (1952). A sociopsychiatric nursing approach to intervention in a problem of mutual withdrawal on a mental hospital ward. *Psychiatry, 15, 193–217.*

Wand, T., & White, G. (2007). Progression of the mental health nurse practitioner role in Australia. *Journal of Psychiatric and Mental Health Nursing, 14*, 644–651.

Watson, J. (1988). New dimensions in human caring theory. *Nursing Science Quarterly, 1*(4), 175–181.

Watson, J. (1999). *Postmodern nursing and beyond.* New York, NY: Churchill Livingstone.

Watson, J. (2008). Nursing: *The philosophy and science of caring* (rev. ed.). Denver, CO: University of Colorado Press.

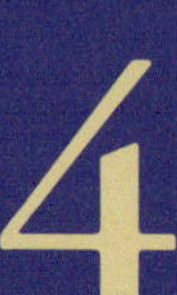

4

Self-awareness and the mental health nurse

LORNA MOXHAM, PAUL ROBSON AND TIM HEFFERNAN

KEY TERMS

LEARNING OUTCOMES

After completing this chapter, you will be able to:

1. Understand the emerging peer workforce and the need for strong workforce partnerships.
2. Explain why self-knowledge and self-reflection are important in mental health nursing.
3. Discuss the concept of personal integration and its relationship to mental health nursing practice.
4. Identify qualities that enable mental health nurses to practise the artful use of self.
5. Describe how the concepts of blame and control affect therapeutic practice.
6. Foster culturally competent care for people with mental illness health disorders by understanding the influence of your own sociocultural background on your nursing practice.
7. Understand the use of empathy in mental health clinical practice.
8. Maintain a respectful attitude towards people for whom you provide care and work with.
9. Discuss the importance of self-care.

LIVED EXPERIENCE

As Australian mental health service settings and workforces move towards true recovery-orientation, mental health nurses will find themselves working in new ways, in new places, with new people. A significant emerging workforce is the peer workforce, so the traditional nursing care provider relationship with individuals will now need to transform into a more equal and collegial relationship. Much of the literature suggests a resistance by some clinicians to peer support workers, so it is important for mental health nurses to engage in critical discussions around the potential implications for the mental health workforce as peer workers become an increasingly established component of the workforce.

Peer workers are employed by public mental health services as advocates, consultants, mentors, educators and peer support workers. Peer workers work with nurses and with voluntary and involuntary consumers in a variety of settings—inpatient, forensic, emergency department, community, education and rehabilitation.

The recent National Mental Health Commission (2014) recommendation around building workforce capacity to support systems changes is to 'improve supply, productivity and access for mental health nurses and the mental health peer workforce'.

We are all in this together!

INTRODUCTION

Throughout this text, you are encouraged to think about the mind–body–spirit of the people for whom you are providing nursing care. This chapter explores some dimensions of self-awareness and self-knowledge, through the examination of personal integration and recurring problems that pertain to the nurse's identity, the personal qualities on which the artful use of self in therapeutic relationships is based, and strategies for taking care of your own mind–body–spirit. It is important to pay significant attention to your own stressors and health (mental and physical) as you practise the art and craft of mental health nursing.

Practice example

Jess: 'I just can't take it. I feel myself getting confused about who is the person with a mental illness. There seems to be such a fine line sometimes. Sometimes I think it could be me.'

Eric: 'I hated mental health—it just didn't seem like nursing to me. I really like to keep busy. When you change someone's dressing, you really feel like you've helped them. Here, it's all so uncertain.'

Makayla: 'What I kept thinking about was that a lot of the people had really unusual thoughts. This one dude thought he had a wire in his brain that had been implanted by the government when he slept. He kept saying that the government were capturing all his thoughts. He was really distressed, and I was upset for him. I didn't know what to say—what if I said the wrong thing?'

PERSONAL INTEGRATION

Many students and clinicians, faced with relating to people whose behaviour they view as challenging, frightening, curious or socially inappropriate, find that their personal attitudes, expectations, myths and values make it difficult for them to fulfil their professional roles. This was the case for Penny.

Practice example

Penny, a second-year nursing student, had a clinical placement at a community-based drug and alcohol service. Despite her initial interest, she developed a pattern of absences from the clinical placement. When her facilitator discussed this with her, Penny blurted out that, much to her own surprise, she was unable to attend the group meetings for pregnant women with substance addictions. The thought of addicting babies before they were born—babies whom she felt would ultimately 'suffer because of their mothers' self-indulgence'—horrified Penny. She found herself negatively judging the women constantly, and avoiding interaction with them. She said they made her 'angry'. 'I feel like they should be jailed instead of given support and sympathy.'

For many nurses, confrontation with people who are perceived as different reinforces a personal sense of stability. Others feel threatened by such confrontation.

Recall the Practice Example of how the nurse described 'Crazy Helen' on page 4 in Chapter 1. Working with people whose personal integration is fragmented, dissolving, divided or alienated puts the nurse's own identity on the line as well. To respond with the compassion necessary to be effective, health professionals must confront their own identity, separate it from the consumer's identity (detached concern), which may indeed be dissolving, and finally integrate different values and behaviours comfortably within the therapeutic relationships they develop.

Detached concern is the ability to distance oneself in order to help others. It is an essential quality, not only in avoiding *burnout* or *compassion fatigue,* a problem discussed later in this chapter, but also in using appropriate *assertiveness* when collaborating with colleagues, and in maintaining *empathic abilities* in highly stressful situations.

Creating a common ground

Because people are constantly building and protecting their own self-images, they try to get others to see their preferred image of themselves. However, it is impossible to see another's self-image or worldview exactly as that person experiences it. Despite this fact, psychiatry has traditionally attempted to have certain people (the consumer) assume the perspective of certain other people (*mental health professionals*).

Given recovery-oriented practice should be the focus, the creation of common ground, of a mutually understood, negotiated reality or shared perspective, should be the approach used. Nonetheless, despite common ground, everyone still brings with them their own conceptions, feelings, attitudes and images of each other and themselves. In many instances, the nurse's image of the person with a mental illness—how it is expected they will act or feel—is not the same as the person's self-image. This can be confusing, and hinders attempts to establish therapeutic relationships and communicate effectively.

Searching for meaning

Mental health nurses work with people in a search for 'meaning'. Nurses therefore need to understand and establish their own personal meaning and integration of self, as these are key resources for practice. In order to be effective, nurses must strive to possess the personal skills to deal with the person's symptoms. And we must be personally working through any problems that might affect our practice. For example, if you want to be liked and admired by everyone you meet, you are likely to find it difficult to set reasonable and rational limits.

Feelings: the affective self

The ultimate effectiveness in terms of relating to and communicating with others depends on how well people know themselves (**self-awareness**), and develop the ability to be sensitive to and care about others. In the following Practice Example, Josh's limited self-awareness hampers his clinical work.

Self-awareness and caring go hand-in-hand. At the root of social interaction is people's ability to understand and care about each other's attitudes and feelings. Because each human

Practice example

Josh is a middle-aged man who sought out nursing as a career. Although he is highly proficient in technical skills, and charming and engaging in relationships with most people, he has discovered a surprising intolerance for some of the behaviours that people with depression may exhibit. He finds himself responding to them with admonitions to stop it, to bite the bullet, to grow up. He personally has seldom allowed himself to experience his own sadnesses, and jokingly characterises himself as a firm believer in repression and denial. The need to empathise with a severely depressed person unable to control their feelings evokes discomfort, and he is unable to work with such people.

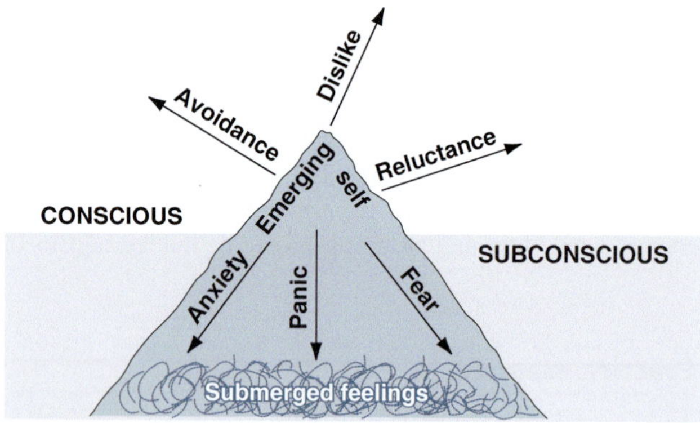

FIGURE 4.1 ■ Self-awareness of feelings. Superficial feelings are visible; deeper feelings are submerged.

being is unique, this ability, called *empathising*, can be difficult and challenging. (Empathy is discussed in greater detail later in this chapter, and empathy as a communication skill is discussed in Chapter 9.) One way to develop this ability is to practise it. Learning to be aware of your responses to the expression of feelings from another person is a starting point. The film *Harry Potter and the Deathly Hallows* illustrates the importance of self-awareness.

Self-awareness of feelings

Feelings are like icebergs: only the tips stick up into consciousness, and the deeper parts are submerged. One such feeling, illustrated in Figure 4.1 ■, is fear. The conscious part may be experienced as dislike, avoidance or reluctance. At a deeper level, the feeling is reported as anxiety. Even deeper, the person may acknowledge 'I feel scared.' Deeper yet, the person may experience genuine panic. Such an iceberg may well explain Josh's attitude towards tearful people with depression. His annoyance, irritation, sarcasm and disdain may represent the tip of the iceberg of Josh's fear of depression. The iceberg comparison also applies to other feelings, such as love, hurt and guilt.

Nurses may put up rigid defences aimed at denying their personal feelings because of the emotional demands of their role. For example, some procedures actually require the nurse to violate a person's emotional or physical state (probing personal questions, injections, dressings). Defending against feelings becomes a way for the nurse to cope with inflicting pain on another person. Dealing effectively with the feelings of others depends on the extent to which you explore your own feelings.

Difficulties associated with submerged feelings

One characteristic of icebergs of feeling is that at the tip of the iceberg feelings lose their experiential quality and are translated into impulses to act. For example, a person with submerged guilt may express it by frequent worrying, but may

MENTAL HEALTH IN THE MEDIA

Harry Potter and the Deathly Hallows

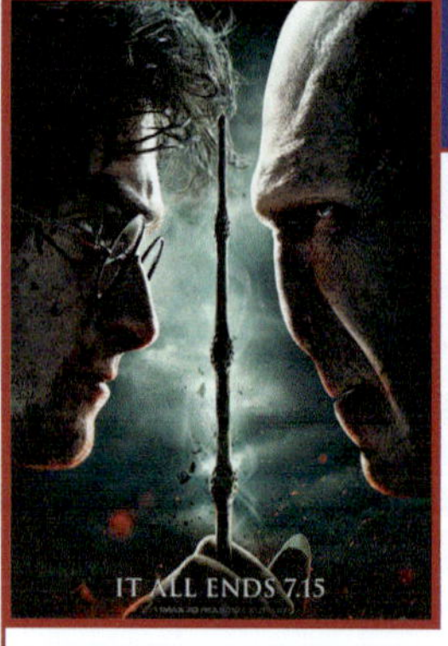

For the main characters in the Harry Potter film series, the battles never seem to end. In this film, Harry, Ron and Hermione battle Voldemort, Dementors and various other villains. But how about their own internal battles? From the first film in 2001, *Harry Potter and the Sorcerer's Stone,* the personality traits with the potential to hinder Harry, Ron and Hermione were evident.

The circumstances of Harry's early life were not the best. His mother and father were killed while he was still an infant. Brought up by his aunt and uncle in an abusive household, Harry was forced to live in a small closet beneath the stairs, he carried out the household chores, and he was treated either as if he did not exist or as if he was an immense bother. And not only that, there is a powerful villain with many disciples bent on killing Harry. Yet, despite these events and the anxiety and depression they engender, Harry is remarkably self-confident and balanced. Kind teachers, hard work and steadfast friends help him to face fearsome challenges.

Ron was born into a household in which he was the last in a long line of boys, and could be easily overlooked or overshadowed by his successful older brothers and his cute and perky little sister. Ron's insecurities and low self-esteem are often dealt with by joking behaviour—perhaps fearing that his opinions are unimportant or will be disregarded—and continually plague Ron in all of the films. His reluctance to talk about his feelings distances himself from others. Yet Ron always overcomes his doubts and fears. He seems to hold it together well enough to save both Harry and Hermione on a number of occasions.

Hermione is fastidious, a workaholic and often at the head of her class in the school of wizardry. However, she sets such high standards for herself that she often feels unfulfilled and unsuccessful. She sometimes seems unable to recognise the effect of workaholism on her health, and continues to try to please her friends as well as her teachers. Her stubbornness and need to control cause interpersonal difficulties. But, because she is steadfast in her determination, and is smart, skilful, brave and willing to use her talents to benefit others, Hermione helps Harry and Ron overcome obstacles.

The Harry Potter films help to educate others about hardiness and resilience in the face of untoward circumstances. A common thread is the value of self-awareness and the means by which self-knowledge can enhance the quality and nature of one's relationships with others.

Photo courtesy of Newscom.

be completely unaware of the underlying feelings. The behaviour is the only outward manifestation.

People lose touch with their feelings over time as they shape their sense of self. They hear such messages as 'boys don't cry' or 'girls are too sensitive', and incorporate these injunctions into their emerging self-system (explained in Chapter 5). Not being sufficiently aware of one's feelings has several disadvantages:

- What people don't know *can* hurt them. Repressed feelings may reappear in behaviours that are difficult to alter. For example, hidden anger may emerge in migraine headaches or the use of sarcasm.
- People who are not aware of their feelings can find it difficult to make decisions. It is hard to tell a 'should' from a wish. Without some awareness of their real wants, they may have trouble saying no or requesting something they need. They are more likely to rely on others—experts, authorities, rules and regulations, and so forth—for guidance.
- People like Josh, who are not in touch with, or are unaware of, their feelings, may find it difficult to be really close to and empathic towards others. Intimacy and empathy demand the expression of here-and-now feelings, whether positive or negative.

As a professional, you appreciate the value of thinking clearly. You understand that it is a learned ability and takes practice. Feeling clearly (authentically) is just as important as thinking clearly. It, too, can be practised and learned.

Dominant emotional themes

In order to be effective, we need to explore the dominant emotional themes in our personalities. If you find that you respond to many situations with the same feelings, you are probably narrowing your range of potential feelings, much as Michelle, Joanne and Ed in the following Practice Example.

Practice example

Whatever the occasion, Michelle was tired or bored. Fatigue and chronically depressed states were routine for her. Holidays, vacations, dinner engagements all evoked the same predictable response.

Joanne was afraid of everything. When she met her brother at the airport, her first question was 'Aren't you afraid of flying?' She was afraid of driving home from the airport. The prospect of starting back to school also frightened her.

Regardless of the circumstances, Ed always questioned the intentions of his wife, his children, his co-workers and his friends. According to Ed, the motives for their behaviour were always up for debate.

People who feel the same way in a variety of situations may be missing a lot of what is happening in those situations. They perceive only what will fit a narrowed range of feelings. Becoming aware of limited emotional themes is a way to begin to widen one's range of feelings.

Acceptance of feelings

Most people have been taught to block off awareness and the expression of certain feelings. Children are taught that being rude or ungrateful or angry is rarely acceptable. To retain love and approval, they usually comply, not by stopping the feelings, but by acting as if they didn't have them. Nursing students can also get similar messages from their lecturers. That is, it is not acceptable to find a person in their care repulsive, to dislike someone who is sick and dependent, or to express anger at or criticism of the teacher or peers. Positive feelings of attraction and love may also seem unacceptable. Failure to recognise these feelings can interfere with interactions.

Recognising and accepting our own feelings make us less vulnerable to other people's ideas about how we should feel. Nurses often feel guilty when they don't feel what others imply they 'should' feel. Nurses who can allow themselves the right to their own feelings can also allow the people in their care the right to have and express theirs.

Beliefs and values

Our personal values are the 'shoulds' that direct our behaviour. Beliefs and values take three major forms:

1. Rational beliefs are beliefs that are supported by available evidence.
2. Blind belief is belief in the absence of evidence.
3. Irrational belief is belief held despite available evidence to the contrary.

Blind and irrational beliefs can cause problems in relationships with others, including our relationships with people who have mental illness.

Dogmatic belief

Dogmatic belief (opinions or beliefs held as if they were based on the highest authority) includes both blind belief and irrational belief. Dogmatically held beliefs are not based on personal experience. Operating on the basis of dogmatically held beliefs often causes us to distort our personal experiences of the world to fit our preconceptions. Box 4.1 has examples of some strongly held beliefs about behaviours that are labelled 'mental illness'.

Box 4.1 Blind and irrational beliefs about mental illness

About mental illness

- Most people in mental health units are dangerous.
- People who seek counselling are mentally ill.
- If parents loved their children more, there would be less mental illness.
- When a person has a worry, it is best not to think about it.
- Many people become mentally ill just to avoid the problems of life.
- People would not become mentally ill if they controlled bad thoughts.
- Anyone who is in a hospital for a mental illness should not be allowed to vote.
- To have a mental illness is to become a failure in life.
- One of the main causes of mental illness is a lack of moral strength.

Issues of blame and control

Inherent in these strongly held beliefs about mental illness are issues of *blame* and *control*. Believing that people cause their own problems involves the issue of blame. Believing that people are responsible for solutions to their problems involves the issue of control. Your assumptions about personal responsibility affect the way you go about your clinical work. For artful therapeutic practice, you need to be aware of your beliefs about blame and control, as well as the person's orientation. The help you offer may not be effective if the person desiring help and the person offering help have different views on personal responsibility.

Most research on strongly held beliefs indicates that people usually know more about the things they believe than about those they don't believe. By staying ignorant about anything they don't already agree with, they can avoid changing. This position cuts off personal growth and learning that could be derived from the unknown. Obviously, people are better served by nurses who are aware of their own dogmatically held beliefs and then challenge those beliefs.

Attitudes and opinions

A feeling is a transitory experience. A feeling held over a period of time is called an *attitude*. An attitude linked to an idea or belief becomes an *opinion*. An opinion, then, involves both thinking and feeling. Research in this area has shown that people are more comfortable when their beliefs are consistent with their attitudes. People do several things to keep their attitudes and beliefs consistent:

- They repress any belief or attitude that seems inconsistent.
- They distract their awareness from conflict, either physically (such as by leaving the room) or psychologically (such as by daydreaming).
- They distort their perceptions to fit an existing attitude or belief.

These strategies take place in an attempt to keep actions consistent with attitudes or beliefs.

Arriving at values

Every day, each person meets life situations that call for thought, opinion-forming, decision-making and action. At every turn in our personal and professional lives, we are faced with choices. Our choices are based on the values we hold, but often those values are not really clear. People actively value something to the degree that they are willing to put energy into doing something about it. Their values are demonstrated in their interests, preferences, decisions and actions, as shown in the next Practice Example.

The distinction in the above examples is between *cognitive values* and *active values*. Susan verbally subscribes to values, but fails to act on them. These are cognitive values. Mal's actions demonstrate that he gives more than lip service to the idea of the dignity of all living beings. He follows active values. Mal 'walks the talk', Susan 'talks the talk'.

Practice example

In talking with colleagues, Susan, a mental health nurse, claims to value interacting with people more than doing paperwork. Yet a quick assessment of how she spends her time—sitting at the nurse's station talking with colleagues, filling out forms, doing her online shopping and checking Facebook—reveals that she acts on other values.

Mal, a nurse working in a setting that cares for profoundly cognitively disabled children, says that he believes the children have feelings, despite their uncommunicative, immobile state. He demonstrates this value in the hours he spends trying to communicate his presence and concern for them, using acupressure and touch performed slowly and with genuine feeling.

Culture and social class

Cultural and social class differences between you and others may impede your best intentions. Gaining awareness of sociocultural differences requires that you first come to understand your own background and the influence of that background on your practice. Nurses are better able to meet the sociocultural needs of others when they acknowledge that a culture and a society influence their own beliefs, values, attitudes and behaviour. Quality nursing care is culturally sensitive; that is, aware of the cultural issues that are important to the person in their care, and that may affect response to treatment.

In planning nursing interventions, plan care that is culturally competent for each person. For example, if a teenage girl is obese and wants to lose weight, you would not hand her a printed 1000-calorie diet plan, but would work with her to plan a diet based on the foods she prefers. If a Buddhist person wants time each day to meditate, you would allow for that time in the care plan. Taking a person's culture into consideration when planning care takes mutual collaboration, time, patience, insight, creativity and respect.

Sociocultural heritage

The questions in the following Self-awareness feature are designed to facilitate acknowledgment of your own sociocultural heritage. Answering these questions honestly and completely will help you understand which sociocultural factors impact your ability to communicate in a culturally sensitive way.

Avoiding misdiagnosis

Clients from different cultures may be misdiagnosed by Western health care providers. Culturally competent nurses play an important role in assessing social, psychological and behavioural symptoms in light of the person's own cultural norms. For example, a psychiatrist may diagnose a man who talks to the dead as having schizophrenia, but for someone from Puerto Rico who believes in *espiritismo*, talking to the dead is a common practice. Someone who is a charismatic Christian may lapse into an altered state of consciousness and speak in tongues. To interpret these behaviours as evidence of psychosis is inappropriate. Obtaining a cultural profile helps prevent misdiagnosis.

SELF-AWARENESS
Influence of sociocultural heritage

Answer the following questions:

- What ethnic group, socioeconomic class, religion, age group and community do you belong to?
- What experiences have you had with people from ethnic groups, socioeconomic classes, religions, age groups or communities different from your own?
- What were those experiences like? How did you feel about them?
- When you were growing up, what did your parents and significant others say about people who were different from your family?
- What things about your ethnic group, socioeconomic class, religion, age or community do you find embarrassing or wish you could change? Why?
- What sociocultural factors in your background might contribute to your being rejected by members of other cultures?
- What personal qualities do you possess that will help you establish interpersonal relationships with persons from other cultural groups?
- What personal qualities do you have that may be detrimental?
- What cultural assumptions do you hold about the people who populate our world?

TAKING CARE OF THE SELF

Knowing who you are is just a beginning. Providing care to others requires that nurses respect and care for themselves. Those who have the quality of hardiness or resilience (see Chapter 1) rise to meet challenges, and pace themselves in order to sustain the effort needed to deal with stress and strain (Fletcher & Sarkar, 2013). This section on assertiveness, the need for solitude, maintaining physical health, attending to cues of personal stress, and avoiding burnout will help you to pace yourself and preserve your personal integration.

Solitude

Most people need time alone to assimilate what has happened in time spent with other people. They also need it for relief from responding to the demands of others. Aloneness need not mean physical distance. People can be alone in a crowd. The crucial factors are that they are making no demands on others and that no one is making demands on them.

After a sanctioned time away, most people return refreshed to their relationships, work and usual circumstances. Planning for time alone is highly preferable to reaching a breaking point and then running away from issues and others.

Physical health

An important way of taking care of oneself is to look after your physical health. A proper diet, adequate rest and exercise rejuvenate and restore the body. All of these activities potentially make nurses more resilient and better able to share themselves with other people. As students, you are also coping with pressures to study, to prepare for clinical experiences and to complete assignments, as well as performing other roles that are important to you. So what are you doing about your own physical health? Remember, also, that nurses are role models to others with regard to health. Do you smoke? Are you overweight?

Sleep deprivation and shift work disorder

Sometimes we manage pressures by sleeping less. However, being chronically sleep-deprived works against maintaining physical health. Research has identified negative consequences of sleep-related fatigue on performance and client outcomes (Doman, Connelly & Spence, 2015). Take the quiz to see if you could be sleep-deprived.

SELF-AWARENESS
Are you sleep-deprived?

Answer the following questions:

- Do you usually fall asleep within five minutes after you turn off the lights?
- Do you struggle to stay awake in lectures?
- Do you 'get by' all week and then try to catch up by sleeping in on the weekend?
- Do you do shift work?
- Do you often wake up with a headache?
- Do you have trouble getting going in the morning?
- Do you push yourself to keep going?

If you answered 'yes' to more than two of these questions, you may not be getting as much sleep as you need.

More than 1.4 million Australians work evening, night or rotating shifts—such as nurses, bakers, pilots, train drivers, truck drivers, police officers, firefighters, factory workers, hospitality industry employees, miners. As you might expect, shift work—in which the 24-hour sleep–wake schedule is disturbed—is a major source of circadian rhythm disruption for nurses (Kang, Miao, Tseng et al., 2015) and other shift workers, as demonstrated in the Practice Examples.

Practice examples

Years after he had retired from his bakery business, Joseph continued to wake very early in the morning. This pattern further complicated a sleep disorder related to his medical condition of Parkinson's disease.

Jane was working rotating shifts in an intensive care unit. She noted that she had worsening insomnia and feared that her judgment would be affected by her increasing sleep deprivation.

There are several behavioural and physical effects of shift work. Lack of sleep has been associated with general psychomotor slowing and diminished cognitive performance, decreased alertness and vigilance, and a decline in mood (Klumpers et al., 2015). This can lead to an impaired ability to function at work and home, increased vehicle accidents from the impaired ability to drive safely, and increased stress on personal relationships. Even a few days of sleep deprivation have been reported to increase appetite and caloric intake, increase levels of pro-inflammatory cytokines, decrease parasympathetic and increase sympathetic tone, increase blood pressure, increase evening cortisol levels, as well as elevate insulin and blood glucose (McEwen & Karatsoreos, 2015). The impact of shift work and sleep deprivation on sleep patterns and sleep disturbance often extends beyond the period of shift work.

Suggestions for obtaining a good sleep despite a shift work schedule can be found at http://www.goodsleep.com.

Attending to internal stress signals

Nursing students who read about various illnesses in their textbooks commonly begin seeing in themselves or their friends and/or family the 'symptoms' about which they are learning. It is important to recognise and respond to our own genuine stress signals. It is difficult for most people to acknowledge difficulties with coping. All people have times in their lives when they may become very upset at small disturbances or see things out of proportion to their ultimate importance. These feelings are significant warning signals that one may not be coping adequately with stress.

Times of stress can be important turning points in people's lives. They are strong messages that change is needed. It is unwise to ignore these messages. In their daily lives, nurses are often tempted to handle their own symptoms of stress by suppressing them or using unhealthy strategies to cope, like drug or alcohol consumption. They could serve themselves better by really paying attention to their mind and body, and attending to what the signals are saying. As Shinde and Hiremath (2014, p. 231) suggest, nursing students have 'numerous stressors that affect their daily grind', so using the strategies that they recommend can help you manage stress and ease tension.

Pain, suffering and distress are sources of some of the most intensely experienced stresses in life. Events such as the death of loved ones, divorce, illness, separation from loved ones, and failure, are all part of the cycle of life's experience. When people are told to pull up their socks or to look around because they really don't have it so bad, this does not help people cope with pain, suffering and distress. People want to continue what *was* instead of living with what *is*. They need to find ways of managing their distress without being overcome by it. Some people need to replace what they have lost with something similar. Others need to explore a new dimension in their lives. Classmates, friends and family members can be great sources of support. Being able to both give and receive support strengthens the individual.

Realising that difficult and challenging times are part of what it is to be a human being makes the pain a bit easier to accept. It is important to attend to genuine feelings about loss or prospective loss. The alternative to experiencing distress is to live on the surface, out of touch with the joyful experiences in life as well as the painful ones. A more life-enhancing approach is to experience all aspects of life, but to have strategies to cope with the difficult parts.

Burnout

The nurse in the following Practice Example verbalises one of the possible consequences of working intensely with distressed people.

Practice example

'After hours, days, and months of listening to other people's problems, something inside you can go dead and you don't care anymore. That's when you'd rather sit in the nurse's station and do the paperwork than be out talking to people on the floor.'

Burnout is the name given to this phenomenon, but it is sometimes also called *compassion fatigue*. It is a condition in which health care professionals lose their concern and feeling for consumers, and come to treat them in detached or even dehumanised ways. Burnout happens to some, but not all, health professionals. Lawyers, social workers, police officers, clinical psychologists, childcare workers, prison personnel and others who struggle to retain both their objectivity and their concern for the people with whom they work can burn out. Burnout involves physical, mental and emotional exhaustion that is attributed to long-term involvement in emotionally demanding situations. Burnout is a less healthy and problematic attempt to cope—by distancing oneself—with the stresses of intense interpersonal work. It hurts not only those they work with, but also themselves, in that they become ineffective and dissatisfied.

In many cases, burning out involves not only thinking in derogatory terms about people, but also believing that somehow they deserve any problem they have. Benner and Wrubel, nursing theorists who have studied both caring and burnout, caution us to avoid making the mistake of thinking that caring is the cause of burnout, and thus trying to prevent burnout by protecting ourselves from caring (1989). According to them, the 'sickness' is the loss of caring, and the return of caring is the recovery. (Benner's work is discussed further in Chapter 3.)

There is little doubt that burnout plays a major role in the poor delivery of mental health care. It is also a key factor in low staff morale, absenteeism and high job turnover.

Cues to burnout

Cues to burnout can be found in the language health professionals use to describe people. Burnout victims may refer to the people in their care as 'frequent flyers' or by diagnosis, such as 'he's just a PD'. Another cue is a lack of involvement with those under their care. Some nurses stay in the nurses' station to avoid interacting. Some openly reject bids for human contact. 'Going by the book/policy' rather than considering the unique factors in a situation is a way of minimising personal involvement with people. By rigidly applying the rules, one can avoid thinking about the person's specific problems. Be careful and be self-aware: burnout can transform an original and creative nurse into a mechanical bureaucrat.

Another cue to burnout is supposedly joking put-downs, such as those in the Practice Example, which make mental health work seem less frightening and overwhelming.

Practice example

When the nurse is asked where Mr Grant is, he laughingly reports that Mr Grant is taking a shower in preparation for his personality inventory test. Everyone in the nurses' station cracks up laughing.

In a discharge conference, the psychiatrist says she'd like to discharge Earl, a young man with a history of violent outbursts. The nurse replies 'With or without a baseball bat?', and everyone chuckles.

Reducing burnout

Research indicates that the causes of professional burnout are rooted not in the permanent psychological characteristics of individuals, but rather in the social context of their work; specifically, lack of resources and workload pressures. Most nurses usually expect the presence of negative conditions, such as large care-coordination loads, time pressures and daily confrontation with distress. Positive factors, like a sense of significance, rewarding interpersonal relationships, the appreciation of others, challenge and variety, are protective factors (Todaro-Franceschi, 2013). The strategies listed in the following Your Intervention Strategies feature can be used to reduce and modify the occurrence of burnout.

YOUR INTERVENTION STRATEGIES

Reducing and modifying the occurrence of burnout

- Address staff–consumer ratios. Giving more attention to each person enables time to focus on the positive, non-problematic aspects of the person's life.
- Recognise that no one is perfect. The people to whom you provide care deserve the best you can provide; it may not always be perfect care, and it isn't 24-hours-a-day, 7-days-a-week care.
- Take sanctioned breaks rather than guilt-provoking escapes from the work situation.
- Talk over your problems to get advice and support when you need it. Clinical supervision is important for mental health nurses.
- Express, analyse and share your feelings about burning out. This lets you get things off your chest, and gives you the chance to get constructive feedback from others and perhaps a new perspective as well.
- Understand your own motivations in pursuing a mental health nursing career, and recognise your own expectations for working with consumers. Deal with the issues of the people you are caring for, not your own.
- Listen to and then attend to your own internal stress signals.
- Pursue happiness and satisfaction in your personal life, through things you enjoy and being around positive people.
- Work with a peer support worker to get a different recovery perspective.

EVIDENCE-BASED PRACTICE

Improving practice and avoiding burnout

You and a colleague work in the medication clinic of a community mental health centre. Both of you have talked about your increasing dissatisfaction with your job. You feel burdened. There are too many consumers and too little time. You feel that you don't get enough feedback on your performance from management. The improvements you would like to make—medication education groups for family members, for example—are impossible to implement given the workload. Neither you nor your colleague feels that you are doing the best you can for the service users and their families. You decide to approach management to discuss the following:

1. consideration of ways to decrease the workload
2. regularly scheduled time for clinical supervision
3. an additional weekly medication education group for family members
4. consideration of working in partnership with a peer worker.

Your requests are based on the following types of research:

Drury, V., Craigie, M., Francis, K., Aoun, S., & Hegney, D. G. (2014). Compassion satisfaction, compassion fatigue, anxiety, depression and stress in registered nurses in Australia: Phase 2 results. *Journal of Nursing Management, 22*(4), 519–531.

Hegney, D. G., Craigie, M., Hemsworth, D., Osseiran-Moisson, R., Aoun, S., Francis K., . . . Drury V. (2014). Compassion satisfaction, compassion fatigue, anxiety, depression and stress in registered nurses in Australia: Study 1 results. *Journal of Nursing Management, 22*(4), 506–518.

Hurley, J., Cashin, A., Mills, J., Hutchinson, M., & Graham, I. (2016). A critical discussion of peer workers: Implications for the mental health nursing workforce. *Journal of Psychiatric and Mental Health Nursing, 23*(2), 129–135.

Wilkinson, S. (2014). How nurses can cope with stress and avoid burnout. *Emergency Nurse, 22*(7), 27–31.

CRITICAL THINKING QUESTIONS

1. What relationship do you see between your experience at the medication clinic and the issue of burnout?
2. How do you deal with feeling that you are not doing the best you can for the people for whom you provide care and their families?
3. What are the essential elements to keep in mind when approaching management to discuss your ideas?

QUALITIES THAT ENHANCE THERAPEUTIC RELATIONSHIPS

Self-awareness, empathy and moral integrity all enable mental health nurses to practise the use of self in therapeutic relationships. Some characteristics of artful therapeutic practice are respect for the person, availability, spontaneity, hope, acceptance, sensitivity, vision, accountability, advocacy, spirituality, empathy, critical thinking and self-disclosure. These personal characteristics will enhance your therapeutic relationships. The therapeutic relationship with individual consumers is the subject of Chapter 2.

Respect for the consumer

Respect emerges from the belief that human beings have inherent worth and dignity. The behaviour of some of the people you care for may indicate a loss of self-respect. Some may appear as though they don't care about their personal appearance. Others may plead, beg or cry. Still others may try to physically harm themselves or others. A relationship where there is unconditional positive regard, and where messages of respect from you are forthcoming, is of immeasurable value. Suggestions for how you can convey respect are listed in Your Intervention Strategies. Expressions of joy and assessments of abilities, talents and capabilities are often neglected. Focusing on strengths is an essential and respectful element of therapeutic practice.

> **YOUR INTERVENTION STRATEGIES**
> **Conveying respect**
>
> Keeping the following principles in mind will help you to convey respect:
>
> - Hold personal judgments in check.
> - Take the time and energy to actively listen.
> - Take care not to invalidate the person's experience of their world with comments such as 'It's not so bad', 'Don't be that way', 'Time heals all wounds' or 'Keep a stiff upper lip'.
> - Give people as much privacy as possible during assessments and treatments.
> - Minimise experiences that strip people of their identity. Facilitate people to make as many of their own choices and be in control of as much of their own lives as possible.
> - Be honest with people about medication, treatment, length of stay, and so on, even when the truth may be difficult to handle.
> - Create an atmosphere that conveys acceptance for the person to express distress as well as joy and pleasure.
> - Hold an inherent but realistic belief in the person's abilities and talents.
> - Ensure that you encourage the person to maintain agency in their life.

Availability

Of all the members of the mental health team, with the exception of peer support workers, the nurse has the richest opportunity to be available to consumers when needed. Because nurses are with those in their care on a relatively constant basis, they are responsible for:

- creating a nurturing, healing milieu
- assisting people to meet their basic human needs
- working with people in a collaborative recovery-focused way to achieve the best outcomes.

Spontaneity

Some nurses believe that therapeutic relationships require them to be stiff, stilted robots uttering clichés from a list of unnatural-sounding communication 'techniques'. Nurses who are comfortable with themselves, aware of therapeutic goals and flexible about using a repertoire of possible interventions find that being natural and spontaneous, while keeping therapeutic goals uppermost in their minds, is their most effective 'technique'. Consumers experience such nurses as authentic; that is, showing their real selves, rather than hiding behind the role of nurse. You are unique, and necessarily bring your own personal style to practice. Everyone has different ways of putting words together to convey to people that we accept and care about them. Sometimes we say it with non-verbal behaviour: keeping promises, being on time, touching and staying with a person who needs someone. We need to trust our own natural styles, combined with sound communication principles such as those discussed in Chapter 9, in working towards therapeutic goals.

Hope

Effective mental nursing practice is characterised by hope and optimism. A positive mental health nurse sees that, no matter how debilitated a person may present, they have the capacity for growth and change. Even people whose most marked deficits are chronicity and deterioration can be worked with to develop an optimal level of wellbeing. The Practice Example here shows a nurse who believes in possibilities, and one who is willing to search for strengths on which to build.

> **Practice example**
>
> Jamie, a creative nurse in a rehabilitation unit, encouraged David, a consumer, to partner with him to assist less-able people towards self-care. Jamie believed that this strategy—increasing the connectedness between himself and David and between David and other consumers—would decrease David's feeling of aloneness while emphasising David's ability to manage his own illness and his capacity to help others.

A key role in mental health nursing is to help people maintain and engender hope, the cornerstone of recovery. The primary obstacle to instilling hope is stigma. Keep in mind that many people lead fulfilling lives despite fairly disabling mental illness. You can have a negative impact on someone if you fail to believe in the person's recovery; if you fail to see them as a person; if you fail to lobby to reduce stigma in both the public and the health care communities; or if you fail to persevere with them in their journey of recovery.

Acceptance

There is a distinction between acceptance and approval. Acceptance means refraining from judging and rejecting a person who you personally dislike or who behaves in a way that makes you uncomfortable, as in the Practice Example that follows.

Practice example

Joan, a staff nurse on an acute inpatient unit, considered herself a faithful Christian who followed the teachings of the Bible. Two people often provided challenges to Joan's ability to accept them. Mary frequently cursed and swore. Sinesa bragged about her sexual prowess and her sexual encounters. Joan overcame these challenges by reminding herself that her place was not to impart moral judgments, and that behaviour can be influenced by illness.

Consumers can feel offended and demeaned if they perceive the nurse as rejecting them. Therapeutic work requires that people be able to examine, explore and understand their coping mechanisms without feeling the need to cover up or disguise them to avoid negative judgments or punishments. Nurses who tell consumers what they should say, or do or feel, deny people the acceptance they need to explore their problems.

Sensitivity

Genuine interest and concern provide the basis for a therapeutic relationship. People recognise the falseness of memorised phrases and assumed postures. You convey general interest and concern by trying to understand the person's perspective, working with them on mutually formulated goals, and persisting even when breakthroughs and improvements are subtle and slow, instead of dramatic and quick. Understanding their perceptions and concerns helps us to connect, acknowledges their importance and facilitates the therapeutic relationship.

Assertiveness

Assertiveness is the ability to express one's feelings, thoughts and beliefs openly, even if doing so is emotionally difficult or personal risk is involved. Assertiveness is a style of interacting with others that protects your rights without depriving others of theirs. It involves standing up for yourself in a non-destructive manner, even if your stance is unpopular.

Being assertive in a therapeutic context means that you are able to take advantage of opportunities to make interpersonal contact with consumers. Confident nurses are assertive nurses, and they recognise that assertiveness and caring are compatible.

Often, people are either so timid that they do not get what they want, or so aggressive and belligerent that they offend and alienate others. Being assertive in one's professional life builds upon being assertive in one's personal life. **Assertive behaviour** is asking for what one wants or acting to get it in a way that respects other people. It is midway between **passive behaviour** (timid holding back) and **aggressive behaviour** (inconsiderate, offensive aggression).

Compare the passive, aggressive and assertive behaviours listed in the Self-awareness feature, below, to see which descriptions best characterise your behaviour with others. Fortunately, old behaviours can be unlearned, and new behaviours can be learned.

Passive behaviour

Fear tends to be the major feeling in passive responses—fear of being embarrassed, of disappointing someone or making someone angry. Because of fear, passive people frequently say 'yes' at the expense of their own happiness or well-being, even when they want to say 'no'. To these individuals, everyone else's feelings and needs are more important than their own. Imagine what could happen if four passive individuals arrive at a four-way traffic stop at approximately the same time. Believing that the others have more important things to do and places to be, no one takes the initiative.

SELF-AWARENESS
Comparing your own passive, aggressive and assertive behaviours

Determine which of the following descriptions most closely match your behaviour. Once you have finished, develop a personal plan for adopting a wider range of assertive behaviours in both your personal life and your professional life.

Passive	Aggressive	Assertive
'I'm not angry (but I am scared)!'	'I'm not scared (but I am angry)!'	'I'm both angry and scared!'
'I always do everything wrong.'	'They always do everything wrong.'	'Neither one of us is perfect, and there's nothing wrong with that.'
'I'll try to make it (but I don't intend to, because I'm resentful of your demands).'	'Get over yourself. I'm not coming. Who do you think you are?'	'We should spend some time together and talk about our relationship.'
'I never achieve my goals.'	'The only way I can achieve my goals is by forcing others to agree with my way of thinking.'	'I almost always achieve the goals I set for myself.'
'I wish someone else would speak up.'	'Be quiet and let me speak. You always monopolise the conversation.'	'We can both have a chance to speak.'

All are fearful of angering or insulting the others. They sit there, waving one another on. People who consistently give up control are often left with resentment in their interpersonal relationships.

Aggressive behaviour

Aggressive responses are at the other end of the continuum of interaction. The three hallmarks of aggressive behaviour are:

1. the major feeling is anger
2. the person says 'no', even when 'yes' could, or should, be said
3. the aggressive person believes that their feelings are more important than the feelings of others.

Collegial aggression among nurses is not uncommon (Edward, Ousey, Warelow & Lui, 2014). Generally speaking, people who feel in the least control can be the most aggressive. Some examples are: a bully, a subordinate at work with little control over others, or someone who shouts angrily, talks over others and insists that there is only one way to do something. Imagine what could happen if four aggressive individuals arrive at a four-way stop simultaneously. Each believes that they have the right to go first. Each is angry with the others and attempts to be the first to cross the intersection. Perhaps all four crash in the middle of the intersection.

Assertive behaviour

People who focus on neither anger nor fear, respect their own and others' feelings, and say 'yes' and 'no' appropriately, behave assertively. Imagine what could happen if four assertive individuals arrive at a four-way stop at the same time. Recognising traffic rules and the rights of others, each allows the person on the right the opportunity to proceed first.

Everyone has assertiveness potential, but not everyone has learned how to be assertive. You can teach people how to behave assertively by incorporating the guidelines in the Collaborative Care feature on page 333 in Chapter 15.

Vision

Mental health nurses facilitate recovery by enhancing quality of life. As such, you need to come to terms with a personal and professional vision of what 'quality of life' means. Some conditions of life associated with high quality are influence or power, freedom, accountability, self-determinism, openness to gratifying experience, action, mastery, a sense of purpose or meaning, privacy, hope, stability, non-violence and intimacy. Mental health nurses facilitate opportunities for these life conditions.

Accountability

According to Peplau (1980), the need for personal accountability—professional integrity—is greater in mental health practice than in any other type of health care. People in mental health settings are often more vulnerable and defenceless than people in other health care settings, particularly because their thinking processes and their relationships with others may be compromised.

You are accountable for the nature of the effort you make on behalf of those in your care, and answerable for the quality of your efforts. As Peplau put it, 'Personal accountability is an attitude—a quality of the heart and mind of those professionals who are competent and determined that every psychiatric patient will have the best problem-resolving assistance possible' (1980, p. 133).

Mental health nurses are also accountable to themselves, their peers, their profession and the public in the following ways:

- Accountability to self involves bringing personal behaviour under conscious control so that the nurse becomes the person-as-nurse that they want to be.
- Accountability to peers involves engaging in peer review with nursing colleagues to give and receive feedback intended to improve the quality of care. Clinical supervision helps with this.
- Accountability to the profession involves clarifying the role of the mental health nurse, keeping current with changes in the field, and encouraging self-regulation to protect the public and enhance the quality of care. The Australian College of Mental Health Nurses (ACMHN) is the peak professional organisation for mental health nurses in Australia (see: www.acmhn.org).
- Accountability to the public requires keeping abreast of knowledge in the field, becoming credentialled according to level of competence, applying the ACMHN standards of mental health nursing practice, and protecting the rights of the people in your care and their families.

The personally accountable mental health nurse will insist on clinical supervision, which is a means of professional development (Moxham & Gagan, 2015). Supervision provides novice and experienced nurses with the opportunity to learn therapeutic techniques and attitudes. It enables them to receive validation, insight and support during challenging times, and enables them to analyse how they affect the outcome of relationships.

Advocacy

Throughout history, mental health nurses have been ardent supporters of a neglected, ignored and forgotten population—people who live with mental illness. In the 21st century, there is a need for new energy and political activism. In the era of mental health care reform, there is an especially important concern—ensuring that the consumer is at the centre of, or ideally leading, their own planning, evaluating care and treatment. Collaborative recovery is paramount, with the national review of mental health services indicating that working with consumers is vital, and Hurley et al. (2016) talking about the implications for the mental health nursing workforce.

Nurses are more politically aware than ever before. A newly energised political activism calls for you to be a strong advocate for those people to whom you provide care and work with.

Successful advocacy is a positive experience for nurses as well as for consumers. Everyone derives a benefit, and being an agent of change is part of the role of a mental health nurse.

Be aware, however, that not all advocating will be successful. Sometimes, despite our most earnest and well-intentioned efforts, we fail in our attempt to advocate for positive change.

Spirituality

Spirituality, the search for meaning and purpose in life through a connection with others, Nature and/or a belief in a higher power, is at the core of each person's existence. Spirituality varies in strength from person to person. Some people already have a meaningful philosophy of life. Others, on a spiritual journey, search for life's meaning and purpose. Still others experience hopelessness, despair and spiritual distress. Helping people find meaning and purpose in their lives empowers them.

For some people, their spirituality becomes a focus in their recovery. They may attempt to resolve internal conflicts or conflicts with others through religious rituals or practices. Other people have behaviours that involve religiosity rather than spirituality (Sessanna, Finnell, Underhill, Change & Peng, 2011). To differentiate between religiosity and spirituality, see Box 4.2 on spirituality.

Research indicates that the connection between mind, body and spirit is complex, and that spirituality is influenced by culture. You need to be aware of the person's source of hope and strength. Helping someone in their search for meaning and purpose is possible when nurses have beliefs that sustain them rather than beliefs that are sources of conflict. Meeting your own spiritual needs will enhance the relationships that you have with others. Take the time to carefully consider the questions in the Self-awareness feature on spiritual growth to determine whether you meet your own spiritual needs.

Box 4.2 Spirituality: helping others rediscover their spiritual path

Spirituality is the third part of the triad known as mind–body–spirit in the holistic practice of nursing. In ancient times, spirit meant breath—as essential to life as air. Spirituality is that part of every person that yearns to share the beauty, love and joyfulness of the universe.

Our spirituality comes from many sources: Nature, a belief in a higher being and a connection to other people. Although many of these sources are incorporated into organised religions, spirituality is not religion, nor is religion spirituality. Religion is the organisation of a set of beliefs, practices and rituals, whereas spirituality is a reflection of one's 'spirit' and its relationship to the rest of the universe. People develop their spirituality in different ways, and people can also lose their spiritual path.

Helping someone rediscover their spiritual path is a fulfilling role for mental health nurses. You can help someone find out who they really are, beyond, for example, simply husband, father, lover, police officer or a mental illness diagnosis. Identifying sources of inner energy is empowering. Spirituality is, though, a deeply personal inner experience, as opposed to a set of behaviours tied to an externally imposed doctrine or ritual. By offering a simple spirituality inventory, such as that in the Spiritual Health Assessment box in Chapter 10 on page 207, you encourage the person to look at the strength of their faith, which will help them on their recovery journey. Faith is a way of being, it is about being open to possibilities, and to healing. It provides hope.

SELF-AWARENESS
Spiritual growth assessment

To help you on your personal journey of spiritual growth, contemplate the following:

1. What gives the greatest meaning or purpose to your life?
2. How do you express your spirituality or your philosophy of life?
3. What do you do to show love for yourself?
4. What brings joy and peace to your life?
5. How do you heal your spirit?
6. What art, music or literature nurtures your spirit?
7. How does your spirituality affect your practice as a nurse?

Empathy

Comprehension of, and ability to use, the process of empathy is one strategy for responding to the feelings of aloneness often experienced by people who have a mental illness. Perhaps the most important function of empathic understanding is to give the person the very precious feeling of being understood and cared about.

Empathy is a pervasive phenomenon in the life experience of all people. **Empathy** can be defined as the ability to feel what others feel, and to respond to and understand the experience of others on their terms. A nurse who empathises with someone momentarily abandons the personal self and relives the emotions and responses of that person. People in everyday life tend to empathise most with those to whom they feel closest. In mental health work, seeking to empathise with those from whom we feel most separate, or whose closeness threatens our own sense of integration, is important.

The capacity for empathy relies on personal integration. A firm sense of self is necessary for a person to be a good empathiser. As we continue to interact with others, we learn to be sensitive to others without losing our own integration. The role of empathy in facilitating communication is discussed in Chapter 9.

Critical thinking

Critical thinking aids in the transfer of nursing knowledge into clinical practice. It is a purposeful mental activity in which ideas are produced and evaluated, and judgments are made. A critical thinker analyses information before drawing conclusions about it. **Critical thinking** can be defined as purposeful, reasonable, reflective thinking that drives problem-solving and decision-making, and aims to make judgments based on evidence.

The ability to think critically is crucial for mental health nurses, because the complexity of care makes critical-thinking skills urgent. Critical thinking mobilises intrapersonal, interpersonal, perceptual, moral/ethical, experiential, practical, scientific and contextual knowledge, all of which are elemental in providing safe and effective care (Rubenfeld & Scheffer, 2015).

Critical thinking challenges occur throughout this text. To develop effective critical-thinking habits, implement the strategies suggested in Your Intervention Strategies, below.

YOUR INTERVENTION STRATEGIES Promoting critical thinking

Strategy	Rationale
Anticipate questions others might ask, such as 'What will my Nurse Unit Manager (NUM) or facilitator want to know?'	This helps identify a wider scope of questions that must be answered to gain relevant information.
Ask 'What if . . . ?' questions like 'What if something goes wrong?' or 'What if we try?'	This helps you to be proactive and creative.
Look for flaws in your thinking. Ask questions like 'What is missing?', 'Have I recognised my biases?', 'How could this be made better?'	Such questions help you evaluate your thinking and make improvements.
Ask someone else to look for flaws in your thinking.	You are usually too close to your own work to be objective; others bring a fresh eye and possibly new ideas and perspectives.
Develop 'good habits of inquiry' (habits that aid in the search for the truth, such as always keeping an open mind, verifying information and taking enough time).	These habits can make critical thinking more automatic.
Develop interpersonal skills, such as conflict resolution and getting along with those who have different communication styles.	If you do not have good interpersonal skills, you are unlikely to get the help or information you need to think critically.
Replace 'I do not know' and 'I am not sure' with 'I will try'.	This demonstrates you have the ability to find answers, and mobilises you to locate resources.
Turn errors into learning opportunities.	We all make mistakes; they are stepping stones to maturity and new ideas.

LIVED EXPERIENCE

Most people who have received voluntary and involuntary treatment will have memories of nurses who made a difference in their recovery. I remember a nurse, whom I now work with in my role as a peer support worker, who cared for me during my last admission, in 2005. I recall her real interest in me as a person, a father, a husband, a teacher, and I valued the therapeutic, empathetic relationship that we built. She still works in much the same way today! I remember another nurse, during an admission in 1985, who was a beacon of compassion on a ward characterised by coercion, sedation and seclusion. Unfortunately, I also remember another nurse on that same ward who threatened and acted on his threats.

A beautiful account of the power of nursing in personal recovery can be found in Kate Richard's *Madness: A memoir* (2013). Kate, now a doctor and an award-winning Australian writer, experienced years of psychotic depression, where abusive voices would cause her to inflict horrific self-harm. Her recovery was aided by medication and a long-term relationship with her psychotherapist, but she also recounts two inpatient stays when her primary nurse made significant contributions to her recovery.

She writes of one nurse, Damien: 'We talk about hope. He has an extraordinary faith that I'll recover, and as I do get better, I hold onto him, like we are together clutching the strings of a balloon . . . Damien and I talk about the business of getting better. We talk about the importance of space and time and the importance of being heard.'

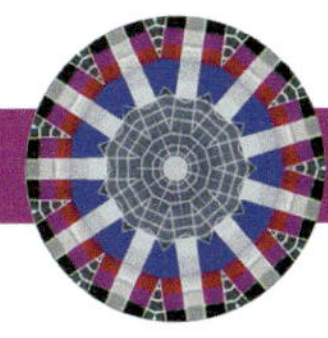

REFERENCES

Benner, P., & Wrubel, J. (1989). Coping with caregiving. In P. Benner & J. Wrubel, *The primacy of caring: Stress and coping in health and illness* (pp. 365–406). Menlo Park, CA: Addison-Wesley.

Domen, R., Connelly, C. D., & Spence, D. (2015). Call-shift fatigue and use of countermeasures and avoidance strategies by certified nurse anesthetists: A national survey. *AANA Journal*, *83*(2) 123–131.

Drury, V., Craigie, M., Francis, K., Aoun, S., & Hegney D. G. (2014). Compassion satisfaction, compassion fatigue, anxiety, depression and stress in registered nurses in Australia: Phase 2 results. *Journal of Nursing Management*, *22*(4), 519–531.

Edward, K.-L., Ousey, K., Warelow, P., & Lui, S. (2014). Nursing and aggression in the workplace: A systematic review. *British Journal of Nursing*, *23*(12), 653–659.

Fletcher, D., & Sarkar, M. (2013). Psychological resilience: A review and critique of definitions, concepts and theory. *European Psychologist*, *18*(1), 12–23.

Hegney, D. G., Craigie, M., Hemsworth, D., Osseiran-Moisson, R., Aoun, S., Francis, K., & Drury, V. (2014). Compassion satisfaction, compassion fatigue, anxiety, depression and stress in registered nurses in Australia: Study 1 results. *Journal of Nursing Management*, *22*(4), 506–518.

Hurley, J., Cashin, A., Mills, J., Hutchinson, M., & Graham, I. (2016) A critical discussion of peer workers: Implications for the mental health nursing workforce. *Journal of Psychiatric and Mental Health Nursing*, *23*(2), 129–135.

Kang, J.-H., Miao, N.-F., Tseng, I.-J., Sithole, T., & Chung, M.-H. (2015). Circadian activity rhythms and sleep in nurses working fixed 8-hr shifts. *Biological Research for Nursing, 17*(3), 348–355.

Klumpers, U. M. H., Veltman, D. J., van Tol, M.-J., Kloet, R. W., Boellaard, R., Lammertsma, A. A., & Hoogendijk, W. J. G. (2015). Neurophysiological effects of sleep deprivation in healthy adults, a pilot study. *PLoS ONE*, *10*(1), e0116906. doi:10.1371/journal.pone.0116906

McEwen, B. S., & Karatsoreos, I. N. (2015). Sleep deprivation and circadian disruption: Stress, allostasis and allostatic load. *Sleep Medicine Clinics*, *10*(1), 1–10.

Moxham, L., & Gagan, A. (2015). Clinical supervision as a means of professional development in nursing. *Australian Nursing and Midwifery Journal*, *23*(2), 37.

National Mental Health Commission (NMHC). (2014). Contributing lives, thriving communities: Report of the national review of mental health programmes and services, NMHC. Sydney, Australia: NMHC.

Peplau, H. E. (1980). The psychiatric nurse—accountable? To whom? For what? *Perspectives in Psychiatric Care*, *18*(3), 128–134.

Richards, K. (2013). *Madness: A memoir.* Melbourne, Australia: Penguin Books.

Rubenfeld, M. G., & Scheffer, B. K. (2015). *Critical thinking tactics for nurses* (3rd ed.). Burlington, NY: Jones and Bartlett.

Sessanna, L., Finnell, D. S., Underhill, M., Chang, Y.P., & Peng, H. L. (2011). Measures assessing spirituality as more than religiosity: A methodological review of nursing and health-related literature. *Journal of Advanced Nursing*, *67*(8), 1677–1694.

Shinde, M. B., & Hiremath, P. (2014). Stressors, level of stress and coping mechanism adopted by undergraduate nursing students. *International Journal of Nursing Education*, *6*(2), 231–234. doi: 10.5958/0974-9357.2014.00640.0

Todaro-Franceschi, V. (2013). *Compassion fatigue and burnout in nursing*. New York, NY: Springer.

Wilkinson, S. (2014). How nurses can cope with stress and avoid burnout. *Emergency Nurse*, *22*(7): 27–31.

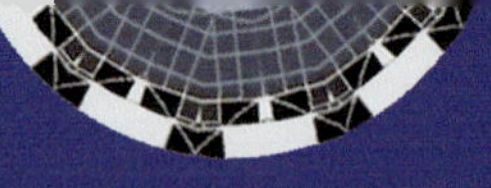

5

Theories for interdisciplinary care in mental health

MIKE HAZELTON AND SIMON SWINSON

KEY TERMS

castration anxiety *82*
client-centred therapy *86*
cognitive-behavioural theory *82*
conditioned response *82*
conditioning *83*
conscious *80*
ego *81*
Electra complex *82*
general systems theory *87*
holistic *78*
humanism *77*
id *81*
interpersonal theory *84*
negative reinforcement *83*
Oedipus complex *82*
operant conditioning *83*
penis envy *82*
positive reinforcement *83*
psychoanalysis *80*
psychoanalytic theory *80*
psychobiology *78*
recovery *75*
reflected appraisals *84*
reinforcement *83*
self-actualisation *86*
self-system *84*
shaping *83*
superego *81*
symbolic interactionism *76*
token economy *83*
unconditional positive regard *86*
unconscious *80*

LEARNING OUTCOMES

After completing this chapter, you will be able to:

1. Discuss the principles of recovery-oriented mental health practice.
2. Discuss the major ideas of interactionism.
3. Discuss the major principles of humanism.
4. Describe the influence of recent knowledge development in psychobiology.
5. Explain how the premises of human interactionism and psychobiology relate to psychiatric–mental health nursing.
6. Compare and contrast the assumptions and key ideas of medical-psychobiological, psychoanalytic, cognitive behavioural, and social-interpersonal theories.
7. Discuss the implications of each theory for the practice of psychiatric–mental health nursing.

LIVED EXPERIENCE

For me, medications are not 'magic bullets', which is what both my family and I thought initially. My improvement was so slow and gradual that medication proved to be a steadying influence, contributing to the possibility of recovery over time. However, it was still necessary for me to work hard on myself, which has involved years of therapy, especially interpersonal psychotherapy.

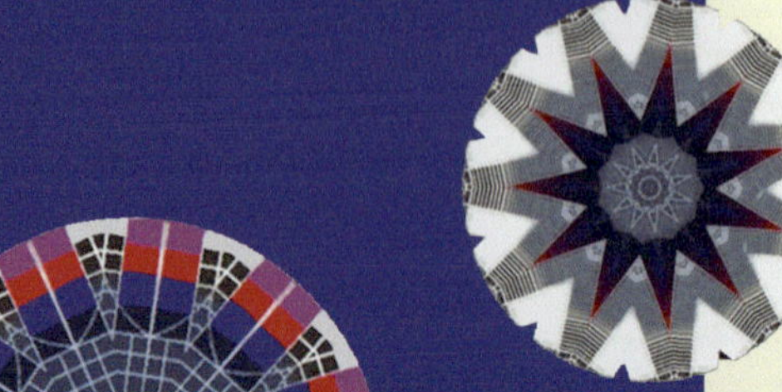

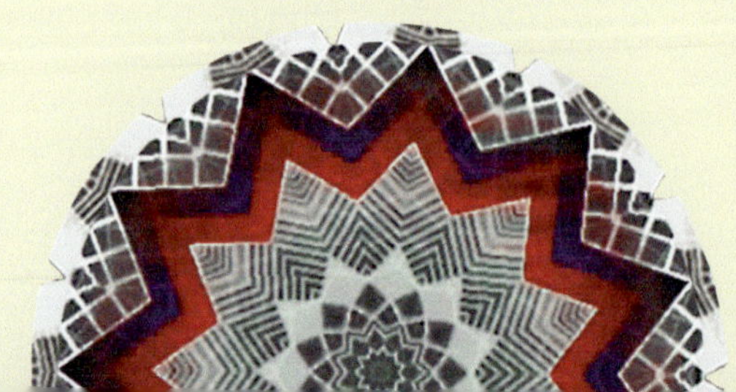

INTRODUCTION

To practise psychiatric–mental health nursing humanistically, you must devote yourself to understanding what makes people human, how they express their joy of living, their sadness, their desire to love, their hopes for growth. Understanding these phenomena becomes even more crucial when trying to explain how the joy of living may turn into the desire to die, how love of self and others may turn to violence and hate, how the hope for recovery may turn to withdrawal and despair, and how alterations in the brain might relate to these human experiences.

This chapter introduces you to a holistic philosophy that includes humanism, interactionism, knowledge development in psychobiology, and the rise to prominence of the concept of recovery in mental health care. In this chapter, we also compare the basic assumptions and implications for practice in the dominant theories for interdisciplinary mental health care, considering these in relation to the key values of recovery-oriented mental health practice. These are as follows:

- medical-psychobiologic theory
- psychoanalytic theory
- cognitive behavioural theory
- social-interpersonal theories.

Clinicians often say they are *eclectic*; that is, they choose one or a combination of these theories in determining what information to assess about people living with mental illness, what intervention outcomes and approaches to recommend, and what ultimate evaluation criteria to set. We believe that clinicians *should* be eclectic, where possible choosing strategies based on scientific evidence about their effectiveness for any given person they are working with. The best strategies based on the best available evidence are reviewed in every chapter of this book. However, this evidence on what works best in mental health treatments must be balanced against what is preferred by the person who must live with the illness and the treatments recommended for the illness. It is in this lived experience context that recovery has become the most important aspect of mental health thought and practice.

Your approach to understanding the experience of people living with mental illness is influenced by your philosophy. We believe, further, that humanistic interactionism is the philosophy that provides the best starting point for psychiatric–mental health nursing goals, especially if approached in relation to recovery principles. Theories such as those discussed in this chapter provide the conceptual tools to formulate that understanding, and to interpret mental health-related clinical data and lived experience. Blend an understanding of these theories with the nursing theories discussed in Chapter 3, and especially the psychiatric–mental health nursing theory of Hildegard Peplau, which is discussed in Chapter 2.

RECOVERY-ORIENTED MENTAL HEALTH PRACTICE

Tondora, Miller, Slade and Davison (2014: 1) suggest that **recovery** involves living a fulfilling life in the context of facing the challenges associated with mental illness. Various approaches have been proposed for understanding the main characteristics of recovery in mental health. Leamy, Bird, Le Boutillier, Williams and Slade (2011) have suggested that for many people the experience of recovery involves at least the following:

- refusing to define self-worth by the experience of mental illness
- participating in the community as a family member, worker, neighbour, friend, citizen
- taking responsibility for and making decisions about one's own life
- engaging with a personal and social support network beyond the mental health system
- celebrating the strengths and capabilities gained from living with and recovering from mental illness
- maintaining hope and optimism for the future.

While policy-makers and health professionals have been criticised for approaching recovery in ways that are often tokenistic (Hamer, Finlayson & Warren, 2014), the concept has become central to mental health policy and practice in many countries, including Australia. For instance, the Commonwealth Department of Health and Ageing (2013) has released a *National framework for recovery-oriented mental health services*. The influence of the recovery movement now even extends into considerations of the types of research that are consistent with the principles of recovery-oriented practice (Gordon & Ellis, 2013).

SCOPE OF PSYCHIATRIC–MENTAL HEALTH NURSING PRACTICE

All nurses are concerned with the quality of human life and its relationship to health. The psychiatric–mental health nurse is especially concerned with the relationship between the individual's optimal psychobiological health and feelings of self-worth, personal integrity, self-fulfilment and creative expression. Just as important are the satisfying of basic living needs, comfortable relationships with others, and the recognition of human rights.

Our scope of practice is broad enough to include issues such as alienation, identity crises, sudden life changes and troubled family interactions. It may deal with poverty and affluence, the experiences of birth and death, the loss of significant others, or the loss of body parts. It is concerned with sustaining and enhancing the individual and the group. Yet it also must address basic life issues shared by people living with mental illness—eating, sleeping, grooming and hygiene. This broad-ranging, humanistic, interactional and psychobiological view of the scope of psychiatric–mental health nursing is different in important ways from the medical or behavioural science orientations of the past 50 years.

Psychiatric–mental health nurses are concerned with the care of people living with mental illness. However, our concerns extend to the wide range of human responses to mental distress, disability and disorder. For example, a parent living with addiction may not only suffer from shame, unemployment and abusive outbursts of anger, but may also lose a sense of purpose and meaning, and experience a disturbed self-concept and spiritual distress. These responses may have detrimental effects on the health of children, partners and other significant people in the person's life.

Like many concepts in the human sciences, the concept of mental disorder lacks a definition that covers all situations. Faced with such a diverse array of human problems, the psychiatric–mental health nurse is challenged to synthesise a holistic philosophy for practice that can be the basis for care.

HUMANISTIC INTERACTIONISM AND PSYCHOBIOLOGY: THE MIND–BODY–SPIRIT CONNECTION

The classic psychiatric and psychological approaches have described and classified signs and symptoms of *illness*, then accounted for it by individual psychological dynamics such as character disorder, weak ego or failed defence mechanisms. The basis for this text is a synthesis of psychosocial and psychobiological knowledge required for practice in the 21st century.

Basic premises of interactionism

One central idea in the approach we advocate has come to be known as **symbolic interactionism** (Hewitt & Shulman, 2011), a term that describes an approach to the study of human conduct. It is based on the philosophical premises identified in Box 5.1.

Box 5.1 Symbolic interactionism: philosophical premises

1. People act with plans and purposes in mind, and have the capacity to think of new ways to act by finding alternative goals and alternative methods.
2. Human beings act towards things (other people, events) on the basis of the meaning that the things have for them; that is, meaning is a basis for behaviour. Life experiences may have different meanings for different people.
3. The meaning of things in a person's life arises from, and is transformed by, the social interactions that person has with others. We learn meanings during our experiences with others.
4. People handle and modify the meanings of the things they encounter through an interpretive process. They come to their own conclusions.
5. People want to regard themselves favourably and to maintain and enhance their self-esteem.
6. When human beings encounter situations they have not faced before, they must find new meanings, new purposes and new methods to deal with these novel situations.
7. As human beings, we inherit a society and a culture within which we live; however, we do not have to reproduce it.

Implications for psychiatric–mental health nursing practice

Interactionism offers psychiatric–mental health nursing a perspective of human beings as having purpose and control over their lives, even if they must live with altered brain structure and chemistry and stressful environments. Interactionism as interpreted in this chapter provides the premise for a philosophy of caring with a strong humanistic cast, such as that described in Evidence-based Practice. Interactionism acknowledges the interaction of psychology, psychobiology and sociocultural contexts.

EVIDENCE-BASED PRACTICE

Strategy of protective empowering

Ellen, a clinical nurse consultant working in a residential rehabilitation service is working with Rebecca, a 35-year-old woman living with schizophrenia. In addition to schizophrenia, Rebecca has a history of amphetamine and cannabis dependence, gambling, pathological stealing, adult antisocial behaviour, relationship issues and Hepatitis C. Rebecca has had multiple hospital admissions and has been in prison for shoplifting. Given this history, little hope was held for her recovery by most members of the treatment team. However, Rebecca stated that she wanted to get control of her life; she agreed to work with Ellen using dialectical behaviour therapy (DBT)—especially distress tolerance, mindfulness and radical acceptance skills. After six months of DBT skills work, it was felt that the progress Rebecca had made offset the risks of her living in the community. She was discharged from hospital to her own unit. In the 12 months since being discharged, Rebecca has not resumed substance use, and regularly participates in a community rehabilitation program. The approach to working with Rebecca outlined above has much in common with the strategy of protective empowering outlined in the following grounded theory research:

Chiovitti, R. F. (2011). Theory of protective empowering for balancing patient safety and choices. *Nursing Ethics, 18*(1), 88–101.

CRITICAL THINKING QUESTIONS

1. How does protective empowerment fit with the basic premises of humanistic interactionism?
2. How does protective empowerment fit with the basic premises of psychobiological theory?
3. How does protective empowerment fit with the basic premises of cognitive behavioural theory?
4. How does protective empowerment fit with the principles of recovery-oriented practice?

The first premise: behaviour is purposeful People act with plans and purposes in mind. That is, human conduct is directed towards some goal or purpose. However, once people set their conduct in motion they may be deflected from their intended paths by obstacles or more appealing objects. Goals and purposes are not fixed and final—they emerge and change as we go about our lives. Behaviour arises from, and is affected by, our interactions with others.

The second premise: different meanings for different people All behaviour has meaning. To understand the actions of people with lived experience, you must identify the meanings those actions have for them. Be wary of interventions that ignore, discount or discredit the meaning an experience has for a person in favour of your own definition of the situation. Thus, you must develop skill in observing, interpreting and responding to the person's lived experiences in the hope of arriving at a common ground of negotiated meanings and authentic communication.

The third premise: meanings arise in one's social world Meanings arise in the *process* of interaction with others. It is essential, therefore, that psychiatric–mental health nurses take into account the social and cultural environment of each person. A holistic assessment of a person living with mental illness accounts for the interaction patterns in that person's social world. People living with mental illness may purposefully choose to dress contrary to the expectations of the health professional staff involved in their care and treatment. Tattoos, unconventional hairstyles, colourful modes of dress may all represent statements of belonging and cultural expression.

The fourth premise: meaning is individually interpreted People come to their own conclusions. You need to keep this premise in mind when responding to an expression of human distress. People handle situations in terms of what they consider vitally important about the situation. Avoid saying 'I wouldn't worry about it' or 'Don't feel that way', 'You are reacting inappropriately' or 'It's not so bad.' Such clichés are not usually helpful, not because they are inherently non-therapeutic, but because voicing them invalidates the basic premise that people interpret the world in their own way.

The fifth premise: self as a valued object Human beings want to regard themselves favourably and to attach a positive value to the self. Human beings desire to act in ways that will develop and sustain coherent images of themselves. They also wish to find a sense of security and place—a sense of social identity—by integrating themselves into group life. They take themselves—their feelings, their interests and their images of self—into account as they act.

The sixth premise: new ways of being It is within interpersonal interaction that people can learn new definitions for life situations and new repertoires for action; indeed, this would seem at the heart of contemporary notions of recovery. This is the heart of the psychiatric–mental health nurse's therapeutic and caring role. The sensitive, intelligent and humanistic use of self within interpersonal relationships is a key part of the psychiatric–mental health nurse's skill. You have the potential for helping people redefine their experiences in more satisfying ways, learn new patterns of coping with stress, and generally enhance the quality of their lives and social worlds. Such is the essence of psychiatric–mental health nursing.

The seventh premise: culture shapes conduct People are born into an already existing society and culture, and are surrounded by others who define reality for us. Human beings are not required to keep cultural definitions set by others. Culture is an environment in which we all live. However, we do not have to reproduce the society and culture that we inherit. In many instances, our survival depends on coming to terms with the culture we have inherited.

Basic premises of humanism

One of the purposes of this chapter is to specify a philosophical basis for subsequent chapters. The seven premises of interactionism provide us with a basic orientation. A theory of life centred on human beings, called **humanism**, adds to the philosophical perspective. The humanistic perspective views human nature as basically 'good', emphasises present conscious processes, and places strong emphasis on people's inherent capacity for self-direction (Butcher, Mineka & Hooley, 2010). It pays less attention to the unconscious processes and past causes emphasised by some of the theories (see, for example, psychoanalytic theory) discussed later in this chapter. It first arose as a reaction against the psychoanalytic and behaviourist perspectives (Ciccarelli & White, 2009).

The central concept of humanism is that the chief end of human life is to work for wellbeing within the limitations of life in today's world. Humanism is a philosophy of service to benefit humanity through reason, science and democracy. The humanistic perspective has seven central propositions (Lamont, 1967) identified in Box 5.2.

Box 5.2 Humanistic perspective: philosophical premises

1. The human being's mind is indivisibly connected with the body.
2. Human beings have the power or potential to solve their own problems.
3. Human beings, while influenced by the past, possess freedom of creative choice and action, and are, within certain limits, masters of their own destinies.
4. Human values are grounded in life experiences and relationships, and our highest goal must be the happiness, freedom and growth of all people.
5. Individuals attain wellbeing and a high quality of life by harmoniously combining personal satisfactions with activities that contribute to the welfare of the community.
6. We should apply reason, science and democratic procedures in all areas of life.
7. We must continually examine our basic convictions, including those of humanism.

Implications for psychiatric–mental health nursing practice

As a philosophy underlying psychiatric–mental health nursing practice, a humanistic perspective means devotion to the interests of human beings wherever they live and whatever their status or culture. It reaffirms the spirit of compassion and caring towards others. It is a constructive philosophy that wholeheartedly affirms the joys, beauty and values of human living. If nurses and other health professionals approach their work in ways that acknowledge and support the autonomy, dignity and complexity of individuals and groups, such caring practices are strengthening possibilities for humanisation (Todres, Galvin & Holloway, 2009).

The subsequent chapters in this text show how these basic premises can be put to use in psychiatric–mental health nursing practice. Some fundamental concepts are described briefly in the following sections.

A holistic view of the mind–body relationship A humanistic interactional view proposes that physical and mental factors are interrelated, and that a change in one may result in a change in another. For example, anger may result in increased blood pressure. An invading organism, a decrease in a neurotransmitter, or a structural change in the body can alter thought processes. Low self-esteem can result in hunched shoulders and skeletal muscle contractures.

There are important implications for psychiatric–mental health nursing in such an approach. Healing and caring must be approached in a **holistic** manner, recognising physical and psychosocial needs and preferences. That is, the psychiatric–mental health nurse deals with the biological aspects of a primarily psychological or emotional pattern, and the psychological or emotional aspects of biological experiences, as in the following Practice Example.

Practice example

Kate, a prominent television personality who wants to remain anonymous, is admitted to the private mental health unit where you are working. She weighs under 40 kilograms, which is extremely thin for her 170-centimetre frame, and is dehydrated, malnourished and preoccupied with getting back to work and looking good in an industry in which the majority of women news presenters are thin.

As a nurse educated to recognise both her physical and psychosocial needs and strengths, you are challenged to work with Kate and other members of her treatment team to formulate a holistic, integrated care plan.

What you will learn in this text is relevant not only in mental health care settings. You can use the philosophies, theories, concepts and principles in the care of any person, no matter the setting, even if their immediate problems are primarily physical.

An expanded role for nurses The humanistic interactional perspective on mental illness implies an expanded role for psychiatric–mental health nurses. We believe that nurses should be prepared to work for change within social and political systems. Psychiatric–mental health nursing must not be limited to activities designed to merely control psychiatric symptoms and increase the capability of people living with mental illness to adjust to prevailing social conditions. Instead, psychiatric–mental health nursing must be involved in social goals that advance health holistically and support recovery. Because psychiatric–mental health nursing has political consequences, it is essential that you begin to develop a philosophical and ethical framework to guide and evaluate the political outcome of therapeutic intervention (Hazelton & Rossiter, 2016). Joining a professional organisation such as the Australian College of Mental Health Nurses (www.acmhn.org/) provides opportunities to become engaged in wider professional and political activities relevant to psychiatric–mental health nursing.

Negotiation and advocacy In this textbook, the model for intervention and change is one of negotiation and advocacy. The responsibility for change remains with the person who engages with psychiatric help or consultation as part of pursuing recovery. As with all citizens, people living with mental illness retain accountability for their own actions. They are not the passive recipients of care given by mental health professionals. Instead, they are empowered in the process of developing new perspectives, and encouraged to weigh alternatives and make self-directed choices. They and their families are educated about their mental illness and its treatment.

Basic premises of psychobiology

The past decades have seen major developments in knowledge about the brain, the mind, the spirit and behaviour. Many of these advances have taken place in a field of study called **psychobiology** or behavioural neuroscience. Research has generated new understandings of how genetics, immunology, biorhythms, brain structure and brain biochemistry might influence mental disorders (discussed in Chapter 6).

New imaging techniques make it possible to view what has never been seen before. Neuroscientists have found that our thoughts, sensations, joys and aches consist of physiological activity in the 100 billion neurons in the tissues of the brain. They can tell a lot about what people are thinking from the blood flow in their brains; whether a person is thinking about a face or a place, or whether the person is looking at a bottle or a shoe.

Medications that seek to correct biochemical imbalances in the brain are now being prescribed. Psychobiological interventions, such as exposure to bright light and white noise, and the restriction of nutrients and non-nutrients believed to affect behaviour, have become commonplace.

Implications for psychiatric–mental health nursing practice

Some authorities argue that psychiatric–mental health nurses should continue to focus on the human aspects of care as psychiatry moves towards 're-medicalisation'. The fear is that by embracing the biological sciences we will diminish the art of psychiatric–mental health nursing. Others contend that, to bring a contemporary holistic perspective to psychiatric–mental health nursing care, we must integrate the rapidly accumulating knowledge in psychobiology. We should not give up our humanistic, psychosocial and interactional premises simply because we recognise the value of the advances being made in psychobiology. Instead, as we redefine the traditional art of psychiatric–mental health nursing care and caring in contemporary society, our practice and research must integrate 'high tech' and 'high touch', nature and nurture, the biological sciences and the behavioural sciences, all within the context of recovery-focused care.

THEORIES FOR INTERDISCIPLINARY MENTAL HEALTH CARE

Dominant social attitudes and philosophical viewpoints have influenced the understanding of, and approaches to, mental disorder throughout history. Concepts and theories that we consider modern may have roots in earlier eras. (See Chapter 1 for a discussion of the history of social attitudes towards mental illness and Figure 1.2 on pages 12–13 for a timeline illustrating these shifts in viewpoints.)

Table 5.1 ■ compares the major features of the medical-psychobiological, psychoanalytic, cognitive behavioural, and social-interpersonal theories discussed next. While the approaches suggested by these theories appear to be very different, it is up to the individual psychiatric–mental health nurse to draw upon helpful aspects of each approach in clinical practice. For example, a biologically-oriented clinician can see the value of psychotherapy or cognitive behavioural therapy, as well as medication, for a person who has a fear of flying, and a cognitive-behavioural therapist can appreciate the anxiety-reducing effects of medication for the person.

Medical-psychobiological theory

The medical-psychobiological model in psychiatry originated in the era of classification. The classification of mental disturbances brought the emotional and behavioural aspects of people into the domain of the medical doctor, during a period when the systematic observation, naming and classification of symptoms were emphasised.

Emil Kraepelin's monumental descriptive diagnostic classification system of mental disorders is acknowledged as the first comprehensive medical model (Wallace & Gach, 2011). He noted that certain patterns of symptoms occurred with enough frequency to be considered as specific types of mental disorders. Kraepelin described these types of mental disorders and worked out a classification scheme that is the basis of our present system, the *Diagnostic and statistical manual of mental disorders (DSM-5)* published by the American Psychiatric Association (2013). The DSM classification system is reproduced in Appendix A, and is discussed in Chapter 10 and throughout the text.

Kraepelin also formulated the notions that the cause of mental illness was organic, that it was located in the central nervous system, that the disease followed a predictable course and that treatment should be based on accurate diagnosis. Contemporary research findings in the field of psychobiology lend support to some of these early ideas, but advance them and make them specific in important ways.

Assumptions and key ideas

Medical-psychobiological theories view emotional and behavioural disturbances like any physical disease. Thus, abnormal behaviour is directly attributable to a disease process, a lesion, a neuropathological condition, a toxin introduced from outside the body, or (most recently) a biochemical abnormality of neurotransmitters and enzymes or a genetic predisposition. The medical-psychobiological position is summarised in Box 5.3.

Box 5.3 Medical-psychobiological views

- The individual suffering from emotional disturbances is sick and has an illness.
- The illness can, at least presumably, be located in some part of the body (usually the brain's limbic system and the central nervous system's synapse receptor sites). Factors related to mental disorders include, but are not limited to: excesses or deficiencies of certain brain neurotransmitters; alterations in the body's biological rhythms, including the sleep–wake cycle; and genetic predispositions.
- The illness has characteristic structural, biochemical and mental symptoms that can be diagnosed, classified and labelled.
- Mental diseases run a characteristic course and have a particular prognosis for recovery.
- Mental disorders respond to physical or somatic treatments, including drugs, chemicals, hormones, diet or surgery.
- Psychobiological explanations of mental disorders can reduce the stigma often associated with them, and can discourage claims that mental disorders result from a lack of willpower or moral character.

TABLE 5.1 ■ Comparison of major features of traditional psychiatric theories

Theory	Assessment base	Problem	Goal	Dominant interventions
Medical-psychobiological	Individual consumer symptoms	Disease	Symptom management; cure	Psychopharmacology and other biological therapies
Psychoanalytic	Intrapsychic; unconscious	Conflict	Insight	Psychoanalysis
Cognitive behavioural	Behaviour; cognition	Learning deficit	Behaviour change; cognitive change	Behaviour/cognitive modification or conditioning
Social-interpersonal	Interactions between individual and social contexts	Interpersonal dysfunction	Enhanced awareness and quality of interpersonal interactions	Group, family and milieu therapies

Implications for psychiatric–mental health nursing practice

Nurses who were first involved in the care of people diagnosed with mental illness were primarily responsible for the person's physical wellbeing. Their responsibilities included administering medications prescribed by the physician, and caring for people undergoing treatments, such as insulin shock therapy, electroshock therapy, hydrotherapy or psychosurgery (see Chapter 1).

Psychobiological theories are the conceptual basis for the continued use of biological therapies in the care of people living with mental illness, the hospital as the setting for care, research into the genetic transmission of mental illness, research on biochemical and metabolic variables among people with diagnosed conditions, and the dominance of the medical practitioner—the psychiatrist—in the mental health team. As long as people living with mental illness are admitted to, and reimbursed for, care according to medical diagnoses, knowledge of this framework is crucial. Furthermore, as long as psychobiological knowledge expands, psychiatric–mental health nurses will have a role in translating that knowledge into care practices that recognise the biological factors related to mental disorders. Chapter 6 of this text provides an outline of contemporary psychobiological knowledge. Advances in psychobiological theory and research are also integrated throughout specific disorders and interventions chapters.

It should be noted, however, that the importance given to biological explanations of mental illness is disputed by many people living with mental illness. For those arguing from this contrary position, the dominance of bio-medicine has led to natural human responses to emotional trauma and adverse experience being pathologised into disorders of brain chemistry.

Psychoanalytic theory

Psychoanalytic theory is usually credited to the Viennese physician Sigmund Freud (Figure 5.1 ■). Freud believed that all psychological and emotional events, however obscure, were understandable. For the meanings behind behaviour, he looked to childhood experiences that he believed caused adult neuroses that interfered with productive and satisfying living. Freud's work shifted the focus of psychiatry from classification to a dynamic view of mental phenomena.

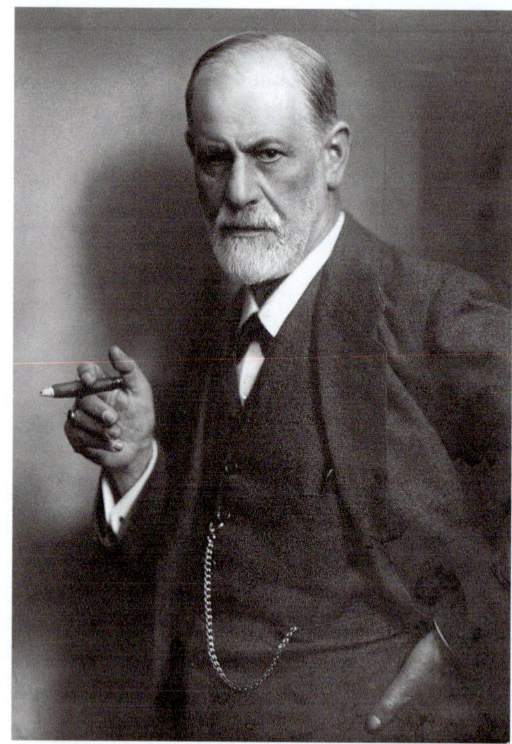

FIGURE 5.1 ■ Sigmund Freud, founder of psychoanalysis.
Photo courtesy of Alamy SZ Photo/Scherl.

Assumptions and key ideas

There are several basic principles that are central to psychoanalytic theory.

Psychic determinism Psychic determinism states that no human behaviour is accidental. Each psychic event is determined by the ones that preceded it. Events in people's mental lives that seem random or unrelated to what went before are only apparently so. Thus, psychoanalysts never dismiss any mental phenomenon as meaningless or accidental. They always search for what caused it, why it happened. For example, people commonly forget or misplace things. They usually view this as simply an accident. Psychoanalysts seek to demonstrate that the accident was caused by a wish or intent of the person involved. Psychoanalysts also view dreams as subject to the principle of psychic determinism, each dream and each image in each dream bearing some relationship to the rest of the dreamer's life.

Role of the unconscious The distinction between conscious and unconscious thought was made famous by Freud. Some kinds of information in the brain—your plans for the day, the faces of the people near you, your pleasures and your pains—are **conscious**. You think about them, discuss them and let them guide your behaviour. Others—the control of your heart rate and the sequence of muscle contractions that allow you to turn the pages of this book—are **unconscious**. They are in your brain someplace, but are sealed off from your planning and reasoning circuits. Likewise, any mental event that occurs outside of conscious awareness represents the unconscious region.

Significant unconscious mental processes occur frequently in normal as well as abnormal mental functioning. Much of what goes on in people's minds is unknown to them, and this accounts for the apparent discontinuities in their mental life. According to psychoanalytic theory, if the unconscious motivation of behavioural symptoms is discovered, the apparent discontinuities disappear, and the connection becomes clear.

Psychoanalysis The most well-known method for studying the unconscious is the technique that Freud evolved over several years called **psychoanalysis**. The basic logic behind psychoanalysis is discussed in Box 5.4.

Box 5.4 The basic logic behind psychoanalysis

1. The person underwent a *traumatic experience* that stirred up intense and painful emotion.
2. The traumatic experience represented to the person some ideas that were incompatible with the dominant ideas constituting the ego. Thus, the person experienced a *neurotic conflict*.
3. The incompatible idea and the neurotic conflict associated with it force the ego to bring into action *defence mechanisms*. (Chapter 8 describes in detail common defence mechanisms.)
4. Therapy is directed towards resolving the conflict by uncovering its roots in the unconscious. If the person is able to release the repressed feelings associated with the conflict, the symptoms disappear.

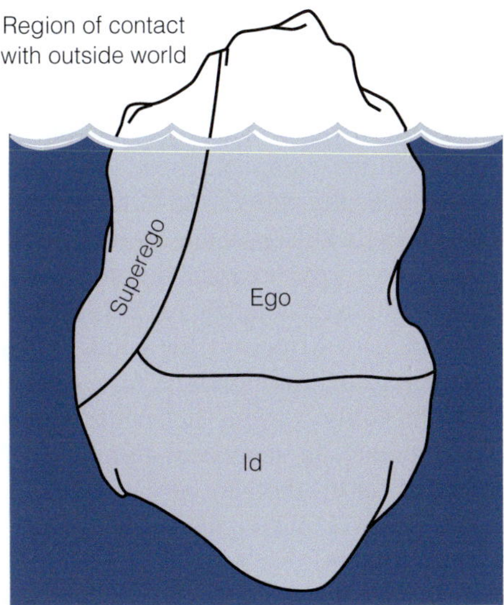

FIGURE 5.2 ■ Levels of awareness in relation to id, ego and superego. In this image, the id is completely below the water's surface, and the superego is partially below and partially above the surface. In comparison to the superego, the ego is more fully above the surface in the realm of conscious awareness.

Strategies used in psychoanalysis are hypnosis, the interpretation of dreams, and *free association*, in which the person is encouraged to express every idea that comes to mind—no matter how insignificant, irrelevant, shameful or embarrassing—ignoring all self-censorship and suspending all judgment.

Structure of the mind With the publication of *The ego and the id* in 1923, Freud introduced the *structural model* of the mind (1962). The structural model of the mind contends that there are three distinct entities: the id, the ego and the superego. The **id** is a completely unorganised reservoir of energy derived from drives and instincts. The **ego** controls action and perception, controls contact with reality, and, through defence mechanisms, inhibits primary instinctual drives. One of its fundamental functions is also the capacity for developing mutually satisfying relationships with others. The **superego** is concerned with moral behaviour. Frequently, the superego allies itself with the ego against the id, imposing demands in the form of conscience or guilt feelings. The relationship between Freud's levels of conscious and unconscious awareness, and his concepts of id, superego and ego, are often depicted as an iceberg (see Figure 5.2 ■).

The id operates according to what Freud called the *pleasure principle*: the tendency to seek pleasure and avoid pain. This is not always possible, so the demands of the pleasure principle have to be modified by the *reality principle*. The reality principle is a learned ego function by which people develop the capacity to delay the immediate release of tension or achievement of pleasure.

Instinctual drives Freud believed that psychic energy was derived from drives. He used the word *cathexis* to refer to the attachment of psychic energy to a person or a thing. The greater the cathexis, the greater the psychological importance of the person or object.

Freud accounted for the instinctual aspects of a person's mental life by assuming the existence of two drives, the *sexual drive* and the *aggressive drive*. The former gives rise to the erotic component of mental activity, and the latter gives rise to the destructive component. The sexual drive came to be known as the *libido*. According to Freud, we all pass through five stages of psychosexual development from infancy through puberty (see Table 5.2 ■). Each stage is characterised by a dominant mode of achieving libidinal (sexual) pleasure.

TABLE 5.2 ■ Freud's psychosexual stages

Stage	Age span	Task	Key concept
Oral	0–18 months	Satisfaction and anxiety management from oral activity	Oral activity gives pleasure and is a source for learning
Anal	18 months–3 years	Learning muscle control for toilet training	Delayed gratification and rule internalisation
Phallic	3–6 years	Gender identification and genital awareness	Repression of attraction to the opposite-sex parent (Oedipus and Electra complexes), leading to same-sex identification
Latency	6–12 years	Repression of sexuality	Oedipal conflict resolved with a shift to other interests and friends
Genital	12 years–young adult	Channelling sexuality into relationships with members of the opposite sex	Re-emerging sexuality to motivate behaviour

The Oedipus complex and the Electra complex Freud believed that each person must resolve the conflicts that arise in each psychosexual stage of development in order to avoid later fixations. He termed one of the most important conflicts the **Oedipus complex**. Freud believed that each young boy symbolically relives the Greek myth, in which Oedipus unknowingly kills his father and marries his mother, in the phallic stage of psychosexual development. However, the young boy, although longing for his mother sexually, fears that his father will cut off his penis as punishment. This fear, termed **castration anxiety**, forces the young boy to repress his hostility towards his father and his sexual desire for his mother. In successful resolution, the young boy has affection for his mother (but not sexual desire) and is able to channel his sexual impulses into relationships with other potential partners.

The **Electra complex** is the female counterpart, and is also drawn from Greek mythology. Freud believed that young girls desire to replace their mothers in order to possess their fathers. It is at this stage that young girls experience what Freud termed **penis envy**, the wish to be more like one's father or brothers.

Decline of Freudian psychoanalysis

We have seen a steady decline in the reliance on psychoanalytic theory and psychoanalysis as a treatment measure. The most frequently cited criticisms are that psychoanalytic theory is based on inferences (not proof) from clinical experiences, no single verifiable cure exists, and psychoanalysis is the costliest and most time-consuming treatment, often requiring expensive weekly meetings with a psychoanalyst for years (Crews, 1998; Webster, 1995).

In addition, because it requires a person to be relatively well-functioning, introspective and financially secure, psychoanalysis would not typically be accessible to many people living with mental illness. It has often been thought that people living with psychotic disorders or personality disorders would be unlikely to benefit from this type of psychotherapy. However, as you will see later in this chapter, variations on Freudian theory have led to the development of various insight-oriented therapies, such as those described in the section on social interpersonal theories. Most psychiatric–mental health clinicians continue to use several relevant psychoanalytic concepts—the structure of the mind, the role of the unconscious, defence mechanisms (discussed in Chapter 8), dream interpretation, and the three concepts of resistance, transference and countertransference (discussed in Chapter 2)—to understand mental processes and the process of the therapeutic relationship.

Implications for psychiatric–mental health nursing practice

Psychoanalytic theory has historically provided a limited treatment role for the nurse. People undergoing psychoanalytic treatments are usually seen in the analyst's office as private patients. However, with the emergence of psychoanalytically-oriented hospital treatment settings, nurses became more involved. In these settings, nurses shared at least in the psychoanalytic language, concepts and speculations about psychosocial dynamics and personality development, but usually not in a psychotherapeutic treatment role.

Cognitive behavioural theory

Cognitive behavioural theory focuses on the present rather than the past. Behaviourist theory in psychiatry has its roots in psychology and neurophysiology. The term *behaviour therapy* has largely been replaced by the term *cognitive behaviour therapy*. The specifics of cognitive behavioural therapy are discussed in Chapter 25.

To the behaviourist, symptoms associated with neuroses and psychoses are clusters of learned behaviours that persist because they are somehow rewarding to the individual. One of the most important contributions to this framework was made by Ivan Pavlov (1849–1936), who in 1902 discovered a phenomenon he called the **conditioned response** in a famous experiment with a dog and a bell (Figure 5.3 ■). The basic principle of the conditioned response is described as follows:

1. A response is a reaction to a stimulus.
2. If a new and different stimulus is presented with, or just before, the original stimulating event, the same response reaction can be obtained.
3. Eventually the new stimulus can replace the original one, so that the response occurs in reaction to the new stimulus alone.

The conditioned or learned response is viewed as the basic unit of all learning, the unit on which more complex

MENTAL HEALTH IN THE MEDIA
Psychoanalysis in the films of Woody Allen

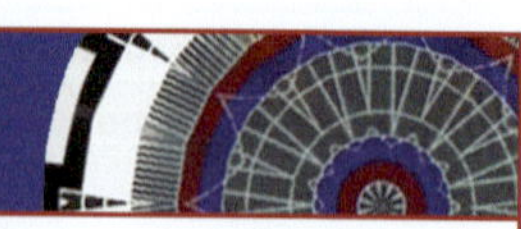

Psychoanalysis and psychoanalysts have long featured as topics in the films of New York film-maker and actor Woody Allen. Examples include *What's Up, Tiger Lily?* (1966), *Bananas* (1971), *Annie Hall* (1977) and *Zelig* (1983). Many of Allen's films address aspects of human distress and emotional dysregulation, as well as the psychotherapeutic techniques for treating the stresses and strains of urban existence. While there is an element of criticism in Allen's often comic treatment of psychoanalytical techniques and therapists, the need for such treatments and therapists is not denied or demeaned. Woody Allen's biographers and movie critics have often noted that his preoccupation with emotional conflict and psychoanalytic treatment parallel the many years in which he has also been receiving psychoanalysis.

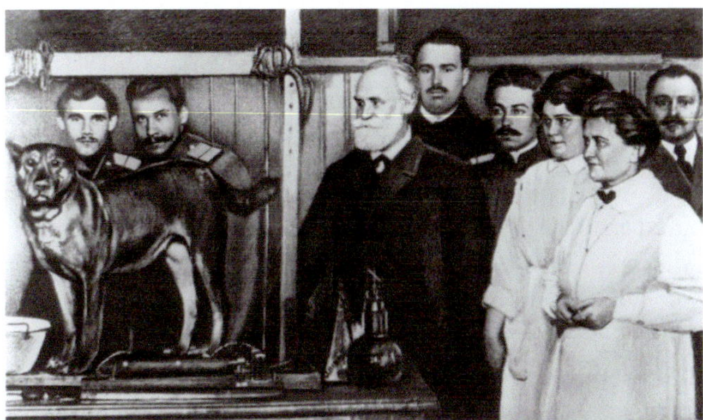

FIGURE 5.3 ■ Pavlov's famous experiment demonstrated the part that conditioning plays in behaviour. Pavlov is shown here with the staff and some of the apparatus used to condition reflexes in dogs.
Photo courtesy of Photo Researchers, Inc.

behavioural patterns are constructed. Such construction occurs through a process called **reinforcement**, in which behaviours are rewarded and persist. Pavlov's theories have influenced contemporary cognitive behavioural therapists, and are valued for their simplicity, concreteness and objectivity. Some behaviourists see them as the key to understanding and controlling the whole range of undesirable human behaviour.

Assumptions and key ideas

The fundamental premises of cognitive behavioural theory are presented in Box 5.5. Both Joseph Wolpe (1956) and B. F. Skinner (1971) are associated with psychiatric treatment approaches that represent one form of **conditioning** (using a specific stimulus to elicit a specific response) and reflect the assumptions in Box 5.5.

Box 5.5 Fundamental principles of cognitive behavioural therapy

- The self in humans is the sum or repository of past conditionings or simply the behavioural repertoire. Therapists can know the people with whom they work only by their behaviours.
- Behaviour is the way in which a person acts. It can be observed, described and recorded.
- There is no autonomous person. People are what they do and what they are reinforced for doing by conditions in their environment.
- The self is a structure of stimulus–response chains or hierarchies of habit. It is possible to know and predict the conditions under which behaviour will occur.
- The symptoms of a mental disorder are, in fact, the substance of that person's troubles. There is no hidden motive, no underlying cause, no internal pathogenic process. There is only the symptom or the behaviour, and the aim of cognitive behavioural therapy is to change the behaviour.
- The therapist, together with the person undergoing therapy, determines what behaviour should be changed and what plan should be followed. Change comes about by identifying events in the person's life that have been critical stimuli for the behaviour, and then arranging interventions for *extinguishing* those behaviours. A changed way of acting precedes a changed way of thinking, according to behaviourist theory.

Wolpe defined *neurotic behaviour* as unadaptive behaviour acquired in anxiety-generating situations. He based his therapeutic method on the introduction of a response that inhibits anxiety when situations occur that ordinarily evoke anxiety. Relaxation, for example, was considered incompatible with anxiety and, therefore, effective in inhibiting it. Thus, Wolpe would direct his intervention to a counter-conditioning technique, usually putting the person under hypnosis and using various techniques for gradual desensitisation. For example, a man afraid of dying might gradually attempt to overcome his anxiety at seeing a coffin, attending a funeral, and so on, by trying to relax in these situations.

Skinner's approach, called **operant conditioning**, emphasises discovering why the behavioural response was elicited in the first place and what actively reinforces it. The key concept in operant conditioning is reinforcement. Skinner originally used the term **positive reinforcement** to describe an event that increases the probability that the response will recur—a reward for behaviour. A **negative reinforcement** was defined as an event likely to decrease the possibility of recurrence because it penalises the behaviour.

The term for an intervention designed to change a person's behaviour is **shaping**. It is a procedure of manipulating reinforcement to bring the person closer to the desired behaviour. According to Skinner, there are times in a person's life when responses are accidentally reinforced by a coincidental pairing of response and reinforcement. This accidental pairing may play a role in the development of phobias (irrational fears) and other distressing and/or dysfunctional behaviours.

In addition to these classics, contemporary cognitive behavioural therapists use a vast array of techniques based on basic psychological science and developed out of psychological research, and validated in thousands of treatment outcome studies. Building upon earlier behavioural work, Aaron Beck (1975) has come to be regarded as the father of cognitive behavioural therapy.

Implications for psychiatric–mental health nursing practice

In many institutional environments, people undergoing treatment follow prescribed schedules for daily living that include a **token economy**. This involves people being rewarded for desired behaviour by token reinforcers, such as food, verbal approval and even money. The use of this approach raises issues of control, responsibility for behaviour, and the morality of using negative or punitive stimuli in a therapeutic context, to name only a few. Mental health professionals who successfully resolve such basic philosophical issues have designed and implemented successful treatment plans for working with children who display overtly aggressive behaviour, people who live with developmental disability, people displaying self-destructive behaviour and people who live with persistent mental illness.

The movement towards community-based psychiatric treatment has made plain some of the shortcomings and economic realities of therapies aimed towards resolving everyone's intrapsychic conflicts. The movement has instead attempted to replace maladaptive behaviour with behaviour that allows people to function effectively within their natural environment. When parents or others in the environment of the person living with mental illness are taught to implement behaviour change procedures, therapy moves away from the artificial situation of the therapist's office into the environment of the person concerned. It no longer requires the presence of highly trained, often expensive experts, and thus makes treatment more accessible and affordable. One area of recent development is e-mental health, in which evidence-based interventions, often using clinician-moderated cognitive-behavioural techniques, are delivered via the internet (Christensen & Petrie, 2013; Jorm, Morgan & Malhi, 2013).

Psychiatric–mental health nurses have had a special role in teaching cognitive behavioural principles to people with little training so that they can act as change agents. Non-professional staff can be taught the effective use of cognitive behavioural principles to modify enduring maladaptive thoughts and behaviours. Hyperactive children or children with borderline intelligence can be treated in the home by their parents when the parents are taught to use approaches such as frequency counts on specific behaviours to be modified, time-outs (short periods of isolation) for undesired behaviour, and the bestowal of attention, praise and affectionate physical contact as rewards.

Cognitive behavioural interventions focus on the individual—what that person feels, thinks and assigns meanings to—and empower people to learn new skills. How psychiatric–mental health nurses can use cognitive behavioural strategies, such as behavioural contracting, in their clinical practice is the subject of Chapter 25.

Social interpersonal theories

Social interpersonal theories of psychiatry grew out of a general dissatisfaction with approaches that account for mental illness in terms of either intrapersonal mechanisms (the symptoms of a disease) or individual personality dynamics, such as anxiety, ego strength and libido. Advocates of this perspective assert that other theories neglect the crucial social processes and cultural variation involved in the development, identification and resolution of disturbed human responses.

Assumptions and key ideas

Two separate but philosophically congruent schools of thought contribute to social interpersonal theories. These are the interpersonal psychiatric (Harry Stack Sullivan, Abraham Maslow, Carl Rogers and Erik Erikson) and the general systems approaches (von Bertalanffy, Menninger). The assumptions and key ideas of each are discussed next.

Interpersonal psychiatric theory: Harry Stack Sullivan Psychiatrist Harry Stack Sullivan (1953) made significant contributions to social interpersonal theory in the first half of the 20th century, and greatly influenced the work of Hildegard Peplau (see Chapter 3). Sullivan is viewed as one of the least reductionist of the psychiatric theorists, and emphasises **interpersonal theory** (the person's past and present relationships with others and modes of interaction) as the real focus of psychiatric inquiry. Sullivan's views were influenced by his teacher, Alfred Adler (1971), who defected in 1911 from the dominant psychoanalytic viewpoint of his teacher, Sigmund Freud. Sullivan became the theoretical and ideological leader of the interpersonal school of psychiatry.

One concept that plays a crucial role in the organisation of behaviour, according to Sullivan, is **self-system** or *self-dynamism.* Self-system enables people to deal with the tasks of avoiding anxiety and establishing security. The self is a construct built from the child's experience, and initially develops in the process of seeking satisfaction of bodily needs and safety. To feel secure, the self essentially requires feelings of approval and prestige as protection against anxiety.

The self-system is comprised of **reflected appraisals**—that is, the view of ourselves that we learn in interactions with significant others. Rewarding appraisals from others yield what Sullivan calls the *good-me* aspect of the self. Anxiety-producing appraisals result in the *bad-me* aspect. The *not-me* aspect exists normally in dreams and in aspects of experience that are poorly understood, and are later experienced as dread, horror and loathing among mentally disordered people.

In summary, Sullivan emphasises the pervasive interaction between the organism and the environment as well as the developmental tasks of the personality (Table 5.3 ■).

TABLE 5.3 ■ Sullivan's stages of interpersonal development

Age	Stage	Task/key concept
Birth–18 months (to appearance of speech)	Infancy	Experiences anxiety in interaction with mother figure; learns to use maternal tenderness to gain security and avoid anxiety
18 months–6 years (from first speech to need for playmates)	Childhood	Learns to delay gratification in response to interpersonal demands; uses language and action to avoid anxiety
6–9 years	Juvenile	Develops peer relationships and uses environment outside the family to shape self
9–12 years	Pre-adolescence	Develops a caring relationship with same-sex peer, chum relationship
12–14 years	Early adolescence	Develops interest in opposite-sex relationships
14–21 years	Late adolescence	Has satisfying relationships; directs sexual impulses
21 years +	Adulthood	Establishes a love relationship

Nonetheless, Sullivan has little to say about the impact on behaviour of specific variations in the social or cultural scene.

Like Sullivan, other advocates of the interpersonal school of psychiatry, such as Karen Horney (1950) and Erich Fromm (1941), stressed the general climate in the immediate family. The interpersonal school of psychiatry in general takes a developmental–interpersonal view of the self.

Hierarchy of basic human needs: Abraham Maslow The *self-actualisation* and hierarchy-of-needs theories of Abraham Maslow (1962) belong squarely in this school (Figure 5.4 ■). Maslow was one of the early humanistic psychologists who rejected the dominant views of psychoanalysis and behaviourism in favour of a more positive view of human behaviour.

Maslow proposed an order, or hierarchy, of basic human needs. According to Maslow, there are eight categories of needs (Maslow & Lowery, 1998). First, we must meet elemental and basic physiological needs for food and water. Once these needs have been met, second-tier or safety needs come next. After safety needs are belongingness and love needs, needs for friends and companions. See the Practice Example below for a discussion of what a person might experience when there are problems meeting these first three levels.

Practice example

Basic biological, safety and belonging needs

In mental illness, many people describe feeling 'disconnected' from their families, their friends, the universe itself and from their faith. For example, depression has sometimes been described as similar to being in a grey or black tunnel, with a profound sense of disconnectedness.

Imagine what it would be like to go for 24 hours or longer without sleep. How would you look? Would you feel disconnected or disoriented? Ask someone who has experienced mania what that's like. Have you ever awakened suddenly and not known where you are? How would it be to feel like that for an hour, a whole day or a month? Ask someone living with schizophrenia what that's like. Perhaps you have driven down the road and realised that you are confused about where you are and how you got there. And what if you had voices inside your head at the same time? Would this be frightening? Would you feel disconnected?

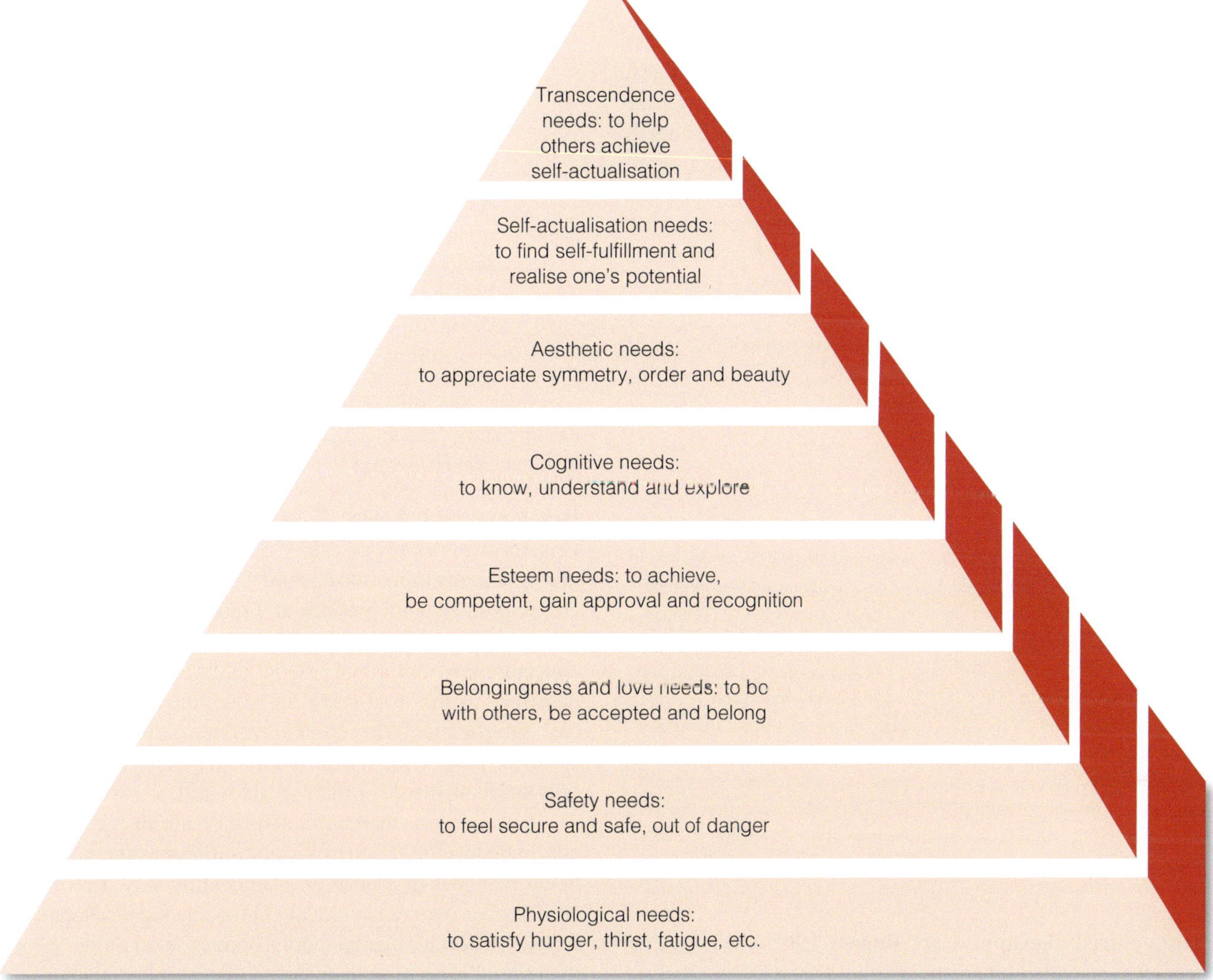

FIGURE 5.4 ■ Maslow's hierarchy of needs. The most basic needs for survival, which must be met first, are at the bottom, and the highest needs are at the top.

Source: Ciccarelli, S. K., & White, J. N. (2009). *Psychology.* Upper Saddle River, NJ: Pearson, p. 367.

LIVED EXPERIENCE

Shortly after experiencing a major psychotic episode in 1999, after I had stopped hearing voices, but before being prescribed an effective regime of antipsychotic medication, I got lost—completely lost—about three blocks from my parents' house. I was unable to recognise signs or other landmarks. I felt very frightened and used my mobile to call a taxi to take me to their house. My mother was astonished that I needed to take a taxi. That was the only occasion on which I experienced a complete loss of direction. I am sure now that the experience was related to psychosis; while frightened, I do not recall being overly disturbed by the experience. I have since thought that it might be similar to getting lost with dementia.

The self-esteem need is the need to feel that one has accomplished something good and earned the esteem of others. Next comes the cognitive needs—the need to gather knowledge so that one can know and understand the world. Aesthetic needs have to do with appreciating beauty and expressing oneself artistically. It is not until all of these needs have been met that one can concern oneself with **self-actualisation** or reaching full human potential. The times that we achieve self-actualisation are called *peak experiences*. The highest need—transcendence—involves helping others achieve their full potential.

Moving up and down the pyramid, and then back up, is quite common. A shift in life circumstances, such as that described in the Practice Example, may require a shift to a lower need.

Practice example

Donna had been retired for several years from her job as an engineer. When she was actively employed, Donna was highly regarded in her field. She often travelled to undertake work in countries such as Thailand, Indonesia and Malaysia. When Donna's husband, Jim, died after a long battle with cancer, Donna found herself in some financial difficulty. The situation became worse when she became unwell and found that her health insurance did not cover a number of the expensive treatments required. Donna's health has now improved, but she continues to struggle financially; in the last year she has sold the family home and moved into a unit and has downsized her motor vehicle. Her children and close friends have been very supportive, ensuring that Donna remains socially connected and active.

Client-centred therapy: Carl Rogers Like Maslow, Carl Rogers was an early humanistic psychologist who emphasised human potential, the ability of each person to become the best they could be. Rogers is probably the first to use the term *client,* rather than 'patient', for the person seeking counselling or mental health services. **Client-centred therapy** focuses on the client as the healer, rather than the therapist.

Rogers identified four elements as key in successful therapeutic relationships:

1. *Reflection.* Rogers believed that it was important to allow the ideas coming from the person undergoing therapy to flow freely in order to attain insight. To this end, he believed that therapists should not interfere with their own interpretations and biases. Reflection is literally a mirroring of the person's statements. Reflection as a therapeutic communication technique is discussed in Chapter 9.
2. *Unconditional positive regard.* Therapists should be warm and accepting, and provide an uncritical atmosphere for the people undergoing therapy. Having **unconditional positive regard** means that therapists respect those with whom they are working, and their feelings, values and goals, even if they differ from those of the therapist.
3. *Empathy.* Empathy is the ability to understand people by acknowledging what they are feeling and experiencing. Empathic therapists listen closely to what is being said, and try to feel what the person they are working with feels without getting their own feelings mixed up with those of the other person.
4. *Authenticity.* Authenticity is the ability to be open, genuine and honest in response to the person undergoing therapy. Being authentic means not hiding behind the role of therapist. It means that the therapist treats the person as a partner in the counselling process.

Like Maslow, Rogers believed in helping people in therapy move towards self-actualisation. Rogers was also an influence on Hildegard Peplau and her work.

Developmental theory of personality: Erik Erikson Erik Erikson also formulated a developmental theory of personality that took much more into account than just biological instincts. He elaborated and broadened Freud's psychosexual stages into more socially, culturally and interpersonally oriented concepts. For example, Erikson believed that, in what Freud described as the 'oral stage' in which the child is focused on oral gratification, the child's real development centres on issues of basic trust. The child develops either a 'basic trust' or a 'basic mistrust' of their social world.

Erikson described eight stages of life in which crises or conflicts develop. Each crisis or conflict has the potential for being resolved in a healthy or unhealthy way. Resolution of each stage is required in order to move forward developmentally. Erikson's developmental theory is considered more optimistic than Freud's, because he believed that people in therapy could return to a developmental task that had not been accomplished previously and relearn it (Erikson, 1963). Erikson's eight developmental stages are discussed in Table 5.4 ■.

TABLE 5.4 ■ Erikson's eight developmental stages

Age	Stage of development	Task/area of resolution	Concepts/basic attitudes
Birth–18 months	Infancy	Trust versus mistrust	Ability to trust others and a sense of one's own trustworthiness; a sense of hope; withdrawal and estrangement
18 months–3 years	Early childhood	Autonomy versus shame and doubt	Self-control without loss of self-esteem; ability to cooperate and to express oneself; compulsive self-restraint or compliance; defiance, wilfulness
3–5 years	Late childhood	Initiative versus guilt	Realistic sense of purpose; some ability to evaluate one's own behaviour; self-denial and self-restriction
6–12 years	School age	Industry versus inferiority	Realisation of competence, perseverance; feeling that one will never be 'any good', withdrawal from school and peers
12–20 years	Adolescence	Identity versus role diffusion	Coherent sense of self; plans to actualise one's abilities; feelings of confusion, indecisiveness, possibly antisocial behaviour
18–25 years	Young adulthood	Intimacy versus isolation	Capacity for love as mutual devotion; commitment to work and relationships; impersonal relationships, prejudice
25–65 years	Adulthood	Generativity versus stagnation	Creativity, productivity, concern for others; self-indulgence, impoverishment of self
65 years to death	Old age	Integrity versus despair	Acceptance of the worth and uniqueness of one's life; sense of loss, contempt for others

General systems theory General systems theory was pioneered by Ludwig von Bertalanffy (1968), a biologist. In **general systems theory**, every entity, or system, from the atom to rapid-transit systems, are maintained by the mutual interaction of its parts; that is, every system is a subsystem of larger systems. A system is more than the sum of its parts—when things are organised into a system, something new emerges (Nichols, 2010). When applied to living systems (people), general systems theory provides a conceptual framework for integrating the biological and social sciences with the physical sciences. In psychiatry, it offers a resolution of the mind–body dichotomy, an integration of biological and social approaches to the nature of human beings, and an approach to psychopathology, diagnosis and therapy. The most common application of general systems theory today is in understanding how families function (see Chapter 24).

Karl Menninger (1963) views normal personality functioning and psychopathology in terms of general systems theory. His work addresses four major issues, as follows:

1. adjustment or individual–environment interaction
2. the organisation of living systems
3. psychological regulation and control, known as *ego theory* in psychoanalysis
4. motivation, which is often called *instinct* or *drive* in the psychoanalytic framework.

A salient point of Menninger's theory is the idea of *homeostasis* (equilibrium). He asserts that the greater the threat or stress on a system, the greater the number of system components involved in coping with or adapting to it. Therefore, pathology can exist at various levels, as follows:

- The cell and organ level: An example might be the behavioural changes that follow cellular alterations due to addictive drugs, a blood clot or a tumour.
- The group level: An example is family violence.
- The community level: Examples are overpopulation, pollution, homelessness and poverty.

In general systems theory, all represent abnormalities or stresses on matter–energy processes, and would be included within the domain of psychiatric professionals.

In Menninger's view, a system's wellbeing depends on the amount of stress on it, and the effectiveness of its coping mechanisms. He asserts that mental illness is an impairment of self-regulation in which comfort, growth and production are surrendered for the sake of survival at the best level possible, but at the sacrifice of emergency coping devices. Therapists using the general systems approach emphasise current conflicts, restoration of impaired systems of functioning and subsequent reintegration of the restored function into future coping strategies.

Implications for psychiatric–mental health nursing practice

Social interpersonal theories give independent and collaborative psychiatric–mental health nursing clear theoretical direction and support. Nursing roles are associated with shifts in the delivery of psychiatric services, variously termed *care coordination, social psychiatry, community psychiatry, psychoeducation, milieu therapy* and *recovery-oriented mental health care.* According to these orientations, all social, psychological and biological activity (including research developments in psychobiology) that affect the mental health of the population is important to professionals in community psychiatry. Therapeutic interventions may include programs for social change, political involvement, community organisation, social planning, family support groups, and education about medications, symptom management, genetic risk and family environment. Many implications for practice can be derived from this theoretical model, which are reflected in the following examples:

- People are approached in a holistic way, reflecting the interrelationship and interaction between the biophysical, psychological and socioeconomic–cultural dimensions of human life.
- Definitions of the 'consumer' must include the concept of the 'consumer system'. A family, a couple, an aggregate or even a community may collectively constitute 'the consumer'.
- Intervention strategies include primary prevention achieved through psychoeducation, social change and research.
- Therapy focuses on helping people in distress gain a useful perspective on their lifestyle and social environment.
- Therapy also focuses on helping people in distress develop coping skills and resources, rather than repressing and controlling their symptoms.
- Psychiatric–mental health nurses must synthesise psychobiological knowledge with psychosocial rehabilitations skills and psychoeducation.
- Psychiatric–mental health nurses must be prepared to function as autonomous members of the mental health team, and to assume more responsibilities in the shift away from the dominance of the physician in decision-making and towards diffusion of roles.

Once people are viewed as becoming distressed in the context of unhealthy or problem-filled interpersonal relationships, establishing healthy, constructive interpersonal relationships becomes important in their care. Psychiatric–mental health nurses can apply concepts of milieu therapy, primary prevention, social psychiatry, community psychiatry and psychobiological interventions to implement this fundamental idea. The Practice Example on this page and the discussion that follows demonstrate how these concepts can be applied in clinical practice.

Practice example

Mrs Dominguez is a 67-year-old Philippino-Australian woman in good physical health. She has become increasingly untidy, forgetful, reclusive, sad and suspicious since the death of her domineering husband from a heart attack six months ago. She recently sold the large house where she had lived for the past 45 years and moved into a two-bedroom apartment in a nearby retirement village. Because of the rules of the retirement village, she was unable to take her 12-year-old cat. She felt compelled to sell the family home, because her husband had said to do so if anything happened to him. (He had made all of the family decisions while he lived.) Mrs Dominguez has taken to skipping meals, often eating only toast and jam because she must rely on a friend to drive her to the grocery store. (Her husband believed she did not need to learn to drive.) Her younger sister (aged 59), seeking advice about Mrs Dominguez's behaviour, contacted the local community mental health team at the suggestion of the family's general practitioner.

The community mental health nurse assessing this situation would tend not to view Mrs Dominguez's symptoms as psychological conflicts reflecting her ambivalence towards her dead husband or as manifestations of a mental disorder, such as major, single-episode depression. Instead, the nurse would focus on the way Mrs Dominguez is functioning in her current interpersonal situation, and her holistic human responses to it. In this analysis, the nurse would not view Mrs Dominguez's illness as being biologically based and thus in need of a somatic treatment such as medication.

Instead, treatment consists of helping Mrs Dominguez develop strategies for coping with her new situation and satisfying her needs. The nurse would seek out the younger sister and other family members in an attempt to enhance Mrs Dominquez's social support network. Efforts may be directed towards mobilising other environmental forces (including the nurse) to provide company, stimulation and proper nutrition for Mrs Dominguez, since the absence of all three contributes to her symptoms and discomfort. The clinical situation would possibly reinforce the nurse's political efforts to point out the potential consequences of lifelong passive dependence for some adult women. The nurse may also become involved in a professional organisation or community organisations working for better services for older people.

The shifts in the delivery of psychiatric services towards a social psychiatry or community psychiatry view are associated with efforts to provide psychiatric services more efficiently to large groups of people (particularly those previously neglected), and attempts to counteract the debilitating effects of long-term institutionalisation. Social psychiatry or community psychiatry are associated with a movement to address social context in providing mental health care for a person.

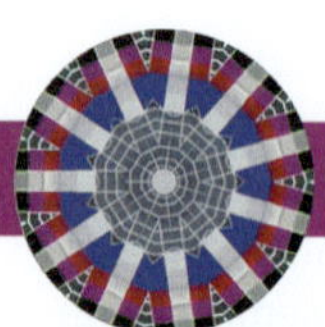

REFERENCES

Adler, A. (1971). *The practice and theory of individual psychology.* New York, NY: Humanities Press.

American Psychiatric Association (APA). (2013). *Diagnostic and statistical manual of mental disorders* (5th ed.) (DSM-5). Washington, DC: APA Publishing.

Beck, A. T. (1975). *Cognitive therapy and the emotional disorders*. Madison, CT: International Universities Press.

Butcher, J. N., Mineka, S., & Hooley, J. M. (2010). *Abnormal psychology* (14th ed.). Boston, MA: Allyn & Bacon.

Chiovitti, R. F. (2011). Theory of protective empowering for balancing patient safety and choices. *Nursing Ethics*, *18*(1), 88–101.

Christensen, H., & Petrie, K. (2013). Information technology as the key to accelerating advances in mental health care. *Australian and New Zealand Journal of Psychiatry 47*(2), 114–116.

Ciccarelli, S. K., & White, J. N. (2009). *Psychology* (2nd ed.). Upper Saddle River, NJ: Pearson.

Commonwealth Department of Health and Ageing (2013). *A national framework for recovery-oriented mental health services.* Retrieved from www.health.gov.au/internet/main/publishing.nsf/.../recovgde.pdf (Accessed 2015, December 9.)

Crews, F. C. (1998). *Unauthorised Freud: Doubters confront a legend.* New York, NY: Viking Press.

Erikson, E. (1963). *Childhood and society* (2nd ed.). New York, NY: Norton.

Freud, S. (1962). *The ego and the id.* New York, NY: Norton.

Fromm, E. (1941). *Escape from freedom.* New York, NY: Irvington.

Gordon, S., & Ellis, P. (2013). Recovery of evidence-based practice, *International Journal of Mental Health Nursing 22,* 3–14.

Hamer, H., Finlayson, M., & Warren, H. (2014). Insiders or outsiders? Mental health service users' journeys towards full citizenship. *International Journal of Mental Health Nursing 23*, 203–211.

Hazelton, M., & Rossiter, R. (2016). 'Talk about trouble': Practitioner discourses on service users who are judged to be resisting, contesting or evading treatment. In M. O'Reilly & J. Lister (Eds.), *The Palgrave Handbook of Adult Mental Health* (pp. 419–440). Houndmills, England: Palgrave Macmillan.

Hewitt, J. P., & Shulman, D. (2011). *Self and society: A symbolic interactionist social psychology* (11th ed.). Boston, MA: Allyn & Bacon.

Horney, K. (1950). *Neurosis and human growth.* New York, NY: Norton.

Jorm, A. F., Morgan, A. J., & Malhi, G. S. (2013). The future of e-mental health. *Australian and New Zealand Journal of Psychiatry, 47*(2), 104–106.

Lamont, C. (1967). *The philosophy of humanism.* New York, NY: Frederick Ungar.

Leamy, M., Bird, V., Le Boutillier, C., Williams, J., & Slade, M. (2011). Conceptual framework for personal recovery in mental health: Systematic review and narrative synthesis. *British Journal of Psychiatry 199*, 445–451.

Maslow, A. (1962). *Toward a psychology of being.* New York, NY: Van Nostrand.

Maslow, A., & Lowery, R. (1998). *Toward a psychology of being* (3rd ed.). New York: Wiley & Sons.

Menninger, K. (1963). *The vital balance.* New York, NY: Viking Press.

Nichols, M. P. (2010). *Family therapy.* Boston, MA: Allyn & Bacon.

Skinner, B. F. (1971). *Beyond freedom and dignity.* New York, NY: Prentice Hall.

Sullivan, H. S. (1953). *The interpersonal theory of psychiatry.* New York, NY: W. W. Norton.

von Bertalanffy, L. (1968). *General systems theory.* New York, NY: Braziller.

Todres, L., Galvin, K., & Holloway, I. (2009). The humanization of healthcare: A value framework for qualitative research. *International Journal for Qualitative Studies on Health and Wellbeing, 4*, 66–77.

Tondora, J., Miller, R., Slade, M., & Davidson, L. (2014). *Partnering for recovery in mental health.* Chichester, England: Wiley.

Wallace, E. R., & Gach, J. (2011). *History of psychiatry and medical psychology.* New York, NY: Springer-Verlag.

Webster, R. (1995). *Why Freud was wrong: Sin, science, and psychoanalysis.* New York, NY: Basic Books.

Wolpe, J. (1956). Learning versus lesions as the basis of neurotic behaviour. *American Journal of Psychiatry, 112*, 923–931.

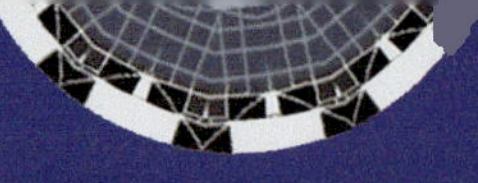

6

The biological basis of behavioural and mental disorders

MERRILEE HARRIS, SIMON SWINSON AND MIKE HAZELTON

KEY TERMS

LEARNING OUTCOMES

After completing this chapter, you will be able to:

1. Understand the basic structures of the brain that are believed to affect thought, behaviour, memory and emotions.
2. Describe the structure and function of a neuron, and the role of neurotransmitters and neuromodulators in neuronal communication.
3. Understand the concept of neuroplasticity and its role in the development of, and recovery from, mental illness.
4. Identify ways in which the endocrine and immune systems are thought to affect a person's neuronal development and mental health.
5. Describe ways in which genetic variation and epigenetic changes might contribute to the development of mental illness.
6. Partner with people living with mental illness and their families to teach the biological implications of psychiatric illnesses.
7. Analyse how your own personal feelings, opinions or beliefs about psychobiology can enhance or diminish your ability to be a support person and advocate for people living with mental illness and their families.

LIVED EXPERIENCE

In the early stages of my journey with schizophrenia, science was one source of information about what I was experiencing; I did this through reading and attending conferences on mental illness (to the surprise and alarm of my doctor!). My interest in the scientific explanations of mental illness waned for a time, as I was unable to make headway in understanding an increasingly complex field. I was fortunate that my sister-in-law is a senior health professional, and through her I have been able to keep up with developments in how schizophrenia is understood and treated. At times science has also played an important role in helping me maintain hope. Being able to discuss treatment options in an open, informed and trusting way with my doctor has been very important; nowadays I have a much better understanding of the medications I take and this has influenced my decision to keep taking them.

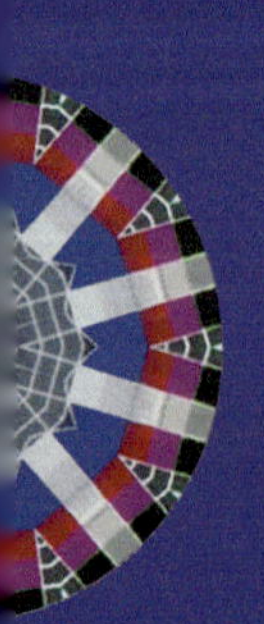

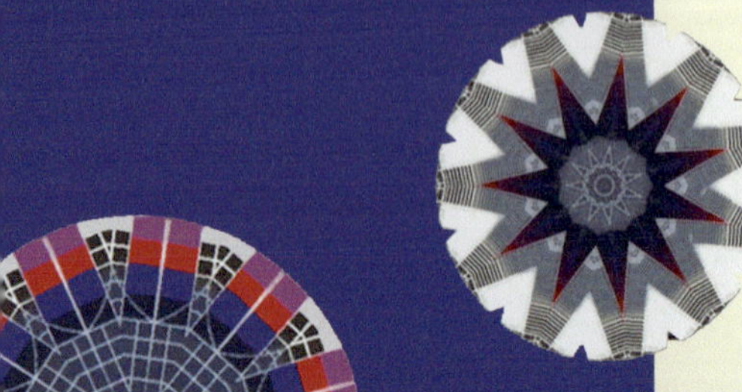

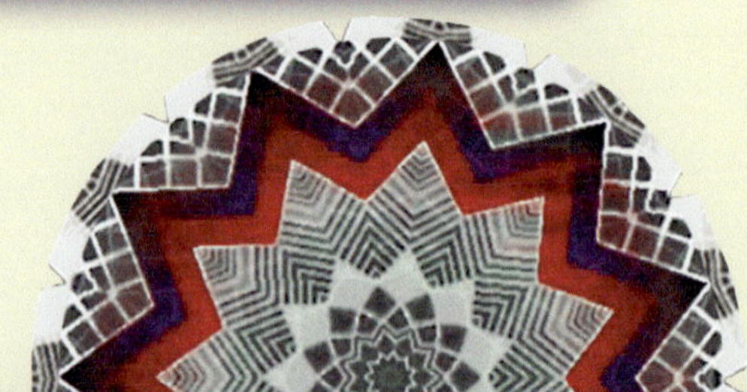

INTRODUCTION

The brain is an extraordinarily complex organ that determines our thoughts, personality and behaviour. The concept of the mind has existed since the birth of humankind, and has been a subject of philosophers' discussions for at least 2000 years. However, only since the mid-20th century has the field of behavioural neuroscience, or psychobiology, begun to deliver a broader understanding of the possible biological basis of the mind and behaviour. Current knowledge about the biological components of behaviour contributes not just to psychiatry, but also our view of behaviour, temperament and mental illnesses, and their treatment. Nevertheless, in our understanding of thought and brain function, more remains unknown than known.

The field of behavioural neuroscience encompasses an enormous amount of information and current research. It includes the study of brain structures, biochemical foundations, molecular and genetic influences on cognition, mood, emotion, affect and behaviour, and the interactions among them. This comprehensive view takes into consideration both internal and external influences across a person's lifespan, including genetics, the effects of other body systems such as the endocrine and immune systems, temperament, resilience in the face of stress, and the environment.

While the scope of this chapter curtails how much psychobiology we can explore, the aim is to provide sufficient knowledge to enable integration of the latest neuroscience concepts into excellence-based psychiatric–mental health nursing practices, as part of your holistic professional care for people with mental illness and their families. We first examine the structure and function of the brain, including genetic and environmental factors that influence brain function, before examining the possible biological basis of specific mental illnesses. Although the anatomical terminology of neuroscience can be confusing, the major brain regions include: the *brainstem*, which controls subconscious vital functions and transmits all incoming sensory and outgoing motor signals; the *limbic system*, our emotional turbo-charger, which mediates motivation, fear and reward; and the *cerebrum*, a cognitive supercomputer, which mediates conscious thought, intelligence, sensory perception and motor function. When all regions of the brain are functioning in an integrated, balanced fashion, the brain is capable of amazing feats of creativity, imagination and critical analysis. However, when brain function becomes unbalanced—for example, hyperactivity in the fear circuits with the cognitive brake of reason reduced—we become susceptible to bouts of mental illness that can be debilitating.

Our increasing understanding of the pathogenesis of mental illness, and how brain function changes at the biological level in response to our thoughts and experiences (neuroplasticity), brings hope for more effective treatment for people with mental illness. Teaching people (as well as their families) about the possible biological aspects of the disorder increases their understanding of the illness and its treatment, and can increase their motivation to continue to seek appropriate treatment and adhere to medication regimens. Clear scientific explanations for psychiatric symptoms can also help dispel long-held myths that parenting styles and lack of character, for example, are, in and of themselves, responsible for mental illnesses. Thus, understanding the working hypotheses of psychobiology is important for combating the guilt and stigma often associated with mental illness.

BRAIN, MIND AND BEHAVIOUR

Communication is a vital aspect of psychiatric–mental health nursing. Through neurobiological discoveries, we now know that communication, behaviours and thought patterns have a molecular, anatomical and chemical basis. Who we are originates from order or disorder at any of these levels.

The brain encodes or decodes information through the complex interactions of neuro-messengers, chemical processes and anatomic systems. When people living with mental illness ask about their symptoms, you can provide useful information using current neurobiological theory and research. For example, a person who has panic attacks certainly feels like they are real, but may not know why they occur. You can bring an understandable scientific explanation of how panic attacks seem to be related to the triggering of an over-reactive alarm centre in the brain. It is thought that this trigger sends a message of fear via the release of a **neurotransmitter**, causing thoughts and feelings associated with anxiety, as well as other physiological symptoms, such as racing heart and shortness of breath.

Neuroanatomy

The brain is the part of the central nervous system (CNS; that also includes the spinal cord) encapsulated by the skull. The brain is the core of our humanity. Intercommunication among different parts of the brain yields the experiences of love, hate, joy, fear, silliness and sadness. The brain provides the underlying biology for will, determination, hopes and dreams, as well as the ability to problem-solve, to establish memory, and to learn and use acquired knowledge productively.

These functions are performed by some 100 billion neurons, communicating via 100 trillion connections. Neurons are cells specialised for communicating with each other using electrochemical 'messages' (see Figure 6.1 ■). Neurons with similar roles are grouped together in specific regions of the brain. The major structural and functional regions of the brain discussed here are the cerebrum, limbic system, diencephalon, cerebellum and brainstem (see Figure 6.2 ■). It is important to realise that neurons in different brain regions work together in a complex interplay to achieve specific actions. These networks of interconnected neurons are called *neural circuits*.

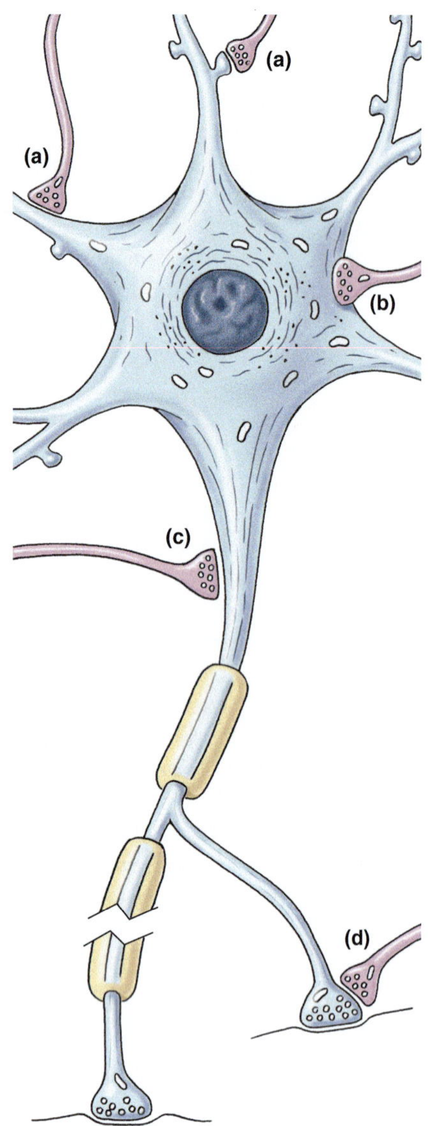

FIGURE 6.1 ■ Synaptic contacts. A neuron is capable of making many different types of synaptic contacts. Shown here are: (a) a synapse contact on a dendrite, called *axodendritic contact*; (b) a contact on the soma, called *axosomatic contact*; (c) a synapse contact on another axon, called *axoaxonic contact*; and (d) an area where signals are sent and received, called *axosynaptic contact*.

Source: Smock, T. K. (1999). *Physiological psychology: A neuroscience approach*. Upper Saddle River, NJ: Prentice Hall, p. 23.

It is the complex, carefully synchronised firing patterns of thousands of neurons in many interacting regions of the brain that determine how we perceive sensory information, how we behave, our memories and thoughts.

Despite its complex functional regionalisation, if you were to dissect the brain you would see homogenous-looking tissue distinguishable only as areas of grey matter and white matter. The darker grey matter contains mostly *neuronal cell bodies* (also called the 'soma') and *dendrites*, structures specialised for receiving and integrating messages from other neurons (Figure 6.1). The white matter contains *axons*, the neuronal structures specialised for sending electrochemical messages to neurons in other areas of the brain (Figure 6.1). Axons are often surrounded by a fatty, insulating substance called *myelin* that gives the white appearance. In order to 'see' the functional regionalisation and workings of the brain, we need to use neuroimaging techniques. Electroencephalograms (EEGs), computerised tomography (CT) scans, magnetic resonance imaging (MRI), and positron emission tomography (PET) scans all give us a glimpse of how the brain works. Figure 6.3 ■ shows these imaging techniques.

Cerebrum

The cerebrum includes the following structures and functions:

- cerebral hemispheres
- conscious thought processes and intellectual functions
- memory storage and processing
- conscious and subconscious regulation of skeletal muscle contractions.

The **cerebrum** comprises the largest part of the human brain. It is divided into two *cerebral hemispheres*, whose surface area is maximised by having a walnut-like appearance with ridges of tissue called *gyri* (singular—gyrus) separated by shallow grooves called *sulci* (singular—sulcus) or deeper fissures. The deep furrow that divides the hemispheres is called the *longitudinal fissure*. The *corpus callosum* contains bundles of axons (also called 'tracts' or 'fibres') that connect the two hemispheres and allow communication between them. In the past, scientists believed that each hemisphere had separate functions, such as logic or creativity and spatial accommodation. With technologies such as positron emission tomography (PET), it is now possible to assess metabolic activity in the brain as it occurs (see Box 6.1 on page 94). Scientists are now able to observe brain activity, and have concluded that creative as well as logical activities require input from both cerebral hemispheres.

The cerebral hemispheres are each divided into five paired lobes: the frontal, parietal, temporal and occipital lobes are named after the parts of the skull under which they lie, and the insular lobe (or insula) is folded deep within the lateral sulcus (see Box 6.2 on page 95). The outermost layer of each of the lobes contains grey mater (neuronal dendrites and cell bodies), and is collectively called the *cerebral cortex*. The cortex contains our conscious mind. Much like the central processing unit (CPU) of a computer, the cortex is the part of the brain that makes sense out of volumes of input. It processes and synthesises information, thought, reasoning, will and choice. Our dreams come from the cortex. Neurons with specific common functions are localised to discrete areas of the cortex, thus each lobe has unique functions that contribute to a person's ability to move, process information, and have thoughts and feelings.

Frontal lobes The frontal lobes contain the primary motor cortex, whose neurons control the voluntary movement of our skeletal muscles, as well as other motor areas controlling speech and voluntary eye movement. The frontal lobes, especially the prefrontal cortex, are also responsible for cognitive control; the ability to purposefully control and direct our thoughts and behaviour. Thus, they are primarily responsible for higher cognitive skills, including planning,

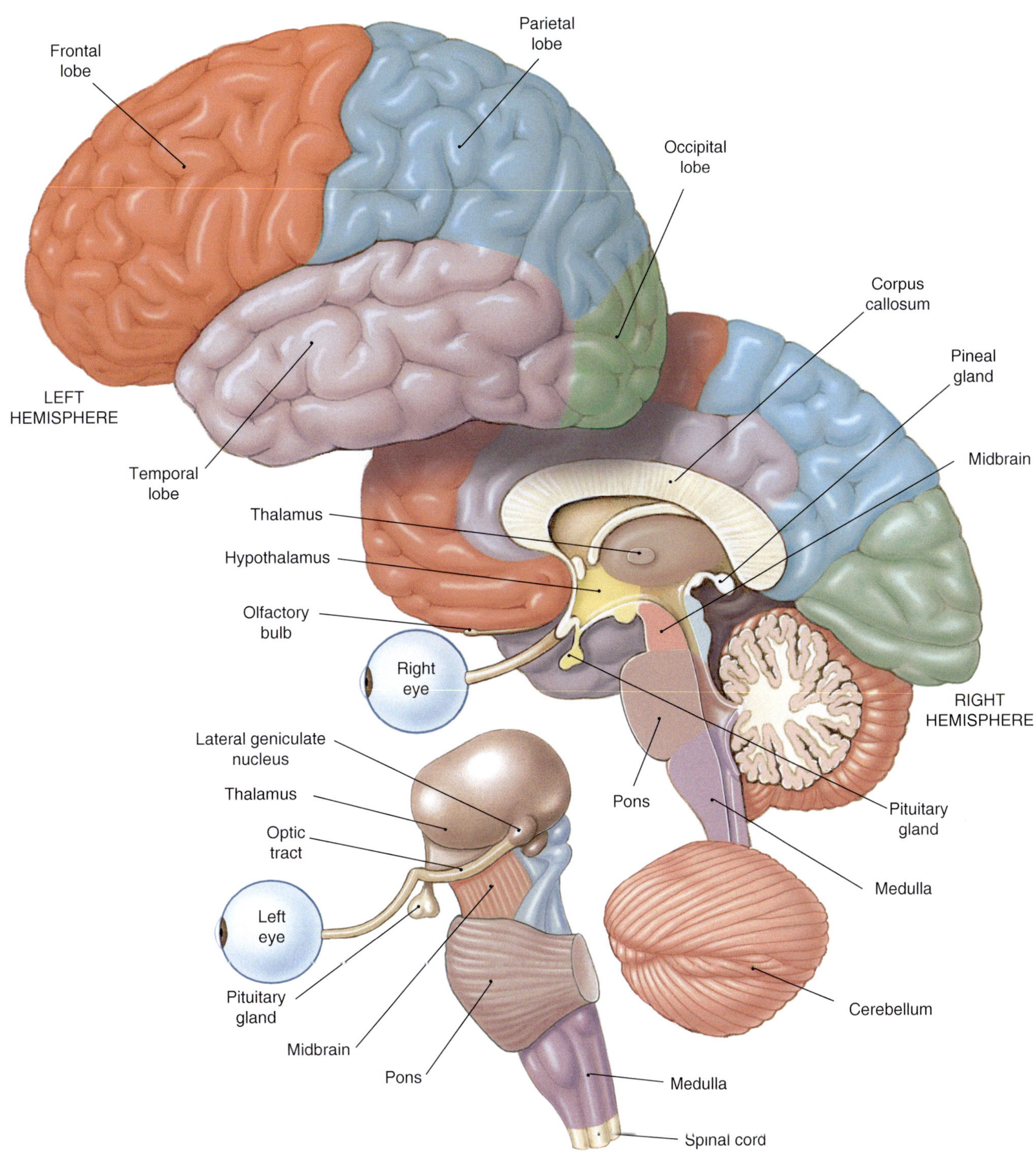

FIGURE 6.2 ■ Structures of the human brain seen in cross-section.
Source: Smock, T. K. (1999). *Physiological psychology: A neuroscience approach*. Upper Saddle River, NJ: Prentice Hall.

concentration, working memory, problem-solving, organising and intelligent behaviour. To achieve these functions, the frontal lobes are extensively connected with all of the other brain regions. They receive external sensory information and internal emotional information, and send information to motor control areas to effect behaviour. Thus, the practical impact of frontal lobe damage or a lesion can be extensive (see Box 6.3 on page 95).

Temporal lobes The cortex of the temporal lobes functions in memory association and formation, cognition and the conscious perception of smell and auditory stimuli (particularly language). It contains some structures of the limbic system, including the amygdala and hippocampus, which are involved in emotions, memory and thought patterns. The limbic system has a central role in many mental illnesses, so will be covered in more detail later in this chapter.

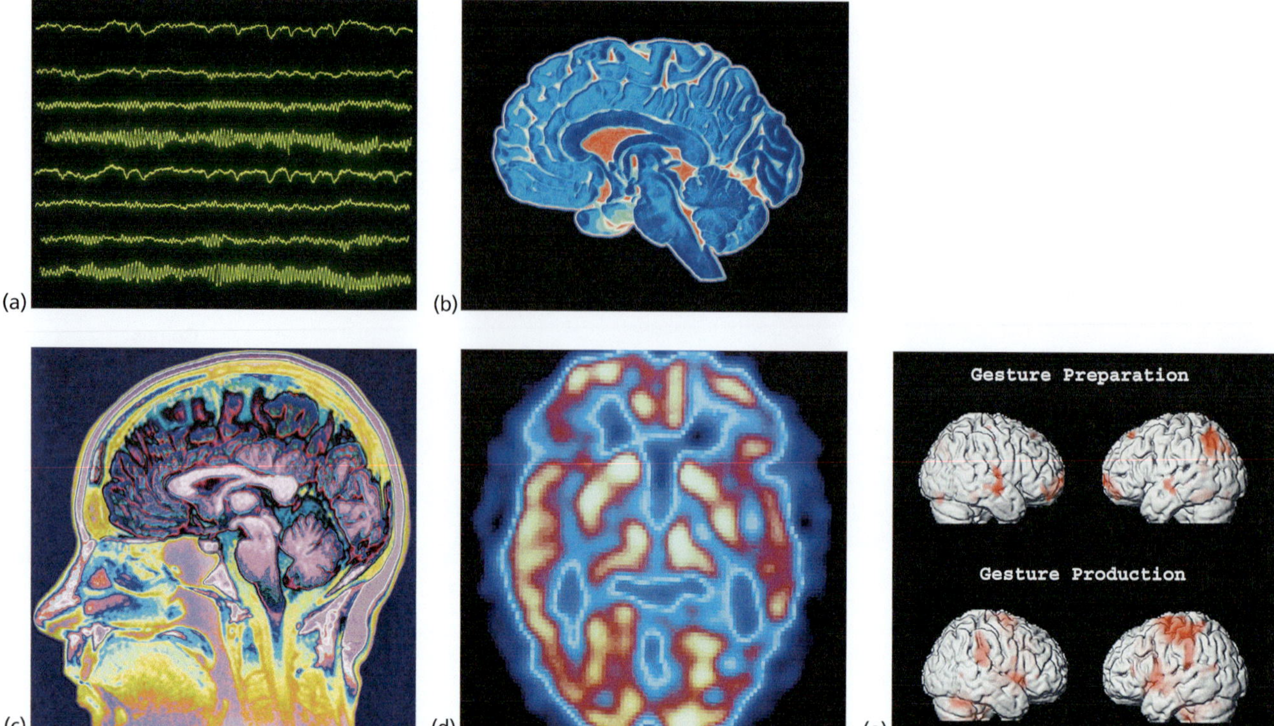

FIGURE 6.3 ■ Studying the brain. These are four methods researchers use to study the brain: EEGs, CT scans, MRIs and PET scans. (a) An example of an EEG readout. (b) A CT scan (coloured by a computer) showing the detail of a centre cross-section of the brain. (c) An MRI (coloured by a computer) showing enhanced detail of the same view of the brain as in the CT scan. (d) A PET scan showing activity of the brain, using colours to indicate different levels of activity; areas that are very active are white, whereas areas that are inactive are dark blue. (e) An fMRI tracking the oxygen levels in the brain shows the difference between brain activity when preparing to make a gesture and brain activity when actually making the gesture.

Source: Ciccarelli, S. K., & White, J. M. (2009). *Psychology* (2nd ed.). Upper Saddle River, NJ: Pearson Education, p. 66.

Photos courtesy of: (a) SPL/Photo Researchers, Inc.; (b) Alfred Pasieka/Photo Researchers, Inc.; (c) © Pete Saloutos/Corbis; (d) Tim Beddow/Photo Researchers, Inc.; (e) Corbis.

Box 6.1 Tools of psychobiology

Brain imaging

- ***Computed tomography (CT).*** An X-ray beam (radiation exposure) is passed through serial sections of the brain to look at structural images.
- ***Magnetic resonance imaging (MRI).*** Reconstructs detailed images of cerebral anatomy from multiple perspectives, including subcortical structures, using radio frequency signals emitted by relaxing hydrogen atoms. It delineates grey and white matter. New instruments image elements other than hydrogen, allowing an MRI to be used for structural imaging. An fMRI (functional MRI) is used to detect the functional and metabolic processes under review. This procedure is contraindicated for people with any metal objects in their bodies, such as pacemakers, due to the presence of a magnetic field.
- ***Positron emission tomography (PET).*** Imaging of active neurochemical substrates and physiological processes; regional localisation of metabolic functions through the measurement of radioactive labels or tags attached to molecules as glucose; density of neuroreceptors; regional cerebral blood flow (rCBF) of the brain. It operates on the principle that blood rushes to the busiest area of the brain to deliver oxygen and nutrients to the active neurons.
- ***Single photon-emission computed tomography (SPECT).*** Measures rCBF; visualises and measures the density of neuroreceptors, using tracer isotopes such as: xenon, a gas; iodine 123; or technetium.

Neurophysiological techniques

- ***Electroencephalogram (EEG).*** Measures electrical activity patterns of the brain from leads connected to surface electrodes placed on the scalp and nasopharyngeal area.
- ***Polysomnography (sleep EEG).*** Measures electrical brain activity data during all-night sleep.
- ***Brain electroactivity mapping (BEAM).*** Extends the EEG by generating computerised maps of brain electrical activity to produce images; permits visualisation of the brain performing tasks or specific functions. Useful with children.
- ***Event-related potential (ERP).*** Repeated auditory or visual stimuli associated with tiny electrical events in the cerebral cortex or subcortical structures, measured by surface electrodes.

(*continued*)

Box 6.1 *(continued)*

Molecular genetics

- ***Linkage map.*** A genetic map that represents the relationship between two genes, often revealed by the inheritance of traits in families, to determine the relative position of genes on a given chromosome.
- ***Next-generation sequencing.*** High-throughput methods of simultaneously sequencing thousands of DNA fragments. Generates hundreds of megabases to gigabases of nucleotide sequence reads in a single instrument run. Has enabled a drastic increase in available sequence data, and fundamentally changed genome sequencing approaches in the biomedical sciences.
- ***Genome wide association studies.*** An examination of many common genetic variants in different individuals to see if any variant is associated with a trait. Typically focuses on associations between single-nucleotide polymorphisms (SNPs) and traits like major diseases.

Box 6.2 Functions of the cerebral lobes

Frontal lobes

- Responsible for movement; the right frontal lobe controls the left side of the body's movements, the left controls the right-sided movements
- Contain the premotor cortex, which organises complicated movement
- Contain prefrontal fibres with capacities for planning and problem-solving; also responsible for social judgment, volition, attention, learning, spontaneity, thinking and affect
- Responsible for executive functioning, which determines how information is interpreted; starting and stopping certain functions (such as verbal exchanges); and filtering and screening out extraneous information

Parietal lobes

- Contain the sensory cortex, which interprets contact sensations such as touch and pressure
- Facilitate spatial orientation

Temporal lobes

- Involved in hearing, memory, language comprehension and emotions
- Connect with the limbic system (the 'emotional brain') to allow for the expression of emotions, such as rage, fear, sexual and aggressive behaviour, and possibly love; damage to the temporal lobes is sometimes seen as extreme and inappropriate expressions of these feelings

Occipital lobes

- Facilitate the interpretation of visual images and visual memory
- Involved in language formation
- Collaborate with many other brain structures in the formation of memory

Insular lobes

- Interpretation of taste and pain
- Interpretation of visceral sensations
- Generation of social emotions, such as guilt, humiliation and lust
- Fast intuitive assessment of complex social situations

Box 6.3 Practical impacts of frontal lobe damage or lesion

The frontal lobe organises various aspects of everyday interactions and functioning. Examples of the effects of damage to this lobe are as follows.

Speech

- In a slow-moving supermarket line, someone with frontal-lobe damage might curse and shout at others in line in a way not typical of that person prior to the injury.
- The capacity to restrain or inhibit expressions of strong emotion may be impaired, regardless of the circumstances. The person will make inappropriate sexual comments, ask rude questions, or say things that others may think but do not say, such as 'You're not too bright, are you?' or 'Your breath really stinks.'
- The person may have difficulty comprehending a moderately abstract idea, such as an assignment to oversee an area or a process, and would not be likely to tell you when they were feeling overwhelmed.

Motor and voluntary movement

- There will be considerable trouble using a straw, groping for objects and gripping objects (objects are often dropped).

Drive and motivation

- There will be a noticeable loss of energy to participate in activities.
- Hygiene activities are neglected or not completed.

Thinking

- Reactions occur without trying to think it through, because it is too demanding.

Planning

- The person has difficulty developing and keeping to a schedule.
- Arranging any type of transportation (bus schedules, calling for a ride) is challenging.

(continued)

Box 6.3 *(continued)*

Concentration

- The person will have regular and remarkable forgetfulness.
- Someone with a frontal lobe problem will not be able to track events that occur in the environment.

Ability to sort out what is happening in the environment

- Stimuli, both internal and external, are disorganised and affect the ability to react.
- The person is easily overwhelmed.

Shifting from one mental activity to another

- The person will have difficulty making the shift from, for example, watching TV to talking to another person.

Behaviour

- The person demonstrates an easy loss of self-control and has temper tantrums.
- Mood changes are common.
- The person is apathetic (not caring about events or ideas).

Parietal lobes The parietal lobes integrate information from many other areas to coordinate complex motor and cognitive skills, such as spatial visualisation and analysis, mathematical calculation, and hand movement control in space (e.g. reaching). The parietal lobes also contain the primary somatosensory area receiving sensory input, including touch, pain and temperature, relayed via the thalamus—you know what your body is trying to tell you because the parietal lobes are working.

Occipital lobes The occipital lobes are involved in the perception and recognition of visual information (Ankney & Colbert, 2011). Different regions of the visual cortex process different aspects of the complex visual information, such as colour, movement and edge definition.

Insula The insula integrates and interprets complex social situations, as well as sensory information, including taste, pain and visceral sensations and smell. It also gives rise to social emotions, such as guilt, disgust, pride, humiliation, trust, love and lust.

White matter (axons) underlies the cortex of the cerebral lobes. The white matter increases with age, while grey matter decreases with age. The *corpus callosum*, a white-matter structure,grows in size about 1.8 per cent each year between the ages of 3 and 18 years. As this structure integrates the activity between the left and right cerebral hemispheres, the increase in corpus callosum may be a sign of an increased ability for problem-solving (Boyd & Bee, 2012). See Mental Health in the Media for an excellent example of what happens when a person does not have a corpus callosum.

The brain in general, and the cerebral hemispheres in particular, are well protected not only by the skull, but also by a protective fluid, called *cerebrospinal fluid (CSF)*, which circulates around and within the brain. Deep within the brain are three spaces, or ventricles, which aid in the circulation of CSF. Normal CSF volume is about 125 mL in an average adult, and is replaced approximately four times in 24 hours. The CSF reflects the neurochemical activity of the brain, and is one method for studying *in vivo* (within the living organism) communication. The purposes of spinal taps are to measure the volume and pressure of the CSF; to look for trauma, blood or infection; and to measure metabolites, which are the products or substances produced from the breakdown of metabolic processes of the brain's neuro-messengers.

Limbic system

The **limbic system**, often called the *emotional brain*, is involved in the creation of our emotional states, drives, and behaviours associated with feelings and motivations. It also functions in memory storage and retrieval, some aspects of attention, and integration of our conscious cerebral cortex functions with subconscious and autonomic brainstem functions. Interconnections between the limbic system and the prefrontal cortex link our feelings with our thoughts. Thus, while the cerebral cortex enables us to perform complex

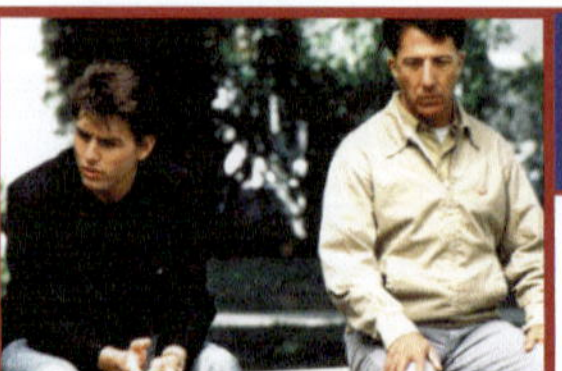

MENTAL HEALTH IN THE MEDIA

Rain Man

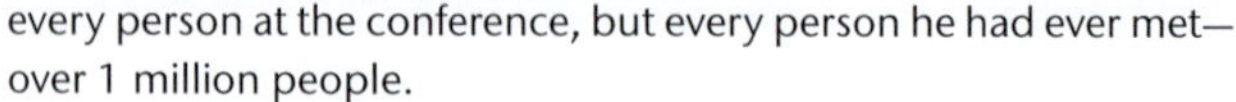

The dichotomy between the deficits of autism and the skills called *savant skills* were displayed in the film *Rain Man*. The real-life inspiration for the brother living with autism depicted in the movie was Kim Peek (who recently died). Mr Peek had limited social skills and was taken care of by his father for his day-to-day needs. When Mr Peek and his father educated people on autism, he demonstrated one of his many extraordinary skills at the beginning of every conference. Typically, he was introduced to each person in the audience as they entered the auditorium or conference centre. During the talk, Mr Peek demonstrated that he remembered not only the name of every person at the conference, but every person he had ever met—over 1 million people.

The neuroanatomical and biological difference between Mr Peek and most other people is that he did not have a corpus callosum. Because he had access to his entire brain without the mediating influence of the corpus callosum, Mr Peek could think and remember very quickly and completely. This contributed to his great memory, in that not only could he remember people, but he could also quote dialogue from any movie, and tell you the day of the week for any date you selected. Despite these unique abilities, problem-solving was always a challenge for him.

Photo courtesy of Alamy.

cognitive tasks, it is the limbic system that motivates us to want to do them.

The limbic system is not a cohesive structure located in one place in the brain; it is a functional grouping rather than an anatomical one. The limbic system forms the border that encircles the upper part of the brainstem. It consists of cerebral hemisphere gyri (ridges) that sit above the corpus callosum, and curve down through the cerebellum and temporal lobes. It also includes nuclei of the *diencephalon*, a part of the brain that connects the cerebrum and midbrain. In neuroanatomy, a nucleus is a cluster of densely packed neuronal cell bodies (grey matter) located deep within the cerebral hemispheres and brainstem. The fornix and other axon fibre tracts link limbic regions together. See Box 6.4.

The following two limbic structures play an especially important role in how emotions and memories are generated:

1. amygdala
2. hippocampus.

Learning and memory are two aspects of the interaction between the amygdala and the hippocampus.

The limbic structures also include the olfactory area. If the olfactory sensors determine a scent, the memory of the event will include this cue. For example, does the smell of baking cookies trigger a pleasant memory of being in a kitchen when cookies are being baked? This is the combined effect of amygdalar and hippocampal functions using the cue of the aroma of cookies as the stimulus for the memory.

Amygdala The amygdalae (singular—**amygdala**; one amygdala in each hemisphere) are integration centres for emotions, emotional behaviour and motivation. They serve as the behavioural awareness centres that determine appropriate emotional and behavioural responses, such as fear and aggression (in response to threats), sexual desire, rage and appetite. Through circuits connecting to the hypothalamus and brainstem, they produce the visceral responses to emotion, such as increases in heart rate, blood pressure and respiration.

Hippocampus The **hippocampus** is also involved in emotional reactions and in learning. It helps process, store and retrieve information in our memory. It provides new information for permanent storage. Hallucinations may, in part, originate from hyperexcitability of psychomotor effects of olfactory, visual, auditory and tactile stimulation in this region (Brown, 2010). Weak stimuli in the hippocampus can cause epileptic seizures.

The limbic system has numerous functions beyond those addressed here, and the neuronal connections are so widespread and intricate within the brain that their complex interactions involve many different areas. Other neuronal groups that participate with the limbic system are the thalamus, hypothalamus and pituitary gland.

Box 6.4 Structures of the limbic system

Cerebral components

Cortical areas: Limbic lobe (cingulate gyrus, dentate gyrus and parahippocampal gyrus)
Nuclei: Hippocampus, amygdalae
Tracts: Fornix

Diencephalic components

Thalamus: Forward (anterior) nuclear group
Hypothalamus: Centre for emotions, appetites (thirst, hunger) and related behaviours

Other components

Reticular formation: Network of nuclei throughout the brain stem

Basal ganglia

The basal ganglia are collectively a set of structures that include the striatum (caudate nucleus, putamen, globus pallidus) and substantia nigra. Their functions include refining movements, planning motor activities, mediating hallucinations and delusions, and processing emotions and memories. The basal ganglia have a high concentration of dopamine receptors, acetylcholine, gamma-aminobutyric acid (GABA), and peptides. A deficit of dopamine in this area is associated with Parkinson's disease. Parkinson's disease is characterised by rhythmic tremors of the extremities, slurred speech and an unchanging facial expression. Former boxer Muhammad Ali, who demonstrated all of these symptoms, sustained numerous blows to his head during his career, which resulted in damage to the basal ganglia.

The basal ganglia, along with the cerebellum, play major roles in the subconscious control of movement through their connection to extrapyramidal motor neurons in the spinal cord involved in reflexes, locomotion, complex movements and postural control.

Reticular activating system The reticular activating system (RAS) is an ascending nerve pathway in the reticular formation of the brainstem that sends continuous impulses to the cerebral cortex to keep it alert and conscious. The RAS also screens out unnecessary or weak sensory stimulation from the environment, sending only important or strong information to the cortex for conscious perception. This enables us to attend or concentrate on important information. The RAS also permits us to not pay attention for a period of time, allowing us to sleep. During sleep, the excitatory neurons of the RAS gradually become more and more excitable because of prolonged rest, while the inhibitory neurons of the sleep centres become less excitable because of overactivity, leading to a new cycle of wakefulness. This helps explain the rapid transitions between sleep and wakefulness. Arousal, as experienced by people living with mental illness, can be the insomnia that occurs when a person's mind becomes preoccupied with a thought. In states of mental disorder, there is obviously some biological disequilibrium of the RAS, because it involves motivation and levels of arousal. However, the details of this imbalance are not yet well understood.

The reticular formation also contains a network of interconnected nuclei throughout the brainstem that send axons to many regions of the brain to regulate their activity (see Figure 6.4 ■). These reticular nuclei include the ventral

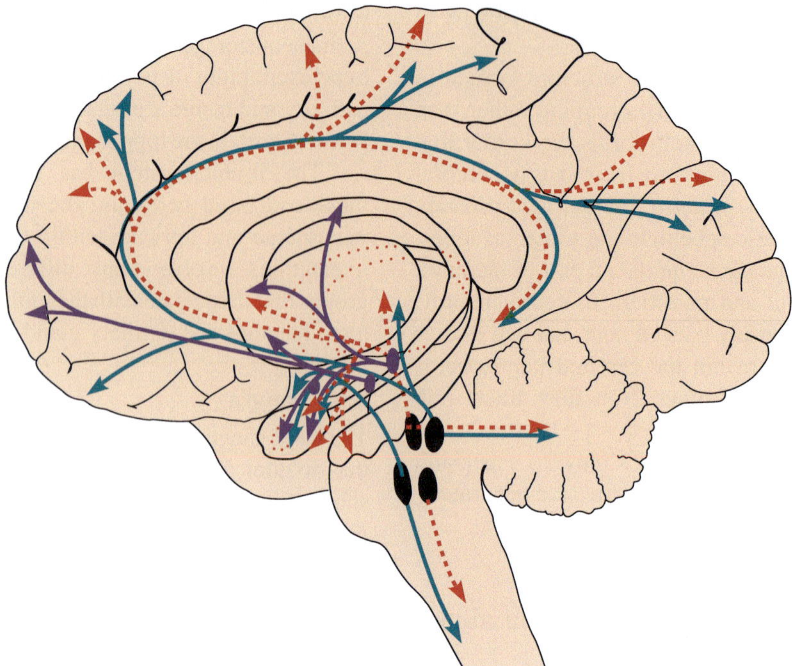

FIGURE 6.4 ■ Common neurotransmitter pathways. Purple = DA, black = NE, dashed line = 5-HT. The dotted line indicates the pons.

tegmental area, whose axons release dopamine to influence motivation and decision-making. Antipsychotics block dopamine activity. Raphe nuclei axons release serotonin throughout the cerebrum and have profound effects on mood. Antidepressants act to prolong the serotonin effects on the cerebrum. Descending pathways and motor nuclei effect subconscious muscle tone for posture control, as well as visceral motor tone (see the extrapyramidal system, on the next page).

Diencephalon

Diencephalon structures sit above the brainstem, and include the thalamus, hypothalamus and epithalamus (which contains the pineal gland). The thalamus functions as a relay and processing centre for sensory information. The hypothalamus controls emotions, autonomic functions and hormone production.

Thalamus The thalamus receives impulses from the spinal cord, brainstem and cerebellum. It acts as a relay station, determining what information is sent to which area of the brain. With the aid of numerous connections in the cerebral hemispheres and cortex, the thalamus regulates activity and movement, sensory experience (except smell) and emotional expression.

Hypothalamus The **hypothalamus** is the link between the nervous and endocrine systems, and thus between the mind and body. Through its endocrine function, it mediates the body's physical response to thoughts and emotions. It weighs approximately 4 grams, and accounts for less than 1 per cent of the total volume of the brain. Its size, however, is not a good indication of its importance. The hypothalamus regulates many of the body's activities critical to homeostasis, including hormone levels, appetite (hunger), body temperature (thermoreceptors), sex drive (libido), water balance (thirst), circadian rhythms, pleasure and pain. See Figure 6.5 ■ for a graphic representation of the hypothalamus as a hub.

The hypothalamus is the critical link between the cerebral cortex, the limbic system and the endocrine system. It serves as a pipeline to the brainstem, and controls the activation of the autonomic nervous system. The mammillary bodies, located at the back of the hypothalamus, help transfer information about the activities of the hypothalamus to other parts of the brain. The amygdala controls hypothalamic impulses due to

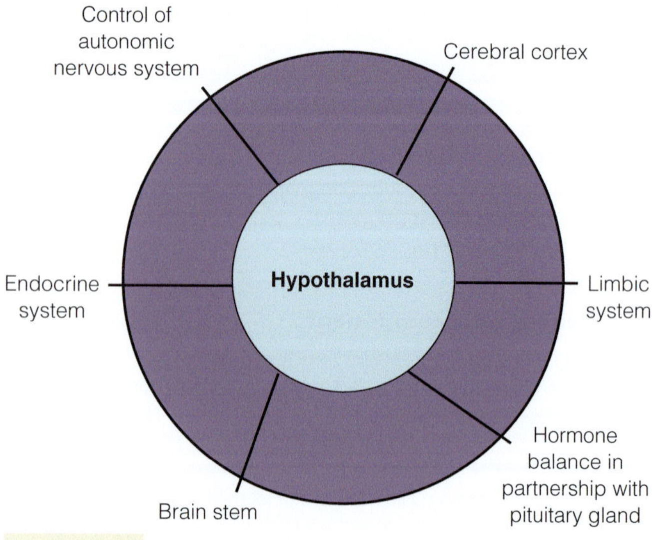

FIGURE 6.5 ■ The hypothalamus hub.

the direct neurological connection. This control is important in the regulation of hunger, thirst, sexual behaviour, rage and/or pleasure.

The infundibulum, a narrow stalk, connects the hypothalamus to the pituitary gland, a part of the endocrine system. The hypothalamus is involved in hormonal balance, along with the pituitary gland. Significant for many mental illnesses is the hypothalamic control of the stress response, whereby cortisol is released from the adrenal glands by the hypothalamic–pituitary axis (Ankney & Colbert, 2011). The thalamus and hypothalamus, as well as the pituitary gland, are illustrated in Figure 6.2.

Pituitary gland

The pituitary gland, under the direction of the hypothalamus, secretes hormones. These hormones are carried through the bloodstream and trigger the activities of other endocrine glands. The pituitary also receives input from the fornix, and includes connections to the thalamus, which in turn communicates to and from the frontal cortex.

Cerebellum

The **cerebellum** lies below the posterior section of the cerebrum. It is our second largest brain structure. Like the cerebral hemispheres, the cerebellum has an outer layer of grey matter and is mainly composed of underlying white matter. The main function of this highly specialised part of the brain is movement, posture, balance and sensory–motor coordination. The hand–eye coordination of a diamond cutter, the fluid movements of a ballerina, and the success of a quarterback's moves all depend on cerebellar functions. The cerebellum also coordinates complex somatic motor patterns, and adjusts the output of other somatic motor centres in the brain and spinal cord.

Brainstem

Beneath the structures in the limbic system is the **brainstem**. The brainstem consists of three smaller structures: the medulla oblongata, the pons and the midbrain.

Medulla oblongata The medulla oblongata relays sensory information to the thalamus and other portions of the brain stem. As the connecting piece of tissue between the brainstem and the spinal cord, it functions as the autonomic centre for the regulation of visceral function (cardiovascular, respiratory and digestive system activities). It is less than 5 centimetres long, but is responsible for controlling many vital functions, including respiration, regulation of blood pressure, and partial regulation of heart rate. It also controls vomiting, swallowing, some aspects of talking, and the perception of pain. Incoming fibres from the spinal cord cross over in the medulla; thus, the left cerebral hemisphere controls the right side of the body, and vice versa.

Pons The pons (Latin for 'bridge') contains conduction paths between the spinal cord and the brain, relaying sensory information to the cerebellum and thalamus, and serving as a visceral and motor centre. It has a role in regulating sleep and controlling rapid eye movement sleep. It also contains reflex centres that mediate sensations of the face, chewing, abduction of the eyes, facial expressions, balance and the regulation of respiration. Located within the pons is the *locus ceruleus*, a tiny oval structure that contains 70 per cent of the neurons (nerve cells) that release noradrenalin, a neurotransmitter affecting the entire brain. One projection of the pons is to the amygdala, resulting in emotional and cardiovascular control. Activation of the locus ceruleus is associated with fear, pain and alarm.

Extrapyramidal system The extrapyramidal system (so labelled because it lies alongside the outer aspects of the pyramidal system) consists of tracts of motor neurons from the brain to parts of the spinal cord. This system has complex relays and connections to areas of the cortex, basal ganglia, cerebellum, brainstem and thalamus. The tracts play an important role in the subconscious control of gross movements and responses of emotional tone, such as smiling and frowning. Antipsychotic medications create side-effects that affect the extrapyramidal system and are called *extrapyramidal side-effects (EPSE)*. A complete discussion of EPSE is in Chapter 7.

Midbrain The midbrain, also called the *mesencephalon*, is located above the pons and below the cerebral hemispheres. The midbrain processes visual and auditory data, and is a reflex centre for the regulation of eye movement, visual accommodation, and the regulation of pupil size. The midbrain is also essential for relaying impulses to the cerebral cortex, generating reflexive somatic motor responses (sending behaviour-producing messages back to the rest of the body), and maintaining consciousness.

Autonomic nervous system Within the brainstem is an area of the autonomic nervous system (ANS) known as the parasympathetic division. In stressful emotional circumstances, the sympathetic division of the ANS (also called the *sympathetic nervous system*), located in the spinal cord, prepares for fight or flight; the parasympathetic initiates the relaxation response with the aid of the endocrine system.

Box 6.5 Mental health skills in practice

As a teacher, researcher and (sometimes) practitioner, I am heavily reliant on scientific understandings of why the symptoms of mental illness occur and what might help to mitigate them. Of course science is only part of the story, but it is a very important part. For me, the challenge in providing effective help for people living with mental illness is how to identify the most effective forms of help, and use these in ways that do not lose sight of the humanity and rights of the people with whom we are working. We also face the challenge of translation—we know a lot about what is likely to help with many forms of mental illness, but unfortunately treatments with demonstrated effectiveness are still not widely available to people living with mental illness.

Mike Hazelton

Neurons, synapses, receptors and neurotransmission

Neurons are specialised cells able to detect and transmit electrical signals. These electrical signals are generated by the movement of charged ions, such as sodium ions Na^+, potassium ions K^+, chloride ions Cl^-, and calcium ions Ca^{2+}, through specialised receptors and channels in the neurons plasma membrane. Communication across the gaps (called 'synapses') that connect adjoining neurons usually occurs via the release of specific chemicals called *neurotransmitters*. Our thoughts, emotions, memories, dreams and hopes result from the complex interplay and patterns of electrical and chemical communication between CNS neurons in response to stimuli from our environment.

As illustrated in Figure 6.1, each neuron has a cell body that contains cytoplasmic organelles and a nucleus. Neurons also have two specialised types of extensions: branched dendrites that detect and receive electrical signals triggered by the binding of neurotransmitters released from adjoining neurons; and an axon that rapidly transmits electrical signals, called *action potentials*, along its length to trigger the release of neurotransmitter from the axon terminal to communicate with the next neuron. Many axons are covered with a white myelin sheath, which increases the speed of action potential transmission, and are visualised as the white matter of the brain and spinal cord. Other cells in the nervous system, collectively called *glial cells*, support the neurons by guiding their growth, forming the blood–brain barrier and controlling the chemical environment around the neurons, forming myelin sheaths, providing protection from microorganisms and producing the cerebrospinal fluid.

Neurons can be classified according to the direction in which they conduct impulses. Sensory neurons, also known as *afferent neurons,* send messages from the peripheral body parts to the brain. For example, if you place your foot into a tub of scalding water, the message that the water is too hot is sent to your brain via sensory neuron pathways. Interneurons in the spinal cord and brain integrate the incoming sensory information and determine the appropriate response. Motor neurons, or *efferent neurons*, then carry messages out of the CNS to effect behavioural change and movement in the peripheral body parts. When your foot is in the hot water, the message from your brain is to remove the foot quickly; this message travels via motor neuron pathways, causing your foot to jerk out of the water.

Synaptic transmission

The dendrites and cell bodies of a single neuron can have between 1000 and 10 000 synaptic connections with other neurons. The axon terminal of a neuron contains many membrane bound sacs called *synaptic vesicles*, which store chemicals called neurotransmitters (NTs). When an action potential arrives at the axon terminal of a presynaptic neuron, it triggers the release of neurotransmitter from the vesicles into the synapse. The released neurotransmitter diffuses across the synapse between the two neurons, and binds to specific neurotransmitter receptors located on the surface of the dendrites and cell body of the postsynaptic neuron (Ciccarelli & White, 2009). The binding of a neurotransmitter to its receptor on the postsynaptic neuron changes the shape of the receptor, which either directly opens a membrane channel allowing rapid movement of a specific ion into or out of the cell (*ionotrophic receptors*), or triggers the activation of a second messenger system that indirectly opens specific ion channels and also alters metabolic activity and gene transcription within the neuron (*metabotrophic receptors*). Thus chemical neurotransmitters (discussed further below) result in the transmission of electrical signals (charged ion flow) to the next neuron.

The effect of neurotransmitter binding on the postsynaptic neuron can be either:

- *excitatory*—making it more likely that an action potential is triggered in the axon of the postsynaptic neuron, or
- *inhibitory*—making it less likely that an action potential is triggered in the axon of the postsynaptic neuron.

Whether neurotransmitter binding is excitatory or inhibitory depends on what type of ion channel is opened by the receptor. Unstimulated, resting neurons have more negative charges on the inside surface of the plasma membrane compared to the outside surface, which is measured as a resting membrane potential (charge difference) of approximately –70 mV. The concentration of sodium ions Na^+, calcium ions Ca^{2+} and chloride ions Cl^- is higher in the extracellular fluid on outside surface of a neuron's plasma membrane, whereas potassium ions K^+ and proteins (which usually have a net negative charge) are more concentrated on the inside surface of the plasma membrane. Opening neurotransmitter-activated ion channels (also called ligand-gated receptors) allows specific ions (and thus electrical charge) to flow across the neuronal plasma membrane down their concentration gradient. Thus dopamine binding to a receptor that opens a sodium ion channel would result in positive charge flowing into the neuron, making the membrane potential less negative (e.g. –30 mV membrane potential). Dopamine binding to a different type of receptor might open a potassium channel, allowing positively charged potassium ions to flow out of the neuron, making the inside of the plasma membrane even more negative with respect to the outside (e.g. –90 mV membrane potential).

The combined influence (net ion flow across the membrane) of all neurotransmitter signalling across potentially thousands of synapses triggers an action potential(s) only if the membrane potential at the start of the axon (axon hillock) reaches a specific threshold voltage (e.g. –55 mV). Reaching this threshold voltage triggers the opening of voltage-gated receptors that allow a rapid influx of sodium ions, and thus a large electrical signal (action potential) that is propagated rapidly, without diminishing along the entire length of the axon. In the motor neurons leading to your toes, this can be a distance greater than a metre.

Therefore, neurotransmitters are excitatory if their binding brings the membrane potential closer to the –55 mV threshold of voltage-gated channels (allow Na^+ inflow, K^+ outflow), and inhibitory if they move the membrane potential further away from –55 mV. This enables the synapses to act as regulation points for neuronal communication. For example, stepping on a thumb-tack usually triggers action potentials in withdrawal reflex neurons that cause you to automatically withdraw your foot. However, you can consciously decide to override this withdrawal reflex, in which case inhibitory neurotransmitter signals from neurons in the cerebral cortex make the triggering of action potentials in the withdrawal reflex neurons less likely. Similarly, neurons involved in cognition, such as those in the prefrontal cortex, can exert inhibitory control over limbic pathways, enabling you to suppress your instinctive fear of snakes, for example. Some mental illnesses involve overactivity in the limbic areas of the brain involved in fear and anxiety, for example, and a reduced cognitive ability to inhibit these emotions.

After release, neurotransmitters are quickly removed from the synapse to ensure that the synapse is ready to convey the next message. There are three mechanisms via which a neurotransmitter is removed from the synapse. It can be reabsorbed back into the presynaptic neuron for recycling (called *reuptake*) by specific reuptake transporters embedded in the membrane of the axon terminal. Neurotransmitters can be broken down by enzymes in the synapse (e.g. the enzyme monoamine oxidase degrades dopamine and serotonin). Some neurotransmitters may diffuse out of the synapse and be absorbed by surrounding glial cells called *astrocytes*. Some psychiatric medications act to slow the removal of specific neurotransmitters from the synapse in order to increase the influence of these neurotransmitters on different brain circuits. For example, selective serotonin reuptake inhibitors (SSRIs) block the reuptake transporter, while monamine oxidase inhibitor medications slow the enzymatic breakdown of monoamines.

Other substances are able to modify the sensitivity of neurons to the effects of neurotransmitters. These substances include neuromodulators such as endogenous opioids and cannabinoids, which helps to explain the effects of illicit opiates and cannabis. Many hormones also exert modulatory effects on neuronal activity in the CNS, either by affecting ion channels or changing gene expression.

It is important to realise that the body uses a limited number of neurotransmitters, but has many different types of receptors for each neurotransmitter. For example, there are five different dopamine receptor subtypes and 14 serotonin receptor subtypes, allowing different messages (excitatory or inhibitory) to be passed to different parts of the brain, depending on the receptor type present. These neurotransmitters and receptors are also used in other parts of the body, not just the brain. In addition to the postsynaptic receptors that act to 'pass on the message' in the next neuron, there are also autoreceptors on the presynaptic neuron. These homeostatic autoreceptors monitor the amount of neurotransmitter in the synapse. If there is too high a concentration of neurotransmitter in the synapse, the autoreceptor will activate a second messenger that turns off further neurotransmitter release. Antipsychotic medications have wide ranging side-effects because they block numerous types of dopamine and other neurotransmitter receptors in all parts of the brain and body.

LIVED EXPERIENCE

Over the years I have experienced a range of sometimes very distressing side-effects, and these can make it difficult to stick to medication that has been prescribed. I prefer to understand as much as I can about the side-effects that might occur with particular medications, and in my experience this is so for many people who live with mental illness. Unfortunately, many of the health professionals I have seen over the years have not been good at telling me what to expect regarding side-effects. I have often wondered if they know themselves.

Neurotransmitters

Neurotransmitters include three classes—monoamines, amino acids and peptides—as well as dissolved gases and a number of other compounds. They control the activity, and thus function, of postsynaptic neurons. It is now known that individual neurons can secrete only one or a number of different neurotransmitters. Neurotransmitters are discussed in Table 6.1 ■.

The monoamines are synthesised from amino acids in neurons of brainstem nuclei. Figure 6.4 illustrates the basic pathways of three of the major monoamines. They regulate the function of the many brain regions into which they are released. Only a small percentage of CNS neurons secrete monoamines; however, many of the currently available psychiatric medications target these neurotransmitters.

Dopamine ***Dopamine*** (DA) is released in many areas in the brain, where it influences how we interact in the world. It is synthesised from the essential amino acid tyrosine, which must be obtained from the diet. Overactive dopamine signalling in some limbic regions may mediate the psychotic symptoms of schizophrenia. Psychoactive drugs like cocaine and LSD inhibit the removal of DA from synapses, leading to excitatory impacts on limbic reward and motivation neurons, and the 'high' associated with their use. Autoimmune damage to dopamine axons that innervate the basal ganglia leads to Parkinson's disease. See Table 6.2 ■ for specific DA areas and functions.

Noradrenalin **Noradrenalin (NA)** is also called *norepinephrine*, and the synapses that release NA are *adrenergic synapses*. Noradrenalin is produced by locus coeruleus nuclei in the pons of the brainstem. Receptors for the neurotransmitter noradrenalin are widespread in the brain (Table 6.3 ■). NA plays a major role in mediating alertness, mood and anxiety. Regulation of noradrenalin has been examined closely in the treatment of mood and anxiety disorders, and has contributed to the development of current pharmacological interventions. See Tables 6.1 and 6.3.

TABLE 6.1 ■ The major known neurotransmitters

Neurotransmitter	Function
Monoamines	
Acetylcholine (Ach) Precursor: choline	Attention; memory; promotes preparation for action; conserves energy; thirst; defence and/or aggression; sexual behaviour; regulates mood; REM sleep; voluntary movement of the muscles; stimulates parasympathetic division of the ANS; controls muscle tone in balance with DA in the basal ganglia
Dopamine (DA) Precursor: tyrosine	Integrates thoughts and emotions; regulates pleasure and reward-seeking stimuli; controls complex movements; motivation; cognition; stimulates hypothalamus to release hormones affecting adrenal, thyroid and sex hormones
Histamine (H) Precursor: histidine	Mediates arousal and attention, smooth muscle constriction; stimulates gastric acid secretion; role in biorhythms and thermoregulation; role in second-messenger transmission; mediates allergic and inflammatory responses
Noradrenalin (NA) or norepinephrine Precursor: Tyrosine	Stimulates sympathetic division of the ANS; role in stress response; fluctuates with sleep and wakefulness; role in attention and vigilance, arousal, ability to focus or learn, feeling of reward, and regulation of mood and anxiety
Serotonin (5-HT) Precursor: Tryptophan	Inhibits activity and behavior; role in level of arousal; increases sleep time; reduces aggression, play, sexual, and eating activity; regulates temperature; controls pain; controls mood states; role in circadian rhythms; regulates senses; helps focus the brain; regulates pituitary
Amino acids	
Aspartate	Excitatory
Gamma-aminobutyric acid (GABA), also written as γ-aminobutyric acid Precursor: Glutamic acid	Reduces aroused aggression, anxiety and excitation; sedation; motor behaviour; anticonvulsant and muscle-relaxant properties
Glutamate	Excitatory; role in learning and memory; neural degeneration
Glycine Precursor: serine	Inhibitory; spinal reflexes; motor behaviour
Peptides (Neuromodulators)	
Cholecystokinin (CCK)	Role in schizophrenia; eating and movement disorders; panic disorder
Corticotropin-releasing hormone (CRH)	Stress, mood, memory and anxiety
Neurotensin	Role in schizophrenia
Opioids: endorphins and enkephalins	Alter emotional behaviour; pain control; hallucinations; pleasure; motor coordination; water balance
Somatostatin	Mood disorders; Alzheimer's disease; negative feedback control of thyrotropin secretion; role in positive symptoms of schizophrenia; excites limbic neurons
Substance P	Excitatory; role in pain syndromes, mood and movement disorders
Vasopressin	Role in mood disorders

TABLE 6.2 ■ Dopamine location and function

Area/location	Dopamine is associated with	
Basal ganglia area	The control of complex movement	
Limbic system	Memory Mood Reward	Pleasure Motivation
Hypothalamic tract	Endocrine functions Circadian rhythms	Food and water intake Temperature
Frontal cortex pathway	Insight Judgment Problem-solving	Inhibition Social awareness

TABLE 6.3 ■ Noradrenalin location and function

Area/location	Noradrenalin is associated with	
Pons, specifically locus ceruleus	Stress response Arousal	Alertness
Cerebral cortex	Cognitive functioning	
Limbic system	Emotional responses Ability to focus or learn Reward	Regulation of mood Pleasure
Hypothalamus	Endocrine functions Temperature	Appetite Biological rhythms

Serotonin Serotonin (also referred to as 5-HT for its chemical name 5-hydroxytryptamine) neurons arise in the raphe nuclei in the brainstem, and project to virtually all areas of brain, like the NA pathways. Serotonin is synthesised from the essential amino acid tryptophan. Brain serotonin levels can be lowered significantly by insufficient dietary tryptophan intake in grains, meat and dairy. Serotonin plays a role in sleep, appetite and mood. Drugs that block the serotonin reuptake transporter relieve anxiety and depression.

Acetylcholine Acetylcholine (Ach) is released by all motor neurons that control skeletal muscles, and by some neurons in the autonomic nervous system. However, acetylcholine neurotransmission to the cortex and hippocampus has a role in attention, learning and memory. Reduced acetylcholine levels in the hippocampus are associated with Alzheimer's disease.

Histamine Histamine (H) mediates a wide range of cellular responses, including allergic and inflammatory reactions, gastric acid secretions, and neurotransmission. In the CNS, histamine is involved in wakefulness, appetite control, learning and memory. The sedation, weight gain and drowsiness side-effects of some tricyclic antidepressants and antipsychotics occur because they block histamine receptors (Preskorn, 2011).

Amino acids The amino acid neurotransmitters are used by the overwhelming majority of neurons in the brain. Although these non-essential amino acids are abundant in our diet and body, their passage across the blood–brain barrier is tightly controlled or restricted.

The amino acid gamma-aminobutyric acid (GABA) is the most prevalent inhibitory neurotransmitter. GABA neurons are widely distributed in the CNS, and play a prominent role in arousal. GABA interneurons constitute 25 per cent of the cerebral cortex, and provide the local constraint over cortical circuits. Benzodiazepine, barbiturates and alcohol increase the inhibitory flow of chloride ions through GABA receptors. Hence, drugs like benzodiazepine are used to help manage conditions where too much CNS activity occurs, including: epilepsy, insomnia, pain, anxiety and mania. Glycine, also an inhibitory neurotransmitter, exists primarily in the brainstem, spinal cord and cerebellum.

Glutamate is the major excitatory neurotransmitter. It is used by over 50 per cent of CNS neurons, primarily located in the cerebral cortex and hippocampus, and has a role in long-term memory and learning. Without glutamate, the brain would not function. Alterations in glutamate neurotransmission have been implicated in a number of mental illnesses, including schizophrenia. However, the fact that too much glutamate is neurotoxic has restricted the development of safe drugs targeting this neurotransmitter. Aspartate may also function as an excitatory neurotransmitter; however, its function remains controversial.

Effects of neuropeptides, hormones and stress on the brain

Neuropeptides are small chains of amino acids, which constitute a broad spectrum of molecules with diverse effects on the brain and body. They include substance P, endogenous opioids and neurohormones secreted by the hypothalamus and pituitary. In the brain, neuropeptides often act as modulators, increasing the effects of the classical neurotransmitters described above. However, many can act as neurotransmitters, modulators or hormones, depending on the tissue, synapse and frequency of action potential stimulation. Some of the best understood neuropeptides are summarised in Table 6.1.

Substance P is an 11-amino acid peptide that has a role in signalling the intensity of pain. It may also contribute to changes in the CNS that predispose individuals to anxiety and depression. Endogenous opioids (e.g. endorphins and enkephalins) inhibit CNS neurons involved in the perception of pain, and are predominantly localised to the spinal cord, hypothalamus and some brainstem nuclei.

The hypothalamus is the major link between the brain and the endocrine system. The hormone-secreting activity of the hypothalamus is stimulated by direct neuronal inputs from the cerebral cortex (inhibitory control), hippocampus (inhibitory control), amygdala (excitatory control) and thalamus. Via its control of the pituitary gland, the hypothalamus controls the major homeostatic and hormonal systems of the body. In turn, many hormones exert effects on the brain via feedback control loops. These effects take time to develop, because hormones tend to modulate the effects of neurotransmitters, change neurotransmitter receptor levels, or alter neuronal metabolism (thyroid hormone) or gene expression (sex hormones).

Dysregulation of the hypothalamus–pituitary–adrenal (HPA) axis is particularly relevant to the development of mental illness (Figure 6.6 ■). The normal response to a threat or stressful situation is the hypothalmic activation of the sympathetic nervous system (liberating adrenalin) and the HPA axis (liberating cortisol) to bring the body and brain to an alert fight-or-flight orientation. Cortisol mobilises energy, increasing cerebral glucose, and turns down non-essential functions (e.g. digestion). The brain becomes more focused and vigilant to help deal with the threat.

Normally, cortisol then participates in negative feedback control loops that turn down the HPA axis and brain hypervigilance when the threat is resolved. However, when stress levels are chronically elevated, the negative feedback loops malfunction, and the brain is unable to turn down the HPA axis, exposing the brain and body to excess cortisol. The pathological consequences of heightened sympathetic activity and HPA activation include hypertension, diabetes, ulcers and impaired immune function. In the brain, the most dramatic negative effect involves the hippocampus, where increased cortisol causes the loss of dendritic connections, reduced brain-derived neurotrophic growth factor (BDNF), decreased neurogenesis and neuroplasticity, and may ultimately lead to neuronal death and shrinkage of the hippocampus. Reduced functioning of the hippocampus then impairs memory and learning. In the prefrontal cortex, prolonged exposure to high levels of cortisol also reduces the number of dendritic and synaptic connections between neurons, and the death of pyramidal neurons. This impairs the cognitive functioning of the prefrontal cortex. In contrast, chronic stress and elevated cortisol

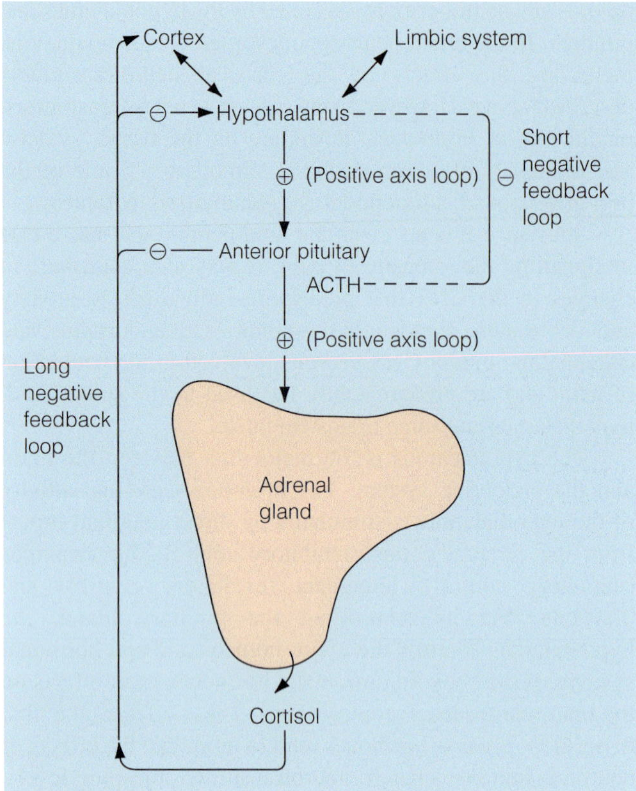

FIGURE 6.6 ■ Example of neuroendocrine feedback. The positive loop in the axis is depicted by the hypothalamus. Upon stimulation from the cortex or limbic system, the release of trophic peptide CRH (corticotropin-releasing hormone) tells the pituitary gland to signal the adrenal cortex, via the ACTH (adrenocorticotropic hormone), to release the glucocorticoid cortisol. Cortisol released into the bloodstream provides negative feedback to the hypothalamus or anterior pituitary. Additionally, ACTH can provide negative feedback to the hypothalamus.

stimulate the amygdala, enabling it to become hyperactive and increase fear and anxiety responses. Dysregulation of the HPA axis and neuroendocrine function have been linked to depression, postpartum psychosis, schizophrenia, panic disorder, obsessive–compulsive disorder, anorexia nervosa, dementia of the Alzheimer's type (DAT), and circadian rhythm disorders.

Brain development and neuroplasticity

The brain is not static or 'hardwired'. Instead, the structure and function of the brain constantly changes in response to its experiences, a phenomenon termed **neuroplasticity**. Thus thinking, talking and acting actually changes the brain, allowing it to adapt to its experiences and environment.

During development, the vast majority of new neuron growth, called neurogenesis, occurs *in utero* and in early childhood. Thus the majority of your neurons are as old as you are! Uterine brain development is predominantly determined by genetics, but is influenced by environmental factors, such as uterine nutrition, maternal stress and toxins. Misguided positioning or connections during uterine neurogenesis may contribute to susceptibility to mental illnesses such as autism and schizophrenia. Neurogenesis continues in early childhood when there is also extensive growth of each neuron's dendrites and axon, with the aim of making new connections. An enriched environment promotes neurogenesis and positive neuroplasticity. Stresses inhibit neurogenesis and promote negative neuroplasticity. During adolescence and early adulthood, extensive refinement of the neuronal connections occurs, where dendrites are pruned and synapses are eliminated. Some axonic connections are strengthened by increased myelination, allowing more rapid propagation of action potentials. This enables the brain to make better, more efficient connections and eliminate excessive connections. People with autism have an increased brain volume, and it has been proposed that excessive connections and insufficient pruning may contribute to this condition. Conversely, schizophrenia, which usually develops in late adolescence, is associated with reduced grey matter (dendrites and cell bodies). Excessive neuronal pruning may play a role in this condition. In adulthood, neurogenesis is restricted, predominantly to the hippocampus, which is involved in memory storage. Growth factors, such as brain-derived neutrophic factor (BDNF), that promote neurogenesis and the maintenance of existing neurons, are increased by physical exercise and learning.

Yet hope remains for your old adult cerebral cortex, because all neurons remain plastic! Existing neurons and their connections remain modifiable throughout life. This neuroplastic change occurs via a number of mechanisms. The sensitivity of synapses to neurotransmitters can be altered, because the activation of metabotrophic receptors alters metabolic activity and gene expression in the target neuron, which can change the number of receptors produced and inserted into the plasma membrane. The number of dendrites, and thus

LIVED EXPERIENCE

I have had a lot of psychotherapy over the years, with mixed results. One of the best experiences was with a therapist I saw for about six years, who helped me a lot. I stopped seeing this person about four years ago, and haven't been able to make the same kind of connection with several therapists I have seen since. Nowadays I try to be my own therapist, or at least my own coach. I fill my days with meaningful activities—involvement in a hearing voices group, studying languages at university, casual teaching at university, writing my contribution to this textbook and many others. I think of such activities in terms of positive neuroplasticity.
At the same time I try to avoid things that might contribute to negative neuroplasticity, such as damaging relationships, stressful experiences and the like.

synaptic connections, a neuron has can be modified. Increased myelination of frequently used axons makes communication more rapid. Neurons can be re-tasked so that more neurons are dedicated to frequently performed tasks, and less to little-used functions. Thus the structure and activity in our neural circuits can be increased or decreased by our experiences and thoughts. Positive neuroplasticity is promoted by learning, a nutritious diet, exercise and by building the activity in circuits that increase our mental wellbeing. Neuroplasticity that is detrimental to our mental wellbeing is promoted by factors such as trauma, illicit drug use, alcohol abuse, infection and chronic stress.

Genetics and epigenetics in mental health

Most mental illnesses are complex, heterogeneous conditions in which no two people present with the same symptoms or personal history. Not surprisingly, genetic studies have found that no single defective gene causes a mental illness, as is the case for conditions like Down's syndrome. Nevertheless, high concordance rates in identical twins with mental illnesses indicate that inherited **genetic variation** does play a significant role in predisposing people to the development of these conditions. Recent studies of schizophrenia, for example, have identified over a hundred different genes potentially linked to this illness. It is generally thought that a complex interplay of susceptibility genes and environmental stressors (e.g. traumatic experiences) are necessary for the development of mental illness. In this context, environmental stress refers to both physical and social stress.

Our genes are comprised of deoxyribonucleic acid (DNA), which is a double-chain polymer of four different nucleotides. Individual nucleotide structure is distinguished (and denoted) by which of four different nitrogen-containing bases they contain: adenine (A), thymine (T), guanine (G) or cytosine (C). A gene sequence is a long specific sequence of these four nucleotides which encodes the amino acid sequence of a specific protein. The average length of a human gene is 15 000 nucleotides, but varies enormously. We all inherit two copies of each gene (alleles), which may differ slightly in nucleotide sequence, one from our mother and one from our father. The nucleotide sequence of a gene encodes the amino acids sequence of its protein, which in turn determines the protein's physical and biological properties.

Variations in the nucleotide sequence, or genetic code, can occur when the DNA is copied in preparation for cell division and gamete production. This variation can be thought of as 'spelling mistakes' made when copying the sequence of 3 billion nucleotides, including those encoding 25 000 different genes, in human DNA. This variation is a rare but normal part of DNA replication that contributes to our individuality and evolution, but also to our disease susceptibility if the variation is deleterious to protein function. Insertions, deletions or substitutions of a single nucleotide within a gene sequence are called *single nucleotide polymorphisms* (SNPs—pronounced 'snips'). However, large-scale errors can also occur through the insertion, deletion and duplication of large sections of DNA many thousands of nucleotides long. These errors are called *copy number variants* (CNVs), because they can encompass the sequence of numerous genes. To date, some 128 common SNPs and at least 15 rare CNVs have been identified that are thought to contribute to a person's susceptibility to developing schizophrenia (Kotlar, Mercer, Zwick & Mulle, 2015). Some of these genes are involved in processes such as supporting synaptic plasticity and memory consolidation and glutamate signalling via N-methyl-D-aspartate (NMDA) receptors.

Gene expression, and thus protein production within a cell, can also be influenced by factors that don't change the actual nucleotide sequence of DNA, but instead alter the ability of the cell's molecular machinery to 'read' the gene sequence. The expression of specific genes can be turned on or off (gene silencing) by the addition or removal of chemical groups (e.g. methyl groups—a carbon molecule with three hydrogens attached) to the DNA or DNA-associated proteins (e.g. histones). These reversible chemical modifications alter access to the nucleotide sequence, or the ability of nucleotides to form stable bonds with complementary nucleotides (base-pairing) and thus be replicated. Importantly, these epigenetic changes have been shown to be altered by environmental factors, providing an important mechanism via which our environment and experiences alter gene expression. For example, maternal neglect in rats and child abuse in humans have been shown to increase the methylation of a specific gene encoding a stress hormone receptor (glucocorticoid/cortisol receptor) in the hippocampus. Reduced expression of this receptor protein is thought to interfere with the regulation of the stress response and make affected individuals more sensitive to stress (reviewed Albert, 2010). Genetic and epigenetic variations have now been associated with susceptibility to all of the major mental illnesses, and it is hoped that this expanding knowledge will improve our understanding and treatment options.

BIOLOGICAL BASIS OF MENTAL ILLNESS

This section examines current hypotheses about the biological basis of schizophrenia, major mood disorder, generalised anxiety disorder, obsessive–compulsive disorder and dementia of the Alzheimer's type (DAT). These illnesses are complex disorders that may involve alterations in many parts of the brain and neuronal communication patterns. The exact causative mechanisms have not been established, and theories used to explain the development of these disorders remain controversial and the subject of intensive research. They are not the result of simple imbalances in neurotransmitter levels, such as serotonin, dopamine and noradrenalin, as has come to be surmised by many members of the public in response to pharmaceutical interventions. They tend to be associated with functional imbalances in the relative activity of different regions of the brain. Some of these functional imbalances can be influenced by pharmaceutical drugs and psychotherapies.

Schizophrenia

Schizophrenia is a clinically heterogeneous illness. People living with schizophrenia contend with a broad range of symptoms that may include positive symptoms (e.g. hallucinations, delusions, disorganised speech/behaviour), negative symptoms (e.g. apathy, flattened emotional expression, poverty of speech) and cognitive impairments (problems with executive function, attention and memory). Inheritance studies suggest that genetic variation contributes 50–80 per cent of the risk of developing the illness; however, it is increasingly apparent that many genes contribute to a person's genetic susceptibility. People who are genetically at risk for schizophrenia are then more sensitive to environmental stressors leading to the development of illness.

People with lived experience of schizophrenia, including children with early-onset schizophrenia, consistently have subtle reductions in total brain volume and grey matter volume. The most obvious sign of these reductions in brain size is a corresponding increase in the size of the ventricles (cerebral spinal fluid-filled spaces) within the brain. This may be associated with a loss of neurons in some areas such as the hippocampus and thalamus. However, in the cortex the loss of grey matter appears to be caused by a reduction in the number of dendritic branches that individual neurons have, rather than a reduced number of neurons. The loss of dendritic density, and thus inter-neuronal connections, is thought to contribute to deficits in information-processing. It affects almost all areas of the cerebral cortex, highlighting the fact that schizophrenia involves many regions of the brain.

Disrupted myelination of the axon tracts that connect different regions of the cortex, and the cortex to underlying brain structures, may also contribute to the poor neuronal communication seen in schizophrenia. Disrupted myelination slows or stops the propagation of the action potential along the axon. Some disrupted neuronal connectivity is likely to occur during brain development before or shortly after birth as a result of the interplay between susceptibility genes and environmental factors, such as poor maternal nutrition, maternal stress and obstetric complications. However, during adolescence the neuronal connections of the brain are further modified by the processes of dendritic pruning and apoptosis. The development of schizophrenia in late adolescence or early adulthood may result from the interplay of genetic factors, such as excessive dendritic pruning and poor synaptic plasticity, and environmental stressors, such as trauma, dysfunctional family interactions and dendritic atrophy caused by elevated cortisol levels.

How could poor connectivity between neurons and neuronal circuits produce the symptoms of schizophrenia? The cognitive impairments associated with schizophrenia implicate reduced functioning of the prefrontal cortex, and indeed reduced blood flow/metabolic activity in the prefrontal cortex has been demonstrated in people living with schizophrenia during cognitive challenge tests. Atrophic, disconnected neurons in the prefrontal cortex are the likely cause of cognitive impairment. Increased rates of dendritic pruning in the prefrontal cortex have also been associated with the development of psychosis. The psychotic or positive symptoms of schizophrenia, such as hallucinations and delusions, can be described as an inability to test reality. Auditory hallucinations in schizophrenia have been associated with reduced dendritic connections in the auditory cortex, which registers external sounds in the temporal lobe, and also with alterations in the white matter circuits that send auditory information from the auditory cortex to the prefrontal cortex for interpretation. People may experience auditory hallucinations because their dysfunctional auditory cortex and its communication circuits are unable to distinguish between a voice generated by external sound and one generated by internal speech/self-talk thoughts. In the prefrontal cortex and hippocampus, disruption of the balance between the activity of excitatory glutamate neurons and inhibitory GABA neurons may contribute to the pathophysiology of schizophrenia. In these areas, the activity of excitatory neurons that use glutamate signalling on NMDA receptors is controlled by inhibitory GABA inter-neurons. Disruption of the inhibitory GABA signals received by the glutamate neurons allows them to increase their activity (action potential output). Correct signalling and control between these neurons are important in working memory, and the experience-dependent synapse plasticity involved in learning and memory. They also function in assigning the 'context' and source to thoughts and retrieved memories. For example, determining if something was actually perceived or imagined, or distinguishing between an experience and a belief, i.e. reality monitoring. It is therefore possible that disruptions of the excitation–inhibition balance in the prefrontal cortex and hippocampus may lay the foundation for the development of psychotic symptoms. Thus, schizophrenia appears to be a disorder of widespread disruption of the connections and signalling between neurons.

Alterations in the excitation–inhibition balance in the prefrontal cortex may in turn change the amount of dopamine released in other areas of the brain (Cannon, 2015). The 'dopamine hypothesis' was originally proposed based on the observation that antipsychotic medications, which block dopamine receptors, blunt (but do not cure) psychotic symptoms. Increased dopamine activity in the mesolimbic pathway has been associated with positive symptoms, whereas decreased dopamine activity in the mesocortical pathway may contribute to the negative symptoms.

Dopamine has a central role in reward and reinforcement. It contributes to determining the 'wanting' or desirability response to sensory input and thoughts. Thus dopamine mediates the conversion of the neural representation of an external stimulus (or internal thought) from a neutral and cold bit of information into an attractive or aversive entity. In particular, the mesolimbic dopamine system is seen as a critical component in the 'attribution of salience', a process whereby events and thoughts come to grab attention, drive action and influence goal-directed behaviour, because of their association with reward or punishment.

Excessive dopamine in the striatum/mesolimbic pathway may lead to the persistent and inappropriate assignment of salience and motivational significance to stimuli. This state of aberrant salience is proposed to lead to inappropriate associations being formed in response to sensory inputs and internal thoughts/memories, and the development of positive symptoms. People living with schizophrenia might begin by assigning significance or importance to an incidental, neutral stimulus and, over a period of time, build up a complex delusion as a way of explaining why this unimportant object/detail/thought has taken on such great meaning. Delusions are therefore a cognitive effort to make sense of these aberrantly salient experiences, and they reflect a maladaptive update of the person's worldview. Similarly, hallucinations may be experiences that result from aberrant salience being applied to internally generated stimuli/perceptions/memories.

Antipsychotic drugs are major tranquilisers that block neurotransmitter receptors, especially dopamine receptors. However, they do not cure psychotic symptoms, they merely reduce them. This has been termed 'dampening salience'. They reduce the significance attributed to stimuli, and therefore their ability to control and direct behaviour. People with lived experience of psychotic symptoms might describe this as their delusions/hallucinations 'not bothering them as much anymore'. Thus antipsychotics provide only symptomatic control, and psychotic symptoms return in most cases if treatment is stopped. They stop people from feeling.

Changes in *sensory gating* have also been identified in people with schizophrenia. Sensory gating continuously monitors and modulates sensory and cognitive information to allow us to selectively attend to important (gated-in) stimuli while ignoring redundant, repetitive and trivial (gated-out) stimuli. Sensory gating is known to occur in all incoming sensory systems (olfactory, somatosensory, visual and auditory). People with schizophrenia appear to be less able to gate-out information, which may contribute to difficulties in sustaining attention and inhibiting distractions. Sensory gating involves complex interactions of excitatory and inhibitory neuronal circuits using multiple neurotransmitters.

It should be acknowledged that many people with lived experience of auditory hallucination reject biological explanations such as those outlined above. The Hearing Voices Movement argues that hallucinations are real and have evolved from what has happened to the person, rather than anything that is wrong with them.

Major depressive disorder

Major depressive disorder is a complex and variable illness diagnosed on the basis of persistent disturbance of mood (e.g. sadness), or loss of interest in/or pleasure derived from most activities (anhedonia). Additional symptoms can include sleep disturbance, guilt, loss of energy, impaired concentration, psychomotor agitation or retardation, and suicidal ideation. Despite its high prevalence (one in seven Australians will experience depression), and considerable burden on individuals and society, the biological basis of depression remains controversial. The monoamine hypothesis has been the dominant biological explanation of depression for the past 50 years. It postulates that depression is associated with relative deficiencies in monoamine neurotransmitters, particularly serotonin and noradrenalin, in functionally important areas of the brain. However, the fact that approximately 40 per cent of patients do not respond to antidepressants targeting these monoamines indicates that the pathophysiology of depression is more complex (Willner, Scheel-Krüger & Belzung, 2013).

People living with depression have profoundly negative views of themselves, the world and their future. This arises from negative biases in attention, interpretation and memory that increase elaboration and focus on automatic negative thoughts producing pathological rumination. A complex interplay of multiple risk genes and early life experiences establish a person's vulnerability to depression. Psychological and biological factors interact to convert adverse childhood experiences, such as poor parental care, criticism and abuse, into characteristic negative styles of processing information in relation to ideas of 'self'. Later in life, a stressful event precipitates the first episode of depression in susceptible people. The stressful trigger can be an internal event, such as hormonal change, a major interpersonal loss, such as bereavement, or an accumulation of chronic stresses, such as poverty and family disharmony. Recurrent episodes of depression sensitise the brain so that weaker and weaker stressors are required to trigger depression.

Structural and functional changes observed in the brain of people living with depression seem to correlate with the

COLLABORATIVE CARE

Teaching about genetics and schizophrenia

At present there is no definitive test for schizophrenia—no blood test or biopsy result that would render a diagnosis—so genetic testing for schizophrenia takes place in research settings. A reliable test using blood and other body cells might be a significant breakthrough in the treatment of schizophrenia. Talking about genetics with people living with schizophrenia and their families may help them to better understand the nature of the illness, treatment options and risk reduction.

If the people with whom you work and their family members have the opportunity to be involved in genetic or other forms of mental health-related research, participant information documents and other informed-consent requirements for participation in these studies will explain what is being tested, the procedures being used and how long the data collected will be kept following the research. People living with mental illness and their family members should know that research does not necessarily help the participants involved in a study. However, the knowledge gained will contribute to a better understanding of the type of mental illness being investigated and/or the development of more cost-effective treatments. An important area of schizophrenia research is the development of a clearer picture of whether the genetics of the disorder does shape what happens to future generations of people who develop schizophrenia or whether the 'illness' is more associated with environmental and social causes.

neurotoxic effects of chronic stress and dysregulation of the HPA axis as described above. The degree of reduced dendritic connections and BDNF in the hippocampus is correlated with the severity of the depression and memory loss. Antidepressants reverse stress-induced hippocampal changes by increasing BDNF, increasing the growth of dendrites and stimulating neurogenesis, and thereby elevate mood. It has been speculated that the neurogenesis promoted by antidepressants supports new learning of more adaptive cognitions and behaviours.

Changes in the balance of activity between different regions of the prefrontal cortex and the circuits that link them with limbic structures are also observed in people with depression. The activity of different regions of the prefrontal cortex is effected by the reduction of dendritic connections and neuronal atrophy associated with stress. A ventral affective circuit that links the ventral and orbital prefrontal cortex with the amygdala, striatum, anterior cingulate cortex, insula and hippocampus, functions in identifying the emotional significance of stimuli, the production of affective states and autonomic regulation in response to emotional situations. Hyperactivity in this affective circuit in depression is likely to give rise to the negatively biased emotional state (sadness and anhedonia), and is associated with increased punishment sensitivity, anxiety and depressive ruminations. A dorsal cognitive circuit that links the dorsolateral prefrontal cortex with the dorsal anterior cingulate cortex and hippocampus, functions in executive control, including selective attention, planning and effortful regulation of affective states. Reduced activity in this cognitive circuit during depression is associated with reduced cognitive capacity, psychomotor retardation, apathy and decreased attentional capacity. Successful treatment with antidepressants (especially those increasing serotonin neurotransmission), electrical stimulation or behavioural therapy improve the balance of activity in these circuits (Singh & Gotlib, 2014; Willner et al., 2013).

Anxiety disorders

The neurobiology of both **anxiety** and mood disorders, and the subtypes of these illnesses, share overlapping and disorder-specific structural, functional and neuroendocrine alterations. Dysregulation of the HPA axis is a common to many of these disorders.

Generalised anxiety disorder (GAD) is characterised by chronically excessive and uncontrollable worry and anxiety in response to a variety of events and situations. It is accompanied by physical symptoms of anxiety, including insomnia, poor concentration, irritability and muscle tension. In people who develop GAD, worrying may become established as a cognitive strategy to avoid perceived threats. In the brain, apprehensive expectations induce hyperactivity in the amygdala, but poor connectivity in emotional regulation circuits between the amygdala and the dorsolateral prefrontal cortex and anterior cingulate cortex mean that the worries are perceived as uncontrollable, and the HPA axis and cortisol secretion become chronically activated. Ensuing dysregulation of the HPA axis further diminishes the functional connectivity between the amygdala and prefrontal cortex, exacerbating the anxiety and further reducing emotional regulating capacity (Hilbert, Lueken & Beesdo-Baum, 2014).

> **LIVED EXPERIENCE**
>
> I have often thought of myself as having an anxiety-prone personality; this has often meant excluding myself from social interactions; worrying over things, such as whether the landlord is going to come around; or struggling with thoughts, such as am I going to burn down the unit. Anxiety has also contributed to sleep problems and a heightened sensitivity to noise. The medications I take to help with anxiety also contribute to problems such as weight gain. I feel better able to tolerate and manage anxiety nowadays, and attribute that largely to positive neuroplastic changes I have made in my life, such as maintaining healthy relationships and high levels of social engagement, and avoiding high-stress situations. I also regularly use guided meditations and find these effective.

Obsessive–compulsive disorder

Obsessive–compulsive disorder (OCD) is characterised by anxiety-provoking thoughts or images (obsessions) and repetitive behaviours that are performed to reduce anxiety (compulsions). People living with OCD have increased activity in the orbital frontal cortex (part of the ventral prefrontal cortex), the striatum (part of the basal ganglia) and the orbitofrontal–striatal–thalamic circuit that connects these brain regions. The orbital frontal cortex enables individuals to adapt their behaviour in response to expected rewards or adversities by anticipating whether some course of action will evoke positive or negative emotions, both immediately and in the future. The striatum (and the orbitofront–striatal–thalamic circuit) supports the automatic or habitual processing of information and patterning of behaviour.

For people with OCD, obsessions and compulsions become excessively automatic/habitual patterns of thought and behaviour, while other cortical cognitive circuits that consciously/critically assess thoughts and behaviours are underactive, making it difficult for people to change their behaviour. The repetitive thoughts and behaviours become linked with the limbic circuits, causing considerable anxiety. Successful treatment with antidepressants or cognitive behaviour therapy normalises the overactivity in the orbital frontal cortex, striatum and orbitofront–striatal–thalamic circuit.

Dementia of the Alzheimer's type (DAT)

Dementia of the Alzheimer's type is a slowly progressing neurodegenerative disorder that is the most common form of dementia in late adult life. It is characterised by progressive

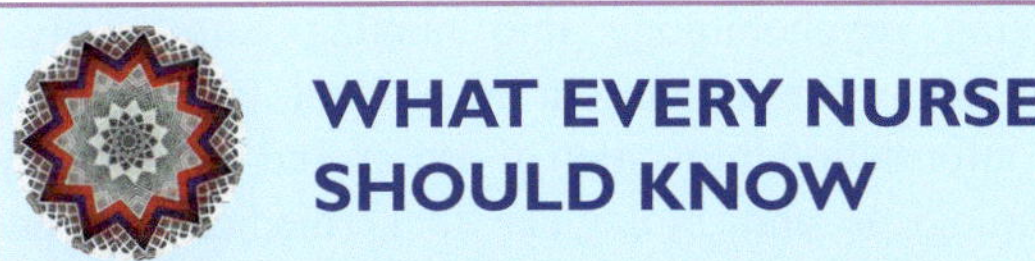

WHAT EVERY NURSE SHOULD KNOW

A person living with schizophrenia who is agitated

Imagine that you are the psychiatric–mental nurse working on a community mental health team. The team receives a call about a very agitated man who has a history of paranoid delusions and hallucinations. You and the other team members approach the man, who is on his verandah mumbling to himself and acting in a very agitated manner.

Your knowledge of the psychobiology of schizophrenia supports the strategy of having only one person speak clearly and simply to this man so as not to overwhelm him. His executive functioning, and therefore his ability to process incoming information, is challenged when symptoms are acute. You interact with him in a calm, straightforward manner, asking what the problem could be. When he answers you in a loud, menacing tone that he must 'strike before the irons have cooled beyond their colouration', you ask him to tell you what he wants you to do. In the conversation that follows, you discover that he has not been eating or sleeping, that he becomes very distressed when people interrupt him (to ask him to eat or try to get some sleep), and that he is exhausted from days of trying to accomplish a task associated with his delusional thinking.

When it is apparent that a person such as this man is experiencing severe symptoms, stabilisation is needed to protect him and others. Stabilisation can be achieved through providing a combination of safe environment, psychopharmacology and compassionate care to help him through this trauma. Chiovitti's (2011) concept of protective empowering provides a useful framework for how situations such as this can be managed.

cognitive decline, the accumulation of amyloid protein plaques outside the neurons that impair synaptic communication, neurofibrillary tangles inside the neurons, and inflammation leading to neuronal cell death and cortical atrophy (Mufson et al., 2015).

Alzheimer's disease has a long preclinical stage of up to 20 years prior to the emergence of clinical symptoms. There is also a high degree of inter-individual variability in the onset of dementia, with some individuals having a high degree of pathology (plaques and tangles) but minimal cognitive impairment. This suggests that neuroplastic alterations in brain synaptic connections and circuits are able to counteract the disease-related changes in the initial stages. Neural degeneration begins in the entorhinal cortex of the medial temporal lobe and proceeds to the hippocampus. The entorhinal cortex–hippocampus system plays an important role in spatial memory, including memory formation and memory consolidation. As hippocampal cells lose their synaptic connections and die, memory starts to falter. However the hippocampus is capable of neurogenesis and significant neuroplasticity, and compensates for neurodegenerative changes in the early stages of Alzheimer's disease. Degenerative changes then spread to the cerebral cortex, leading to greater difficulty with language and judgement.

Neurodegeneration leads to disruptions in neurotransmitter balance in different areas of the brain. Neurotransmitters commonly affected include serotonin, noradrenalin and acetylcholine, with acetylcholine being the most affected and decreasing by up to 90 per cent. The gradual death of cholinergic brain cells contributes to the progressive and significant loss of memory, cognitive and behavioural function. Soluble beta-amyloid protein disrupts the production and release of acetylcholine, and interferes with the actions of a nerve growth factor involved in maintaining the structure and function of cholinergic neurons. The progression of Alzheimer's disease can be modestly slowed by the therapeutic administration of acetylcholinesterase inhibitors, which stop the release of the enzyme acetylcholinesterase that breaks down acetylcholine in the synapse. However, they do not stop the destruction of cholinergic neurons, although they may temporarily boost the cognitive performance of people with the illness; their main advantage is that they slow the progression of decline by keeping acetylcholine levels as high as possible in the early stages. The only other medication currently available for the treatment of moderate to severe Alzheimer's disease is memantine, which blocks the NMDA receptor for glutamate. This slows the excitotoxic damage associated with excessive glutamate release from degenerating neurons and astrocytes.

At its core, Alzheimer's disease is a protein misfolding disorder centered on amyloid precursor protein, a membrane protein located in the synapse that has an integral role in neuronal plasticity. Genetic mutations involved in the metabolic pathways of amyloid precursor protein have been associated with an early-onset, genetically-inherited form of Alzheimer's called 'familial Alzheimer's disease'. The amyloid cascade hypothesis proposes that the pathophysiology of Alzheimer's disease is initially associated with the abnormal enzymatic conversion of amyloid precursor protein into beta-amyloid protein. An imbalance in the production and clearance of beta-amyloid protein by both neurons and astrocytes (a glial cell) (Kumar & Ekavali, 2015) allows high concentrations of the beta-amyloid proteins to spontaneously aggregate into soluble beta-amyloid oligomers, which then further coalesce into insoluble fibrils (abnormally folded amyloid protein polymers) that are eventually deposited in diffuse senile plaques outside the neuron. The beta-amyloid oligomers promote additional neuronal cell damage by causing oxidative damage, abnormal hyperphosphorylation of tau proteins (a neuron structural protein) leading to neurofibrillary tangles, the destruction of myelin, toxic effects mitochondria and the destruction of synapses.

The insoluble amyloid plaques are not deposited outside the neurons and into the cerebral blood vessels until a late stage in the development of the disease. However, when they are deposited, they attract and activate microglia, which sets off an inflammatory cascade of events in which cytokines released by the microglia stimulate the production of more soluble beta-amyloid oligomers, exacerbating the extensive neuronal and vascular damage seen in the brains of people with advanced Alzheimer's disease.

PSYCHOBIOLOGY AND NURSING

Throughout this text you are frequently reminded that linking body, mind, brain and behaviour is the essence of holistic psychiatric–mental health nursing practice. Integrating psychobiological principles enhances that goal. To function effectively as a health care professional, it is important to be aware of any personal feelings, opinions or beliefs that you have that may diminish your ability to be an advocate for, and support person to, people living with mental illness and their families.

Your attitude about the underlying neurobiology of behaviour can influence therapeutic outcomes. It is important to consider how treatment outcomes are potently influenced by both the style of, and knowledge incorporated into, interventions. If comprehensive assessment, interpretation of the assessment, mental health teaching and evaluation of the intervention are based on knowledge of the biological, cognitive, behavioural and social factors that affect a person, there is greater opportunity for successfully reducing the symptoms being experienced by that person. If, however, you are ambivalent about the value of biological or somatic therapies, it is possible that this attitude will be communicated to the person and their family, and your interventions may not be as effective as they could be. Remember, you integrate your own viewpoint into the mental health teaching you undertake, and its expression can hinder or help the people with whom you are working and their families.

Integrating psychobiology into nursing care involves our skills as nurses throughout our assessment, integration of assessment information into a plan of action, and interventions with psychological and biological foci (medications and physiological-based strategies). It enables the nurse to fine-tune assessments, diagnoses, interventions and evaluations of treatment response patterns. The synthesis of this critical thinking provides quality, cost-effective care for people living with mental illness and their families.

Being a nurse provides many opportunities to be flexible, creative and a visionary. It can be a helpful professional strategy to keep a diary of how your work with a person contributed to their recovery. Was there a biological aspect to your work with this person? Reflect on the approach you used in trying to make a difference, and link it with cost-effective care. The psychobiologically-informed therapeutic relationship remains the core of your nursing practice.

The exact biological determinants for psychiatric disorders and behaviours are yet to be discovered. To date, there is no definitive biological test to identify any psychiatric disorder. We still rely on professional observations and assessment. However, multifocal and multi-disciplinary care that incorporates psychobiological dimensions advances our ability to offer informed, more effective assessments and interventions for people living with mental illness.

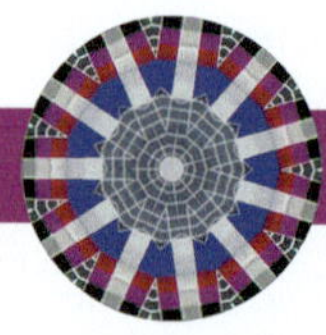

REFERENCES

Albert, P. R. (2010). Epigenetics in mental illness: Hope or hype? *Journal of Psychiatry and Neuroscience, 35*(6), 366–368.

Ankney, J. J., & Colbert, B. J. (2011). *Anatomy and physiology for health professions: An interactive journey* (2nd ed.). Upper Saddle River, NJ: Prentice Hall.

Boyd, D. A., & Bee, H. L. (2012). *Lifespan development* (6th ed.). Upper Saddle River, NJ: Pearson.

Brown, S. A. (2010). Implementing a brief hallucination simulation as a mental illness stigma reduction strategy. *Community Mental Health Journal, 46*(5), 500–504.

Cannon, T. D. (2015). How schizophrenia develops: Cognitive and brain mechanisms underlying onset of psychosis. *Trends in Cognitive Sciences, 19*(12), 744–756.

Chiovitti, R. F. (2011). Theory of protective empowering for balancing patient safety and choices. *Nursing Ethics, 18*(1), 88–101.

Ciccarelli, S. K., & White, J. N. (2009). *Psychology* (2nd ed.). Upper Saddle River, NJ: Pearson Education.

Hilbert, K., Lueken, U., & Beesdo-Baum, K. (2014). Neural structures, functioning and connectivity in generalized anxiety disorder and interaction with neuroendocrine systems: A systematic review. *Journal of Affective Disorders, 158,* 114–126.

Kotlar, A. V., Mercer, K. B., Zwick, M. E., & Mulle, J. E. (2015). New discoveries in schizophrenia genetics reveal neurobiological pathways: A review of recent findings. *European Journal of Medical Genetics, 58,* 704–714.

Kumar, A., & Ekavali, A., S. (2015). A review on Alzheimer's disease pathophysiology and its management: An update. *Pharmacological Reports, 67,* 195–203.

Mufson, E. J., Mahady, L., Waters, D., Counts, S. E., Perez, S. E., Dekosky, S. T., . . . Binder, L. I. (2105). Hippocampal plasticity during the progression of Alzheimer's Disease. *Neuroscience, 309,* 51–67.

Preskorn, S. H. (2011). CNS drug development: Part III: Future directions. *Journal of Psychiatric Practice, 17*(1), 49–52.

Singh, M. K. & Gotlib, I. H. (2014). The neuroscience of depression: Implications for assessment and intervention. *Behaviour Research and Therapy, 62,* 60–73.

Willner, P., Scheel-Krüger, J., & Belzung, C. (2013). The neurobiology of depression and antidepressant action. *Neuroscience and Behavioral Reviews, 37,* 2331–2371.

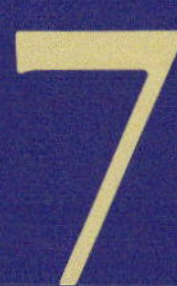

7

The science, practice and experience of psychopharmacology

MIKE HAZELTON AND SIMON SWINSON

LEARNING OUTCOMES

After completing this chapter, you will be able to:

1. Explore developments in psychiatric–mental health nursing since the introduction of psychopharmacological medications in 1958.
2. Incorporate psychotropic medications into treatment for various groups of people living with mental illness.
3. Apply the biological impacts of medications to the care of people living with mental illness.
4. Identify two manifestations that require you to differentiate psychiatric symptomatology from medication side-effects.
5. Describe how you would document the positive and negative impacts of psychiatric medications on behaviour.
6. Compare and contrast the general classifications of medications used for particular symptoms of mental illness.
7. Explain the psychobiological mechanisms important in psychopharmacology.
8. Teach people living with mental illness and their families about the effects and uses of psychotropic medications.
9. Explore the experience of psychotropic medication use of people living with mental illness.

LIVED EXPERIENCE

Medications used in psychiatry have made it possible for me to maintain a relatively positive outlook on life and good mental health for over a decade. I credit the medications with stabilising my thinking and mood. I also believe they have played an important role in preventing what once would have been called 'breakdowns'. This has had the consequence of radically improving my quality of life. I am in the pro-medications camp and would not consider ever ceasing my treatment. At the same time, these benefits have been accompanied by weight gain and reduced physical health. However, in recent years I have felt well enough to tackle these medication side-effects. For instance, in the past 12 months I have shed about 12 kilograms through being more conscious of diet and engaging in increased physical activities, such as walking. Overall, I feel psychotropic medication has been an important part of my recovery journey.

KEY TERMS

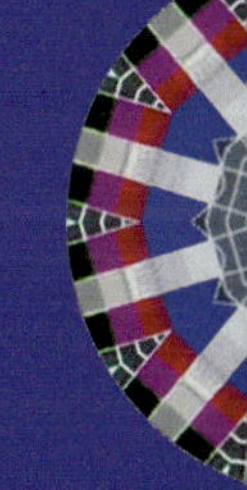

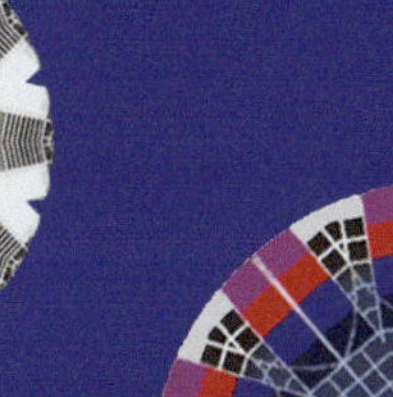

INTRODUCTION

This chapter explores the science, practice and lived experience of the psychopharmacological agents used to treat symptoms of mental disorders and disabilities. The categories and main effects of these medications are detailed here, as well as some rationales for certain medication choices. The chapter also addresses ways to help people manage their medications and the side-effects they may experience. The science, practice and experience of psychopharmacology are intertwined; however, this chapter's discussion of the basics of the major medication groups used in psychiatric–mental health nursing can help you create a useful platform on which to build your therapeutic interactions.

Psychopharmacological nursing interventions deal with the side-effects, drug interactions, psychosocial implications, and education activities involving you, the people living with mental illness with whom you work, and their families. Psychotropic medications are an important part of the work undertaken by psychiatric–mental health nurses, and over time have contributed to the development of the practice of the profession.

As can be seen in the psychopharmacological timeline in Figure 7.1 ■ on pages 114–115, in the years prior to the 1950s (when psychopharmacology became available and widely used), the focus was on behavioural interventions and sedative substances. In the past six decades, considerable progress has been made in treating many of the symptoms of mental illness. While disputed by commentators within the critical psychiatry movement (O'Reilly & Lester, 2016), it is held that mental illness can be understood (in part) as an imbalance of brain chemicals that to some extent can be addressed or corrected with medications. This way of thinking about mental illness and its treatment has much in common with understandings of physical health problems, such as the endocrine disorder diabetes which responds to treatment with insulin.

It has sometimes been argued that developments in biological psychiatry triggered the dramatic decrease in psychiatric inpatient numbers since the inception of psychopharmacology. While such developments were undoubtedly important in shifting the focus of mental health care from institutions to the community, public concern over the neglect and mistreatment of patients in psychiatric hospitals was also significant (Lewis, 1990).

Psychopharmacology is an important part of psychiatric–mental health nursing care, and requires nurses to monitor treatment response as well as identify problems or side-effects. This is a holistic function, which incorporates the person's life, likes and dislikes, and activities, along with symptomatology, into a comprehensive view of treatment. One of the aims of psychopharmacological interventions is to teach people about their medications, including over-the-counter medications and supplements, and the likely impact of these medicines and supplements.

PSYCHOPHARMACOLOGY AND NURSING

The knowledge base of psychopharmacology continues to grow as a result of research and clinical expertise. Psychiatric–mental health nursing has similarly grown, and our responsibilities to people living with mental illness include psychopharmacological expertise. It is important that nurses are able to use neuroscientific and pharmacological knowledge to provide safe and effective clinical management for people taking these medications.

Every nurse is responsible for maintaining an updated knowledge base in psychobiology and pharmacology to draw upon during clinical work. The National Strategy for Quality Use of Medicines (Commonwealth of Australia, 2002) aims to make the best possible use of medicines to improve health outcomes for all Australians, by improving the way health care providers prescribe and administer medications; treatment prescriptions are adhered to by people receiving treatment; and all stakeholders (practitioners, consumers, service managers, industry representatives) are committed to, and collaborate in, improving the quality of medication use. Nurses are important players in ensuring the safe and effective use of medication, and this is especially true in psychiatric–mental health nursing, in which the goal of psychopharmacological interventions is to promote the person's physiological stability, as part of working towards recovery. See Your Intervention Strategies, on the next page, for ideas regarding how to help people prescribed psychotropic medications to adhere to the treatment regimens.

The word *drugs* conjures up a variety of powerful positive and negative images. Media messages depict the devastating negative effects of IV drug use, alcoholism and methamphetamine use. They also give a picture of people leading productive lives, professionals working to achieve the relief of symptoms, and schoolchildren being inoculated against diphtheria, polio and pertussis. All of these images are powerful, and each is backed by truth. But every media representation, positive or negative, must be viewed critically, because misunderstanding and outright ignorance about psychiatric disabilities can lead to inaccurate portrayals of symptoms and treatments. Powerful media messages can influence and interfere with effective care.

It is important that health professionals such as nurses reflect on their attitudes about medications, in particular psychiatric medications. A good starting point would be for you to look at the following Self-awareness box. Exploring your personal feelings will be a healthy challenge throughout your psychiatric–mental health nursing practice, and psychopharmacology could evoke very strong feelings in either direction for you. It is important that you are aware of your biases and have well-informed opinions, so that you are able to provide the best possible care for the people with whom you are working.

YOUR INTERVENTION STRATEGIES Enhancing adherence to medication

The following are ideas that you can use to help people maintain their prescribed medication regimen:

- Discuss their health behaviours with the person and their families.
- Use atypical antipsychotic medications—they have a lower side-effect profile, and can increase adherence because they tend to be easier to tolerate.
- Try another medication with a different neurotransmitter action that may have a different or more tolerable side-effect profile.
- Use role-playing and assertiveness techniques in practice sessions to teach people how to report the range and severity of side-effects.
- Discuss the side-effects of the medication, and teach the person how these can be managed to make them more tolerable (e.g. gum or sweets for dry mouth, pillowcase protectors for night-time drooling).
- Simplify the medication regimen.
- Discuss expectations of medication use. This should include whether the medication use is likely to be temporary or longer-term.
- Use practical, easy-to-use education tools—pamphlets, booklets, workbooks, videos, posters, computer-assisted resources.
- Enhance the person's control over the treatment regimen by offering real choices.
- Teach the person how to self-administer medications.
- Involve the person in planning for problem-solving, as well as learning how to problem-solve.
- Consider the use of depot medications, so that the person does not have to remember to take pills daily.
- Suggest the use of reminders to serve as cues to remembering (e.g. wearing a rubber band or similar on the wrist as a visual cue that 'when I see this I need to take my pills'; calendars, to-do-lists, pre-setting alarms on clocks or phones).
- Recommend the use of pillboxes for medications that can be taken out of their original containers.
- Keep all medications and product information in one cool, dry place—not in the bathroom, or by a sink or dishwasher in the kitchen.
- Encourage the person to be hopeful regarding their ability to manage the medications and any associated side-effects.
- Discuss safe ways of reducing and coming off the medication if the person feels it is impairing their recovery, or their physical or mental wellbeing. This should include the importance of first discussing changes in medication usage with the person who prescribed the medication.

SELF-AWARENESS
Your views on psychopharmacology

Your cultural experiences have an influence on your attitudes towards medications. These attitudes have an impact on one of the major interventions in psychiatry—psychopharmacology. Which of these views do you hold about medications? How will they affect the care you provide to people living with mental illness?

- They will make me healthier.
- This stuff will kill me.
- It is only for a short time.
- They are addictive.
- I will take medications only if my life depends on it.
- Isn't modern pharmacology a wonderful thing?
- I take the right medication for the problem.
- Taking the medications will mean I am a bad/weak person, because I couldn't battle my disorder on my own.
- Medicine is made from herbs—it is the same thing, so I would rather take the herbs.
- Medications are too strong for me, so they are too strong for everybody.
- I cannot contaminate myself with these chemicals.
- If I take psychiatric medications, people will think I am crazy.
- What if the people at work find out I am taking these pills? They will think I cannot do my job.
- I am flawed because I need medication.
- People are more sophisticated these days. They would understand that I am taking the exact same medications as a well-known public figure.

Neuroleptics and psychotropics

The complexities of psychiatric disorders and the desire to address the challenges faced by people who experience symptoms have resulted in the development of a number of medication regimens. Research has further expanded our knowledge, and a clearer understanding of the pros and cons of these compounds is emerging. Many medications have multiple indications beyond their original ones, which have necessitated more global terms to describe the medication. Classification names such as 'antipsychotic' and 'antidepressant' are still in use; however, this is changing, and some medications are labelled 'neuroleptic' or 'psychotropic', with the understanding that they can be used across a number of diagnostic groups.

One example of this phenomenon is fluoxetine, used originally as an antidepressant, but now also indicated in the treatment of obsessive–compulsive disorder. A second example is risperidone, an atypical or newer antipsychotic, now also indicated for use in stabilising the manic phase of bipolar disorder, but also used for behavioural disturbance in dementia. A term that is sometimes applied to the use of medications outside their approved indications is 'off-label' use. A recent Australasian clinical practice guideline recommends careful documentation supporting the off-label use of medication, and also advocates that the reasons for such prescriptions are explained to the people taking the medications, including the possibility of additional costs due to lack of third-party payer subsidy (Galletly et al., 2016). It should also be noted that there are risks associated with the use of psychotropic medications

Important dates in the treatment of mental disorder with psychopharmacology

Before psychopharmaceuticals

164BCE to 1951CE

- Olive oil infused with narcotics, opium, morphine or other sedatives was used to medicate 'insane' and 'deranged' people.

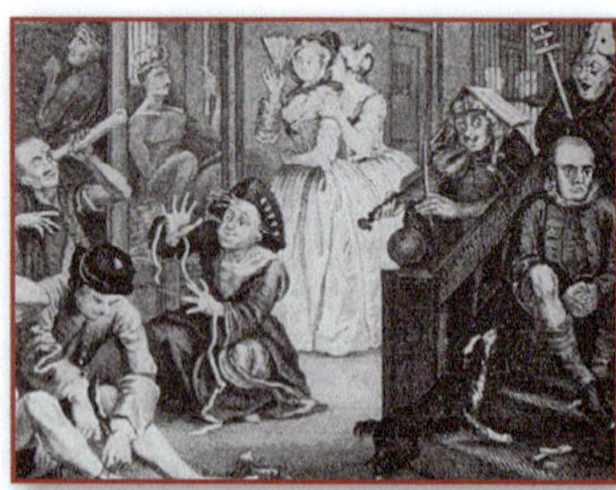

Conventional antipsychotics

1950s

- Quite by chance, chlorpromazine was first used to treat schizophrenia in 1952 after it was observed that its use as an antihistamine also calmed preoperative patients. It changed forever the face of psychiatry, dramatically decreasing the number of inpatients and gave birth to modern notions of psychiatric treatment.

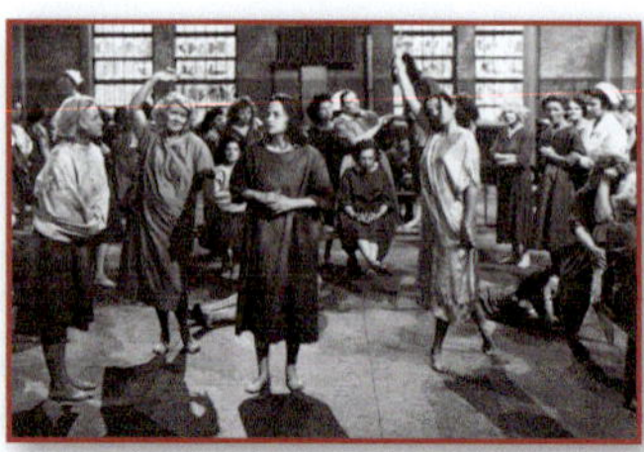

- In this decade, other antipsychotics, trifluoperazine, perphenazine and thioridazine, were developed.

Psychopharmaceuticals for the new millenium

2000s

- Nonbenzodiazepine anxiolytic, ramelteon, used to treat anxiety.
- The first sedative–hypnotic for long-term treatment of insomnia, eszopiclone, is released.
- Synaptic action developments lead to antidepressant SSRI medications sertraline, paroxetine and citalopram.

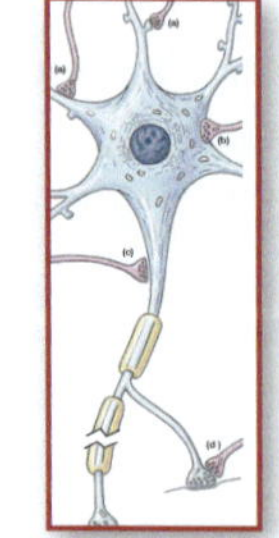

- Antidepressants called serotonin and norepinephrine reuptake inhibitors desvenlafaxine and duloxetine—which treat depression and pain—are developed and released or newly indicated for depression.
- Atypical antipsychotics ziprasidone, aripiprazole, paliperidone and asenapine add to treatment options.
- The first long-acting atypical antipsychotic, Risperdal Consta, provides long-acting antipsychotic without the side-effects of the conventional antipsychotic. This leap forward in treating psychosis was followed by other long-acting atypical antipsychotics Zyprexa Relprevv and Invega Sustenna.
- Acetylcholinesterase inhibitor medication, galantamine, is developed and released.
- The first medication for dementia modifying the brain's glutamate pathway, memantine, pioneers alternative modes of dementia treatment.

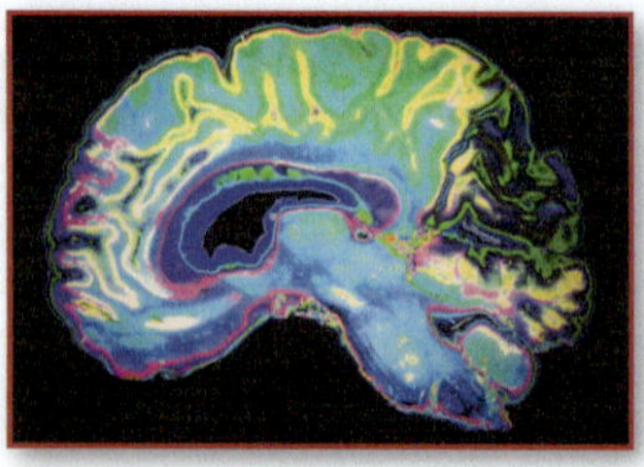

FIGURE 7.1 ■ Important dates in the treatment of mental disorder with psychopharmacology.

First generation antipsychotics and anxiolytics

1960s–1970s

- Other antipsychotics such as haloperidol are made available.
- During this period, antianxiety agents were developed to relieve anxiety and induce sleep. Meprobamate was the first antianxiety agent in common use.
- Medications help people move out of institutions into less restrictive settings and homes.

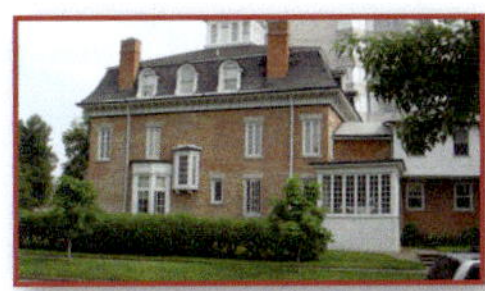

- Long-acting injections of haloperidol and fluphenazine allow consumers to maintain steady levels of antipsychotic without depending on oral formulations. Injections can be given every 2, 3 or 4 weeks.

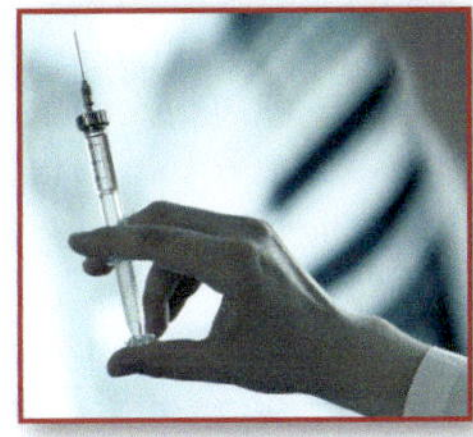

Advances in the decade of the brain

1990s

- Atypical antipsychotic clozapine is re-released after extensive research to establish safety and use in North America. Becomes the 'gold standard' in managing a treatment-resistant or treatment-refractory psychosis. Different dopamine action has decided impact on both negative and positive symptoms of schizophrenia.

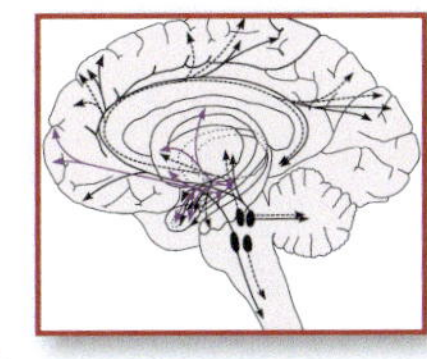

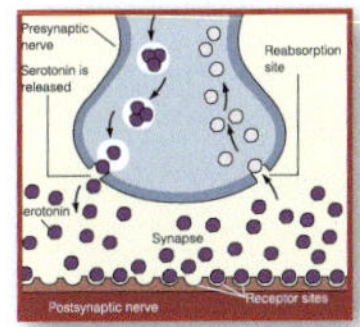

- Atypical antipsychotics risperidone, olanzapine and quetiapine are developed and released, and have the advantage of being easier on the body, have fewer side-effects due to advances in neurotransmitter effects, and do not require blood monitoring.
- Antidepressant SSRIs sertraline, paroxetine and citalopram are made available.
- Acetylcholinesterase inhibitors donepezil and rivastigmine are developed and released.
- The first nonbenzodiazepine anxiolytic, zolpidem, is developed, followed by zaleplon.

2010s

Contemporary developments

- Development and release of the National Strategy for Quality Use of Medicines, which aims to make the best use of medicines to improve health outcomes for Australians.
- Atypical antipsychotic lurasidone is synthesised, adding yet another compound to treat psychosis.

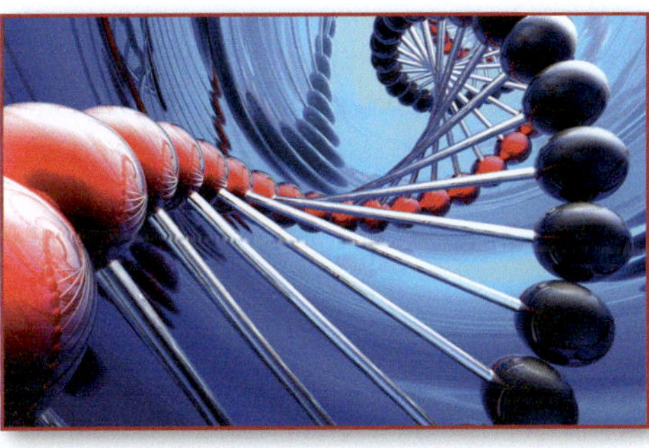

- Genetic phenotypes and variations, as well as the effects of ethnicity on psychiatric pharmacology (ethnopharmacology), are being explored so that someday soon we may be able to have exactly the right medication to help a consumer reach stability and recovery.

LIVED EXPERIENCE

When I was first commenced on antipsychotic and antidepressant medication, one of the first questions I asked my psychiatrist was whether I could become addicted to these drugs. His response was that the available evidence suggested this was unlikely. My concerns were prompted by the hostility some of my close friends displayed towards psychiatric medications; the implication was that the adverse effects caused by these drugs would outweigh any benefits. It was also implied, I felt, that taking medications was a sign of weakness. Over time, through meeting other people living with mental illness who were taking medications, I came to realise that those who adhered to prescribed treatments did better than those who did not. Most of the people I knew who relapsed had stopped taking their medication.

outside their approved indications. A recent example is risperidone (referred to earlier in this paragraph) which in the past decade has been the subject of a series of class-action lawsuits in the United States, some of which have already been concluded in favour of the plaintiffs. The cases brought against the pharmaceutical company producing risperidone have included fraudulent marketing, obscuring dangerous side-effects such as substantial weight gain, increased risk of diabetes and stroke, and gynaecomastia in men.

The clinical application of non-psychiatric medications to treat a psychiatric diagnostic group or a set of psychiatric symptoms also occurs. The complexity of the brain's involvements in physical and emotional problems indicates the need for overlapping and interwoven treatments. One of the most apparent examples is the anticonvulsant class. Sodium valproate, carbamazepine and lamotrigine are all used as mood stabilisers as well as for their original indications.

Ethnic and cultural considerations in psychopharmacology

It is possible that the effects of medications will vary between ethnic groups. For instance, people of East Asian background may require lower doses of psychotropic medications and be more at risk of developing extrapyramidal side-effects (Ormerod, McDowell, Coleman & Ferner, 2008). It is also important to consider cultural factors, and to negotiate these when working with a person to decide the best approach to medication and other forms of treatment. This is of critical importance for nurses and other health professionals who work with Aboriginal and Torres Strait Islander people. It is essential that non-Indigenous clinicians are familiar with the key policy documents pertaining to the health and wellbeing of the Indigenous people of Australia (National Aboriginal and Torres Strait Islander Health Council, 2004), and seek and accept the advice of Indigenous non-clinicians to ensure that symptoms are not misunderstood or incorrectly attributed to cultural factors. The communication styles of non-Indigenous practitioners may also need to be reviewed when working with people of Aboriginal and Torres Strait Islander background. See Box 7.1, Recommendations for Working with Aboriginal and Torres Strait Islander People.

Box 7.1 Recommendations for working with Aboriginal and Torres Strait Islander people

- Cultural awareness training should be mandatory for all mental health clinicians.
- Cultural consultants should be available within mainstream services, ideally matched for gender, language and cultural group.
- Mainstream health services should create an atmosphere of cultural safety using culturally adapted resources.
- Mental health services should use engagement strategies that recognise cultural attitudes to mental illness.
- Consideration should be given to arranging for a family member or cultural consultant to act as a mediator.
- An appropriate manner of communication (e.g. narrative 'yarning', less direct questioning style, open-ended questions) should be adopted.
- Provision of comprehensive treatment, recognising the roles of substance use, stress and trauma in complicating assessment and management.
- Careful sharing of knowledge, to enable informed choices and support concordance with treatment.
- Awareness of increased risk of side-effects, especially cardiometabolic syndrome with psychotropic medications such as antidepressants and antipsychotics.
- Awareness that Aboriginal and Torres Strait Islander people with mental illness have an elevated risk of suicide.

Source: Adapted from Galletly et al., (2016) and Mahli et al., (2015).

ANTIPSYCHOTIC MEDICATIONS

Antipsychotic medications are those used to treat hallucinations, delusions, disorganised thinking and other psychiatric and non-psychiatric conditions and symptoms. The discovery of the first antipsychotic medications, such as chlorpromazine, is a prime example of the role of chance in the history of psychopharmacology. Chlorpromazine was initially synthesised as an antihistamine to facilitate operative procedures, and was not tried as a tranquiliser for people living with schizophrenia until 1952. Its effects on the behaviour, thinking, affect and perception of people living with schizophrenia were sufficiently positive that information about chlorpromazine's properties was rapidly disseminated, and it became widely used within three to four years.

Chlorpromazine's effects on the hospital practice of psychiatry were considerable. Its use contributed to steadily reducing inpatient populations in psychiatric institutions in many countries, including Australia, New Zealand, the United Kingdom and the United States. It is often thought that the availability of chlorpromazine initiated modern notions of psychiatric treatment—unlocked wards, milieu treatment, occupational and recreational therapy, psychiatric rehabilitation and supervised-living environments. However, it is now recognised that the introduction of antipsychotic medications such as chlorpromazine was one of a number of important developments that eventually led to the transfer of mental health care to the community (Lewis, 1990). While antipsychotic medications may have made it possible for most people living with mental illness to live outside an inpatient facility, the infrastructure and support necessary to live in the community also needed to be established, including the provision of secure accommodation, income support, education and employment opportunities. Unfortunately, services in many of these areas remain under-developed (Carr, Whiteford, Groves, McGorry & Shepherd, 2012).

In the decades since the discovery of chlorpromazine, much has been learnt about which medications work under which circumstances. While the research has not always been unequivocal, there is evidence indicating that, for most people, taking antipsychotic medication is more effective than taking no medicine, and that taking it regularly is important to the long-term treatment of schizophrenia. We know that medications alone are not sufficient to cure the illness, but they can play an important part in managing it. These medications may also help people obtain better results from psychosocial interventions. Decades of experience demonstrate how psychopharmacology can assist people in managing anxiety, stress and other symptoms, so nurses and other health professionals can intervene with education about coping strategies and developing or strengthening support systems.

A good place to learn more about the effectiveness of the various medications used in mental health care is clinical practice guidelines, such as those on the management of schizophrenia and related disorders (Galletly et al., 2016) and mood disorders (Mahli et al., 2015), that have recently been published by the Royal Australian and New Zealand College of Psychiatrists. Selected evidence-based and consensus-based recommendations from these clinical practice guidelines are set out in Box 7.2.

Understanding the psychobiology of antipsychotic medications requires a basic knowledge of the functions of the central nervous system. Chapter 6 provides an inside look at the psychobiological mechanisms that are important in psychopharmacology. Here is an overview of the basic mechanisms of action.

Basic mechanisms of action

Generally, neuroleptics (medications that work on the central nervous system) work by blocking a variety of central nervous system (CNS) receptors. Most medications work on more than one neurotransmitter system. Therefore, it is likely that several types of neurotransmitters and neuromodulators are affected by the administration of a single medication. While most neuroleptics have an affinity for several types of neurotransmitters, others are more specific and work more selectively. These differences account for the effects of the

Box 7.2 Recommendations on the medication management of schizophrenia and related disorders and mood disorders

Major depressive disorder (MDD)

Antidepressant therapy for MDD

1. An adequate trial of antidepressant therapy for MDD should be a minimum of three weeks at the recommended therapeutic dose using a suitable medication (EBR 111).
2. When commencing antidepressant therapy, clinical response and side-effects should be closely monitored from the outset (CBR).

Combination therapy for MDD

1. A combination of psychological and pharmacological therapy should be considered, when response to either modality alone has been suboptimal or unsuccessful (CBR).

First-episode psychosis

1. The management plan should be discussed fully with the individual and their family/carers, wherever possible. The benefits and risks of drug therapy should be explained in a non-coercive manner (EBR 11).
2. Medication should be used in combination with psychosocial interventions, including strategies to encourage adherence to medications (EBR 11).
3. The choice of antipsychotic medicines should be based on (EBR 1):
   a. the person's preference after risks and potential benefits have been explained
   b. the person's prior response to the medicine (if known)
   c. clinical response to adequate treatment trial
   d. individual tolerability
   e. potential long-term adverse effects.
4. The lowest effective antipsychotic dose should be used to establish treatment acceptance and minimise side-effects (EBR 11).
5. Prescribe only one antipsychotic agent at a time, unless it has been clearly demonstrated that the person's symptoms are resistant to monotherapy (EBR 11).
6. Prescribe antipsychotic medicines at doses that are adequate to prevent relapse, suppress symptoms and optimise the person's subjective wellbeing (EBR 11).
7. Provide an adequate duration of treatment. Monitor treatment and adverse effects appropriately (EBR 11).
8. Consider the use of long-acting injectable antipsychotic medicines if (EBR 11):
   a. the person prefers a long-acting injectable medicine
   b. adherence has been poor or uncertain
   c. there has been a poor response to oral medication.
9. Treatment with clozapine should be considered early if appropriate pharmacological interventions are ineffective (EBR 1).

- **EBR** denotes evidence-based recommendation
- **1, 11, 111** denotes level of evidence, where 1 = systematic review of randomised control trials (RCTs); 11 = a RCT; 111 = a pseudo RCT
- **CBR** denotes consensus-based recommendation (consensus by a group of experts in the field)

Source: Galletly et al., (2016) and Mahli et al., (2015).

various neuroleptic medications. Blockade of postsynaptic dopaminergic receptors (in other words, receptors that are designed specifically for dopamine are prevented from receiving dopamine) is one way these medications can have their main effect. Other pathways and mechanisms may also contribute. The side-effects that result from this mechanism are consistently dry mouth, blurred vision, constipation, urinary retention and Parkinsonian side-effects.

Major effects

The beneficial effects of antipsychotic medications have been demonstrated for all psychotic disorders. Multiple and varied criteria have been used to measure improvement. These medications have been shown to be at least partly effective when used with people experiencing delusional thinking, hallucinations, confusion, motor agitation and motor retardation. Antipsychotic medication is also used to treat thought disorder, blunted affect, bizarre behaviour and social withdrawal, although the extent of improvement that can be linked specifically to the medication usage remains controversial.

The most common disintegrative condition treated with antipsychotic medication is the group of symptoms traditionally labelled *schizophrenia* (see Chapter 14). The problem of assessment is complicated by the fact that many illnesses can cause syndromes with features similar to those of schizophrenia. For example, delusions may indicate a variety of DSM conditions, including schizophrenia, bipolar mania and dementia of the Alzheimer's type. All people experiencing psychotic symptoms should have a thorough review of their medical history and a physical examination to rule out treatable medical illnesses, many of which are accompanied by behaviours considered psychotic or psychobiological in nature. It is worth reflecting on the clinical and ethical implications of treating a person's symptoms with neuroleptic medications when a basic physical examination might have determined that the problem was a result of infection or a tumour.

The choice of a specific medication

There are currently a range of older ('typical' or 'first-generation') antipsychotic medications and newer ('atypical' or 'second-generation') antipsychotic medications on the market in Australia. Some of the newer antipsychotics come in a long-acting injectable form. Medications have varying success rates, because individual responses frequently dictate use. The choice of a particular medication depends on its pharmacological properties and likely side-effects, the person's or a family member's history of response to that medication, and the prescriber's experience with various medicines. It is important to take into account the person's past experiences with specific medications, a history of allergies, a history of serious or intolerable side-effects, and their current ability to manage a medication schedule. Some medications may have side-effects such as sedation, which, while not necessarily desired by the prescriber, may nevertheless prove helpful in treatment. A certain amount of trial and error can be expected with each clinical application.

Tables 7.1 ■ and 7.2 ■ list the major antipsychotic medications used in Australia. The list is extensive and growing, and it makes sense for each member of the treatment team to become familiar with at least a few representative medications, their predictable effects and their common side-effects. As the nurse, you will likely be a resource for the other non-medically trained team members in this regard (that is, social workers, rehabilitation counsellors and psychologists). Some characteristics of these medications are discussed in the sections that follow.

A number of distinct chemical classes of antipsychotic medications are in use in Australia and other countries. As a result, there are choices in terms of side-effects and potential treatment responsiveness. A person who is unresponsive to one class may respond to another that circumvents a problem in absorption, accumulation at neurotransmitter receptor sites, or metabolism. However, there are many people for whom the available medications are not especially helpful, or, if major symptoms are addressed, the side-effects reduce the overall benefit of the medication. You will see in the course of your career, whether it is as a psychiatric–mental health nurse or in any other specialty practice, that more choices are still needed.

Tables 7.1 and 7.2 show the wide range among antipsychotic medications in milligram-per-milligram potency. This fact is most relevant when treating people who require larger doses. In such cases, a more potent medication is often considered.

Newer antipsychotics

The newer antipsychotics (also called *atypical antipsychotics* or *second-generation antipsychotics*) have a different

TABLE 7.1 ■ Common oral antipsychotic agents

Agent	Daily starting dose	Maximum recommended daily dose
Amisulpride	100 mg	1200 mg
Aripiprazole	10 mg	30 mg
Asenapine (sublingual)	10 mg (5 mg twice daily)	20 mg
Chlorpromazine	75–100 mg	800 mg
Clozapine	12.5 mg	900 mg
Haloperidol	0.5 mg	10 mg
Lurasidone	40 mg	160 mg
Olanzapine	5 mg	20 mg
Paliperidone (control-release)	3 mg	12 mg
Pericyazine	10 mg	75 mg
Quetiapine	50 mg	800 mg
Risperidone	0.5–1 mg	6 mg
Trifluoperazine	2 mg	15–20 mg
Ziprasidone	80 mg (40 mg twice daily)	160 mg (80 mg twice daily)
Zuclopenthixol hypdrochloride	10–20 mg	75 mg

Source: Galletly et al., (2016).

TABLE 7.2 ■ Long-acting injectable antipsychotic agents

Agent	Usual dose range	Usual interval between injections	Notes
Aripiprazol	300–400 mg	4 weeks	Supplement with oral antipsychotic for 2 weeks during initiation
Flupenthixol	20–40 mg	2–4 weeks	Give second dose after 4–10 days, then space out to every 2–4 weeks. Higher doses (up to 100 mg) have been used for treatment resistance
Fluphenazine	12.5–100 mg	2–4 weeks	An oral dose of 20 mg of fluphenazine hydrochloride is equivalent to fluphenazine decanoate 25 mg (1 ml) every 3 weeks
Haloperidol	25–200 mg	4 weeks	Initiate at a lower dose (maximum 100 mg) and adjust dose upward as required. There is limited clinical experience with doses greater than 300 mg per month
Olanzapine	300–400 mg	2–4 weeks	Post-injection delirium/sedation syndrome can occur in about 1% of recipients, so appropriate monitoring is required
Paliperidone	25–150 mg	4 weeks	Loading dose can be given Formulation with a duration of action of 3 months may become available soon
Risperidone	25–50 mg	2 weeks	Supplement with oral antipsychotic for at least 3 weeks during initiation
Zuclopenthixol	200–400 mg	2–4 weeks	Short-acting form (zuclopenthixole acetate), lasting 2–3 days, is also available as a second-line treatment of acute behavioural disturbance in schizophrenia

Source: Galletly et al., (2016).

physiological action than do the traditional or conventional antipsychotics. Conventional antipsychotics primarily affect the positive symptoms of psychotic disorders, with little or no effect on the negative or cognitive symptoms. Their mechanism of action is thought to occur through non-selectively blocking the neurotransmitter dopamine D_2 receptors in the brain. To be clinically effective, these medications occupy between 70 per cent and 90 per cent of the D_2 receptors, while the advent of extrapyramidal side effects (EPSEs) occurs at above 80 per cent occupancy (Veselinovi et al., 2011; Müller et al., 2010). The newer antipsychotics have a much reduced affinity, or attraction, for D_2 receptors, and they all have an affinity for the serotonin receptors, a profile that appears to lessen EPSEs and can improve the negative symptoms of psychotic disorders.

The newer antipsychotics offer a wider range of options for the care and treatment of people experiencing psychotic conditions. Research into psychopharmacological treatments for the psychoses is ongoing. If medications can be developed that provide relief from symptoms without undue side-effects, people will be more likely to continue taking them, and will therefore have fewer symptoms of their illness and stay healthier longer.

Uncomfortable side-effects are reasons many people do not continue taking any prescription medication. If someone with a severe mental illness such as schizophrenia stops taking an antipsychotic without first consulting a health professional, there is a high risk of becoming very sick and losing the ability to function effectively. Mental Health in the Media, below, provides one such example.

There is a variety of atypical antipsychotics, including clozapine, risperidone, paliperidone, olanzapine, asenapine and lurasidone. An overview of two examples follows.

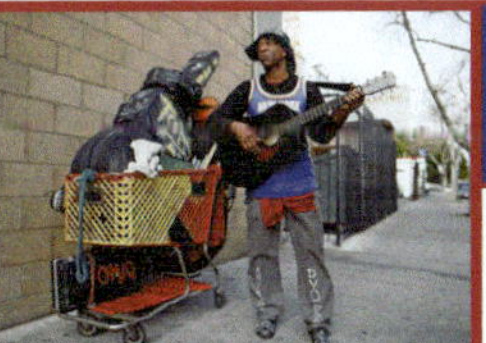

MENTAL HEALTH IN THE MEDIA

The Soloist

The movie *The Soloist* is based on the true story of a homeless musician with schizophrenia, Nathaniel Ayers (played by Jamie Foxx), befriended by a *Los Angeles Times* correspondent, Steve Lopez (played by Robert Downey Jr), who wrote a series of articles that brought the plight of the homeless and the seriously mentally ill to attention. Nathaniel, a cello prodigy at Juilliard, dropped out of the prestigious music school and ended up on the streets when he was no longer able to handle the voices in his head. An accomplished musician, Nathaniel also plays the violin, French horn, clarinet and oboe. The movie shows Nathaniel sleeping each night on one of Skid Row's filthy, rat-infested streets, in which thousands of homeless, mostly mentally ill, people sleep. *The Soloist* is essentially the story of the ups and downs, and bumps in the road, in a friendship between a person with schizophrenia who has the right to refuse treatment, such as medications, and a person who tries to help from his own frame of reference. The movie does not end with Ayers magically getting better and rejoining mainstream society. In 2009, Ayers was honored by the National Association on Mental Illness in the United States for decreasing the stigma associated with being mentally ill. The friendship between Ayers and Lopez continues to this day.

Source: LUCY NICHOLSON/Reuters /Landov.

Clozapine

The first atypical antipsychotic on the market in Australia was clozapine. Clozapine is an antipsychotic medication with an unusual pharmacological and clinical profile. It was used in Europe for several years, and is now generally used in Australia with people who cannot tolerate the EPSEs of other antipsychotics, or who have a treatment-resistant or treatment-refractory psychosis, as is the case with some people who live with schizophrenia. Reviews of studies regarding the effectiveness of clozapine have demonstrated its beneficial effects on positive symptoms, and suggested possible improvements in negative symptoms.

Serious side-effects Despite its capacity to ameliorate some very recalcitrant symptoms for people, clozapine has some serious side-effects. The most serious is **agranulocytosis** (a marked decrease in granulated white blood cells), which occurs in less than 1 per cent of people taking this medication. It is, therefore, essential to monitor the white blood cell count (WBC) and absolute neutrophil count (ANC) of people taking clozapine. Immediately discontinuing the medication when agranulocytosis is detected and before signs of an infection develop will usually resolve the episode. There are specific guidelines for treating a person who experiences agranulocytosis as a result of using clozapine; in Australia, this includes strict monthly monitoring for adverse effects.

There is a risk for agranulocytosis with other psychotropic medications (conventional antipsychotics, benzodiazepines, anticonvulsants); however, there is a higher risk with clozapine. There have been reported rates of agranulocytosis at significantly lower levels than the currently estimated 1 per cent (that is, 0.25 per cent, according to Snowdon & Halliday, 2011). One of the important questions for clozapine treatment remains: is there a specific risk period for agranulocytosis, and, if there is, when does it occur? The risk period establishes the frequency of blood monitoring, which can be an impediment to the initial and continued use of the antipsychotic.

Currently, it is estimated that this rare side-effect of agranulocytosis may occur up to a year following initial treatment with clozapine, although the vast majority of cases appear within five months. As a result of these data, blood monitoring for agranulocytosis is completed weekly for the first six months of therapy. If WBC levels remain normal and regular use is not interrupted throughout those six months, then blood monitoring can be reduced to biweekly frequencies. After another six months of regular use and normal blood results, monitoring can be done monthly. Because the medication stays in the system for some time after discontinuation, blood monitoring must continue for four weeks following the discontinuation of clozapine regardless of where the person being treated is in this schedule.

Another serious side-effect is the potential for seizure, which seems to be dose-related at over 600 mg/day. Less acute, but nonetheless important, side-effects include sedation, tachycardia, sialorrhea (drooling), weight gain and hypotension.

Risperidone

Risperidone became available in the mid-1990s. It was the first of a new class of antipsychotics—benzisoxazole derivatives—that does not clinically relate to any existing antipsychotic medication. An important feature is the relative absence of EPSE at the therapeutic dosing level. It addresses the positive, negative and affective symptoms of schizophrenia, and may also alleviate depression and anxiety. Side-effects similar to those experienced with haloperidol are seen in doses above the maximum recommended daily dosage of 6 mg.

Recommended dosage for orally-administered risperidone commences with 0.5–1 mg daily, and is slowly increased according to the person's tolerability and response, The maximum recommended daily dose is 6 mg (Galletly et al., 2016). Dosage at above the maximum daily dosage increases the risk of EPSE.

Risperidone has been very useful in the treatment of psychotic symptoms, and the clinical knowledge gained from using it regularly has been valuable. Note, however, the class action lawsuits brought against the pharmaceutical company producing and marking risperidone, referred to earlier in this chapter (see page 116). Risperidone is now available in depot injection form. (**Depot injection** is a term used to describe the slow release of a long-term medication given by intramuscular or subcutaneous injection using the body as a temporary storage device for the entire dose.) This form of the medication is injected every two weeks. This additional administration mode for risperidone offers another choice in the array of treatments for psychotic symptoms. (See Unique Routes of Administration, page 122.)

Other uses for risperidone include the treatment of acute mania in bipolar disorder, behavioural problems in dementia, and behavioural symptoms in children and adolescents living with autism.

LIVED EXPERIENCE

When I was diagnosed in 1999, I was commenced on the second-generation antipsychotic risperidone, when I perhaps should have been initially trialled on a first-generation antipsychotic. I have been on this medication ever since—some 16 years. There has been one attempt to phase it out, but when the dosage was halved my sleep pattern was adversely affected, and so with my GP's agreement I returned to the originally prescribed dose. In addition to the medication suppressing positive symptoms, such as delusions, the sedation effects have helped me to sleep soundly throughout those years. More recently, a newer antipsychotic has been added with good effect. At present I feel the best I have ever felt in my adult life. I have long considered that adhering to treatment has been important to my recovery.

Dosage

Dosage ranges for antipsychotic medications vary widely among the people for whom they are prescribed. Medications must be titrated against the psychotic target symptoms and the appearance of side-effects. The standard approach for administering oral antipsychotic medications is to 'start low and go slow', meaning that a person is commenced with the lowest recommended dose, and this is gradually increased within the recommended dosage range, with careful attention being paid to symptom improvement and the emergence of side-effects. Most of the older 'typical' antipsychotic are high-potency medicines, and often cause debilitating EPSEs. The evidence is not clear regarding whether the newer 'atypical' antipsychotics are more effective than the older 'typical' antipsychotics in treating the positive symptoms of schizophrenia. However, the newer medications (in oral form) may be more effective in relapse prevention, and in possibly improving negative symptoms (Galletly et al., 2016).

The type of presentation often influences the medication regimen used. The pharmacological management of acute behavioural disturbance in psychosis in an emergency department setting may require intramuscular administration of olanzapine (10 mg repeated every 2 hours to a maximum of 30 mg in 24 hours) until the person settles. In other settings, such as inpatient mental health units, administration of antipsychotic medication would typically commence with the recommended starting dose and be increased gradually. In either of the cases referred to above, the person undergoing treatment would be carefully monitored for symptom improvement and the emergence of side-effects (Galletly et al., 2016).

In the past few decades, the newer 'atypical' antipsychotics have largely replaced the older drugs, such as chlorpromazine, as first-line treatments for schizophrenia and related psychoses. It is thought that the more recently available medicines, such as risperidone, aripiprazole and olanzapine, are effective in ameliorating behavioural and cognitive symptoms while avoiding some of the more troublesome side-effects associated with the older antipsychotics. Given a generally more benign side-effect profile, atypical antipsychotics are considered to be more likely to be tolerated by the people for whom they are prescribed, thus reducing the risk of treatment non-adherence.

After maximum clinical improvement has been obtained, antipsychotic medications are generally reduced in a gradual manner. Continuing to give a person maintenance doses of an antipsychotic following a psychotic episode lowers the chances of relapse and re-hospitalisation. Rehabilitation and recovery interventions (Chapters 14 and 25) are especially helpful for individuals who have psychiatric symptomatology. Psychotherapy with people living with schizophrenia may not be particularly effective without maintenance medications in conventional treatment settings, but it is thought to improve psychosocial functioning in people who are also taking maintenance medications. It is generally believed that people should be kept on doses of antipsychotics sufficient to suppress symptoms for at least 12 months before cessation of medication is considered. After that interval, the severity of illness experienced by the person, risk factors, individual and family history and circumstances, and the availability of health professional support and monitoring in the community should be taken into account. Some people will make a good recovery from a psychotic episode. For others, the illness may follow a deteriorating course with recurrent episodes of psychosis. Preventing relapse is clearly important, and linked to the safe and effective use of antipsychotic medications.

The decision to use a medication

The following principles provide guidance in the use of antipsychotic medication:

- Medications are given to treat target symptoms of schizophrenia or other psychotic disorders.
- Initial treatment may require parenteral doses or rapidly dissolving forms. These are changed to oral forms, such as pills, as the behavioural disturbance subsides.
- Total dosages are tailored to individual needs; wide variations exist among people.
- For medications with sedating side-effects, divided doses are changed as soon as is practical to a single dose, given at bedtime to maximise the medication's sedative properties.
- Most people with an enduring course require maintenance doses for sustained improvement, and to reduce the risk of relapses.

Other considerations for using a particular medication include the use of adjunctive therapies. Adjunctive treatment may be necessary when an available compound has a necessary, but insufficient, impact on symptoms, and another medication using different pathways or different mechanisms is able to provide an additional and sufficient impact. This package of two or three medications can work in concert for the person receiving treatment. The ever-present danger with this practice is called *polypharmacy* where too many medications are used without careful consideration of when medications can and should be discontinued from the mix (Mojtabai & Olfson, 2010). As a general principal, it is advisable for a consultant psychiatrist to be involved in decision-making surrounding the use of more than one antipsychotic medication.

Do the medications needed to treat one problem blend well with any or all of the other medications the person may need? People living with schizophrenia often have more than a single mental disorder. Comorbid diagnoses require more complex treatment regimens, including pharmacotherapy. See Your Assessment Approach on the next page for antipsychotic medication interactions with other medications and substances to which the person with whom you are working may be exposed.

Special considerations

The following special considerations apply to the use of antipsychotic medication.

YOUR ASSESSMENT APPROACH Antipsychotic medication interactions

Combining one of these	With one of these antipsychotics	May lead to these problems
Antacids	Phenothiazine antipsychotic	Decreased phenothiazine effect
Anticholinergics	Clozapine	Potentiated anticholinergic effect of clozapine
	Antipsychotic	Increased level of neuroleptic in the system, with extrapyramidal side-effects
Benzodiazepines	Clozapine	Respiratory arrest, circulatory difficulties
Carbamazepine	Haloperidol	Decreased effect of either medication
	Clozapine	Additive bone marrow suppression
CNS depressants such as: narcotics, anxiolytics, alcohol, barbiturates or antihistamines	Antipsychotic	Additive CNS depression
Coffee, tea, milk or fruit juices	Phenothiazine antipsychotic	Decreased phenothiazine effect

COLLABORATIVE CARE

Teaching about antipsychotic medications

The teaching plan that follows outlines the major areas to be addressed when educating people about antipsychotic medications. The teaching plan can be individualised to address such issues as: the person's specific medication(s), responses to medication, side-effects, and the person's and their family members' abilities and interests in learning. Documentation of the education provided can be in the form of a narrative note or a check-list of the topics discussed.

'What does this medication do?'

'Antipsychotic medications help to treat the emotional and thinking problems of schizophrenia or psychosis. It helps organise thinking, keeps you in touch with reality and reduces the symptoms of your illness. It is not a cure. If you stop taking the medication, the benefits may wear off over time, and you could start to experience these problems again, possibly at a more distressing level.'

'How should I take this medication?'

'The medication should be taken as prescribed on a regular basis. If you feel that you cannot or do not want to continue, it is important to notify your doctor or your care coordinator.'

'What should I do if I miss a dose?'

'Take the dose as soon as you remember if it has only been a few hours. But if it is almost time for your next dose, do not take double or extra doses.'

'What other medication does not mix with this antipsychotic medication?'

Tailor your response to this question to the specific medication prescribed. Mention the major drug interactions with prescribed medications, over-the-counter substances, alternative and complementary supplements, and alcohol and recreational drug use. There may also be interactions with caffeine, nicotine and food items, and these should be addressed in detail.

'What side-effects can I expect?'

The discussion should address the person's previous experience with side-effects from the medication in question. While it is important to avoid overwhelming the person with excessive information, it is important that they know what actions to take when side-effects occur. Ordinary and extraordinary side-effects should be addressed, as well as the actions that can be taken in response to these side-effects. Commonly occurring side-effects should be addressed, including dystonia, akathisia, agitation, confusion, sensitivity to sunlight, and changes in sexual interest and performance.

'Where can I keep my medication?'

'In a safe place at room temperature. Do not keep it in the bathroom where there is a shower or bathtub, in the kitchen where there is a dishwasher, or above or right next to the kitchen sink. Do not keep medications in a motor vehicle, because temperatures can reach extreme levels within such an enclosed area. Moisture, light and heat can affect your medication.'

'What can I do if I have a problem?'

Give the person and family with whom you are working the names and contact details of health care providers they can call upon for questions and in emergencies.

Unique routes of administration

A number of typical and atypical antipsychotic medications are available in long-acting injectable form. These medications are gradually released over an extended period of time, two to four weeks. These long-acting injectable (or depot) antipsychotics can be helpful in managing non-adherence and reducing relapse rates in schizophrenia (Kishimoto et al., 2013). It is important that careful consideration should be given to establishing the acceptability of this mode of administration to the person receiving the medication. However, achieving an optimal dose may be less straightforward in long-acting injectable antipsychotics compared to the oral form of the medication; in some long-acting agents, it may take up to four months for optimal plasma concentrations to be achieved.

With all long-acting injectable antipsychotics, it is important that the oral form be given first to ensure the person tolerates the medication. With the long-acting injectable form of olanzapine there is a risk of post-injection delirium/sedation, necessitating careful observation for two hours after each injection. The main advantages of depot forms are that they may reduce a person's ambivalence about taking medication, eliminate the need for constant medication-taking, and can help people who have illness-related cognitive impairments. Memory and concentration difficulties are often found among those with executive functioning deficits, one of the major impairments that must be overcome by people who have schizophrenia. (Chapter 6 discusses executive functioning.) Making sure people have a steady level of medication in their system minimises the fluctuations in blood level seen in non-parenteral forms of medication administration. A fluctuating blood level leads to more difficulty managing symptoms, especially if the person is sensitive to minor fluctuations. A depot antipsychotic with relatively fewer side-effects has the potential to prolong antipsychotic medication use and minimise dissatisfaction with, and discontinuation of, treatment.

Pharmaceutical companies have explored better routes for medication administration for many years. As a result, there is yet another way to give a number of antipsychotic preparations. A number of atypical antipsychotics are also available in orally disintegrating tablet and wafer formulations. These tablets and wafers begin disintegrating in the mouth within seconds, so they can be swallowed with or without liquid, thus reducing problems with swallowing and concealing behaviours, and offering a more discreet option for taking medication during activities. This vehicle for administering full doses of medication promotes adherence.

In the future we are likely to see a variety of innovative technologies for enhancing the administration and absorption of psychiatric medications. Currently, research is investigating the following:

- multiphase, multi-compartment capsules using gelatin, natural hydroxypropyl methylcellulose and alternative capsule materials
- quick-dissolving strips and films
- inhalers
- implanted pumps.

These opportunities for medication-delivery platforms, coupled with research for new compounds to treat disorders, may help normalise psychiatric disorders—that is, they are treated just as all other physical disorders are treated—and provide more options. Over the course of your career in nursing, you are likely to see innovative absorption-enhancing delivery systems and routes for the administration of medications to treat and improve the quality of life for the people with whom you will work.

Potential side-effects of antipsychotic medications

Continuous contact with people living with mental illness gives nurses an advantage over other professionals who may see a person only every other day or, at best, once a day. Both the dangerous and the more uncomfortable side-effects frequently have a rapid onset and need prompt attention.

The side-effects of antipsychotic medications that nurses must recognise can be divided into the following classes:

- autonomic nervous system
- extrapyramidal
- other central nervous system
- allergic
- blood
- skin
- eye
- endocrine
- weight gain

These will now be considered in greater detail.

Autonomic nervous system side-effects

All antipsychotic medications possess anticholinergic and anti-adrenergic side-effects; that is, they interfere with the normal transmission of nerve impulses by acetylcholine and epinephrine, in both central and peripheral nerves. Anticholinergic side-effects are the most common and are generally drying to the various tissues. They are usually more pronounced in older adults. Anticholinergic side-effects include:

- nervousness, drowsiness, headache
- tachycardia
- blurred vision
- dry mouth, constipation, nausea, vomiting (less frequently paralytic ileus)
- urinary hesitancy/retention
- cognitive functioning impairment and hallucinations (especially in older adults).

Constipation Constipation can be a side-effect of many psychotropic medications. Medications and supplements that can cause constipation include opioids, anticholinergics, tricyclic antidepressants, antispasmodics, calcium channel blockers, iron supplements, some antacids, and antiemetic, chemotherapeutic and anti-Parkinsonian medications (Bliss, Savik, Jung, Whitebird & Lowry, 2011). Strategies for managing this common and uncomfortable side-effect can be found in nursing fundamentals texts.

Orthostatic hypotension Orthostatic hypotension, also known as *postural hypotension*, is a common anti-adrenergic effect. The main danger here is injury from a fall. People receiving parenteral medication should have their blood pressure monitored, both lying down and standing, before and after each dose. Advice should be given to rise from the supine position gradually, and to sit down if the person feels faint. Support stockings and keeping up fluid intake may be indicated. Orthostatic hypotension is less significant with oral medication, although it is important to record both baseline and routine vital signs. This establishes the person's tolerance for medications without the untoward side-effects of orthostatic hypotension and subsequent falls. The technique for measuring orthostatic blood pressure can also be reviewed in your nursing fundamentals text.

Extrapyramidal side-effects

Another common and sometimes frightening group of side-effects results from the effects of antipsychotics on the extrapyramidal tracts of the central nervous system, which are involved in the production and control of involuntary movements. This group of reactions is known as **extrapyramidal side-effects (EPSEs)**. Your Assessment Approach, right, details each EPSE.

The first-generation, conventional or typical antipsychotics, such as haloperidol, trifluoperazine and chlorpromazine, tend to be harsher on the body and cause significant EPSEs. Although the majority of people prescribed antipsychotic medication are now taking second-generation antipsychotics, some respond well to first-generation antipsychotics and thus continue to take these. Managing the EPSEs as a long-term treatment option involves careful interventions and education for both the people taking the medications and their families. Four major types of EPSEs are discussed in the following section and in Your Assessment Approach; each EPSE has distinguishing clinical characteristics and times of onset after the initiation of drug therapy.

There are several different types of EPSEs that take unique and distinctive forms. They are discussed next. It is important to be aware of the frequency with which these syndromes complicate treatment. Any suspicious signs or symptoms ought to be promptly reported to the health professional who has prescribed the medication.

Acute dystonic reactions The earliest and most dramatic EPSEs are the *acute dystonic reactions*, which are forms of dystonia. These occur in the first few days of medication treatment, sometimes after a single dose of medication. They involve bizarre and severe muscle contractions. These reactions can be physically painful and are often frightening to the individual. They are reversible. The term 'dystonia' describes the experience of the side-effect. The prefix *dys-* typically means bad, and *-tonia* means muscle tone; essentially these are muscle spasms.

Dystonic movements can occur abruptly and co-occur with other EPSEs (Fontenelle, Oostermeijer, Harrison, Pantalis & Yucel, 2011). Treatment to resolve the EPSEs is effective in many instances, although the impact on the person is taken into account. Continued experiences that are painful and unpredictable tend to shatter trust in psychopharmacology, and discontinuing the medication may be necessary.

Parkinsonian syndrome Parkinsonian syndrome, or drug-induced Parkinsonianism (so named because of its resemblance to true Parkinson's disease) commonly occurs after a week or two of the medication therapy. It is as a result of dopamine blockade caused by psychiatric medications. Treatment with oral medication is usually sufficient. Your accurate observation of the course of therapy can promote prompt recognition and proper interpretation of EPSEs. If care is not taken, the health care provider may misinterpret the increasing

YOUR ASSESSMENT APPROACH
Extrapyramidal side-effects (EPSEs)

Acute dystonic reaction, or dystonia

- Usually begins within 48 hours after beginning treatment, but may occur at any time.
- Described by the consumer as 'sometimes my back tightens up', or 'I get tongue-tied when I try to talk'.
- Characterised by abnormal tonic contracts of muscle groups.
- Characterised by odd posturing and strange facial expressions, such as torticollis (twisting of the neck and back, forcing the back to arch and the neck to bend backward), and oculogyric crisis (a fixed gaze that cannot return to lateral once raised vertically).
- Is more common in young males.
- Treated prophylactically by anticholinergics. Some people may experience a 'high' from this treatment.

Parkinsonian syndrome, or drug-induced Parkinsonism

- Usually occurs after three or more weeks of treatment.
- Characterised by rigidity (cog-wheeling), tremor, or regular rhythmic oscillations of the extremities, particularly the distal parts, and in the hands (a pill-rolling movement of the fingers).
- People are more susceptible to aspiration or to injury by falling.
- Treatment consists of decreasing the medication dosage or administering anticholinergics.

Akathisia

- Usually occurs after three or more weeks of treatment.
- Described by the consumer as 'my nerves are jumping' or 'I feel like jumping out of my skin'.
- A subjective need or desire to move, not a type of pattern or movement.
- Mild akathisia: vague feelings of apprehension and irritability.
- Severe akathisia: an inability to sit (or the feeling one cannot sit) for more than a few seconds, resulting in running, rocking or agitated dancing.
- Not always responsive to anticholinergics: lowering the medication dosage may be necessary.
- There is an associated dysphoria not treated by anticholinergics or benzodiazepines.

Tardive dyskinesia

- Late onset during the course of treatment with antipsychotics, with frequently irreversible abnormal movements or a neurological syndrome.
- Characterised by coordinated, arrhythmic, involuntary movements (lip smacking, tongue protrusion, rocking, foot tapping).
- Complications include inability to wear dentures, impaired respirations, weight loss, and impaired gait and posture.
- Treatment is primary prevention through careful initial assessment of the person's needs, as well as continuous evaluation of the course of treatment.

withdrawal, emotional blunting, apathy and lack of spontaneity (observations of Parkinsonian syndrome) as an increase in the severity of psychotic symptoms.

Akathisia Another reversible EPSE is **akathisia**. The word 'akathisia' is derived from the Greek word *kathisia*, meaning 'ability to sit' (the prefix *a-* indicates 'not' or 'without'; hence 'inability to sit still'). Akathisia is a motor restlessness perceived subjectively by the person affected, and experienced as an urge to pace, a need to shift weight from one foot to the other, or an inability to sit or stand still. Akathisia can occur weeks to months into the course of therapy.

Akathisia can also be mistaken for psychotic agitation, and this error in interpretation may lead to a mistaken increase in medication, which will aggravate the condition. People experiencing akathisia require a reduction in the dose of the offending agents and/or treatment with an anti-Parkinsonian drug.

Tardive dyskinesia The most severe EPSE is **tardive dyskinesia**, which can often be irreversible. Tardive dyskinesia frequently appears after years of antipsychotic drug treatment, although it can occur earlier. It usually appears after a maintenance dose is discontinued or reduced, and it can be masked—but not treated—by reinstituting the medication or increasing the dosage, or by switching to another drug. The term 'tardive dyskinesia' is formed from the word *tardive*, meaning 'late onset' or 'slow' (from the root for 'tardy' and 'retardation'); the prefix *dys-*, and the word *kinesia*, meaning movement. It is essentially late-arriving bad movement. Tardive dyskinesia is a neurological syndrome involving the innervation of muscle groups. Typical tardive dyskinesia movements include thrusting the tongue outside of the mouth and facial grimacing.

It is generally thought that atypical antipsychotics cause less tardive dyskinesia, although it remains a risk, especially when higher doses of medication are prescribed. Early detection through regular examinations (at least every six months) is recommended.

There is no known cure for tardive dyskinesia. The recommended intervention is to stop all medication to see whether the syndrome resolves spontaneously. This option must be weighed against the consumer's need for medication and the likelihood of relapse into psychosis.

Sedation and reduction of the seizure threshold

The central nervous system (CNS) side-effects of antipsychotic medications are sedation and a reduction of the seizure threshold. Because antipsychotics vary in their sedative effects, these side-effects are troublesome, but can be managed by changing to a less sedating agent. Seizures are not a contraindication for using these medications; however, their use in the presence of seizures requires close observation.

Allergic effects

The main allergic manifestation of the antipsychotics is cholestatic jaundice. This is much less common now, and is usually a benign and self-limiting condition. Older medications such as chlorpromazine and the tricyclic antidepressants can cause cholestatic jaundice, which is not always thought to be an allergic reaction. It is thought that chlorpromazine may exert a direct toxic effect on the bile secretary mechanisms of the liver. Other side-effects can sometimes be mistakenly reported by consumers as allergic reactions. It is important that all such reports are carefully considered, as the reactions experienced may turn out to be very serious; for instance, neuroleptic malignant syndrome (discussed below) or a dystonic reaction. Failure to carefully scrutinise reports of allergic reactions may also result in the mistaken withdrawal of effective medications.

Cardiac effects

Antipsychotics can have an impact on the length of time it takes the heart to go through its electrical and muscular cycle. This cycle is abbreviated as the QT complex, referring to the length of the interval between the first wave identified in an ECG—there are Q, R, S and T waves—and the last wave. A standardisation of the length of the cycle is referred to as the QTc (a corrected QT interval). An interval longer than 450 to 500 msec can indicate a cardiac problem. An elongated QT interval can lead to arrhythmias and a drug-induced cardiac condition called torsades de pointes. High doses of antipsychotics can contribute to the prevalence of QT-interval abnormalities. Medications with the potential for QT prolongation include the typical antipsychotic haloperidol and the atypical antipsychotic aripiprazole. However, the incidence of cardiac side-effects is low, and the increased risk of QTc abnormalities can be managed (Hough et al., 2011).

Blood, skin and eye effects

The most serious side-effect in this category is *agranulocytosis*. It is both potentially fatal and rare (Barnes & Patten, 2011). In this condition, the body is not producing enough of the particular white blood cell called 'granulocytes' (grainy cells), which are needed to fight infection. Usually the person acquires an infection and deteriorates rapidly or begins to bleed spontaneously, requiring emergency medical attention.

Skin eruptions, photosensitivity leading to severe sunburn, blue-grey metallic discolouration over the face and hands, and pigmentation changes in the eyes are all potential side-effects. Consumers are generally advised to avoid prolonged exposure to sunlight or to use a sunscreen agent when outdoors. These conditions usually remit. An important feature of skin eruptions for people living with psychosis is what it means to them. Delusions may be exacerbated as a result of eczema, rashes or other eruptions. They can be frightening to someone who has paranoia, or can be perceived as punishment by someone who is experiencing unrealistic guilt.

Endocrine effects

Lactation in females and gynaecomastia and impotence in males are some of the distressing endocrine changes that can occur with antipsychotic drug treatments. Hyperprolactinemia is a common side-effect that will affect many aspects of a consumer's sex life. Difficulties with libido, arousal, excitation, orgasm, male ejaculatory volume and overall performance can occur to a disturbing degree with hyperprolactinemia. It is not difficult to imagine the impact of these side-effects with the regular or long-term use of the medication. Hyperprolactinemia is also responsible for oligomenorrhea or amenorrhea in women, galactorrhea in women and sometimes in men, and, in cases of prolonged hyperprolactinemia, osteoporosis (Veselinovic et al., 2011).

Another endocrine problem is diabetes in people living with schizophrenia. The baseline occurrence of diabetes is elevated in schizophrenia, and seems to be further escalated by endocrine changes associated with psychotropic medication use. Although weight gain increases the risk of diabetes, some studies show diabetes occurring in people who have not gained significant weight. The particular medicine used may be a contributing factor.

Weight gain

Weight gain is a significant side-effect that affects self-esteem and poses health serious health risks for the person taking various psychotropic medications. Certain antipsychotics, antidepressants, lithium, anticonvulsants and others classes of drugs can cause an increase in weight. As mentioned above, an increase in weight can increase the risk for health problems such as diabetes, hypertension and coronary artery disease. The impact of weight gain can be more distressing to people than EPSEs. Over time, this side-effect can be a devastating blow to long-term treatment and quality of life. Paying careful attention from the inception of treatment can help in the recognition and management of this particular side-effect.

Neuroleptic malignant syndrome

Neuroleptic malignant syndrome (NMS) (muscle rigidity, hyperpyrexia, altered consciousness and diaphoresis) is a severe and potentially life-threatening side-effect of all psychotropic medications. This condition is believed to be the result of either dopamine blockade in the striatum of the brain or dopaminergic antagonism in the CNS (Thompson & Johnson, 2011). NMS occurs in a very small percentage of people taking psychotropic medications, with more men being affected than women; younger people seem to be more susceptible than older ones (Seitz & Gill, 2009). NMS typically occurs within the first two weeks of treatment with a new medication or a return to a previously used medication, or when a dosage has been increased. There are also reports of NMS occurring months after the commencement of a new medication regimen. Nurses are in the best position to monitor and assess for this serious condition. Treatment for NMS includes discontinuing all psychotropic medication immediately, and prompt commencement of medical management. If cooling and rehydration are not achieved quickly, the person may die. The pathology of NMS is complex, and not well understood beyond the knowledge that the major symptoms are caused by blockade of the dopamine receptors.

Metabolising psychiatric medications

A liver enzyme called cytochrome P_{450} (abbreviated as CYP) is responsible for metabolising most psychiatric medication out of a person's system. The two main directions that can influence how the people with whom you are working metabolise psychiatric medications are called *inhibition* and *activation* (or *induction*). Inhibition of the enzyme allows the medication and its metabolites to remain in the system longer than usual, accumulating and causing higher blood levels, enhanced effects of the medication, and greater side-effects. Imagine a jammed parking lot or gridlock on a city street, as the medication is unable to flow out of the system easily.

Induction (or activation) of the enzyme speeds the medication and its metabolites out of the system faster than usual. When a medication does not have enough time to take full effect, it may appear that symptoms are not being competently addressed. The medication is considerably less effective in this case than if it had the time to be fully utilised by the body. Picture the medication being washed out of the system faster than intended.

Other co-administered medications, the person's genetics, foods eaten and cigarettes smoked are some of the factors that can induce or inhibit cytochrome P_{450}. The field of study on CYPs is extensive, covering the intricacies of medication interactions, metabolism and co-administration cautions.

> **LIVED EXPERIENCE**
>
> Over the years, I have experienced a range of side-effects of psychotropic medication, most notably weight gain. Within three months of commencing on risperidone I had significant weight gain, and this has been a struggle ever since. I also take lithium and often experience headaches, especially if I am not drinking enough water; I usually drink about 3 litres of water daily. I also frequently feel slow and lethargic, and put this down mainly to the medication I am taking. Despite the impact of such daily medication-related experiences, I would be reticent to interfere with my current treatment because it has brought stability to my life for a considerable period of time.

ANTIDEPRESSANT MEDICATIONS

Classes of **antidepressant medications** (pharmaceutical compounds used to treat the symptoms of depression) that currently exist include: **tricyclic antidepressants (TCAs)**, **monoamine oxidase inhibitors (MAOIs)**, **selective serotonin reuptake inhibitors (SSRIs) serotonin and norepinephrine reuptake inhibitors (SNRIs)** and atypical antidepressants (so-called because of their variety of formulation and actions). For a look at some of the variety of antidepressant medications currently available from different classes with differing actions, see Table 7.3 ■.

TABLE 7.3 ■ Antidepressant medications

TCA	Other	SSRI	MAOI	SNRI
Amitryptyline	Mirtazapine	Citalopram	Phenelzine	Venlafaxine
Clomipramine	Mianserin	Escitalopram	Tranylcypromine	Duloxetine
Dothiepin	Bupropion	Fluvoxamine		Desvenlafaxine
Imipramine	Moclobemide	Fluoxetine		
Nortryptiline		Paroxetine		
Doxepin		Sertraline		

Similarly to antipsychotic medications, the original antidepressant medications were discovered accidentally. In the case of imipramine, the first of the tricyclic antidepressants, investigators were actually searching for effective antipsychotics similar to chlorpromazine. The 'tri-' in *tricyclic antidepressants* refers to the triple chemical rings at the centre of each of the medications. Iproniazid, a MAOI, was discovered when people with tuberculosis who were regularly treated with a similar medication, isoniazid, became less depressed. Antidepressants have played a part in the development of a better understanding of the biochemical mechanisms of the brain in both normal and abnormal emotional expression.

Psychobiological considerations

Knowledge about the pharmacology of antidepressant medications has led to a theory of the biochemistry of depression. Basically, all of the true antidepressants make the neurotransmitters norepinephrine (NE) and serotonin (5-HT) more available to the synaptic receptors in the central nervous system. Tricyclics block the reuptake of these substances into the neuron after their release, thereby postponing their degradation. MAOIs interfere with the enzymes responsible for the actual breakdown of the neurotransmitter molecules. Because both are antidepressants, these observations have led to the theory that NE and 5-HT shortages in the brain cause depression, at least the type of depression that responds to medication therapy.

The initial distinction to be understood in the psychopharmacology of depression is between true antidepressants and stimulants or euphoriants. TCAs and MAOIs are not stimulants and do not induce euphoria in healthy people. In a single dose they have a sedative effect. Amphetamines and methylphenidate (Ritalin), on the other hand, are stimulants but not antidepressants in the pharmacological sense. They can induce an increased sense of wellbeing in certain individuals, but do nothing to combat depression on a lasting basis.

Tricyclic antidepressants were the 'first generation' of antidepressant medications; that is, they were among the first medications identified as effective in the treatment of depression. New developments and ideas in chemical motivations to help treat symptoms of depression are labelled as subsequent generations.

Since the introduction of the first antidepressants, a number of medications have been developed to treat the symptoms of major depression and the depressive features of schizoaffective disorder. Among these medications are the MAOIs, the SSRIs, the SNRIs and a number of atypical antidepressants with a variety of neurotransmitter actions.

Bupropion is an oral antidepressant medication that is not a TCA, and is unrelated to other known antidepressants. Bupropion has been well tolerated in people who experience orthostatic hypotension when taking TCAs. This medication has the potential to cause seizures to a greater extent than other antidepressants, depending on the dose. It has few anticholinergic side-effects, and essentially no important cardiovascular effects. Bupropion is also indicated for use as an aid to smoking cessation. For smoking cessation, the medication is used for up to 14 weeks.

As each new group of medications becomes available, there can be a tendency for practitioners to use the new medications to the partial exclusion of the old. When a person is not responding to a medication, it is helpful to have an array of choices from which to select further treatment. The side-effect profiles of antidepressants remain one of the linchpins of successful care. If sedation is a side-effect and the person is sleeping at a higher-than-preferred level, then a class of medications with less sedating side effects may be a better choice. Experience suggests that a number of treatment and medication options are necessary to effectively treat psychiatric disorders; therefore, all categories of antidepressants remain useful.

Tricyclic antidepressants (TCAs)

Tricyclic antidepressants (TCAs) were named for their consistent triple-ringed chemical structure. Compared to selective serotonin reuptake inhibitors (SSRIs), TCAs have a greater side-effect burden and toxicity in overdose, and are thus nowadays considered a second-line treatment. However, compared to other antidepressants, TCAs may be more effective in treating severe depressive symptoms, especially if melancholia is present (Mahli et al., 2015).

Monoamine oxidase inhibitors (MAOIs)

Monoamine oxidase inhibitors (MAOIs) are effective antidepressants, but nowadays are not recommended as first-line treatments due to the risk of **hypertensive crisis** (severe elevation in diastolic blood pressure) if the person taking the medication does not adhere to strict diet and drug interaction restrictions. They must avoid ingesting foods that contain the amino acid tyramine and sympathomimetic medications (see Collaborative Care: Teaching About a Low-tyramine Diet, below). MAOIs may be used as second-line or third-line treatments for melancholia, presentations with atypical symptoms or treatment-resistant depression. Phenelzine and Tranylcypromine are two MAOIs in use in Australia. The potential to have an antidepressant interact with other medications is explored in Your Assessment Approach: Antidepressant Medication Interactions on the following page.

Further development of antidepressants has been the result of a scientific search for medications with fewer toxic side-effects and greater biological predictability in the treatment of depression. Newer antidepressants are believed to be more neurotransmitter-specific, and better able to treat conditions related to dopamine, serotonin or norepinephrine dysfunctions.

The earlier antidepressants have certain disadvantages. Uncomfortable and sometimes intolerable side-effects and a number of use restrictions with certain populations, combined with the dietary restrictions of the MAOIs, make these medications inappropriate for many people.

Selective serotonin reuptake inhibitors (SSRIs)

The next class of antidepressant medications developed was the selective serotonin reuptake inhibitors (SSRIs). While chemically different, SSRIs inhibit the reuptake (and thus the deactivation) of the neurotransmitter serotonin, allowing for the increased availability of serotonin at the synapses. The first SSRI developed was fluoxetine. There are now a number of potent and highly specific medications with this action. An important difference with this group of medications is that they are considered to be safer and to have more tolerable side-effects.

The SSRIs shed light on the workings of the synapses. For the first time, psychiatric–mental health nurses were able to see the direct impact of changing neurotransmitter concentrations. Figure 7.2 ■ shows the structure of the synapse.

An important consideration for people taking SSRIs is the proximity of the administration of MAOIs. Fluoxetine and a MAOI together may cause serious and fatal interactions. The half-life of fluoxetine is such that there must be a five-week

COLLABORATIVE CARE

Teaching about a low-tyramine diet

MAOIs combined with certain foods and medications may produce a significant increase in blood pressure, which can be a health hazard. In general, foods that cause this reaction are those that have been ***pickled, fermented, smoked or aged***. The list below includes the main foods, fluids and medications that should be avoided while taking a MAOI and for at least two weeks after discontinuation of a MAOI. It should be noted that preservatives in foodstuffs and beverages can change over time, and thus dietary restrictions should be updated regularly.

Foods and beverages to avoid completely

Meats and fish: Pickled herring, dried fish, aged/dried/cured meats, unrefrigerated fermented fish, liver, caviar, fermented sausage (salami, pepperoni), fermented oyster sauces used in Asian dishes, jerky, meat extracts, miso, soy sauce, teriyaki sauce.

Vegetables: English broad beans, Chinese pea pods, fava beans, banana peels, Italian or broad green beans, fermented cabbage, lentils, lima beans, sauerkraut, overly ripe fruits, peanuts, spinach.

Dairy products: Yoghurt, many types of cheese (e.g. English Stilton, mozzarella, Parmesan).

Beverages: Chianti, aged wines, imported beers, aged beers.

Combination foods: Breads made with aged cheeses, and meats, or yeast extracts; homemade or high-yeast breads; pizza; lasagna; macaroni and cheese; quiche; liver pâté; Caesar salad; all yeast products (e.g. brewer's yeast, yeast extracts such as Vegemite and Marmite).

MSG: MSG is frequently used in Asian dishes as a meat tenderiser and flavour enhancer; many prepared and processed foods also use MSG (e.g. canned soups, packaged noodle meals, frozen prepared meals, salad dressings).

Medications: Cough and cold medications, nasal decongestants (tablets, drops, sprays), hayfever and allergy medications, weight-reduction preparations, anti-appetite medications, asthma inhalants.

Foods and beverages that can be taken in small amounts

Dairy products: Most processed cheeses bought in a supermarket.

Fruits: Raisins, prunes, bananas, avocados, plums, canned figs.

Caffeine sources: Coffee, chocolate, colas.

Beverages: Domestic red wines; domestic beers, ales, stouts; sherry. (Note: alcohol is a CNS-depressant, and so should be avoided by individuals in treatment for depression.)

Allowed foods

Beverages: White wines. (Note: alcohol is a CNS-depressant, and so should be avoided by individuals in treatment for depression.)

Baked goods: Raised with yeast, but not high in yeast.

Dairy products: Cottage cheese, cream cheese, milk, cream, ice cream.

Additional information

St John's wort: This naturally occurring MAOI, less potent than pharmaceutical grade; is not regulated and may cause inconsistent access to the active ingredient. It has the same dietary and medication restrictions as pharmaceutical-grade MAOIs.

YOUR ASSESSMENT APPROACH Antidepressant medication interactions

Combining one of these	With one of these antidepressants	Can lead to these problems
Antiarrhythmic	TCA	Additive antiarrhythmic effect, myocardial depression
Anticholinergic	TCA	Additive anticholinergic effect
Anticonvulsant	TCA	Decreased TCA effect, lower seizure threshold
Antihypertensive	TCA	Hypertensive crisis
Antipsychotic	TCA	Increased TCA effect, confusion, delirium, ileus
CNS depressants such as: Alcohol Antihistamines Anxiolytics Barbiturates Narcotics	TCA	Decreased TCA effect, additive CNS depression
Foods or medications containing tyramine	MAOI	Hypertensive crisis
Levodopa	MAOI	Hypertensive crisis
MAOI	SSRI	Serotonin syndrome, serious adverse reactions
MAOI	TCA	Hyperpyrexia, severe excitation
Nicotine	TCA	Decreased TCA serum level
St John's wort (herb)	SSRI	Sedative–hypnotic intoxication
SSRI	TCA	Increased TCA serum levels, elevated nortriptyline serum levels with adverse effects

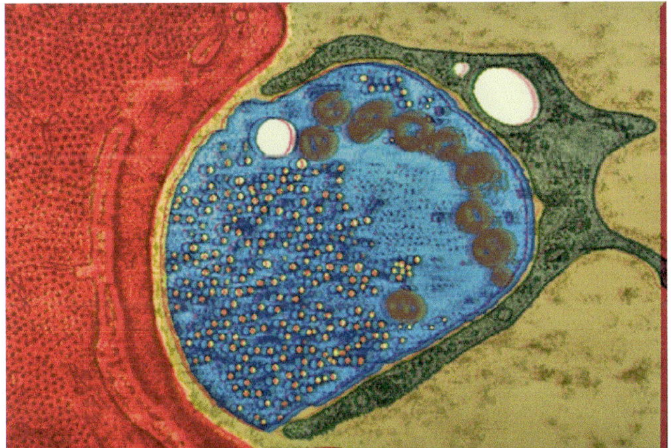
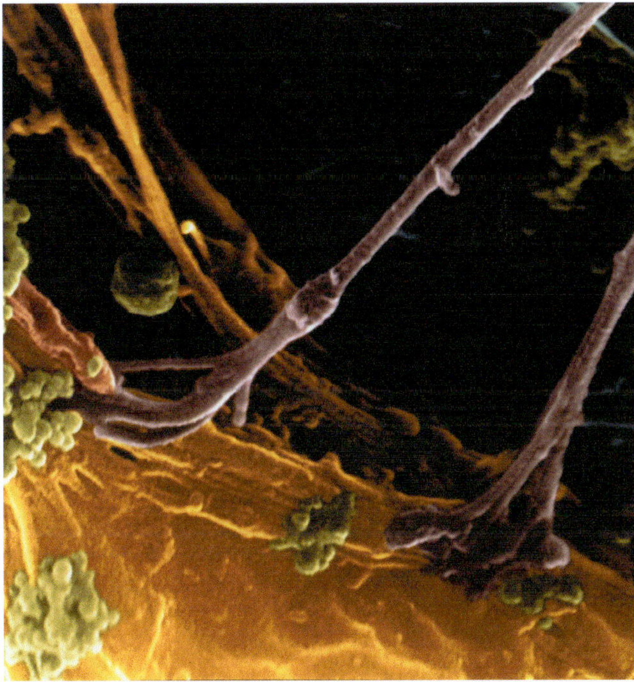

FIGURE 7.2 ■ Structure of the synapse: The synapse at the left has many specialised characteristics. On the right, the electron micrograph shows the vesicles containing the synaptic transmitter, the abundance of mitochondria necessary for energy production, and the abundance of protein in the presynaptic and postsynaptic densities. On the left are incoming axons (purple) contacting dendrites (yellow) with non-neural cells nearby (green).
Photo courtesy of (left) Photo Researchers, Inc., Don W. Fawcett; (right) Photo Researchers, Inc.

gap between taking fluoxetine and taking a MAOI, and vice versa. Sertraline, paroxetine, citalopram and escitalopram have shorter half-lives, and there must be gap of up to two weeks (both directions) between taking these medications and taking MAOIs. It is also important to note that St John's wort is a naturally occurring MAOI and, although as a botanical it

LIVED EXPERIENCE

I first commenced on an SSRI about 12 years ago for major depression. For me, depression is currently the worst symptom I experience, and the SSRI in combination with lithium has substantially contributed to my improved outlook on life and how I view myself. My mood is much more stable nowadays, and I experience far fewer days of feeling down than once would have been the case. I have always felt that the SSRI allowed me to more effectively engage with talking therapy, and the combination of medication and psychological work has benefited me greatly. However, as is often the case with psychotropic medications, the benefits come with costs. For me this has included sedation, weight gain, lethargy and dry mouth; if I miss a dose for even a few days, I start having nightmares and my nights become restless.

is much less potent than a pharmaceutical-grade compound, it can also interact with an SSRI and cause a negative episode for the person taking these agents. Figure 7.3 ■ illustrates the process of serotonin neurotransmission, which is so important to the effectiveness of SSRIs. Imagine the movement of neurotransmitters back and forth across the synapse—this is the movement that SSRIs affect.

Of note is the cross-diagnostic use of medications initially indicated for other conditions. Fluoxetine is an antidepressant and was the first SSRI developed. This compound is approved for another treatment regimen. It may also be used to treat the mood and physical symptoms of premenstrual dysphoric disorder (PMDD), which is differentiated from depression and other mental disorders. The dosing is flexible, and is usually 20 mg/day.

Serotonin and norepinephrine reuptake inhibitors (SNRIs)

Venlafaxine was the first in a class of new-generation antidepressants called serotonin and norepinephrine reuptake inhibitors (SNRIs). They have two mechanisms of action: inhibiting the reuptake of both serotonin and norepinephrine. Anticholinergic-like side-effects may occur. Other SNRIs include desvenlafaxine and duloxetine. A time buffer is also necessary when a SNRI is used in conjunction with MAOIs: a 14-day gap after discontinuing a MAOI before starting the SNRI, and at least a seven-day gap after discontinuing an SNRI and before starting a MAOI. SNRIs appear to be more effective than SSRIs in treating severe depressive symptoms and melancholia. However, side-effects such as headache, sexual dysfunction, sweating and gastrointestinal symptoms often limit SNRIs to second-line treatment. Duloxetine

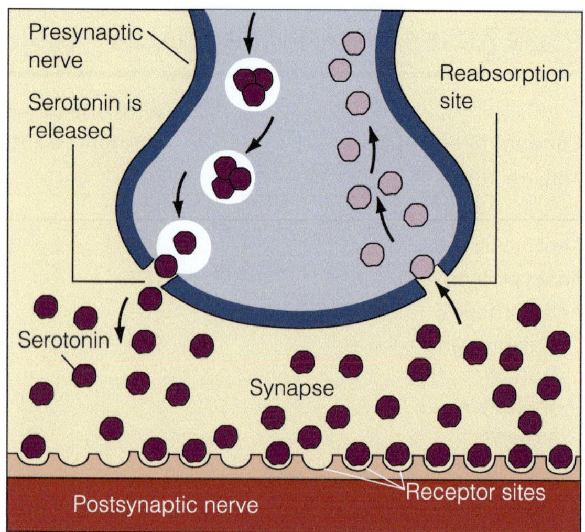

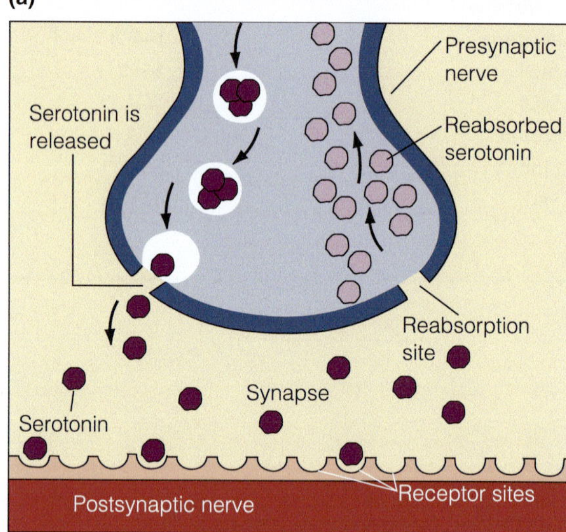

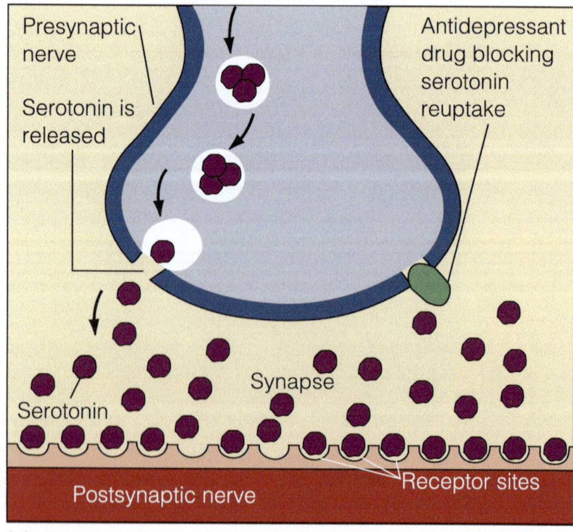

FIGURE 7.3 ■ Serotonin neurotransmission. (a) A highly schematic model of normal serotonin (5-HT) neurotransmission. (b) In depression, there may be a shortage of 5-HT in the synapse. (c) The action of an antidepressant medication blocking 5-HT reabsorption (reuptake).

may enhance the effects of benzodiazepines, but does not seem to enhance the effects of alcohol (Knadler, Lobo, Chappell & Bergstrom, 2011).

YOUR ASSESSMENT APPROACH
SSRI discontinuation syndrome

- Withdrawal from an SSRI is characterised by symptoms including dizziness, light-headedness, insomnia, fatigue, anxiety or agitation, nausea, headache and sensory disturbances. Other possible problems include hypomania, worsening of mood, aggressiveness and suicidality.
- A possible cause of the syndrome could be a hyposerotonergic state, because the long-term use of SSRI medication may downregulate (or de-sensitise) the postsynaptic serotonin receptors. Abrupt continuation may restore or even enhance serotonin reuptake, resulting in a depletion of synaptic serotonin. It may take two to three weeks for these systems to readapt.
- Mild, transient symptoms, such as jitteriness, sleep disturbance and heart palpitations, have been reported in newborns whose mothers received SSRIs during pregnancy.
- Short-acting SSRIs cause more numerous symptoms that appear earlier after discontinuation and typically last up to three weeks.
- Abrupt discontinuation or 'drug holidays' should be avoided with short-acting SSRIs.
- Short-acting SSRIs should be slowly tapered if discontinued.
- If symptoms appear, the taper needs to be more gradual.

Other medications used for depression

Stimulants, such as amphetamines and methylphenidate, and the phenothiazines are less commonly used antidepressants. Stimulants are not a proven treatment. Phenothiazines may be particularly useful in the presence of agitation. Some clinicians and researchers believe that major depressive episodes with psychotic features (delusional depressions) respond better to a combination of an antidepressant and an antipsychotic agent or to electroconvulsive therapy (ECT) than to antidepressants alone. Others simply recommend higher-than-usual doses of antidepressants.

Age-related considerations

Antidepressant use has raised the concern that children, adolescents and adults might, as a result of certain medications, demonstrate an increased risk of suicidal behaviour. This has not been fully established by the data. However, it is important that health practitioners are at all times vigilant for the possibility that people being treated for depression with antidepressants may experience an increase in energy prior to resolution of depressive and suicidal thinking. People who are being commenced on antidepressant medications should be assessed for clinical worsening, changes in behaviour, or suicidality. See Chapter 19 for more information on this topic.

COLLABORATIVE CARE

Teaching about antidepressants

Psychoeducation can enhance the effectiveness of medication and can help make the difference between adherence and non-adherence to a medication regimen. Medication-related education begins when a person commences on a drug and is repeated throughout the period of hospitalisation, if the person is an inpatient. It is a good idea to provide information both orally and in writing. Including family and significant others is also important, especially if they are going to be involved in supervising medication administration at home.

Initiating antidepressant therapy

- Make sure the person knows the name and dose(s) of the medication being taken. (*Rationale: This is basic information that every person taking medication should know.*)
- Advise the person to rise slowly from a sitting or lying position, and to sit on the side of the bed before standing up. (*Rationale: This allows the body time to compensate for medications that have postural hypotension as a side-effect.*)
- Encourage the use of ice blocks, sugar-free gum, sugar-free sweets and increased fluids. (*Rationale: Alleviates dryness of mouth.*)
- Advise the person and their family that it may take two to four weeks to see a therapeutic response to antidepressant therapy. (*Rationale: Prevents discouragement and impatience.*)
- Monitor for urinary retention or constipation, and take necessary amelioration actions. (*Rationale: These problems may result from the anticholinergic effects of some antidepressants.*)
- Advise the person to take their medication early in the day if insomnia occurs as a side-effect. (*Rationale: Some antidepressants have a stimulating effect.*)
- Advise the person to take their medication later in the evening if sedation occurs as a side-effect. (*Rationale: Some antidepressants have sedating side-effects.*)
- Monitor and record sleep patterns. (*Rationale: Normalisation of sleep patterns should occur.*)
- Avoid giving TCAs, or SSRIs and MAOIs concurrently. (*Rationale: To reduce the risk of a hypertensive crisis, give them two to three weeks apart.*)
- Observe the person for skin rashes, photosensitivity, weight gain and signs of infection. (*Rationale: These are adverse side-effects that should be evaluated.*)

(*continued*)

COLLABORATIVE CARE *(continued)*

- Advise the person that drowsiness, blurred vision, dry mouth, and jittery feelings should diminish after a few days on the medication. (*Rationale: Sedation and anticholinergic effects [except dry mouth] tend to diminish over time. However, they may recur if the dosage is raised.*)
- Monitor the person for suicide risk, particularly as depression begins to lift. (*Rationale: People who are profoundly depressed lack the energy to plan and implement suicide. As they begin to improve and become more energised, but are still profoundly depressed, their suicide risk increases.*)
- People on high doses of TCAs should be closely monitored for seizures. (*Rationale: High-dose tricyclics lower the seizure threshold.*)

People on SSRIs

- Depressive symptoms may begin to resolve within one week. (*Rationale: SSRIs tend to work more quickly than TCAS and MAOIs.*)
- Taking more than the prescribed dose will not resolve depressive symptoms more quickly. (*Rationale: More SSRI than prescribed will not hasten recovery.*)
- There may be feelings of restlessness, headaches, gastrointestinal upset, and vivid or disturbing dreams when first taking an SSRI. These are often temporary side-effects. (*Rationale: The side-effects may resolve within three weeks.*)
- There are no dietary restrictions with SSRIs. However, they cannot be taken simultaneously with MAOIs or with St John's wort (which is a naturally occurring MAOI). (*Rationale: Co-administered SSRI and MAOI can cause CNS depression from ataxia and slurred speech to coma and death.*)

People on MAOIs

- Supervise the person's intake, and make sure no tyramine-rich agents are offered. (*Rationale: Tyramine may precipitate hypertensive crisis.*)
- Monitor the person closely for headaches and elevated blood pressure. Withhold medication and report these signs to the prescribing health professional immediately. (*Rationale: These may be early signs of hypertensive crisis.*)
- Should severe hypertension occur, this should be treated as a medical emergency. (*Rationale: Hypertensive crisis requires prompt medical treatment and close monitoring.*)
- Observe people who are diabetic closely for hypoglycaemia. (*Rationale: MAOIs promote hypoglycaemia.*)

Prior to discharge

- In collaboration with the person, work out a time schedule that fits the person's lifestyle. (*Rationale: This will increase the likelihood that the person will adhere to the medication regimen.*)
- Advise the person to take the medication as ordered, and to avoid using alcohol or other central nervous system depressants during therapy. (*Rationale: Varying the dosage impairs the maintenance of therapeutic blood levels. Alcohol and other CNS depressants have a potentiating effect on antidepressants and may cause sedation, and in extreme cases stupor or coma.*)
- Teach the person and their family members about possible adverse reactions, and measures to initiate if they occur. (*Rationale: Promotes comfort and safety.*)
- Advise the person against operating dangerous equipment, driving a motor vehicle or engaging in tasks requiring mental alertness if drowsiness persists. (*Rationale: Promotes safety.*)
- Advise the person against not discontinuing the medication abruptly. (*Rationale: Antidepressant dosage should be gradually decreased to avoid withdrawal symptoms, such as nausea, dizziness, insomnia and headache.*)
- People on MAOIs should be provided with a list of tyramine-containing substances, and efforts should be taken to ensure that the person and their family understand the risks of consuming tyramine-rich products (*Rationale: Promotes safety.*)
- Accurately record the medication-related education that has been provided for the person and their family. (*Rationale: Documenting medication-related education proves information to other members of the health care team and legal defence in the event of an adverse reaction.*)

MOOD STABILISERS

The earliest discovery of a mood-stabilising medication was made in 1948 by Australian physician John Cade. Cade found that lithium worked to subdue wild behaviour in animals, and, to the surprise of his colleagues, went one step further and gave lithium to humans.

The psychopharmacological treatment of conditions collectively labelled *mania* used to be virtually synonymous with lithium carbonate therapy in countries such as Australia and the United States. Many well-controlled clinical studies indicated that lithium was initially the most effective agent for treating the vast majority of acute manic and hypomanic episodes. In addition, because of the absence of sedative side-effects, the people being treated felt much more connected to their environment and able to function normally while under the influence of lithium.

In recent decades, other medications have been added to the list of pharmacological treatments for bipolar disorder. The first was carbamazepine, used to control bipolar symptoms in people who either could not take lithium or did not respond therapeutically to it. Recognising the potential effectiveness of carbamazepine in certain mood disorders, other anticonvulsant medications such as valproate have also been adopted as mood stabilisers.

Pharmacological treatments for bipolar disorder have expanded, and are a substantial improvement over the clinically efficacious choices available in previous decades. New guidelines for bipolar treatment have been created, and have thus expanded our ability to care for people living with bipolar disorder. The Australian and New Zealand College of Psychiatrists released an updated clinical practice guideline for mood disorders (including bipolar disorder) in late 2015 (Mahli et al., 2015). (See Chapter 15 for more information on treating mood disorders.) In general, the pharmacological treatment for bipolar disorder should involve:

- use of a mood stabiliser in all phases of treatment
- use of an atypical antipsychotic if antipsychotic treatment is indicated
- avoidance of antidepressants if symptoms of mania are present
- avoidance of antidepressants if there is a history of rapid cycling and/or a high level of mood instability.

Lithium is the foundation of acute-phase and preventive treatment for mania. An additional treatment feature is the use of atypical antipsychotic medications in the acute manic phase of the disorder. The Practice Example on the following page provides a description of a manic episode with psychotic features. The medications that are effective during the acute manic phase are also used for the long-term prevention of mania. Bipolar depression may necessitate the use of lithium to stabilise people in monotherapy for depression.

The various treatments for bipolar disorder necessitate an in-depth view of medication interactions. See Your Assessment Approach, below, for examples of potential problems.

Dosage

The management of an acute manic episode involves the rapid initiation of the selected mood stabiliser, increased to substantial doses during the first week of treatment. Lithium is available only in oral form. Because lithium is an ion, its concentration can be measured in the blood. In the acute phase, the blood level must usually attain a concentration of 0.8 to 1.2 mmol/L, reducing to 0.6 to 0.8 mmol/L once the person's mood has moderated. A short-term benzodiazepine and an antipsychotic may also be added if the acute symptoms of mania are accompanied by behavioural or cognitive disturbance (Mahli et al., 2015).

The basic principles for lithium medication therapy are as follows:

- blood levels must be monitored after each dosage increase
- blood levels are checked every two to three months, or sooner if there is evidence of mood instability.

For symptoms of breakthrough depression seen with bipolar depression, the dosing of a mood stabiliser should be maximised before other stabilising or antidepressant agents are added to the regimen. After that episode resolves, the doses of the antidepressant medication are tapered slowly over the following two to six months. Careful assessment is required during the tapering process to detect any resurgence of depressive symptoms.

YOUR ASSESSMENT APPROACH Mood stabiliser medication interactions

Combining one of these	With one of these mood stabilisers	Can lead to these problems
Aminophylline	Lithium	Increased lithium secretion
Benzodiazepines	Valproate	Excessive CNS depression
Carbamazepine	Lithium	Increased effect of lithium, lithium toxicity
Carbamazepine	Topiramate	Decreased topiramate level
Chlorpromazine	Valproate	Valproic acid toxicity
Clozapine	Carbamazepine	Additive bone marrow suppression
CNS depressants	Topiramate	Possible topiramate-induced CNS depression as well as other adverse cognitive and neuropsychiatric effects
Diuretics	Lithium	Increased lithium levels and potential lithium toxicity (monitor electrolytes, especially sodium)
Haloperidol	Carbamazepine	Decreased effectiveness of either compound
Lamotrigine	Valproate	Increased lamotrigine levels, decreased valproic levels
MAOIs	Lithium	Increased depressant and anticholinergic effects
Marijuana	Lithium	Increased lithium levels and potential lithium toxicity
Neuroleptics	Lithium	Encephalopathy
NSAIDs	Lithium	Increased effect of lithium, lithium toxicity
SSRIs	Lithium	Increased effect of lithium, lithium toxicity
Tetracyclines	Lithium	Lithium toxicity
Thyroid hormones	Lithium	May induce hypothyroidism

The length of treatment with medication for bipolar disorder is a debated issue. Clinical practice suggests prophylactic use of a mood stabiliser, preferably the compound effective during the acute phase of treatment, for at least two years. Stopping or reducing treatment without the advice of a health professional and monitoring runs the risk of relapse with no guarantee that the medications that supported mood stabilisation will be successful if reintroduced after cessation. The following Practice Example illustrates the use of medication in the case of a person with bipolar disorder.

Practice example

Chris, a 32-year-old office worker, was brought to the emergency department by her sister after losing her job. She had been arguing constantly with other workers in the office, and stood on a meeting-room table, loudly telling people how to do their jobs. She had not slept in three days, and was so irritable that she pushed and swore at her manager when approached about seeking help. Her sister stated that Chris was grandiose, spoke very quickly, moved from topic to topic in a rapid-fire manner and demeaned everyone around her. The family was very concerned. She had not taken any prescription or recreational compounds so far as the family knew. In the past five years she had been prescribed lithium, which seemed to help; however, Chris refuses to take it now, because it leaves a metallic taste in her mouth.

On interview, Chris spoke about having special powers, such as bringing people back from the dead because she was a 'sanctioned angel'. Her episodes in the past did not include delusional thinking, and this was the first time her family could not contain her. Chris had some awareness that her behaviour had frightened her family. She was told she had bipolar disorder with delusions. She was commenced on lithium 500 mg at night, and risperidone 1 mg twice daily, to control the mania and the psychosis. Chris was not hospitalised because her family agreed to supervise her care. After a week, the Chris's behaviour was beginning to stabilise.

The use of anticonvulsants as mood stabilisers has its own unique set of effects and termination-of-treatment issues. Some anticonvulsants, such as carbamazepine, have sedation, gastrointestinal (GI) disturbances and dizziness as side-effects. The body needs time to adapt to the medication; therefore, some side-effects are temporary. However, dosage adjustments can minimise the impact of these side-effects so that the quality of life is not shifted downward.

Important teaching points when using anticonvulsants as mood stabilisers are twofold. When using an anticonvulsant as a mood stabiliser, the initial dose may be too low to address symptoms, and must be gradually increased to prevent negative cognitive impacts. The result is less-than-optimal symptom control until a therapeutic dose is reached. People receiving treatment and their significant others need to be prepared for this stage. The other relevant and vital issue is the body's inability to handle the abrupt discontinuation of these medications. Frank discussions must highlight the increased chance of having a seizure, even if the person has never had one, if the dose is not tapered slowly to discontinuation.

Remaining on a mood stabiliser can be a challenge for people living with bipolar disorder, but effective interventions and medication teaching can promote adherence. The success seen with maintenance medication for someone with bipolar disorder is described in Mental Health in the Media, below. Even the stressors and pressures of a life in the Arts can be managed with the help of psychopharmacology.

Psychobiology of lithium

The psychobiology of bipolar disorder remains unclear, but much can be said about the psychobiology of lithium. Lithium is a salt that occurs naturally in our bodies. People who live with bipolar disorder and respond to lithium do not have a deficit of lithium in their systems. Lithium, not unlike the antidepressants, affects the neurotransmitters, especially norepinephrine and serotonin. In short, lithium aids in the reduction of neurotransmitter release into the synapse and enhances its return, yielding a lower overall amount of the neurotransmitter in the synapse. Behaviourally, these biological changes can be observed as an absence of mania or depression. What is unclear is why lithium takes up to a few weeks to be fully effective, when its effects can be observed on synaptic activity almost immediately. Also, why do some people with bipolar disorder *not* respond at all to lithium therapy? Many psychobiologists believe that lithium's effects are likely to be based on neurocellular changes that occur over weeks or months after a person begins lithium therapy. A similar explanation may hold true concerning the effectiveness of other mood stabilisers.

MENTAL HEALTH IN THE MEDIA

Patty Duke Aston

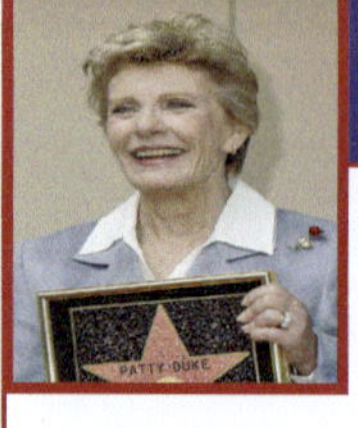

Patty Duke Aston was an actress who shared her story of bipolar disorder and how she struggled, and succeeded, over the years. An actress with her own show, *The Patty Duke Show*, Patty Duke had pressures and responsibilities at a very young age. She also had remarkable symptoms of bipolar disorder that few recognised, and some took advantage of, for the benefit of the fast-paced world of entertainment. Once Patty Duke finally received treatment after years of bizarre behaviour and outrageous stunts, she was able to reach stability and share her story. She spoke at professional conferences, did public speaking to explain mental illness and established The Patty Duke Online Center for Mental Wellness. She was an example of how stability, recovery and rehabilitation are not only possible, but highly probable with proper treatment. Patty Duke Aston was well known to Australians watching television in the late 1960s and 1970s. She passed away in March 2016.

Photo courtesy of Alamy.

> **YOUR INTERVENTION STRATEGIES**
> **Lithium maintenance considerations**
>
> To maintain stable lithium levels, nurses, people prescribed lithium and their family members should know the following:
>
> - stabilise the dosing schedule (through sustained-release formula or divided doses)
> - if a dose is missed, take it within two hours; if more than two hours has elapsed, skip the one dose
> - ingest adequate dietary sodium
> - maintain hydration
> - replace fluids and electrolytes lost during exercise, exertion or GI illness
> - monitor for side-effects and lithium toxicity.
>
> Watch for events that may cause lithium levels to increase:
>
> - change in hydration status
> - increase in other medications
> - cannabis use
> - lithium overdose
> - decreased sodium intake
> - diuretic medication use
> - medical illness
> - nonsteroidal anti-inflammatory medication use
> - tetracycline use
> - fluid and electrolyte loss through fever, sweating, diarrhea, vomiting or dehydration.

ANXIOLYTIC MEDICATIONS

Medications in this class are used to treat a variety of problems, from high levels of anxiety and panic to insomnia.

Effects

Anxiolytic medications, or anti-anxiety agents—sedatives and hypnotics—have very similar pharmacological attributes. All can be used in small or moderate doses to relieve anxiety, and in larger doses to induce sleep. Although they share the major clinical effect of tranquilisation or **disinhibition** (loss or reduction of an inhibition) of fear-induced behaviour, their side-effects, including their addictive potential and overdose sequelae, make certain medications in this category more suitable for routine use, and others better reserved for limited, special circumstances.

Anti-anxiety medications are sometimes called *minor tranquilisers*, but this is a misleading term. Their effects on anxiety have qualities that are different from those of the 'major tranquilisers' or antipsychotic medications, but the quantity of the impact is the same.

Meprobamate

Meprobamate was the first anti-anxiety agent to gain popularity, in the 1960s. The results of controlled studies of the effects of meprobamate compared to placebos were generally favourable, but not overwhelmingly convincing. This, and the addictive and fatal overdose potentials of the medication, prompted investigators to develop more effective and safer medications, and meprobamate is no longer available in many countries, including Australia.

Benzodiazepines and non-benzodiazepines

Benzodiazepines and non-benzodiazepines are widely used today in the management of anxiety. This group, which includes alprazolam, diazepam and others, accounts for a high percentage of all the psychoactive medications prescribed in Australia. This fact usually evokes a mixed response in professional circles. The easy distribution of medications for such a ubiquitous human phenomenon as anxiety fosters the development of a pill-oriented and pill-dependent society, say critics. If someone's anxiety level is low to moderate and they are unable to learn how to effectively cope with anxiety, or the person is unaware that they could develop the skills in therapy, then taking a pill seems like a logical course of action. Using a medication instead of a skill leaves the individual vulnerable to distress when the medication is not available or is no longer effective. Sympathisers focus on the proven effectiveness of the medications, which help people achieve higher levels of functioning, more pleasurable experiences, and even more productive psychotherapies in some instances.

The dosing and timing of an anti-anxiety medication determine whether the treatment of anxiety is effective or interferes with a person's ability to learn how to cope. These are two entirely different pathways in the treatment of anxiety. Anxiety is a normal human response to threats of varying intensities, and is not necessarily an experience to be avoided. At low to moderate levels, anxiety can be motivating and instructive, and helps one to be more aware of one's environment. Treatment is not needed for this entirely healthy human reaction. But when anxiety passes these stages and becomes excessive, high anxiety and panic can occur. Extreme feelings of anxiety and panic are not motivating—in fact, they are immobilising and make learning very difficult (see Chapter 8). Treatment with psychotherapy, and possibly also medication, would be introduced at that point, because anxiety has surpassed a normal-level reaction and become a symptom.

The clinical application and purpose of anti-anxiety medications is primarily to support people through episodes of stress and anxiety at moderate to high levels. Medicating so that higher levels of anxiety are reduced allows the individual to have a lower level of anxiety that can be managed with the coping skills taught by nurses and other health professionals, and to gauge the effectiveness of their coping skills. If anti-anxiety medications are given without regard for the actual anxiety level and the individual's need to learn coping skills, it is possible to avoid the need to learn to cope. Instead, the person learns to rely on the medication to become less anxious. Having taken the medication and with anxiety in check, the person would not be motivated to do anything. The lesson that will have been learned is: when anxious, take pills. For a list of currently available benzodiazepines and non-benzodiazepines, see Table 7.4 ■.

TABLE 7.4 ■ Benzodiazepines and non-benzodiazepines

Benzodiazepines	Nitrazepam
Alprazolam	Oxazepam
Bromazepam	Temazepam
Clonazepam	**Non-benzodiazepines**
Diazepam	Buspirone
Flunitrazepam	Zopiclone
Midazolam	

New medications

In recent years, anxiety-related research has expanded tremendously, and several new anxiolytic medications have been introduced. The newer benzodiazepines give prescribers a wider range of therapies to target the often idiosyncratic manifestations of anxiety. Some of the new medications have more rapid onsets and shorter half-lives, while others have the usual benzodiazepine onset time and an extended half-life.

With what we know now about psychobiology, a variety of benzodiazepine medications can be used in the treatment of a number of disorders. Benzodiazepines may be used for the following:

- anxiety disorders
- sleep disorders
- mood disorders
- anxiety associated with medical illness
- psychotic symptoms and disorders
- convulsive disorders
- involuntary movement disorders
- spastic disorders and acute muscle spasms
- intoxication and withdrawal from alcohol and other substances
- pre-anaesthesia
- nausea and vomiting associated with chemotherapy
- anxiolytic, sedative and amnestic effects in a wide range of stressful diagnostic procedures.

Uses for anxiolytics

There is no question that, when used carefully, benzodiazepines offer a rapid, effective and safe treatment for the emotional state commonly known as anxiety. Caffeine interferes with the effectiveness of these medications, both pharmacologically and as an irritant to the person's mood and systems.

These medications are absorbed much more rapidly and completely from the gastrointestinal tract than from intramuscular injection, and so are almost always administered orally. Exceptions are the intramuscular injections of lorazepam or diazepam. Peak levels of diazepam are reached in the bloodstream one to two hours after ingestion.

The major side-effects of benzodiazepines are related to their sedative qualities. People may complain of excessive drowsiness, and must be cautioned against driving a car or operating other machinery.

Other medications used to treat anxiety, generally less effectively, include the beta-blocker propranolol.

Another common use of benzodiazepines, for instance diazepam, is in the detoxification of individuals who are alcohol-dependent.

Psychobiology of anxiolytic medications

Antianxiety medications probably work through a process of synaptic activity involving the neurotransmitter gamma-aminobutyric acid (GABA) in the brain and spinal cord. Benzodiazepines most likely potentiate GABA, producing muscle relaxation. This mechanism involves a complex process of presynaptic and postsynaptic receptor activity. The anti-anxiety effectiveness seen with these medications is related to their impacts on GABA receptors. Recent research has yielded information about the presence of a postsynaptic receptor called the *benzodiazepine receptor*. As the term implies, benzodiazepines bind perfectly and with great specificity to these receptors, allowing for the sensation of relaxation. Two types of benzodiazepine receptors have been identified in the CNS. Type 1 receptors are located in parts of the brain responsible for sedation, and non-benzodiazepines bind exclusively to the Type 1 receptors. This makes non-benzodiazepines a good choice for the treatment of sleep disturbances. Type 2 receptors are positioned in parts of the brain responsible for cognition, memory and psychomotor functioning. Benzodiazepines bind with either Type 1 or Type 2 receptors.

Researchers are working to develop next-generation benzodiazepines by adjusting the chemical design to deliver a more selective main effect that avoids the many unwanted

YOUR ASSESSMENT APPROACH Anxiolytic medication interactions

Combining one of these	With one of these anxiolytics	Can lead to these problems
Cimetidine	Alprazolam	Decreased alprazolam clearance
CNS depressants	Anxiolytics	Increased CNS depression, increased risk of apnea
Digoxin	Oxazepam	May increase serum digoxin level, digoxin toxicity
Kava (herb)	Alprazolam	May cause coma
MAOIs	Buspirone	Elevated blood pressure
TCA	Alprazolam	Increased TCA plasma level

side-effects. Your Assessment Approach points out potential medication interactions between existing anxiolytics and other medications and substances.

TREATMENT FOR INSOMNIA

The pharmacological management of insomnia presents an interesting and challenging clinical problem. Many of the hypnotic medications tend to have undesirable effects, including physiological dependence, fatal overdose potential and dangerous interactions with other medications because of liver enzyme induction. The first principle of treatment is to assess whether the insomnia is related to one of the major mental disorders, such as schizophrenia or major depression. If so, the insomnia can and should be treated as part of the larger problem, and sedative antipsychotics or antidepressants may be given at bedtime for this purpose.

In the management of simple insomnia without an associated major mental disorder, sedative–hypnotics are indicated for short-term treatment. Overall, the available sedative–hypnotics include certain antidepressants, benzodiazepines, non-benzodiazepines, over-the-counter (OTC) medications, barbiturates and some miscellaneous substances, such as alcohol (Adams, Holland & Urban, 2011; Samuel, Zimovetz, Gabriel & Beard, 2011). Prescription medications are more effective than OTCs, while barbiturates are rarely, if ever, prescribed, due to safety and substance-dependence problems.

The rapid absorption of non-benzodiazepines, along with efficient elimination and the minimal hangover effects of sedation the following day, makes them useful in the treatment of insomnia. One such medication is Zolpidem. It was hoped that fast-acting, effective sleep-inducing, and quickly-eliminated medications such as Zolpidem, would avoid the difficulties associated with other commonly used compounds. However, clinical reports of unusual side-effects from the non-benzodiazepines include sleep walking, sleep eating and other behaviours that the individual does not remember. It is important that people using these medications are informed about these and other side-effects.

Sleep hygiene is an important topic for nurses to discuss with people who are being treated for sleep problems. Behavioural and pharmacological circumstances can affect sleep as well as interfere with effective treatment. See What Every Nurse Should Know on the next page about relevant information for medications that affect sleep.

TREATMENT OF DEMENTIA

A group of medications that is used to treat some of the behavioural symptoms of dementias are atypical antipsychotics. They are common choices for treating the delusions, hallucinations, aggression and agitation sometimes seen with people who have dementia. Lower doses of these medications than would be used in the treatment of younger people with psychotic disorders are usual.

There is ongoing debate about whether the adverse effects of atypical antipsychotics offset the advantages. As these concerns are explored, atypical antipsychotics offer good symptom control with far fewer side-effects than haloperidol, the antipsychotic previously used to treat the symptoms of dementia.

ACETYLCHOLINESTERASE INHIBITORS

The class of medications with specific abilities for dementia treatment is **acetylcholinesterase inhibitors**, also called *cholinesterase inhibitors*. The title of this class describes how these compounds affect the CNS. The enzyme responsible for the breakdown of a particular neurotransmitter is inhibited from acting by the medication. The enzyme is acetylcholinesterase, and the neurotransmitter it specifically works on is acetylcholine. The cholinergic system is involved in memory, the ability to logically progress from one step to the next in problem-solving, and the identification of objects and people in the environment, among other skills. People with dementia of the Alzheimer's type (DAT) have acetylcholine neurotransmitter deficits at the root of some of their problems. When the breakdown of acetylcholine is slowed, it allows more of the neurotransmitter to remain in the synapse, thus promoting acetylcholine's function—transmitting information from one cell to another. In mild to moderately affected individuals, when there is more acetylcholine in the CNS, cognitive functioning and memory improve. This is essentially the path by which these medications slow the progression of the memory deficits in people with early-stage DAT.

Acetylcholinesterase inhibitors are best utilised early in the process of dementia when deficits are still mild to moderate in scope. But the best timing and the most effective use of the compounds are frequently thwarted by the realities of human nature. Instituting treatment at early stages may be difficult, because many people are not aware that they are in the early stages of dementia. Frequently they are unable to grasp their own level of symptomatology, and lack information on the early signs, symptoms or issues of dementia. Confabulation or denial prevents the person or loved ones from noting deficits or recognising the implications of low-level difficulties. For example, a woman who is unable to tie her shoes may ask her husband to do that for her; both of them attribute her difficulty to arthritis, musculoskeletal problems or the side-effects of medications. Another example is the man who stops balancing his bank accounts, ostensibly because the bank has always been correct, when in reality he has lost the basic maths skills required.

Think of this medication class as a treatment for specific symptoms, not a cure. Acetylcholinesterase inhibitors do not alter the course of the underlying disease process or have an impact on the progressive nature of the disease. They are a way to temporarily improve neurotransmission and thus ameliorate memory deficits. The first of the acetylcholinesterase inhibitors was tacrine. Although its effectiveness was controversial, it was the first step in the direction of active treatment for a major portion of people with dementing processes. Problems with this medication included liver toxicity, which could be controlled, and several common side-effects including GI disturbances and headache. From this beginning, other compounds were developed. Donepezil and rivastigmine are

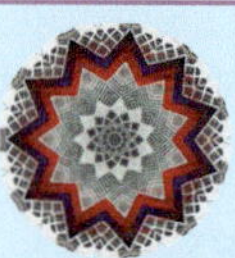

WHAT EVERY NURSE SHOULD KNOW

Medications that affect sleep

Type	Examples	Comments
Antidepressants	Tricyclic antidepressants such as amitriptyline	Induce drowsiness to varying degrees; effect on insomnia associated with depression usually occurs earlier than antidepressant effect; suppress REM
	Selective serotonin reuptake inhibitors such as fluoxetine	Generally decrease total sleep time, increase wakefulness, may induce vivid dreaming
Antiepileptics	Phenytoin	Sedation common, less so with newer seizure-control medications
Antihistamines	Cyproheptadine, promethazine and pseudoephedrine compounds	Induce drowsiness to varying degrees
Antimanic medications	Lithium	Improves sleep, but may cause daytime sleepiness initially
Anti-Parkinson medications	Levodopa	Low doses may improve sleep, but generally persons on medication for Parkinson's have poor sleep with insomnia, vivid dreaming
Antipsychotics	Traditional antipsychotics such as chlorpromazine and haloperidol	Chlorpromazine very sedating, haloperidol less so
	Atypical antipsychotics such as clozapine, risperidone	High incidence of sedation with clozapine, less so with risperidone
Anxiolytics	Benzodiazepines such as temazepam	May be used as hypnotics to induce and sustain sleep (note differences between short- and long-acting types)
	Buspirone	Little effect on sleep and alertness
Caffeine	Additive to some pain and headache remedies, coffee, tea, colas	Increases wakefulness, effects may last 8–14 hours
Cardiovascular medications	Antihypertensives such as propranolol, clonidine (Catapres)	Insomnia, sedation and nightmares, less so with captopril and other angiotensin-converting enzyme inhibitors
Corticosteroids	Prednisone	Generally disturb sleep, especially if taken late in the day; suppress REM sleep
Hypnotics	Zopiclone	Effective for sleep-onset insomnia because of rapid absorption

acetylcholinesterase inhibitors with improved impacts and fewer difficulties from side-effects. Donepezil is indicated in the treatment of all degrees of severity of DAT. GI disturbances occur at a much lower level than with the original compound, and headaches are reported at only a slightly higher level than with clients taking a placebo. There is hope that these medications can play a role in preventing individuals with cognitive deficits from converting to DAT. See Chapter 12 for a discussion of DAT and its progression.

GLUTAMATE PATHWAY MODIFIER

Another approach to address the memory difficulties in the pathologic process of DAT involves looking at glutamate. Glutamate is a primary excitatory neurotransmitter in the brain, and glutamate receptor activity is associated with information processing, storage and retrieval. Glutamate triggers *N*-methyl-D-aspartate (NMDA) receptors to allow calcium to flow into a nerve cell, creating the chemical environment required for information storage. Too much glutamate overstimulates the NMDA receptors to allow too much calcium into the nerve cells, leading to the disruption and death of the cells. It may be that overexcitation of these receptors contributes to the impaired cognition and memory in DAT.

The medication memantine is the first glutamate pathway modifier, and is used to mitigate the impacts of DAT on functioning. Its job is to moderate the glutamate such that it does not overexcite the NMDA receptors. As a result, nerve cells are not negatively impacted or destroyed, and degradation is minimised over time. While the mechanism of action of memantine in DAT is not known, the principal pharmacological actions at a therapeutic dose are inhibition of NMDA receptors. Memantine can reverse the decreased metabolic activity associated with DAT, possibly accounting for its beneficial effects on cognition and global functioning. Memantine also has neuroprotective properties and can inhibit amyloid-beta-induced toxicity and neurodegeneration.

MEDICATION COUNTERFEITING

Medications available through prescription can be, and are, counterfeited and sold through non-prescription means. Counterfeit medications are illegal and inherently unsafe, and are a growing public health problem in Australia and internationally. A counterfeit medication is a fake medication. It may be contaminated or contain the wrong—or no—active ingredient, be made with the wrong amount of ingredients, or be packaged in phony packaging. Typically, a person who cannot afford a particular medication may purchase it over the internet and unknowingly receive a counterfeit medication instead, with unintended and possibly serious consequences.

The World Health Organization (WHO) has the International Medical Products Anti-Counterfeiting Taskforce, or IMPACT, to protect people from counterfeit medicines. Regulation and technology are being employed to try to minimise this public health problem. To ensure the people with whom you are working are receiving safe medications, it is important that you advocate that they obtain medications only from a licensed pharmacy. In Australia, the Therapeutic Goods Administration (TGA) investigates the manufacture and supply of counterfeit medications and medical devices. More information about this aspect of the work of the TGA is available on the following website: www.tga.gov.au/counterfeit-medicines-and-medical-devices.

HERBAL MEDICINES

Herbal medicines are widely used as an alternative or complementary therapy. A significant proportion of prescription medications and hundreds of OTC medications are derived from plants. Herbs and plants generally take longer to act than pharmaceuticals, and few have the potency of a prescription medicine. However, many herbal agents have powerful medicine-like actions and side-effects.

One of the key features of safe and effective nursing care is communication about complementary and alternative treatments. It is important to keep in mind the variety of terms used to describe these treatments: complementary, alternative, botanical, nutriceutical, herbal medicine; home remedy, natural remedy, homeopathic remedy; health food, vitamin therapy, dietary supplement, phytomedicine, supplements, herbal tea, and others.

The concomitant use of herbal medicines with psychiatric pharmaceuticals can be accomplished safely only when health providers know what agents are being used, and when the safety and effectiveness for the person's specific condition have been thoroughly appraised. It is important to assess whether and how a person is using herbal medicines.

There are many benefits to using alternative substances. For example:

- self-treatment can be empowering
- the very low concentrations of these substances could be helpful and might not be harmful for those who are sensitive to even low doses of pharmaceutical compounds
- some people feel safer using 'natural' products, and distrust chemical formulations
- standard labelling and dosing are possible.

However, there are potential problems with the use of alternative substances in psychiatry, even though these substances have lower potencies. A number of alternative substances are widely used as lay therapies for mental health problems and psychiatric disorders; for instance, St John's wort for depression and *Ginkgo biloba* for dementia. You may encounter people using ma huang for general malaise, kava for anxiety and stress, and ginseng, SAMe or St John's wort for depression. Careful assessment is required to identify the potential for difficulties with alternative substances. Problems with using herbs may include:

- contamination of the product
- dosing inconsistencies
- delayed absorption of other co-administered medications
- worsening of high blood pressure, potassium imbalance and coagulation problems
- side-effects, such as nerve damage, kidney damage and liver damage
- advertising of unproven claims
- aggravation of allergic reactions
- interference with breastfeeding
- believing that one is treating the problem, when in reality the symptoms could continue to worsen, making effective treatment much more difficult.

Assessing herb consumption

Many people do not tell health care providers about their herbal use for fear of being ridiculed or criticised. How do you find out what alternative therapies a person is taking? Good interviewing skills—tolerance, a nonjudgmental stance and carefully considered questions—will bring much of the person's life into the light. See Communication for examples of a conversation about this topic. Questions such as 'Do you do anything to improve your health?' or 'What do you buy

COMMUNICATION

Communicating with a person about herbal medicines

CONSUMER: 'I do not like taking all these chemicals. It is not natural.'

NURSE RESPONSE 1: 'Are you more comfortable taking medicine to help you when you know it is natural?'

(*RATIONALE:* This question gathers more data about what the person needs in order to feel better, and raises the possibility of alternative substance use.)

NURSE RESPONSE 2: 'Have you had bad experiences with anything in particular?'

(*RATIONALE:* This response makes the connection for the person between the idea and a possible result. It may also encourage discussion of recreational substance use.)

at the grocery store or health food store besides food?' can open the subject.

It is important to be aware of the person's need to talk to a knowledgeable professional. The person may tell you about someone else who is taking alternatives while watching for your reaction. A nonjudgmental response would include questions about what the person thinks about it, whether it has helped or whether the person would consider using this particular treatment. Not knowing about the person's use of botanicals risks dangerous medication interactions or costly and painful tests or treatments when a herb causes an unrecognised side-effect.

Psychopharmacology is an important aspect of the treatment of people who live with mental illness. As you develop an understanding of the science, practice and experience of pharmacology, your confidence and skills as a psychiatric–mental health nurse will grow. This will influence how you go about teaching people about medications as a vital part of psychiatric treatment, promoting self-care, and advocating for the best possible outcomes.

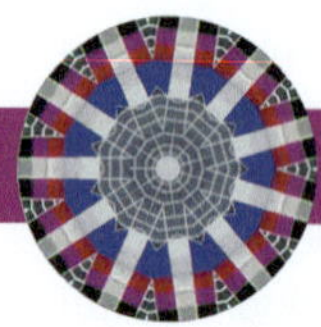

REFERENCES

Adams, M. P., Holland, L. N., & Urban, C. Q. (2011). *Pharmacology for nurses: A pathophysiologic approach* (3rd ed.). Upper Saddle River, NJ: Prentice Hall.

Barnes, T. R. E., & Patten, C. (2011). Antipsychotic polypharmacy in schizophrenia: benefits and risks. *CNS Drugs, 25* (5), 383–399.

Bliss, D. Z., Savik, K., Jung, H.-J. G., Whitebird, R., & Lowry, A. (2011). Symptoms associated with dietary fiber supplementation over time in individuals with fecal incontinence. *Nursing Research, 60*(3S), S58–S67.

Carr, V., Whiteford, H., Groves, A., McGorry, P., & Shepherd, A. (2012). Policy and service development implications of the second Australian National Survey of High Impact Psychosis (SHIP). *Australian and New Zealand Journal of Psychiatry, 46*(8), 708–718.

Commonwealth of Australia (2002). *The National Strategy for Quality Use of Medicines*. Canberra, Australia: Department of Health and Ageing.

Fontenelle, L. F., Oostermeijer, S., Harrison, B. J., Pantelis, C., & Yucel, M. (2011). Obsessive–compulsive disorder, impulse control disorders and drug addiction: Common features and potential treatments. *Drugs, 71*(7), 827–840.

Galletly, C., Castle, D., Dark, F., Humberstone, V., Jablensky, A., Killackey, E., . . . Tran, N. (2016). Royal Australian and New Zealand College of Psychiatrists clinical practice guidelines for the management of schizophrenia and related disorders. *Australian and New Zealand Journal of Psychiatry, 50*(5), 410–472.

Hough, D. W., Natarajan, J., Vandebosch, A., Rossenu, S., Kraner, M., & Eerdekens, M. (2011). Evaluation of the effect of paliperidone extended release and quetiapine on corrected QT intervals: A randomized, double-blind, placebo-controlled study. *International Clinical Psychopharmacology, 26*, 25–34.

Kishimoto, T., Agarwal, V., Kishi, T., Leucht, S., Kane, J., & Correll, C. (2013). Relapse prevention in schizophrenia: A systematic review and meta-analysis of second-generation antipsychotics versus first-generation antipsychotics. *Molecular Psychiatry, 18*(1), 53–66.

Knadler, M. P., Lobo, E., Chappell, J., & Bergstrom, R. (2011). Duloxetine: Clinical pharmacokinetics and drug interactions. *Clinical Pharmacokinetics, 50*(5), 281–294.

Lewis, M. (1990). *Managing madness: Psychiatry and society in Australia 1788–1980*. Canberra, Australia: Australian Institute of Health, AGPS.

Mahli, G., Bassett, D., Boyce, P., Bryant, R., Fitzgerald, P., Fritz, K., . . . Singh, A. (2015). Royal Australian and New Zealand College of Psychiatrists clinical practice guidelines for mood disorders. *Australian and New Zealand Journal of Psychiatry, 49*(12), 1087–1206.

Mojtabai, R., & Olfson, M. (2010). National trends in psychotropic medication polypharmacy in office-based psychiatry. *Archives of General Psychiatry, 67*(1), 26–36.

Müller, D. J., Zai, C. C., Sicard, M., Remington, E., Souza, R. P., Tiwari, A. K., . . . Kennedy, J. L. (2010). Systematic analysis of dopamine receptor genes (DRD1-DRD5) in antipsychotic-induced weight gain. *Pharmacogenomics Journal*. Advance online publication. doi:10.1038/tpj.2010.65

National Aboriginal and Torres Strait Islander Health Council (2004). *National Strategic Framework for Aboriginal and Torres Strait Islander, 2003–2013: Framework for action by governments*. Canberra, Australia: National Aboriginal and Torres Strait Islander Health Council.

O'Reilly, M., & Lester, J. N. (2016). Introduction: The social construction of normality and pathology. In: M. O'Reilly & J. N. Lester (Eds.), *The Palgrave handbook of adult mental health* (pp. 1–19). Houndmills, England: Palgrave MacMillan.

Ormerod, S., McDowell, S., Colemen, J., & Ferner, R. (2008). Ethnic differences in the risks of adverse reactions to drugs used in the treatment of psychoses and depression: A systematic review and meta-analysis. *Drug Safety, 31*(7), 597–607.

Samuel, S., Zimovetz, E. A., Gabriel, Z., & Beard, S. M. (2011). Efficacy and safety of treatments for refractory generalized anxiety disorder: A systematic review. *International Clinical Psychopharmacology, 26*, 63–68.

Seitz, D. P., & Gill, S. S. (2009). Neuroleptic malignant syndrome complicating antipsychotic treatment of delirium or agitation in medical and surgical patients: Case reports and a review of the literature. *Psychosomatics, 50* (1), 8–15.

Snowdon, J., & Halliday, G. (2011). A study of the use of clozapine in old age psychiatry. *International Clinical Psychopharmacology, 26*(4), 232–235.

Thompson, J. W., & Johnson, A. C. (2011). Acute lithium intoxication: Properly directing an index of suspicion. *Southern Medical Journal, 104*(5), 371–372.

Veselinovic, T., Schorn, H., Vernaleken, I. B., Schiffl, K., Klomp, M., & Gerhard Grunder, G. (2011). Impact of different antidopaminergic mechanisms on the dopaminergic control of prolactin secretion. *Journal of Clinical Psychopharmacology, 31*(2), 214–220.

Stress, anxiety and anxiety disorders

8

DEB O'KANE AND ANN SMITH

LEARNING OUTCOMES

After completing this chapter, you will be able to:

1. Explain how stress and anxiety affects an individual, and how it can relate to anxiety disorders.
2. Discuss the biopsychosocial theories of stress, and their contribution to understanding stress and coping.
3. Identify the sources of anxiety, and describe the methods people use to cope with stress and anxiety.
4. Discuss the distinctive characteristics of anxiety disorders.
5. Identify the relevant theories associated with causal factors in anxiety disorders.
6. Describe a comprehensive assessment of a person experiencing anxiety disorders.
7. Describe a plan of care for intervening into mild, moderate, severe and panic levels of anxiety.
8. Educate people with anxiety and their families about the pharmacological and nonpharmacological measures for anxiety disorders.

LIVED EXPERIENCE

Living through chronic anxiety, I survived a living hell

Just another Monday, so I thought. It was a Monday that changed my life's journey. I started work at 8.30am as a happy-go-lucky, fun-loving employee, a mother, wife, foster mother, daughter, sister, friend, neighbour and student with a promising future. At 8.45am, all this came to an end. I was no more.

I was sucked deeper and deeper into a terrifying fear, the feeling of being pushed with great force into a corner with no escape. The stench of fear, the fetid taste, dry mouth, pounding heart, burning heat rising in waves, nausea, diarrhoea, stomach cramps, restlessness, irritability, excess weight loss, hair falling out, inability to sleep . . . I could not remember the day or time, everyday noise sent me into a panic and the need to flee, or into a rage where I feared for my children's safety. 'Don't touch me!' 'Leave me alone!'

I would run and run until I was exhausted. The world became too fearful and unsafe. Nowhere to hide; nowhere to escape the panic, the terror within, a living hell for both me and my family. I just wanted it to stop! I was detained to a high-security inpatient unit as a high suicidal risk on many, many occasions.

(continued)

KEY TERMS

LIVED EXPERIENCE (*continued*)

One day I just decided I could not live my life this way, nor could I continue to cause such harm and sorrow to my husband and children, and I decided to regain control of my life and myself. The beginning of a very hard, arduous, long journey.

This experience had to be for a reason. I trained as a consumer representative, and advocate and peer worker, to enable me to assist those who had no voice of their own and who were also lost.

In 2008, I was awarded the Margaret Tobin Award of Excellence; in 2014, I was honoured with an Order of Australia for advocating for people who experience mental health issues. In 2015, I was included in the Who's Who of Australian Women. So people do recover and overcome their demons.

Am I the same person who started out on this journey? No. There is a deep underlying sadness and grief for the loss of those years of my life, and for the significant impact on my husband's and children's lives. As I write a very brief history, which spanned over a quarter of a decade, tears roll down my face.

INTRODUCTION

How do we handle the ups and downs of life? Our brains have built-in chemical circuit-breakers that shut off stress hormones, and networks of nerves whose job it is to calm us down. The circuit-breakers and the nerves require us to take regular breaks from our everyday routines—that is, we have a biological need to periodically disengage. Consider how advances in technology have affected our lives: mobile phones, text messaging, social media, tablets, laptops . . . With instant messaging we are on call 24/7/365. When exploring the possible negative health impact of using mobile phones, Thomée, Härenstam and Hagberg (2011; 2012) found that young adults accepted that they would be contactable daily, and one in four reported that they were expected to be available 24 hours a day. Instant communication technology makes it harder, not easier, to get away, to relax or to disengage, particularly at times when we require stress relief. In addition, personal and professional expectations have risen exponentially in a culture that favours constant, measurable productivity. At work, we feel that we must reach the benchmarks that are set for us. Then there is the driver who cut you off this morning, the argument with your partner and the newest workload increase at university. The global condition keeps us on edge every day: terrorist attacks; wars in Iran, Syria and Afghanistan; threats of bird and swine flu; medication-resistant strains of *Staphylococcus*; and earthquakes and other natural disasters.

Insurance claims for stress, job burnout and depression are among the fastest-growing disability categories in developed countries. Are our nervous systems designed to take this kind of beating?

The study of stress raises other questions:

- Why is the same event stressful for one person but not another?
- Is change always stressful?
- How do people typically cope with stress?
- How does stress affect psychological and physical health?

In this chapter, we show how the traditional view of stress as a purely biological phenomenon has given way to a biopsychosocial model. That is, stress is caused by a complex interaction of biological, psychological and sociocultural factors. The chapter then leads on to explore how stress and the ways in which people cope can impact on an individual's health, particularly the experience of anxiety disorders. People with these disorders have one thing in common: anxiety is so disabling that their functioning is adversely affected. The functional disabilities they have may affect all dimensions of life, including physical, emotional, cognitive, sociocultural and spiritual, as well as social, work and family relationships

Practice example

Joanne and Rebecca are highly-paid employees for a national bank. Rumours of pending redundancies had been circulating among the employees, creating an atmosphere of high anxiety for the two of them.

The bank has offered employees opportunities to undertake free training to upskill and gain further qualifications. Joanne has taken advantage of the training and qualified as a business analyst, meanwhile concentrating on personal debt reduction and savings.

Rebecca refused training opportunities, extended her mortgage to take the family on a cruise, took out a personal loan and purchased a new car, and increased the limit on her Visa card.

Rebecca and Joanne were advised last week that their employment was to be terminated, and were given a month's notice. Rebecca responded with anger and tears, and took days off work, blaming the bank for her current perilous financial situation. Joanne was very tearful and verbalised concerns over her future, but immediately updated her resumé and engaged an employment agency.

1. In your opinion, which employee proactively managed their anxiety?
2. Does everyone react in the same way to stress? And anxiety? How do you manage your own stress levels?
3. What strategies do you believe are more effective for handling stress and anxiety? In what way?

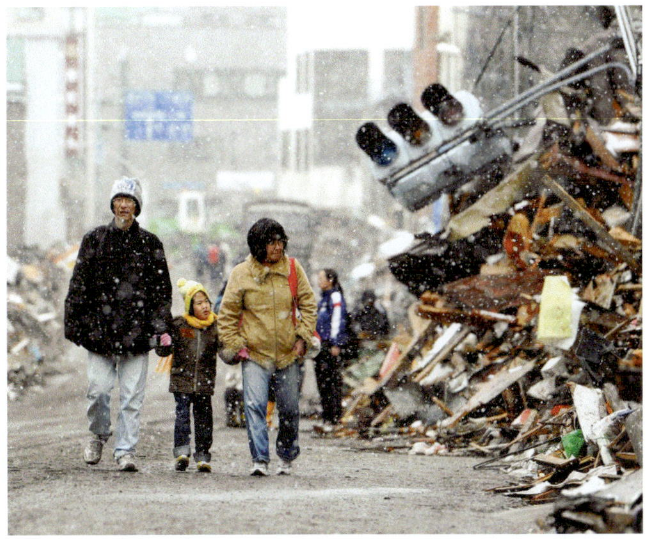

FIGURE 8.1 ■ A family is shocked at the devastation caused by the powerful earthquake in their hometown in Fukushima Prefecture, Japan, on 11 March 2011. The stressed and anxious family has an additional worry—the state of emergency at the nearby Fukushima nuclear power plant, which was damaged by the earthquake and its strong aftershocks.
Photo courtesy of Photoshot Holdings.

STRESS

Stress is part of being alive. Standing erect stresses the muscles and bones, which must work together to keep the body erect; eating stresses the digestive system, which must produce enzymes and absorb nutrients; and breathing stresses the respiratory system, which must exchange carbon dioxide and oxygen. Facing a demanding situation is stressful. While the word 'stress' is recognisable to the majority of people, the word can be used differently for individuals depending on their description. For example, a person may use the word stress to describe a stimulus, whereas another person may use it to describe their response. For the purpose of this chapter, we define 'stress' more broadly and holistically as an interaction. Stress is what happens when threats, such as demanding situations or daily challenges, are greater than our coping abilities or resources, and upset our balance. The threats may be to physical safety, long-range security, self-esteem, reputation, peace of mind or other things that one values.

This broader definition fits more closely with the humanistic perspective of this textbook. In this view, stress is a person–environment interaction. That is, our interpretation or perception of what is happening to us. The source of the stress, the demanding situation, is known as a **stressor**. Most people recognise this as producing an internal state of tension, anxiety or strain. This has been called 'distress', or negative stress. See Figure 8.1 ■ for an example of stress as a person–environment situation. In contrast to this, psychologists Lazarus and Folkman (1984) have identified that stressors can also be positive, in that they motivate you, focus energy and provide excitement. This is identified as 'eustress' (Barkway, 2103). Examples of this positive reaction to stress include starting a new job, planning a wedding or winning the lottery. Whether we feel distress or eustress in a situation is determined by how we perceive the situation in the first instance.

Among stress theorists and researchers, there is no one universally accepted definition of 'stress'. However, an interactional view of stress, such as the one given earlier, is consistent with how nurses view human experiences. The theories of stress that follow in this chapter are those in common use. Although they do tell us a great deal about responses to stressful situations, these explanations are not necessarily consistent with nursing's orientation. The causes, the situational context in which the stressful event occurs, and the psychological interpretation of the demanding situation must be considered in a holistic, humanistic approach to the person in your care. These and other important factors related to stress are illustrated in Figure 8.2 ■. The DSM-5 (American Psychiatric Association [APA], 2013) offers some general parameters for assessing the severity of stress. The DSM-5 is discussed in Chapter 10.

Conflict as a stressor

The concept of conflict is useful in helping to identify the stresses that may cause ineffective coping patterns. Conflict can be interpersonal, involving other people, or intrapersonal, occurring within an individual's own mind. It can often explain avoidant behaviours, such as hesitation, indecision, delaying and fatigue.

Conflict—having opposing desires, feelings or goals—is frequently seen in the behaviour of anxious people, who may have difficulty making even the simplest decisions.

The following conflicts are the most likely to cause stress:

- conflicts that involve social relations with significant people
- conflicts that involve ethical standards
- conflicts that involve meeting unconscious needs
- conflicts that involve the problems of everyday family living.

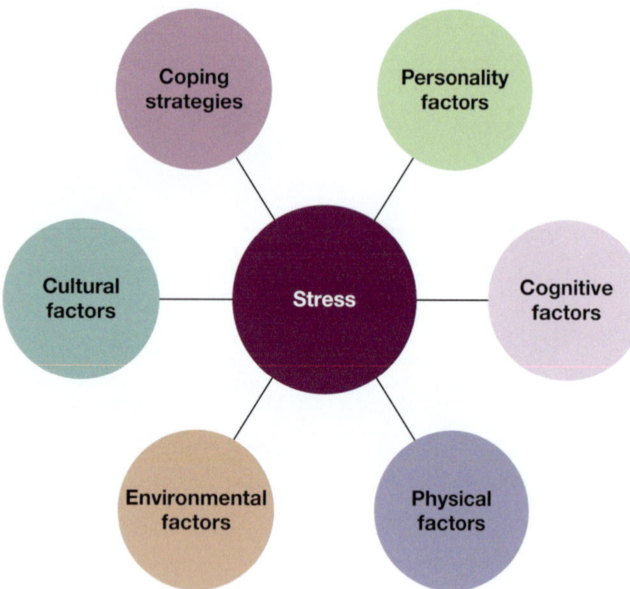

FIGURE 8.2 ■ Factors involved in stress. Several important factors are involved in understanding stress. They include personality factors (such as how we handle anger), cognitive factors (such as whether we perceive an event as a challenge or threat), physical factors (such as how the body responds to stress), environmental factors (such as fog, fire, drought or snow), cultural factors (such as our learned beliefs about religion, health and family), and coping strategies (such as what we do to manage stress).

A conflict proceeds according to the following four steps:

1. The person holds two goals simultaneously.
2. The person moves in relation to both of the goals, using approach–avoidance, avoidance–avoidance or approach–approach movements.
3. The person shows hesitation, indecision, blocking or fatigue.
4. Resolution occurs either temporarily or permanently.

Approach–avoidance conflict

When a person is faced with a single goal that has both attractive and unattractive aspects, the person is in an 'either/or' situation. If the person chooses one goal, the other goal is rejected or abolished automatically. The following is an example.

Practice example

Mrs Reynolds wants to talk her nurse about her fears of going back to work. At the same time, she wants not to be perceived as weak or 'a bother'. Mrs Reynolds makes a movement in relation to her goal—talking to the nurse—by walking up to her. When the nurse stops and turns towards her, Mrs Reynolds asks some superficial question about the time of their next meeting. In this way, she avoids discussing her real concerns. When the nurse offers an opening to talk further, Mrs Reynolds avoids the conversation she needs by saying she wants to rest. An hour later, she approaches the nurse with an apologetic but vague question about her medication.

Vacillation appropriately describes Mrs Reynolds's behaviour. Vacillation is the inability to choose between different actions or towards a desirable goal. Mrs Reynolds demonstrates this when first she talks to the nurse, then moves another way to avoid what is undesirable; that is, being perceived as weak or as a bother.

Avoidance–avoidance conflict

In avoidance–avoidance conflict, a person is faced with two undesirable or unattractive goals at the same time. This is the sort of situation we find ourselves in when we say we are 'between a rock and a hard place'. The person attempts to avoid the nearer of these two goals, but with the retreat from the nearer goal, the tendency to avoid the second goal increases. Unless the tendency to avoid one of the goals overpowers the tendency to avoid the other goal, resolving the conflict is rarely resolved, and can be a source of anxiety or other common responses, such as indecisiveness and complete inaction. Obviously, avoidance–avoidance conflicts are most unpleasant and highly stressful, posing most risk to the development of physical and psychological problems, such as depression and alcohol dependence (Wong & Moulds, 2011).

Practice example

Robert and Terry have been best friends since high school. Recently, Robert and Terry's wife, Cath, started working together in a local manufacturing company. Robert is finding himself increasingly attracted to Cath, and believes he may be falling in love. He wants to pursue the relationship, but simultaneously wants to remain best friends with Terry. By pursuing his relationship with Cath, he knows he would lose the friendship of Terry, but remaining in the workplace and seeing Cath on a daily basis would be too emotionally taxing. Both decisions are equally unattractive; therefore, it is easier for Terry to avoid both by leaving his current job, despite enjoying his work.

Approach–approach conflict

In an approach–approach conflict, a person must make a choice between two desirable goals, as described in the next Practice Example. The old saying 'six on the one hand, half a dozen on the other' describes this conflict nicely.

Practice example

Niesha is shopping at the mall for a dress to wear to the school formal. She has narrowed her choices down to two dresses that she really likes—an indigo blue chiffon dress with a bouffant skirt and spaghetti string straps, and a slinky red dress with one shoulder strap. She cannot afford both, and must decide which one to buy.

Among the three types of conflict, approach–approach conflict tends to be the least stressful. Deciding which of two equally beautiful dresses to buy is not usually exhausting. However, approach–approach conflicts may sometimes be troublesome, especially if the alternative not chosen represents a loss of sorts. For example, stress may be increased when having to deciding between two future career opportunities.

BIOPSYCHOSOCIAL THEORIES OF STRESS

Each of the theories discussed in this section contributes to our understanding of stress and coping. However, none is complete in and of itself. Psychoneuroimmunology, the final theory discussed in this section, offers a comprehensive framework for understanding the immune system and the nervous system, and the relationship between the two. It takes the best of what other theories offer, and integrates them with the increasing body of evidence on how stress can alter immunological functioning and, consequently, disease susceptibility and pathology.

The fight-or-flight response to stress

Beyond the routine and essential stress of everyday life, humans risk encountering undesirable or excess stress that threatens wellbeing and may even be life-threatening. They cope with such threats through either a fight (aggression) or a flight (withdrawal) response. The **fight-or-flight response** was first discussed by the physician Walter Cannon in 1932, when he identified stress as an actual cause of disease. The fight-or-flight response is mediated by the sympathetic division of the autonomic nervous system which controls blood vessels, muscles and glands.

Consider the following situation of extreme stress: a woman is walking down a dark, deserted street when a man with a knife emerges from the shadows just in front of her. Does she try to defend herself? Does she run away? Whichever action she takes is a result of a variety of physiological responses to extreme danger. The following signs of adrenaline rush are likely to happen when a person faces such a situation:

- the heart beats strong and fast to circulate the blood more quickly
- the airways in the lungs dilate, so that the extra blood becomes oxygenated
- glucose is released into the blood by the liver
- the blood vessels dilate to permit the oxygen-rich blood to get to where it is needed most
- the pupils of the eyes dilate, making vision more acute
- peristalsis in the gastrointestinal system is inhibited, so that the energy peristalsis would consume becomes available for other purposes
- norepinephrine-containing cells in the central nervous system are active
- the palms of their hands become sweaty; the mouth becomes dry.

Although these physiological responses seem appropriate, imagine the wear and tear on the body if humans responded to all stress in all of these ways each and every day.

Many specialists in the field of behavioural medicine believe the fight-or-flight response to be unhealthy. For example, some forms of hypertension are caused or made worse by the chronic activation of the heart, due to either an excessive amount of stress or an excessive response to stress.

Selye's stress–adaptation theory

Hans Selye, a Canadian endocrinologist and the most well-known and widely recognised stress researcher, developed a response-oriented framework for understanding the effects of stress on the human body (1956). He disputed the idea that only serious disease or injury causes stress. Instead, Selye believed that any emotion or activity requires a response or change in the individual. Stressors can be physical, chemical, physiological, developmental or emotional. Playing in a tennis competition, going out in the rain without an umbrella, having an argument, and getting a promotion are all examples of stressful events. Life itself is basically stressful, because it involves a process of adaptation to continual change. Although the experience of adaptation is stressful, it is not necessarily harmful. Indeed, it can be exciting and rewarding under certain circumstances; and, although we cannot avoid the stress of living, we can learn to minimise its damaging effects.

Selye observed that, regardless of the diagnosis, most physically ill people had certain symptoms in common; they lost their appetite, they lost weight, they felt and looked ill, they were anxious and fatigued, and they had aches and pains in their joints and muscles. A long series of experiments led to more objective evidence of actual body damage: enlargement of the adrenal glands; shrinkage of the thymus, spleen and lymph nodes; and the appearance of bleeding gastric ulcers. Feelings of anxiety, fatigue or illness are subjective aspects of stress.

Although stress itself cannot be perceived, Selye found that it can be objectively measured by the structural and chemical changes that it produces in the body. These changes are called the **general adaptation syndrome (GAS)**, because when stress affects the whole person, the whole person must adjust to the changes. The GAS occurs in three stages: alarm, resistance and exhaustion. The three stages of the GAS are illustrated and summarised in Figure 8.3 ■.

Selye's theory has stimulated extensive research on the neuroendocrine mechanisms underlying stress. However, the consequent research into psychoendocrinology brought Selye's model into question, since it focuses only on the physiological process and omits to consider how a person cognitively appraises a situation. Now classical research has demonstrated that neuroendocrine response differs for different stressors, and that there is individual variance in the sensitivity to psychosocial stimuli (Lazarus & Folkman, 1984). In addition, a response based model of stress such as Selye's is not consistent with our view that each individual is unique and people respond differently to similar situations. For instance, Selye's model makes reference only to the responses an individual makes to actual stress, whereas we now know that when a person anticipates a stressor the response can be just as stressful (Barkway, 2013; Taylor, 2015). For instance, a person with agoraphobia can be immobilised for long periods of time in their place of safety, usually their own home, because of their anticipated fear of experiencing a panic attack or severe anxiety.

Life changes as stressful events

Most people are accustomed to thinking of untoward events as stressful, but they do not realise that desirable events, such as job promotions, vacations, parenthood or outstanding personal

Alarm stage
Sympathetic nervous system is activated by adrenal glands

Resistance stage
Inability to produce glucocorticoids Failure of electrolyte balance

Exhaustion stage
Cumulative structural or functional damage to vital organs

Forehead, neck, shoulder, arm, and leg muscles contract
Pupils enlarge
Breathing is frequent and shallow
Blood pressure remains high
Liver runs out of sugar
Sugar is released into the bloodstream for energy
Accelerated heart rate increases blood flow to muscles; blood pressure increases
Hormones from adrenal glands are released into bloodstream
Prolonged muscle tension causes fatigue

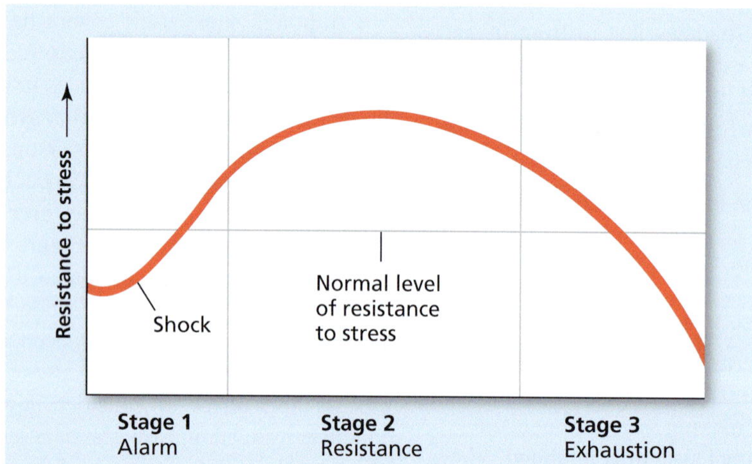

FIGURE 8.3 ■ Selye's general adaptation syndrome. The diagram at the top shows some of the physical reactions to stress in each stage. The diagram at the bottom shows the relationships of the stages to the individual's ability to resist a stressor. In the alarm stage, resistance drops at first as the sympathetic nervous system quickly activates. But resistance then rapidly increases as the body mobilises its defence systems. In the resistance stage, the body is working at a much increased level of resistance, using resources until the stress ends or the resources run out. In the exhaustion stage, the body is no longer able to resist, because resources have been depleted. At this point, disease and even death are possible. The third stage of exhaustion may be reversible if the total body is not affected and if the person can eventually eliminate the source of stress.
Source: Adapted from Ciccarelli, S. K., & White, J. N. (2009). *Psychology* (2nd ed.) Upper Saddle River, NJ: Prentice Hall, p. 445.

achievements, may also prove stressful. Holmes and Rahe (1967) studied life changes—noticeable alterations in one's living circumstances that require readjustment—as stressful events, and devised the Social Readjustment Rating Scale (SRRS) as a way to measure the amount of stress in a person's life. Unlike the models of 'psychological stress' that had been developed at a similar time by theorists such as Lazarus (1966), and which attempted to explain how different individuals react differently to a stressful situation, Holmes and Rahe (1967) placed no emphasis on the person's psychological meaning, emotion or perceived salience connected to the event. The SRRS was solely designed to measure objective changes in the pattern of events.

Similar to Seyle's earlier notion that the more people experience life changes, the more predisposed they become to illness, the authors Holmes and Rahe also believed that frequent life events require us to utilise coping behaviour, and thus decrease a person's ability to handle subsequent stress and make the person more susceptible to illness. Although there has been a long-held belief of the relationship between stress and many illnesses, such as cardiovascular disease, obesity, autoimmune diseases, diabetes and depression, it is only recently that research is beginning to find physical evidence to support the link between the two (Cohen et al., 2012; Heidt et al., 2014).

Holmes and Rahe's research assigned ratings to 43 different life changes, called *life change units (LCUs)*. They asked subjects to indicate what life changes had occurred in the past year, and then to add up the points assigned to each one (some life changes have higher ratings than others). According to these researchers, a low score indicated that the subject was not likely to have an adverse reaction. A 'mild' score meant that there was a 30 per cent chance that the person would manifest the impact of stress through physical symptoms. People in the 'moderate' category had a 50 per cent chance of a change in health status, and a 'high' score meant an 80 per cent chance of major illness in the next two years. High LCU scores also correlated with an increased probability of accidental injury. The following Practice Example demonstrates the LCU model.

Practice example

Marcia Montes, a 22-year-old woman, had recently been divorced from her husband (LCU 73) after attempting to achieve a marital reconciliation (LCU 45). Marcia's pregnancy (LCU 40) earlier in the year was uneventful, and the couple's healthy son was born on 2 June (LCU 39). At six weeks of age, the child suddenly and unexpectedly died in his crib (LCU 63). The couple began to argue frequently (LCU 35) before they made the decision to divorce. After the divorce, Marcia found herself short of funds (LCU 38) and went to work as a waitress in a pizza restaurant (LCU 36). She found it necessary to move to a less-expensive apartment (LCU 20). In the period of one year, Marcia accumulated an LCU score of 389 and was in the high-risk group.

Critics of the life event theory suggest factors such as personality, socioeconomic status and social support should be considered when looking at the health impact for individuals (Paykel, 1978). More recent research in this field has adopted these recommendations, and as a result is closing the gap between the psychological approaches and the theoretical bases of life events in the study of stress (Moloney, Weston, Qu & Hayes, 2012). Despite this, the SRRS has been modified over the years and remains widely cited in research exploring stress. For instance, in Australia, a modified version of the list of items was used in the Household, Income and Labour Dynamics (HILDA) report, which examines a wide range of aspects in the lives of Australian residents (Wilkins, Warren, Hahn & Houng, 2011).

Application to clinical practice

This model is based on several assumptions that depict a person as a passive recipient of stress caused by life changes. At present, there is little reason to believe that change in itself is inherently or inevitably stressful. To understand the effects of life changes on health, you need to identify what each individual perceives as stressful. Only then can you help people become aware of the stress they face in their lives and plan for the future. In the Practice Example that follows, we return to the example of Marcia Montes, who had accumulated an LCU score of 389.

Practice example

During the course of therapy, Marcia shared her desire to return to university and complete the midwifery program in which she had been enrolled before her marriage. To do so, she would have to make a number of changes: move to an apartment close to the university, because she could not afford to own a car, change her working hours or job so that she could attend classes, change her sleeping habits, change her recreational and social activities, and reduce her other expenses to pay higher-education costs. The changes required would add almost 200 LCUs to her score.

In therapy, Marcia was able to consider this information and re-evaluate her goals. She decided to delay her return to higher education until she could get on her feet financially. She chose not to make any other changes in her life for the present time.

Consumers can identify the life change events in their lives, much as Marcia did, to help decide when it might be advantageous or disadvantageous to engage in a life change. This knowledge helps them make conscientious decisions about the directions their lives will take. Collaborative Care: Teaching About Life Changes includes some strategies based on the interrelationship between life changes and stressful events.

COLLABORATIVE CARE

Teaching about life changes

You can assist people by incorporating the following guidelines:

- help recognise when a life change occurs
- encourage them to think about the meaning of the change, and identify some of the feelings associated with the change
- discuss the different ways they might best adjust to the event
- encourage them to take their time in arriving at decisions
- if possible, anticipate life changes and plan for them well in advance
- encourage them to pace themselves—it can be done, even if they are in a hurry
- encourage the person to consider the accomplishment of a task as a part of daily living, and to avoid looking at such an achievement as a stopping point or a time for slowing down.

Stress as a transaction

Richard Lazarus, a pioneering theorist and researcher in stress, coping and health, is known for his transaction-based approach to understanding stress. He believed that measuring major life events misses the point. Instead, the constant minor irritants or hassles that go on in a person's life, day in and day out, are more important than large or landmark changes. His view is reflected in the definition of stress given at the beginning of this chapter, and his transactional model—stress is a process of complex interplay among the perceived demands of the environment and the perceived resources one has for meeting these demands (Lazarus & Folkman, 1984)—is consistent with nursing's holistic approach.

In the Lazarus model, perceived threat—what the person appraises as taxing or exceeding their resources and endangering their wellbeing—is the central characteristic of stressful situations, because it threatens a person's most important goals and values (Monat & Lazarus, 1991). Once a person has perceived a threat, the person evaluates it by thinking about it. This process is termed *cognitive appraisal.* According to Lazarus, the process works like this:

1. The person assesses the potential for benefit, harm, loss, threat or challenge in a situation. This is called *primary appraisal.*
2. The person who has identified a threat or a harmful effect then evaluates their coping resources and options in the situation. This is called *secondary appraisal.*
3. The person applies the coping resources and options at their disposal. This is called *coping.*
4. The person engages in ongoing reinterpretation of the situation based on new information. This is called *reappraisal.*

Lazarus believes that stress depends not only on external conditions, but also on the person's physical vulnerability and the adequacy of that person's coping styles.

Cognitive appraisal and coping style are influenced by the person's culture. Providing culturally competent care requires understanding the client's perspective and recognising that a client's cognitive appraisal of a situation may, and probably will, differ from your own.

Psychoneuroimmunology framework

The most comprehensive framework for understanding the relationship between stress and disease and the biopsychosocial nature and complexity of the stress process is the **psychoneuroimmunology (PNI)** framework. In simple terms, psychoneuroimmunology studies the relationship between the immune system and the nervous system. It is concerned with interaction among the neurological, endocrine and immune systems, and takes into account the nature of the influence of psychosocial factors on immune function and health outcomes. In other words, the PNI framework integrates the person–environment transactions of the stress process with the psychological and pathophysiological processes involved in stress. An important key area that has surfaced in some of the recent research on stress and prodromal psychosis (Holtzman, Shapiro, Trotman & Walker, 2012; Pruessner, Iver, Faridi & Malla, 2011) is the importance of improving resilience. Resilience is defined and discussed in Chapter 1.

What is emerging is a complex picture of the body's response to stress that involves several related pathways. Over the past few decades, corticotropin-releasing factor (CRF) signalling pathways have been shown to be the main coordinators of the endocrine, behavioural and immune responses to stress (Stengal & Taché, 2010). Cortisol—as well as adrenaline (recall the signs of adrenaline rush described earlier on page 145 that helps us to either take flight or to fight in the presence of immediate danger)—is a stress hormone. Cortisol, however, is produced more slowly, and lingers longer in the bloodstream. Because it is primarily immunosuppressive, cortisol contributes to reductions in lymphocyte numbers, function and NK-cell activity (natural killer lymphocytes that attack infected cells and tumour cells in the body). Neuropeptides, the chemical messengers that are the links between the mind and the body, are produced in the brain and in the endocrine and immune systems. In summary, the interrelationship between these pathways—i.e. the immunity, endocrine functions, thoughts and emotions—can have a huge influence on health and behaviour as they send messages to each other (Barkway, 2013).

In addition to the physiological research, 40 decades of sociological research tell us that stressors have measurable damaging impacts on physical and mental health (Thoits, 2010). Caring for the mind and spirit is an example of the multi-faceted nature of the psychoneuroimmunology framework.

Self-healing personalities

Neuropeptide manufacture is activated by positive mental states, and suppressed by negative mental states. Several stress and coping-related studies have suggested that some people have *self-healing personalities*, while others have *disease-prone personalities*. Self-healers are emotionally stable people who bounce back from stressful situations. These are people whom others describe as enthusiastic, joyful, secure, energetic, alert and content. They are likable and have close, warm relationships with others. The nurse-theorist Jean Watson, whose nursing theory identifies the centrality of caring, also stresses people's self-healing potential (Friedman & Kern, 2014).

Hardiness, resilience and health

A now-classic study on hardiness and health found that individuals who have strong feelings of confidence in their ability to control circumstances, a willingness to see life events as challenges rather than as obstacles, and a strong commitment to the experiences and demands of daily living, have fewer illnesses than those who lack these qualities (Kobasa, 1979). Although the term was originally coined by Abraham Maslow, Martin Seligman (2011) stands today as the father of positive psychology. He has spent 30 years researching failure, helplessness, optimism and resilience, with a recent development of the PERMA model of Flourishing (Seligman, 2011). This model has been taken up internationally by various organisations, ranging from education to business management, with the focus on developing 'wellbeing' in people across various settings. See the following Practice Example.

Practice example

Some studies have recently been examining the relationship between personality and health (Vedhara et al., 2015). A person is often described by their personality traits, such as being referred to as an extrovert, introvert, conscientious or neurotic. Despite the recent literature in the area, the question whether personality traits affect how our bodies respond to illness, or whether it's the immune system that manipulates a person's behaviour, still remains largely unanswered. We do know, however, that wars wage within our bodies every minute of every day. We have evolved legions of specialised cells that silently battle to keep us healthy, but on some occasions, such as when we are tired or stressed, these bodily defences are penetrated, and we develop a cold, the flu or something worse. Why did I catch a cold from the sick toddler on the airplane when the woman next to me did not? Why didn't you come down with the flu when your roommate was sick? Why do only some of the people exposed to HIV develop the disease? Why do some people with cancer die within a year or two while others have survived? We don't, as yet, have all the answers to these questions.

While we cannot promote the idea that people are in total control of the disease process and the state of their health, or that the mind or the spirit can cure disease, we can and should teach those in our care the self-care and self-nurturing behaviours that long-term survivors of illness such as HIV and cancer are using to maintain their health. Relaxation and mindfulness techniques have been proven to be worthwhile in alleviating stress and helping recovery from both mental and physical illness. For instance, living day-to-day, being mindful of everyday occurrences, such as making a cup of coffee or getting out of bed, can help us accept the present moment and remove the peripheral elements from our lives that may cause us stress and anxiety (Broadbent et al., 2012; Sundquist et al., 2014). By assessing a person's level of stress, quality of social support, and mood factors that influence their quality of life, nursing interventions can help people enhance neurological, immunological and cognitive functioning by focusing on improved nutrition, adequate sleep–wake patterns, hygiene, stress reduction, and social and spiritual support.

ANXIETY

Although **anxiety** is a universal experience, people vary in their ability to tolerate anxiety and anxiety-producing situations. Anxiety, a subjective feeling experienced in response to stressors, is a normal response that usually helps people cope with threatening situations. There are four levels of anxiety: mild, moderate, severe and panic. Mild anxiety serves as a catalyst for change, and is an ideal time for learning to occur. In the moderate level of anxiety, the perceptual field is narrowed, and the individual is able to attend to selected stimuli. People experiencing severe and/or panic levels of anxiety have varying levels of functional impairments. It is essential that a person experiencing extreme anxiety be closely monitored for safety reasons (see Figure 8.4 ■). Common coping behaviours of individuals experiencing anxiety include withdrawal, acting out, avoidance, somatisation and problem-solving.

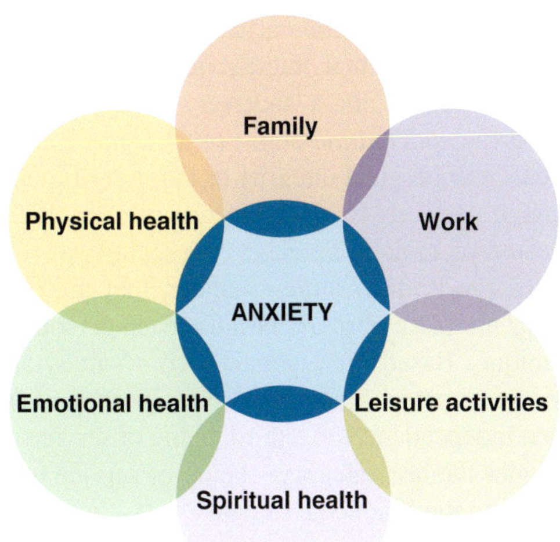

FIGURE 8.4 ■ The holistic impact of anxiety.

Current and accurate estimates of the prevalence for anxiety in Australia and New Zealand varies, although all agree that anxiety disorders remain one of most prevalent mental conditions in today's society. According to the Slade et al. (2009), 14.4 per cent of the adult population will experience an anxiety-related problem at some point in their life, with post-traumatic stress disorder being the most common disorder for both men and women. It is also one of the most treatable mental health problems in Australasia. You will encounter people with anxiety disorders in every clinical practice setting, including primary care and general hospital settings, not just mental health facilities. Anxiety disorders affect people of every socioeconomic status. It is also relatively common for a person to have one anxiety disorder co-exist with another, such as depression. You can readily apply what you learn about anxiety disorders in this chapter to any area in which you choose to work.

Sources of anxiety

Anxiety is an inevitable result of the attempt to maintain equilibrium in a changing world. People experience anxiety in many different situations and interpersonal relationships. However, the general causes of anxiety have been classified into two major kinds of threats, discussed in Box 8.1. It is

Box 8.1 General causes of anxiety

1. Threats to biological integrity: actual or impending interference with basic human needs such as the needs for food, drink or warmth.
2. Threats to the security of self and self-identity:
   a. unmet expectations important to self-integrity
   b. unmet needs for status and prestige
   c. anticipated disapproval by significant others
   d. inability to gain or reinforce self-respect or gain recognition from others
   e. guilt, or discrepancies between self-view and actual behaviour.

crucial to understand that *either* actual *or* impending interference may cause anxiety; actual interference with a biological or psychosocial need is not a necessary condition. All that is necessary is the *anticipation* of one of these major threats.

Threats to biological integrity or to the fulfilment of such basic human needs as food, drink, warmth and shelter are a general cause of anxiety. Threats to the security of self are not as easily categorised. In some instances, they are obvious; in others, they are more obscure, because each person's sense of self is unique. Based on a person's core values and belief systems, to one person, power and prestige may be essential; to another, independence; to a third, being of service to others.

Consider the last category—being of service to others—as displayed in the Practice Example.

Practice example

Mrs C, a nurse, is convinced that a person in her care would feel much better if he expressed his fears to her. But no matter how often she provides the opportunity, he insists, 'This is not the time to talk about it,' and thwarts her attempt. She is not able to help him in a way that is important to her sense of self. In addition, she believes that the unit's nurse manager (whose skills she admires) expects her to have been successful in this endeavour.

Mrs C is worried and anxious. When unmet needs or expectations related to essential values (such as being of service to the person in her care) are coupled with the actual or anticipated disapproval of others who are important (the nurse manager), anxiety is generated.

Anxiety as a continuum

Many theorists conceptualise anxiety as a continuum (Figure 8.5 ■). Mild to moderate anxiety can be functionally effective, in that it helps us focus our attention and generates energy and motivation. Thus, anxiety is an aspect of problem-solving, in that it alerts us to the need to concentrate our resources. However, severe anxiety and panic narrow our attention to a crippling degree. Under these conditions, alertness is greatly reduced and learning does not usually take place.

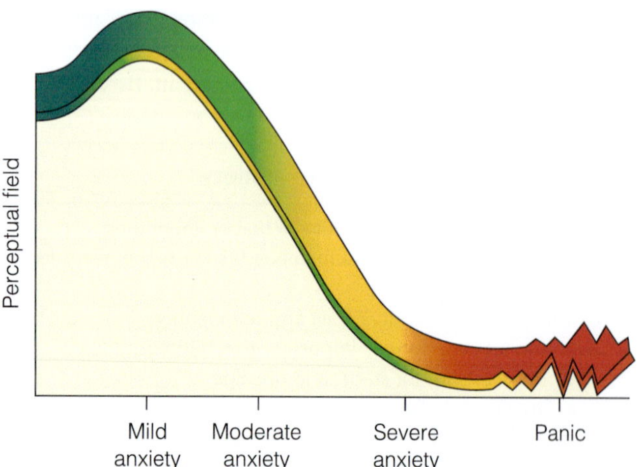

FIGURE 8.5 ■ The effect of anxiety on the perceptual field. Notice that the perceptual field is increased in mild anxiety, becomes increasingly constricted as anxiety increases, and is completely disrupted at the panic level.

Mild anxiety

Mild anxiety helps one deal constructively with stress. A mildly anxious person has a broad perceptual field, because mild anxiety heightens the ability to take in sensory stimuli. Such a person is more alert to what is going on, and can make better sense of what is happening with others and the environment. The senses take in more; the person hears better, sees better and makes logical connections between events. The person feels relatively safe and comfortable. Because learning is easier when one is mildly anxious, mild anxiety helps people learn, for instance, how best to administer their own insulin. Mild anxiety can also help a nursing student review psychiatric–mental health nursing before a final examination.

Moderate anxiety

In moderate anxiety, a person remains alert, but the perceptual field narrows. The moderately anxious person shuts out the events on the periphery while focusing on central concerns.

Practice example

A nursing student who is moderately anxious about the final examination may be able to focus so intently on studying that they are not distracted by an argument between roommates, loud music on the stereo and a rousing chase scene on the television. The student shuts out the chaos in the environment and focuses on what is of central personal importance—preparing for the exam.

This process of taking in some sensory stimuli while excluding others is called **selective inattention**.

People also use selective inattention to cope with anxiety-provoking stimuli. This phenomenon may account for the anxious preoperative person who fails to remember what the nurse said about postoperative pain, or about the need to cough and breathe deeply after surgery.

Although the perceptual field is narrowed and the person sees, hears and grasps less, there is an element of voluntary control. Moderately anxious individuals can, with direction, focus on what they have previously shut out.

Severe anxiety

In severe anxiety, sensory reception is greatly reduced. Severely anxious people focus on small or scattered details of an experience. They have difficulty in problem-solving, and their ability to organise is also reduced. They seldom have the complete picture. Selective inattention may be increased and may be less amenable to voluntary control. The person may be unable to focus on events in the environment. The person may experience new stimuli as overwhelming, which may cause the anxiety level to rise even higher.

The sympathetic nervous system is activated in severe anxiety, causing an increase in pulse, blood pressure and respiration, as well as in epinephrine secretion, vasoconstriction and even body temperature. A multitude of physiological changes may be observed, which are described in the following sections.

Panic

The panic level of anxiety is characterised by a completely disrupted perceptual field. Panic has been described as a disintegration of the personality experienced as intense terror. Details may be enlarged, scattered or distorted. Logical thinking and effective decision-making may be impossible. The person in panic is unable to initiate or maintain goal-directed action. Behaviour may appear purposeless, and communication may be unintelligible.

Assessing anxiety

Anxiety can be assessed in the physiological, cognitive, emotional and behavioural dimensions, since it is a multi-dimensional phenomenon involving every aspect of the person. Selective inattention can interfere with the person's awareness of anxiety and ability to provide accurate information; therefore, nursing observations and families' and carers' contributions may be critical to provide an accurate assessment.

Physiological dimension

Observations of a person's physiological state are likely to indicate autonomic nervous system responses, particularly sympathetic effects. Sympathetic nervous system dominance is associated with arousal as occurs during anxiety or as the body's response to a physical emergency. The parasympathetic nervous system maintains normal, smooth functioning. Various organs may be affected, such as the adrenal medulla, heart, blood vessels, lungs, stomach, colon, rectum, salivary glands, liver, pupils of the eyes, and sweat glands. Figure 8.6 ■ illustrates the sympathetic and parasympathetic nervous systems in detail.

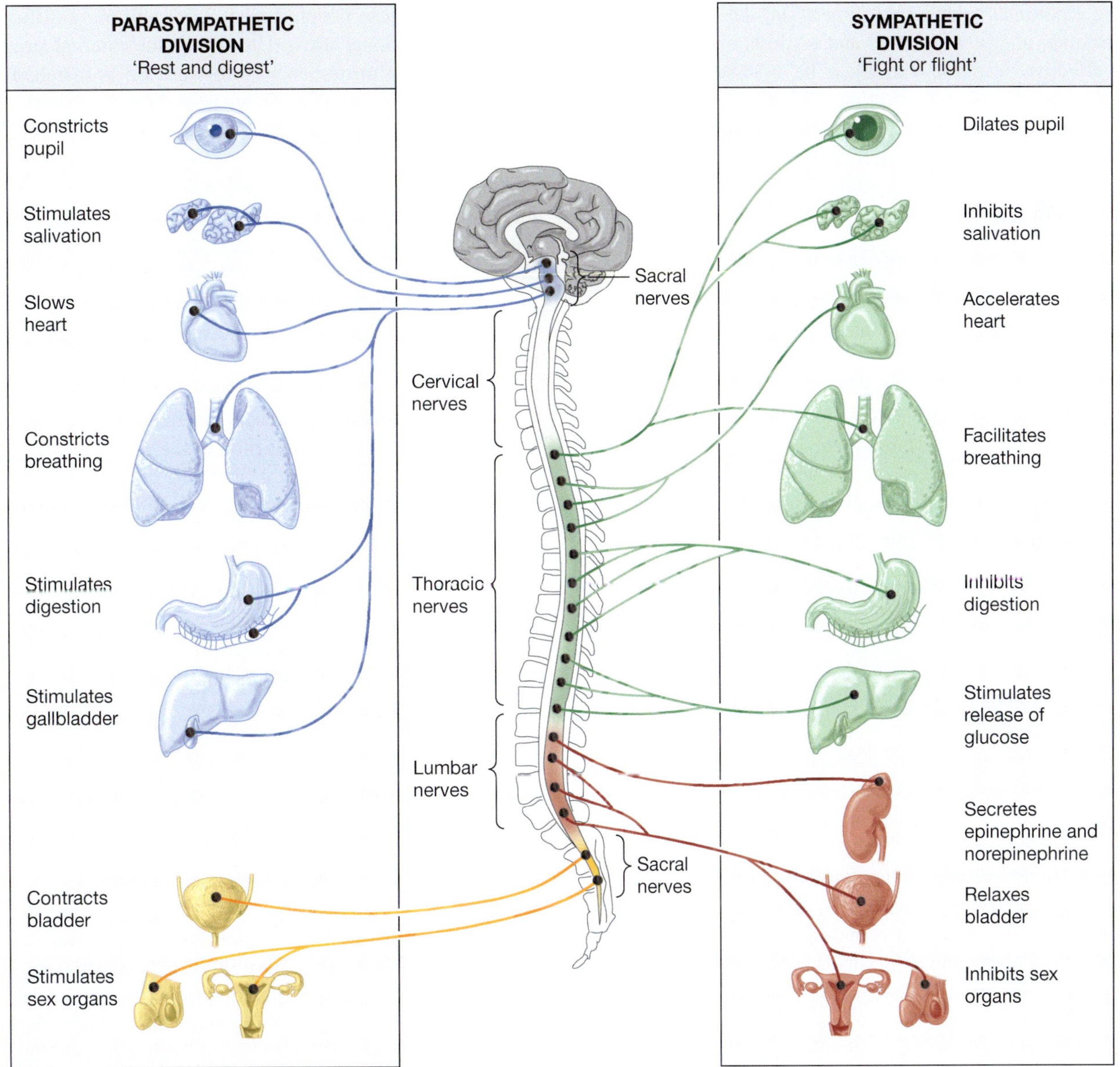

FIGURE 8.6 ■ Involuntary control of bodily functions. The autonomic nervous system has two divisions, the sympathetic and the parasympathetic, which exercise automatic control over the body's organs, generally in opposing ways. The parasympathetic generally has inhibitory or relaxing effects, while the sympathetic has stimulatory effects. Axons of the parasympathetic division emerge not only from the spinal cord, but from the brain as well.
Source: Krogh, D. (2000). *Biology: A guide to the natural world.* Upper Saddle River, NJ: Prentice Hall, p. 515.

An anxious person may have an increased heart rate, increased blood pressure, difficulty breathing, sweaty palms, trembling, dry mouth, 'butterflies in the stomach' or a 'lump in the throat', as well as other symptoms.

Cognitive dimension

Assessment of cognitive function may indicate difficulty in logical thinking, narrowed or distorted perceptual field, selective inattention or **dissociation**, lack of attention to details, difficulty concentrating, or difficulty focusing. The level of anxiety determines the extent to which cognitive function is affected. Mild, moderate, severe or panic-level anxiety is assessed according to the descriptions earlier in this chapter.

Emotional/behavioural dimension

In the emotional/behavioural dimension, the consumer may be irritable, angry, withdrawn and restless, or they may cry. The affective response can often be assessed through the client's subjective description. People may describe themselves as 'on edge', 'uptight', 'jittery', 'nervous', 'worried' or 'tense'. They may feel dizzy or faint, and may experience a feeling of impending doom as if something terrible were about to happen.

COPING WITH STRESS AND ANXIETY

Reactions to threatening situations can be divided into two general categories: task-oriented responses and defence-oriented responses.

When we feel competent to deal with stress and the situation is not too threatening to our sense of self, our behaviour tends to be *task-oriented*. Task-oriented behaviour is geared towards problem-solving, whereas *defence-oriented* behaviour is used as a protective measure when we feel inadequate to cope with stress and the situation is extremely threatening to our sense of self. Such behaviour becomes harmful only when it is the predominant means of coping with stress. In such cases, problem-solving and reality-based behaviours are continually avoided.

Everyday ways of coping with stress

Coping strategies are a set of behaviours people under stress use in struggling to improve their situation. Everyday coping strategies offer an immense repertoire of defences to maintain control and balance in the face of stress. A person can cope on different levels, including physical, social, cognitive and emotional levels. However, the devices people choose to cope with stress depend on many factors. Among them are the external circumstances, the suddenness and intensity of the stress, the resources available to the person, and the person's predisposition to certain coping patterns, established over the course of one's development. One man who is late for an appointment because he gets caught in a traffic jam may react with a furious outburst of anger. Another may begin to daydream and forget where he is going. A third may use the time to solve the problem.

Most often, individuals use behaviours that have worked well for them in the past. Sometimes they behave in a certain way because it is the only method they have of coping with stress, or because other coping strategies have failed to work. Some people learn to turn to others for protection and nurturance; some learn to turn to drugs and alcohol or food; some rely on self-discipline and keeping a stiff upper lip; others feel better after expressing their feelings through venting; some withdraw physically and/or emotionally; still others exercise or talk the problem out.

Defence-oriented ways of coping: defence mechanisms

The above coping strategies are considered normal. They are simply ways of getting along. In some people, however, what passes for a normal adjustment is actually a very tenuous one, with few outlets for controlled aggression, little chance for loving relationships, and few opportunities for satisfaction and growth. These people find it more and more difficult to cope with additional stress. Ultimately, the external stress the person is trying unsuccessfully to ward off is matched by a mounting internal stress. The person suffers both from increased anxiety and from the strain on overworked stabilisers.

When a person is unable to ward off stress or reduce tension in the usual way, anxiety mounts as the person feels increasingly inadequate to cope with the situation. Under these circumstances, the person is more likely to engage in *defence-oriented behaviour*. Defence-oriented behaviour is not a specific attempt to solve a problem; it consists of using mental mechanisms to lessen the uncomfortable feelings of anxiety and to prevent pain, regardless of cost. These characteristic mental mechanisms are commonly called **defence mechanisms**. Defence mechanisms are automatic psychological processes that protect the self by allowing the person to deny or distort a stressful event, or to restrict awareness and reduce the sense of emotional involvement. Defence mechanisms are mostly unconscious and often inflexible coping patterns that protect a person through intrapsychic (coming from within) distortions that are really self-deceptions. The person usually has little awareness of what is happening or even less control over events.

Although these reactions may help keep the lid on anxiety, they also limit the ability to grow from and savour the experience, they interfere with rational decision-making and the ability to work productively, they can easily become a substitute for addressing the underlying cause, and they impair and erode interpersonal relationships. Even adaptive devices can go wrong. Being unable to ward off stress is at the heart of the film discussed in Mental Health in the Media.

You will notice that some of the various defence mechanisms have similar associated behaviour, as the same observed behaviour may often be explained by more than one type of defence. In addition, people do not use one method of defence at a time; they usually rely on a combination of defences. The more common defence mechanisms include: **repression, regression, suppression**, dissociation, **identification, introjection, projection**, denial, fantasy, **rationalisation**, reaction formation, displacement, undoing and intellectualisation. They are summarised in Table 8.1 ■.

EVIDENCE-BASED PRACTICE

Psychoeducation for managing stress

As the nurse in a psychiatric day unit for older people, you are especially aware of the difficulty some of the consumers have in handling stress. Most of the people attending are diagnosed with a psychotic disorder or post-traumatic stress disorder and have difficulty maintaining relationships with friends and family, and finding or keeping a job. Thus, most have become marginalised, and the day unit has become the core of their daily activities.

You understand that it is important to strengthen life control among those who have become marginalised. People who are in charge of their lives have a sense of coherence. They are more likely to be able to cope with stressful situations in ways that decrease, or even eliminate, their distress. To help your clients develop a sense of coherence and strengthen their resilience to stress, you develop a psychoeducation program for them, focusing on the following:

1. achieving understanding of the internal environment (what thoughts, feelings and wishes drive the individual)
2. achieving understanding of the external environment (what forces affect what an individual is able to accomplish)
3. exploring human relationships to include client–family, client–client, client–employer, client–staff and other active relationships or potential relationships in the individual's life
4. identifying personal strengths, resources and abilities
5. exploring the meaning of present events; that is, focusing on the here-and-now, rather than the there-and-then, to gain an understanding of what the stressors are in the lives of the individuals
6. partaking in a program of regular physical activity that includes flexibility training and walking in place.

The psychoeducation program you have developed is based on the following research citations:

Böttche, M., Kuwert, P., & Knaevelsrud, C. (2012). Posttraumatic stress disorder in older adults: An overview of characteristics and treatment approaches. *International Journal of Geriatric Psychiatry, 27*(3), 230–239.

Chan, D., Fan, M. Y., & Unutzer, J. (2011). Long-term effectiveness of collaborative depression care in older primary care patients with and without PTSD symptoms. *International Journal of Geriatric Psychiatry, 26*(7), 758–764.

CRITICAL THINKING QUESTIONS

1. What actual activities would help clients to understand their internal environment and explore human relationships?
2. What does it mean to explore the meaning of present events by focusing on the here-and-now?

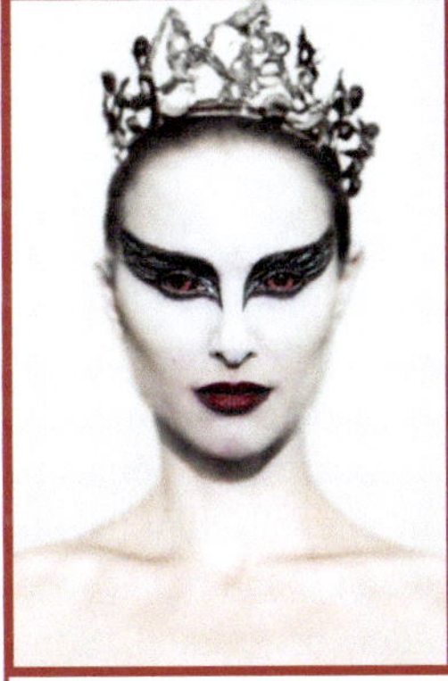

MENTAL HEALTH IN THE MEDIA

Black Swan

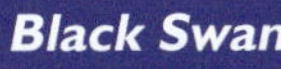

Desperately wanting the lead in a production of *Swan Lake*, Nina is a fragile ballerina in the stressful world of a prestigious New York dance company. Kept in a state of perpetual childhood by a hovering, unfulfilled and controlling mother, she has dedicated her life to the pursuit of her art, obsesses over being perfect and lacks the coping resources that help people deal with a stress-laden life. Her journey begins with tension and anxiety, and moves rapidly to purging, drugs and self-injury. Her all-consuming drive to become the best leads to growing paranoia and hallucinations, and she becomes increasingly unstable. Nina achieves her goal as the Black Swan, but dies on stage as the result of her self-injury. A very dark movie, *Black Swan* emphasises Nina's inability to cope that leads to an inevitable tragic ending.

TABLE 8.1 ■ Common defence mechanisms

Name	Definition	Example
Denial	Blocking out painful or anxiety-inducing events or feelings	A manager tells an employee he may have to fire him. On the way home, the employee shops for a new car.
Displacement	Discharging pent-up feelings on people less dangerous than those who initially aroused the emotion	A student who has received a low grade on a term paper blows up at his girlfriend when she asks about his grade.
Dissociation	Handling emotional conflicts, or internal or external stressors, by a temporary alteration of consciousness or identity	A woman has amnesia for the events surrounding a fatal automobile accident in which she was the speeding driver.
Fantasy	Symbolic satisfaction of wishes through non-rational thought	A student struggling through graduate school thinks about a prestigious, high-paying job she wants.

(continued)

TABLE 8.1 ■ *(continued)*

Name	Definition	Example
Identification	Unconscious assumption of similarity between oneself and another	After hospitalisation for minor surgery, a girl decides to become a nurse.
Intellectualisation	Separating an emotion from an idea or thought because the emotional reaction is too painful to be acknowledged	A man learns from his doctor that he has cancer. He studies the physiology and treatment of cancer without experiencing any emotion.
Introjection	Acceptance of another's values and opinions as one's own	A woman who prefers a simple lifestyle assumes the materialistic, prestige-oriented values of her husband.
Projection	Attributing one's own unacceptable feelings and thoughts to others	A man who is quite critical of others thinks that people are joking about his appearance.
Rationalisation	Falsification of experience through the construction of logical or socially approved explanations of behaviour	A man cheats on his income tax return and tells himself it's alright because everyone does it.
Reaction formation	Unacceptable feelings disguised by repression of the real feeling and by reinforcement of the opposite feeling	A woman who dislikes her mother-in-law is always very nice to her.
Regression	Reverting to an earlier stage of development	A man who is hospitalised may start bedwetting again.
Repression	Unconsciously keeping unacceptable feelings out of awareness	A man is jealous of a good friend's success, but is unaware of his feelings.
Suppression	Consciously keeping unacceptable feelings and thoughts out of awareness	A student taking an examination is upset about an argument with her boyfriend, but deliberately puts it out of her mind so she can finish the test.
Undoing	Attempting to take back an unconscious thought or behaviour that is unacceptable or hurtful	A young woman realises that she has just insulted her boyfriend, and spends the rest of the evening complimenting him on his looks and his athletic ability.

ANXIETY-RELATED DISORDERS

Anxiety disorders are characterised by a mixture of physiological, psychological, behavioural and cognitive symptoms. Anxiety disorders affect individuals across the entire lifespan. Baxter, Scott, Vos and Whiteford (2013) report that, globally, the prevalence of anxiety disorders ranges from 4.8–10.9 per cent, with European and Anglo cultures in some instances being reported at 15.5 per cent. The Australian Bureau of Statistics (ABS) (2008) reports that 2.3 million (14.4 per cent) of the population aged between 16 and 85 have had an anxiety disorder for 12 months or longer and, along with depression, alcohol abuse and personality disorders, anxiety disorders account for almost three-quarters of the total of non-fatal disease burden in Australia (National Mental Health Commission, 2012).

Even though each anxiety disorder has its own distinct characteristics, they all have the common theme of excessive, irrational fear and dread. It can be challenging for the nurse to differentiate between normal anxiety and an anxiety disorder; therefore, it is important to ensure that a full health assessment is undertaken, particularly when some of the symptoms mimic those of physical conditions, such as cardiac problems, diabetes and electrolyte imbalance.

In anxiety disorders, the source of anxiety can be either identifiable or unidentifiable. For instance, in generalised anxiety disorder the source is unknown, and the person may persistently worry over several areas in their lives, such as finances and health. This is known as '**free floating**'. For some people, the source of their anxiety is very clear and can be identified as a specific situation, object or idea which results in avoidance behaviour, as the person attempts to master the symptoms (as in confronting the dreaded object or situation in a phobic disorder).

People in anxiety states experience anxiety both as a subjective emotion and as a variety of physical symptoms resulting from muscular tension and autonomic nervous system activity. When acute, anxiety drives the individual to seek help. When chronic, anxiety can lead to a number of somatic discomforts or disabilities (e.g. heartburn, epigastric distress, diarrhoea and constipation). Chronic muscular tension can lead to a variety of musculoskeletal aches and pains.

The onset of anxiety may be sudden or gradual. Some people experience an unexpected, incapacitating outbreak of acute anxiety, as in panic disorder. In other people (especially those with generalised anxiety disorder), anxiety may express itself through relatively mild somatic symptoms in which the existence of underlying anxiety is overlooked. Therefore, it is necessary to specifically assess the client's level of anxiety. There are several types of anxiety disorders, and these will be discussed in the following section.

Panic disorder

A common disorder, **panic disorder**, is characterised by recurrent attacks of severe anxiety lasting a few moments to an hour. These attacks are not a response to a specific stimulus, but instead seem to occur suddenly and spontaneously. They may, however, become associated with certain situations, such as going to a shopping mall or driving a car.

LIVED EXPERIENCE

'The terror is just as real'

If you have ever witnessed a dog terrified by a thunderstorm or fireworks, the animal may be panting heavily, shaking, with eyes wide open and rolling, running wildly trying to find a way to escape, lose bladder or bowel control, be either barking or whimpering, and be unable to hear or respond to calming voices or a soothing touch, due to the pure terror of a situation they have no control over or understanding of—not dissimilar to a person experiencing a panic attack. Only a person is less likely to be treated with the same understanding as an animal, and instead is more likely to be questioned 'What is the matter with you?' or told to 'pull yourself together'. The terror is just as real, the physical symptoms not dissimilar to those of the dog, but the response from fellow humans is considerably different, less tolerant, less understanding and less empathetic.

The person usually experiences physical symptoms, such as palpitations, nausea, diarrhoea, dyspnea, rapid pulse, and a feeling of choking or suffocation. The pupils are dilated and the face is flushed. The person may feel dizzy or faint, and often has a sense of impending doom or death. Restlessness is acute, and the person may make pleading, apprehensive appeals for help.

In its most advanced state, panic may create a group of symptoms that mimic myocardial infarction and mitral valve prolapse. Thus, the diagnosis of **panic disorder** is often not made until a full medical assessment has been taken. The following Practice Example describes Jo-Ann, who is experiencing a panic disorder.

Practice example

Jo-Ann, a 35-year-old single parent of two small children and the owner of a beauty salon, went to the emergency department stating, 'I can't breathe! Help me! I feel like I'm smothering and going to die.' Jo-Ann has been treated for similar symptoms in this emergency department three times over the past year. You, the registered nurse, overhear another staff member say that JoAnn is a 'frequent flyer who is making up her symptoms. She just wants attention.'

1. Do you think this staff member's comments are valid? Why, or why not?
2. How do you respond to the staff member?
3. Why is it important that a complete physical assessment be done on Jo-Ann, even if health care providers believe her symptoms are of psychogenic origin?

When panic attacks occur frequently and interfere with the person's functional abilities at work, school or in the family, the condition is called *panic disorder*. People who have repeated attacks, or persistently worry about having another attack, are diagnosed with panic disorder. Anticipatory fear of helplessness or of losing control during a panic attack is a common occurrence. The individual frequently avoids situations that induce the fear, sometimes developing a phobic avoidance reaction. The next Practice Example shows the impact of panic attacks on the person's functional abilities.

Practice example

Jo-Ann's panic attacks persisted, gradually increasing in frequency and severity. She noticed that her symptoms seemed to begin every time she entered the local shopping mall. Jo-Ann began to avoid shopping, telling her family she was sick, and thus avoided all activities with friends whenever a social event may require shopping.

Panic disorder is usually first noted in late adolescence or early adulthood. It may be limited to a single brief period, lasting several weeks or months, recur several times or become chronic. Physical disorders such as hypoglycaemia, hyperthyroidism, and amphetamine or caffeine intoxication must be ruled out before a diagnosis of panic disorder can be made.

Phobic disorders

A **phobia** is a persistent and irrational fear of a specific object, activity or situation, which results in a compelling desire to avoid the dreaded object or situation. Most people will experience panic when in contact with the phobic situation. The fear is recognised by adults or adolescents as unreasonable in proportion to the actual danger. However, children do not always identify their fears as unrealistic.

In the development of phobia, it is believed that fear arises through a process of displacing an unconscious conflict onto an external object symbolically related to the conflict. Thus, in becoming phobic, the individual fears a specific external object rather than an unknown internal source of distress. The phobic person can then control the intensity of the anxiety by avoiding the object with which the anxiety is associated.

A diagnosis of phobic disorder is generally made when the avoidance behaviour becomes extreme or the problem so pervasive that it interferes with the person's normal functional ability. Phobic disorders are classified into three main types: agoraphobia, social anxiety disorder and specific phobia. They are described next.

Agoraphobia

Individuals with **agoraphobia** often fear leaving the safety of their home, worrying that they might develop an incapacitating symptom, such as dizziness, loss of bowel or bladder control, or cardiac distress. Normal activities are increasingly curtailed as the fears dominate the person's life. Agoraphobic people often limit travel and need a companion when away from home. Those who endure the phobic situation experience intense anxiety.

Agoraphobia and panic disorder used to be linked together for diagnosis in DVM IV-TR (American Psychiatric

Association, 2000), believing agoraphobia without panic attacks was relatively rare; however, current thinking recognises the two disorders as different, and that people with agoraphobia do not always experience panic symptoms. Most people with agoraphobia have a history of generalised anxiety or anxiety attacks at the onset of the phobic behaviour. Onset of this disorder usually occurs in the middle to late twenties. Agoraphobia is more frequently diagnosed in women than in men. Separation anxiety in childhood and sudden object loss appear to be predisposing factors. Depression, anxiety, rituals, minor checking compulsions and rumination are frequently associated features of agoraphobia.

The prognosis for people with agoraphobia is variable. Some less severely disturbed individuals experience intermittent symptoms and may have periods of remission. Those who are more severely impaired may experience lifelong disability.

Social anxiety disorder

Social anxiety disorder (also called *social phobia*) is thought to affect 1 in 10 people at some point in their lives. It is characterised by persistent fear and avoidance of situations in which the person may be exposed to scrutiny by others. The person especially fears being humiliated or embarrassed. Examples of social anxiety disorders are an extreme fear of performing or speaking in public, of making complaints, or writing or eating in front of others. Other common anxieties include fear of interacting with members of the opposite sex, superiors or aggressive individuals.

According to the ABS (2008), 4.7 per cent of Australians are affected by social anxiety disorders, making it one of the most prevalent of all of the anxiety disorders. Familial pattern and predisposing factors are unknown, and the incidence is evenly distributed between men and women. Other anxiety disorders may also co-exist with social anxiety disorder. Similarly, mood disorders, avoidant personality disorder and substance use disorder must be taken into account when assessing for social anxiety disorder, since there is substantial evidence of comorbidity between social anxiety disorder and other mental health problems (NICE, 2013). Often appearing in late childhood or early adolescence, it is possible for people to make a complete recovery in the absence of treatment, whereas for those whose symptoms continue into adulthood, a full recovery without intervention is rare (NICE, 2013).

Specific phobia

More common than any other type of phobic disorder, a **specific phobia** is an isolated fear focused on one situation or object, such as darkness, heights or animals. This category of phobic disorders encompasses all phobias not included in agoraphobia or social anxiety disorder. Many specific phobias begin in childhood and subsequently disappear as the person ages. Phobias that persist into adulthood rarely go away without treatment. Specific phobia is more often diagnosed in females than in males. School phobia, which affects some children, may result in academic failure, impaired social relationships and self-esteem problems.

Specific phobias generally cause minimal impairment if the phobic object is rarely encountered and easily avoided; for example, a fear of snakes does not seriously impair an individual living in a high-rise condominium. The phobia can, however, be incapacitating if the phobic situation is frequently encountered and not easily avoided. A fear of heights or elevators would seriously incapacitate a person living or working in a high-rise building. A specific phobia may lead to lifestyle restrictions that vary in severity according to the degree of anxiety.

Significant changes to the DSM-5 (APA, 2013) now mean that agoraphobia, specific phobia and social anxiety disorder must be present for a minimum of six months prior to diagnosis. This prevents the over-diagnosis that has occurred in the past. Factors such as environment, context and situation are now taken into account to assess whether the anxiety is 'out of proportion' to the real danger posed, rather than the anxious person recognising their own symptoms as unreasonable or excessive, since evidence suggests that people will often exaggerate the danger when faced with their phobic situation.

Generalised anxiety disorder

Generalised anxiety disorder (GAD) is considered less specific and less debilitating than panic disorder and phobic disorder. GAD is characterised by pervasive, persistent anxiety of at least six months' duration, but without phobias, panic attacks, or obsessions and compulsions. The person experiences chronic feelings of nervousness and apprehension for no apparent reason, and is unable to control the worry. The worry is greatly exaggerated in relation to the probability that the event will actually occur.

People with GAD are unable to stop worrying, even though they realise that their anxiety is more intense than the situation warrants. Overall, those with GAD are unable to relax. The excessive worries usually lead to insomnia and/or impaired quality of sleep, and are associated with physical symptoms such as muscle tension, headaches, sweating, hot flashes, headaches, shortness of breath and dizziness. Irritability is a common psychological manifestation of GAD. In order to accurately diagnose GAD, a thorough physical examination must be done to determine the presence of any medical conditions (e.g. hyperthyroidism) or effects from having taken a substance that could lead to similar symptoms.

There is little generally accepted information about age of onset, predisposing factors, cause of illness, prevalence, familial pattern or sex ratio, although there appears to be a more equal sex ratio than in panic disorder. Associated mild depressive symptoms are not uncommon in individuals with GAD.

Obsessive–compulsive disorder

The DSM-5 (APA, 2013) recently removed **obsessive–compulsive disorder (OCD)** from its section on anxiety disorders due to increasing evidence of a relationship with other disorders, such as hoarding, body dysmorphic disorder and excoriation disorder based on preoccupation and repetitive behaviour. Despite this distinction, there remains a close link with anxiety, as symptoms presented are often related to extreme anxiety when an individual tries to resist an obsession or compulsion.

An **obsession** is a recurring thought that cannot be dismissed from consciousness. These intrusive thoughts are sometimes trivial or ridiculous, often morbid or fearful, and always distressing and anxiety-provoking. Other common obsessive thoughts have to do with violence or contamination.

A **compulsion** is an uncontrollable, persistent urge to perform certain acts or behaviours in order to relieve an otherwise unbearable tension. Most compulsive acts are attempts to control or modify obsessions, because the person either fears the consequences or is afraid they will not be able to control the primary impulse. Although compulsions are attempts to reduce tension, they eventually increase tension, because the individual becomes increasingly agitated, unable to decide whether to stop or continue the compulsive actions.

Typical compulsive acts are endless handwashing, checking and re-checking doors to see if they have been locked, and elaborate dressing rituals. Such compulsive acts are defences used to contain, neutralise or ward off the anxiety related to the primary impulse. Compulsive acts such as counting and elaborately checking routine duties are frequently associated with the fear of failing or making a mistake, or with the need to be perfect. The following Practice Example describes the progression of obsessive thoughts to compulsive behaviours.

Practice example

Edward's inability to get the nursery rhyme 'snips and snails and puppy dog tails' out of his mind is an example of a strange but trivial obsession. Even though Edward tried to distract himself with activities, he found the rhyme running through his mind at work and at home, especially when he was trying to sleep at night. In turn, Edward developed a compulsion that involved ritualistic handwashing, to ward off the anxiety generated by his apparently silly obsession.

Melinda's obsession was much more ominous. She could not stop thinking that she must kill her children in order to prevent a worldwide race war. In turn, Melinda, obsessed with thoughts about killing her children, and engaged in symbolic rituals of touching religious objects to repel evil influences through magical interventions by the saints.

People with OCD usually fear that they will harm someone or something. They rely heavily on avoidance, and are best understood in terms of their control needs. Individuals who develop obsessive–compulsive symptoms have a great need to control themselves, others and their environment. OCDs and compulsions have the following features in common:

- an idea or impulse persistently intrudes into the person's awareness
- a feeling of anxious dread accompanies the primary manifestation, and often leads the person to take counter-measures against the forbidden thought or impulse
- both the obsessions and the compulsion are ego alien—that is, they are foreign to one's self-perception
- no matter how compelling the obsession or compulsion, the person has enough insight to recognise it as irrational and experience it as a significant source of distress.

According to the Australian National Survey of Mental Health and Wellbeing (2007), the prevalence of OCD in Australia over a 12-month period is 2.7 per cent. Although symptoms usually occur in late adolescence or adulthood, some can commence in childhood, affecting both males and females (McEvoy, Grove & Slade, 2011).

Table 8.2 ■ lists some common obsessions and compulsions.

Trauma and stress-related disorders

Trauma and stress-related disorders, such as PTSD and acute stress disorder, have distinct differences from anxiety disorders. This has led to the DSM-5 and the upcoming edition of the International Classification of Mental and Behavioural Disorders (ICD) recognising trauma and stress-related disorders in their own right as a diagnostic category (Maercker et al., 2013; Stein et al., 2014). However, since they also share similar symptoms with anxiety disorders (e.g. distress, lack of concentration and avoidance), they will be briefly explored in this chapter.

Post-traumatic stress disorder (PTSD) is the experience of a significant stressor or trauma, outside the range of usual experience, which is followed by recurrent subjective re-experiencing of the trauma. The types of trauma that precipitate PTSD are varied, including military combat, criminal attack (i.e. assault, rape), child abuse (especially incest), terrorist

TABLE 8.2 ■ Common obsessions and compulsions

Behaviour	Related compulsion	Related obsession
Repetitious handwashing	Urge to wash, scrub or clean	Fear of disease or contamination
Returning home often to make sure appliances are turned off	Need to re-check related to self-doubt	Fear of disaster
Hoarding junk mail, receipts and all types of papers	Need to keep everything	Fear of losing things
Ritualistic counting of the number of stairs climbed	Urge to count repeatedly	Belief that counting will yield control and thus prevent making mistakes
Avoiding stepping on seams of tiles, carpets, sidewalks	Need for order and routine	Belief that order and routine will negate all anxiety

attack (i.e. bombing, skyjacking) and natural catastrophes (i.e. earthquakes, tornadoes, hurricanes). Children who have witnessed violence in their families, schools or communities are also vulnerable to developing PTSD. First-responders (e.g. paramedics) and other health care providers, especially those who work in critical care areas and trauma centres, are at risk of developing PTSD as a result of witnessing extreme suffering. The trauma that precipitates the development of PTSD has to be extreme; therefore, the client's cultural context must be considered in the diagnostic process.

The psychological effects of trauma affect individuals throughout their lifetimes. For example, a child who observes domestic violence (especially repeated episodes) is at risk for developing PTSD as an adult. The violence associated with rape, whether experienced or witnessed, is severe enough to precipitate the onset of PTSD. Within the Australian Defence Force the prevalence is substantially more than in the general population, standing at 8.3 per cent and 5.2 per cent, respectively (McFarlane, Hodson, Van Hooff & Davies, 2011). The following Practice Example provides a description of combat-related PTSD.

Practice example

Joe is a veteran of military action in Afghanistan and Iraq. He attends a PTSD program at a veterans' hospital outpatient clinic. Upon returning home from combat, he continued to relive his experiences through recurrent nightmares about improvised explosive devices. Joe experienced insomnia, had trouble concentrating and took no pleasure in previously enjoyed activities. He felt guilty about the actions he had to take in order to survive when other men in his unit died.

A common manifestation in individuals with PTSD is hyperarousal while re-experiencing the traumatic event. As a result, the person is unable to relax; hypervigilance occurs, and the person is always 'on edge'. Another common feature of PTSD is dissociation, in which emotions about the traumatic event are blocked. The individual becomes emotionally numb, and experiences impaired social relationships. People with PTSD may also avoid the stimuli associated with the traumatic event. For example, a woman who is raped in an elevator may avoid using any elevator—an example of how PTSD can restrict daily functioning. A significant complicating problem is the person's use of alcohol or other substances in an attempt to maintain control and soothe emotions.

The course of PTSD is variable. Most people who have suffered a significant stressor tend to have an acute reaction from which they recover spontaneously. In others, however, the reaction may be delayed or prolonged, and eventually become chronic. PTSD can occur in people of any age, thus the DSM-5 includes separate diagnostic criteria for children six years and younger.

Following a traumatic event, it is important to thoroughly assess everyone, including physical, psychological, sociocultural and spiritual domains. Across the lifespan, associated symptoms of anxiety, increased irritability and high rates of comorbidity, such as depression and substance abuse, are common.

Acute stress disorder

Acute stress disorder (ASD) is the development of anxiety and dissociative symptoms that occur within one month of an extremely traumatic event. The precipitating stressors of ASD are similar to those of PTSD, but with greater emphasis on dissociative symptoms. They include exposure to a trauma in which the individual experienced or witnessed event(s) that involved actual or threatened injury or death, and were accompanied by feelings of intense helplessness, fear or horror. As in PTSD, the precipitating event must be a trauma that is outside the usual human experience. The traumatic event may be a natural disaster or a human-induced event (e.g. rape, terrorist bombing). One type of trauma that often triggers ASD is disasters that affect entire communities. Individuals feel overwhelmed as a result of the trauma, and are unable to cope effectively.

Although it is similar to PTSD, ASD can be differentiated in the following ways:

- the duration is shorter
- the interval from the trauma to the development of symptoms is shorter
- the person has at least three of these dissociative manifestations: sense of detachment or numbing, depersonalisation, derealisation, dissociative amnesia, decreased awareness of surroundings (being in a daze)
- the dissociative symptoms interfere with effective coping.

Individuals with ASD may experience depression accompanied by despair and helplessness. Thus, there is a very real danger of suicide. They may feel that they are responsible for the outcome of the trauma. For example, if another person was killed in the traumatic event, survival guilt frequently occurs. People affected by ASD often neglect safety precautions and the basic needs for daily living. First-responders and other emergency personnel are at high risk for developing ASD. The next Practice Example describes the onset of ASD as a response to a natural disaster.

Practice example

William was a member of a team of firemen from rural Victoria who volunteered to help with rescue efforts following several catastrophic bush fires. William and his fellow volunteers worked through rubble and ash, at first looking for survivors, then removing bodies. William's symptoms of acute stress disorder began one week after returning home from the traumatic event.

BIOPSYCHOSOCIAL THEORIES

There are several schools of thought regarding the causes of anxiety disorders. These theories include biological, genetic, psychosocial, behavioural and humanistic, which are discussed in the next section.

Biological factors

Refresh your understanding of the biological basis of anxiety disorders by referring to Figure 8.7 ■, which illustrates the physiological responses in anxiety disorders in relationship to

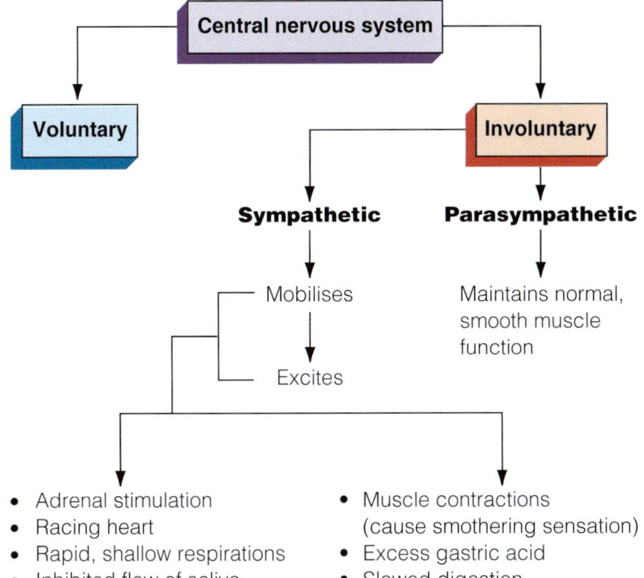

FIGURE 8.7 ■ Physiological responses in anxiety disorders.

the sympathetic and parasympathetic divisions of the central nervous system. Notice that they are the same as the fight-or-flight response described earlier in this chapter. A major research question that remains unanswered is: are the physiological imbalances a *cause* or a *result* of the anxiety disorder?

Recent research findings point to biological changes in the brains of individuals experiencing anxiety disorders. For instance, functional MRIs showed that individuals with generalised anxiety disorder experienced irregular activity in the medial prefrontal and anterior cingulated regions of the brain (Paulesu et al., 2010). Another study indicates that the medial prefrontal cortex is activated in people with excessive anxiety levels (Etkin, Prater, Hoeft, Menon & Schatzberg, 2010). Many substances can also increase anxiety levels. Caffeine stimulates the central nervous system (CNS), as can nicotine, by increasing the same physiological arousal response experienced with exposure to stress.

Genetic theories

We now know that genes play a significant role in the extent to which anxiety disorders run in families. The traits people pass down and others inherit will impact on an individual's behavioural response to stress. Research evidence indicates that a familial predisposition for anxiety disorders may exist particularly in panic and phobic disorders. First-degree relatives of people with panic disorder are four to seven times more likely to develop panic disorder, and in approximately 25 per cent of individuals with GAD there is a family history of the disorder (Sadock & Sadock, 2010). The results of such studies have clearly demonstrated increased risk of anxiety disorders among first-degree relatives, and can help explain why some people exposed to stress develop anxiety and others do not. Although we still have a way to go, genetic research offers an opportunity to unravel the molecular basis of anxiety in the future, and help identify pathognomonic markers from which a diagnosis of anxiety disorder can be made.

Psychosocial theories

Psychoanalytic theory views anxiety as a sign of psychological conflict resulting from the threatened emergence into consciousness of forbidden or repressed ideas and/or emotions. The individual fears expressing the forbidden impulses; anxiety is an outcome of repressing such impulses. Other analytic views, sometimes called *neo-Freudian,* evolved from the work of Freud and differ on the nature of anxiety. Rank (1952) believed that anxiety can be traced back to birth trauma. According to the psychoanalytic model, the unconscious conflict must be brought into conscious awareness through psychoanalysis so that the real source of anxiety can be discovered and resolved.

Social interpersonal theorists, such as Sullivan (1953), stressed the importance of the early relationship between the mother and the child, and the transmission of the mother's anxiety to the child. In the interpersonal model, treatment takes the form of the less time-consuming psychodynamic psychotherapy.

Behavioural theories

Behavioural learning theorists view anxiety as a learned response that can be unlearned. For example, behaviourists believe that the cause of phobias is traumatic exposure to the avoided object, situation or activity. According to this theory, during the development of obsessions an original neutral obsessive thought evokes anxiety because it becomes associated with an anxiety-provoking stimulus. In compulsions, a person discovers that a certain action relieves the anxiety associated with the obsessive thought. The person repeats the action to achieve relief, until eventually the act becomes a learned pattern of behaviour. Compulsive behaviour is viewed as a maladaptive attempt to alleviate anxiety.

Behavioural approaches are often effective in the treatment of anxiety, and are widely used for modifying symptoms in phobic disorder and obsessive–compulsive disorder. Behavioural therapists believe it is unnecessary to use insight-oriented psychotherapy to help clients cope with the anxiety. Instead, clients need only face the anxiety repeatedly until it becomes manageable. Behavioural treatment approaches are often used in treating phobias, because the methods are more efficient, less costly, and less time-consuming than insight-oriented psychotherapy.

Humanistic theories

The humanistic perspective is particularly important in understanding anxiety disorders. Environmental stressors, biological factors and intrapsychic fears or conflicts cannot be adequately dealt with separately, but only as they interact with one another. For example, those suffering from a phobic disorder experience shame and helplessness as they attempt to cope with fears of annihilation in the presence of the dreaded object or situation. The result may be interpersonal withdrawal and functional impairment, which create long-lasting disability.

This perspective has given rise to a multi-faceted approach to the care of those with anxiety disorders. Humanistic treatment approaches are integrative, and may include a range of psychotherapeutic interventions, including psychotherapy (cognitive, behavioural and/or dynamic), measures to develop effective social support systems, measures to reduce environmental stress, and psychopharmacological treatment.

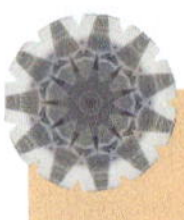

NURSING PROCESS
Caring for the person with anxiety

Mental state assessment

Consumers with anxiety disorders have impaired psychosocial and physiological function. The emotional disturbances and physical and intellectual changes that take place as a result of extreme or chronic anxiety affect the person's work, school and social functioning, and frequently impair or threaten previously meaningful interpersonal relationships.

The occurrence of acute anxiety and its related symptoms is common to a number of physical conditions and acute medical emergencies. Therefore, a careful evaluation should always be conducted to initiate appropriate treatment quickly. A history and physical examination should rule out such conditions as hyperthyroidism and other endocrine problems, Ménière's syndrome, brain disorders, caffeine intoxication, mitral valve prolapse and medical emergencies (such as myocardial infarction).

Differentiation from other psychiatric diagnoses is difficult when anxiety and depression are mixed. The question of which one predominates can puzzle many practitioners, and necessitates ongoing thorough assessment. Some ways to differentiate anxiety and depression are listed in Table 8.3 ■. Anxiety is part of many other clinical conditions, such as schizophrenia and mood disorders; therefore, diagnosis may be made on the basis of the dominant, most debilitating symptom.

TABLE 8.3 ■ Comparison of anxiety and depression

Clinical manifestations	Anxiety	Depression
Affect	Fear and/or dread	Sadness, despair, helplessness and/or hopelessness
Insomnia	Initial difficulty in falling asleep	Early morning awakening followed by difficulty returning to sleep
Motor activity	Agitation	Retardation (slowing)
Negativism	Limited to specific areas	Global

YOUR ASSESSMENT APPROACH
Person with an anxiety disorder

Use the questions that follow as guidelines for assessing people with anxiety disorders.

Physiological assessment

- How often do you experience palpitations (heart pounding)?
- Do you have difficulty breathing?
- Do you experience muscle tightness? If so, where, and how long does it last?
- How often do you experience changes in bladder or bowel function?
- How do your symptoms affect your sleep?

Psychological assessment

- How do you feel? What are your feelings about the future?
- How often do you lose your temper?
- Do you enjoy being with other people?
- How often do you criticise yourself?

Cognitive assessment

- How often do you think about the same things over and over?
- How frequently do you have trouble concentrating on important activities?
- How often do you worry about the past or the future?
- What activities that were pleasurable for you in the past do you still enjoy?

During assessment, determine not only whether the person is anxious (and, if so, to what extent), but also the possible source of the anxiety. Knowing the source will help you plan and implement effective care. It is important to assess the person's perception of threat; the greater the perceived threat, the more intense the anxiety. For extremely anxious individuals, suspend formal data-gathering in favour of immediate, direct action to reduce anxiety.

Subjective information

People with an anxiety disorder may report a variety of physical and emotional symptoms. It is important to encourage them to describe the symptoms in their own words, and to explain how the symptoms affect their daily activities. They may report emotional distress, cognitive and perceptual changes, somatic discomforts, and/or role impairments.

They may reveal a number of distressing emotional feelings, such as the following examples:

- 'I feel like something terrible is going to happen.'
- 'I feel helpless for no reason at all!'
- 'I just can't seem to enjoy life—everything bothers me.'

Anger, guilt, feelings of worthlessness and anguish frequently accompany anxiety. When the anxiety is acute or extreme, as in panic disorder or PTSD, the person feels in immediate danger and may seek protection and reassurance from others. If the anxiety is too severe, however, they may become immobilised and unable to report their terrifying

YOUR ASSESSMENT APPROACH
Client with panic attack

To determine the psychological effects of panic on the person in your care, ask them:

- How do you feel right now?
- When did you start feeling this way?
- Did this feeling start gradually, or all at once?
- How well are you able to concentrate?
- How do you feel about the future?
- Do you sometimes feel out of control?

To determine the somatic effects of panic on the person in your care, ask them:

- Are you having chest pains or shortness of breath?
- Have you felt dizzy or faint?
- Can you hold your hands steady, or do they shake?

feelings at all, or they may refuse assistance and run away or become physically aggressive.

Sometimes consumers with anxiety disorders may deny the existence of anxious feelings. They try to protect themselves by dissociating these feelings. It is important to recognise the anxiety despite their denials. In such instances, assessment requires an especially careful observation of objective data.

Cognitive and perceptual changes

People experiencing anxiety frequently have difficulty concentrating and making decisions. Some people report feeling as if they are 'going in circles', unable to think through a problem in order to make an effective decision. They may worry about their effectiveness at work, and fear they will lose their job as a result of attention and judgment problems. In the clinical situation, they may ask staff members to make decisions for them. At the same time, however, they may express difficulty following through with suggestions, finding many loopholes or possible problems with the plan of action. Others may become forgetful or misinterpret what they hear.

In extreme anxiety, as in a panic attack, the person is often unable to assess a situation accurately and realistically, and requires immediate attention from, and orientation by, you.

For those who experience somatic symptoms, complaints of nausea, indigestion, headache, decreased appetite and a constant feeling of fatigue can occur. They may relate these somatic disturbances to having 'bad nerves', or they may be unaware of any psychological component of their discomfort.

People with OCD who engage in repetitive activity, such as compulsive handwashing or hair-pulling, may report special health problems (tissue breakdown or hair loss) as a result. You must compare the psychological benefits to the physical consequences of the person's compulsive rituals when determining appropriate interventions.

Those with PTSD may report fitful sleep, terrifying nightmares and a fear of returning to sleep. The subsequent sleep loss becomes an additional physiological stressor. Be sure to assess the sleep pattern of consumers with PTSD.

Others may be aware of the impact that emotional, cognitive/perceptual and somatic changes have on their social, family and work roles. They report worry about losing their jobs or being unable to continue caring for their families. This worry only exacerbates the underlying anxiety, and sets up a vicious cycle of worry compounding anxiety, which adds to the worry. The next Practice Example describes two people who are experiencing interpersonal difficulties as a result of anxiety.

Practice example

Kathy despairs that she is unable to take her daughter to the playground because her phobias prevent her from leaving the house.

Abe, a middle-aged accountant, obsessed about tallying his firm's financial data, is unable to put his job aside for the weekend, and misses his son's football game. He experiences anger, guilt and self-recrimination as a result.

Objective data

In addition to noting the general signs and symptoms of anxiety, as discussed earlier, other specific physical, emotional, cognitive and role-performance changes may be observed in those experiencing an anxiety disorder. Look for indicators of hypervigilance, such as guarding and suspiciousness; these are common occurrences in people experiencing PTSD.

YOUR ASSESSMENT APPROACH
Person with PTSD

The person's answers to the questions that follow will help you to assess for PTSD.

- When was the last time you struck out in anger?
- Are you able to laugh and cry at appropriate times/situations?
- How would you describe your mood right now? Happy? Sad? Depressed?
- How much time do you spend thinking the same thing over and over?
- Describe how you relax.
- When was the last time you lost your temper? Or said something without thinking first?
- How do you sleep at night? Any nightmares or repetitive dreams?
- How is your memory?
- Are you able to finish tasks?

Physical findings

Some people may experience a panic reaction and show extreme discomfort. Look for acute physical changes, such as breathing difficulty, sweating, trembling and/or vomiting, during these incidents. During a panic episode, the person may be incoherent or unable to verbalise what is happening. They may be so frightened that they refuse help at that moment, and may require firm reassurance and protection until the episode subsides.

The person with an ongoing anxiety disorder may develop long-term physiological effects, such as susceptibility to viral infections or the development of ulcers, hypertension or asthma. Substance abuse may develop as they try to alleviate their anxiety through chemical means, and can become a serious complicating problem. Substance use (discussed in Chapter 13), which frequently occurs in individuals experiencing PTSD, may be an attempt to avoid traumatic memories by self-medicating. Other physical findings may be the effects of ritualistic or compulsive activity—skin lesions in someone who obsessively picks at their skin, for example.

Emotional changes

Family and friends of a person with PTSD may report personality changes in the person, including increased irritability, suspiciousness, angry outbursts, and a tendency to blame others and to withdraw emotionally. Remember to pay attention to your own feelings when interacting with highly anxious clients. Because anxiety can be transmitted interpersonally, use self-awareness to determine the source of your own anxiety when interacting with people experiencing anxiety.

Cognitive deficits

An unrealistic or distorted perception of a situation is common in anxiety states. During panic attacks, a person may distort or exaggerate details. They may complain about some seemingly insignificant detail. People may lose their ability to take in other pertinent data, and thus make errors in judgment. In assessment interviews, consumers with anxiety disorders are often forgetful and unable to concentrate or attend to details. Errors in calculation and grammar are also common.

Impact on role function

The symptoms of anxiety disorder affect social, work and family relationships. It is important to understand the possible effects of anxiety symptoms on interpersonal relationships. Obsessive–compulsive acts, for instance, may become so pervasive that they take the place of relating to other people. Sometimes, a person may use obsessions and compulsions to negotiate social interactions and social roles. Nurses who plan intervention strategies for people with anxiety disorders should first assess the impact of the symptoms on the family system. In the following Practice Example, the person, Vanessa, knows that her compulsive cleaning is irrational, but is unable to stop the behaviour. Vanessa does not connect the excessive need for cleaning to an attempt to negate her sense of decreased control over her family members.

Practice example

Vanessa's house is so clean and orderly that you could literally 'eat off the floor'. Vanessa spends a large amount of her time after work and on weekends making sure that the house is sparkling clean. She prepares to-do cleaning lists for her young adult children to follow when they visit. When Vanessa's husband comes home after travelling on business, he is often met with his own to-do list. Family social activities are put on hold until Vanessa's lists have been accomplished. Vanessa's husband and children complain about having to clean an already clean house. Vanessa is upset that her children are visiting less often, and that her husband seems to be spending more and more time travelling on business.

Reports from the person and/or their family that they are having trouble at work are additional evidence of role impairment. The person with anxiety may be in jeopardy of losing their job because of poor performance. A person with PTSD, for example, may be fired for absences, drug or alcohol abuse, or outbursts of temper.

Mental state examination

As discussed in Chapter 10, when undertaking a mental state examination there are some fundamental areas to be assessed. For the person experiencing anxiety, important areas to cover within the domains of the mental state examination are fear, anxiety, ineffective coping, ineffective role performance, impaired verbal communication, risk for trauma, disturbed thought processes and disturbed sensory perception, and insomnia. We shall now look at these separately.

Fear

Fearful responses to anxiety can occur on a continuum, ranging from slight apprehension to paralysing terror. One anxious person may state 'I'm scared', whereas another may be filled with alarm and unable to verbalise their feelings of panic. In extreme cases of anxiety, panic is communicated through behavioural responses rather than verbalisations. Behaviours such as being immobilised with fear or striking out at others are often exhibited by individuals experiencing panic.

Anxiety

Apprehension and tension are emotional experiences common to people with anxiety disorders. A person may worry excessively, ruminating about what might go wrong in the future. They may express anxiety through worry about their physical wellbeing; somatic preoccupation or hypochondriasis may develop. Sexual drive or behaviour may also be inhibited by anxiety. The potential for substance abuse is high, and suicidal potential is increased.

Ineffective coping

Excessive anxiety can cause alterations in conduct and impulse control. Some people, such as those with PTSD or panic disorder, manifest unpredictable behaviours in an attempt to cope with their overwhelming fears. Individuals with OCD are unable to alter behaviours, even though they may recognise the behaviours as harmful or irrational. In an attempt to cope, a person may begin to self-medicate with alcohol or other drugs, which results in disordered conduct and impaired impulse control.

Ineffective role performance

Anxiety disorders impair performance in the family, at school and at work. People who are anxious may become less efficient and accurate at work or school because of distractibility or other perceptual and cognitive difficulties. A person may withdraw emotionally from formerly important and meaningful relationships, or they may become overly dependent on others for help. They may isolate themselves and avoid previously enjoyed activities and recreation. Excessive need for reassurance, decreased productivity, reduced creativity, impaired hygiene and impaired home maintenance are all possible outcomes for the person experiencing severe anxiety.

Impaired verbal communication

People with anxiety disorders can often have difficulty communicating. They may speak too quickly or too loudly, may over-elaborate, or may talk about too many subjects at once. Easily distracted, anxious people may have trouble understanding explanations or retaining information. Written communication may also be impaired.

Risk for trauma

Impairments in motor behaviour are often related to hyperactivity and restlessness, which may place the person at risk for accidental injury. Wringing of the hands, poor coordination and startle reaction are motor behaviours associated with anxiety disorders. Those with OCD may perform bizarre repetitive acts, such as repeatedly washing their hands, which can often result in broken and dry skin.

Disturbed thought processes and disturbed sensory perception

Anxiety disorders affect perception and cognition, and reduce a person's ability to solve problems. Judgment, concentration, abstract thinking and attention are impaired. They are indecisive, but at the same time may make decisions impulsively in an attempt to relieve tension. In panic disorder, the person may become disoriented, misinterpret reality, and distort the meaning of situations or events. Loss of self-esteem and a lowered self-concept often result because they are unable to use skills that were previously helpful in coping.

Insomnia

Insomnia is a frequent response to anxiety; a majority of people with anxiety disorders have trouble sleeping. Sleep may be further disturbed by nightmares or night terrors, as experienced by people with PTSD.

Planning and implementation

When planning and implementing care for an anxious person, remember that anxiety is communicated interpersonally and often affects the person's family and friends, other consumers, and staff members as well.

When developing a nursing care plan, it is essential for the person and their carers to be involved in the process when possible. This shared-decision approach means each plan of care is individualised according to the person's symptoms, needs and priorities. The following list provides goals that generally apply to people experiencing anxiety disorders in the community or in a hospital setting:

- Demonstrate a reduction or absence of the level of anxiety experienced.
- Identify indicators of own anxiety, and be able to recognise symptoms of increasing anxiety.
- Explore feelings of anxiety with an identified health professional.
- Seek assistance when anxiety becomes difficult.
- Participate in the use of self-management strategies—such as relaxation, controlled breathing and positive visualisation techniques—that can help manage the anxiety.
- Demonstrate positive health behaviours.

Nursing interventions for people with anxiety disorders should be geared towards effective coping skills, such as problem-solving, identifying early warning signs and education.

Reducing fear

Fear and anxiety usually co-exist, in that a person who is fearful is generally anxious as well. The clinical manifestations of fear and anxiety are very similar. Thus, when dealing with a person who is afraid, nursing interventions for reducing anxiety are appropriate (see the following).

Reducing anxiety

Because anxiety is such an uncomfortable feeling, we learn early in life to reduce it or diminish its effects as soon as possible. Although individuals use a variety of behaviours, the most common automatic responses to anxiety are anger, withdrawal and somatisation. Automatic responses are limiting, rigid and inflexible, and therefore prevent a creative response to the stressor.

Intervening with people who are extremely anxious or in a panic state These situations require immediate, direct and structured intervention. During an acute panic attack, perception and personality are disrupted to such a degree that the person cannot solve problems or discuss the source of anxiety. Your first goal is to reduce the person's immediate anxiety to more moderate, tolerable and manageable levels. The anxious person's family needs counselling about how to respond therapeutically, because they are often present during a panic episode. The interventions listed in the next Your Intervention Strategies can help alleviate the person's panic.

LIVED EXPERIENCE

Family involvement

Unfortunately my family were never involved or educated, but hopefully things are changing now. If family and friends do not know how to respond to an acute panic attack, and cannot de-escalate the person's rising anxiety, they can unwittingly add fuel to the fire, particularly if they themselves are becoming anxious. The end result can be both parties engaging in a fierce argument, and days of ill feeling towards one another disrupting the entire household. An ounce of prevention is worth a pound of cure.

YOUR INTERVENTION STRATEGIES
Person experiencing panic

Strategy	Rationale
Stay with the person	Being left alone may further increase the anxiety
Maintain a calm, serene manner	Prevents transmission of anxiety from nurse to the individual
Use short, simple sentences	Disruption of the perceptual field causes difficulty in focusing
Use a firm and authoritative voice	Conveys your ability to provide external controls
Take the person to a quieter, smaller, less-stimulating environment	Prevents further disruption of the perceptual field by sensory stimuli
Focus the person's diffuse energy on repetitive or physically tiring task	Repetitive tasks or physical exercise help reduce excess energy
Administer anti-anxiety medications if prescribed	Anti-anxiety medications may help reduce anxiety by altering brain chemistry

Intervening in less severe anxiety You can frequently detect subtle indications of increasing anxiety and intervene early to prevent escalation. Some people are adept at covering up their anxiety, even though their behaviour usually transmits cues to the sensitive observer. Anxiety may make people excessively demanding. Your response to the person's demands should always consider the possible effects of your response on their anxiety. In some cases, it may be reassuring to set limits and deny the request. In other cases, such a response may place further stress on the individual.

The intervention strategies for those who suffer from prolonged anxiety are intended to help people use their anxiety to learn about themselves and their coping strategies. This requires the person to endure the anxiety while searching out its causes, and to develop more effective and satisfying coping strategies to replace the maladaptive ones. To help people learn to cope more effectively with anxiety, first detect the anxiety and then make thoughtful observations and responses that facilitate learning. Refer to the following Your Intervention Strategies for the person experiencing anxiety.

It is important that you avoid reinforcing a person's justifications for their usual coping patterns. Often, people try to give plausible explanations for their ineffective anger, withdrawal or somatisation. However, these rationalisations do not explain the relief in terms of the factors that caused the anxiety. The relief afforded by the usual coping patterns does not last long, because the needs or expectations that originally caused the symptoms still exist. The underlying needs may become even more intense. The person experiencing anxiety can begin to change disturbed coping patterns only when they understand what their unmet needs are, what they did instead of fulfilling these needs, and their subsequent feelings.

YOUR INTERVENTION STRATEGIES
Person with anxiety

Strategy	Rationale
Use a quiet, calm, firm approach	Minimises the interpersonal transmission of anxiety Role-models expected behaviour
Observe the person's verbal and non-verbal behaviour	Anxiety is manifested verbally and non-verbally Early detection of cues promotes prompt intervention to prevent escalation of anxiety
Encourage verbalisation of feelings	The act of talking is cathartic, and therefore reduces the anxiety level Identification of a problem is the first step in the problem-solving process
Teach relaxation techniques when the anxiety is at a mild level	People with moderate, severe or panic-level anxiety are unable to process new information. Maximum learning is possible at the mild anxiety level
Encourage the use of relaxation techniques as needed	The relaxation response counters the hyperarousal of anxiety states

People with anxiety disorder have two alternatives. They can change their hopes and expectations, or they can try new tactics or resources to get their needs met. Discuss these options with the person, and negotiate a plan to work on one or both goals. Acting on either option involves problem-solving. Simple physical activities often help reduce anxiety to more tolerable levels. Encourage adaptive mechanisms that work, such as the activities that promote relaxation or mindfulness. Examples of activities that promote relaxation can be found in Your Intervention Strategies on the next page.

You can use a variety of techniques and skills in intervening with people who experience anxiety. Cognitive behavioural therapy helps individuals face their fears in order to cope. Progressive muscle relaxation, meditation to activate the relaxation response, thought-stopping techniques, and guided imagery may teach new ways to reduce the disturbing affect. Other methods include helping people test reality, because their sense of danger is often out of proportion to actual danger. Developing goal-oriented care plans may help reduce a person's sense of inner chaos by providing structure and direction, and actively involves the person in their own healing process. This involvement increases their sense of control, thereby alleviating feelings of powerlessness.

LIVED EXPERIENCE

Starting the journey towards recovery

I have always had a problem with goal-oriented care plans; they seem to be more for the worker than the person. If you are unable or simply do not want to achieve these goals, then the worker needs to redirect the focus onto what your hopes, dreams and ambitions were before you became unwell, and onto how you can again work towards recapturing a sense of the past and bringing it back to the present, and start the journey to fulfil aspects of former expectations for your life. I would have preferred information, education, and learning how to understand myself and how to make sense of the intense fear I was experiencing, and a helping hand to guide me to keep moving forward. To have high expectations, and not settle for the 'no hope of recovery' written across the first page of my medical record.

YOUR INTERVENTION STRATEGIES

Activities that promote relaxation

Passive behaviours	Active behaviours
■ Soak in a warm bath.	■ Take a long walk.
■ Listen to soothing music.	■ Ride a bicycle.
■ Have a back rub or massage.	■ Phone someone and discuss your feelings.
■ Perform progressive muscle relaxation.	■ Organise your desk, pantry or closet.
■ Take slow deep breaths, to counter the effects of hyperventilation.	■ Garden or mow the lawn.
	■ Engage in an activity such as painting.

LIVED EXPERIENCE

Practice and persistence

The most effective tool to de-escalate rising anxiety for me was the firm and authoritative voice of a psychiatrist who commanded me to focus on my breathing—slow, deep breaths while counting to 10. I still experience episodes of anxiety, but I have now mastered the skill to listen to his authoritative voice in my head: 'Ann, you need to focus on your breathing—slow, deep breaths while you count to 10.' It works every time now, but took a great deal of practice and persistence.

Educating the person experiencing anxiety about medications

Part of people learning about their anxiety is to discuss all of the possible treatment options available to manage their anxiety. This includes teaching people the major medications used to manage acute anxiety, their limitations and possible side-effects. MIMS, a comprehensive and authoritative medicine database, can be accessed online, and offers valuable information about the pharmaceuticals available in Australia.

Antidepressants and anti-anxiety medications (also known as *anxiolytics*) are frequently used to treat anxiety. Anxiolytics consist of benzodiazepines and non-benzodiazepines. Particular attention should be paid to the use of benzodiazepines, since long-term use can cause dependence. They therefore are not usually a first-line treatment and, if prescribed, should be within a short timeframe and used cautiously and sparingly.

Selective serotonin reuptake inhibitors (SSRIs) are generally the first antidepressant medication of choice for treating anxiety disorders, because they exert fewer side-effects than other medications.

It is worth noting that some antipsychotic medications may have a paradoxical effect and trigger the development of anxiety disorders. This is especially true of clozapine, a precipitant of OCD in some individuals. When used to treat anxiety disorders, medications are started at a low dosage level and gradually increased until a therapeutic level is achieved. Inform people that it may take up to two to four weeks before they begin to feel better. This information is crucial in helping individuals continue to take the medication. These medications are discussed more fully in Chapter 7.

Although medications may alleviate the symptoms of anxiety, they do nothing to help an individual understand the source of their anxiety. Other interventions should also be considered, such as mindfulness techniques, cognitive behavioural therapy and relaxation, since they have all proved effective in relieving anxiety symptoms. Ideally, if medication is used, it should be used for the short-term treatment of anxiety—days, weeks or months, instead of years. However, some people may require longer-term treatment, depending on the degree of anxiety relief. Thus, it is necessary to closely monitor each person and determine the efficacy of medication. Treatment of anxiety should not be solely reliant on medication.

Promoting effective coping

Coping skills can be taught to clients with every type of anxiety disorder. In addition to anxiety alleviation, there are other therapeutic benefits to using previously learned coping skills, such as increased self-esteem, improved self-efficacy and more effective problem-solving. You need to demonstrate patience in order to project a sense of calm when working with anxious people. Coping skills can vary for each person, but may include problem-solving, self-help groups, exercise and talking to someone. Box 8.2 provides examples of some therapeutic techniques.

Promoting effective communication

Nursing interventions that reduce anxiety are important measures to promote more effective communication and

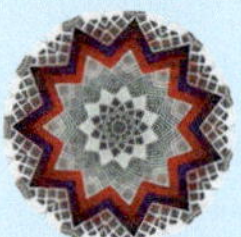

WHAT EVERY NURSE SHOULD KNOW

Anxious person in an emergency department

Imagine that you are a nurse in an emergency department:

- When a person enters your emergency department, it is important to assess their level of anxiety, just as you assess every person's vital signs and pain level.
- Knowing a person's level of anxiety will help determine your next action.
- Approach the person experiencing anxiety with a calm, reassuring manner to help them feel less threatened and more secure.
- Involve the person in their own care as much as possible. This will increase their sense of control, as they will understand 'why' things are happening.
- Protect the safety of the person whose anxiety is escalating, as well as the safety of other others and yourself.
- Call for help from team members immediately if your interventions have not de-escalated the person's anxiety.

behaviour. Often, simply offering the opportunity to acknowledge and discuss feelings of anxiety helps a person regain control. People are more likely to share their concerns if you have taken the first step in demonstrating genuine interest and concern.

While encouraging the person to express their feelings, be sure to listen attentively. Fear, anger, sadness, disappointment or alienation may be expressed, and it may be difficult for you to hear about the individual's pain. Some nurses feel helpless in the face of a person's catharsis, and think they should be able to provide ready answers. Instead, ready answers are more likely to interfere with the communication process. Genuine, concerned listening, without judgment or giving advice, is an effective intervention in itself.

Explanations should be simple, clear and concise. Be careful not to overload severely anxious people with more information than they can handle. If anxiety has contributed to knowledge deficit, reduce the anxiety before trying to teach about health or provide information. If their perceptual field is narrow or disrupted, it is unlikely the person will be unable to assimilate information.

Box 8.2 Therapeutic techniques for people with anxiety, trauma and stressor-related disorders

- ***Cognitive restructuring:*** Provides new, less-threatening interpretations of events. Includes techniques such as thought stopping and thought substitution (see Chapter 26 for specific cognitive therapies).
- ***Education:*** Provides an explanation of the dynamics of the anxiety disorder and of treatment modalities.
- ***Exercise and nutrition:*** Strengthens the body's adaptive resources.
- ***Family conference/counselling:*** Provides support to the person by encouraging their family to work on resolving the many psychosocial effects evoked by the trauma.
- ***Group therapy:*** Provides support and reinforces new coping skills.
- ***Individual therapy:*** Provides important ego-supportive and/or cathartic benefits.
- ***Relaxation training:*** Focuses on developing new skills that the person may use when faced with their fear, anxiety or memories of the traumatic event.

LIVED EXPERIENCE

What works for one may not work for another

Personally, I found relaxation training wasn't for me. I dreaded these groups! What did help me was the informal group sessions held between the patients: we talked, problem-solved, offered each other solutions and strategies that we had used to cope, provided information and education, and understanding, without judgment of one another. We gave each other comfort and support. I have always said it was the other patients' insight and life experiences which significantly contributed to my recovery.

Those with anxiety require patience and an unhurried attitude, especially with regard to details and ruminations. If you use the techniques of paraphrasing and reflecting, these people will say you did not get the details right. They will then

COLLABORATIVE CARE

Teaching about medications for anxiety disorder

- Drowsiness is a common side-effect. Avoid activities requiring mental alertness, such as driving or important decision-making, until you know how the medication will affect you.
- Do not consume alcohol while taking this medication. Check labels on over-the-counter drugs and toiletries (e.g. mouthwash), because many contain alcohol.
- Because drinking caffeine decreases the effect of your medication, use decaffeinated beverages.
- Do not take other medications without first discussing it with your health care provider. Many drugs interact negatively with others.
- Do not increase the dosage or stop taking the medication without checking with your health care provider.

COMMUNICATION

Person with social anxiety disorder

PERSON: 'I just had to get out of that room. I couldn't stand it with all those people looking at me. I thought I was going to die!'

NURSE RESPONSE 1	NURSE RESPONSE 2
NURSE RESPONSE 1: 'That sounds very frightening. Tell me more about this.' *RATIONALE:* This response demonstrates reflection of the person's affect, and encourages them to continue verbalising their feelings.	**NURSE RESPONSE 2:** 'Think of other times when you have felt that way. What helped you feel less frightened?' *RATIONALE:* This response asks the person to identify specific coping methods that were helpful in a similar situation. Such methods can then be used in anticipatory planning for future anxiety-provoking situations.

go on to correct, qualify and clarify. This striving for accuracy produces greater vagueness and confusion. It is as if parallel conversations are going on simultaneously. Some people will hear only themselves repeating and correcting insignificant details, and completely lose the overall meaning of the message. Developing patience in listening, and skill in providing well-timed, simple direction, is crucial to working effectively with anxiety disorders. See the example in the Communication feature.

Promoting safety

Lack of coordination, tremors and impaired concentration can make those experiencing anxiety prone to accidents. Counsel people not to perform potentially dangerous activities, such as driving a car, when anxiety is high. Advise them to move more slowly, or to repeat instructions carefully when they undertake new tasks or use tools and/or equipment that are potentially dangerous. Advise the person to speak with family before making any life decisions, such as those involving finances or employment. Provide this same instruction to those receiving anxiolytics, which can also affect their ability to perform potentially dangerous activities and make sound decisions.

Promoting effective sensory perception and thought processes

To function more effectively and independently, the anxious person needs to know about normal anxiety and anxiety disorders. Providing accurate information at the right time and in an appropriate manner is an essential nursing responsibility. Other nursing strategies to promote effective perception and cognition include the following:

- use adjuncts to verbal communication, such as visual aids or role-playing, to enhance the retention of information
- practise problem-solving vignettes to improve judgment and insight
- identify misperceptions that a person may hold as a result of a narrowed perceptual field—begin with comments such as 'I wonder if you've considered this possibility . . . ?' or 'Perhaps if we tried . . .'
- help the person perform a reality test—that is, explore their opinions in the light of validated experience, rather than emotional needs that block accurate perception.

See Table 8.4 ■ for further information on cognitive behavioural techniques.

Promoting sleep

Nonpharmacological nursing measures to promote sleep should be used before medications. Such measures may include a variety of relaxation techniques. One effective method is the use of music that promotes a relaxing atmosphere; listening to the sounds of Nature is soothing and induces sleep in some people. Other suggestions include reading a book, drinking warm, decaffeinated liquids, or taking a warm bath before retiring. See those listed in Collaborative Care on the next page.

TABLE 8.4 ■ Cognitive behavioural techniques for treating phobias

Technique	Description	Example
Systematic desensitisation (exposure therapy)	A person is exposed to a series of increasingly anxiety-provoking situations, beginning with the least threatening. The person gradually becomes desensitised to each stimulus in the series, until the stimulus that induced the most anxiety is no longer threatening.	A man who is terrified of earthworms might first talk about earthworms until the topic no longer evokes the same level of anxiety. Then he might be shown pictures of earthworms, until he masters that level of closeness. Over time, he will progress to holding a live earthworm in his hand without experiencing severe or panic-level anxiety.
Reciprocal inhibition	The anxiety-provoking stimulus is paired with another stimulus associated with an opposite feeling strong enough to suppress the anxiety.	Through the use of meditation, yoga, biofeedback training, hypnosis or anti-anxiety medications, people can learn how to induce a calm state.
Cognitive restructuring	This intervention is based on the belief that anxiety stems from erroneous interpretations of situations. The person learns to reframe (or relabel) a frightening situation, object, activity or event, so that it becomes less threatening.	A woman who fears she is going to die if she leaves her apartment learns to change her perception to one that is more reality-based, by saying, 'I may feel uncomfortable, but I will not die. I can do this.'

COLLABORATIVE CARE

Teaching about improving sleep quality

1. Think about the kind of sleep schedule that seems to fit you best.
2. Make a list of things that help you get to sleep (how dark you like it to be, what temperature, how you get ready for bed).
3. Jot down all the 'rules' and 'suggestions' you have heard about how to get better sleep. Cross out the ones that don't seem to fit. (Some people sleep better by not having a bedtime snack; other people sleep better after having a snack. Do what feels best for you. If you aren't sure, try an experiment doing it one way for a week, and then the other way for the next week.) Put a question mark by the rules and suggestions you have never really tried, and underline the ones you think are important for you.
4. Consider what you could change to get an extra half-hour of sleep each night.
5. Keep a sleep diary for two weeks. For the first week, just keep track of your usual pattern (time you went to bed and got up, number of hours of actual sleep, how you felt in the morning, etc.). At the end of the first week, review the diary and your responses to items 1 through 4. In the second week, experiment with one change you think would be helpful to you.
6. Carry on the process a bit longer if you like, but remember:
   - you can manage on very little sleep if you have to
   - you know better than anyone else what works for you
   - your needs and preferences regarding sleep may change as you get older or take on different roles and activities.

(Adapted from Centre for Clinical Interventions, 2008)

Evaluation

Evaluation is used to determine a person's response to interventions. In other words: is the anxious person demonstrating progress? Are the anxiety-related symptoms decreasing? Are coping skills being used effectively? In addition to these questions, it is also important to evaluate progress in the following areas: role performance, communication, safety, thought processes, perception and sleep.

COMMUNITY-BASED CARE

Individuals with anxiety disorders are usually aware that their behaviours are problematic to themselves and others. However, insight alone does not necessarily result in behavioural changes. Or, when change does occur, it is a very gradual process. As a result, people with anxiety disorders are often treated in the community—in mental health clinics, community centres and medical centres. Some people may be visited by nurses who provide care in the home environment in order to improve social interactions and shape behaviour.

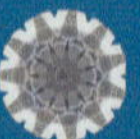

NURSING CARE PLAN: A PERSON WITH PANIC DISORDER WITH AGORAPHOBIA

Identifying information

Mrs Randolph is 43 years old, married and the mother of four daughters in their late teens and early twenties. She was referred to the mental health outpatient clinic for follow-up counselling by the emergency department of the local general hospital, where she had been seen on the previous day with symptoms of a panic attack.

History

At the time of the panic attack, Mrs Randolph believed she was having a heart attack and feared she was dying. She reported racing heartbeat, sweating and feeling faint. She could not identify any events, thoughts or feelings that precipitated the incident; it seemed to her to occur 'out of the blue'. She felt unable to cope with the severity of the symptoms of the attack: 'I tried to talk myself out of it, to tell myself it would go away, but it only got worse.'

Mrs Randolph reported that she had had similar attacks over the years, and that she had always been reassured of her medical and cardiac health, but when these attacks occurred she 'feared the worst' and 'lost all perspective'. The previous attacks had lasted from two minutes to two hours. Her daily routine had become quite restricted, because she now sought to have one of her daughters or her husband with her when she went out of the home, due to fear of an attack. She did not feel comfortable when alone in her home, and could not go to sleep if the other family members were not home. She felt ashamed and angry about her growing disability, and often tried to cover up her fears to friends and family.

By interviewing the family, the nurse was able to gather information about a number of significant recent life events preceding the panic episode:

- Recent major surgery: Mrs Randolph had had a hysterectomy four weeks earlier.
- Loss of employment due to her hospitalisation: She was abruptly terminated from her position at a new job because of too many absences.
- There is an upcoming anniversary of her father's sudden death from a heart attack.

Mrs Randolph had never been hospitalised for a mental health condition, although she had been to the emergency department on three prior occasions with symptoms of panic attack. She had seen a therapist years ago when the attacks first occurred—'about the time I left home to marry.' She did not follow up with the therapist, however, saying she felt ashamed ('I've always been a strong and effective person!'), that the episodes were not so severe at that time, and that she found relief from panic attacks after she had the children.

Both of Mrs Randolph's parents had died within the past six years. She was especially close to her father, and the second anniversary of his death was approaching. Mrs Randolph's mother was considered a

(continued)

NURSING CARE PLAN: A PERSON WITH PANIC DISORDER WITH AGORAPHOBIA *(continued)*

'homebody'; she rarely left the house and took part in social activities only if they occurred at the family home. Mrs Randolph wondered if her mother had 'these fears', too. She reported that she had also begun to curtail social and recreational activities, preferring to stay at home where she was most comfortable.

Mrs Randolph described her relationship with her husband as emotionally warm and supportive. Although she sometimes resented his being away from her, she recognised this as part of her 'problem' with being alone. Her primary relationships had been with her husband and children. She talked of facing the 'empty nest' as her daughters, one by one, left for work or higher-education opportunities.

With the exception of chronic gynaecological problems leading to the recent hysterectomy, Mrs Randolph reported a history of good health. She had no allergies or other chronic illnesses. Her only other hospitalisations were to have her children. The recent hospitalisation had been more physically taxing than she had expected, and the fact that she was not allowed to return to work after her recovery had come as a blow.

Current mental status

Mrs Randolph is an attractive, carefully groomed woman who looks her stated age. She sits erect in the office chair, appearing somewhat tense. She answers questions by engaging with conversation, but at times with some hesitation, as if expecting criticism or judgment from the interviewer.

She is oriented to time, place and person. Her memory is intact, and her recall good. She has no difficulty with calculations. Her judgment is unimpaired. During times of panic, however, sensory and perceptive awareness are greatly impaired.

Affect appears normal, with occasional evidence of anger in the form of irritability and light sarcasm. Mood is within normal limits.

Speech is normal in flow and volume. It appears pressured at times, when she attempts to correct an impression she believes the interviewer holds. Posture is at times rigid, but she relaxes as she becomes more comfortable during the interview.

There are no delusions, ideas of reference or hallucinations. Obsessive worry about the occurrence of panic episodes and her safety is present. Embarrassment and shame over her symptoms are apparent. Suicidal or homicidal thoughts are denied. Associations and abstractions are appropriate, and there is no evidence of thought-process disorder or difficulty in concentration, except during acute panic, at which times concentration is impaired and thought processes are disorganised. Some guardedness towards the interviewer is noted. Insight into the meaning of the current situation is minimal.

Other clinical data

Mrs Randolph is considering the use of anti-anxiety medication, despite 'hating the idea' of medication.

It is important to note that the following care plans are a snapshot of the identified issues, focusing on possible short-term goals. A care plan should always have a recovery focus, reflect the consumer's needs, and be extended to include the strengths and resources the consumer has identified as part of their own experience. See Chapter 26 for further information on care planning.

Issue identified: Frequent increased-anxiety levels preventing completion of daily chores, such as leaving the house, shopping, employment.

Expected outcome: Mrs Randolph will be in control of her anxiety levels as evidenced by her ability to complete activities such as walking outside and going to the local shops.

Short-term goals	Interventions	Rationales
Demonstrate skills in managing anxiety symptoms to allow the completion of walking outside	Maintain calm manner	A calm approach prevents escalation of anxiety by role-modelling control of the situation
	Stay with Mrs Randolph during periods of severe anxiety, and reassure her that she is safe	Mrs Randolph's panic is alleviated in the presence of others, and this will ensure her safety
	Use short, simple sentences	Simple language facilitates a person's ability to concentrate and follow direction
	Direct Mrs Randolph's attention to a repetitive or physical task	Distraction serves as an outlet for anxious energy
	Administer prescribed anti-anxiety medication	To provide temporary relief due to their relaxing and calming effects
	Teach relaxation exercises	Muscle relaxation counters the stress response, and will enable Mrs Randolph to feel more in control of her breathing
	As Mrs Randolph's anxiety subsides, explore the antecedents preceding the increasing anxiety levels, and the link between thoughts, feelings and behaviour	Recognising the relationship between emotions, thoughts and behaviour will help develop alternative responses

(continued)

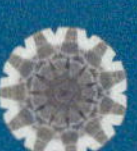

NURSING CARE PLAN: A PERSON WITH PANIC DISORDER WITH AGORAPHOBIA *(continued)*

Issue identified: Ineffective coping related to overwhelming fears.
Expected outcome: Mrs Randolph uses actions/behaviour to manage stressors that tax her personal resources.

Short-term goals	Interventions	Rationales
Demonstrate effective coping as evidenced by employing behaviours to reduce stress	Review coping skills used in the past	To identify useful and existing strengths and resources, and transfer them to the current situation
	Identify healthy ways to deal with anxiety	To be aware of alternative actions that can promote effective coping, such as problem-solving and distraction
	Spend time with Mrs Randolph on each shift, encouraging her to explore and articulate her fears and anxieties	Verbalisation of thoughts and feelings reduces anxiety levels by the process of catharsis
	Provide education materials associated with anxiety	For Mrs Randolph to understand the anxiety process and know why she is reacting in certain ways, which will in turn enable her to independently manage her anxiety levels
	Identify triggers for anxiety and early warning signs	Awareness of early warning signs will allow the opportunity for Mrs Randolph to implement appropriate coping skills

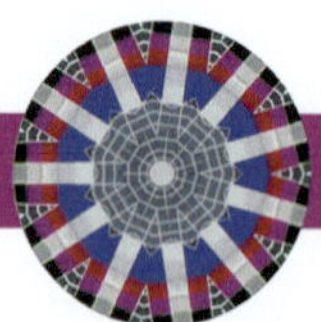

REFERENCES

American Psychiatric Association (APA). (2000). *Diagnostic and statistical manual of mental disorders* (4th ed., Text Revision) (DSM-IV-TR). Washington, DC: APA Publishing.

American Psychiatric Association (APA). (2013). *Diagnostic and statistical manual of mental disorders* (5th ed.; DSM-5). Washington, DC: APA Publishing.

Australian Bureau of Statistics (ABS). (2008) *National Survey of Mental Health and Wellbeing: Summary of results, 2007.* Cat. No. 4326.0. Canberra, Australia: ABS.

Barkway, P. M. (2013). *Psychology for the health professionals* (2nd ed.). Sydney, Australia: Elsevier.

Baxter, A. J., Scott, K. M., Vos, T., & Whiteford, H. A. (2013) Global prevalence of anxiety disorders: A systematic review and meta-regression. *Psychological Medicine*, *43*(5), 897–910.

Böttche, M., Kuwert, P., & Knaevelsrud, C. (2012). Posttraumatic stress disorder in older adults: An overview of characteristics and treatment approaches. *International Journal of Geriatric Psychiatry, 27*(3), 230–239.

Broadbent, E., Kahoekehr, A., Booth, R. J., Thomas, J., Windsor, J. A., Buchanan, Hill A. G. (2012). A brief relaxation intervention reduces stress and improves surgical wound healing response: A randomised trial. *Brain, Behavior, and Immunity*, 26, 212–217.

Centre for Clinical Interventions. (2008). *Sleep hygiene*. Perth, Australia: Department of Health, Government of Western Australia.

Chan, D., Fan, M. Y., & Unutzer, J. (2011). Long-term effectiveness of collaborative depression care in older primary care patients with and without PTSD symptoms. *International Journal of Geriatric Psychiatry, 26*(7), 758–764.

Ciccarelli, S. K., & White, J. N. (2009). *Psychology* (2nd ed.) Upper Saddle River, NJ: Prentice Hall.

Cohen, S., Janicki-Deverts, D., Doyle W. J., Miller, G. E., Frank, E., Rabin, B. S., & Turner, R. B. (2012). Chronic stress, glucocorticoid receptor resistance, inflammation, and disease risk. *Proceedings of the National Academy of Sciences of the United States of America, 109*(16), 5995–5999.

Etkin, A., Prater, K. E., Hoeft, F., Menon, V., & Schatzberg, A. F. (2010). Failure of anterior cingulate activation and connectivity with the amygdala during implicit regulation of emotional processing in generalized anxiety disorder. *American Journal of Psychiatry, 167*(5), 454–554.

Friedman, H. S., & Kern, M. L. (2014). Personality, well-being and health. *Annual Review of Psychology, 65*, 719–742.

Heidt, T., Sager, H. B., Courties, G., Dutta, P., Iwamoto, Y., Zaltsman, A., . . . Nahrendorf, M. (2014). Chronic variable stress activates hematopoietic stem cells. *Nature Medicine*, *20*(7), 754–758.

Holmes, T. H., & Rahe, R. H. (1967). The social readjustment rating scale. *Journal of Psychosomatic Research, 11*, 213–218.

Holtzman, C., Shapiro, D., Trotman H., & Walker, E. (2012). Stress and the prodromal phase of psychosis. *Current Pharmaceutical Design, 8*(4), 527–533.

Kobasa, S. C. (1979). Stressful life events, personality, and health: An inquiry into hardiness. *Journal of Personality and Social Psychology, 37*, 1–11.

Krogh, D. (2000). *Biology: A guide to the natural world.* Upper Saddle River, NJ: Prentice Hall.

Lazarus, R. S, (1966). *Psychological stress and the coping process*. New York, NY: McGraw-Hill.

Lazarus, R. S., & Folkman, S. (1984). *Stress, appraisal, and coping*. New York, NY: Springer.

Maercker, A., Brewin, C. R., Bryant, R. A., Cloitre, M., Reed, G. M., van Ommeren, M., . . . Saxena, S. (2013). Proposals for mental disorders specifically associated with stress in the International Classification of Diseases-11. *Lancet, 381*, 1683–1685

McEvoy, P. M., Grove, R., & Slade, T. (2011). Epidemiology of anxiety disorders in the Australian general population: Findings of the 2007 Australian National Survey of Mental Health and Wellbeing. *Australian and New Zealand Journal of Psychiatry;45*, 957–967.

McFarlane, A. C., Hodson, S. E., Van Hooff, M., & Davies, C. (2011). Mental health in the Australian Defence Force: 2010 ADF Mental Health and Wellbeing Study: Full report. Canberra, Australia: Department of Defence.

MIMS Australia. (2015). Available http://www.mims.com.au/index.php/products/mims-online (Accessed 2015, March 30.)

Moloney, L., Weston, R., Qu, L., & Hayes, A. (2012). *Families, life events and family service delivery: A literature review* (Research Report No. 20). Melbourne, Australia: Australian Institute of Family Studies.

Monat, A., & Lazarus, R. S. (1991). *Stress and coping* (3rd ed.). New York, NY: Columbia University Press.

National Mental Health Commission. (2012). *A contributing life: The 2012 national report card on mental health and suicide prevention.* Sydney: National Mental Health Commission.

NICE. (2013). *Social anxiety disorder: Recognition, assessment and treatment.* NICE clinical guideline 159. Retrieved from www.nice.org .uk/guidance/cg159 (Accessed 2015, March 25.)

Paykel, E. S. (1978). Contribution of life events to psychiatric illness. *Psychological Medicine, 8*, 245–253.

Paulesu, E., Sambugaro, E., Torti, T., Daneli, L., Ferri, F., Scialfa, G., & Sassaroli, S. (2010). Neural correlates of worry in generalized anxiety disorder and in normal controls: A functional MRI study. *Psychological Medicine, 40*(1), 117–124.

Pruessner, M., Iver, S. N., Faridi, K., & Malla, A. K., (2011). Stress and protective factors in individuals at high risk for psychosis, first episode psychosis and healthy controls. *Schizophrenia Research, 129*(1), 29–35.

Rank, O. (1952). *The trauma of birth.* Philadelphia, PA: Robert Brunner.

Sadock, B. J., & Sadock, V. A. (2010). *Kaplan & Sadock's pocket handbook of clinical psychiatry* (5th ed.). Philadelphia, PA: Lippincott Williams & Wilkins.

Seligman, M. (2011). Flourish: A new understanding of happiness and wellbeing—and how to achieve them. London, Nicholas Brealey Publishing.

Selye, H. (1956). *The stress of life.* New York, NY: McGraw-Hill.

Slade T., Johnston, A., Teesson, M., Whiteford, H., Burgess, P., Pirkis, J., & Saw, S. (2009). *The mental health of Australians 2. Report on the 2007 National Survey of Mental Health and Wellbeing.* Canberra, Australia: Department of Health and Ageing.

Stein, D. J., McLaughlin, K. A., Koenen, K. C., Atwoli, L., Friedman, M. J., Hill, E. D., . . . Kessler, R. C. (2014). DSM-5 and ICD-11 definitions of posttraumatic stress disorder: Investigating 'narrow' and 'broad' approaches. *Depression and Anxiety, 31*, 494–505.

Stengel, A., & Taché, Y. (2010). Corticotropin-releasing factor signaling and visceral response to stress *Experimental Biology and Medicine, 235*, 1168–1178.

Sullivan, H. S. (1953). *The interpersonal theory of psychiatry.* New York, NY: Norton.

Sundquist, J., Lilja, A., Palmer, K., Memon, A., Wang, X., & Johansson, L. (2015). Mindfulness group therapy in primary care patients with depression, anxiety and stress and adjustment disorders: Randomized controlled trial. *British Journal of Psychiatry*, 206(2), 128–135.

Taylor, S. E. (2015). *Health psychology* (9th ed.). New York, NY: McGraw-Hill.

Thoits, P. A. (2010). Stress and health: Major findings and policy implications. *Journal of Health and Human Behavior, 51*(Suppl), S41–S53.

Thomée, S., Härenstam, A., & Hagberg, M. (2011). Mobile phone use and stress, sleep disturbances, and symptoms of depression among young adults—a prospective cohort study. *BMC Public Health, 11*, 66.

Thomée, S., Härenstam, A., & Hagberg, M. (2012). Computer use and stress, sleep disturbances, and symptoms of depression among young adults—a prospective cohort study. *BMC Psychiatry, 12*, 176–189.

Vedhara, K., Gill, S., Eldesouky, L., Campbell, B., Arevalo, J., Ma, J., & Cole, S. (2015). Personality and gene expression: Do individual differences exist in leukocyte transcripome? *Psychoeuroendocrinology, 52*, 72–82.

Wilkins, R., Warren, D., Hahn, M., & Houng, B. (2011). *Families, incomes and jobs: Vol. 6: A statistical report on waves 1 to 8 of the Household, Income and Labour Dynamics in Australia Survey.* Melbourne, Australia: Melbourne Institute of Applied Economic and Social Research, University of Melbourne.

Wong, Q. J., & Moulds, M. I. (2011). The relationship between maladaptive self-beliefs characteristic of social anxiety and avoidance. *Journal of Behavior Therapy and Experimental Psychiatry, 42*(2), 171–178.

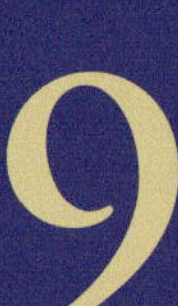

9

Therapeutic communication

DEB O'KANE AND ANN SMITH

KEY TERMS

LEARNING OUTCOMES

After completing this chapter, you will be able to:

1. Describe the factors that influence the process of human communication.
2. Explain why non-verbal communication is important in interpersonal relationships.
3. Outline the models of human communication, and explain why they are essential to understanding therapeutic relationships.
4. Describe strategies for improving your personal ability to communicate therapeutically.
5. Explain how therapeutic communication skills foster relationships and communicating in a mental health care setting.
6. Identify the principles of cultural competence within the process of communication.
7. Understand the perspective of people with mental health problems when communicating with them.

LIVED EXPERIENCE

'It was a conversation, not an interrogation'

I instantly knew this counsellor understood, explanation was unnecessary; we were fully engaged in conversation, not a question-and-answer affair, exploring what I knew and understood, how I felt and did I understand 'why I felt this way'? As we talked, he built on what I already knew, he offered options, alternative ways of coping, ways of dealing with the challenges of a person with dementia. It was a very pleasant experience for both of us, we learnt from each other, we learnt about each other (not in a personal sense). I left, feeling a sense of 'thank goodness, he has the skill and knows how to help me through this difficult time'.

I felt confident in his ability to guide, teach and listen, and hear and understand what I was saying; he was honest and open, we were both relaxed. It was a conversation, not an interrogation, between equal partners. He was a gentle, calm, quiet person. He listened.

Practice example

You are about to embark on your first clinical mental health placement. You feel anxious because, although you have read about the therapeutic communication techniques described in this chapter, you feel uncomfortable about using them. They seem artificial, stilted and 'not you'.

1. What can you do to decrease your discomfort and anxiety and help make your mental health nursing experience a positive learning experience, for you as well as for those whom with you are working?
2. How would you modify the therapeutic communication techniques discussed in this chapter to match your own personal style?
3. What problems could you run into by overusing a communication technique?
4. How can therapeutic communication techniques be useful when communicating with classmates? Friends? Family members?

INTRODUCTION

The mechanism for establishing, maintaining and improving human contacts is interpersonal communication. Communication is a very special process, and the most significant of human behaviours. Moreover, it is the foundation of an effective nurse–consumer relationship. When people tell 'their story', they explain themselves, the events of their lives and the circumstances they face. As mental health nurses, we help the consumer tell their story, explore the circumstances of their lives, and move in a more satisfying and mentally healthier direction.

For many students, like the student in the Practice Example that follows, the instruction to use one's self therapeutically is mysterious jargon quite unlike the clear-cut step-by-step procedures for some physical treatments.

Because the process of human communication is complex and has many dimensions, it cannot be reduced to a few simple steps that you can simply memorise and perform. However, there are some principles and techniques that we will teach you to use so that you can be comfortable and therapeutic at the same time. Effective communication is the cornerstone for all mental health nursing practice. Two other chapters correlate closely with this chapter on communication. Chapter 2 discusses the actual structure and process of the one-to-one relationship. Chapter 4 discusses the nurse's personal characteristics that are a basis for therapeutic use of self.

Practice example

I found myself closely watching my preceptor and the staff on the unit when they talked with consumers. Somehow I thought that by imitating the things that they did or said, I would figure out what 'being therapeutic' was supposed to mean. I knew it had something to do with things the nurse said or didn't say when she talked with people. But it all got very fuzzy to me, beyond that very elementary grasp of it. I used to latch onto ideas like 'Agreeing is untherapeutic. So is giving advice or opinions.' The only entries I felt safe putting down in my learning journal were stiff-sounding reflections like 'You sound angry.'

THE PROCESS OF HUMAN COMMUNICATION

As you will see in this chapter, communication is an ongoing, dynamic and ever-changing series of events. Some people mistakenly believe that communication is simply the transfer of information or meaning from one human being to another. The truth is that meaning *cannot* be transferred; it must be mutually negotiated, because meaning is influenced by a number of significant factors.

Role of perception

A person's perception of the world is an essential element in communicating. The term **perception** refers to the experience of sensing, interpreting and comprehending the world in which one lives. Perception is a highly personal and internal act.

People process through their senses all of the information they have about the world around them. However, seeing is not always believing. Communication specialists have discovered that because of human physiological limitations, the eye and brain are constantly being tricked into seeing things that are not really what they seem; these are called **illusions.** Before continuing to read, stare at Figure 9.1 ■ for 20 seconds. The illustration will appear to swing back and forth. You can verify that the movement is an illusion by checking your visual perception against your tactile sensations.

What people 'see' or sense is strongly influenced by many factors. For example, past experiences have prepared us to see

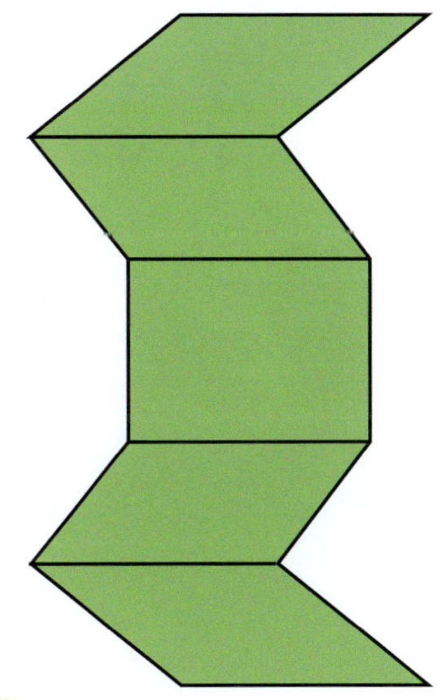

FIGURE 9.1 ■ A perceptual illusion.

things, people and events in particular ways. Also, we tend to observe more carefully when a purpose guides the observation. The nurse in an intensive care unit observes a cardiac surgery patient differently than how a family member does.

Finally, when understandings differ, you and I can look at the same object and see different things. Our mental set helps determine how and what a person perceives based on previous perceptions and how we have responded in the past. Before you read any further, look at the picture of the young woman in Figure 9.2 ■. Do you see the silhouette of a young woman? Do you also see the face of an elderly woman? (Remember: stop here and look at Figure 9.2.) Using the phrase 'the picture of the young woman in Figure 9.2' encouraged you to perceive the illustration in a particular way. Now you should also be able to see the elderly woman in the illustration.

As the illustrations demonstrate, the old axiom might be better stated: 'Believing is seeing.' Because we tend to perceive in terms of past experiences, expectations and goals, perceptions may be a prime obstacle to communication. No two individuals perceive the world in exactly the same way, and the meanings of events differ because people's perceptions of them differ. Perceptions of other human beings are of particular importance, because human communication is inevitably affected by how we perceive one another. To see others at all as they are, people need to know themselves and to know how the self affects their perceptions of others.

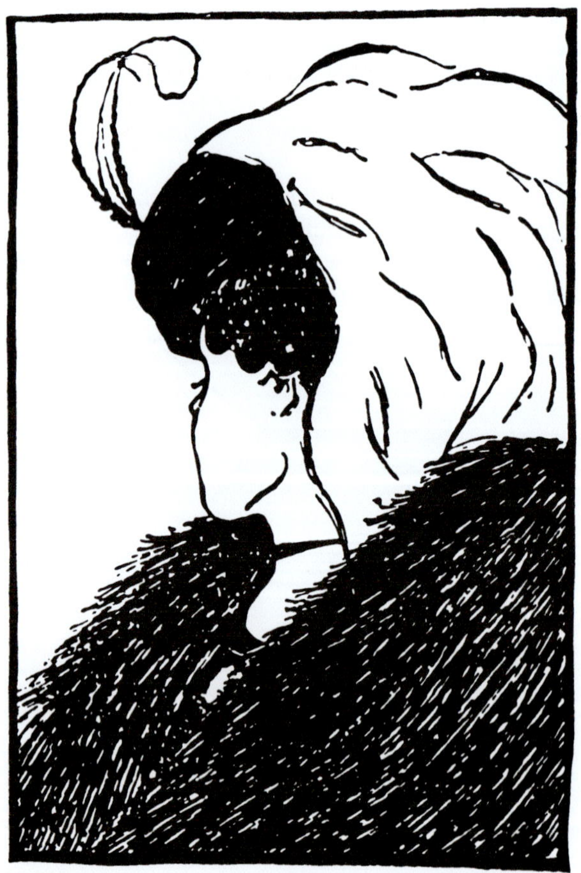

FIGURE 9.2 ■ The influence of mental set on perception.

Role of values

Values are concepts of the desirable. People value what is of worth to them. Values influence the process of communication, because people's values, like their perceptions, differ.

Value systems differ for a number of reasons. Age is one. Children's values shift when they become teenagers. School or work experience generally influences values in yet other directions. Marrying or being a parent or grandparent may cause other value changes or shifts.

Being aware of our own values and other people's is helpful to avoid any conflict that may expose a person to uncertainty and confusion. Consider the following Practice Example.

Practice example

The parents of a 15-year-old girl were upset to find a small plastic bag of marijuana in her dresser drawer. She had been playing hooky from school and wore low-slung jeans that her parents considered too sexy. After a series of lengthy, angry discussions with her parents, she was confined to her room. During this period she refused to eat or drink. When the teenager was seen by a mental health assessment team, the members' opinions were divided. Some said that her behaviour signalled an emotional disturbance. They labelled her antisocial, depressed and anxious. Others believed the parents were old-fashioned and too rigid in attempting to force her to accept their values.

Here, we see contrasting values influencing the team's understanding of the situation. The daily roles people take also influence their values. In any one day, a man may be a student, husband, father, nurse, citizen, speaker, artist, son and teacher.

These examples make it obvious that communicating with meaning requires that the participants take culture into account. How people communicate with others who do not share similar histories, heritages or cultures is of critical importance in humanistic mental health nursing practice.

When English is not a person's first language and you are a monolingual clinician, it will help if you select the words you use carefully, avoiding buzz words, slang and technical or medical jargon. Show respect by speaking clearly and directly

LIVED EXPERIENCE

Valuing communication

If someone does not feel that they are being heard, regardless of whether the correct words have been used, if the meaning and feeling they are trying to impart is being dismissed as irrelevant, unimportant, ignored or misunderstood, the result will be that the person you are trying to help will not engage or trust you. This is why it is of utmost importance that all communication be respectful and valued, even if the listener judges the conversation to be meaningless.

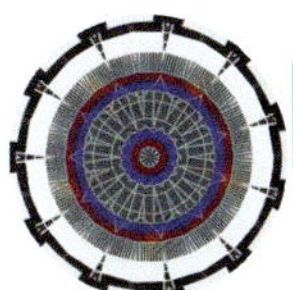

DEVELOPING CULTURAL COMPETENCE

Role of culture

Each culture provides its members with notions about how the world is structured and what it means. These preconceptions, learned at an early age, are so subtle that they often go unrecognised. They nonetheless set limits on communication and interaction with others. Relying on culturally determined generalisations or stereotypes can have profound effects on one's relationships with others.

Communication is culture-bound in a wide variety of ways. The culture and the **subculture** (the culture within the culture) teach people how to communicate through language, hand gestures, clothing and even in the ways they use the space around them. In some cultures, belching after dinner is a compliment to the host. In other cultures, belching may be considered uncouth or an insult. Other interesting examples of cultural differences in communication are discussed in the following paragraphs.

Australia is home to a growing population of people with diverse cultural and linguistic needs, including both Indigenous and immigrant groups. It is therefore important to take this into consideration when establishing a therapeutic relationship. Being culturally sensitive to an individual's needs and participating within a framework of cultural safety embraces the principles of respect, acceptance and genuineness.

Cultural differences in communication

We know, from research, that people interpret communication from their unique cultural perspectives. For example, facial expressions that convey sadness, happiness, anger, disgust and surprise seem to be shared in most cultures. However, rules for displaying emotions may vary. In Japanese culture, the show of negative emotions is discouraged—it is more important to 'save face' for one's self and others than it is to express a negative emotion. There seems to be more eye contact between Arabs, South Americans and Greeks than between people from other cultures. The 'thumbs-up' gesture made by forming a closed fist and extending the thumb upwards usually indicates a sign of approval in Australia, but has sexual connotations in some Middle East and South American countries. Similarly, the 'okay' sign made by forming a circle with the thumb and finger in some countries, such as Russia, Germany or Brazil, can be a highly offensive gesture, referring to a bodily orifice.

People from Greece, Italy and South America come from high-contact cultures. They prefer closer distances, exhibit more touching behaviour and expect more touching behaviour than people from Australia and New Zealand. Men tend to require more space around them than women, and are more likely to use gestures, while women smile more often than men. Women also use their voices to communicate a wider range of emotions than do men.

CRITICAL THINKING QUESTIONS

1. What are the rules in your culture for the expression of emotion?
2. How might your preferences for interpersonal distance and touching behaviour influence your nursing care?

to the person, pacing yourself to be neither too fast nor too slow. Words that are slurred, have many syllables in them or are too technical make communication more difficult. Speaking too fast may overload a person and make it difficult for them to follow. Speaking too slowly may lose their attention.

Select the gestures you use with care, using your non-verbal behaviour to underscore your words and your actions. The proper use of gestures can clarify a message; however, be careful because, as discussed earlier in this chapter, not all gestures mean the same thing in all cultures, and so some body language may be offensive or misunderstood.

Listen to an individual's words and watch their gestures carefully. Do your best to understand and validate the meaning they have for you. Listening carefully to the person and their carers helps you avoid focusing on what you will say or do next, and demonstrates your genuine concern for a person's distress. The use of drawings, diagrams or written communication can be helpful to support the message you are trying to convey (Arnold & Boggs, 2015).

If a person attempts to speak English, their thoughts may appear distorted when language is the real problem. There have been a number of documented instances in which people have been diagnosed as mentally disordered and confined to a mental hospital because mental health professionals erroneously diagnosed a language problem or value difference as disordered thinking or psychosis. Use open-ended questions and rephrase them in several ways to obtain accurate information.

An interpreter may be necessary if language is a barrier, or you may be able to enlist the aid of a bilingual staff member. For the sake of confidentiality and privacy, avoid using family members as interpreters, as people may not want family members privy to personal information (Martin & Nakayama, 2012); for example, sexual preference, drug or alcohol use, or the content of hallucinations (what the voices say). Health and social services departments, Aboriginal liaison officers or cultural centres will often know of people who are willing to volunteer as interpreters. Most health care facilities have contracts with interpreter services using a variety of technologies (three-way phones, computers and videophone, etc.). Remember to always speak directly to the person and not to the interpreter.

Being aware of cultural phenomena that affect etiquette will be appreciated by the people you work with and can improve the therapeutic relationship. Spector (2009) suggests the following strategies:

1. Use the proper form of address for a given culture.
2. Know the ways by which people from that culture welcome one another; that is, when a handshake or embrace is expected, as well as when physical contact is prohibited.
3. Be aware of when smiling indicates friendliness or is taboo, and when eye contact is a sign of respect or aggression.
4. Remember that gestures do not have universal meaning.

Emphasising similarities can help to form a therapeutic relationship. Differences may serve as topics for discussion. An open, ongoing dialogue is beneficial for both parties, because it promotes understanding.

The culture of disability

When exploring cultural competency you will find little attention is given to those people with a disability, yet it is highly likely that within your practice you will encounter a person with disability, such as hearing loss, sight impairment, or intellectual or physical disability. For instance, figures show us that one in six Australians may experience some degree of hearing loss, with a projection that by 2050 this will have increased to one in four (Access Economics, 2006). When working with people with a disability, it is important to remember that each person will have different needs, and it is your responsibility to observe the uniqueness the person brings to the therapeutic relationship. It may be that a person who is sight-impaired is attuned to your voice, tone and noises in the surrounding environment, detecting subtle changes that a sighted person may not pick up. Similarly, the person who is hearing-impaired may be more focused on your non-verbal communication to convey information to them. If you fail to recognise and compensate for a person's disability, you risk miscommunication and a breakdown in the therapeutic relationship.

The following are some suggestions for communicating with a person who is deaf or hard of hearing, based on the work of Queensland Health (2008):

1. Choose an environment that is free of competing noise, such as television sets, radios and so on.
2. Provide continuous eye contact to keep the person engaged in the conversation. It can be construed as rude if eye contact is not maintained when communicating with a person who is deaf or hard of hearing.
3. Place yourself so that the person can see you clearly, preferably with light on your face.
4. Make sure your lips and face are visible throughout the communication, so that lip patterns and facial expressions can be observed.
5. Be aware of your facial expressions and body language, and use them freely to convey information.
6. Speak at a natural rate. People comprehend faster than they speak, so it is not necessary for you to slow down unless the person does not understand.
7. Make use of visual aids to help reach a shared understanding of what is being said.

The spoken word

Problems arise when we discover that words mean different things to different people. That is, *words* do not 'mean' something; *people* do. If communication between yourself and the person you are caring for is to be mutually negotiated in order to be understood by both of you, then you must understand the four concepts discussed next.

Denotation and connotation

A *denotative meaning* is the literal or restrictive meaning of the word. It is one that is in general use by most people who share a common language. A *connotative meaning* usually arises from a person's personal experience. That is, it has a personal and subjective meaning. While all Australians are likely to share the same general denotative meaning of the word *pig,* the word may have a completely different positive or negative connotation for a farmer, a consumer of meat, a person of the Muslim faith, someone who is Jewish, and a prisoner. For instance, '*pig*' used to be seen as an insult to police officers in Australia, yet many younger officers now place a positive connation on the word, and use it to describe the qualities pride, integrity and guts (P.I.G.) (Australian Federal Police, 2015).

Private and shared meanings

For communication to take place, meaning must be shared. People can use private meanings to communicate with others only when the parties agree about what the word means. The private meaning then becomes a shared meaning. It is common for families, friends or members of larger social groups (military personnel, drug users, adolescents) to use language in highly personal and private ways. Problems arise when the assumption is made that people who are outside the group share these meanings. For example, if you are not familiar with Australian slang, you will not know that 'crook' refers to a person being seriously ill, 'firies' is a term used for firefighters, and 'snags' refers to sausages. In Australia, contemporary slang between young people often derives from British and American counterparts in terms of idiom, due to the wide dissemination of pop culture, including movies, TV shows and music.

People with schizophrenia (refer to Chapter 14) may use language in an idiosyncratic way or may use a private, unshared language referred to as neologisms. Such people are unaware that others don't share this use of language. People who use neologisms, such as the young man in the following Practice Example, expect to be understood and may become upset when they are not.

In trying to make private meanings shared, make an effort to reach a mutual understanding of the person's message. It is insufficient, and quite possibly inaccurate, to attach meaning based solely on your (or the other person's) interpretation of an event, a word or phrase, or a gesture.

Practice example

A young man who was hospitalised at a mental health assessment unit complained to other consumers and staff members that he had been 'odenated', and he became increasingly frustrated and anxious when it became apparent that he wasn't being understood. Rather than simply writing him off as confused, his primary nurse recognised that 'odenated' most likely had a private meaning. With some help, he was able to explain that he was upset about having been moved to a different room. The room was, he said, so dark and dingy that it looked like a cave. Animals live in caves that are called 'dens'. In his view he had been o-den-ated—put into a cave.

Non-verbal messages

Most researchers agree that **non-verbal communication** channels carry more social meaning than spoken words. That is, chances are that people are making inferences about you based on your non-verbal communication (Stein-Parbury, 2013).

There is a wide variety of non-verbal channels: body movements, including facial expressions and hand gestures; the pitch, rate and volume of the voice; the use of personal and social space; touch; and the use of cultural artefacts (such as clothing, jewellery and cosmetics). Non-verbal cues help us judge the reliability of verbal messages more readily, especially in the presence of a **mixed message** (inconsistency between the verbal and non-verbal components), because non-verbal messages are the way we communicate our feelings and attitudes.

Body movement

The study of body movement as a form of non-verbal communication is called *kinaesics*. Facial expressions, gestures and eye movements are the most common categories.

Facial expressions are the single most important source of non-verbal communication. They generally communicate emotions. The silent-film comedians—blank-faced Buster Keaton and comic Charlie Chaplin—and the great mime Marcel Marceau communicate not only isolated acts but complete sequences of behaviour with kinaesics alone.

Body movements and gestures provide clues about people and about how they feel towards others. For example, hand gestures can communicate anxiety, indifference or impatience, among other things. Foot shuffling and fidgeting may express the desire to escape.

Body position gives cues about how open one person is to another person, or how interesting and attractive one person is to another. People tend to position their bodies according to their feelings about the person with whom they are communicating. Choosing to stand or sit close to another usually indicates attraction, whereas creating greater physical distance may signify an attempt at interpersonal distance.

Eye contact is another very important cue in communicating, and in most Western cultures several common but unstated rules about eye contact are as follows:

- Interaction is invited by staring at another person on the other side of the room. If the other person returns the gaze, the invitation to interact has been accepted. Averting the eyes signals a rejection of the looker's request.
- A person's frank gaze is widely interpreted as positive regard.
- Greater mutual eye contact occurs among friends.
- People who seek eye contact while speaking are usually perceived as believable and earnest.
- If the usual short, intermittent gazes during a conversation are replaced by gazes of longer duration, the person looked at is likely to believe that the person gazing considers the relationship between the two people to be more important than the content of the conversation.

It is good practice to keep in mind that non-verbal messages are often moderated by culture, in particular eye contact. For example, in some Aboriginal and Torres Strait Islander cultures, making direct eye contact can be disrespectful or confronting (O'Toole, 2012). The same is true for Maori and Pasifika cultures. Similarly, the cultural artefacts we observe when interacting with people can function as non-verbal stimuli: clothes, cosmetics, perfume, deodorants, jewellery, eyeglasses, body piercings, wigs and hairpieces, beards and mustaches, and so on.

Think about what information is communicated through artefacts such as a full-length mink coat, hair that is dyed purple, a gold band on the third finger of the left hand, or a military uniform.

Voice quality and non-language sounds

Voice quality, such as pitch and range, and non-language vocalisations, such as sobbing, laughing or grunting—noises without linguistic structure—are other components we use to make inferences about other people.

Vocal cues can differentiate emotions. Who hasn't heard the injunction: 'Don't speak to me in that tone of voice!'? Sometimes people use vocal cues to make inferences about personality traits. For example, people who increase the loudness, pitch, timbre (overtones), and rate of their speech are often thought to be active and dynamic. Those who use greater intonation and volume and are fluent are thought to be persuasive. Status cues in speech are based on a combination of word choice, pronunciation, grammar, speech fluency and articulation, among other factors.

Personal and social space

Being aware of your own and other people's personal space will help you build the therapeutic relationship. Individuals usually have some sense of their own personal space and when a person has overstepped these boundaries. This is often influenced by culture (O'Toole, 2012). Knowing something about proxemics—the study of how people use space—is useful, for example, in planning the physical space in which communication is to occur. You can arrange furniture to increase or decrease interpersonal distance. A cozy, open seating arrangement encourages interaction; chairs in a row that face the front of a room discourage interaction. It is important to be especially sensitive to the constraints imposed on communication by physical objects. An understanding of proxemics, coupled with paying attention to how others use interpersonal space, will enhance your ability to decipher verbal communication.

Practice example

Norma was an avid bingo player. She played at the same bingo hall almost every day. Norma always carved out her territory. She put her purse on the chair to her left, her bingo cards in the middle of the table, her snacks and beverages on the left side of the table, and her bingo markers on the right side of the table. In essence, Norma secured for herself the space normally shared by three people.

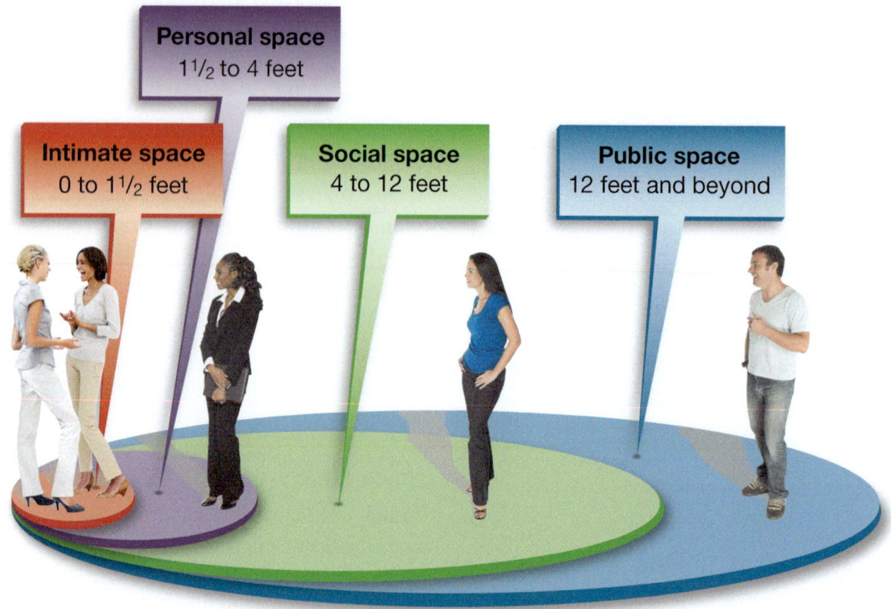

FIGURE 9.3 ■ Edward T. Hall's four zones of space.
Source: Beebe, S. A. (2011). *Interpersonal communication: Relating to others*. Upper Saddle River, NJ: Pearson Education, Figure 7-1, p. 200.

Figure 9.3 ■ illustrates the various relationships between intimacy and personal space.

Touch

Touching behaviours, because they tend to personalise communication, are extremely important in emotional situations. In Australian society, the use of touch is governed by strong social norms (Euson, 2012). Unwritten guidelines control who, when, why and where people touch. For example, Australian men are more uncomfortable with being touched by other men than women are with being touched by other women. Some people are high-touch-avoidance individuals—they simply do not like to be touched.

Most of the taboos against touching seem to stem from the sexual implications of touching behaviour. However, although touching is a physical act, it may or may not be sexual in nature. A realisation of the importance of touch, and an understanding that touching is not necessarily a sexual behaviour, may make this channel of communication available to more people. It is equally important to be sensitive to the other person's disposition towards touching, so as not to alienate another by infringing on the person's right not to be touched. The use of touch in therapeutic work is discussed in Chapters 2 and 4.

> **LIVED EXPERIENCE**
>
> **The kindness of human touch**
>
> There was a time when I was so very unwell, afraid of the world, very frightened that I would never be me again. At this time I was under the care of a young male consultant psychiatrist. One day when I was extremely distressed, he simply rested his hand on my shoulder, gave a gentle squeeze and said, 'All will be well, I will keep you safe.' That simple kindness of human touch spoke volumes—that I was cared about, he would be my protector and had my best interests at heart.

Verbal and non-verbal links

The verbal and non-verbal elements of human communication are inextricably linked. Six different ways in which verbal and non-verbal systems interrelate are discussed here.

1. A non-verbal cue may *repeat* a verbal cue, but in a different way. The deep-sea fisherman who verbally describes the size of the snapper he caught may also extend both hands to indicate its length. The gesture repeats the idea.
2. Non-verbal behaviour may also *contradict* verbal behaviour. Consider the woman who meets a college roommate she hasn't seen for some time. She says, 'You haven't changed a bit', but her tone of voice and facial expression convey sarcasm. When verbal and non-verbal cues contradict one another, it is usually safer to put more faith in the non-verbal cues.
3. Non-verbal messages may *add to or modify* verbal messages. When a man says he is a 'little' irritated about being kept waiting, his tone of voice and body actions may indicate a more profound anger.

4. Certain non-verbal cues *accent or emphasise* verbal cues. A woman shrugs her shoulder when she says she doesn't really care which movie she and her companion see. A master of ceremonies holds up his hand when he asks for quiet. These gestures and body movements emphasise the words.
5. Cues that *regulate,* such as those that tell people when to start talking or when to stop talking, are usually non-verbal. A woman who keeps opening and closing her mouth briefly while others are talking is indicating that she wants a turn to speak, too.
6. Sometimes non-verbal cues are used to *substitute* for words. A wave from a friend at a distance replaces 'hello'. Applause at the end of a play tells the actors that they have pleased the audience.

BIOPSYCHOSOCIAL THEORIES AND MODELS OF HUMAN COMMUNICATION

Communication takes place on at least three different levels: intrapersonal, interpersonal and public (such as communication through the mass media or giving a public speech). Mental health nurses are more concerned with intrapersonal and interpersonal communication. **Intrapersonal communication** occurs when a person communicates within themselves. It is a way for a person to reflect or clarify things within their own mind. When you walk into a consumer's room and think 'That jug of water is almost finished. I'd better get a fresh one', you are communicating intrapersonally. **Interpersonal communication**, which this chapter discusses in depth, takes place between two or more people. This level of person-to-person communication respects each other's role and what they offer to the communication process. Within a best practice framework, this is at the heart of mental health nursing.

One of the easiest ways to illustrate the nature and process of human communication is through a model, or visual representation. Models of communication continue to evolve from the 1960s, but there remains great value in exploring some of the classic communication models to highlight key issues in interpersonal communication.

People use models frequently for many purposes. They might use a map or their navigation system, which are visual representations of a geographical location, to find their way to the community mental health centre they plan to visit. However, models provide an incomplete view—a map does not show all of the trees, buildings or park statues in the area. It is important to keep this in mind when looking at models. They sometimes make a process look simpler than it is.

Symbolic interactionist model

A symbolic interactionist model, named by Herbert Blumer in 1969 (Heath & Bryant, 2013), is based on a transactional perspective. It views human communication on the social–interpersonal level, and accounts for the whole persons involved in the process. Communication is viewed as a process of simultaneous mutual influence, rather than as a turn-taking event. The participants are products of their social system and integral parts of it. In the communication, some events take place *within* the participants (they are intrapersonal), and some take place *between* the participants (they are interpersonal).

Participants are who they are in relationship to the other person with whom they are communicating. For example, in this dyadic (two-person) communication event between Jeff and Sarah, there are at least *six* perceptions involved:

1. Jeff's perception of himself
2. Jeff's perception of Sarah
3. Jeff's impression of the way Sarah sees him
4. Sarah's perception of herself
5. Sarah's perception of Jeff
6. Sarah's impression of the way Jeff sees her.

Therefore, in addition to the *content* message, a *relationship* message also exists. Suppose Jeff passes Sarah in the corridor and Jeff says, 'Hi, how are you?' Sarah answers, 'Just fine, thanks', but moves down the corridor and away from Jeff as quickly as possible, and without reciprocating the greeting. Their subsequent communication will be affected by whether Jeff perceives Sarah as walking away because she wanted to get home before a rainstorm, or because he believes that Sarah is angry with him and her behaviour is a comment on their relationship. The transactional model of the communication process illustrated in Figure 9.4 ■ helps explain what takes place between Jeff and Sarah.

A transactional approach is based on systems theory, which was discussed in Chapter 5. Recall that a system is a set of interconnected elements in which a change in any one element affects all of the other elements. Therefore, in a transactional model of human communication, a change in any aspect of the communication system can influence all of the other elements in the system. Note in Figure 9.4 that both individuals are the source of communication as well as the receiver of communication, and that messages involve feedback (the response to the message) as well as context (the psychological as well as the physical environment for communication). Note, also, that both individuals send and receive messages at the same time. Their communication is not linear and it is complex, because all of the components occur simultaneously. Every element of communication is connected to every other element of communication.

Let us say that Jeff is attracted to Sarah and would like to get to know her better. Jeff first scans the information about himself and others (Jeff enjoys movies and remembers hearing Sarah tell a friend that she'd really like to see one particular movie), and then mentally rehearses possible actions to take (*role-playing*), and possible reactions of the other (*role-taking*). This gives Jeff the chance to think of four or five different ways to approach Sarah. In this rehearsal phase, Jeff decides what to say, how to say it, and even whether to send the message to Sarah at all. His decision is to ask Sarah to the movie.

Jeff's message ('Would you like to go to the movie with me?') serves as a stimulus for Sarah. Sarah thinks about Jeff's invitation, decides whether she wants to go to the movie with him, and considers what response to make to Jeff. Sarah's response provides feedback and serves as a stimulus for Jeff, and the interaction continues. Feedback (Sarah's response)

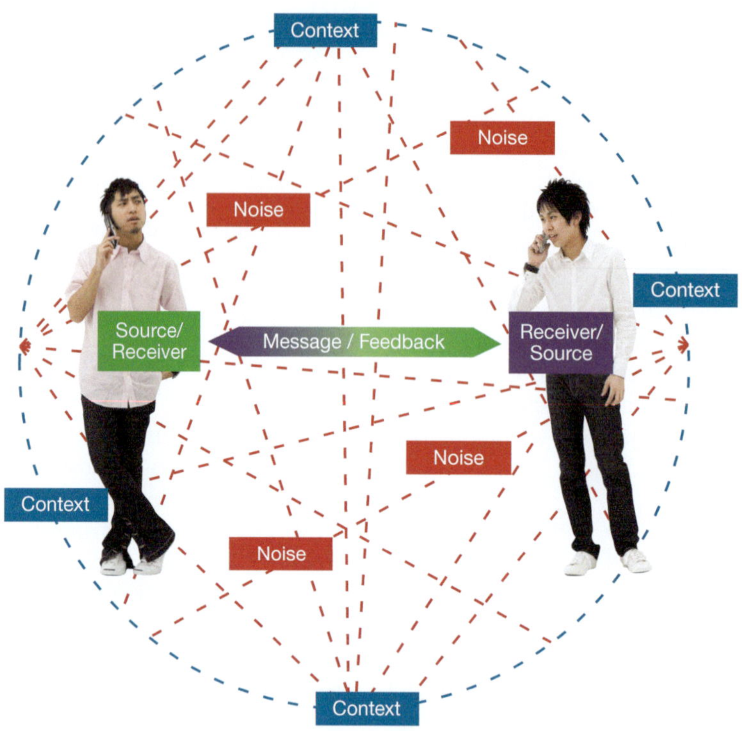

FIGURE 9.4 ■ A model for communication as a mutual transaction.
Source: Beebe, S. A. (2011). *Interpersonal communication: Relating to others*. Upper Saddle River, NJ: Pearson Education, Figure 1-3, p. 11.

allows the person an opportunity to determine whether they have made an error in the approach to the other, and to make appropriate corrections. Jeff carefully considers Sarah's response. He listens to what she says and watches her behaviour towards him. If her response is less than enthusiastic, he will try to determine what went wrong and how to correct it.

In summary, the transactional view of communication includes the following concepts:

- People run through a series of internal trials in the process of organising a message.
- People select and transmit the message that will, in their view, have the highest probability of success.
- Success depends on the accuracy and completeness of the cognitive map, and the accuracy and efficiency of the intrapersonal and interpersonal feedback loops.
- Communication is a dynamic (ever-changing) process that is unrepeatable and irreversible.
- Communication is complex.
- The meaning of messages is not transferred; it is mutually negotiated. Communication is, at the very least, a very complicated process.

Neurobiological factors

Looking at communication in its broadest sense requires us to go beyond the spoken word, the written word and motor activity to the molecular level. In this broad view, communication can also be thought of as the movement of neurotransmitters within a synapse between neurons. Communibiology researchers, such as Beatty and McCrosky, believe that energy and movement at the molecular level may be the root of all brain functioning, including communication (Littlejohn & Foss, 2011).

The neuron, the functional unit of the brain, differs from other cells in the body in that it is specialised for the function of information processing. The flow of information from one nerve cell to another involves the passage across the cell membrane of the neuron of electrically-charged chemical particles—sodium, potassium, calcium and chloride. Neurotransmitters released by the presynaptic membrane of the axon cross the synaptic cleft, and bind to their receptors on the postsynaptic membrane of the dendrite of the target cell. This process is more fully described in Chapter 6.

Therefore, brain activity can also be thought of in terms of messages and receptors. It makes sense to acknowledge that when communication is disrupted at one level—for example, when a crucial chemical in the brain undergoes an alteration—the end result can be felt at other, more obvious communication levels of the individual (such as verbal and non-verbal communication, and intrapersonal and interpersonal communication). To put this into perspective, your understanding of the words on this page is related not only to your understanding of written English, but also to the chloride ion channel activity on the membranes of millions of your brain cells.

The neurobiology of human communication is very complex and not yet fully understood. For example, we know that there is a speech circuit in the brain between the auditory cortex on the left, which passes to Wernicke's area in the temporal cortex, and from there to Broca's area in the left frontal lobe via the arcuate fasciculus (a pathway composed

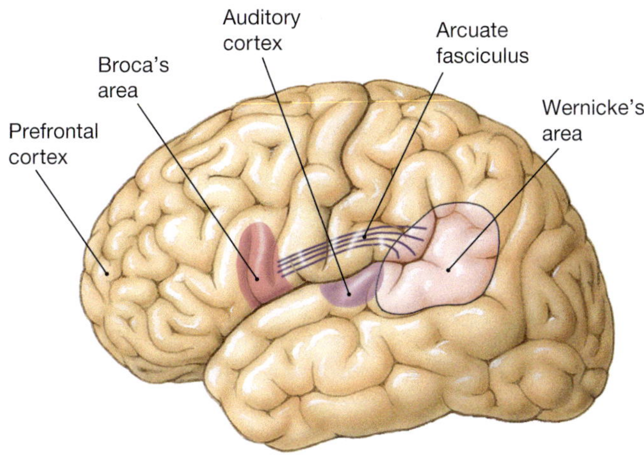

FIGURE 9.5 ■ The speech circuit.
Source: Smock, T. K. (1999). *Physiological psychology: A neuroscience approach.* Upper Saddle River, NJ: Prentice Hall.

mainly of axons that synapse with other neurons). This speech circuit is detailed in Figure 9.5 ■.

However, knowing about the speech circuit does not go far enough in explaining the complexities of the neurobiological basis of human communication. Some elements of the communication process are distributed more widely in the brain than was previously believed. To add to the complexity, these areas are not the same in all of us. Therefore, there is no specific map of the brain that can locate specific communication functions with absolute certainty. Nor does it mean that damage in a specific region will necessarily cause a deficiency in a function thought to be contained in that region.

Therapeutic communication theory

In the view of psychiatrist Jurgen Ruesch (1961), communication includes all of the processes by which one human being influences another. Ruesch's theory takes into account the perceptions and interpretations that influence one person's view of the other. Further, Ruesch assumes that, to survive, the individual must communicate successfully.

According to Ruesch, communication is one of the most difficult human skills to master. It takes a long time to learn because it occurs in a series of steps, each building on the previous one. To communicate effectively requires decades of continuous practice. It is believed that interference hampers development and leaves an indelible mark.

Basic concepts

The basic concepts of Ruesch's theory are as follows:

- Communication occurs in four different settings: intrapersonal, interpersonal, group and societal.
- The ability to receive, evaluate and transmit messages is influenced by perception, evaluation (which involves memory, past experiences and value systems), and the transmission quality of messages (amount, speed, efficacy and distinctiveness).
- Messages achieve meaning when they are mutually validated or verified between the two parties.
- Correction through feedback is basic to adaptive, healthy behaviour and successful communication.

Successful versus disturbed communication

The four formal criteria for successful communication are efficiency, appropriateness, flexibility and feedback. When these criteria are not met, communication is disturbed (Ruesch & Bateson, 1968).

Efficiency

Simplicity, clarity and correct timing are all components of efficient messages. Mental health nurses and other health professionals may find themselves using complex and scientific words or health jargon to convey messages that without a shared meaning do nothing to promote understanding of the message (O'Kane, 2013a). Obscure or clumsy language and irrelevant or useless information may also prevent others from understanding a message. Clear messages give a sense of order or structure, and reduce ambiguity by narrowing the number of possible interpretations of meaning.

Proper timing is also important. It is best to give messages when the other person is able to 'hear' them, when there are no intervening noises or inputs, and when the other person can interpret them without undue haste. Problems occur if the interval between the messages is either too short or too long.

Appropriateness

Messages are appropriate when they are relevant to the situation at hand, and when there is mutual fit of overall patterns and constituent parts. Communication is inappropriate when it does not fit the circumstance, is irrelevant or is misconstrued.

Communication can also be inappropriate in amount. Because every individual has both high and low tolerance levels for stimulation, a person's ability to cope with ideas, make decisions and act is affected by the amount and rate of sensory input received. Exceeding a tolerance level is called **overload**. A person who is overloaded by too many messages or by messages too closely spaced cannot handle incoming messages. **Underload** occurs when a delay or lack of information interferes with a person's ability to comprehend the message of another. Check out the example of 'overload' as explained in Lived Experience on the following page.

The **tangential reply** is another example of inappropriateness. A tangential reply to a statement disregards the content of the message, and is directed towards an incidental aspect of the initial statement, the type of language used, the emotions of the sender, or another facet of the same topic. It indicates that the other person is not attending to your message.

Flexibility

People cannot always be sure how a message will be received, because each person with whom they communicate is unique and changing. Because they cannot expect constancy from others, people need to be flexible. In communication, lack of flexibility manifests itself as either exaggerated control or exaggerated permissiveness. Both extremes increase the likelihood of frustrating, ungratifying, disturbed or ineffectual communication.

LIVED EXPERIENCE

'I became completely overwhelmed'

Recently, I was put in the position of making the decision to lodge an application for guardianship for a family member to the South Australian Civil and Administrative Tribunal (SACAT) due an extremely high level of family conflict. The tribunal refers applications to the Office of the Public Advocate (OPA) for family mediation. I was extremely anxious about lodging an application, as having been under guardianship under the SA Mental Health Act I am strongly opposed to forced care. At the SACAT office, I had to deal with a number of different people, all giving me different information and instructions. I became completely overwhelmed. I became so anxious I ceased to be able to make any sense of the interactions and the process I was required to follow.

Maintaining flexibility can be difficult if doing so requires a person to abandon or temporarily lay aside a carefully planned goal. To be flexible, a person must have the ability to set new priorities and to move to meet immediate goals. Nurses who practise humanistic and person-centred care will achieve flexibility in their relationships with those they care for and for their carers, and with colleagues.

Feedback

Feedback is the response to the message (Beebe, 2011). It is the process by which performance is checked and malfunctions corrected. It performs a regulatory function in the communication process. One example of how feedback can help to correct a system malfunction is illustrated in Evidence-based Practice. Feedback allows people to decide which messages have been understood as intended. It requires the cooperation of two people—one to give it and one to receive it. Giving helpful feedback is discussed further later in this chapter.

Under certain circumstances of ineffective communication, feedback either fails or functions poorly. When messages do not get through or are distorted, appropriate replies cannot be obtained, and corrective feedback does not occur. Content that elicits anxiety, fear, shame or any of several other strong emotions is likely to hamper feedback.

EVIDENCE-BASED PRACTICE

Feedback helps create a more human setting

Julie Pilatapa, a registered nurse in the emergency department of a large hospital, has been concerned because of the unfavourable evaluations left in the comment box by visitors to the department. Although the waiting room has been newly remodelled and has comfortable seating, visitors to the department feel they are ignored for long periods of time while waiting to be seen. Their view of the staff is that staff members are very busy and seem to be working very hard. This doesn't seem to make up for the visitors' feelings that nurses and other staff are emotionally distant or 'just there to do a job'. The majority of visitors believe they have waited longer to be seen than what the documented records show; for them, time seems to pass very slowly.

Julie believes the emergency department staff should be rated as highly as the physical environment. To achieve this goal, Julie has come up with the following plan, which she presented to her colleagues in their weekly meeting:

1. Provide a staff member presence at intermittent intervals—a nurse attuned to the person's needs and concerns related to their condition or to their care, and a volunteer to assist visitors with other questions or concerns, such as those relating to waiting times, transportation, hospital admission and so on.
2. Provide relaxing music, educational videos, books and puzzles, magazines and newspapers, and games for visitors' use.

   The volunteer would be responsible for maintaining these activities.

Julie's rationale for her proposal is that providing more than a physical presence in the waiting room avoids the perception that staff members are emotionally distant or just there to do a job and, in conjunction with the additional activities, transforms a technical, potentially impersonal setting into a more human place. Her rationale is based on knowledge she has gained from several research articles, including:

Bost, N., Crilly J., & Wallen, K. (2014). Characteristics and process outcomes of patients presenting to an Australian emergency department for mental health and non-mental health diagnoses. *International Emergency Nursing, 22*(3), 146–152.

Broadbent, M., Moxham, L., & Dwyer T. (2014). Implications of the emergency department triage environment on triage practice for clients with a mental illness at triage in an Australian context. *Australasian Emergency Nursing, 17*(1), 23–29.

Shafiei, T., Gaynor, N., & Farrell, G. (2011). The characteristics, management and outcomes of people identified with mental health issues in an emergency department, Melbourne, Australia. *Journal of Psychiatric and Mental Health Nursing, 18*(1), 9–16.

CRITICAL THINKING QUESTIONS

1. What personal steps could busy nurses take to reduce the emotional distance between themselves and consumer and/or themselves and carers?
2. Consumers and carers waiting to be seen in an emergency department often feel anxious. If anxiety is interpersonally communicated, what staff behaviours in this example could add to their anxiety?
3. Which verbal and non-verbal therapeutic communication skills are likely to help reduce their anxiety?

Behavioural effects and human communication theory

Watzlawick, Beavin and Jackson (1967) base their theory of human communication on the assumption that communication is synonymous with interaction. These authors maintain that, in the presence of another, all behaviour is communicative. This theory is concerned with the pragmatics, or the behavioural effects, of human interaction. What makes this theory particularly useful to you is its conception of human communication as a reciprocal process.

Communication levels

According to this theory, one cannot *not* communicate. Both activity and inactivity, verbalisations and silences, convey messages. This communication occurs on two levels. The *content level* of a communication is the report aspect, in which information is conveyed. The *relationship level* is communication about a communication.

All interchanges can be viewed as either *symmetric* (based on equality) or *complementary* (based on difference). In symmetric relationships, the partners usually mirror each other's behaviour, thus minimising difference. Complementary relationships, in contrast, maximise difference.

Communication disturbances

Communication can be disturbed when a person attempts *not* to communicate. As an example, in this framework, the basic dilemma occurs when a person attempts not to communicate. However, because it is impossible not to communicate, the attempt to not communicate is a communication in itself.

Another disturbance occurs when a person communicates in a way that invalidates the messages sent to or received from the other person. Such communications, called *disqualifications,* include a wide range of behaviour such as self-contradictions, inconsistencies, subject switches, incomplete sentences and misunderstandings.

A person may communicate in a way that confirms, rejects or *disconfirms* the other person's view of self. Confirmation of one person's self-view by another is thought to be the greatest single factor in ensuring healthy mental development and stability. Rejection of the other's definition of self essentially conveys this message: 'You're wrong.' Disconfirmation causes others to value themselves less by conveying this message: 'You don't exist.' Disconfirmation questions the other's authenticity. Disconfirmation leads to alienation, and has been found to occur with some regularity in the experiences of people with schizophrenia.

Although all relationships are necessarily either symmetric or complementary, *runaways* (exaggerations to the point of disturbance) may occur in either of the patterns. For example, the danger of competitiveness is ever-present in symmetric relationships. Symmetric interactions that lose their stability may enter a spiral in which each individual attempts to be just a little bit 'more equal' than the other. Runaways are seen in quarrels between people or wars between nations, behaviours that are relatively open. Rejection of the other's self generally occurs when a symmetric relationship breaks down. Breakdowns in complementary relationships, however, are generally characterised by disconfirmation of the other. For this reason, they are usually viewed as more serious (Watzlawick, Beavin Bavelas, Jackson & O'Hanlon, 2011).

Neurolinguistic programming theory

Neurolinguistic programming (NLP) is a communication model developed in the early 1970s by Richard Bandler and John Grinder. The model is derived from theory in linguistics, neurophysiology, psychology, cybernetics and psychiatry (Bandler, 1993).

Bandler and Grinder concluded that people take in, or *access,* information via their sensory modalities, but have a preferred representational system, usually involving one of the following three principle senses:

1. visual
2. auditory
3. kinaesthetic.

These are often referred to as 'VAK'. Further, each person prefers one mode over the others. Sounds may facilitate communication with one person, while sight or touch may be more effective with another person. In addition, people process information, or make sense out of it, according to the representational system (the NLP phrase for 'sensory modality') through which they receive it (O'Connor & Seymour, 2011).

Bandler and Grinder also found that the expert communicators they observed were able to adapt themselves to match a person's representational system, and to imitate the client in a natural and respectful way. They theorised that, by tuning into and then using the other person's preferred sensory mode, one could greatly enhance the ability to establish rapport. The most effective communicators, according to NLP theory, are those who can use all three modalities and easily move from one representational system to another.

Determining the sensory modality

To determine whether a person's representational system or sensory modality is auditory, visual or kinaesthetic, one identifies the person's:

- preferred predicates (verbs, adjectives, adverbs that tell something about the subject)
- eye-accessing cues
- gross hand movements
- breathing pattern
- speech pattern and voice tones.

Preferred predicates A necessary first step before attempting to link words with non-verbal behaviour is observing a person to see which set of predicates is preferred. A sample of preferred predicates of the auditory, visual and kinaesthetic types is listed in the following Your Assessment Approach.

Eye-accessing cues Eye-accessing cues correlate with an individual's thinking process. People who are visualising generally turn their eyes upward or look straight ahead,

YOUR ASSESSMENT APPROACH

Preferred predicates

Auditory	Visual	Kinaesthetic
Argue	Appear	Attach
Chant	Bright	Breathless
Debate	Colourful	Calm
Eavesdrop	Glimpse	Excite
Hassle	Image	Fondle
Hear	Observe	Hurt
Listen	Pretty	Rough
Overhear	Scan	Sharp
Praise	Sight	Soft
Quiet	Spy	Sore
Scream	Stare	Support
Silent	Ugly	Tension
Tell	View	Throw
Whine	Watch	Touch
Whisper	Wink	Warm

focusing on nothing. Someone processing auditory information usually moves the eyes from side to side. A person engaging in intrapersonal communication usually focuses the eyes down in the direction of the non-dominant hand. A person in the kinaesthetic mode looks down towards the dominant hand when experiencing sensations or emotions.

Gross hand movements Gross hand movements also give clues to an individual's sensory mode. People have a tendency to point towards or touch the sense organ that matches their current sensory mode. The person in a visual mode often points towards the eye, and the person in an auditory mode often points towards or touches the ear.

Breathing pattern Assessing the breathing pattern helps the observer understand a person's representational model. Shallow, thoracic breathing is often associated with visual accessing. Even breathing or prolonged expiration is associated with auditory accessing, and deep abdominal breathing is associated with kinaesthetic accessing.

Speech pattern and voice tones Visual accessing often correlates with quick bursts of words that are high-pitched, strained or nasal. Auditory accessing is often associated with a clear, mid-range voice tone, or with a rhythmic tempo and clearly enunciated words. Kinaesthetic accessing is associated with a slow voice and a low volume or deep tone, or with a breathy tone and long pauses.

Therapeutic use of NLP

Using NLP theory in mental health nursing practice can enhance our interactions with the people we are caring for and their carers (Thomson & Menzies, 2010). It gives us yet another way to empathise with individuals by 'trying on' their style. People tend to be less anxious with the familiar. Those of us who mirror the consumer's sensory mode are likely to be experienced as more comfortable and safer to be with, conditions that facilitate rapport.

We can use mirroring to help a person follow our lead. For example, with a person experiencing anxiety, we might begin by mirroring the behaviours that indicate their anxiety and then shift into a more relaxed posture and less anxious behaviours. It is easier to lead an individual from a more anxious state to a less anxious state by employing the NLP principles discussed here; however, there is little research to evidence the use of NLP and its effects on health outcomes (Sturt et al., 2012).

An important benefit of the NLP approach is that it allows us to assess a person's style and preferred sensory mode, and to communicate more effectively by using both verbal and non-verbal communication in an individual's preferred mode. The following examples express the same nursing intervention with different predicates, depending on the person's preferred mode:

Visual—'Yes, I can *see* that you are much better. You *look* good, your eyes are *clear,* your *appearance* has certainly changed.'

Auditory—'Yes, I can *hear* from the *sound* of your voice that you are better. *Talking* with you today is quite different from yesterday.'

Kinaesthetic—'Yes, you do seem to be *feeling* much better today—you are *holding* your head up, and your *grasp* is certainly *firmer* than yesterday.'

By expanding our abilities to communicate with people in all three modes, we can become more effective communicators.

FACILITATING COMMUNICATION AND BUILDING A RELATIONSHIP

Therapeutic communication aims at initiating, building and maintaining fulfilling and trusting relationships with other people. Communicating ideas and feelings with clarity, efficiency and appropriateness helps a person to be interpersonally effective. In reading the rest of this chapter, try to relate the therapeutic communication principles and practices discussed earlier to these ideas about facilitating communication.

Don't forget about using appropriate non-verbal skills. Your verbal and non-verbal messages should be consistent with one another. Non-verbal messages should enhance, not detract from, verbal messages. Self-awareness, next page, presents some guidelines for you in achieving this goal.

Superficiality versus intimacy

Most relationships between people begin at the level of social superficiality. In a nurse–consumer relationship, we try to develop therapeutic intimacy. This differs from the social intimacy you experience with partners, family and friends. For example, the interdependence that characterises the social relationship is greatly reduced. In social relationships, participants may 'tell their stories' to one another. In relationships that have therapeutic goals, only the consumer

SELF-AWARENESS
Guidelines for improving non-verbal communication

1. ***Relax.*** The simple act of relaxing makes it easier for others to be relaxed and more open. Remember, anxiety is interpersonally communicated. Take some deep breaths, do a quick body scan, and allow the tension to flow out of your body (see Chapter 8 for further information on relaxation techniques).
2. ***Use facial, hand and body gestures judiciously.*** Non-verbal gestures that are used indiscriminately lose their effectiveness. Overdoing a gesture—constantly smiling, constantly nodding your head—may become annoying to others and make it more difficult for them to talk with you.
3. ***Ask for feedback on your non-verbal communication.*** Your classmates, colleagues and instructors are sources of feedback. Ask them to comment on the facial expressions and body gestures that you use when you converse with them. Consider being videotaped so that you can see for yourself any mannerisms or gestures that intrude on your ability to be an effective communicator.
4. ***Practise.*** Once you have identified any intrusive facial expressions or body gestures, practise blending your verbal message with appropriate non-verbal cues, such as hand gestures, body posture, facial expression and tone of voice. Then role-play with your classmates, and ask them to comment on your effectiveness.

is engaged in storytelling with the nurse. The process is specifically focused. The person not only explains themselves, the events of their lives and the circumstances they face, but they do so with a purpose in mind—understanding the circumstances through exploring them and moving to improve their lives.

LIVED EXPERIENCE
The eyes are the mirrors of the soul

When unwell and heavily medicated, it is not always possibly to find the words to express your feelings and concerns. Medication also blunts facial expressions, slows thoughts and impacts on one's thinking and flow of speech. However, a person's eyes will express anger, sadness, fear, disinterest, comprehension, confusion, distrust and dislike—all emotions which cannot be controlled or hidden. Communication occurs on many different levels. A consumer experienced with the counselling process will have the knowledge and skill to manage their tone of voice, facial expressions, and hand and body movements, but the eyes are 'the mirrors of the soul'.

Movement towards therapeutic intimacy may be difficult at first. For one thing, such intimacy violates certain social taboos. For example, at a party it may be socially incorrect to comment on a person's anxiety, stuttering or facial tic. When communication has a therapeutic goal, all messages, including these non-verbal ones, are heeded and may be discussed. Therapeutic intimacy also requires that the participants move beyond social 'chitchat' into meaningful areas of concern for the person seeking help. Therapeutic intimacy requires high involvement and commitment.

Facilitating intimacy

Several interpersonal principles and practices are essential to facilitating intimacy.

Responding with empathy

Most theorists believe that empathy is the most important dimension in the helping process. Without a high level of empathic understanding, nurses have no real basis for helping. Empathy facilitates interpersonal exploration, as listening alone is often not enough. Empathic understanding not only increases your grasp of a person's difficulties, but also helps you offer feedback on how the person affects others. Empathy can best be understood as a process through which people feel with one another. They are able to sense the feelings of another because they have evoked in themselves the attitude of the person to whom they are relating (in other words, they have engaged in role-taking). Central to learning the skill of empathising is embracing the idea that what the person has to say or what the person feels is important (to them) and deserves acknowledgment. A recent study of what it means to individuals with mental illness to be understood revealed that understanding their perspective is central to forming a relationship. It promotes a connection with the person, and validates their importance (Gerace, O'Kane, Hayman, & Muir-Cochrane, 2012).

Empathic involvement with troubled consumers can have a number of stressful consequences. Problems can arise at any phase in the empathy process. The obstacles to achieving an empathic concern for people can be understood as a failure to cope with one of the four phases of achieving empathy. These four phases are discussed in Box 9.1. Be careful not to over-identify and lapse into sympathy for the person. By doing so, you may fail to incorporate the individual's feelings and instead project personal ones. Bypassing the reverberation phase and substituting gut-level intuitions for rational problem-solving can be another problem. Be sure to guard against over-distancing or burnout.

The term *empathy* is often mistakenly used synonymously with *sympathy*. Empathy contains no elements of condolence, agreement or pity. When we sympathise rather than empathise, we assume that there is a parallel between our feelings and those of the person. The perceived similarity makes professional judgment and objectivity difficult. Sympathy can also be an appropriate response given the right circumstances. What Every Nurse Should Know discusses how to respond appropriately with sympathy.

Box 9.1 Phases of therapeutic empathising

According to Reik (1949), the process of empathic understanding has four phases:

1. ***Identification.*** Through the relaxation of conscious controls, we allow ourselves to become absorbed in contemplating the person and their experiences.
2. ***Incorporation.*** We take in the experiences of the person rather than attribute our own experiences and feelings to the situation.
3. ***Reverberation.*** We interplay the internalised feelings of the person and our own experiences or fantasies. While fully absorbed in the person's identity, we still experience ourselves as separate personalities.
4. ***Detachment.*** We withdraw from subjective involvement and totally resume our own identity. We use the insight gained from the reverberation phase, as well as reason and objectivity, to offer responses that are useful to the person.

(Clark, 2014)

Responding with respect

Responding with respect demonstrates that you value the integrity of the person, and have faith in their ability to solve problems, given appropriate help. By encouraging them to put forward possible plans of action, you convey respect for their ability to take charge of their own recovery. Giving advice, by contrast, conveys a directly opposite message.

Responding with genuineness

Genuineness refers to the ability to be real or honest with another. To be effective, genuineness must be timed properly and based on a solid relationship. Honesty is not always the best policy, especially if it is brutal or if the person or their carer is not capable of dealing with it. You cannot pretend to be genuine, since your behaviour, mannerisms and non-verbals will come across as patronising, false and insincere. The nurse who is genuine is more likely to deal with and eventually help the person they are caring for resolve all problems, rather than just those that are safe or socially acceptable.

Responding with immediacy

Responding with immediacy means responding to what is happening between the person and yourself in the here-and-now. Because this dimension may involve the feelings of the person towards you, it can be one of the most difficult to achieve. For example, the person or their carer may confront you with overt or implied criticism of your role or competence. If you respond in a defensive or evasive way, the relationship may be threatened. If you are open, reasonable and concerned, the relationship may be strengthened.

Responding with warmth

Warmth is so closely linked with empathy and respect that it is seldom communicated as an independent dimension. It is important, however, to note some additional points about the expression of warmth. Effusive, chatty, 'buddy-buddy' behaviour should not be confused with warmth. Warmth is most often conveyed in communications of respect and empathy.

Be aware of, and accept, a person's right to maintain distance (refer back to Figure 9.3 on page 178). Warmth and intimacy cannot be forced. Initially, high levels of warmth can be counterproductive for people who have received little warmth from others in their lives, are suspicious, or have been taken advantage of by others. Warmth alone is insufficient for building a relationship and solving problems.

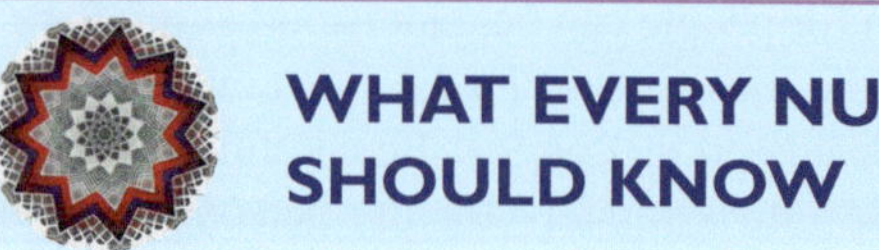

Expressing sympathy to the bereaved

Although empathising is preferable to sympathising when you are serving in a professional role, there are occasions in which sympathy is not only appropriate, but helpful. One such example is when someone in your care dies, or a friend, colleague or acquaintance has just lost a loved one, and you wish to reach out and offer support to the bereaved individual or family. Many people worry about finding the right words, or worry that they will say the wrong thing. It is hard to go wrong if you are sincere in offering support. Remember that non-verbal messages enhance verbal messages, and your sincerity when acknowledging the bereaved person's feelings will temper any words that are not quite perfect.

THERAPEUTIC COMMUNICATION SKILLS

Think of the communication techniques presented here as having the potential to foster effective communication. These are often referred to as *micro-skills*. You must make them your own and adapt them individually for each human encounter. Blend them with the understanding you have gained from the interpersonal communication principles and practices discussed earlier in this chapter, and the dimensions of self-knowledge that you examined in Chapter 4.

Be aware that using a set of communication skills as a sort of relationship 'magic' will probably doom you to failure. Relationships, and the people in them, are unique and much too complex to rely on a communication formula that can be applied to all people and all situations. Remember that a holistic approach is inconsistent with the rigid, inflexible application of communication techniques.

Active listening

Most of us assume that we are good listeners. The truth is that **active listening** requires *mindful* listening, which is more difficult than you might think. Mindfulness is the ability to consciously think about what you are doing and experiencing. It is more than being quiet while the other person talks—it requires paying undivided attention to what each person says, does and feels, by putting aside your own judgments and ideas long enough to really hear. Mindful listening requires intention—that is, when you intend to really hear what another is saying, the better you can understand that person and their needs. If you don't listen mindfully, you won't be able to comprehend the message. If you don't comprehend the message, you will not be able to effectively use the therapeutic communication techniques that follow.

There are several blocks to listening that may prevent you from hearing what a consumer is saying, and instead convey the message that what they are saying is not very important:

1. *Rehearsing:* Being too busy planning what you are going to say next.
2. *Being concerned with yourself*—your intelligence, your level of competence, your feelings or your accomplishments.
3. *Assuming:* Thinking that you know what a person 'really means' because of your assumptions and hunches.
4. *Judging:* Framing what you hear or what you see in terms of your judgment of an individual as being wrong, immature, anxious, paranoid or depressed.
5. *Identifying:* Focusing on your own similar experiences, feelings or beliefs when what the person says triggers your own memories or concerns.
6. *Getting off track:* Changing the subject or making light of it when you become uncomfortable, bored or tired.
7. *Filtering:* Tuning out certain topics or hearing only certain things, perhaps because of anxiety, regardless of what else is said.

Mindful listening is best accomplished when environmental distractions are minimised. Consider finding a quiet place, turning off the television, or closing the door if it is appropriate and safe. Avoid taking notes, but if necessary make sure you make brief notes so that you don't take your attention away from the person for too long and miss some of what is being said on the verbal level and being done on the non-verbal level.

Face the person, use eye contact, show interest and listen objectively, while minimising your own personal responses. Remaining silent while people express themselves is a sign of respect and interest. Avoid interrupting because you feel the need to say or do something. Specific circumstances in which it is appropriate, for therapeutic reasons, to interrupt the person or steer the conversation in another direction may be required when trying to collect particular information or require a person to focus on a specific question.

When listening, pay attention not only to what a person says (the verbal communication) but also to what the person does and how the person looks (the non-verbal communication). Non-verbal cues often shed light on what is being said. Although listening enables you to observe an individual's non-verbal messages, it does not follow that you will necessarily interpret the non-verbal cues accurately. You should validate non-verbal cues with the person to clarify meaning and understanding.

Using silence

Do not feel obligated to respond after every statement a person makes. *Using silence* goes beyond mindful listening and can be a very effective therapeutic technique. Remaining silent and not responding can encourage a person to continue speaking, can provide time to ponder what has been said, allowing the person to make possible connections, allows time for them to collect their thoughts, and to consider alternatives. Looking interested while maintaining an open posture or a questioning look will encourage the person you are working with to use the time effectively.

If a silence becomes uncomfortable, then it advisable to take a break and analyse what might be occurring in the therapeutic relationship. You would not want the person to become increasingly anxious or resistive. (See Chapter 2 for suggestions on handling resistance.)

Remember, silence is an effective communication technique only when it is used as an appropriate and purposeful therapeutic intervention. For example, people experiencing depression and feeling pressured to interact will benefit from your silent, undemanding presence. Nurses who are silent because they are uncomfortable, or because they lack the knowledge or the skill to communicate effectively, must seek an experienced clinical supervisor to help them analyse their own personal and professional needs.

Paraphrasing

The only way to know whether or not you have understood another person's message is to check your understanding of the facts and ideas by paraphrasing your understanding. In *paraphrasing,* you assimilate and restate in your own words what an individual has said. Paraphrasing the *content* of the message basically repeats a person's statement, allowing an opportunity for the consumer to hear and mull over what they have told you. It encourages a shared understanding of what is being said, and a chance to correct any misunderstandings. Following are some examples:

- 'In other words, you're fed up with being treated like a child.'
- 'I hear you saying that when people compliment you, you feel embarrassed. If they knew the real you, they'd stay away.'

Paraphrasing gives you the opportunity to test your understanding of what a person is attempting to communicate, and can dramatically reduce misunderstandings. It is reflective in nature, in that it lets the person know what you heard, and how you understand what has been said. It also gives the person the opportunity to clarify content or feelings. People are more likely to trust and value those who paraphrase the content and their feelings (Beebe, 2011).

Paraphrasing is perhaps one of the most misused and overused methods in mental health counselling. Use it judiciously. It loses its effectiveness when used for lack of other choices, and can be seen as patronising.

Reflecting feelings

Reflecting *feelings* is verbalising the implied feelings in a person's comment. Remember to respect an individual's right to their opinion and feelings, even when you may disagree with them. Following are some examples:

- 'Sounds like you're really angry at your brother.'
- 'You're feeling anxious about being discharged from the hospital.'

In reflecting feelings, you attempt to identify latent and connotative meanings that may either clarify or distort the content. Reflection is useful because it encourages the person to make additional clarifying comments (Blonna, Loschiavo & Watter, 2011).

Imparting information

Imparting information helps the communication process by supplying additional data. This encourages further clarification based on new or additional input. Following are some examples:

- 'The ward round will be held on Tuesday afternoon from 1.30 until 3.00.'
- 'I am a nursing student.'

It is not constructive to withhold useful information from a person, or to reply 'What do you think?' to a straightforward, information-seeking question. However, be careful not to cross the line between giving information and giving advice, or giving information as a way of avoiding an area of interpersonal difficulty (Waugh, McNay, Dewar & McCraig, 2014). Also, by giving personal, social information, you will likely move out of the realm of therapeutic intervention (see the discussion of self-disclosure in Chapter 2). Information that is important to disclose to a consumer includes your title and position. Resist the temptation to deny you are new to the field—it may only cause mistrust.

Remember that an individual's participation in decision-making begins when they take in and understand information about their own condition. This is part of the process in delivering person-centred care, and is central to developing and maintaining a therapeutic relationship (O'Kane, 2013b). The goal of imparting information should be to provide effective education that empowers the person and their carers, and enables the person to have a voice in their recovery. The person involved in the own recovery is more likely to achieve positive mental health outcomes, and less likely to need admission or readmission to an acute care facility.

Avoiding self-disclosure

Self-disclosure in nursing refers to when the nurse imparts personal information to a person and their carers. Although used regularly in personal relationships, there are boundaries in its use within therapeutic relationships. Self-disclosure must be used cautiously, so that the professional boundaries between the nurse, the person in their care and their carers do not become blurred. The use of self-disclosure can be helpful in some situations and strengthen the relationship, as it helps people perceive the nurse with humanity and warmth rather than being evasive and rude. The skill is to know when it is appropriate to self-disclose, to whom, and for what purpose (Henretty & Levitt, 2010). Any form of self-disclosure that serves the needs of the nurse rather than the person they are caring for is unacceptable (O'Kane, 2013a).

There may be times when you choose to avoid self-disclosure (such as those discussed in the section on self-disclosure in Chapter 2), and several communication techniques may be helpful. For instance, a carer might ask you to disclose your marital status, home address, religious affiliation or a pressing personal problem. The following list offers practical and therapeutic ways to deflect a request for self-disclosure:

- *Use honesty:* 'I don't share my home address with the people I am caring for or their carers.'
- *Use benign curiosity*: 'I wonder why you're asking me this today?'
- *Use refocusing*: 'You were talking about how your father treats you. I wonder why you changed the topic? You were saying that . . .'
- *Use interpretation*: 'I notice that every time you talk about your father, you change the subject and ask me a question.' (pause)
- *Seek clarification*: 'You keep asking me my home address. I wonder what concerns you might have about me today.'
- *Respond with feedback and limit-setting*: 'I'm really uncomfortable when you ask me about my partner. Talking about my partner isn't part of our agreement to work together.' Adding 'The last time we met, you were deciding if you were going to call your boss on the phone . . .' helps restructure the situation.

Use these communication techniques in the context of the therapeutic relationship, and assess and evaluate received responses in an ongoing manner with senior clinicians or your clinical supervisor.

Clarifying

Sometimes, even though you have listened carefully, you are still not totally clear. In this situation, it is important to ask for clarification. *Clarifying* is an attempt to understand the basic nature of a person's statement. The following are some examples:

- 'I'm confused about exactly what is upsetting to you. Could you go over that again, please?'
- 'You say you are feeling anxious now. What's that like for you?'

Asking a person to give an example to clarify a meaning helps you understand the intended message better. A person who describes a concrete incident is more likely to see the connections between it and similar occurrences. Illustrations or examples are also very useful qualifiers.

Checking perceptions

Checking perceptions means sharing how one person perceives and hears another. After letting a person know what your perceptions of their behaviours, thoughts and feelings are, ask the person to verify the perception. Asking someone to confirm your perception actively demonstrates that you are committed to understanding their behaviour. It gives the other person the opportunity to correct inaccurate perceptions, and allows you to avoid actions based on false assumptions. The following are some examples:

- 'Let me know if this is how you see it, too.'
- 'When I see you fidgeting in your chair and tapping your foot, I get the feeling that you're uncomfortable when we're silent. Does that seem to fit?' or 'I know you said it doesn't matter, but when you frown, won't look at me, and fold your arms across your chest, it seems as if you're upset. Are you feeling angry?'

Perception checks are equally important in relationship to non-verbal behaviour. When you observe a person's eye contact, posture, facial expression, gestures or tone of voice, you interpret what you think the person is expressing. Be sure to check the validity of your interpretation with the person by asking whether it is accurate.

Questioning

Questioning is a very direct way of speaking with people. But when used to excess, questioning controls the nature and range of a person's responses. Questions can be useful when you are seeking specific information as in a structured mental health assessment (see Chapter 10) or when you are assessing a consumer for suicidal ideation (see Chapter 19). When your intent is to engage someone in meaningful dialogue, however, you should limit questions.

When you do use questions, it is best to make them open-ended rather than closed. An *open-ended question* focuses the topic but allows freedom of response, encouraging people to respond in more than a few words. The following are some examples:

- 'How were you feeling when your mother said that to you?'
- 'What's your opinion about . . .?'

Asking a *closed-ended question* limits a person's choice of responses, generally to 'yes' or 'no' ('Were you feeling angry when your mother said that?'). Closed-ended questions limit therapeutic exploration. On some occasions, however, within mental health practice, there may be people experiencing a mental illness whose thinking is disorganised and needs to be guided by closed-ended questions. Closed-ended questions are helpful when you require specific information (Ivey, Ivey & Zalaquett, 2014).

'Why' questions can be both useful and, if not used carefully, a hindrance. They are often impossible to answer, and can make a person feel interrogated. Alternatively, if used appropriately and in the right context, they can enhance understanding of a situation. Try reframing 'why' questions with questions that include 'who', 'what', 'when' and 'how' (Ivey et al., 2015).

It is also advisable when questioning not to steer a person to answer in a certain way. For example, 'You don't drink alcohol to excess, do you?' suggests that the consumer should answer 'no'.

LIVED EXPERIENCE

Active listening

When I was employed as a peer worker on an mental health unit, I was ask to speak with a middle-aged woman who had a long history of severe and enduring mental illness due to trauma resulting from severe childhood abuse. During this admission, she had been particularly anxious, agitated and distressed; not normally how she presented. Any conversation was jumbled and didn't appear to make sense. By listening attentively, though, it became apparent that all of the conversations had the same theme, such as 'I would have been a good mother, I would have protected, cared and loved my child. Children should be precious and protected.' It then became clear that this lady was grieving over her missed chance of being a mother due to the onset of menopause.

Structuring

Structuring is an attempt to create order or evolve guidelines. It helps the individual become aware of problems and the order in which to deal with them. The following are some examples:

- 'You've mentioned that you want to improve your relationships with your wife, your sister and your manager. Let's put them in order of priority.'
- 'No, I won't be giving you advice, but we can discuss some possible solutions together.'

Structuring is particularly useful when people introduce a number of concerns in a brief period and have little idea of where to begin. Use structuring not only to explore content, but also to de-limit the parameters of the nurse–consumer relationship, and to identify how you will participate in the problem-solving process.

Pinpointing

Pinpointing calls attention to certain kinds of statements and relationships. For example, you may point to inconsistencies among statements; to similarities and differences in the points of view, feelings or actions of two or more people; or to differences between what one says and what one does.

- 'So, you and your wife don't agree about how many children you want.'
- 'You say you're sad, but you're smiling.'

Linking

In *linking*, you respond in a way that ties together two events, experiences, feelings or people. You can use linking to connect past experiences with current behaviours. Another example is linking the tension between two people with current life stress, as shown in the following examples:

- 'You felt depressed after the birth of both your children.'
- 'So, the arguments didn't really begin until after you got your promotion.'

Giving feedback

Giving *feedback* is telling the other person your reaction to what they have said. It helps people become aware of how their behaviour affects others, and how others may perceive their actions. Responding with feedback is therapeutic self-disclosure on your part. It allows you to offer constructive information that makes them aware of their effect on others. However, total self-disclosure by the nurse is inappropriate in the nurse–consumer relationship. It places a burden of interdependence on the consumer, and limits the time and energy available to work on the consumer's concerns.

Effective feedback should be immediate (given as soon as possible), honest (giving your true reaction), and supportive (given in ways that are tolerable to hear and not hurtful or brutal). The following are some examples:

- 'When you wring your hands, I feel your anxiety.'
- 'Sometimes when you turn your head away from me, I think you're angry.'

It is important to give feedback in a way that does not threaten a person and result in increased defensiveness. The more defensive the person, the less likely they will hear and understand the feedback. Feedback that is harsh, hurtful or cruel, or appears to reject the person, creates barriers between yourself and the person within the therapeutic relationship. You want to do your best to prevent a person from experiencing your feedback as a personal rejection. Your Intervention Strategies lists strategies and rationales for giving helpful, non-threatening feedback.

Be aware that people will express not only information about themselves when they interact with you, but also information about how they perceive you. Cues about how your words and your behaviour affect others are there if you look for them. Be open and receptive to these unsolicited cues—the person's or their carer's feedback to you—that can help you to become a more effective mental health nurse. The Self-awareness feature on the next page will help you to engage in self-reflection.

Confronting

Constructive and empathic confrontations often lead to productive change. *Confronting* is a deliberate invitation to examine some aspect of personal behaviour that indicates incongruity between what the person says and what the person does. It can be described as challenging a person in a supportive manner (Ivey, Ivey & Zalaquett, 2015). Confrontation

YOUR INTERVENTION STRATEGIES Giving helpful, non-threatening feedback

Strategy	Rationale
Focus feedback on behaviour, rather than on the person.	Refer to what a person actually does, rather than how you imagine the person to be.
Focus feedback on observations, rather than inferences.	Refer to what you actually see or hear the person do; inferences refer to conclusions or assumptions you make about individuals.
Focus feedback on description, rather than judgment.	Report what occurred, rather than evaluating it in terms of good or bad, right or wrong.
Focus feedback on 'more or less', rather than 'either/or' descriptions of behaviour.	'More or less' descriptions stress quantity rather than quality (which may be value-laden).
Focus feedback on here-and-now behaviour, rather than there-and-then behaviour.	The most meaningful feedback is given as soon as it is appropriate to do so.
Focus feedback on sharing information and ideas, rather than advice.	Sharing ideas and information helps a person make decisions about their own wellbeing; giving advice takes away a person's freedom to be self-determining.
Focus feedback on exploration of alternatives rather than answers or solutions.	Focusing on a variety of alternatives for accomplishing a particular goal prevents premature acceptance of answers or solutions that may not be appropriate.
Focus feedback on its value to the person, rather than on catharsis it provides you.	Feedback should serve the consumer's needs, not your own.
Limit feedback to the amount of information a person is able to use, rather than the amount you have available to give.	Overloading will decrease effectiveness of feedback.
Limit feedback to the appropriate time and place.	Excellent feedback presented at an inappropriate time may be ineffective or harmful.
Focus feedback on what is said, rather than why it is said.	Focusing on why things are said or done moves away from observations and towards motive or intent (which can only be assumed, unless verified).

SELF-AWARENESS

Reflecting on feedback from consumers and carers

Input—both positive and negative—from consumers, carers, classmates, tutors, staff, family and friends can help you to become aware of your 'blind spots', the characteristics about yourself that you ignore, deny or defend. Protecting oneself through self-deception interferes with both relating and communicating. To become more self-aware, do the following:

- think about a recent interaction with a consumer and how they responded to you
- identify the positive/negative elements in the interaction
- try to determine what the consumer was telling you about yourself in this interaction (i.e. What characteristic(s) do you have that enables people to openly express their thoughts and feelings? What characteristic(s) do you have that prevents people from openly expressing their thoughts and feelings?)
- discuss the interaction and your interpretation of it with a supervisor
- ask for feedback on your behaviour from others—family members, classmates, staff, friends.

requires careful attention to non-verbal communication, and the discrepancies between non-verbal and verbal messages or the mixed messages being received.

Confrontations may be informational or interpretive, and they may be directed towards both the strengths and the limitations of a person. It is your job to point out the incongruities being observed or heard, and support the person to resolve them. An *informational confrontation* describes the visible behaviour of another person. The following is an example:

- 'You say you're "the dummy in the family", yet none of your brothers or sisters went to university like you did.'

An *interpretive confrontation* expresses thoughts and feelings about the other's behaviour, and draws inferences about the meaning of the behaviour. The following is an example:

- 'Ever since your mum and dad criticised the way you looked, you haven't spoken to them. It looks like you're feeling angry.'

Six skills to be incorporated in constructive confrontations are as follows:

1. use of personal statements with the words *I*, *my* and *me*
2. use of relationship statements expressing what you think or feel about the person in the here-and-now
3. use of behaviour descriptions (statements describing the visible behaviour of the person)
4. use of description of personal feelings, specifying the feeling by name
5. use of responses aimed at understanding, such as paraphrasing and perception checking
6. use of constructive feedback skills (see Your Intervention Strategies).

Summarising

Summarising highlights the main ideas expressed in an interaction. It shows the person that you understand. Both you and the person benefit from this review of the main themes of the conversation. Summarising is also useful in focusing an individual's thinking and aiding conscious learning. Following are some examples:

- 'The last time we were together, you were concerned about . . .'
- 'You had three main concerns today.'

You can use this technique appropriately at different times during an interaction. For example, it is useful to summarise the previous interaction in the first few minutes you and the person spend together. Early summarising helps the person recall the areas discussed, and gives them the opportunity to see how you have synthesised the content of a previous session. Summarising is useful because it keeps the participants directed towards a goal.

Injudicious use of summarising is a common pitfall. You may rush to summarise despite other, more pressing and immediate, consumer concerns. In this instance, summarising is likely to meet your needs for structure, but does nothing to address the person's here-and-now concerns and needs.

Processing

Processing is a complex and sophisticated technique. Process comments direct attention to the interpersonal dynamics of the nurse–consumer experience—in the content, feelings and behaviour being expressed within the therapeutic relationship between the two parties involved.

- 'It seems that important things that need to be taken care of come up in the last five minutes we have together.'
- 'Today is the first day our time together has started out with silence. Last week it seemed there wouldn't be enough time.'

As you can see, processing is an advanced skill. It is most useful when therapeutic intimacy and mutual engagement have been achieved. It can deepen and enhance the relationship, providing an opportunity for a person to become more self-aware, and apply what they learn in the therapeutic relationship to other relationships in their lives (Hill & Knox, 2009)

COMMON MISTAKES

When we are experiencing discomfort or strong negative feelings, it becomes difficult to empathise and to communicate with people in a therapeutic way. Some common mistakes to guard against are as follows:

- *Giving advice:* Giving advice ('You should . . .', 'Why don't you . . .', 'It would be better if you . . .') carries the implicit message that a person is incapable of solving their own problem.
- *Minimising or discounting feelings:* Telling a person that they are over-reacting, that there is nothing to be afraid of, or not to worry, are attempts at reassurance that minimise and discount the person's feelings.

- *Deflecting:* Hearing a person express their pain can be anxiety-provoking. Changing the subject or making a joke are attempts to move to something less painful. This is not a positive shift of focus—rather, it gives the message that you cannot or do not want to cope with the pain the person is feeling.
- *Interrogating:* Asking a barrage of questions implies that you are more interested in gathering information than you are in listening to a person's story.
- *Sparring:* No matter what a person says, you know better. Debating or disagreeing with a person prevents you from actively listening.

HOW I WILL USE MY MENTAL HEALTH SKILLS IN PRACTICE

Belinda's story: I have known for five years that I want to be a mental health nurse. When I served in the Australian Defence Force, I was trained as a field medic and did two tours of duty in Afghanistan, and then worked at an army hospital's outpatient clinic. In both places, I saw several soldiers who had big problems—they couldn't relax, they couldn't sleep, they had nightmares all the time. A lot of the veterans we saw started drinking too much and too often. They moved from marijuana to harder drugs, and some lost their jobs and their families. That's when I made up my mind to go to nursing school and learn as much as possible about stress and how it affects people. I have one more semester to go, and when that's done I'm going back into the service. I'll be joining the Army Nurse Corps and go to Officer Training School in Canberra.

PRACTISE, PRACTISE, PRACTISE!

Practising and nurturing these micro-skills to establish and maintain a therapeutic relationship is the cornerstone to your role as a mental health nurse. The experiences of the people you care for and their carers will be greatly influenced by how you meaningfully implement communication skills in practice to enhance the recovery journey. Effective communication starts with you, and is the key to establishing, maintaining and safely terminating therapeutic relationships.

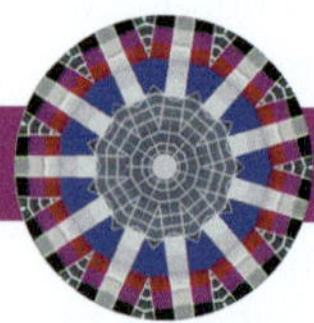

REFERENCES

Access Economics. (2006). *Listen hear! The economic impact and cost of hearing loss in Australia: A report by Access Economics Pty Ltd.* East Melbourne, Australia, CRC for Cochlear Implant and Hearing Aid Innovation: Vicdeaf.

Arnold, E. C., & Boggs, K. U. (2015). *Interpersonal relationships: Professional communication skills for nurses*. London, England: Elsevier Health Sciences.

Australian Federal Police. (2015). Retrieved from: http://www.afp.gov.au/media-centre/publications. (Accessed 2015, April 18.)

Bandler, R. (1993). *Time for a change*. Denver, CO: Meta Publications.

Beebe, S. A. (2011). *Interpersonal communication: Relating to others*. Upper Saddle River, NJ: Pearson Education.

Blonna, R., Loschiavo, J., & Watter, D. (2011). *Health counseling: A microskills approach for counselors, educators, and school nurses* (2nd ed.). Sudbury, MA: Jones and Bartlett Learning.

Bost, N., Crilly J., & Wallen, K. (2014). Characteristics and process outcomes of patients presenting to an Australian emergency department for mental health and non-mental health diagnoses. *International Emergency Nursing, 22*(3), 146–152.

Broadbent, M., Moxham, L., & Dwyer T. (2014). Implications of the emergency department triage environment on triage practice for clients with a mental illness at triage in an Australian context. *Australasian Emergency Nursing, 17*(1), 23–29.

Clark, A. J. (2014). *Empathy in counseling and psychotherapy: Perspectives and practices*. Hoboken, NJ: Taylor & Francis.

Euson, B. (2012). *C21: Communicating in the 21st century* (3rd ed.). Milton, QLD, Australia: John Wiley & Sons.

Gerace, A., O'Kane, D., Hayman, C., & Muir-Cochrane, E. (2012). 'Hold my hand and walk through the park with me': Empathic relationships in acute care mental health settings. Paper presented at the 12th Annual Conference of the Australian Psychological Society's Psychology of Relationships Interest Group, Adelaide, 8–9 November.

Heath R., & Bryant J. (2013). *Human communication theory and research: Concepts, contexts, and challenges* (2nd ed.). New York, NY: Routledge.

Henretty, J., & Levitt, H. (2010). The role of therapist self-disclosure in psychotherapy: A qualitative review. *Clinical Psychology Review, 30*, 63–77.

Hill, C. E., & Knox, S. (2009). Processing the therapeutic relationship. *Psychotherapy Research, 19*(1):13–29

Ivey, A. E., Ivey, M. B., & Zalaquett, C. P. (2014). *Essentials of intentional interviewing: Counselling in a multicultural society* (8th ed.). Belmont, CA: Brooks/Cole Cengage Learning.

Ivey, A. E., Ivey, M. B., & Zalaquett, C. P. (2015). *Intentional interviewing and counseling: Facilitating client development in a multicultural society* (3rd ed.). Belmont, CA: Brooks/Cole Cengage Learning.

Littlejohn S., & Foss, K. (2011). *Theories of human communication* (10th ed.). Long Grove, IL: Waveland Press.

Martin, J. N., & Nakayama, T. K. (2012). *Intercultural communication in context* (6th ed.). Philadelphia, PA: McGraw-Hill.

O'Connor, J., & Seymour, J. (2011). *Introducing NLP: Psychological skills for understanding and influencing people.* Newbury Port, MA: Red Wheel Weiser.

O'Kane, D. (2013a). Communication in healthcare practice. In P. Barkway (Ed.), *Psychology for health professionals* (2nd ed.) (pp. 182–200). Sydney, Australia: Churchill Livingston, Elsevier.

O'Kane, D. (2013b). Partnerships in health. In P. Barkway (Ed.), *Psychology for health professionals*. (2nd ed.) (pp. 201–221). Sydney, Australia: Churchill Livingston, Elsevier.

O'Toole, G. (2012). *Communication core interpersonal skills for health professionals* (2nd ed.). Sydney, Australia: Elsevier.

Queensland Health. (2008). *Deafness and mental health guidelines for working with people who are deaf or hard of hearing*. Brisbane, Australia: Queensland Health.

Reik, T. (1949). *Listening with the third ear: The inner experience of the psychoanalyst*. New York, NY: Grove.

Ruesch, J. (1961). *Therapeutic communication*. New York, NY: Norton.

Ruesch, J., & Bateson, G. (1968). *Communication: The social matrix of psychiatry*. New York, NY: Norton.

Shafiei, T., Gaynor, N., & Farrell, G. (2011). The characteristics, management and outcomes of people identified with mental health issues in an emergency department, Melbourne, Australia. *Journal of Psychiatric and Mental Health Nursing, 18*(1), 9–16.

Smock, T. K. (1999). *Physiological psychology: A neuroscience approach*. Upper Saddle River, NJ: Prentice Hall.

Spector, R. E. (2009). *Cultural care: Guide to heritage assessment and health traditions* (6th ed.). Upper Saddle River, NJ: Prentice Hall.

Stein-Parbury, J. (2013). *Patient and person: Interpersonal skills in nursing* (5th ed.). Sydney, Australia: Churchill Livingstone/Elsevier.

Sturt, J., Ali, S., Robertson, W., Bourne, C., & Bridle, C. (2012). Neurolinguistic programming: A systematic review of the effects on health outcomes. *British Journal of General Practice, 62*, e757–e764.

Thomson, G., & Menzies, S. (2010). Effective interaction. Interview by Mary-Claire Mason. *Nursing Standard, 24*(31), 25.

Watzlawick, P., Beavin, J., & Jackson, D. (1967). *The pragmatics of human communication*. New York, NY: Norton.

Watzlawick, P., Beavin Bavelas, J., Jackson, D., & O'Hanlon, B. (2011). *Pragmatics of human communication: A study of interactional patterns, pathologies and paradoxes*. New York, NY: W. W. Norton.

Waugh, A., McNay, L., Dewar, B., & McCaig, M. (2014). Supporting the development of interpersonal skills in nursing, in an undergraduate mental health curriculum: Reaching the parts other strategies do not reach through action learning. *Nurse Education Today, 34*(9), 1232–1237.

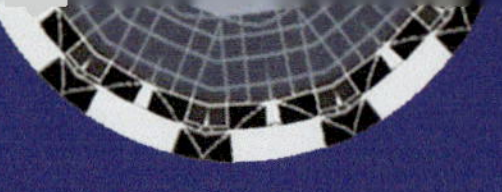

10

Psychiatric–mental health assessment

EIMEAR MUIR-COCHRANE AND FRANKLIN D. BIRTLE

KEY TERMS

Beck Depression Inventory *203*
Global Assessment of Functioning (GAF) *205*
intellectual disability *205*
Mental Status Examination (MSE) *197*
Mini-Mental State Exam (MMSE) *200*
Minnesota Multiphasic Personality Inventory–2 (MMPI–2) *203*
Nurses' Observation Scale for Inpatient Evaluations (NOSIE) *201*
psychiatric history *195*
State–Trait Anxiety Inventory *203*

LEARNING OUTCOMES

After completing this chapter, you will be able to:

1. Undertake an ongoing psychiatric–mental health assessment with people in your care.
2. Determine how and when to apply assessment principles in professional practice.
3. Conduct a mental status examination with a person.
4. Describe the essential components of physiological assessment, neurological assessment, psychological testing and psychosocial assessment.
5. Recognise the person as an expert in their own care and their role in assessment, and the nurse's development in understanding the individual's mental distress.

LIVED EXPERIENCE

My first admission

When I arrived at hospital for the first time, it was a frightening experience. I didn't know anyone or anything about how the ward worked. When a nurse asked me a little bit about who I was, it felt like she was interested. She didn't write anything down when she was talking to me, but I always thought that those were the most simple questions I was asked and that those were the most honest answers I gave on my journey through the mental health system. I imagine that the interaction formed part of my assessment, and was probably the assessment that found out the most about who I was as a person. When I look back on all the different professionals who have assessed me, the nurse who met me as a person that day was probably the most skilful clinician I met.

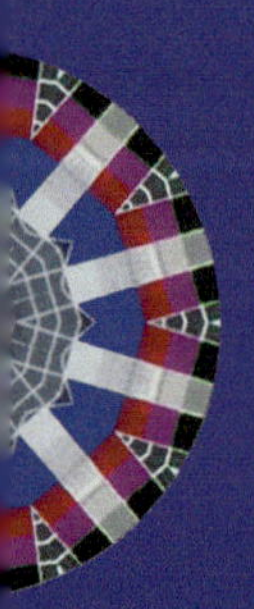

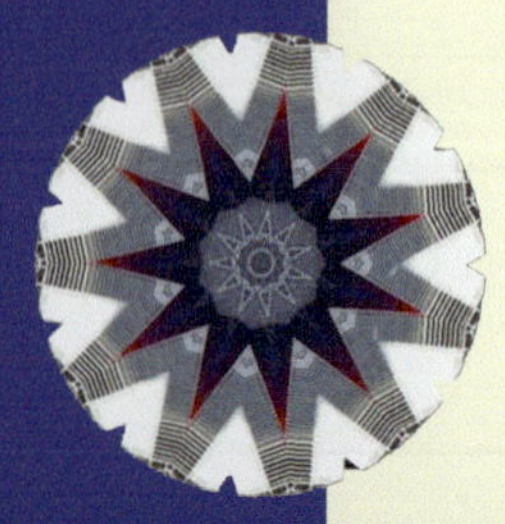

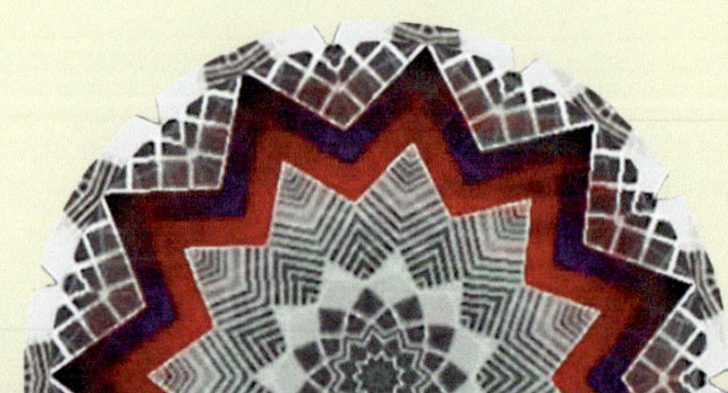

INTRODUCTION

As the preceding Lived Experience describes, the initial engagement between the nurse and the consumer is an opportunity to begin to establish rapport, and demonstrate to the consumer that you can be trusted, care for their welfare and are interested in helping understand their distress. The next section details the nurse's role in mental state assessment.

THE NURSING ROLE IN ASSESSMENT

Practice example

You are responsible for an admission assessment with Jared, who is 35 years old. He is being admitted to inpatient care from an emergency department after driving his car off the road, potentially deliberately. He has no alcohol or drugs in his system. His psychiatric diagnosis is major depression with psychotic features, and he has had prior hospitalisations for self-harming behaviour, as noted in his medical record. Most guidelines for conducting a mental status intake examination emphasise the importance of a suicide assessment, which includes questions such as 'Have you ever thought of ending it all?', 'Have you ever considered suicide?' and 'Do you plan to hurt yourself?', but also recognise the importance of narrative in understanding the potential suicide risk. In your interview, you ask Jared whether he is considering hurting himself again, and he says 'No.'

Jared seems anxious and does express feeling 'down all the time'. He mentions that 'You have better things to do than waste your time on just me.'

1. You consider that he is not actively suicidal at this point in time, so what would your assessment focus on as the next priority?
2. When in your assessment would you discuss the types of antidepressants and other medications Jared is taking?
3. Would you consider Jared's statements evidence of a thought process disorder?

Psychiatric–mental health nurses are required to undertake thorough and systematic mental state assessments in a range of settings, and with persons from across the lifespan. A full assessment includes risk assessment and a complete biopsychosocial assessment.

A comprehensive assessment will enable you to make sound clinical judgments and plan appropriate interventions. The primary sources of data in most instances are the people themselves, and often their families. Nurses' documentation, psychological evaluations and medical tests, and other health professional's records and other secondary data sources, can enlarge, clarify and substantiate data obtained directly from the person.

Your assessment skills are essential, and will be utilised throughout an individual person's care. Because nurses assess on an ongoing basis, the success of a collaboratively planned approach to care in every setting depends on a nurse's continual assessment of the changing needs of an individual through engagement and open communication with them.

Primary mental health nursing skills, including person-centred approaches, collaboration with persons in their care, and valuing each human being as an individual, can support the ongoing assessment and the nurse's role in an individual's recovery journey.

MENTAL STATE ASSESSMENT

Systems of data collection and assessment vary among mental health agencies. The psychiatric examination consists of two parts: the psychiatric history and the mental status examination. It is most often facilitated during initial or early interactions with a person. The traditional psychiatric examination is discussed in this chapter, because it is still used in settings where psychiatric nurses work, and is considered the counterpart of the physical examination and history. Understanding another clinician's perspective in a documented psychiatric evaluation is an important skill that can aid a nurse in developing their own understanding using information from formal assessment and the person's reported experience.

The person and person–clinician perspective on assessment are provided later in the chapter, and challenge elements of the traditional psychiatric examination.

Psychiatric history

The **psychiatric history** gathers information about the person's current condition and previous diagnoses, interventions and treatment, along with a family history.

LIVED EXPERIENCE

The process of assessing my needs

Developing an understanding of my psychiatric history was not a process that happened in one interview. Different people used different scales to understand the presenting experience. It often felt like clinicians would read my notes and think they knew me. The best nursing assessments I experienced were when the nurse was not afraid to hear something new, and then find out when that meant to me and how they could help with the information I shared. Of course, the information might not be the same as the last notes they read, and the nurses with whom I shared information were those who invited me to tell more of the story. The invitation was a great skill that one nurse offered, and it must have given everyone a better understanding of my journey, including me.

Data sources

Not all data gathered during psychiatric history-taking are obtained from the person. There are several other sources. Family, friends, police, mental health personnel and others may contribute data to the psychiatric history. When the sources are varied, the psychiatric history focuses on the perceptions of others: how they see the person and the circumstances of the person's life. Always clearly indicate the sources of the information in the psychiatric history, and their relationship to the person. Review and understand information given by these collateral sources in terms of that relationship.

The psychiatric history generally includes the following categories of data:

- *Complaint:* The main reason the person is having a psychiatric examination. The person may have personally initiated the psychiatric examination, or others may have initiated it (such as courts, hospital staff, family, referral from school or an employer). Record the 'chief complaint' verbatim, and use with quotation marks ('I just don't want to live any longer' or 'I know these are crazy thoughts, but I can't stop them. They're too strong.').
- *Present symptoms:* The nature of the onset and the development of symptoms. These data are usually traced from the present back to the last period of wellness.
- *Previous hospitalisations and mental health treatment:* Information from the person, their medical records and ancillary information.
- *Family history:* Generally, whether any family members have ever sought or received mental health treatment.
- *Personal history:* The person's birth and development; past and recent illnesses; schooling and education; occupation; marital status; the use of alcohol, drugs, caffeine and tobacco; trauma history; and religious, spiritual or cultural practices. The person's description is important, as it will give an understanding of how the person perceives their history, and may give indicators to the reason for the presenting need.
- *Personality:* The person's relationships with others, moods, feelings, interests and leisure activities.

Input from family and friends can give you a better perspective of the person, as well as insight into the psychosocial aspects of the circumstances in which the person lives. This input includes perceptions of the person by others (how they see the person), how symptoms are expressed in that environment, and patterns of interaction. Keep in mind that family and friends have their own perspectives through which they filter events. All information from family and friends is treated as important data to be contributed to the whole assessment, and not necessarily a total picture of the person.

The main purpose of history-taking is to gather information, although skilful history-taking can provide an opportunity to begin the important process of establishing a rapport with the person. The information the person offers will not likely emerge in the exact order of the forms you will complete. You can shape and guide the interview while allowing the person to provide information at a comfortable pace. You can also promote rapport by avoiding an interrogative approach and allowing the person's story to unfold naturally. For the most part, the assessment process involves inserting all collected data for documentation without maintaining a rigid structure.

Assessing for psychological symptoms is not substantially different for nurses in varying specialty areas. It may be more demanding to be an emergency department nurse, and have to assess for emergent physical situations in addition to psychological symptoms; however, the basics remain the same: recognition of the person as an individual with a story to share, and to approach the individual with compassion and humanity. See What Every Nurse Should Know for an example of how you would assess in those circumstances.

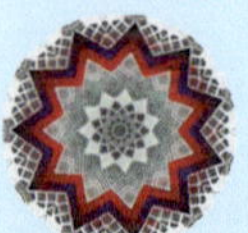

WHAT EVERY NURSE SHOULD KNOW

Assessing a person experiencing mental distress in an emergency department

Bringing a person identified as experiencing mental distress into this fast-paced, noisy and often crowded environment requires adjustments in order to understand the needs and to provide good nursing care.

Verbal interactions are the main approaches appropriate for interacting with a person in the emergency department (ED), as opposed to standard measurements for physical care. Your assessment of a person begins when you first observe them. How are they standing or sitting? What are they wearing? These initial assessments can aid how you will approach them to establish rapport and assess them comprehensively. Your assessment of a person with mental health problems focuses on why the person is in the ED at this time. For that person now to be in the ED, something has happened to make today different from yesterday. Ask questions about the current situation and what has changed for the person.

Other considerations for ED assessments of mentally distressed persons include allowing for greater personal space than you would with someone receiving physical care. Physical contact may be interpreted entirely differently than usual, especially normally supportive gestures such as hand-holding or shoulder-touching; however, they may well continue to be an appropriate and important part of care. Checking with the individuals is the best way to understand their experience.

Keep in mind that speed is not an asset under these circumstances. People who have psychiatric illnesses may have cognitive difficulties, may or may not be able to absorb information quickly, may have trouble concentrating and remembering, and may value a low-stimulus environment. Using your assessment skills in a tempered and deliberate manner will facilitate appropriate planning of care

Mental Status Examination

The **Mental Status Examination (MSE)** is usually a standardised procedure in the agencies that use it. The primary purpose of the MSE is to help the examiner gather more objective data to be used in determining aetiology, diagnosis, prognosis and treatment, and to deal immediately with any risk of violence or harm. The sections of the MSE that deal with sensorium and intellect are particularly important in establishing the existence of delirium, dementia, and amnestic and other cognitive disorders. The purpose of the MSE differs from that of the psychiatric history, in that it identifies the person's present mental status. The categories of information (not necessarily in the sequence presented here) follow in the next section. The MSE is often repeated throughout the care process as a standard ongoing assessment at any given time, and results can be compared for consideration of changes.

General behaviour, appearance and attitude

Provide a complete and accurate description of the person's physical characteristics, apparent age, manner of dress, use of cosmetics, personal hygiene, postures, gait, gestures, facial expression, mannerisms, general activity level and responses to the MSE examiner. Other descriptors that may be used include 'frank', 'friendly', 'irritable', 'dramatic', 'evasive', 'indifferent' and so forth. Details should be sufficient to identify and characterise the person. Note any mannerisms a person may have, their expression, eye contact and ability to follow requests.

For descriptive purposes, we will use excerpts from the MSE of Andrew, a person requesting services at a mental health clinic, as a Practice Example throughout this section.

LIVED EXPERIENCE

Understanding my experience

At the weekly ward round, a nurse would always sit with me and go through how I was. She would then sit in on the ward round with the doctor and repeat what I had just said to her. I never understood why I was not able to speak to the doctor for myself!

Over time I could see whether a format was being followed, and how interested the nurse was to genuinely hear how my mental state was at the time. Then I met a nurse who never asked me the set questions; in fact, she never appeared to be assessing me. That was the greatest skill I experienced in assessment: listening to me and finding out how I felt, even if it didn't fit with the standards questions. After all, I would have thought that assessment would be a process of trying to understand my experience, and listening to the person is a good place to start.

Practice example

Appearance, behaviour and attitude

Andrew, a 35-year-old white male, appears his stated age, dressed in torn, dishevelled jeans. He presents with a tense facial expression, rigid posture and a stiff gait. He is cooperative, and has an elevated activity level, in that he moves quickly and uses abrupt gestures.

Speech

Speech is described in terms of volume and tone (loud, soft, weak, strong, monotone), rate (fast or slow), and quantity (talkative, expansive, paucity, silent), as well as the level of coherence (understandable speech). Fluency refers to the person's speech being slurred or clear, hesitant or aphasic. You may include a sample of the person's conversation in quotation marks.

Andrew's speech is described in the following Practice Example.

Practice example

Speech and language

He was cooperative. His speech was loud, and he used an excessive number of words in his responses. There was some disjointed speech, with a pattern of topic shifts from himself to his ex-wife.

Mood and affect

The person's pervasive or dominant mood or affective reaction is recorded here. Both subjective and objective data are included. Subjective data are obtained through the use of non-leading questions, for instance, 'How are you feeling?' If the person replies with general terms, such as 'nervous', ask the person to describe how the nervousness shows itself and its effect, because such words may have different meanings to different individuals.

Facial expression, motor behaviour, the presence of tears, flushing, sweating, tachycardia, tremors, respiratory irregularities, states of excitement, fear and depression: the attitude of the person towards the MSE examiner sometimes offers valuable clues. Note any hostility, suspiciousness, flirtatiousness, a desire for bodily contact or outspoken criticism. Although a potential sign of underlying mental state, it may be that the individual simply does not want to engage in the process.

If possible, record verbatim the replies to questions concerning the person's mood. The relationship between mood and the content of thought is particularly significant. There may be a wide divergence between what a person says or does and their emotional state as expressed by attitudes or facial expressions.

The distinction between mood and affect in the MSE is subject to some disagreement. For example, Trzepacz and Baker (1993) describe 'affect' as 'the external and dynamic manifestations of a person's internal emotional state' and 'mood' as 'a person's predominant internal state at any one time'. Using this definition, mood is regarded as a current subjective state as described by the patient, and affect as the inferences of the quality of the patient's emotional state as assessed by health professionals, based on objective observation.

Note whether intense emotional responses accompany discussion of specific topics. *Flat affect* is an insufficiently intense emotional display in association with ideas or situations that ordinarily would call for a stronger response. Dissociation or disharmony is often indicated by an inappropriate emotional response, such as smiling or silly behaviour, when the attitude should be one of concern, anxiety or sadness. Persons who are trying to cover up a deep depression may feign cheerfulness and good spirits. Use of Socratic dialogue may elucidate the underlying experience.

The person's emotional reactions may be constant or may fluctuate during the examination. Try to specify the ease or readiness with which such changes occur in response to pleasant or unpleasant stimuli. You can use the following terms to describe intensity of response:

- composed, complacent, frank, friendly, cheerful, boastful, elated, grandiose, ecstatic
- tense, worried, anxious, pessimistic, sad, bewildered, gloomy, depressed, frightened
- aloof, disdainful, distant, defensive, suspicious
- irritable, resentful, hostile, sarcastic, angry, furious
- indifferent, apathetic, dull, affectless.

Pay attention to the influence of content on affect, and note especially disharmony between affect and content. Also important is constancy or change in the emotional state. The following Practice Example continues with Andrew's MSE:

Practice example

Mood and affect

His affect was slightly tense. His mood frustrated. 'I really get upset when she doesn't inform me of stuff.' There was a pessimistic tone to his descriptions, although this may be a recent change to his perspective.

Form of thought

This assessment is based on evidence of the amount of thought, slow thinking or vague expression, and the logical order or flow of ideas. The following types of form of thought exist.

Mutism The person has no verbal response, despite indications that they are aware of your questions.

Circumstantiality The person's speech is cumbersome, convoluted and has unnecessary detail in response to questions.

Perseveration This is a pattern of repeating the same words or movements, despite apparent efforts to make a new response.

Flight of ideas These are rapid, overly productive responses to questions that seem related only by chance associations between one sentence fragment and another; with flight of ideas, you might hear rhyming, clang associations, punning and evidence of distractibility. Be mindful of the stress of an assessment setting, and discern between mental health and situational anxiety.

Blocking *Blocking* is a pattern of sudden silence in the stream of conversation for no obvious reason, but is often thought to be associated with the intrusion of delusional thoughts or hallucinations.

Content of thought

Special preoccupations and experiences, such as *delusions,* illusions or hallucinations, depersonalisations, obsessions or *compulsions,* phobias, fantasies and daydreams are documented here. You can elicit these data by asking such questions as 'Do you have any difficulties with your thinking?' or 'Have you been troubled or ill in any way?' or 'Are there any thoughts or images that you find hard to keep put of your head?'

Delusions are beliefs held by an individual in the face of contradicting evidence or no evidence to external observers. If the person has delusions of someone or something in the environment paying extra attention to them, some of the following questions might reveal them: 'Have you ever been watched or spied on, or singled out for special attention?' 'Do others have it in for you?' If you suspect the person has delusions of being controlled by someone or something, ask the person such questions as 'Do you ever feel your thoughts or actions are under any outside influences or control?' or 'Are you able to influence others, to read their minds, or to put thoughts in their minds?' The use of immediacy can provide a non-threatening expression of the fact that you are not experiencing the content expressed by the person. It can also lead to an improved understanding of how the person views the world, in the way they respond to your not experiencing the same things as they are. Chapter 14 discusses these psychotic symptoms in more detail. See both Communications features in this chapter for examples, and rationales for these interactions.

Hallucinations are not thoughts, but are sensory perceptions that are not able to be experienced by other people. It is often difficult to draw direct links between the individual's experiences and the life events that the hallucinations may relate to. Hallucinations occur with the five senses of hearing, seeing, smelling, tasting or touching. Try to elicit details of the experience—for example, the source of sounds or voices (from outside or inside the head), the clarity and distinctness of the perception, and the intensity. Be mindful that the person may be hesitant to discuss their experiences due to fear of your reaction. Explore potential alternative realities with acceptance and a sense of hope that individuals can maintain autonomy over their experiences. Be interested in what the person thinks is happening to them or what the hallucination means to them.

Obsessions are insistent thoughts recognised as arising from the self. The person usually regards them as absurd and relatively meaningless, yet they persist despite endeavours to get rid of them. *Compulsions* are repetitive acts performed through some inner need or drive, but supposedly against the person's wishes; yet not performing them results in tension and anxiety. *Fantasies* and *daydreams* are preoccupations that are often difficult to elicit from the person. The difficulty may be that the person is not sure what you want in terms of

COMMUNICATION

Assessing the person

Person 'I don't trust you. You are just another one of those cogs in the big wheel meant to crush my spirit.'

NURSE RESPONSE #1: 'You seem uncomfortable, so let's get this done together as soon as we can.' *RATIONALE:* Empathic reflection, redirection, guidance and limit-setting.	**NURSE RESPONSE #2:** 'It sounds as though you see little value in this process. Can we try and work towards understanding your experience, in your words?' *RATIONALE:* Accurate empathy, therapeutic reframing.

COMMUNICATION

Assessing the person

Person: 'They're all out to get me. I can't get a day without being interfered with and manipulated. I hear them talking about me even now.'

NURSE RESPONSE #1: 'You have a sense that others that others have it in for you?' *RATIONALE:* Focus on process, acknowledgment of the individual's experience and ventilation/catharsis of feelings.	**NURSE RESPONSE #2:** 'It sound as if you have been strong to manage these experiences. Tell me the ways you've been coping. I imagine you have found ways that work best for you. Would it be useful for us to discuss how you manage, and see if we can figure out what would be best for you?' *RATIONALE:* Focus on emotional process, seeking details of the person's behaviours and planned actions Recognising the person as being skilful and resourceful.

detail, or they are ashamed to discuss fantasies and daydreams because of their content. Fantasy is discussed in Chapter 8.

Practice example

Content of thought

Although Andrew denied having delusions or hallucinations, he seemed to be distracted during the interview. When asked a question, he would pause and tip his head, mumble indistinctly, then answer the question. Andrew acknowledged the distraction, but stated there were sounds and noises in the room that 'you probably can't hear because I have super-strong hearing'. He denied current and past lethality. Andrew may well be understandably anxious about acknowledging his experiences in depth, for fear of the response by the clinical team. People who experience hallucination, especially verbal auditory hallucinations, are often concerned about being held involuntarily in hospital and medicated, if they articulate their experience. It may also be that voices are telling a person not to express current experiences. It can be a simple as asking the individual about the presence or content of voices that will facilitate them telling you about what they are experiencing.

Orientation

Document the person's orientation in terms of time, place, person and self or purpose; it helps determine the presence of confusion or clouding of consciousness. You may ask: 'Have you kept track of the time?' If so, 'What is today's date?' Ask people who say they do not know to estimate or guess the answer. Many clinicians begin the MSE with these questions, because disorientation would raise the question of the validity and reliability of data obtained subsequently. If you have developed a rapport by this stage and explored wider interests with Andrew, you could use subjects that relate to Andrew's own frame of reference to gain a deeper understanding of his orientation.

Practice example

Orientation

Oriented to person, but not to time (stated the year as two years before), or place (did not know where he was). Reported having trouble because 'I get so mad I get confused', and those incidents were related to mood. Denied alcohol abuse or substance use.

Memory

Attention span and ability to retain or recall past experiences in both the recent and remote past are tests of memory. If memory loss exists, determine whether it is constant or variable, and whether the loss is limited to a certain time period. Be alert to *confabulations*—memories invented to take the place of those the person cannot recall. It is useful to introduce questions relating to memory with some general question, such as 'How has your memory been?' Then you can move on to more specific questions, such as 'Have you had difficulty remembering where you put things or appointments?'

- *Recall of remote past experiences:* Ask for a review of the important events in the person's life. Then compare the response with information obtained from other sources during the history-taking. The person may give different information depending on their experience of developed rapport.
- *Recall of recent past experiences:* Ask for the events leading to the present seeking of treatment.
- *Retention and recall of immediate impressions:* Ask the person to repeat a name, an address or a set of objects (for example, rose, teacup and battleship) immediately, and again after three to five minutes. Another test is to

have the person repeat three-digit numbers at a rate of one per second, or repeat a complicated sentence.

- *General grasp and recall:* You might ask the person to read a story and then repeat the gist of the story to you with as many details as possible. If you plan to do this, consider the literacy of the individual and their ability to undertake the task.

Practice example

Memory

Andrew's memory functions appeared grossly intact. Three objects named at the beginning of session were recalled without difficulty.

General intellectual level

This is a non-standardised evaluation of intelligence. You are exploring the person's ability to use factual knowledge in a comprehensive way.

- *General grasp of information.* The person may be asked to name five recent news events in the media.
- *Ability to calculate.* Ask the person to subtract from 100 by sevens until the person can go no further (serial sevens test).
- *Reasoning and judgment.* A common test of reasoning is to ask what the person might do with a gift of $10 000. Examiners must be particularly careful to correct for their own biases and values in assessing each person's answer.

Abstract thinking

In this section of the MSE, you are asking the person to make distinctions between abstractions; for example, asking what the difference is between poverty and misery, or idleness and laziness. It is common to ask the person to interpret simple fables or proverbs, such as 'Don't cry over spilt milk.'

Insight and judgement evaluation

This section of the MSE determines whether the person recognises the significance of the present situation, whether they feel the need for treatment, and how they explain their symptoms. Often, it is helpful to ask persons for suggestions for their own treatment. It is important to consider that the person's experience may have links to events in their own life, and understanding of these links might constitute insight. You may consider insight to be broader than solely focused on the person having to demonstrate insight into a psychiatric model that may not make sense to them.

Summary

Summarise the important findings and make a tentative diagnosis. Add to the summary any pertinent facts from the medical history and/or physical examination. Remember to assess the person's appetite and sleep for alterations in their normal patterns, as these are often disrupted when a person is emotionally unwell.

PAMSGOTJIMI This is an acronym used to help recall key behaviours during mental state examination. The following provides a summary of Andrew's mental state examination using this acronym:

Perception Denies hallucinations or delusions, but appears distracted. Stated there were sounds and noises in the room that I couldn't hear. Denies any past or current suicidal ideas.
Affect Slighty tense.
Mood Frustrated in reference to his ex-wife; pessimistic tone.
Speech Loud, disjointed, used an excessive number of words in his responses (over-inclusive), topic shifting from himself to his wife and vice versa.
General behaviour Rigid posture, stiff gait, moving quickly around and with abrupt gestures.
Orientation Oriented to person but not time; reports being confused at times.
Thought Appears to be experiencing auditory hallucinations.
Judgment Impaired, unable to answer problem-solving question.
Insight Impaired.
Memory Grossly intact.
Intelligence Not formally assessed.

Australian and New Zealand states and jurisdictions use variations on the core components of a mental state examination, so be prepared for such differences. The mental state examination can be written in the present or the past tense, and it is useful to include quotations to record verbatim what the person said.

Mini-Mental State Exam

The **Mini-Mental State Exam (MMSE)** (Folstein, Folstein & McHugh, 1975) provides a framework for an assessment of cognitive function in older adults.

For the test to be efficient and valid, you must ask the questions in the order they are listed. Box 10.1 shows four sections of the MMSE, and the general area of information the questions address. A total of 11 questions cover the scope of a person's thinking and reactions. Scores are assigned to each question, and the total score indicates the likelihood and level

Box 10.1 MMSE sample items

- *Orientation to time*—'What is today's date?'
- *Registration*—'Listen carefully, I am going to say three words. You say them back after I stop. Ready? Here they are: APPLE [pause], PURPLE [pause], SPOON [pause]. Now repeat those words back to me.' [Repeat up to five times, but score only the first trial.]
- *Naming*—'What is this?' [Point to a wristwatch.]
- *Reading*—'Please read this and do what it says.' [Show examinee a piece of paper with the following instruction written on it, 'Close your eyes.']

Source: Mini-Mental State Examination, by Marshal Folstein and Susan Folstein, © 1975, 1998, 2001 by Mini Mental LLC, Inc. Published 2001 by Psychological Assessment Resources, Inc.

of cognitive decline. The maximum score is 30 points, and the score is represented as a fraction with the actual points scored as the numerator and 30 points as the denominator (e.g. 28/30, 20/30, etc.).

It is important to note that there are limitations to using the MMSE with people who have certain disabilities with sight or motor movement related to writing. If a person is not able to perform one of the activities, it may be necessary to conduct a full MSE or to document the results of the relevant aspects of the MMSE without a score.

Mental illnesses are categorised in two diagnostic classification systems: the *Diagnostic and Statistical Manual of Mental Disorders* (DSM-5) of the American Psychiatric Association (APA), the 5th edition of which became available in 2015; and the International Classification of Diseases (ICD-10) of the World Health Organization, a new 11th edition of which is expected to be released in 2018. Completion of a full psychiatric–mental health assessment provides the data with which to identify the mental illness the person is suffering from. Such classification systems are increasingly criticised for their focus on medicalising a person's experience, but remain the dominant diagnostic tools today, and are discussed later in the chapter.

Nurses' Observation Scale for Inpatient Evaluations

An assessment tool designed specifically for use by inpatient nurses is the **Nurses' Observation Scale for Inpatient Evaluations (NOSIE).** Developed and determined to be a valid and reliable tool in 1966 (Honigfeld, Gillis & Klett, 1966), it has been useful in quickly assessing a person's functioning on positive features and negative features. Because you can complete this by observing and assessing, it is extremely useful with individuals who refuse to divulge information or are so agitated that closer interactions would not be safe or productive. The NOSIE comes in a long version and a short version, and is undertaken within a specific time period, typically within three days of admission.

PHYSIOLOGICAL ASSESSMENT

As the summary of the MSE suggests, carefully consider the possibility that a person's symptoms may have a physiological or, in particular, a neurological basis. Neurological conditions can present with symptoms very similar to those of psychosis, for example. Thus, there is value in careful assessment regarding general health issues and screening for biological disorders. In many community settings, psychiatric–mental health nurses are the only mental health care providers equipped to undertake a biological and neurological assessment and interpret the results.

The objectives of a biological and neurological assessment are as follows:

1. detection of underlying, and perhaps unsuspected, organic disease that may be responsible for psychiatric symptoms
2. understanding disease as a factor in the overall psychiatric disability
3. appreciation of somatic symptoms that reflect primarily psychological rather than physiological problems.

Physical health history-taking

This procedure is among several that can contribute to a fuller understanding of the biological aspects of psychiatric symptoms. Inquire into three primary areas of a person's physical health history:

1. facts about known physical diseases and dysfunction
2. information about specific physical complaints
3. general health history.

Information about previous illnesses may provide essential clues. People with comorbidities of substance abuse and mental disorder can provide the nurse with additional challenges in identifying presenting need. For example, suppose the person's presenting symptoms include paranoid delusions and the person has a history of similar episodes. During each previous episode, the person responded to diverse forms of treatment and demonstrated no residual symptoms. This history suggests a strong possibility of amphetamine- or other drug-related psychosis, and so a drug screen laboratory test may be indicated.

The second area of emphasis is eliciting information from the person about specific physical complaints. Again, it is crucial to consider symptoms in terms of both psychiatric conditions and physical diseases. Symptoms that are atypical of psychiatric disorders are particularly revealing clues. For example, suppose a person with hallucinations and delusions also complains of a severe headache at the onset of the symptoms. All of the symptoms together suggest possible brain disease, and call for careful and repeated neurological assessment and use of brain imaging techniques.

History taking should also include information about any medications the person is currently taking. Digitalis intoxication (from digoxin, a medication to treat heart problems) may result in visual distortions that may be interpreted as hallucinations. Reserpine (a medication to treat blood pressure) may produce symptoms generally considered psychiatric in nature. Complications such as ataxia and slurred speech could arise from combining the antidepressant medication category selective serotonin reuptake inhibitor (SSRI) with a naturally occurring monoamine oxidase inhibitor (MAOI), which is the herb St John's wort (Fontaine, 2011).

If a person has recently been prescribed psychotropic medication and reports ceasing taking it suddenly, the symptoms of psychosis could be related to medication withdrawal.

The third area is the general health history. As mentioned earlier, psychiatric–mental health nurses need to assess for a variety of general health problems, and must therefore have medical/surgical nursing skills. During your assessment of any person, assess for medical problems as well as the psychiatric symptomatology. A good gauge of a person's health and psychiatric status is the person's sleep patterns. Consider asking the questions in the following Your Assessment Approach feature to determine whether a problem exists. Keep in mind that some medical problems are masked by

YOUR ASSESSMENT APPROACH Basic sleep pattern assessment

Sample questions for assessing a person's basic sleep patterns are as follows.

Sleep–wake schedule

What time do you usually go to bed?
How long does it usually take you to fall asleep after you have turned off the light?
What time do you usually wake up?
What is different about your sleep–wake schedule on the weekend/days off?
How often do you take naps? (Be alert here for cultural influence, such as taking siestas, or occupational influence.) Under what circumstances?

Getting to sleep

What helps you to get to sleep?
What makes it difficult for you to get to sleep?

Staying asleep

On average, how many times do you wake up during the night?
What seems to waken you?
How long does it usually take to get back to sleep?
What do you do if you are having trouble getting back to sleep?
Do you experience recurrent nightmares or distressing dreams that wake you?

Waking up

How difficult is it for you to wake up?
How soon after waking up do you usually get up?
How do you feel when you first get up?

Daytime functioning

At what time of day do you usually feel most energetic?
At what time of day do you feel most sleepy?
Would you call yourself a 'morning person' or an 'evening person'?

Satisfaction with sleep; potential problems

How satisfied are you with the sleep you usually get?
Do you think you get enough sleep on average? How do you know?
How has your sleep been during the past two weeks in comparison to what is normal for you?
Are you concerned about any of the following things?

- Getting to sleep
- Waking up too many times during the night
- Waking up too early
- Having to fight sleepiness during the day
- Snoring, restlessness, talking or walking in your sleep
- Bad dreams
- Drinking too much coffee (or other caffeine/nicotine sources)

When do you enjoy sleep the most?

psychiatric symptoms, and that psychiatric symptomatology can be the result of a medical disorder.

Observation

Observation also yields important data bearing on the possible presence of organic disorders. Some examples follow:

- An unsteady gait may suggest diffuse brain disease or alcohol or drug intoxication.
- Asymmetry—dragging a leg or not swinging one arm—might be a sign of a focal brain lesion.
- Inattention to proper hygiene and dress may be a symptom of depression or psychosis, but may also be due to a neurological deficit such as dementia.
- Frequent, quick, purposeless movements are characteristic of anxiety, but they are equally characteristic of chorea and hyperthyroidism.
- Tremors accompanied by anxiety may point to Parkinson's disease.
- Recent weight loss, although often encountered in depression and schizophrenia, may be due to gastrointestinal disease, carcinoma, Addison's disease, and a number of other physical disorders.

Observe skin colour, pupillary changes, alertness and responsiveness, and quality of speech and word production, keeping in mind the possibility of delirium, dementia, substance intoxication or other medical conditions.

NEUROLOGICAL ASSESSMENT

A careful neurological assessment is mandatory for each person suspected of having brain dysfunction. Its goal is to discover signs pointing to circumscribed, focal cerebral dysfunction or diffuse, bilateral cerebral disease.

Brain imaging techniques

As described in Chapter 6, a range of brain imaging techniques are now available for viewing the living brain to: detect seizure activity; evaluate sleep disorders; detect disorders such as multiple sclerosis; detect tumors, trauma and strokes; examine the blood flowing to the brain; and identify cerebral atrophy, cerebral hemorrhage, cerebral infarct, haematomas and abscesses. All of these conditions may present as psychiatric or behavioural symptoms. The most frequently used brain imaging techniques are described in Box 6.1, Tools of Psychobiology, in Chapter 6.

Mental health professionals understand the need for thorough biological and neurological assessment of people seen in psychiatric settings. The psychiatric literature abounds with accounts of people whose symptoms were initially considered exclusively psychiatric but ultimately proved medical, especially neurological. Assessment errors occurred not because the symptoms did not suggest medical disease, but because such symptoms were given too little weight or were misinterpreted. Changes in the DSM-5 (APA, 2013) require that both a medical condition and substance abuse be ruled out as conditions resulting in psychiatric symptoms, before a psychiatric diagnosis is made.

PSYCHOLOGICAL TESTING

Clinical psychologists administer and interpret a wide variety of psychological tests. There are two categories—those concerned with personality, and those concerned with cognitive function. An awareness of these tests is useful for psychiatric–mental health nurses when reading case notes and attending multi-disciplinary team meetings. See the Box 10.2 for some common psychological tests.

Box 10.2 Common psychological tests

- **Minnesota Multiphasic Personality Inventory–2 (MMPI–2)** is a true–false test. There are 10 major clinical scales measured in this test, which include paranoia, schizophrenia, depression, mania and anxiety.
- **State–Trait Anxiety Inventory** is a self-report instrument. It measures state anxiety (a transitory emotional state characterised by consciously perceived feelings of tension and apprehension and heightened autonomic nervous system activity) and trait anxiety (relatively stable individual differences in vulnerability to anxiety) (Spielberger, 1976).
- **Beck Depression Inventory** consists of questions that ask the person to rate the presence and intensity of various symptoms of depression.

LIVED EXPERIENCE

Trying to understand my experience

At times I really wanted to know what my diagnosis was. It felt like it might give me an explanation to understand my experience. In reality, the diagnosis didn't give me the answers.

When I was living in a housing community for people with mental health problems, no one talked about diagnosis much. We talked to one another as equals, as normal people. The nurse who worked at the house never talked about my diagnosis.

Diagnosis is an important part of the journey in some ways, and has a role to play, but when I arrived at the housing project the nurse who met me there simply asked what my hopes were in life and then accepted my answer. She may have been thinking about how my diagnosis might impact on my hopes, but she didn't project those limitations on to me. Those perspectives and limitations, including the diagnosis I had been given, belonged to her in that moment.

PSYCHIATRIC DIAGNOSTIC PRACTICE ACCORDING TO THE DSM: THE PROBLEM WITH TAXONOMIES

As Chapter 1 demonstrated, determining whether someone is mentally ill is often a matter of judgment. Individual perceptions and social contexts influence how we distinguish normality from abnormality. A now classic study that voiced doubts about the validity of psychiatric diagnosis is at least partly responsible for revamping the system of psychiatric diagnosis.

In this study, David Rosenhan (1973) enlisted the assistance of eight pseudo-patients who sought admission to a variety of mental hospitals in five states. The pseudo-patients arrived at the hospitals complaining of one false symptom—hearing voices. Other than this false symptom, they acted as they normally would, and gave accurate information when interviewed for a psychiatric history and mental status examination. All were admitted to the mental hospitals to which they applied. There were a total of 12 admissions (some pseudo-patients did it twice). In all but one case, the admitting diagnosis was schizophrenia.

Once in the hospital, the pseudo-patients stopped simulating the symptom (hearing voices) and behaved in their usual manner. The average length of stay was 19 days; the range was 7 to 52 days. While in the hospital, the pseudo-patients openly took notes on their experiences. Their note-taking was not hidden from the staff or the other persons. An examination of their charts after the study was concluded revealed that the staff viewed the note-taking solely as a symptom of the pseudo-patients' mental disorder. They were discharged with a diagnosis of schizophrenia in remission (indicating that the disorder is currently under control). In other words, the normality of the pseudo-patients was unrecognised even when they were released after ample opportunity for observation by the staff.

Interestingly, the other persons in care recognised the normality of the pseudo-patients more frequently than did the professional staff. Many told them something like, 'You're not crazy. You're a journalist or a professor checking up on the hospital.' On the other hand, the pseudo-patients were impressed by the largely normal quality of the behaviour of the people in care. They also revealed that the staff spent surprisingly little time interacting with them, and concluded that people with mental illness act in a deviant manner only a small fraction of the time. This lack of interaction presumably contributed to the staff's failure to detect that the pseudo-patients were normal.

Rosenhan's study provoked a great deal of controversy. In defence of the hospitals and their staffs, critics of the study argued that it would have been inhumane to turn away an individual who was hearing voices, and that hearing voices made schizophrenia the most probable diagnosis. This is undeniably true. However, it overlooks the fact that the hospital staff did not have to make an immediate diagnosis based on one symptom alone. They could have deferred a diagnosis pending further observation and assessment.

The subsequent revisions of the DSM led to substantial increases in diagnostic consistency, but has also received increasing scrutiny about pathologising behaviours previously seen as normal. Let us look at how this system has evolved into its current form. The American Psychiatric Association (APA) published the first edition of the DSM in 1952. The DSM-5, published in 2013, represents the current state of knowledge about diagnosing mental disorders. The continual evolution of this specialty area is represented in the changes made from the original DSM. It is composed of a list of all the official numerical codes and terms for all recognised mental disorders, along with a comprehensive description of each, and specified diagnostic criteria that must be present in order to make each diagnosis. Each edition contains updated information regarding numerous clinical issues, such as prevalence and comorbidity, among others. (For a complete list of codes and diagnoses according to the DSM-5, see this text's Appendix A.)

The DSM uses a language describing mental health and disorders that is used by many specialty disciplines in psychiatry/mental health. Studies show that 50 per cent of Western populations would now be diagnosed with a mental disorder under DSM-5, says Professor Gordon Parker, the founder of The Black Dog Institute and a University of New South Wales Scientia professor of psychiatry (ABC online, 2013). 'For 50 per cent of the population to now be regarded as having a psychiatric condition strikes me as straining credulity,' Parker said at a recent media briefing. 'We could quibble about and say "well we don't really mean that you are mad or whatever", but it's not without its implications. If you . . . put down that you have had a DSM diagnosis, such as major depression, you will have great difficulty in getting insurance protection and even travel insurance' (ABC online). In Australia, it is one of two diagnostic manuals currently used; the other, as mentioned earlier, is the International Classification of Diseases: Classification of Mental and Behavioural Disorders 10th Revision (ICD-11), which is published by the World Health Organization.

Nurses use the DSM in two primary ways: we use the diagnostic categories to communicate with other professionals using a common framework, and we use the research presented for causes and prevalence in discussions with consumers and their families.

SELF-AWARENESS

Evaluating your own assessment skills

Person-centred theory was developed by Carl Rogers. The core conditions of accurate empathy, unconditional positive regard and congruence can support your approach to assessment, and provide a framework for reflection on the strengths and weakness of your skills. Rogers stated that it was with the use of these conditions that the potential for change occurs. As part of an evaluation of your skills, you could consider the short explanations of the core conditions before reflecting on the questions below:

- **Congruence**
  - 'It has been observed that personal change is facilitated when the therapist is what he is . . . openly being the feelings and attitude which at that moment are flowing.'
- **Unconditional positive regards**
  - The therapist is experiences a warm, positive and accepting attitude towards what 'is' the person in their care. A genuine willingness for them to be whatever feeling they are experiencing at the time.
- **Empathetic understanding**
  - Sensing feelings and personal meanings which the person is experiencing in each moment, and perceive this from the 'inside', as it seems to that person.

(For further reading, see: Rogers C. R. (1967). *On becoming a person: A therapist's view of psychotherapy*. London, England: Constable.)

Evaluate your assessment skills by responding to the following questions, and reflect on the thoughts and feelings that you experience in response to the prompting questions:

1. Can you ask an open-ended question and not anticipate the answer?
   What is it like not to know the answer?
2. Are you able to remain silent during an interview without being uncomfortable?
   How do you feel when you are sitting in silence with another person?
3. Do you accept information given to you without criticism or judgment?
   How do you respond if you feel criticised or judged?
4. Can you show empathy, not sympathy, for others' problems?
   How would you identify the difference between empathy and sympathy?
5. Gauge your tolerance for unusual or abnormal behaviour.
   How do you experience the behaviour of another person effecting you?
6. Evaluate how aware you are of other cultures and their expressions of distress.
   How will you learn to understand other cultural perspectives?
7. What is your skill level for understanding the content of what is said to you as well as the process (how things are said, not said, done, and not done)?
   What is your own expectation of how much you understand?
8. Do you have success getting your message across to others?
   What would you identify as your key skills in how you communicate, and what skills do you think you might need to develop?
9. Rate your skills for assessing someone accurately on a scale of 0 to 10, with 0 being the lowest level and 10 being the highest. (For example, use a brief interaction with a new colleague, and then discuss your assessment with the colleague.) Discover your weak assessment areas and work on improving them (and raising your score). Repeat regularly.
   What are the specific skills that you are rating, and why did you chose to consider those particular skills?

Basic principles of the multiaxial system

In the DSM multiaxial system, every person is evaluated on five axes, each dealing with a different class of information about the person. DSM's multiaxial assessment is congruent with holistic views of people, recognises the role of environmental stress in influencing behaviour, and requires that the clinician collect data about a person's adaptive strengths as well as about symptoms or problems. Although holistic in its outlook—a positive aspect of the DSM multiaxial system—it should be remembered that the diagnostic process lacks evidence and is subjective in nature. There are limited diagnostic tests available to confirm a mental disorder. It is also worth considering whether the idiosyncrasies of human behaviour might be understood through the multiaxial system, but could also be understood by the person as a valid and understandable reaction to life events and not that of a disorder. You might consider how you will manage the dissonance that can be present in the context of diagnosis.

The following Practice Example illustrates the principle behind a multiaxial system.

Practice example

Multiaxial assessment

A 54-year-old woman came to an outpatient mental health clinic for evaluation and treatment of severe fear and avoidance of flying that amounted to a phobia. However, she also had a long-term personality disturbance and had noticeable eczema.

Clinicians are required to assess this woman's problems in each of three different areas of functioning: behavioural or psychological, personality and physical functioning. However, psychiatric–mental health nurses need to be cognisant of this person's perceptions of her problems and what help she is seeking, rather than assuming that she wants to be helped in all three areas.

The DSM multiaxial system includes the five axes described below. Axes I and II include all the mental disorders in the DSM, and therefore might be said to represent the intrapersonal or *psychological* area of functioning. Axis III is for recording general medical conditions related to understanding the cause of psychiatric symptoms and treating the individual, and thus represents the area of physical functioning. Axes IV and V, for identifying psychosocial and environmental problems and the Global Assessment of Functioning (GAF) scale, respectively, include an assessment of social functioning. In this sense, the multiaxial system provides a comprehensive biopsychosocial approach to assessment.

Description of the axes

The following are the components of the multiaxial system.

Axis I: Clinical disorders Axis I includes all of the Adult and Child Clinical Disorders. Axis I also contains other conditions that may be a focus of clinical attention, but it is not universally agreed that these conditions actually constitute clinical syndromes. Nevertheless, the symptoms elucidated in these conditions are observed often enough to warrant their inclusion in the diagnostic array available to clinicians. These include psychological factors that would affect a physical condition, medication-induced movement disorders, and relational problems.

A mental illness is differentiated from other problems as a clinically significant behavioural or psychological syndrome or pattern that occurs in an individual. A psychiatric disorder is associated with either a painful symptom (distress) or impairment in functioning (disability), or with an increased risk of suffering, death, pain, disability or loss of freedom.

Axis II: Personality disorders Axis II contains the personality disorders, usually diagnosed in adults, and developmental disorders including **intellectual disability** (formerly labelled *mental retardation,* and describes impaired cognitive functioning and adapting), diagnosed in children and adolescents. Axis II is also used to report maladaptive personality traits. All of the remaining mental disorders of adults and children and associated conditions are recorded on Axis I.

The classes of disorders on Axis II were given their own axis because their usually mild and chronic symptoms are often overshadowed by a more problematic Axis I condition. Individuals experiencing the distress associated with an Axis II disorder would be unlikely to describe their distress as mild. The nursing assessment and reflection should aim to understand the experience of the individual and their presentation at assessment. DSM clarifies the distinction between Axis I and Axis II by noting that Axis II conditions have an early onset and follow a stable, not episodic, course. Axis II also has options for describing the lack of a diagnosis or condition on the axis.

Axis III: General medical conditions Clinicians use Axis III to record physical disorders and medical conditions that must be taken into account in planning treatment, or that are relevant to understanding the aetiology or worsening of the mental disorder.

Axis IV: Psychosocial and environmental problems Axis IV is used to identify psychosocial problems that may affect the diagnosis and treatment of mental disorders. In addition to identifying the type of problem(s), evaluators should also note in their own words the specific problems they consider pertinent.

Axis V: Global Assessment of Functioning Axis V, the **Global Assessment of Functioning (GAF)**, reports on the person's overall level of functioning. This information is useful in planning treatment and measuring its impact, and in predicting outcomes. You can perform the reporting of overall functioning on Axis V using the GAF Scale. The GAF Scale gives the clinician an opportunity to examine the overall impact of the person's circumstances on psychological, social and occupational performance. The ratings on this scale fall within decile ranges, and track both symptom severity and functional level. When symptoms and functioning are at different levels, the worse of the two is shown through the score. For example, if a person has moderate symptoms and severe problems functioning, the rating would demarcate the severe problems in functioning. If a person's functioning is basically unimpaired but the symptoms experienced are significant, the symptom level would be represented in the GAF rating. Generally, ratings on the GAF Scale reflect the person's current level of functioning, meaning the lowest level of functioning within the previous seven days.

You should always refer to the person to understand the primary difficulty. The individual may identify different priorities to those identified in the GAF Scale.

PSYCHOSOCIAL ASSESSMENT

Psychosocial assessment is a dynamic process. It begins during the initial contact with the person and continues throughout your nurse–consumer experience. Individual psychosocial assessments are an option, as are family or group psychosocial assessments. The value of a psychosocial assessment or wider interest in a person's life is identified in recovery-orientated assessments such as the Maastricht interview schedule of voice hearing, the Tidal Model and The Recovery star. The wider social experience and sense of citizenship is central to recovery, and therefore needs to be considered as part of the psychosocial assessment. Family and group assessments are discussed in Chapter 24. In every case, they begin with the identifying characteristics, such as name, gender, age, marital status, and ethnic and cultural origins. Problem identification and definition are also necessary phases in the assessment process.

Individual assessment

The whole assessment should be focused on the individual as a full citizen seeking to find agency in their own journey. Nursing values are ideally placed to facilitate this assessment, and to understand the needs of the whole person as part of a recovery journey.

> ## LIVED EXPERIENCE
>
> ### Strengths-based assessment
>
> The assessments that genuinely focused on me were those that considered my hopes and dreams, who I am and what has happened in my story. The greatest assessments found strengths and skills in the experiences of my life. Nurses who didn't seek to change me, because that isn't possible, but instead chose to be creative by exploring how the skills I had developed throughout my life could underpin my recovery journey, were the nurses who had the more valuable part to play in my life. I imagine they loved nursing because they would have experienced the value I found in the way they supported my own empowerment by helping me to connect with the person I am, despite the mental distress I experienced.

During the individual assessment, consider the following factors with the person as the centre and focus of the assessment:

1. physical and intellectual
   a. presence of physical illness and/or disability
   b. appearance and energy level
   c. current and potential levels of intellectual functioning
   d. how the person sees their personal world and translates events around self; the person's perceptual abilities
   e. cause-and-effect reasoning (as agreed between the person and the nurse—it is important to avoid personal judgment); ability to focus
2. socioeconomic factors
   a. economic factors—level of income and adequacy of subsistence, and their effect on lifestyle, sense of adequacy, and self-worth; management of personal finances may be related to mental distress but could also be related to how they were or were not taught to manage personal finances, including cultural factors such as gender, culture and socioeconomic identity
   b. employment and attitudes about it
   c. cultural and ethnic identification; sense of identity and belonging
   d. religious identification can be linked to significant value systems, norms and spiritual practices; spirituality and its meaning for the person are a part of the psychosocial assessment; attachment to a system of meaning, whatever that system may be, can be an asset (see the Practice Box on spiritual health assessment for sample questions that you can use during a spiritual health assessment).
3. personal values and goals
   a. presence or absence of congruence between the person's values and their expression in action; meaning of values to the individual
   b. congruence between the person's values and goals and the immediate systems with which the person interacts
   c. congruence between the person's values and the assessor's values; how agreement or divergence regarding values impacts intervention
4. adaptive functioning and response to present involvement—in the case of a person who has been exposed to interruption in their psychological development, adaption may have a perceived positive benefit to the person, and understanding context is important
   a. manner in which the person presents self to others—grooming, appearance, posture
   b. emotional tone, and change or constancy of levels
   c. style of communication—verbal and non-verbal; ability to express appropriate emotion, follow train of thought; factors of dissonance, confusion, uncertainty
   d. symptoms or symptomatic behaviour

   e. quality of relationships the person seeks to establish—direction, purposes, and uses of such relationships by them
   f. perception of self
   g. social roles that are assumed or ascribed; competence in fulfilling these roles
   h. relational behaviour:
      - capacity for intimacy
      - degree of dependence or independence on a continuum from one extreme to the other
5. developmental factors
   a. how role performance equates with life stage
   b. how developmental experiences have been interpreted and used
   c. how past conflicts, tasks and problems have been handled
   d. whether the present problem is unique in the person's life experience.

The place of assessment in practice

Assessment is essential in clinical practice and serves a number of purposes:

- supporting the nurse to understand the needs and goals of the individual in their recovery journey
- identifying the person's motivations, strengths and resources
- identifying forces (both internal and external to the person) that may hinder the team's therapeutic plan
- setting reasonable goals that are identified and led by the person, given who the person is at this time
- determining appropriate intervention strategies in collaboration with the person
- providing continuous evaluation of the recovery experience, and agreeing with the person when an indication of a potentially valuable change in the therapeutic plan arises.

LIVED EXPERIENCE

My spiritual needs

I had always had difficulty working out the spiritual questions that had arisen in my life. Inviting me to explore my spiritual health and recognising the importance to me was important. This included one nurse talking about her own beliefs, not to try and persuade me to share her beliefs, but to demonstrate that she could relate to their importance. That nurse put me in touch with the chaplain at the hospital. The chaplain became a person who supported me throughout my journey. The nurse who took the time to consider my spiritual needs has given me a gift that has gone way beyond treatment of a mental illness. She gave me the opportunity to find out more about myself and how I find meaning in the world.

Practice example

Spiritual health assessment

For these first five statements, indicate whether you *never, sometimes, often* or *nearly always* agree.

1. I trust myself.
2. I feel my life has meaning and purpose.
3. Other people give meaning to my life.
4. I trust other people.
5. I have close friends.
6. I have experienced the following in my life:

   Loss _____ Separation _____ Divorce _____

   Geographic moves _____ Rejection _____ Death _____
7. Do *religion* and *spirituality* mean the same thing to you? If not, what are the differences to you?
8. With 1 being the lowest and 10 the highest, place an X on the following scale to indicate your relationship with your higher power, and circle the place on the scale that you feel would be ideal for your relationship with your higher power. Explain why you chose each of these points.

   (no relationship) (turn only problems over) (turn total self over)

   1 2 3 4 5 6 7 8 9 10
9. My religious upbringing and background can be described as (check as many as apply):

   Nurturing _____ Helpful _____ Strict _____

   Conservative _____ Liberal _____ Punishing _____

   Negative _____ Had very little _____ Had none _____

Assessment is an ongoing, dynamic process that utilises all of your senses and all of your skills in collaboration with the senses and skills of the person in your care. Your observations, combined with all of the information you receive from the person, interdisciplinary team members and collateral sources, provide an opportunity to engage in a partnership based on the mutual definition of problems and goals. If a person says, 'I'd be better off dead', you must assess the lethality risk and intervene to prioritise the person's safety. However, exploration of the statement may broaden your understanding and impact on the sense of risk. If you see physical signs of abuse, such as bruises in various stages of healing without adequate explanation, your assessment warrants a private interview with the person during which you can ask, 'Does anyone ever hurt you?' If treatment does not seem to be addressing the main symptoms, or side-effects from medications seem to cause flagging, focus on continued adherence, assess the person's reactions and discuss options.

Assessment is the solid base upon which you build your practice and perform your interventions. See the following Evidence-based Practice feature for an example of how assessment of the person and the environment are vital to good nursing care. Information and services that help nurses, physicians, persons, other providers and health plans navigate the complexity of the health care system can be found at Web MD (http://www.webmd.com).

EVIDENCE-BASED PRACTICE

Assessment of an older adult and her caregiving family members

Jane is 84 years old, and her 87-year-old husband and other family members provide caregiving services in her home for end-stage heart disease. Even though she enjoys having her family care for her, there are many times when Jane feels stressed by the reactions of her family to the inevitability of her health status. Fatigue and shortness of breath have been the main symptoms Jane experiences, although she has been sad and feeling unsupported lately. Jane has not told anyone about these feelings.

Your assessment of Jane's situation is based on current research results. Your research review highlights quality-of-life issues for end-of-life care, and the contribution of psychological distress for the caregivers when higher levels of care are needed. You learned that Jane, and possibly her husband, will likely have psychosocial symptoms. A discussion with Jane and her husband may help both of them to voice their feelings and consider the interplay of physical and emotional symptoms. Assessing physical and psychosocial symptoms allows a complete picture of the status of a person and directs interventions.

The professional involved in Jane's care discussed the information you gathered during your assessment. The plan is to incorporate feeling identification, support system structures, and ongoing assessment of symptoms of depression into the overall care that Jane receives. Intervening with Jane's caregivers is similarly important.

You should base action on more than one study, but you would find the following research helpful in this situation.

Pinquart, M., & Sörensen, S. (2011). Spouses, adult children, and children-in-law as caregivers of older adults: A meta-analytic comparison. *Psychology and Aging, 26*(1), 1–14.

CRITICAL THINKING QUESTIONS

1. How could you use the Global Assessment of Functioning Scale to develop a plan of care for Jane?
2. Why would you approach Jane and her family members to discuss these issues?
3. What specific communication techniques (based on the information in Chapter 9) would be helpful in obtaining an accurate assessment and encouraging Jane and her family to talk with you about their concerns?

Care plans

Care plans are a means of providing nursing personnel with information about the needs and therapeutic plans for each person. They are of major importance when an agency uses source-oriented documentation, because they provide an ongoing, up-to-date record of goal-directed, individualised nursing care. When problem-oriented documentation is used, nursing care plans may be an outgrowth of that documentation.

Care plans should be clinical presentation of collaboratively agreed plans with the person.

HOW I WILL USE MY MENTAL-HEALTH SKILLS IN PRACTICE

In clinical practice, the use of nursing knowledge and skills underpins the approach to assessment. It does not necessarily mean explicitly employing the many assessment tools and diagnostically-driven concerns of risk and containment. Considering the person as a fellow student of the current experience or mutual therapist can support the process of keeping the person central to the assessment process.

Adopting a nursing model that fits with your personal ethical and philosophical perspectives can be a valuable method of approaching assessment. Many nursing models exist that support both specific aspects of nursing or the more broad approach. Two nursing models that seek to place the human relationships and understanding of the individual's experiences as a primary approach are described briefly here. Models that place emphasis on the relationship between the nurse and the person provide a framework in which you can apply the relevant assessment tools and approaches, described in this chapter, and remain clear about your value base as a nurse.

You may choose to explore other nursing models that resonate with you views and values.

The first model we will look at is Joyce Travelbee's *interpersonal aspects nursing model* (Travelbee, 1971). Also referred to as the *human-to-human model of nursing*, this approach places value on the uniqueness of the relationship that is developed between two individuals. The primary goal in the human-to-human model is to establish a rapport. Travelbee identified that developing rapport may take weeks or months. When rapport is established, then the practical work of mental health nursing can begin: working towards personal meaning with the individual (person) in overcoming suffering.

The second model that is consistent with the value of the human encounter in a nursing intervention is Hildegarde Peplau's *theory of interpersonal relations* (Peplau, 1952). The model is a psychodynamically-orientated approach that places the nurse as a representation of the different challenges the person may have faced in their journey to the point of mental distress. The role of the nurse is to develop a trusting and secure relationship with the person, enabling the person to work through the difficulties that have presented in their life towards resolution of mental distress.

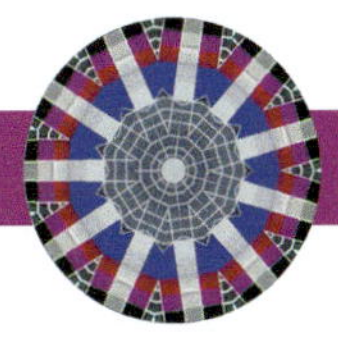

REFERENCES

ABC online. (2013). The Pulse DSM5 Why all the fuss? http://www.abc.net.au/health/thepulse/stories/2013/05/23/3766048.htm (Accessed 2015, August 4.)

American Psychiatric Association (APA). (2013). *Diagnostic and statistical manual of mental disorders* (5th ed.). Washington, DC: APA Publishing.

Folstein, M., Folstein, S., & McHugh, P. (1975). Mini-Mental State: A practical method for grading the cognitive state of patients for the clinician. *Journal of Psychiatric Residents, 12,* 189.

Fontaine, K. L. (2011). Herbs and nutritional supplements. In K. L. Fontaine (Ed.), *Complimentary and alternative therapies for nursing practice*. New York, NY: Pearson.

Honigfeld, G., Gillis, R. D., & Klett, C. J. (1966). NOSIE-30: A treatment-sensitive ward behavior scale. *Psychological Reports, 19,* 180–182.

Peplau, H. E. (1952). *Interpersonal relations in nursing*. New York, NY: G. P. Putnam & Sons.

Pinquart, M., & Sörensen, S. (2011). Spouses, adult children, and children-in-law as caregivers of older adults: A meta-analytic comparison. *Psychology and Aging, 26*(1), 1–14.

Rogers, C. R. (1967). *On becoming a person: A therapist's view of psychotherapy.* London, England: Constable.

Rosenhan, D. I. (1973). On being sane in insane places. *Science, 179,* 250–258.

Spielberger, C. D. (1976). The nature and measurement of anxiety. In C. D. Spielberger & R. Diaz-Guerrero (Eds.), *Cross cultural anxiety* (pp. 3–12). Washington, DC: Hemisphere/Wiley.

Travelbee, J. (1971). *Interpersonal aspects of nursing* (2nd ed.). Philadelphia, PA: F. A. Davis Company.

Trzepacz P. T., & Baker R. W. (1993). *The psychiatric mental status examination.* Oxford, England: Oxford University Press.

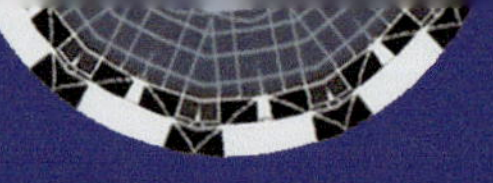

11 Ethics, legal issues and the rights of people with a mental illness

EIMEAR MUIR-COCHRANE, ADAM GERACE AND JANNE MCMAHON

KEY TERMS

competency *219*
discharge *216*
expert witness *222*
fitness to plead *219*
informed consent *217*
involuntary admission *216*
least restrictive setting *223*
mental impairment/illness/ incompetence or insanity defence *220*
Tarasoff decision *223*
voluntary admission *216*

LEARNING OUTCOMES

After completing this chapter, you will be able to:

1. Relate the six principles of bioethics to the practice of psychiatric–mental health nursing.
2. Apply ethical guidelines in reconciling ethical dilemmas.
3. Describe how psychiatric–mental health nurses can avoid indirectly contributing to the stereotypes associated with psychiatric diagnostic categories.
4. Understand the principles of mental health legislation.
5. Deliver psychiatric–mental health nursing care in a manner that preserves and protects peoples' rights, dignity and autonomy, and supports their recovery.
6. Partner with people with a mental illness and their families in developing psychiatric advance directives.

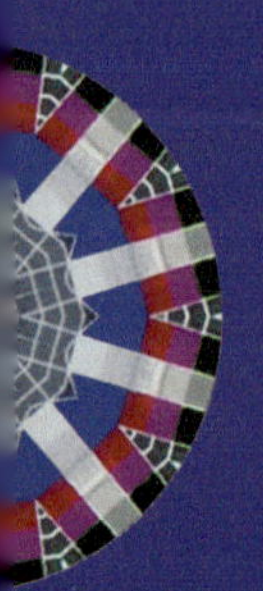

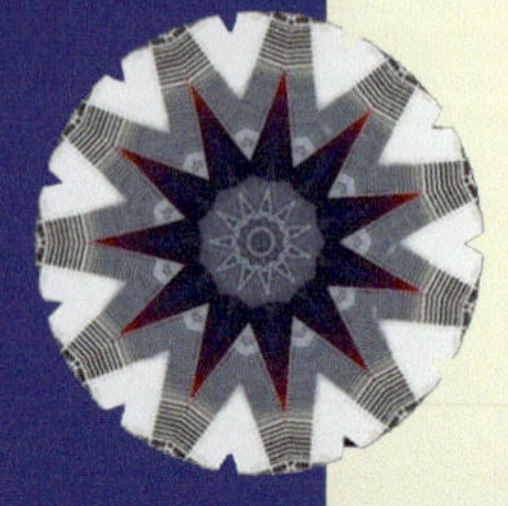

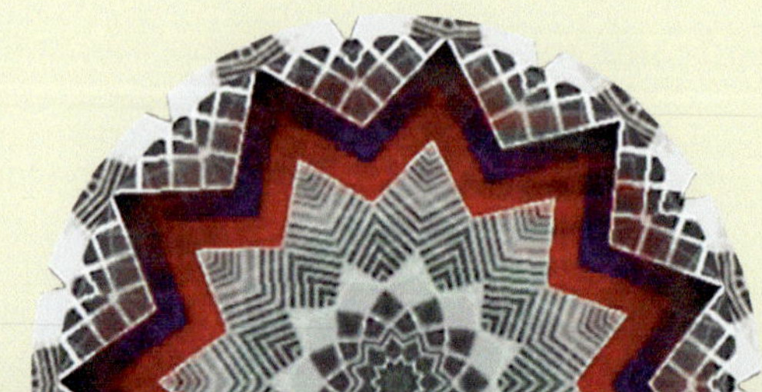

Practice example

Person refusing treatment

Sue Aberdeen is a person attending a mental health community clinic. She was diagnosed with bipolar disorder more than 20 years ago. At one time or another during this period, various mental health care providers have prescribed several different medications for Sue. Most have been only slightly helpful, or ineffective. Most recently, Sue has been taking lithium, which seems to be the most helpful. Her long-time friend has brought Sue to the clinic because Sue has not been taking her medication. She has been unable to sleep, and is distracted and agitated. Sue has been to many different bars during the week, on occasion taking men home to have sex. The nurse assigned to her case has been attempting to persuade Sue to take her lithium. Sue has continued to refuse, and the nurse has continued to explain and cajole. Finally, Sue shouts: 'You just don't get it, do you? You're a bitch!' and stomps out of the clinic.

1. How can you reconcile the desire and duty to help with Sue's refusal of treatment?
2. When do you think it is acceptable for a person to refuse to be treated?
3. What are the options for handling a person's refusal to cooperate with treatment?

INTRODUCTION

Ethical, legal and economic decisions profoundly influence mental health practice, and bring about changes in the understanding and practice of mental health intervention. These changes challenge the psychiatric–mental health nurse to examine such central issues as the following:

- How does one balance the common 'good' and the individual 'good' in health care?
- What are the rights and accountabilities of nurses and people with mental illness?

An examination of these issues generally improves care, but it often confuses the boundaries of ethical behaviour, mental health practice and the law. This confusion entraps mental health care professionals, people with a mental illness, families, lawyers and the public in a muddle of conflicting policies and procedures. In addition, a person's right to privacy, and to receive and refuse treatment, pivots on society's values.

This chapter will bring some clarity to the ever-changing relationship between ethics, the law and mental health services, so that you can practise ethically and with confidence, and also exercise your power as citizens, professionals and advocates to influence the direction of mental health care.

ETHICS

Having a good foundation in ethics is important in psychiatric–mental health nursing. You may find yourself having to identify alternative courses of action, and decide what to do when there is a conflict of rights and obligations between people with a mental illness and their families, between yourself and other mental health care workers, and between yourself and the mental health agency or institution.

Ethics is a branch of philosophy that deals with the values that are related to human conduct, the rightness and wrongness of actions, the goodness and badness of one's motives, and the goodness and badness of the results of one's actions. *Bioethics* is a field that applies ethical reasoning to issues and dilemmas in the area of health care. Ethical conflicts involve complex ethical issues and dilemmas that are tempered by the need to provide culturally congruent care.

Ethical analysis

One of the major difficulties in ethical analysis is that there are no definite, clear-cut solutions to ethical dilemmas. For centuries, moral philosophers—beginning with Socrates, Plato and Aristotle—have struggled with two main ethical questions: 'What is the meaning of "right" or "good"?' and 'What should I do?'

Taking a stand on an ethical issue involves much more than merely accepting the moral position or personal values of another. It requires an understanding of the principles of bioethics. To identify, clarify, define and defend a stand on an ethical issue, we must engage in a process of ethical reasoning. Carefully consider the content in Mental Health in the Media. Which of the following ethical principles may have been violated in the circumstances described there?

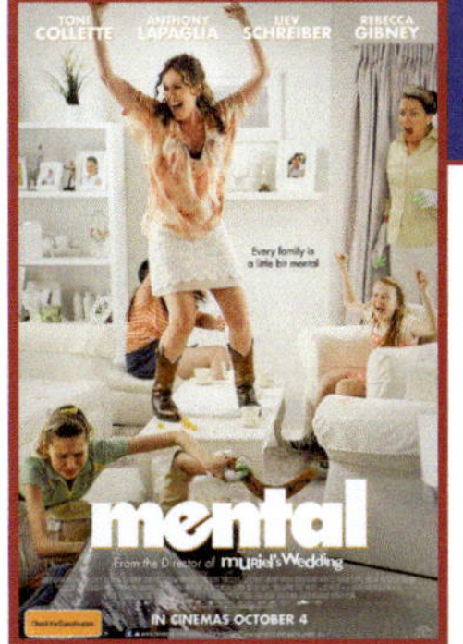

MENTAL HEALTH IN THE MEDIA

Mental

The Moochmores are an unusual family living in a quiet coastal town in Australia. Shirley and her husband have five daughters, who are a handful. Shirley is obsessed with *The Sound of Music*, and when her behaviour is deemed to be 'out of control' she is sent 'on holiday to Wollongong', which is code for involuntary detention in a psychiatric hospital. This is a controversial comedy exploring a number of mental illnesses and other social taboos with irreverence. However, it is also a deeply moving film, and reflects on the nature of the human condition with great clarity. Sheila is hospitalised against her will on more than one occasion, and this is disguised as her going on a 'holiday'. Why do you think her husband deals with her illness in this way? What other strategies would have been more beneficial for Sheila and her family? What positive messages about mental illness does the film portray?

Principles of bioethics

The six principles of bioethics discussed here are autonomy, beneficence, fidelity, justice, nonmaleficence and veracity. Nurses in psychiatric–mental health settings are continually balancing the principles of beneficence and nonmaleficence with autonomy (Chiovitti, 2011).

Autonomy

Autonomy is the freedom to choose a course of action, to act on that choice, and to live with the consequences of that choice. Helping people with a mental illness, and their families and significant others, make choices fosters autonomy. You help a person in care by providing them with the information they need in order to choose, helping them to understand and sort through the information, and supporting their choice, even when that choice is one that you may not have made yourself. Professional autonomy for you, as a psychiatric–mental health nurse, means having to account for and accept the consequences of professional decisions and actions. Nursing professionals must balance the goal of greater autonomy with efforts to achieve what providers and people with a mental illness determine are the common good and the individual good in health care.

Beneficence

Beneficence is the principle of attempting to do things that benefit others or promote the good of others. You operate under the principle of beneficence whenever you help people with a mental illness who cannot decide for themselves, or are incapacitated or incompetent. Protecting people with a mental illness from harming themselves because of thoughts, feelings or behaviours that lead to self-harm is done in a spirit of beneficence.

Fidelity

Fidelity means that you maintain loyalty and commitment to the people with a mental illness in your care, and are faithful to your promises, duties and obligations. Fidelity is crucial to establishing trusting relationships with people with a mental illness, their families and other mental health workers. Fidelity also means that you do not make promises you will not or cannot keep.

Justice

Justice is the principle of treating others fairly and equally. It is the fair and equitable distribution of burdens and benefits. The principle of justice has always been a cornerstone of bioethics, and has become even more important when considered with regard to issues related to health care reform and managed care.

Nonmaleficence

Nonmaleficence is the intention to do no wrong. Your motives for actions should be in the direction of helpfulness based on sound knowledge of psychiatric–mental health theory. Nonmaleficence requires you to be self-aware, and is the principle behind the Self-awareness features throughout this text.

Veracity

Veracity is the intention to tell the truth. Like fidelity, veracity is crucial to establishing trust with people with a mental illness, their families and other mental health care workers. If you cannot be trusted to do what you say you will do, or to tell the truth, you cannot be depended on; what you do and what you say will be open to suspicion.

Ethical guidelines for psychiatric–mental health nurses

Most professions develop guidelines for the behaviour of their members. Ethical guidelines for psychiatric–mental health nurses stem from two sources. The first source is the standards for psychiatric–mental health nursing practice published by the Australian College of Mental Health Nurses (2012). These standards are reproduced and discussed in detail in Chapter 3). Standard Four specifically refers to ethics in health care. Standard Six refers to the role of the psychiatric–mental health nurse in striving to reduce stigma and promote social inclusion for all people with mental health issues, while Standard Eight reflects nurses' responsibilities to the profession's code of conduct and related ethics.

In New Zealand, the New Zealand College of Mental Health Nurses (2012) uphold Standards of Practice for Mental Health Nursing in Aotearoa New Zealand. These standards underpin quality mental health nursing practice for all psychiatric–mental health nurses in Aoteraroa New Zealand. The standard of professional performance that deals specifically with ethics for psychiatric–mental health nurses is Standard Six. Use these sources to make clinical judgments and to engage in ethical reasoning.

In Australia, the Nursing and Midwifery Board of Australia (2013) has established a specific Code of Ethics for Nurses, which details the fundamental ethical values to which all registered nurses are committed. They are as follows:

1. Nurses value quality nursing care for all people.
2. Nurses value respect and kindness for self and others.
3. Nurses value the diversity of people.
4. Nurses value access to quality nursing and health care for all people.
5. Nurses value informed decision-making.
6. Nurses value a culture of safety in nursing and health care.
7. Nurses value ethical management of information.
8. Nurses value a socially, economically and ecologically sustainable environment promoting health and wellbeing.

Clinical judgment and ethical reasoning

Psychiatric–mental health nurses are frequently faced with the following two goals:

1. responding to the therapeutic needs of individuals
2. enacting the *Mental Health Act* to protect society from people who may be at risk to themselves or others due to their mental illness.

Often, these two goals are in conflict, and nurses face the dilemma of placing one above the other, especially in circumstances in which an unwell individual behaves in a threatening or violent manner (Mariano et al., 2011).

Nurses are necessarily guided in their therapeutic work by a belief system—some vision of what kinds of changes would improve the person's life. Nurses are further guided by some moral principles that limit the extent to which they will help a person obtain happiness at the expense of others, and the extent to which they will participate in the oppression of an individual in the interests of societal control. Anyone who is responsible for moral choices is obliged to recognise the reason or principle on which they make a decision. Laws represent yet another source of limits. They are discussed later in this chapter in the section on the rights of people with a mental illness.

Ethical dilemmas in psychiatric–mental health nursing

Ultimately, nurses must reconcile a number of crucial ethical dilemmas with their personal and professional values. Among these issues are the following:

- the stigma of psychiatric diagnostic labels
- psychiatry's right to control individual freedom
- the justification for involuntary treatment
- the use of restrictive treatment interventions
- the person's right to suicide
- the person's right to privacy.

Practising psychiatric–mental health nursing requires ethical responsibility; however, problems arise when there is conflict about the ground rules for behaviour between people with a mental illness and health professionals. As Davis and her associates put it, nurses are agents for both the organisation and the person (Davis, Fowler & Aroskar, 2010). These problems are phrased in the ethical language of right and wrong. Circumstances likely to give rise to such problems include the following:

- The professional and the person with a mental illness are from different cultures and may have different values.
- The voluntary nature of the person's participation is compromised.
- The person's competence to enter into an agreement about intervention is questionable, or the person does not realise that certain interventions are being implemented.
- External factors (lack of time, lack of staff, high demands) prevent the professional from doing what is best for the person with a mental illness.
- There is a dimension of 'power' differential, whether real or perceived.

It has been suggested that having moral insight, virtue and ethics in nursing can be taught through appropriate experience, habitual practice and good role models (Cannaerts, Gastmans & Dierckx de Casterle, 2014). Therefore, it is optimal to look for an experienced nurse mentor who can supervise your ethical practice and serve as a good role model.

Every nursing relationship begins with an unusual burden of ethical responsibility. The following sections explore some of these moral issues.

Neuroethics: an emerging field

The field of neuroethics is emerging from a 21st-century partnership between bioethics and neuroscience. Rapid advances in neuroscience, brought about by brain research, have raised critical ethical, social and legal issues about neuroimaging, psychopharmacology, deep-brain stimulation, which is a form of psychosurgery that can ameliorate symptoms of Parkinson's and sometimes disable obsessive–compulsive behaviours, and ameliorate intransigent depression. Deep-brain stimulation involves the implantation of fine stimulating electrodes into small areas of the brain. The electrodes are then connected to a pacemaker device placed under the skin of the chest. The electrodes electrically stimulate local brain areas to try to modify brain activity that is proposed to be abnormal in a particular disorder. The critical questions revolve around: the prediction of disease (including mental disorders in certain instances); questions of privacy and confidentiality; concerns about the effects on an individual's autonomy; and the influences of neuroimaging, psychopharmacology (Mohamed & Sahakian, 2011) and deep-brain stimulation (Clausen, 2010) on an individual's concept of self and personal identity.

Despite myriad new neuroscience information and the creation of a new journal focusing on neuroscience and ethics in 2008 (*Neuroethics*), the brain remains the most complex and least understood of all the organs in the human body. Mapping the neural correlates of the mind through brain scans, and altering these correlates through surgery, stimulation or psychopharmacologic interventions, can affect people in both positive and negative ways. Neuroscientists and mental health professionals must carefully weigh and actively debate the potential benefits of this knowledge and technology against their potential harm. There are also now emerging centres in neuroethics, such as The Center for Cognition and Neuroethics (CCN), a joint venture between the Philosophy Department at the University of Michigan-Flint and the Insight Institute of Neurosurgery and Neuroscience (IINN), in the United States.

Stigma of psychiatric diagnoses

The list of stereotypes associated with psychiatric diagnostic categories is well known to most nurses. Equally familiar are the consequences to people with these diagnoses. Stereotypes include terms such as 'druggies' and alcoholics, and these individuals acquire a discredited social identity because of the character flaws often associated with these labels. To much of society, the labels used in psychiatry suggest criminality, immorality and wanton disregard for society's values. It is important to consider how and when psychiatric–mental health nurses, while advocating humane treatment for people with a mental illness, indirectly contribute to discrediting a person's social identity by participating in the arbitrary use of oppressive labels. Reflect on the following: do you believe that standardised labels and vocabulary dismiss the unique stories of people with mental health issues and their families?

LIVED EXPERIENCE

Who I am

A psychiatric diagnosis does not define a person. It is vital that the whole person is seen as who they are—that is, a daughter, son, mother, father, sibling and so on; a human being with the same faults and values as other members of society. Having a psychiatric diagnosis does not mean that the person is any less worthy of care than someone with a physical condition or illness.

It does not mean that people are unpredictable or dangerous, nor does it mean that those requiring acute care or those admitted involuntarily do not have the ability to understand. Having a psychiatric diagnosis is not the same thing as having an intellectual disability; rather, many people are quite able to make choices, and these choices should be respected. This is the essence of autonomy. Too often in today's society, labels hurt, and being placed into a category where you lose your identity is not helpful in functioning, awareness or outcome. There is also a parallel position for some people with a mental illness: that being given a diagnosis may provide them with a sense of relief, that the things they experience have a name, thus legitimising their experiences.

People with a mental illness are not a homogenous group, and may be comfortable with a diagnosis and the treatment they receive, while others may have very strong beliefs about how they wish to manage their recovery.

Need for diagnostic labels Diagnosis has considerable value in psychiatric practice, and often dictates a particular course of treatment to facilitate a person's recovery. Diagnostic categories enable nurses to plan comprehensively for person-centred care and to conduct research. However, without a diagnosis people cannot receive treatment from either public or private mental health services. This is problematic from a recovery-oriented approach, where people may wish to receive support and treatment from mental health professionals but do not accept their diagnosis.

Nurses' moral stance on diagnoses Take time to consider carefully how you would answer the following questions:

- Does labelling with psychiatric diagnoses provide psychiatric professionals with some additional sense of control over treatment of people with a mental illness in their care?
- Is it true that a diagnosis gives staff members an increased sense of being able to predict a person's behaviour, and a way of calmly viewing what might otherwise be upsetting behaviour? For example, 'Those behaviours are just a manifestation of paranoid delusions.'

The consequences of psychiatric labels for people with a mental illness and their families, however, raise moral questions about their legitimacy. Nurses have a moral responsibility to question practices that may prevent or reduce opportunities for recovery in people with a mental illness.

Control of individual freedom

Involuntary hospitalisation and treatment of people with a mental illness are usually considered necessary interventions. Yet, any practice that directly and coercively deprives a person of freedom has political implications. In some jurisdictions and in certain circumstances, people with a mental illness have little certainty about the time they may be held involuntarily. Any compulsory inpatient treatment must be justified as necessary to protect the person or others from harm.

Violence against others Psychiatric–mental health nurses are faced with the dilemma of trying to be both carers and agents of social control. Dealing with violent people with a mental illness requires balancing the value of life against the value of liberty.

Suicide Traditionally, nurses have felt that they should do everything possible to preserve life. This imperative has been relied upon to justify intervention in suicide attempts, as well as heroic technical measures to avert impending deaths. Psychiatry, in general, rejects the notion of rational suicide, and assumes that suicidal ideation is an irrational belief resulting from mental disorder. Further, it is assumed that a person without a mental disorder would not choose suicide. Thus, we seek to prevent suicide on the basis that this is what the person would choose if they were mentally capable of choosing. In this, as well as in many areas of psychiatric–mental health nursing practice, there are contested matters and areas of differing opinion.

The treatment given to people dying is often in conflict with the treatment they desire. For example, a physician may disregard a person's protests against treatment. The physician may assert that the person's medical condition is causing them to behave irrationally. There is not necessarily an ethical difference between people dying of physical deterioration and people with a mental illness dying of emotional or mental deterioration. Many of the same ethical questions emerge about the suicidal person, as in the following examples:

- How is *quality of life* defined?
- Is the definition limited to physical factors?
- Who should have the right to make the definition?
- How is rationality to be measured?
- Are people always in conscious control of their choices?

A thorough discussion of suicide is given in Chapter 19.

An individual's right to choose when and how to die is a complex bio-ethical issue. The thoughtful professional nurse needs to clarify the issues, give them careful consideration, and search for a personal position. There are many ways in which people can deliberately shorten or end their own lives. They can take their own lives quickly with fireams or by hanging, or slowly through the chronic use of drugs such as tobacco or alcohol. When is coercive intervention by psychiatric practitioners justified?

Psychotropic medications The discovery that certain medications can radically alter the expression of human emotions has had an enormous impact on psychiatry and society in general. Mental health professionals have associated the advent of psychotropic medications with a new optimism and less fear about working with people labelled mentally ill. Furthermore, it might be argued that medications have helped keep people out of hospital, and have decreased the need for other more dramatic measures, such as restraint and seclusion. Psychotropic medications today can enable people to live productive lives in recovery; however, many people are not relieved of all their symptoms with medication, and some medications cause harm through unwanted and irreversible side-effects, such as metabolic syndrome and cardiovascular disease.

The cautious and judicious use of drugs with the person's consent can be helpful. Decisions about the use of drugs ought be made in the context of the person's social situation and environment. In hospital settings, medications are regularly used to reduce symptoms and make the person's behaviour more manageable. Some staff members justify their use of chemical controls to control violent or bizarre behaviour, as in the Practice Example that follows.

Practice example

After pacing angrily up and down the hall in front of the nurses' station for 20 minutes or so, Carlotta kicks the day-room door. A male staff member shouts to the nurse to get her PRN medication ready and enters the day room telling Carlotta to stop it. Carlotta cries and shouts, and several other staff members rush over to assist. They restrain Carlotta into her room, where she is given intramuscular medication to calm her. She continues to scream and hit out at staff. Finally, staff decide to transfer her to the unit downstairs, where she can be put into a seclusion room. In a report, a staff member describes the incident as: 'Carlotta lost control and needed to be secluded to calm down.'

What other strategies could staff have explored to assist Carlotta to calm down? Was it necessary to place her in seclusion?

Restraints From the perspective of a person with a mental illness, containment in the form of seclusion or forced medication (restraint) has a negative psychological impact, is traumatising, and is perceived as unethical behaviour on the part of staff members (Strout, 2010). Many people view these interventions as forms of abuse, while staff see them as a last-resort management tool, when all other strategies have been exhausted, (McCann, Baird & Muir-Cochrane, 2015).

LIVED EXPERIENCE

Least restrictive environment

There is a political imperative to reduce or eliminate restraint—both physical and chemical—and seclusion in Australia. Why was Carlotta not approached to seek the reason for her agitation? Perhaps with this information the staff member might or ought to have been able to defuse or de-escalate the situation, if Carlotta were approached calmly and with a genuine desire to relieve her agitation or meet her needs. In other words, engage meaningfully with Carlotta first before reaching for medication.

All the judgments made about restraining people with a mental illness involve moral decisions such as:

- What other calming and de-escalation techniques have been tried?
- Is the person obviously out of control?
- How does the nurse decide when restraints are necessary?
- Is the person cognitively compromised?
- What will be the effects on the person of such a dramatic intervention?
- What are the effects on others witnessing restraint?

LIVED EXPERIENCE

Restraint always a last resort

In reality, being restrained does not mean people will become compliant; rather, this is a withdrawal of choice. It is dehumanising, traumatic and has a lasting effect, sometimes for a lifetime. People do not choose to be restrained. Rather, this is something that is forced upon them, mostly in the name of aggression reduction or risk management. There are instances where this is appropriate, but only after everything else has been done to genuinely engage in discussion about what the person is experiencing or about meeting their needs. It is an ethical dilemma: eliminate the harm to self or others by seclusion or restraint, or risk being an agent in the withdrawal of personal freedom. Seclusion or restraint must never be used to punish or force compliance, and should only be used as a last resort when all other alternatives have been tried.

LAW, MENTAL HEALTH AND INVOLUNTARY TREATMENT ISSUES

Each state in Australia has a *Mental Health Act*, which makes provisions for the treatment, care and control of those people with a mental illness. The laws differ between jurisdictions, and it is critical to your practice to be knowledgeable about the statutes and regulations in the jurisdiction in which you practice. In New Zealand, provisions are made through one national mental health Act. Most mental health agencies and facilities maintain copies of these statutes, and the latest versions are readily available on the websites of the Parliamentary Counsel Office in New Zealand and state health departments in Australia.

Admission and treatment order categories

The two major categories of inpatient hospitalisation are voluntary and **involuntary admission**. The procedures for admission and release, as well as the rights of people under these admissions (e.g. to refuse treatment interventions, leave the mental health facility) differ. For people with a mental illness under an involuntary admission, there are different types of treatment orders, with mental health Acts specifying the criteria for enacting various treatment orders, procedures for review of orders, and variation/revocation of involuntary orders. People also have a right to appeal against involuntary hospitalisation and treatment. In both voluntary and involuntary admissions, treatment plans (also named, depending on the specific legislation: treatment and care plans; treatment, support and **discharge** plan) must consider the person's recovery from illness.

Voluntary admission

Voluntary admission involves a person being admitted at their request, or at the request of someone acting on their behalf, such as a guardian, parent or partner, with the person's consent. Authorised medical staff make a determination that the person requires care and treatment in the inpatient setting. The person has the right to leave the psychiatric unit at any time, although during their hospitalisation authorised staff may make an application for an involuntary treatment order if the person wants to leave against the advice of treating staff. In keeping with the objectives of contemporary mental health service provision that care is provided in the least restrictive means, many mental health Acts specify that services be provided as much as possible on a voluntary basis. However, the move towards community-based treatment often means that those people who are most unwell and under an involuntary order make up the largest group of people in inpatient treatment facilities. Staff also face the dilemma of providing care for voluntary patients in such a setting. For example, voluntary patients in units where entry and exit doors are locked would need to ask staff to open the door to allow them to leave (Muir-Cochrane & Gerace, 2014).

Involuntary hospitalisation

Involuntary hospitalisation can come about if authorised medical or mental health practitioners find that the person meets the criteria for an involuntary treatment order. Other designated bodies, such as a court or administrative tribunal, often make the decision that a person fits the criteria for an involuntary treatment order.

Most states and territories provide for more than one involuntary hospitalisation procedure. The criteria vary between jurisdictions according to the type of involuntary hospitalisation. However, all involuntary admission statutes can be expected to include one or more of the following criteria:

- the person has a mental illness or is considered to have a mental disorder
- the assessment has been undertaken by a suitably qualified clinician
- treatment is required to prevent risk of harm to the person or others
- treatment is required to prevent deterioration of the person's mental or physical health or the ability to take care of themselves
- less-restrictive means, such as voluntary admission or treatment in the community under a community treatment order, are not considered appropriate for the required treatment.

In more recent mental health legislation in Australia, the concept of *decision-making capacity* is used as a criterion for an assessment or treatment order. This reflects an increased focus on human rights as set out in conventions and human rights legislation, such as the United Nations Convention on the Rights of Persons with Disabilities (CRPD), which was ratified by both Australia and New Zealand in 2008 (Callaghan & Ryan, 2012). In these mental health Acts, if a person has the ability to understand, remember, use and weigh information, and to communicate their wishes, it is presumed that they have capacity to make an informed decision and provide consent about their assessment and treatment. This does not mean, however, that a person will not be made subject to an order if authorised staff consider this appropriate for their care; and some consider involuntary hospitalisation and treatment a contradiction of the CRPD (Callaghan & Ryan, 2014). More broadly, involuntary hospitalisation can produce an ethical conflict for health professionals—the duty of beneficence towards others versus the removal of personal autonomy (Cherry, 2010).

Types of involuntary orders and specific procedures to be followed differ between jurisdictions in Australia and New Zealand. Involuntary orders can be divided into the following categories:

- assessment or examination orders
- treatment orders
- court treatment orders.

Assessment or examination orders *Assessment* or *examination orders* provide for the compulsory examination of a person at a mental health service to determine whether they meet the criteria for further hospitalisation and an involuntary treatment order. Assessment orders may also be enacted while the person is in the community. Under these orders, treatment is not to be provided unless it is deemed necessary to prevent imminent serious harm to the person or to others. Medical or mental health practitioners make an order for assessment, and this may be based on an application from nurses, police, ambulance officers, guardians or other prescribed persons. Courts may also make court assessment orders for persons who plead guilty or are found guilty of an offence. Many of the same criteria under a mental health Act apply; as well as criteria specified in Acts specific to sentencing those who have committed an offence.

A registered medical or mental health practitioner should have examined the person within a specific period of time designated by the relevant Act before applying for an order, and inform the person of the procedure and the purpose of the examination. The person must be given a statement of their rights and a copy of the order, and relevant persons—such as guardians, carers or those responsible for guardianship—notified. Usually the period a person may be under an assessment period is within 24 hours of them being received at a mental health service. Assessment orders may be longer for persons subject to court assessment orders. Once the person has been examined, the treating psychiatrist may revoke the order. If they believe further examination or treatment is needed, they may apply for further assessment or treatment to be undertaken and a treatment order to be made.

Treatment orders *Treatment orders* vary, depending on where they are enacted, in their length and the procedures to be followed. All state and territory legislation in Australia provides for the involuntary hospitalisation and treatment of a person for a specified period of time. In some states and territories, approved medical practitioners must apply to a tribunal for a treatment order; in other states and territories, a psychiatrist or medical practitioner has the power to confirm or revoke an order. Regardless of who may confirm an order, consideration of the preferences or views about treatment of the person or their carers and guardians must be undertaken. The duration of a treatment order depends on the type of order enacted, with both shorter (e.g. seven days for a South Australian level 1 treatment order) and longer periods (e.g. six months for an inpatient treatment order in Victoria, and a treatment order in Tasmania). In cases where continued hospitalisation is required, authorised psychiatrists make an application for the further treatment of the person. In New Zealand, after preliminary examination and assessment, further assessment and treatment may be undertaken in a first period of assessment and treatment (up to five days), a second period of assessment and treatment (up to 14 days after the initial five-day period), and then, if needed, a compulsory treatment order made (up to six months).

As is the case with an assessment order, the person is given information regarding their rights, a copy of the order, and relevant persons notified. Booklets containing a statement of rights must be provided to the person. Written information explains that the person has the ability to make decisions and provide **informed consent** to treatment, but that treating psychiatrists have the ability to make treatment decisions that differ from the wishes of the person. Consideration should also be given to any advance written statements (often called 'advance directives') that people have made regarding their treatment.

Treatment and care plans developed by staff in consultation with the person specify the treatment that the person is to receive. Certain types of treatment are often specifically governed by legislation and are heavily regulated. For example, in New South Wales, psychosurgery is a prohibited procedure; in Victoria and now Queensland, the person's consent must always be obtained, regardless of admission status, for the use of neurosurgery (including deep-brain simulation). The need for consent for surgery is similarly provided for in New Zealand legislation (referred to in that Act as 'brain surgery'). Mental health Acts also govern the use of electroconvulsive therapy (ECT). For restrictive interventions, such as the use of seclusion and restraint, there are guidelines for their use, and procedures to be followed while the person is restrained or secluded. These include that these measures be used only when there is an imminent risk to the person or others, less restrictive measures have been attempted, and that the person is continually monitored and regularly reviewed. In spite of this, incidents where people with a mental illness have been restrained or secluded for lengthy periods of time are often reported.

Another implication of involuntary treatment orders is the inability to leave the hospital or service without the permission of treating physicians, in the form of approved leave. Such absence without leave, or absconding, is a serious concern, since it interrupts treatment and the person may come to harm (Mosel, Gerace & Muir-Cochrane, 2010).

Court treatment orders *Court treatment orders* are how mental health Acts and criminal law Acts for the states provide for the involuntarily hospitalisation of persons who have been deemed by the courts not fit to stand trial, or not guilty by reason of mental impairment. These will be considered in a later section. There are also provisions in the Acts for the treatment of persons who have pleaded guilty or been found guilty of a criminal offence, and where the court has taken into account mental illness in deciding to put them in hospital. Prisoners may also be transferred under orders to a treatment facility.

Community treatment orders

Moves towards least-restrictive care and treatment in the community mean that treatment for mental illness is often provided outside of the hospital setting. Studies of the numbers of people receiving mental health care in the community under an order in Australia and New Zealand report increased use over time, and higher rates than those found in other countries, such as the United States, Scotland and Canada (Light, Kerridge, Ryan & Robertson, 2012; O'Brien, 2014). Criteria for a community treatment order are similar to those of involuntary inpatient hospitalisation: mainly, the person has a mental illness requiring treatment to prevent risk of harm to others and/or themselves and deterioration of their condition. The legislation provides for the consideration of whether treatment may be appropriately delivered in the community setting. State tribunals make determinations of whether a community treatment order should be enacted. In New Zealand, the courts assess applications for community treatment orders.

A person may be placed under a treatment order while residing in the community. In other cases, a community treatment order may follow discharge from hospital, with the order providing for continued involuntary treatment and monitoring of the person by mental health professionals.

While treatment in the community is considered in some ways less restrictive than treatment in a specialist mental health facility, community treatment orders carry similar requirements of the person. Care and treatment plans may specify particular counselling therapy and rehabilitation, and management of the person's mental illness may require regular medication to be taken. Community orders may be extended or revoked, or it may be deemed appropriate that the person be placed on a treatment order in hospital. It is important, therefore, that mental health professionals consider the ethical dilemmas posed by these orders, including issues of coercion, intrusiveness, autonomy and consent (Light, Kerridge, Ryan & Robertson, 2012).

Health professionals should consider the perceptions and experiences of people with a mental illness being placed under community treatment orders, as well as any inpatient mental health order. Recent studies have raised concerns about the efficacy of treatment orders in reducing inpatient treatment and maintaining wellness (Kisely & O'Reilly, 2015). In both Australia and New Zealand, the presence of Indigenous groups, who have experienced significant dispossession, racism and discrimination, and oppression (Vicary & Westerman, 2004) means that health professionals need to be particularly aware of the ways in which mental health systems operate within Western ideas of what illness is and what therapeutic approaches should be undertaken (Gerace et al., 2015). Participants in one Australian study reflected on inpatient hospitalisation occurring away from family and community. There were also concerns about community treatment such as the prescription of medication, which 'often results in an inability of the individual [under mental health care] to fulfil their roles in the family and community' (Vicary & Westerman, 2004, p. 6).

In a New Zealand study, the number of hospitalisations for people with a mental illness following outpatient treatment for first-episode psychosis was higher for Māori than non-Māori persons (Turner, Boden & Mulder, 2013). Another study in New Zealand investigated the perceptions of Māori and non-Māori people who were under a community treatment order regarding the orders. This research found little difference in perceptions of community treatment orders between Māori and non-Māori participants, or between those Māori people in a mainstream service and those in a specialist Māori mental health service (Newton-Howes, Lacey & Banks, 2014). Cultural identity—not only whether a person is Aboriginal and/or Torres Strait Islander or Māori—is vital to understanding the person's experiences of inpatient and community treatment (Tapsell & Mellsop, 2007).

Ethical dilemmas of involuntary hospitalisation

Involuntary hospitalisation is an exercise of power and, like all forms of power, it can be abused. Because of this potential for abuse, involuntary admission criteria are important. In Australian legislation, *prevention of harm* to the person or others is focused on; while in New Zealand, serious *danger* to self and/or others is a criterion for assessment and hospitalisation. There are problems in both the reliable *prediction* of risk or 'dangerousness', even when validated risk assessment tools are used, and the *prevention* measures used once a person is assessed as high-risk.

People with a mental illness who are assessed as being of a high risk of aggression or violence, for example, but who did not subsequently commit an act of violence (called a *false-positive* categorisation), may have been subject to more coercive treatment and longer admission than necessary (Ryan, Nielssen, Paton & Large, 2010). The opposite may have been true for those patients assessed as being of a low risk of aggression and violence, but who did commit an act of violence (*false-negative* categorisation). Tension between ensuring safety and delivering individualised and person-centred care mindful of the rights of the person exists (Muir-Cochrane et al., 2011), including between risk aversion and the notion of dignity of risk, where a person's recovery involves being able to take calculated risks (Buchanan-Barker & Barker, 2008; Wyder, Bland, Blythe, Matarasso & Compton, 2015).

The case of absconding illustrates another issue. While research has found that male patients and those with schizophrenia abscond in greater numbers than females and those with a mood disorder, an over-focusing on this group may mean that females and those with a depressive disorder (who may be at risk of suicide if they do abscond) are not monitored for this risk. This is reflected in research that has found that nurses grapple both professionally and emotionally with managing the risk of absconding by patients under an involuntary order in an acute inpatient unit (Grotto et al., 2015).

In addition to the problems posed by reliable risk assessment and management, more coercive or restrictive admissions may lead to the stigmatisation of those with a mental health condition, through media reporting of absconding and acts of violence or public perceptions. For example, the locking of psychiatric unit front doors may lead the public to conclude that all of those with a mental illness are dangerous. Another consideration is that, while hospitalisation may reduce the potential for certain harm, other harm such as deprivation of liberty, fear, lack of autonomy, agency and personal control, and aggression on the unit may occur (Callaghan & Ryan, 2014; Muir-Cochrane & Gerace, 2014; Wyder et al., 2015).

The World Health Organization has developed 10 basic principles of mental health care law to guide healthcare practice (see Table 11.1 ■).

Discharge or separation categories

A person can be discharged from a mental health facility in one of three ways: discharge, transfer and absence without leave.

TABLE 11.1 ■ Mental health care law: 10 basic principles (World Health Organization, 1996)

Ten basic principles	Description
1. Promotion of mental health and prevention of mental disorders	Everyone should benefit from the best possible measures to promote their mental wellbeing and to prevent mental disorders
2. Access to basic mental health care	Everyone in need should have access to basic mental health care
3. Mental health assessments in accordance with internationally accepted principles	Mental health assessments should be made in accordance with internationally accepted principles
4. Provision of the least-restrictive type of mental health care	Persons with mental health disorders should be provided with health care which is the least restrictive
5. Self-determination	Consent is required before any type of interference with a person can occur
6. Right to be assisted in the exercise of self-determination	In case a patient merely experiences difficulties in appreciating the implications of a decision, although unable to decide, they shall benefit from the assistance of a knowledgeable third party of their choice
7. Availability of review procedure	There should be a review procedure available for any decision made by official (judge) or surrogate (representative, e.g. guardian) decision-makers and by health care providers
8. Automatic periodical review mechanism	In the case of a decision affecting integrity (treatment) and/or liberty (hospitalisation) with a long-lasting impact, there should be an automatic periodical review mechanism
9. Qualified decision-maker	Decision-makers acting in official capacity (judge) or surrogate (consent-giving) capacity (e.g. relative, friend, guardian) shall be qualified to do so
10. Respect of the rule of law	Decisions should be made in keeping with the body of law in force in the jurisdiction involved, and not on another basis nor on an arbitrary basis

Discharge

People with a mental illness may be discharged, also referred to as *separation*, from a mental health facility when their treatment order expires or is revoked. Alternatively, an application for a further order may be made if the professionals treating the person make a judgment that further hospitalisation is required. The person may require further access to mental health care and follow-up in the community. Any services, support and management that the person requires to continue their recovery are specified in their treatment and care plan. The person may be under a community treatment order on discharge, with adherence to outpatient care, demonstrated ability and willingness to take medications, and the ability to meet the needs of daily living being a few of the many possible prerequisites in their treatment plan.

Transfer

A person may be transferred to another mental health facility if it is deemed appropriate for their care or safety. Most are transfers within mental health systems in the same state or territory. A smaller number are transfers from one state or territory to another.

Absence without leave

A client may decide to terminate the relationship with the facility by informally leaving the hospital grounds. This is commonly referred to as *AWOL* (absent without leave) or *absconding*. Voluntary clients cannot generally be returned to the hospital against their will. However, involuntarily admitted people with a mental illness may be brought back to the hospital against their will with the assistance of the police, ambulance officers or mental health professionals, if necessary. In cases where the person has been away from the hospital for an extended period of time and has not returned or been returned, discharge may be initiated.

PSYCHIATRY AND CRIMINAL LAW

The legal systems in Australia, New Zealand and other countries make provisions for offenders who are determined to not be criminally responsible for their actions as a result of the presence of a mental impairment at the time of the offence. Courts also make decisions, based on statute, regarding a person's mental **fitness to plead** and stand trial. These concepts are known as **competency** and *fitness to plead and/or stand trial* (White, Day & Hackett, 2007).

In a court of law, a person's mental competence and responsibility for their actions, and fitness to engage in court proceedings, is presumed unless proven otherwise. In Australia, both Commonwealth and state and territory legislation addresses competency and fitness. In New Zealand, national legislation is relevant to these matters.

Practice example

Carolyn has a 12-year history of bipolar disorder, and has not been taking her medication since being discharged from a psychiatric hospital. Two weeks prior to the alleged offence, Carolyn began having difficulty sleeping, her behaviour became erratic, and she spent most nights walking up and down the streets in her neighbourhood. Two nights ago, neighbours called the police after they saw her removing items from garages and painting driveways with colourful rainbows. Carolyn was arrested and charged with burglary and malicious mischief.

Determining competency

Legislation in Australia and New Zealand specifies that a person is not responsible and shall not be convicted if they were suffering from a mental impairment at the time they committed the offence. A defence based on mental impairment is variously referred to as a **mental impairment** defence, a **mental illness** defence, an **insanity** defence, or a **mental incompetence** defence. Terminology is very much a reflection of when legislation was drafted, and how recently it has been updated (White et al., 2007).

M'Naghten Rules

In Australia and New Zealand, as well as several other countries, a determination of competence is based on the *M'Naghten Rules,* which were the result of a famous case in England.

Practice example

Daniel M'Naghten (sometimes spelled 'McNaughton' or 'McNaughtan') was a Scottish carpenter who believed that the Jesuits and Tories were tormenting him. He told his family that spies for the government were following him and laughing at him. He was evicted from his boarding house because of his bizarre behaviour. In 1843, he stalked Prime Minister Sir Robert Peel, eventually shot Peel's secretary, Edward Drummond, and was charged with the death. Nine physicians who were experienced in the care of persons with mental disorders testified at the trial (three for the defence, three for the prosecution, and three who listened to the evidence and observed M'Naghten's behaviour in the courtroom). All nine agreed that M'Naghten suffered from monomania (probably paranoid schizophrenia today) and was not legally sane, according to the legal tests at the time. The jury huddled in the courtroom for two minutes, and then found him to be legally insane. He was sent to the local mental institution, Bethlehem Hospital. The public was outraged, believing hospitalisation to be too lenient. The Queen ordered a taskforce in the House of Lords to review the case and come up with a new legal standard. Five abstract questions of law were asked of a panel of judges, and their responses form the M'Naghten Rules.

Subsequent legislation and court decisions (common law) in Australia and New Zealand have further addressed the concepts that arose from this case (Allnut, Samuels & O'Driscoll, 2007). These include the case of *R v Porter* (1933) 55 CLR 182 in Australia, where Bertram Edward Porter was found not guilty on the grounds of insanity of the murder of his child, Charles Robert Porter, in 1932.

A case with much notoriety in the United States involved John Hinckley Jr, who attempted to assassinate President Ronald Reagan in 1981, wounding President Reagan, his press secretary James Brady, police officer Thomas Delahanty, and Secret Service agent Timothy McCarthy. In the Hinckley trial, the prosecution failed to prove that Hinckley was sane beyond a reasonable doubt (the practice at that time in the federal courts). The burden of proving legal insanity shifted to the defence as a result of the *Hinckley case*. Most states now place the burden of proof on the defence. In federal courts, the defence now must prove a defendant's insanity rather than the prosecution having to prove that the defendant is sane.

In the Australian *Criminal Code Act 1995* (Commonwealth), it is specified that:

> A person is not criminally responsible for an offence if, at the time of carrying out the conduct constituting the offence, the person was suffering from a mental impairment (s 7.3).

In the New Zealand *Crimes Act 1961*, under the section 'Insanity', it is specified that:

> No person shall be convicted of an offence by reason of an act done or omitted by him or her when labouring under natural imbecility or disease of the mind (s 23(2)).

Legislation in Australia and New Zealand has different definitions of what types of 'mental impairment' meet the criteria for a competency defence under the Acts. Terminology differ between states, territories and countries, with mental impairment including 'mental illness', 'intellectual disability', 'mental disease' or 'infirmity', and 'senility'. It is important to be mindful of the stigma and associations that may be inherent in certain terminology.

There are generally two provisions based on the M'Naghten Rules in legislation in Australia and New Zealand for a competency defence. Some states and territories in Australia include a third provision (Allnut et al., 2007). It is specified that, as a consequence of mental impairment, the person was unable to:

- understand the nature and quality (what they were doing) of their actions and behaviour
- know right from wrong regarding their conduct
- control their actions and behaviour.

Only a minority of criminal offenders are found to be not guilty of an offence as a result of a mental impairment. In one Australian state, South Australia, a file review of 55 cases where a person was found not guilty on this basis in the District and Supreme Courts between 2006 and 2012 was undertaken. This represented approximately 90 per cent of the total number of cases during this time. The sample had more males (78 per cent) than females (22 per cent). In the sample, 85 per cent of people had a diagnosis of a mental illness prior to the offence, and 47 per cent of people had a diagnosis of schizophrenia, followed by drug-induced psychosis or substance abuse and dependence (24 per cent). The main basis of a finding of mental incompetence in these cases was that the person, as result of mental impairment, was unable to know that their conduct was wrong. This was the main reason in 87 per cent of cases; and in 11 per cent of cases this was involved along with either the person not knowing the nature and quality of their actions, or the person being determined as unable to control their actions (Government of South Australia, 2013).

In a New Zealand study involving the forensic services of Auckland and surrounding rural areas, it was found that 37 of 62 people evaluated from 2007 to 2013 met the criteria for an insanity defence. There were more men (81 per cent) than women (19 per cent) referred for evaluation. Of those who were found not guilty by reason of insanity, 84 per cent had a prior psychiatric diagnosis (offenders could have more than one diagnosis), with 54 per cent having a past diagnosis prior to their offence of a psychotic disorder, followed by a mood disorder (41 per cent), or a substance use disorder (16 per cent) (Li & Friedman, 2015).

The defence may raise the need for an investigation of competence. The prosecution or court may also believe that the defendant's competence should be investigated. This involves hearing relevant evidence and representations by the defence and prosecution. Psychiatrists and other health professionals may be asked to examine and report their professional and expert opinions to the court. The court (judge or jury) reaches a decision of whether it has been established that the person meets the criteria for the defence. This decision is made on the *balance of probabilities*. The judgment of competence is made separately from a determination of whether the objective elements of the offence have been proven beyond a reasonable doubt.

If the decision has been made that the person is not guilty by reason of mental impairment, and the objective elements of the case have been proven, there are a number of options. Assessments of risk of causing harm to others and consideration of the autonomy of the person are undertaken. It is most likely that a supervision order will be made. This can mean that the person is detained in a secure psychiatric facility for treatment. The person may also be released into the community, but with conditions for treatment and supervision. For lesser charges (e.g. those where a custodial sentence would have not been given if a person was found guilty), the person may be released unconditionally. The length of an order is often determined by the length of sentence that would have been received if the person had been found guilty in the absence of mental disorder. In some jurisdictions, a limiting term is not set, with indefinite supervision possible. For these patients, reviews are undertaken at set times to see whether or not the order should still apply (Government of South Australia, 2013). In the South Australian study described above, 64 per cent were released on licence (into the community with conditions), 32 per cent were detained to a facility, and 2 per cent were released unconditionally, with 2 per cent not yet determined (Government of South Australia, 2013). In the New Zealand study, people found not guilty by reason of insanity were hospitalised in a forensic hospital (49 per cent), placed on a community treatment order (38 per cent) or released (14 per cent) (Li & Friedman, 2015).

Fitness to plead and/or stand trial In Australian and New Zealand criminal and mental health legislation, a determination of whether a person is mentally fit to enter a plea and/or stand trial for a crime may be undertaken if it is raised by the defence, prosecution or court. As with a determination of competence, the criteria for assessing fitness differ depending on which country and/or state/territory is involved (White et al., 2007). Some of the criteria included state that a person is unfit to stand trial if disordered or impaired mental processes mean that the person is unable to:

- enter a plea
- understand the nature of the charge
- respond to and answer the charge
- exercise procedural rights (e.g. the right to challenge jurors)
- instruct their counsel
- understand the general nature of the trial and court proceedings
- follow the course of proceedings
- understand the nature of evidence, and the effect of evidence to the trial.

Like a determination of competence, determination of whether the objective elements of the offence have been proven is undertaken. The expert opinions of psychiatrists, psychologists and medical practitioners are sought (van der Wijingaart, Hawkins & Golus, 2015). In New Zealand, court liaison nurses may also provide reports regarding mental state, and issues with comprehension and communication (Sakdalan & Egan, 2014). Professionals make use of interviews as well as tools for assessing fitness. The court (judge or jury) reaches a decision of whether it has been established that the person meets the criteria for the defence. If it is established that the person does, a supervision order will be enacted. The case may also be adjourned if it is the opinion of health professionals and the court that the person will regain mental capacity required to plead and stand trial. Factors associated with a finding of unfitness to plead/stand trial include the presence of psychiatric disorders, intellectual disability and IQ testing scores (Sakdalan & Egan, 2014).

The presence of a developmental disability, symptoms of a mental disorder, or a history of mental disorder does not necessarily preclude one's competence to stand trial. For example, the presence of delusions may or may not have an impact. It depends on whether the delusion is related to the courtroom, the crime or the proceedings. The specific content of the delusion, and the degree to which the symptoms affect the abilities and skills needed to be competent, are the important factors.

Both competency and fitness to plead and/or stand trial have significant implications for a person's treatment, freedom and autonomy. If a person is found unfit to plead/stand trial or not guilty by reason of mental impairment/insanity, they may then be put under supervision orders for significant lengths of time.

FORENSIC MENTAL HEALTH NURSING

Forensic mental health nursing can be defined as the assessment, formulation, planning, implementation and evaluation of nursing care within a therapeutic alliance with individuals experiencing mental illness involved in criminal justice processes. The defendant is the person, and the primary focus of care is to improve the person's mental health in the context of the relationship between the nurse and the person. Forensic mental health nursing is a challenging and rewarding specialty area of mental health nursing, where combinations of scientific and clinical approaches are applied in a legal context. This legal context consists of criminal, correctional, civil and legislative elements. Forensic nurses may also care for survivors of violence.

Forensic mental health nurses practise in a range of settings: high- and low-security forensic inpatient settings, courts of law and court diversion services, prisons and in the community. The treatment they offer focuses on an individual's offending behaviour as well as their mental illness. Their role is to work towards reducing the risk of re-offending, and towards rehabilitation and recovery. Forensic mental health nurses also work with families and carers to assist people's recovery, and play a strong advocacy and education role.

Dimensions of practice

The dimensions of practice in forensic mental health nursing are affected both by the nature of the person and the person's current involvement with the criminal justice system. While the core of practice is psychiatric–mental health nursing, the relationship between the nurse and the person is markedly different from that in the usual psychiatric–mental health nursing role, because of the alternative social context of the situation that precipitates their interaction. In addition, the setting—a crime scene, a courtroom, a forensic treatment setting or a correctional facility—influences the forensic mental health nurse's practice.

In Australia, forensic mental health nursing has established standards set by the Victorian Institute of Forensicare in 2012. The development of these standards involved consultation with mental health nurses, allied health professionals and input from consultants and carer advocates. These 16 standards build on the standards of practice and code of ethics which apply to all nurses, and have a strong advocacy role towards forensic service patients. The term 'patient' is deliberately used by forensic mental health nurses in this context, as the people they are caring for are compulsorily detained due to criminal charges.

Role preparation

The forensic mental health nurse must be highly skilled in interpersonal relations and communication. Developing collegial relationships with other disciplines is central to the role, because of the intersections of practice that overlap with the domain of other disciplines (forensic science, criminal science). The prerequisite to this expanded role is educational preparation—a graduate degree in forensic mental health nursing, or a graduate degree in psychiatric–mental health nursing with additional training in forensic mental health nursing. Colleges and universities offer degree programs, as well as certificate courses, in forensic subspecialties.

Expert witness

Any registered nurse can be subpoenaed to court as a witness of fact. In this role, you testify as to what you personally saw, heard, performed or documented relating to a particular person's care. You are questioned as to these first-hand experiences, and then excused from the courtroom.

An **expert witness** is recognised by the court as having a high level of skill or expertise in a designated area, in order to render an opinion on a legal matter in court. As an expert witness, you will be subpoenaed to court to testify on your involvement with the defendant. You will testify as to the role you performed and to your documentation. At this point, the court will allow you to give additional testimony in the form of your professional opinion, based on your conclusions, as to the defendant's legal sanity, competence to proceed, future dangerousness, or likelihood of committing future felonious acts.

To establish credibility as an expert and to have one's opinion given weight in court, the forensic mental health nurse must have the following:

1. *Expertise:* This is established by your credentials.
2. *Trustworthiness:* This is the degree of honesty exuded in your demeanour and opinion, as perceived by the judge or jury.
3. *Presentation style:* This is how you come across to others. You may be credible, trustworthy and an authority in a specialty area, but, without the ability to communicate in a concise and convincing fashion, the value of your testimony is limited.

THE RIGHTS OF PEOPLE WITH A MENTAL ILLNESS

The current concern for *the rights of people with a mental illness* has been evolving since the 1960s, when there was an increased interest in under-represented minority groups—the poor, women and the mentally ill. The right to participate in care is now a part of the Australian Charter of Healthcare Rights. The United Nations Convention on the Rights of Persons with Disabilities came into effect in 2008. It applies to people who have disabilities secondary to any illness, including mental illness. Article 12 of this Convention is titled 'Equal Recognition Before the Law'. This article says that all people should be assumed to be able to make their own decisions. Article 12 also dictates that if decision-making is taken away from a person—for example, when a person is receiving involuntary treatment under a detention order or a community treatment order—it is still necessary to respect the rights, will (wishes) and preferences of the person. While some decisions that are made may be against a person's wishes, it is likely that many other decisions about treatment can still be made in accordance with what a person wants. For example, a person may be detained in hospital against their will, but still be able to be fully involved in the choice of treatments, both talking therapies and drug treatments. This Convention also underpins supported decision-making, so that a person even though unwell can have some decision-making powers.

For supported decision-making to work, there needs to be a 'supporter'—someone who can be available when the person is unwell, to attend key appointments and help the person make decisions. The supporter may be a family member or friend.

The rights that people with mental illness should have in practice, and that you should consider when planning your interventions, are outlined in Your Intervention Strategies.

The National Standards for Mental Health Services in Australia (2010) determine a set of mental health service

YOUR INTERVENTION STRATEGIES
The rights of people with mental illness

Keep the following rights in mind when planning and implementing nursing interventions:

- the right to informed consent
- the right to treatment
- the right to refuse treatment
- the right to treatment in the least restrictive setting
- the right to communicate with others
- the right not to be subjected to restraint
- the right to privacy
- the right to periodic review of status
- the right to independent psychiatric examination
- the right to participate in legal matters, including making a valid contract, executing a will, marrying or divorcing, voting, driving a motor vehicle, practising a profession, suing or being sued, managing or disposing of property
- the right to habeas corpus
- the right to legal representation
- the right to keep clothing and personal effects
- the right to religious freedom
- the right to education
- the right to self-determination.

standards for all mental health services, public and private, government and nongovernment. In particular, Standard 6 refers to the rights for people to receive comprehensive and integrated mental health care that meets their individual need and achieves the best possible outcome in terms of their recovery. Standard 7 refers to the need for mental health services to respect, value and support the importance of carers in the wellbeing, treatment and recovery of people with a mental illness.

LIVED EXPERIENCE

There are a number of other rights that a person should be afforded. These include the right to participate in all things that affect them, the right to be safe and to be heard, and the right to choose. A fundamental right for people is to speak up against injustice, certainly as they see it in relation to health settings, treatment and care. This might be in conflict with the role of the psychiatric–mental health nurse's duty of care, or the organisation's policies and procedures. Irrespective of personal or moral views, the underlying principles are to provide treatment and care to people with autonomy, respect and dignity.

There is also an expectation that along with rights come responsibilities. The person should be held accountable to treat staff in a respectful manner and comply with reasonable requests regarding their everyday care.

Right to treatment in the least restrictive setting

The idea of the least restrictive setting or the least restrictive alternative has become an important component of consumers' rights movements. The term **least restrictive setting** generally refers to the placement of people with a mental illness in a therapeutic setting that will provide care while allowing maximum freedom. By extension, it also means providing for the least amount of limitation or interference in an individual's thought and decision-making, physical activity, and sense of self, as necessary to provide for safety.

People with a mental illness have the right to the least restrictive treatment when being transported to hospital, and while in hospital. This right emphasises the judicious use of any mechanical restraint or the use of seclusion. Since 2006, the Australian government, like other countries such as New Zealand, has introduced strategies to reduce the use of seclusion and restraint of people with a mental illness. Nevertheless, there is evidence of the use of these containment measures continuing, and in some places, such as emergency departments, increasing (Gerace, Pamungkas, Oster, Thomson & Muir, 2014).

Disclosure to safeguard others

An exception to confidentiality and privilege that has developed from a California Supreme Court decision illustrates the competition between two responsibilities of the mental health care professional: (1) confidentiality to the person, and (2) the protection of the public from a 'violent' person. This landmark case is often referred to as 'the *Tarasoff* decision' among mental health professionals. In the ***Tarasoff* decision**, the court's ruling underlined the mental health care professional's responsibility to balance confidentiality with the 'duty to warn' and the 'duty to protect'. The circumstances that gave rise to the *Tarasoff* decision are discussed in the following Mental Health in the Media.

YOUR INTERVENTION STRATEGIES
When the right to privacy can be breached

The release of information without the person's consent can be made under the following conditions:

- when acting in the person's best interests in an emergency situation
- when acting to protect third parties
- when making a court-ordered evaluation or report
- when reporting child abuse, gunshot wounds or contagious diseases, as required by law
- during criminal proceedings
- in child custody disputes.

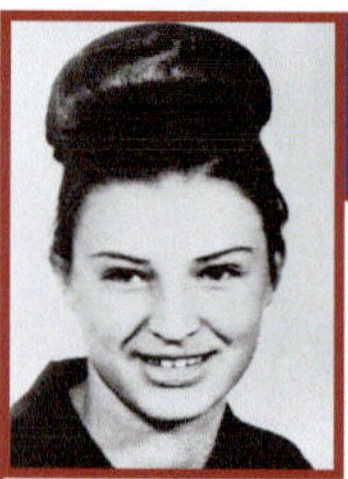

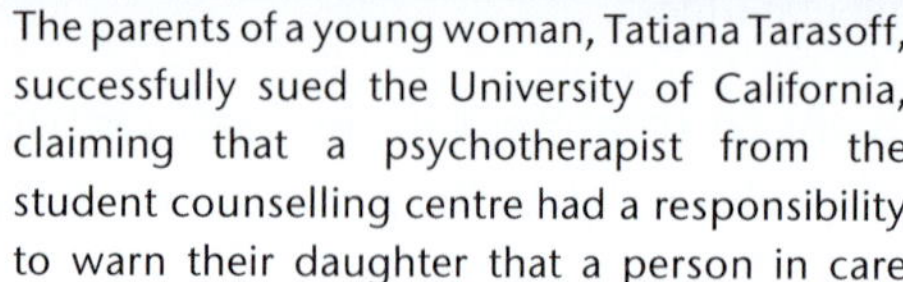

MENTAL HEALTH IN THE MEDIA

The *Tarasoff* decision

The parents of a young woman, Tatiana Tarasoff, successfully sued the University of California, claiming that a psychotherapist from the student counselling centre had a responsibility to warn their daughter that a person in care had threatened to kill her. At the time, the psychologist did notify campus security officers that he believed the person was dangerous and should be involuntarily committed for observation and treatment. However, the man appeared rational to the police, and promised them that he would stay away from the young woman. He then terminated treatment, and two months later killed her.

The California Supreme Court said that, despite the unsuccessful attempt to confine the person, the therapist knew that the person was at large and dangerous, and so had a duty to warn the young woman of the danger. The court recognised the person's right to confidentiality, but said that this must be weighed against the public's need for safety against violent assault, especially when an individual in danger can be identified.

Photo courtesy of AP PHOTO.

MENTAL HEALTH ADVANCE DIRECTIVES

Mental health advance directives are a contemporary way of decision-making and ensuring autonomous behaviour for people who wish to advise what treatment and care they would like to receive (or not) when mentally unwell. In addition, they help engage the person in treatment, increase the person's satisfaction with treatment, and enhance the therapeutic alliance with mental health care providers (Van Dorn, Scheyett, Swanson & Swartz, 2010). While mental health advance directives are becoming more popular (they first came into existence in the 1990s), they are still not in common use.

The Department of Health in South Australia advises that mental health advance directives may have some legal weight under common law if signed by the person and an independent witness and/or the treating team, and should be taken into account when decisions are being made for the person. In South Australia, a Ulysses agreement is an example of an advance care plan which is often signed by the person and the treating team, and guides care and treatment for the person when they become ill.

However, in Australia advance directives cannot over-ride treatment decisions by mental health services when the person is under an order of the *Mental Health Act* (i.e. an inpatient treatment order or a community treatment order). This is a major drawback for people with a mental illness, and it is not surprising that people with a mental illness do not feel empowered by the legal implications of having their autonomy regarding decisions about their care overturned when they are under an order of the *Mental Health Act*. Nonetheless, advance directives can be useful for people with a mental illness to specify what they would like to happen when they are ill, in terms of who they would like to be allowed to visit them in hospital, and what kind of support they would like, or not, when they are in hospital and when discharged to community care.

LIVED EXPERIENCE

Advance directives

Advance directives are an excellent way of allowing people to have some say in their treatment and care. One of the most important aspects is to develop the content for the advance directives when people are well, can make informed decisions, and can choose who they want or don't want involved in their treatment and care.

As with any document of this type, care should be taken to ensure, as far as possible, that the person's wishes are adhered to. Advance directives can also be very useful in documenting who the primary carer is, providing permission to engage with the carer, and to ensure that the carer is involved in all aspects of treatment and care. In recent times, mental health legislation requires a designated carer, 'primary carer' (New South Wales) or 'carer or support person' (Queensland) to be identified. However, under Queensland legislation, communication with the person's carer or support person does not apply if the person requests that communication does not take place. While legislation over-rides advance directives, in this particular situation a clear message is provided that the person wishes their carer or support person to be, or not to be, involved. This provides some comfort for mental health nurses in that confidentiality is not being breached; rather it is the request of the person, documented through the advance directive. Mental health nurses' duty of care to the person and society should always over-ride the advance direction in any situation where harm to self or others is a possibility.

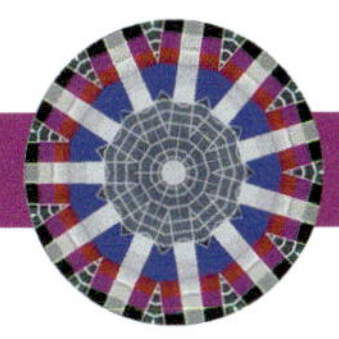

REFERENCES

Allnutt, S., Samuels, A., & O'Driscoll, C. (2007). The insanity defence: From wild beasts to M'Naghten. *Australasian Psychiatry, 15*(4), 292–298.

Australian College of Mental Health Nurses. (2012). Mental Health Nursing Standards. Retrieved from http://www.acmhn.org/career-resources/workforce-standards. (Accessed 2016, March.)

Australian Government Department of Health. (2010). National Standards for Mental Health Services 2010, Commonwealth of Australia. Canberra, Australia: Australian Government Department of Health.

Buchanan-Barker, P., & Barker, P. J. (2008). The tidal commitments: Extending the value base of mental health recovery. *Journal of Psychiatric and Mental Health Nursing, 15*(2), 93–100.

Callaghan, S. M., & Ryan, C. (2014). Is there a future for involuntary treatment in rights-based mental health law? *Psychiatry, Psychology and Law, 21*(5), 747–766.

Callaghan, S., & Ryan, C. J. (2012). Rising to the human rights challenge in compulsory treatment—new approaches to mental health law in Australia. *Australian and New Zealand Journal of Psychiatry, 46*(7), 611–620.

Cannaerts, N., Gastmans, C., & Dierckx de Casterle, B. (2014). Contribution of ethics education to the ethical competence of nursing students: Educators' and students' perceptions. *Nursing Ethics, 21*(8), 861–878.

Cherry, M. J. (2010). Nonconsensual treatment is (nearly always) morally impermissible. *Journal of Law and Medical Ethics, 38*(4), 789–798.

Chiovitti, R. F. (2011). Theory of protective empowering for balancing patient safety and choices. *Nursing Ethics, 18*(1), 88–101.

Clausen, J. (2010). Ethical brain stimulation—neuroethics of deep brain stimulation in research and clinical practice. *European Journal of Neuroscience, 32*(7), 1152–1162.

Davis, A. J., Fowler, M. D., & Aroskar, M. A. (2010). *Ethical dilemmas and nursing practice* (5th ed.). Upper Saddle River, NJ: Pearson Education.

Gerace, A., Oster, C., Mosel, K., O'Kane, D., Ash, D., & Muir-Cochrane, E. (2015). Five-year review of absconding in three acute psychiatric inpatient wards in Australia. *International Journal of Mental Health Nursing, 24*(1), 28–37.

Gerace, A., Pamungkas, D., Oster, C., Thomson, D., & Muir-Cochrane, E. (2014). The use of restraint in four general hospital emergency departments in Australia. Australasian Psychiatry, 22(4), 366–369.

Government of South Australia. (2013). A discussion paper considering the operation of Part 8A of the Criminal Law Consolidation Act 1935 (SA). Government of South Australia. Retrieved from http://www.agd.sa.gov.au/sites/agd.sa.gov.au/files/documents/Initiatives%20Announcements%20and%20News/Discussion%20Paper%20-%20Part%208A%20Criminal%20Law%20Consolidation%20Act.pdf

Grotto, J., Gerace, A., O'Kane, D., Simpson, A., Oster, C., & Muir-Cochrane, E. (2015). Risk assessment and absconding: Perceptions, understandings and responses of mental health nurses. *Journal of Clinical Nursing, 24* (5–6), 855–865.

Kisely, S., & O'Reilly, R. (2015). Reappraising community treatment orders—can there be consensus? *Medical Journal of Australia, 202*(8), 415–416.

Light, E., Kerridge, I., Ryan, C., & Robertson, M. (2012). Community treatment orders in Australia: Rates and patterns of use. *Australasian Psychiatry, 20*(6), 478–482.

Light, E. M., Kerridge, I. H., Ryan, C. J., & Robertson, M. D. (2012). Out of sight, out of mind: Making involuntary community treatment visible in the mental health system. *Medical Journal of Australia, 196*(9), 591–593.

Li, S. S., & Friedman, S. H. (2015). Moral wrongfulness and insanity: A New Zealand sample. *The Journal of Forensic Psychiatry and Psychology, 26*(5), 686–698.

Mariano, M. T., Grace, J. J., Trigoboff, E., Di Stefano, D. J., Olympia, J. O., & Watson, T. H. (2011). Individuals with threatening or violent criminal behavior: Civil commitment or release after incarceration. *Innovations in Neuroscience, 8*(6), 29–34.

McCann, T., Baird, M., & Muir-Cochrane, E. (2015). Nurses' experiences of restraint and seclusion use in short-stay acute old age psychiatry inpatient units: A qualitative study. *Journal of Psychiatric and Mental Health Nursing, 22*(2), 109–115.

Mohamed, A. D., & Sahakian, B. J. (2012). The ethics of elective psychopharmacology. *International Journal of Neuropsychopharmacology, 15*(4), 559–571.

Mosel, K. A., Gerace, A., & Muir-Cochrane, E. C. (2010). Retrospective analysis of absconding behaviour by acute care patients in one psychiatric hospital campus in Australia. *International Journal of Mental Health Nursing, 19*(3), 177–185.

Muir-Cochrane, E., & Gerace, A. (2014). Containment practices in psychiatric care. In D. Holmes, J. D. Jacob, & A. Perron (Eds.), *Power and the psychiatric apparatus: Repression, transformation and assistance* (pp. 91–115). Surrey, England: Ashgate.

Muir-Cochrane, E., Gerace, A., Mosel, K., O'Kane, D., Barkway, P., . . . Oster, C. (2011). Managing risk: Clinical decision-making in mental health services. *Issues in Mental Health Nursing, 32*(12), 726–734.

New Zealand College of Mental Health Nurses. (2012). *Standards of Practice for Mental Health Nursing in Aotearoa New Zealand.* Retrieved from http://www.nzcmhn.org.nz/Publications/Standards-of-Practice-for-Mental-Health-Nursing (Accessed 2016, March).

Newton-Howes, G., Lacey, C. J., & Banks, D. (2014). Community treatment orders: The experiences of non-Maori and Maori within mainstream and Maori mental health services. *Social Psychiatry and Psychiatric Epidemiology, 49*(2), 267–273.

Nursing and Midwifery Board of Australia. (2013) *Code of ethics for nurses in Australia.* Retrieved from http://www.nursingmidwiferyboard.gov.au/Codes-Guidelines-Statements/Professional-standards.aspx

O'Brien, A. J. (2014). Community treatment orders in New Zealand: Regional variability and international comparisons. *Australasian Psychiatry 22*(4), 352–356.

Ryan, C., Nielssen, O., Paton, M., & Large, M. (2010). Clinical decisions in psychiatry should not be based on risk assessment. *Australasian Psychiatry, 18*(5), 398–403.

Sakdalan, J. A., & Egan, V. (2014). Fitness to stand trial in New Zealand: Different factors associated with fitness to stand trial between mentally disordered and intellectually disabled defendants in the New Zealand criminal justice system. *Psychiatry, Psychology and Law, 21*(5), 658–668.

Strout, T. D. (2010). Perspectives on the experience of being physically restrained: An integrative review of the qualitative literature. *International Journal of Mental Health Nursing, 19*(6), 416–427.

Tapsell, R., & Mellsop, G. (2007). The contributions of culture and ethnicity to New Zealand mental health research findings. *International Journal of Social Psychiatry, 53*(4), 317–324.

Turner, M. A., Boden, J. M., & Mulder, R. T. (2013). Predictors of hospitalization two years after treatment for first-episode psychosis. *Psychiatric Services, 64*(12), 1230–1235.

United Nations. (2008). *United Nations Convention on the Rights of Persons with Disabilities.* Office of the High Commission for Human Rights Retrieved from http://www.un.org/disabilities/convention/about.shtml. (Accessed 2016, March.)

van der Wijngaart, S., Hawkins, R., & Golus, P. (2015). The role of psychologists in the South Australian fitness to stand trial process. *Psychiatry, Psychology and Law, 22*(1), 75–93.

Van Dorn, R., Scheyett, A., Swanson, J., & Swartz, M. (2010). Psychiatric advance directives and social workers: An integrative review. *Social Work, 55*(2), 157–167.

Vicary, D., & Westerman, T. (2004). 'That's just the way he is': Some implications of Aboriginal mental health beliefs. *Australian e-Journal for the Advancement of Mental Health, 3*(3), 1–10.

White, J., Day, A., & Hackett, L. (2007). *Writing reports for court: A practical guide for psychologists working in forensic contexts.* Bowen Hills, QLD, Australia: Australian Academic Press.

Wyder, M., Bland, R., Blythe, A., Matarasso, B., & Crompton, D. (2015) Therapeutic relationships and involuntary treatment orders: service users' interactions with health-care professionals on the ward. *International Journal of Mental Health Nursing, 24*(2), 181–189.

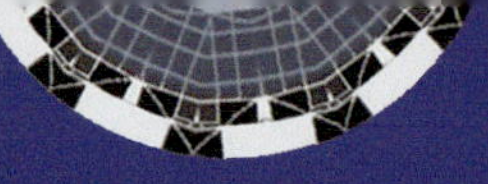

12 Cognitive disorders

LORNA MOXHAM AND HOWARD JAMES STREET (JIM)

KEY TERMS

amnestic disorder *237*
aphasia, expressive *241*
aphasia, receptive *241*
Creutzfeldt–Jakob disease *235*
delirium *228*
dementia *230*
dementia of the Alzheimer's type (DAT) or Alzheimer's dementia (AD) *232*
dementia with Lewy bodies (DLB) *234*
HIV-associated dementia (HAD) *237*
Huntington's disease *235*
new variant Creutzfeldt–Jakob disease (nvCJD) *236*
Parkinson's disease *235*
Pick's disease *235*
pseudodementia *236*
sundowning *242*
traumatic brain injury (TBI) *237*
vascular dementia *235*

LEARNING OUTCOMES

After completing this chapter, you will be able to:

1. Examine current scientific understanding of delirium, dementia, amnestic disorders and other cognitive disorders.
2. Differentiate the various types of cognitive disorders.
3. Understand the differences between delirium, dementia and depression.
4. Identify mental health nursing strategies that support optimal memory and cognitive functioning in the care of people with cognitive disorders.
5. Appreciate the difficulties that carers may face when their family member has a cognitive disorder.
6. Examine your personal feelings and attitudes about people who are cognitively impaired.

LIVED EXPERIENCE

Thoughts from a carer (Jim)

About five years ago it became apparent that Celia, my wife, was having small memory lapses. These were initially put down to getting older. I was also told it could be related to a recent hip replacement that Celia had undergone. However, on advice from a close friend of us both, who was a mental health nurse, professional diagnosis was sought. This took a number of years, with the resulting news revealing our worst fears: Celia had the beginnings of dementia. Over time, myself, our family and our friends have witnessed a steady decline. Medication was prescribed to help ally the condition and slow the symptoms. I put these tablets in a plastic container, a bit like a Webster system, to make it easier for Celia to remember to take her tablets. Despite the container being clearly labelled, Celia has to be constantly reminded to take her tablets each morning, as she is confused as to whether she has taken them or not. Celia constantly asks 'What day is it today?' and 'What month is it?' This unrelenting barrage of the same question is frustrating for both Celia and myself.

I have learned to accept that this is the norm and treat every question, no matter how often it is asked, as if it is the first time that I have heard it. Sometimes the same question can be asked 10 times in 10 minutes. At first, before I understood what was actually happening to her, I was worried that Celia was seemingly becoming 'lazy'; from being a very fussy homemaker, having everything in its place and no dust at all, to largely ignoring all

(continued)

LIVED EXPERIENCE *(continued)*

household chores until I began to do them. She was not at all lazy, never has been. She just didn't remember that chores needed to be done, not until I started to do them. This seems to jog her memory, and she will get out of her chair and help, but now often forgets mid-way what she is meant to be doing. Stuff often gets put away in the wrong cupboards (for which I get the blame). Celia will ask me 'What do you want for lunch?' I might respond with 'a ham sandwich', but unless I supervise her making the lunch, I inevitably don't get what I asked for.

Shopping can be a minefield. Not only with what is needed, but if, for example, Celia needs to use the bathroom, if I am not close at hand she is unable to remember where she left me, where the car is, or what she was last doing. It's frightening for her. If we go on a car journey, I am constantly asked—probably every five to six minutes—'Where did you say we are going?'

It has been suggested that I get someone in sometimes to give me some respite. Celia would recognise this, and she refuses to believe that there is anything wrong. She does tell people that she 'can't remember things' and that she has 'short-term memory loss', but that's the extent of any admission. The last thing I want to do is upset her.

At times she seems to 'switch off' and stare vacantly through the door or fall asleep. Sleeping patterns have changed—she seems to need more and more. Sometimes she can sleep for up to 10 hours. My respite is to go into the garden and enjoy my Japanese Koi carp for which I have won national awards. I also go for a walk very early each morning with a friend, before Celia wakes up. We take holidays sometimes with friends, but Celia's memory of them soon fades. Celia can speak very coherently about long-ago past events, but these conversations are also repetitive. She talks about the same things over and over. Memories include growing up with her brother, her aunt who had 'sleeping sickness', and losing her father at a young age as a result of an operation that went wrong. She also talks about when she swam, and how she was quite good but that she could never tumble-turn.

I try to keep life as normal as possible—for example, Celia has money in her purse and will pay at the supermarket checkout. All activities have to be under a watchful eye, though.

Things will get worse, but Celia is my wife and I am determined to cope. If I had a few keys words to describe life as a carer for a person with a dementia, they would be 'repetition, frustration, tolerance, patience, love, understanding and, last but not least, sorrow'.

INTRODUCTION

As a result of the ageing population, mental health nurses are increasingly in contact with people who have cognitive disorders. People who have these disorders provide a challenge, because they may perceive themselves and their environment differently than others do, and often have problems in receiving communication and expressing themselves. These are similar challenges that mental health nurses face when communicating with someone who is experiencing a florid psychosis. Communicating effectively, comprehensively assessing how the person feels, and planning and implementing quality care are vital nursing skills.

In addition to carers, nurses are also advocates for people with cognitive disorders. Frequently, it is nurses who are the care coordinators, who are in charge of day treatment centres or residential care facilities, or are the facilitators of support groups. Families look to nurses for suggestions to ease their care load, for strategies to cope with difficult behaviour, for education to explain the disorder, and for suggestions and strategies that help them to cope.

Nurses' in-depth knowledge of psychobiology and our holistic person-centred approach to treatment are unique assets essential to providing quality care for people with cognitive disorders. Before the 20th century, all organic brain disorders of older adults were categorised as 'senile dementia'. At the turn of the 20th century, scientists distinguished senile dementia from arteriosclerotic conditions and neurosyphilis. Arteriosclerotic brain disease was then considered the primary cause of confused states in older adults and the result of diseased cerebral vessels.

By the middle of the 20th century a new category, organic brain disease (OBD), was identified. This category was broader, allowing for defects in both the vessels and the brain. The category organic brain syndrome (OBS) then followed, which recognised the need for a diagnosis that included symptoms without a known cause. Some years ago, the term *organic mental syndrome* (OMS) referred to a group of psychological or behavioural signs of unknown or unclear aetiology, while *organic mental disorder* (OMD) referred to a particular syndrome whose aetiology was known or presumed. These older, general terms from psychiatry, referring to many physical disorders that cause impaired mental function, are no longer used. The term *cognitive disorder* is now preferred.

DELIRIUM

Older adults, especially those with dementia, are prone to transient cognitive disorders usually called either *delirium* or *acute confusional state*. Studies suggest that delirium is common in hospitalised older adults, ranging in prevalence from 20 per cent to 50 per cent in general medical-surgical units, and from 70 to 80 per cent in intensive care units (Eubank & Covinsky, 2014). Delirium is associated with poorer in-hospital functional and clinical outcomes, and increased post-discharge mortality (Noriega et al., 2015). Residents over 75 years of age in long-term care facilities are at particular risk, and significant numbers may have a delirium at any time.

Delirium is an abrupt-onset type of confusional state marked by:

1. fluctuations in level of confusion
2. inability to pay attention during interactions
3. disorganised thinking
4. changes in consciousness
5. agitation or quiet and hypoactive behaviour (such as quickly falling back to sleep).

Additional elements include diminution of all mental activity. Rage, depression, fear, apathy and incontinence are also common.

Differentiating delirium from dementia can be a challenge. However, failure to recognise delirium can delay appropriate treatment, with serious health consequences.

Signs of delirium

Detecting delirium involves carefully assessing how the person thinks (cognition), their ability to pay attention, their degree of wakefulness and their psychomotor behaviour.

Cognition

The three components of cognition—perception, thinking and memory—are all disrupted in the person who has a delirium:

1. *Perception.* The person shows a reduced ability to distinguish and integrate sensory information, and to differentiate it from hallucinations, dreams, illusions and imagery.
2. *Thinking.* The thinking process is fragmented and disorganised to the extent that the person is unable to reason, judge, abstract or solve problems.
3. *Memory.* Memory is impaired in all three aspects; the person is unable to form memories or store and retrieve (register, retain or recall) information.

> **DIAGNOSTIC FEATURES**
> **Cognitive disorders**
>
> **Delirium:** Delirium is a disturbance of consciousness with a reduced ability to focus, sustain or shift attention. There is a change in cognition, and the disturbance develops over hours to days, and tends to fluctuate during the day. Medical conditions can also contribute to these difficulties.
>
> **Dementia of the Alzheimer's type (DAT):** DAT involves multiple cognitive deficits, with memory impairment and aphasia, apraxia, agnosia and/or a disturbance in organising. This causes impairment and decreased functioning in important areas. It starts gradually and is progressive, and problems are not due to other sources.

Attention and wakefulness

Attention is impaired in all three areas. The person has difficulty with:

- alertness, or maintaining vigilance
- selectiveness, or the ability to focus and filter out or selectively attend to stimuli at will
- directiveness, or the ability to pull oneself back to a task or direct and focus one's mental processes.

Wakefulness is usually reduced during the day, leading to drowsiness and naps. The person often experiences sleeplessness, restlessness and agitation at night. There is a disturbed sleep–wake cycle, with hour-to-hour variation. Interestingly, delirium and dreaming are both characterised by the same electroencephalographic (EEG) changes. The person with delirium is then caught between dreaming, sleeping and wakefulness.

Psychomotor behaviour

A person with a delirium can be either hyperactive or hypoactive, often alternating between the two extremes. Speech may be slurred and disjointed, with seemingly aimless vocalisations and repetitions. Tremors and irregular spasmodic (choreiform) movements may be present, as illustrated in the following Practice Examples of delirium.

Practice example

Aged 55, Mr Brunner, was in the midst of a difficult divorce and went drinking with his friends. He drank numerous 'straight shots', and shortly thereafter began screaming, crying and acting aggressively. At one point he tried to choke a man, and later he picked up a chair and threw it. The police took him into custody and then, when he began to convulse, he was transported to the nearest hospital.

Mrs Westing, aged 65, was in hospital with renal problems. Although previously alert, she rapidly became agitated and confused about where she was. She was unresponsive to the nurse's efforts to orient her, and refused to cooperate during her morning care. Within hours of this extreme agitation, she lapsed into a stupor and then a coma.

DIFFERENTIATING DELIRIUM FROM DEMENTIA AND DEPRESSION

The following criteria distinguish delirium from dementia:

- *State of consciousness.* People with delirium have fluctuating consciousness, but people with dementia are as attentive as they can be and do not have clouded consciousness until terminal stages.
- *Stability.* In people with delirium, the ability to pay attention and respond changes from hour to hour. People with dementia pay attention and respond at a particular level in a relatively stable manner.
- *Duration.* Delirium can be short-lived; dementia is prolonged.
- *Rate of onset.* Delirium develops rapidly, whereas dementia is usually an insidious, gradual process.
- *Cause.* Delirium may be traced to a recent source, whereas dementia cannot be linked to another cause.

For a summary of the characteristics of delirium and dementia, and the differentiation between them and depression, see Table 12.1 ■. Depression is discussed in detail in Chapter 15.

DEMENTIA

There are more than 342 800 Australians living with dementia, with this number expected to increase to 400 000 in less than 10 years. The story told by Jim about his life with Celia is one such example. By 2050, the number is expected to be 900 000. Each week, there are more than 1800 new cases of dementia in Australia; that is, approximately one person is diagnosed every six minutes. This is expected to grow to 7400 new cases each week by 2050. There are approximately 25 100 people in Australia with younger-onset dementia (a diagnosis of dementia under the age of 65, including people as young as 30). Dementia affects 3 out of 10 people over 85 years of age, and almost 1 in 10 people aged over 65 have dementia. An estimated 1.2 million people are involved in the care of a person with dementia. Dementia is the second leading cause of death in Australia. There is no cure for it, and on average symptoms of dementia are noticed by families three years before a firm diagnosis is made (Alzheimer's Australia, 2016).

The impact of dementia in Australia

Dementia is the single greatest cause of disability in older Australians (aged 65 years and over), and the third leading cause of disability burden overall. By 2029, Australia will have an expected shortfall of 150 000 paid carers for people with dementia. In 2009–2010, health expenditure on people with dementia was $4.9 billion. Dementia will become the third greatest source of health and residential aged-care spending within two decades. These costs alone will be around 1 per cent of gross domestic product (GDP). By the 2060s, spending on dementia is set to surpass that of any other health condition. It is projected to be at least $83 billion, and will represent around 11 per cent of health and residential aged-care sector spending. More than 50 per cent of residents in Australian government-subsidised aged-care facilities have dementia (85 227 out of 164 116 permanent residents), and almost half (44 per cent) of permanent residents with dementia also have a diagnosis of a mental illness (Alzheimer's Australia, 2016).

With statistics like these, you will most likely be involved in the care of someone with a dementia during your nursing career. See Mental Health in the Media for examples of well-known people who had some type of dementia.

Residential care facilities have large populations of people who have dementia. Manifestations include:

- global cognitive impairment, extending to the areas of abstract thinking, judgment, insight, complex capabilities (language, tasks, recognition) and personality change

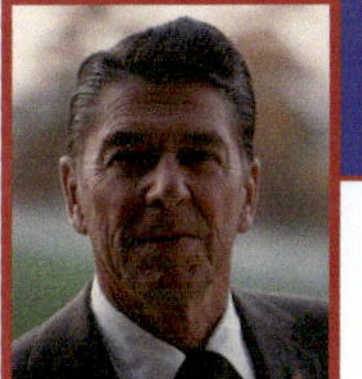

MENTAL HEALTH IN THE MEDIA

Famous people with dementia

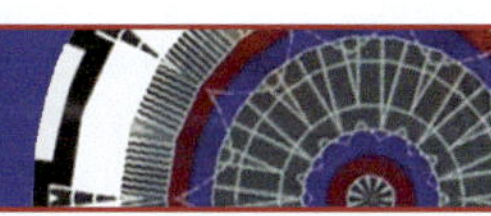

A number of people have been in the news for their struggles with dementia.

- Hazel Hawke—*wife of former Australian prime minister*
- Ronald Reagan—*40th president of the United States*
- Charlton Heston—*American actor*
- Rita Hayworth—*American actor*
- Terry Pratchett—*British novelist*
- Neville Wran—*former NSW premier*
- Malcom Young—*AC/DC guitarist*
- Winston Churchill—*British prime minister*

Photo courtesy of Corbis Images.

- memory impairment
- decline in intellectual function
- altered judgment, in awake and alert states
- altered affect
- spatial disorientation.

Dementia is a disorder involving functional decline in multiple cognitive areas, including memory, along with behavioural and psychological symptoms. Symptoms related to specific areas of brain damage are shown in Figure 12.1 ■.

Dementias are classified according to either the cause or the area of neurological damage (such as cortical or subcortical). Dementia of the Alzheimer's type (DAT) is the classic cortical dementia, whereas Huntington's disease and Parkinson's disease are common subcortical types. The cortical and subcortical types are quite similar. People with subcortical dementias, however, have a higher order of functioning.

Some types of neurological regression may be attributable to reversible causes. Some of these causes include metabolic

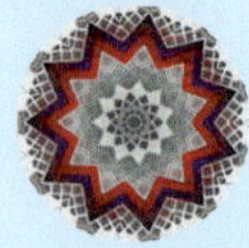

WHAT EVERY NURSE SHOULD KNOW

A family member's cognitive skills

Community health nurses often have contact with older people still living independently in their own homes. When you make a home visit to an older couple to treat the husband's leg ulcers, you notice that his wife is having some difficulty. Her shoelaces are not tied, and when you mention it she looks down and pushes them into the inside of her shoes instead of tying them. Her emotions seem blunted, she has been neglecting her personal hygiene, and her husband is worried about her decreased energy and motivation, and lack of initiative. This, in combination with her difficulties understanding some of your conversation, leads you to think she may be having some cognitive problems. Under these circumstances, an assessment is warranted.

TABLE 12.1 ■ Comparing delirium, dementia and depression

	Delirium	**Dementia**	**Depression**
Diagnostic features	Disturbance of consciousness accompanied by a change in cognition unaccounted for by a pre-existing or evolving dementia. Reduced clarity of awareness of the environment. Impaired ability to focus, sustain or shift attention. Change in cognition may include memory impairment, disorientation to time and/or place, or language disturbance, such as rambling, irrelevant or pressured and incoherent speech. Simple or complex perceptual disturbances may include misinterpretations, illusions or hallucinations.	Multiple cognitive deficits, including memory impairment and either aphasia, apraxia or agnosia; or a disturbance in executive functioning (the ability to think abstractly, to organise, plan, initiate, sequence, monitor and stop complex behaviour). Impairment in occupational or social functioning that represents a decline from earlier level of functioning.	Dysphoric mood, loss of interest or pleasure in usual activities and pastimes, appetite disturbance, change in weight, sleep disturbance, psychomotor agitation or retardation, decreased energy, feelings of worthlessness or guilt, difficulty concentrating or thinking, thoughts of death or suicide or suicide attempts.
Associated features	Emotional disturbance: fear, anxiety, irritability, anger, euphoria, apathy. Disturbance in sleep–wake cycle with daytime sleepiness or night-time agitation and difficulty falling asleep. Disturbed psychomotor behaviour, including groping or picking at bedclothes, sudden movements, or sluggishness and lethargy. Possible extremes of psychomotor activity during the day.	Spatial disorientation, poor judgment, poor insight, violence, suicidal behaviour, disinhibited behaviour, slurred speech, anxiety, mood and sleep disturbances, delusions, hallucinations, vulnerability to physical and psychosocial stressors. Progressive disease that slowly but steadily destroys the neurons of the brain and reduces, among other neurotransmitters, the concentration level of acetylcholine.	Depressed appearance, tearfulness, feelings of anxiety, irritability, fear, brooding, irrational guilt, excessive concern with physical health, panic attacks, phobias. Delusions or hallucinations may be present. In older adults, symptoms suggesting dementia (i.e. disorientation, memory loss, distractibility, apathy, difficulty in concentration, inattentiveness).
Onset	May begin abruptly. Relatively rapid: over hours. Short period of time: a few days. Especially common in children and after the age of 60.	Depends on underlying aetiology. May be rather sudden (e.g. head trauma) or insidious in onset and slow, but progress is relentless over several years (i.e. primary degenerative dementia).	Usually able to date onset with some precision. Onset is variable; symptoms usually develop over a period of days to weeks, but may be sudden. In some instances, prodromal symptoms may occur over several months.
Course	Fluctuates; symptoms usually worse at night; lucid intervals usually in the morning.	Depends on underlying aetiology. May be progressive, stable or (less likely) remitting.	Often not recognised or misdiagnosed in older adults. Need to differentiate from dementia.

(continued)

TABLE 12.1 ■ *(continued)*

	Delirium	Dementia	Depression
Duration	Transient. May resolve in a few hours or a few weeks.	May progress to death over several years. May be slowed.	Can be self-limiting. Median time period is 8 months; may last up to 2 years.
Outcome	Depends on severity. Poorer prognosis with severe delirium. Recovery possible if underlying disease is corrected or self-limiting. If disorder persists, delirium would shift to another more stable organic brain syndrome. May cause death.	Generally irreversible. Slowing of deterioration depends on underlying pathology, timely diagnosis and treatment. The more widespread the structural damage to the brain, the less likely the clinical improvement.	Can be successfully treated if identified and treated. Recurrent depression common in the elderly. Severe depression may end in suicide.
Aetiological factors	Multifactorial. Systemic infections. Metabolic disorders (hepatic or renal disease, hypoxia, hypercapnia, hypoglycaemia, ionic imbalances, thiamine deficiency). Postoperative states. Substance intoxication and withdrawal. Head trauma. Lesions of the right parietal lobe and occipital lobe. Toxin exposure. Anticholinergic effects of medication.	Primary degenerative dementia, Alzheimer's type. Infections of central nervous system. Brain trauma. Virus (i.e. AIDS). Prion (i.e. Creutzfeldt–Jakob disease). Toxic metabolic disturbance. Vascular disease (i.e. vascular dementia). Normal pressure hydrocephalus. Neurological conditions such as Huntington's disease, multiple sclerosis, Parkinson's disease. Post-anoxic or post-hypoglycaemic states.	Situational: bereavement, loss of health, major catastrophic event in person's life, trauma.

Source: Adapted from: Voyer, P., Richard, S., Doucet, L., & Carmichael, P.-H. (2011). Factors associated with delirium severity among older persons with dementia. *Journal of Neuroscience Nursing, 43*(2), 62–69; and Blazer, D., Hughes, D. C., & George, L. K. (1987). The epidemiology of depression in an elderly community population. *The Gerontologist, 27*, 281–287.

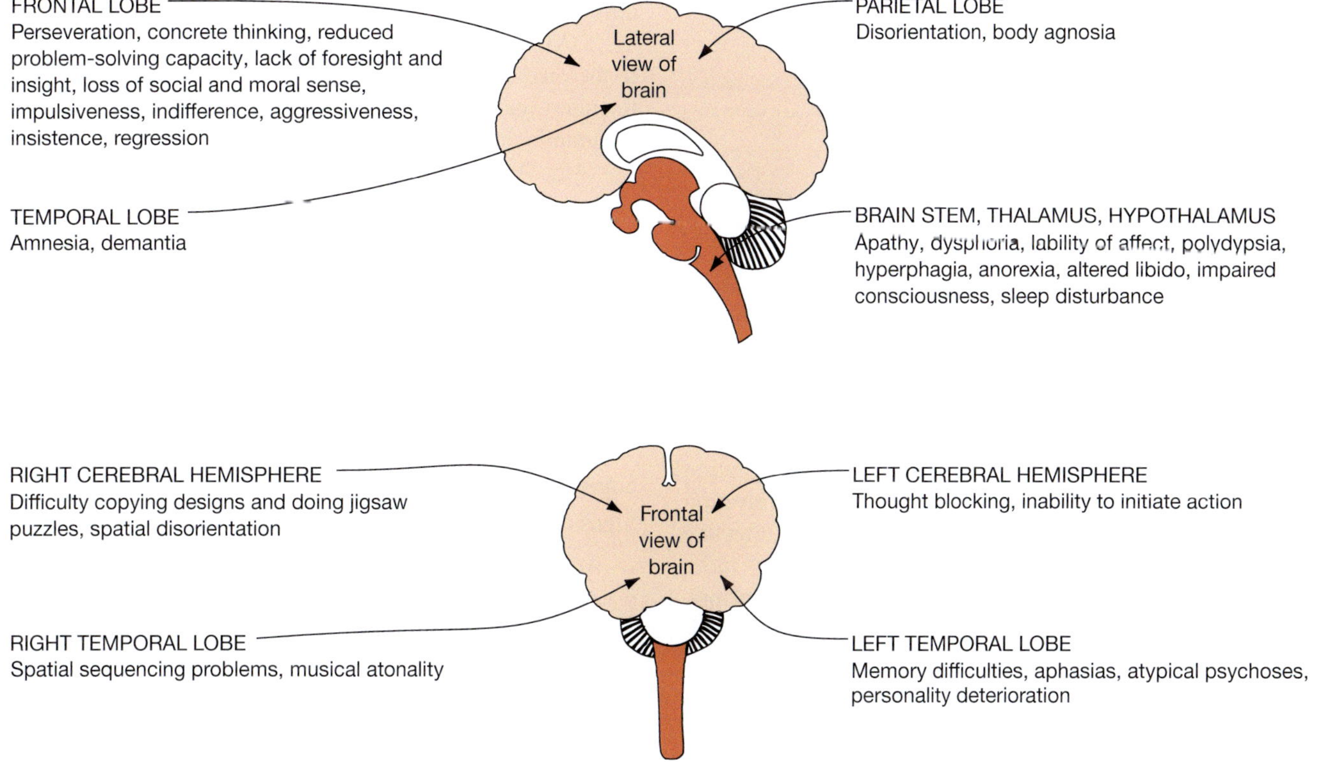

FIGURE 12.1 ■ Behavioural changes related to specific areas of brain damage. Damage to each part of the brain results in specific alterations and deficits in the individual's behaviours and skills.

abnormalities (e.g. hypothyroidism), dementia syndrome due to depression, paraneoplastic disease, or cobalamin C deficiency. (Krueger et al., 2015). How dementia affects function depends on the area of the brain involved in the disease. Different types of dementia have different symptoms. A frequent complication is the presence of mixed dementias. With such a broad array of dementias, establishing a clear diagnosis is complex and time-consuming, but necessary in order to determine appropriate treatment.

Sleep apnoea increases with age, and is being investigated for its association with dementia (Pan & Kastin, 2015). It is important to assess nocturnal breathing patterns in people with dementia. Sleep deprivation can lead to restlessness, reduced concentration and, if prolonged, hallucinations and delusions. Chronic sleep deprivation may exacerbate dementia behaviours, as in this Practice Example.

Practice example

Ellen, an older adult, was hospitalised for management of a medical condition. She was known to have early dementia of the Alzheimer's type (DAT), but had been managing alone in her unit up to this point. Over a period of several days, she became increasingly agitated, demanding cigarettes from nursing staff, other people staying on the ward and visitors. Attempts at distraction or providing unsolicited attention were unsuccessful.

A nursing student began questioning how much sleep Ellen was getting. At that point, the nurse's only cue was the lack of success with other interventions, but the nurse also knew that sundowning is common in people with dementia. The brief chart notes offered scant information. From a neighbour who came to visit, the nurse found out that prior to the hospitalisation Ellen had been phoning the neighbour during the night in an agitated state. The night staff agreed to observe and record the amount of time that Ellen spent sleeping, and the day staff did the same. With this additional data it was soon apparent that Ellen was averaging no more than four hours of sleep per 24-hour period. Meanwhile, her agitated behaviour was increasing.

After a multi-disciplinary team conference in which the nursing student offered her hypothesis of sleep deprivation, the nurse practitioner prescribed a mild, short-acting hypnotic for the next three nights. Nursing staff continued to monitor Ellen's sleep patterns and behaviour. By the end of the three nights, during which Ellen did appear to sleep for longer periods, the agitated behaviour and demands for cigarettes subsided considerably.

The use of hypnotics was not a long-term solution for Ellen, but it broke the escalating cycle of increasing agitation and decreasing sleep. Recognising the role of sleep deprivation in contributing to daytime behaviours can facilitate effective short-term intervention, and create a context for more comprehensive assessment of possible contributing factors, such as fear, relocation stress, powerlessness, or sensory and/or perceptual alterations.

Nurses also need to be aware of how culture plays a significant role in the health care practices of people with dementia and their families. An interesting ethnography on this topic is a book called *Unforgotten love and the culture of dementia care in India* by Bianca Brijnath.

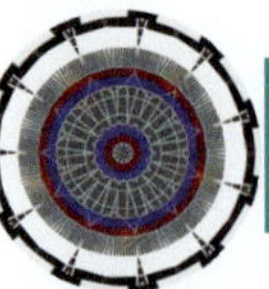

DEVELOPING CULTURAL COMPETENCE

Culture and dementia

Developing cultural competence when working with people who have dementia and their families is important. Cultural factors influence perceptions about what is normal ageing. Look for cultural bias (language, expected response, speed, etc.) in cognitive screening tools, and discuss these biases with colleagues.

Nurses promote effective health practices in the community setting; for example, taking blood pressure, discussing healthy diet, and noticing early symptoms of dementia. Education and outreach to diverse populations can provide support for people with dementia and their families.

CRITICAL THINKING QUESTIONS

1. What are some possible explanations for why different cultures have different attitudes about ageing?
2. Which cultures do you think treat older people with the most respect? Why?

Dementia of the Alzheimer's type (DAT)

Dementia of the Alzheimer's type (DAT), also known as *Alzheimer's disease* or *Alzheimer's dementia (AD)*, is a chronic progressive disorder, and the most common form of dementia among older adults. Reference to this disease with either abbreviation—DAT or AD—is accepted. To keep the distinction clear that this is one of many different types of dementia, and to prevent confusion with the abbreviation AD used to refer to anxiety disorder, it will be referred to as DAT throughout this chapter.

DAT cannot currently be prevented or cured. In addition to the quality-of-life issues for all people involved, there are financial realities that affect the individual, the family, the community and the health care system in general.

Alois Alzheimer first recognised the features of what would come to be called DAT in 1907 while conducting an autopsy on a 51-year-old woman with a four-year history of dementia. He discovered senile plaques in the brain and other pathological lesions that he called *neurofibrillary tangles* (Alzheimer, 1907). Neurofibrillary tangles are illustrated in Figure 12.2 ■. These are now called *Alzheimer-type changes*. This disease may also destroy the neurons that secrete the neurotransmitter acetylcholine, which plays a role in memory and learning.

Signs of dementia of the Alzheimer's type (DAT)

Signs of this disease include:

- *Aphasia:* The loss of language ability.
- *Anomia:* Over time, the person experiences difficulty remembering words.
- *Agraphia:* An inability to express thoughts in writing.
- *Alexia:* An inability to understand written language (eventually, the condition progresses to a loss of all verbal ability).
- *Apraxia:* The loss of purposeful movement without loss of muscle power or coordination in general. The ability to

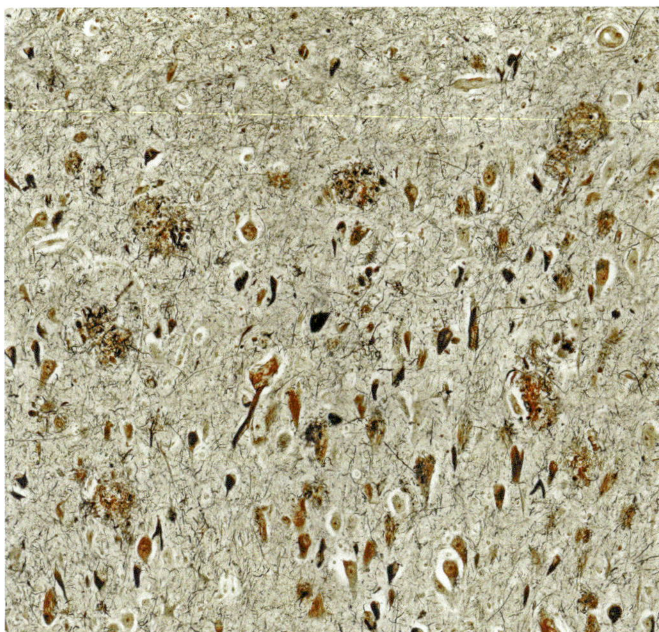

FIGURE 12.2 ■ Neurofibrillary tangles. This photomicrograph of a brain tissue specimen from a person with Alzheimer's shows the characteristic plaques (dark patches) and neurofibrillary tangles (irregular pattern of strand-like fibres).

conceptualise or perform motor tasks deteriorates. People with apraxia may have difficulty carrying out complex tasks.

- *Agnosia:* The loss of the sensory ability to recognise objects. Initially, the person has difficulty recognising everyday objects. In the later stages, people with agnosia recognise neither loved ones nor their own body parts.
- *Mnemonic disturbances:* Memory loss. The inability to remember recent events, especially in new or changing environments, extends to profound memory loss of both recent and past events (American Psychological Association [APA], 2011).

Frequently, symptoms of DAT occur insidiously. Family members may notice that routine tasks cannot be completed or items are placed in unusual places. The movie *Away from her* (see Mental Health in the Media) demonstrates some of the small and odd changes that take place in the beginning stages of DAT.

Hallucinations, more often visual than auditory, can be quite disturbing. Behaviour can become agitated, and will run counter to the person's usual personality and interactional style. Spending time in a health care facility for physical reasons, such as rehabilitation or surgery, can bring some of the symptoms to the attention of health care providers. See Box 12.1 on the next page for the behavioural changes of DAT. The following is a Practice Example of dementia.

Practice example

Therese Thomas, an 81-year-old retired piano teacher, is recuperating from knee replacement surgery at a rehabilitation centre. Nursing staff have noticed slight changes in her interactions over the past two weeks, including refusing to use cutlery during meals, a significant difference from her typically fastidious habits. During an assessment interview, Ms Thomas was asked how her vision and hearing have been lately, because seeing well and hearing well frequently become issues with older adults. She replied that she has been seeing and hearing just fine. These questions can be asked or stated in such a way as to seem more a physical set of questions than an emotional or psychiatric-focused set of questions (e.g. 'Sometimes people may not hear as well as others and words are missed.'). Then the question was asked, 'Sometimes your hearing may be such that you are hearing things that other people don't hear. Does that ever happen to you?'. Ms Thomas admitted she did hear things to which other people were not reacting. When asked to elaborate, Ms Thomas stated that her cutlery had begun speaking to her. When the nurse asked what was being said, Ms Thomas replied, 'Nothing good.'

Progression of dementia of the Alzheimer's type (DAT)

There are three clinically distinct global stages of DAT based on functional and cognitive capacity: Stages 1, 2 and 3. One assessment tool useful in assessing the cognitive capacity in DAT is the Mini-Mental State Exam (MMSE, see Chapter 10). Usually, a score of 18 or higher is seen in the early stages of DAT, between 12 and 18 in moderate DAT, and lower than 12 in severe DAT. The average decline in MMSE scores is approximately 3 points per year.

Functional disability can be assessed grossly through determining competence with activities of daily living (ADLs). When you assess a person for DAT, observe for functional disabilities. There is a correspondence between the stages of central nervous system (CNS) ageing and DAT. Note any

MENTAL HEALTH IN THE MEDIA

Away from Her

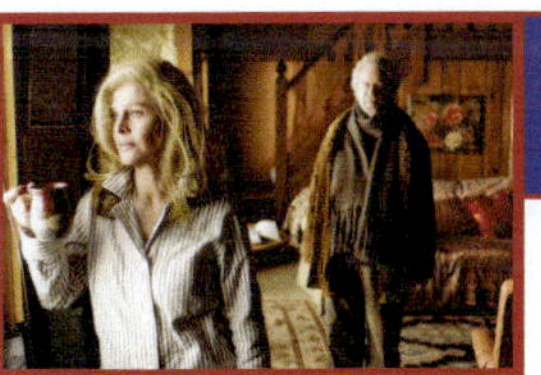

The movie *Away from Her* is the story of a man coping with the institutionalisation of his wife because of DAT. Their wonderful life full of love and adventure is reduced to infrequent and brief glimpses of its former glory as he watches the progression of her disease from putting a frying pan away in the refrigerator to not knowing who he is. The movie brings us along on the waves of his gut-wrenching feelings of loneliness as he leaves her at a specialty facility, sleeping without her for the first time. He faces the unimaginable changes in their relationship as he watches her transfer her affections to another man who also lives at the long-term care facility. Her fear and confusion from DAT are palpable as she tells him she doesn't want to be near him because she doesn't know how to feel.

Both sides of the DAT story are told with frankness and candor while being true to presenting the symptoms of the disease and the practical side of lives changed by DAT.

Photo courtesy © Lions Gate/courtesy Everett Collection.

Box 12.1 Behavioural changes of dementia of the Alzheimer's type (DAT)

DAT has an average course of 5–10 years, with a range of 2–20 years. Early onset often leads to very rapid deterioration.

Stage 1 (2–4 years): Early

Changes in behaviour include:

- Complex tasks become more difficult, related to a recent decline in memory.
- Concentration decreases while distractibility increases.
- Making accurate judgments becomes difficult.
- Disorientation about time occurs, but memory about people and places remains.
- Personal appearance may decline, and the person needs help in selecting appropriate clothing.
- Planning in general is seriously limited, so incomplete verbal or written reports are common at work sites.
- Verbal skills decline, and word finding and object naming become difficult. Speech in noisy, distracting environments is too difficult.
- The person may accuse others of wrongdoing because of transitory delusions of persecution ('You hid my keys'). People recognise their own confusion and are frightened by it. They cover up and rationalise symptoms.
- Poor driving skills because of misperceptions and errors in judgment can lead to accidents. See the Driving and Dementia Decision Aid (DADD) (Andrew, Traynor, Carmody & Erven, 2015).
- *Hypertonia* (an increase in muscle tone) can occur and may result in muscle twitching.
- Anxiety and depression are common, as are frustration, helplessness, apathy and stigma.
- Psychotic symptoms are common.
- Depression worsens the symptoms of dementia, and needs to be treated.

Stage 2 (several years): Middle

Changes in behaviour include:

- Progressive recent and remote memory loss.
- New information cannot be retained.
- Failure to recognise family members or past significant events signals loss of remote memory.
- Behaviour deteriorates rapidly, and is often socially unacceptable.
- Poor impulse control leads to outbursts and tantrums.
- Emotional lability is common—the mood quickly shifts from a flat affect to marked irritability.
- Comprehension of language, interactions and significance of objects is greatly diminished.
- Disorientation occurs to the three spheres of person, place and time.
- Wandering occurs.
- The person has difficulty tracking the sequence of events, especially for bathing, dressing and toileting.
- Psychotic symptoms are common.
- Familiar people are seen as unfamiliar, and vice versa.
- The sleep cycle is impaired, with a decrease in total sleep time and frequent awakenings.
- Accidents are common, especially falls and injuries, because of difficulty in using sharp objects.

Stage 3 (1–2 years): Late

Changes in behaviour include:

- Hyperorality (placing everything within reach into the mouth) and periodic binge eating occur.
- Hypermetamorphosis occurs (the need to compulsively touch and examine every object in the environment).
- Motor skills seriously deteriorate.
- Emotional responses dwindle to non-responsiveness.

cognitive decline and the corresponding functional disability when you formulate your assessments. Movement disorders are a frequent finding in DAT, and an important differential diagnosis (Mercello & Starkstein, 2014).

Treatment for DAT

The available treatment choices for a person with DAT include pharmacological interventions. Chapter 7 discusses the science of psychopharmacology and addresses the medication treatment issues, and this discussion explains how the brain chemistry affects what symptoms you see in people with DAT. The target symptoms are agitation, aggression, psychosis and, to a lesser extent, memory. Two main groups of medications used in DAT are acetylcholinesterase inhibitors, or cholinesterase inhibitors, and a glutamate pathway modifier. These medications can slow the progression of symptoms, but do not treat the disease. The important neurotransmitters altered by the disease, and attempted to be corrected by these medications, are acetylcholine and glutamate.

Acetylcholine is useful in storing and retrieving memories. People with DAT struggle with these issues, so working on increasing the amount of acetylcholine helps memory. The enzyme that breaks down the acetylcholine—acetylcholinesterase—is inhibited when an acetylcholinesterase inhibitor is used. The result is a slight increase in the amount of acetylcholine in the brain. This has the chance to improve memory.

Glutamate is a primary excitatory neurotransmitter in the brain, and glutamate receptor activity is associated with information processing, storage and retrieval. There is a glutamate excitotoxicity hypothesis to DAT, in that too much glutamate causes an over excitation that can lead to toxic effects. This is observed when the person cannot complete a simple task, do a series of steps to a process, such as dressing or hygiene, and has memory difficulties. When the pathway is modified, the person has less toxic effects and can function more competently.

Dementia with Lewy bodies

Dementia with Lewy bodies (DLB) is the second most common late-onset dementia after DAT, accounting for 15–20 per cent of the neurodegenerative dementias. The name of this dementia subtype comes from the pathological feature of Lewy body inclusions. Lewy bodies are abnormal concentrations of protein that develop inside nerve cells and appear as masses that displace other cell components and their function.

One of the main concerns regarding DLB is improving clinical detection (Galvin, 2015) before pharmacological treatment is initiated. This is important because people with DLB are sensitive to many antipsychotic medications prescribed for dementia, and can have a severe and even fatal sensitivity to the extrapyramidal side-effects. People with DLB are at much higher risk of developing side-effects, such as tardive dyskinesia or neuroleptic malignant syndrome, in response to traditional antipsychotics (such as Haloperidol). Although the newer atypical antipsychotic agents are generally less likely to provoke side-effects, people with DLB can be at unacceptably high risk. Quetiapine (Seroquel), however, is an atypical antipsychotic that has a relatively low risk of provoking these side-effects, and people with DLB are often better able to tolerate Quetiapine than other antipsychotics.

Three core diagnostic features of DLB were defined by McKeith and colleagues (1996):

1. spontaneous Parkinsonism or extrapyramidal signs
2. persistent or recurrent visual hallucinations
3. fluctuating cognition.

People with DLB are much less common than those who have a concomitant DAT. Neuropathological studies have found that 20–30 per cent of older adults with degenerative dementia have an overlap of both DAT and DLB. It is also difficult to differentiate DLB that is comorbid with DAT as a unique clinical syndrome. It is also challenging to distinguish these people from those with a Parkinson's disease (PD)–DAT blended syndrome.

An action tremor may precede other Parkinsonian features, and dementia is often heralded by myoclonus and hallucinations. The progression of symptoms of DLB appears to be intermediate, as compared with the progression of symptoms in the PD and PD–DAT subgroups.

In addition to Parkinsonian features, dementia and a frequent tendency to episodic delirium, the syndrome may be clinically indistinguishable from DAT. On autopsy, there will be diffuse involvement of cortical neurons with Lewy body inclusions, and an absence of, or inconspicuous number of, neurofibrillary tangles and senile plaques.

Vascular dementia

Vascular dementia, also known as *ischaemic vascular dementia* (IVD) and formerly known as *multi-infarct dementia,* accounts for about 19 per cent of the dementias. Unlike Alzheimer's disease, vascular dementia is abrupt in onset and episodic, with multiple remissions. The person with IVD demonstrates focal neurological signs, such as one-sided weakness, emotional outbursts and a stepwise—rather than progressive—decline in intellectual functioning, and has a history of hypertension, diabetes or cardiovascular disease affecting other organs.

In IVD, brain tissue is destroyed by intermittent emboli that can range from a few to over a dozen. Individual infarcts may vary by 1 centimetre in diameter. Symptoms are commonly absent until 100–200 cubic centimetres of brain tissue have been destroyed.

Parkinson's disease (PD)

The association between **Parkinson's disease** (PD) and dementia has deepened over the years. Some people with dementia have PD. A subset of people have both PD and DAT. The diagnosis is difficult to determine. There are several varieties of PD, and the cause of classic PD is unknown. Another type, post-encephalitic, has been linked to previous viral infection in the brain.

Huntington's disease

Huntington's disease is a genetic, progressive, degenerative disorder characterised by motor and cognitive changes, chorea and dementia. This disease, one of the more frequently observed types of genetic nervous system diseases, usually begins between the ages of 40 and 50. By the time of diagnosis, the person has often had children, passing this inherited disease to another generation. The movement disorder is thought to be caused by vulnerability to damage and subsequent loss of nerve cells in the brain.

Movement abnormalities slowly increase, ultimately involving all muscle groups. The motor dysfunction is characterised by *chorea:* quick, jerky, purposeless, involuntary movements. The average lifespan after an initial diagnosis is 15 years. Mood disturbances, particularly depression, are common early in the disease, followed by deterioration of cognitive function.

Supplementing with coenzyme Q_{10} (CoQ_{10} or ubiquinone) has been known to replace deficient levels of the enzyme in muscle and decrease cerebellar-based ataxia. The enzyme could have an impact by slowing the disease's progression. As with all diseases, rigorous research is required to explore this issue further.

Pick's disease

Pick's disease is a rare disorder where cerebral atrophy is present in the frontal and/or temporal lobes. These circumscribed pathological changes are different from DAT, where the atrophy is mild and diffuse. The two patterns of behaviour evident in Pick's disease represent the temporal and frontal types of the disease. People with the temporal type are talkative, light-hearted, joyous, anxious and hyperattentive. People with the frontal type often have inertia, emotional dullness and lack of initiative. As the disease progresses, the deterioration becomes more global, affecting memory and language. There is profound atrophy of the frontal and/or temporal lobes. Pick's disease worsens rapidly.

The expected lifespan after original diagnosis is seven years. A higher incidence is seen in some families, suggesting a genetic predisposition. Because language is affected, nurses need to attend to the behavioural messages of people with Pick's disease.

Creutzfeldt–Jakob disease (CJD)

Creutzfeldt–Jakob disease is an infectious, transmissible degenerative dementia affecting the cerebral cortex through cell destruction and overgrowth. It is marked clinically by a very rapid onset and involuntary movements. This profound dementia is evidenced by cerebellar ataxia, diffuse myoclonic

LIVED EXPERIENCE

Celia is the mother of our three boys, all of whom are married with children, and some with grandchildren. Celia cannot remember the names of our grandchildren, she can't recall where they go to school, who belongs to who or how old they are. Despite there being much media coverage of dementia and memory loss, the grandchildren do not understand why she doesn't know them and why she doesn't remember. It is upsetting for everyone, including my wife.

Once, we were having friends around for dinner and I asked Celia to peel some potatoes and cut them up ready for a roast while I got everything else ready. This was something my wife has done a thousand times. Celia was a fantastic cook and very much enjoyed serving her family many delicious meals. What she did was peel the potatoes and then cut them into thin strips, ready for chips. This was repeated a number of times until I stood right beside her to ensure that the task was undertaken successfully. When she looked in the bin and saw quite a lot of potato in there, she admonished me for wasting money and food.

jerks, and other visual and neurological abnormalities. There are distinctive electroencephalographic changes with CJD. The infection is presumed to be caused by a *prion,* a small protein particle that is resistant to treatment and sterilisation procedures. There may be a genetic susceptibility to infection; however, the only definitive spreading mechanism is iatrogenic, as seen after corneal transplantation and after the injection of human growth hormone derived from the pituitary gland of cadavers with the disease. Elevated levels of brain-derived proteins are detected on lumbar puncture. Levels in the cerebrospinal fluid (CSF) may increase over time; therefore, repeated testing—even when the first test is negative—may be diagnostic.

New variant Creutzfeldt–Jakob disease (nvCJD)

Once the disease known as 'mad cow disease' (bovine spongiform encephalopathy [BSE]) became widespread, an unusual presentation of Creutzfeldt–Jakob disease was noted, and since 1996 has been identified as **new variant Creutzfeldt–Jakob disease (nvCJD)**. It appears to be caused by the same agent as BSE, although it is unclear how transmission to humans takes place. There is no blood or tissue test for nvCJD, and it can be transmitted through blood transfusions. Evidence suggests that nvCJD is linked to eating contaminated beef. Usually, CJD occurs in older adults and begins as dementia. This new variation can occur in younger people, and includes unusual spongiform changes in the cerebellum. nvCJD is currently more of a problem in Europe than in Australia or New Zealand, due to varying health codes and standards.

Binswanger's disease (BD)

Binswanger's disease (BD) is a subcortical vascular dementia caused by widespread, microscopic areas of damage to the deep layers of the brain's white matter. As the arteries become more and more narrowed by atherosclerosis, less blood is supplied, and the subcortical areas of the brain are not properly nourished and cannot survive. Changes in the person's behaviour may be sudden, or gradual and then progress. BD often coexists with DAT.

Behaviours and treatments that slow the progression of disease processes, such as high blood pressure, diabetes and atherosclerosis, can lower the likelihood of developing BD. However, there is no specific cure for BD. Consistent use of the proper medication, as well as eating a healthy diet and keeping appropriate activity and rest cycles, and not smoking or drinking too much alcohol, is thought to slow the progression of Binswanger's disease.

Pseudodementia

Affective disorders, particularly depression, can be masked by symptoms suggestive of dementia. Clinical symptoms may include impaired attention and memory, apathy, self-neglect and complaints of depression. The term **pseudodementia** has been used to describe the reversible cognitive impairments seen in depression. It is essential to detect pseudodementia, because, with appropriate treatment, people can recover. Pseudodementia should be suspected when the onset is abrupt, the clinical course is rapid, and the person complains about

LIVED EXPERIENCE

Celia goes swimming in the morning at the local public pool with her brother who is visiting from England. Every day, her friend Helena rings Celia to have a chat. The matter of swimming is raised. 'I haven't been swimming for years,' says Celia, 'although I used to be a good swimmer, but I could never tumble-turn.' Celia swam less than two hours ago, and this conversation is repeated every time Helena calls.

Celia saw me putting the washing on. She wanted to do it, and told me to 'go and do something else'. I left the laundry and went to tend to my Koi carp in the garden. Twenty minutes later, I went back to the laundry. The washing machine was not on, clothes were still in the basket and nothing was happening. Celia was sitting on the lounge. I started to do the washing. Celia came in and told me to 'go and do something else'. After a number of attempts, when Celia went to the bathroom, I loaded the machine, put in the washing powder and turned it on. Celia had no recollection that anything had occurred. When the wash cycle was complete, my wife hung the washing out on the line, again telling me to 'go and do something else'. She had no recollection of anything that had happened at all.

cognitive failures. People with dementia often fail to perceive, or attempt to cover up, their deficits.

Medical conditions affecting cognition

Physiologically-based clinical neuropsychiatric manifestations or disorders are common among adult persons with AIDS (Gannon, Khan & Kolson, 2011). A neurological syndrome or neurocognitive impairment may be the first clinical manifestation of HIV disease. Neurocognitive changes associated with HIV consist of cognitive, behaviour and motor dysfunction. Significant numbers of people with HIV experience neuropsychiatric manifestations for two major reasons:

1. Because the virus is capable of invading CNS tissue, several of the opportunistic infections and neoplasms associated with AIDS also affect the CNS.
2. Prescribed pharmacological treatment may have neuropsychiatric side-effects.

In addition to neurocognitive changes, more ominous changes—delirium, dementia and coma—can occur.

Focal brain processes

The most common focal brain processes are toxoplasmosis (a parasitic opportunistic infection), cryptococcal meningitis (a fungal opportunistic infection), cytomegalovirus (CMV), encephalitis (a viral opportunistic infection), progressive multifocal leukoencephalopathy (PML, a viral opportunistic infection) and CNS lymphoma (a neoplastic process). Signs and symptoms associated with these processes include focal deficits, altered level of consciousness, confusion, memory disturbances, headaches and seizures.

Medication side-effects

Several antiretroviral medications, and medications used to treat associated symptoms and opportunistic infections, cause significant neuropsychiatric side-effects. Adverse reactions can include hallucinations, sleep disturbances including insomnia, vivid dreams and nightmares—and memory impairment. In addition, side-effects can include agitation, anxiety, confusion, delirium, depression, headache and irritability. It is important to know which medication(s) the person is taking in order to accurately assess the presence of neurological and emotional signs and symptoms.

HIV-associated dementia

A syndrome caused by direct HIV infection of the CNS, **HIV-associated dementia (HAD)**, is rare—but the milder form, HIV-associated neurocognitive disorders (HAND), persists in this population. The positive impacts of antiretroviral therapy (ART) on neurocognitive functioning is the result of people adhering to medication regimens.

HAND pathogenesis includes the following:

- persistent systemic and CNS inflammation
- ageing in the HIV-infected brain
- HIV subtype (clade) distribution
- potential neurotoxicity of ART.

HAD is characterised as a progressive dementia with:

- cognitive dysfunction: forgetfulness, loss of concentration, confusion and slowness of thought
- declining motor performance: loss of balance, muscle weakness and deterioration in fine motor skills, such as handwriting
- behavioural changes: apathy, withdrawal, dysphoric mood and regressed behaviour
- other symptoms, such as headaches or seizures.

HAD is often initially confused with depression, but may progress in a period of months to the point at which the affected person is bedridden. People with HAD may also quickly succumb to opportunistic infections because of an inability to care for themselves.

AMNESTIC DISORDER

Amnestic disorder, a relatively uncommon cognitive disorder, is characterised by short- and long-term memory deficits, an inability to recall previously learned information or past events, an inability to learn new material, confabulation, apathy and a bland affect. Impairment ranges from moderate to severe. Possible causes include head trauma, hypoxia, encephalitis, thiamine deficiency and substance abuse. These causes shape the three main types of amnestic disorder, which are briefly described here: those due to (1) a medical condition, (2) a substance, or (3) other causes.

Traumatic brain injury (TBI) is an acquired brain injury, and is frequently associated with amnesia. The cause of the trauma creates a connection between the general medical condition (which includes physical trauma), and the amnestic disorder when this type is diagnosed. The diagnosis of amnestic disorder is supported by the timing of the onset of amnesia (the amnesia is coordinated with physical trauma), an atypical presentation of a memory problem, and the ruling out of other explanations for the disorder. The emotional and behavioural sequelae of a TBI need explicit and intense team efforts for successful treatment (Chung & Khan, 2014).

Substance-induced amnesia persists beyond the immediate effects of the substance and the duration of intoxication or withdrawal from the substance. Deficits can worsen over the years, despite abstinence from the substance.

Amnestic disorder not otherwise specified (NOS) is the diagnosis used when the criteria are not met for the two other types described earlier, or when there is not enough supporting evidence to link a cause to the amnesia.

BIOPSYCHOSOCIAL THEORIES

Theories about the causes of cognitive disorders are as varied as the disorders themselves. Genetics, infection and vascular insufficiency are all believed to be causative factors. Because delirium is usually caused by an underlying systemic illness, investigations are essential for treatable conditions such as dehydration, diabetes, hyponatremia, hypercalcaemia, thyroid crisis, infection, silent myocardial infarction, drug intoxication, or liver or renal failure (Djukic, Wedekind, Franz, Gremke & Nau, 2015). If the cause is treated, complete recovery from delirium can be achieved.

The actual cause of DAT remains unknown, but several factors are believed to play a role. DAT has been correlated with the loss of specific groups of nerve cells and the disruption of communication between nerve cells from acetylcholine and serotonin deficits. Researchers are working to identify a slow-acting, virus-like causative agent. This work has been prompted by the findings of just such an agent in CJD.

Advanced age, family history of the illness, Down's syndrome and a history of head trauma are considered risk factors for DAT. There are linkages between genetic markers and DAT on a number of chromosomes—namely, chromosomes 1, 14 and 21, and one or both alleles coding for the e4 variant of apolipoprotein on chromosome 19 (referred to as APOE e4). People with DAT have four times the family incidence of dementia. Yet in identical and fraternal twins, in only 40 per cent of cases do both get DAT, suggesting that DAT cannot be due to a single autosomal dominant gene. The disease also appears in twins and in various family members at different times, making it difficult to interpret the markers found in genetic studies.

Other possible risk factors are environmental toxins, stroke, thyroid disorder, lower educational status, and female gender. Ongoing research focuses on causes and treatment that can either protect or restore neurons, thereby combating memory loss. Additional studies focus on ameliorating behavioural symptoms. Vitamin B_{12} deficiency in DAT is explained in the Practice Example.

Practice example

Vitamin B_{12} deficiency

There are numerous dementia-related metabolic dysfunctions, such as the imperfect metabolism of vitamin B_{12}. DAT interferes with vitamin B_{12} metabolism, and so vitamin B_{12} deficiency is one way in which DAT affects the body.

People who have the variation of the apolipoprotein-E gene (abbreviated as APOE), variation e4, are at increased risk for developing late-onset DAT. Research suggests people who have the APOE e4 gene are much more likely to be dysfunctional metabolisers of vitamin B_{12}. Vitamin B_{12} deficiency manifests in behavioural disturbances, such as unusual actions and psychotic symptoms, as well as alterations in circadian rhythm patterns and mood disorders. These problems are slightly more frequent in people who have the APOE e4 variation of the gene.

Vitamin B_{12} depletion can occur outside the occurrence of DAT. It is common among older adults because of age-induced changes in the gastrointestinal tract. A lack of vitamin B_{12} causes anaemia, and in time anaemia is accompanied by neurological signs and symptoms, including diminished vibration and position senses, and dementia.

Being up-to-date on information about the whole-body effects of DAT, such as metabolic dysfunction, can prevent a great deal of misery and distress for people and their carers. Attend to the person's food and nutrition.

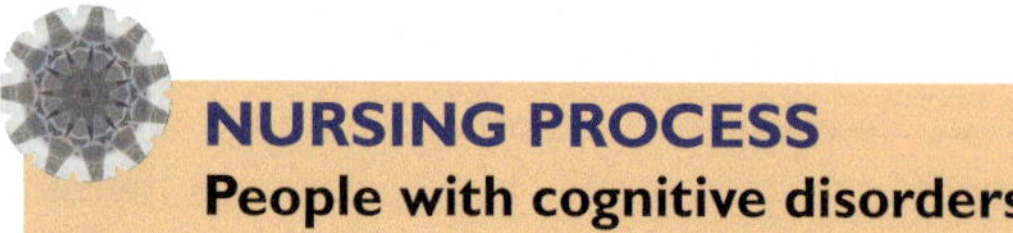

NURSING PROCESS
People with cognitive disorders

The nursing process with all cognitive disorders revolves around the principles of care used in dementia.

Assessment

Accurate assessment of people with cognitive disorders is important for developing and delivering safe and competent care.

Subjective data

Gathering data about people with delirium, dementia, amnestic disorder and other cognitive disorders is difficult. These people are sometimes anxious, defensive and confused, and give unreliable histories. Often, there is no dependable secondary source of information. To maximise efforts, gather all data in a setting that is free from distraction and discomfort:

- Decibel levels of ambient (surrounding) noise must be low.
- Light should be sufficient to dispel shadows.
- Room temperature should be comfortable for the person.

When asking questions, pace them slowly to allow sufficient time for the person to think about them and answer comfortably. Older people can normally process information after receiving it, but may have difficulty taking in information. Placing the person in a situation that interferes with an already compromised sensory apparatus only heightens their anxiety, and seriously compromises attempts to undertake an assessment.

Health history When completing the person's health history, include all past and present medical conditions, and pay special attention to chronic conditions for which the person is being treated, and any recent changes in health status. Ask the person: 'Are you seeing anyone about your health at this time?', 'Why did you seek medical help?', 'What does your nurse or doctor say is the problem?' Infections may present as confusion and other symptoms of dementia before any change in temperature, pulse and respirations is noted.

Sensory impairment Older adults are particularly sensitive to the confusion associated with sensory deprivation. Physiological changes in their sensory apparatus may be directly related to ageing or to pathological processes. Both diminish sensory receptive ability. The changes in sensory apparatus, however, are not clear-cut. The older adult may have difficulty hearing high-frequency sounds, such as consonants. Turning up the volume on the radio may help the person hear one range of sounds, but may also cause sensory overload because the rest of the sounds are too loud. The overall result is deprivation and distortion.

Try to ascertain any possible sensory problems, especially in hearing and vision. To test hearing, stand so that the person cannot see your face, and ask a question in a normal tone of voice. The questions you ask should require more than a yes or no answer, so make them open-ended. Test vision with pictures that the person will easily recognise.

Nutrition When possible, obtain an estimate of the person's food intake. 'What do you usually eat for breakfast? Lunch? Dinner?' Make special note of their protein and vitamin intake. Avitaminosis, pellagra, anaemia and hypoglycaemia have all been associated with reversible brain syndromes. Hydration is also an important factor, so look for signs of dehydration. Dehydration can also cause confusion. Anticholinergic side-effects from typically prescribed medications and over-the-counter (OTC) drugs can also cause dehydration and confusion.

Head trauma Falls are common among older adults. Misjudging distances and not being aware of obstructions also contribute to injuries. Cerebral contusions, midbrain haemorrhage and subdural haematoma may result from a fall. Confusion may be the result of any of these conditions.

Medication Older adults are prone to adverse drug reactions as a result of age-related bodily changes. These factors are compounded by the high consumption of many different medications: more than one-third of all drugs are consumed by the 15 per cent of the population who are older. Older people are particularly susceptible to medications with anticholinergic properties (major tranquilisers, antidepressants, barbiturates, adrenal steroids, atropine, anti-Parkinsonians, antihistamines, antihypertensives and diuretics). Ask the person about both prescription and over-the-counter medications: 'Are you taking any medicines prescribed by your doctor?', 'Do you take laxatives, cold pills, or other medicines that you buy at the chemist or supermarket without a prescription?', 'Have you tried health foods, herbs, supplements or other remedies?'

Alcohol consumption Talk about alcohol consumption. Beyond being another source of dehydration, alcohol is a CNS depressant, and intoxication may mimic symptoms of cognitive disorders. Alcohol ingestion also compromises nutritional status, and may cause withdrawal effects. Ask questions like 'What is your favourite drink?', 'How much alcohol do you drink in one day/week?' and 'Have you ever had periods of not remembering after you have been drinking?' Drinks like cider may be perceived as non-alcoholic or not 'counting' as alcohol consumption. Ask questions about these types of drinks separately from alcohol consumption questions, possibly when discussing nutrition.

Family history Families can be a major source of information and support. In Australia, many older adults have seen one or more relatives in the previous week, and many live within 60 minutes of their nearest child. Common living arrangements include living with a spouse, child or sibling. Family assessment should include the following:

- living arrangements
- care arrangements for the person (e.g. shopping assistance, daily visits, telephone calls)
- family knowledge of the current illness
- family expectations for the future
- special family concerns about care
- family style of coping with stress (e.g. death of a relative, illness)
- the identified spokesperson/decision-maker for the family
- the family's perception of the person's coping abilities.

Throughout the interview, observe the interactions between family members. Do family members support and respect what the person says? Do people listen to one another? What is the atmosphere in the family group? What is the level of intimacy between family members? Do they relate to each other with warmth and affection? Chapter 24 includes an expanded family assessment.

Activities of daily living Carefully and thoroughly assess the person's level of self-care. This is often called a *functional assessment*. What activities of daily living (ADL) can the person do without help? For which activities is help required? What type of help is needed? As cognitive deficits increase, dependence on others for assistance increases. For a study about the ADL needs of the person with DAT, see Evidence-based Practice.

EVIDENCE-BASED PRACTICE

Developing a bathing protocol for a person with a cognitive impairment

You are a nurse in a residential care facility. Eddie, a 76-year-old man with dementia who owned and ran his own business for years, now lives in the facility. His daughter Esther is his guardian, and has been involved in both her father's care and some program development at the facility. Bathing has become an issue with Eddie — it seems to frighten and embarrass him. Discussions with his daughter have revealed this to be a new problem.

The first difficulty arose when staff members entered Eddie's room with bathing equipment and announced it was time to 'have a wash'. This time, what had been a usual routine was not received well. Eddie grabbed a female staff member and murmured that there was no way she was going to see what he needed to keep private, nor could she squeeze the life out of him with 'that stuff'. Calm explanations did not reassure him, and Eddie was determined not to allow bathing.

Eddie needs to exercise some control over the situation, and understand that bathing routines can be designed to be pleasant and comfortable for him. Letting him have a say in when he bathes ('Not now' is an acceptable response) and what gets cleaned (wash his hair first, last or not at all) has immediate positive results. Keep in mind that older skin can be dry, bathing can cause further drying (soybean oil-based no-rinse cleansers promote healthier skin), and arthritis and other conditions make movement painful. A person-centered approach makes bathing more pleasant, more comfortable and safer. Ensure Eddie's privacy is fully maintained.

The approach outlined for Eddie is based on the following research:

Gallagher, M., & Long, C. O. (2011). Advanced dementia care: Demystifying behaviors, addressing pain, and maximizing comfort: Research and practice: Partners in care. *Journal of Hospice and Palliative Nursing, 13*(2), 70–78.

Sheu, E., Versloot, J., Nader, R., Kerr, D., & Craig, K. D. (2011). Pain in the elderly: Validity of facial expression components of observational measures. *Clinical Journal of Pain, 27(7), 593-601.* doi: 10.1097/AJP.0b013e31820f52e1

CRITICAL THINKING QUESTIONS

1. What are the physical and emotional benefits to the person of altering a general routine to meet their specific needs?
2. Staff members derive benefits also. How can altering Eddie's bathing routine help staff?

Community functioning The Comprehensive Functional Assessment (CFA) tool measures the ability to sustain oneself in the community. It covers the basic skills of living, working, relating to others, and recreating in community settings. Assess not only their ability to live independently in the community, but also their degree of social involvement. Does the person belong to any clubs, religious organisations or groups? Do friends visit the person at home? Ask about attendance at senior citizen programs, and the level of participation in activities involving others.

Objective data Evaluating older adults with a cognitive impairment is usually organised into three areas: physical and mental assessment, laboratory assessment and imaging techniques.

Physical and mental assessment A thorough assessment, including a complete neurological examination (evaluation of cranial nerves, motor and sensory systems, and reflexes) and a mental health consultation is important for all older adults with a cognitive impairment. Because older adults with organic illness frequently manifest confusion and depression, clinicians work from the assumption that reversible illness is present. Chest X-ray films and an electrocardiogram are taken.

Laboratory assessment The following tests are routinely ordered for older people:

- complete blood count, including folic acid and vitamin B_{12} levels to detect anaemia
- erythrocyte sedimentation rate (ESR) to detect infection
- SMA (sequential multiple analyser) to detect electrolyte imbalances
- syphilis tests (Venereal Disease Research Laboratory [VDRL])
- thyroid function studies
- serum levels of barbiturates, bromides and digitalis
- liver function studies
- human immunodeficiency virus (HIV)
- serology
- heavy metals
- toxicology
- urinalysis.

Imaging techniques Views of the brain's structure and function can be provided through a computed axial tomographic brain scan (CAT scan) or computed tomographic brain scan (CT scan), positron emission tomography (PET), and single-photon emission computed tomography (SPECT). Figure 12.3 ■ presents PET scan images of a normal brain and the brain of a person with DAT. These tests can be ordered for the person considered high risk; that is, those having acute deterioration in cognitive functioning of recent onset. Acute deterioration is often associated with focal lesions and hydrocephalus.

A number of other diagnostic procedures may be used. However, because of their intrusive nature their use should be carefully considered:

- lumbar puncture
- skull X-ray films
- electroencephalography (EEG)
- magnetic resonance imaging (MRI)
- cerebral angiography
- isotope cisternography.

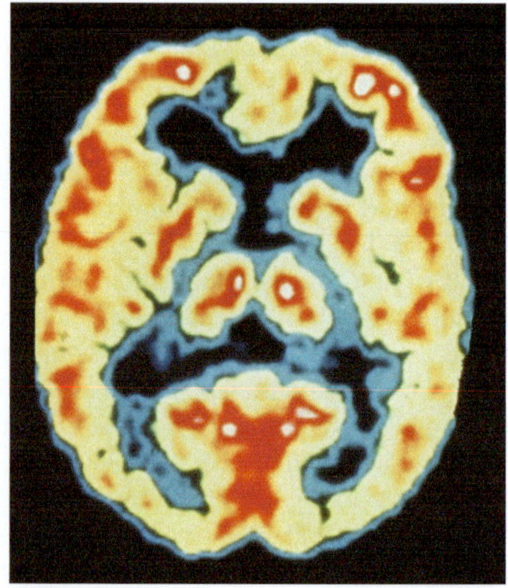

(a)

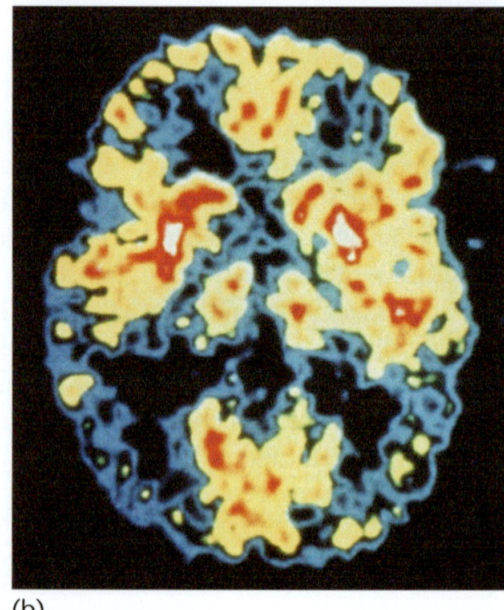

(b)

FIGURE 12.3 ■ PET scan brain images in dementia of the Alzheimer's type. Compare a normal brain scan (a) with the brain of a person with Alzheimer's disease (b). (a) The red and yellow areas indicate normal metabolic rates. (b) Note the blue areas indicating abnormally low metabolism in the parietal and temporal lobes.
Photo courtesy of Dr Robert Friedland/Photo Researchers, Inc.

The amygdala plays a key role in enhancing pleasant and unpleasant memories, and it modulates memory processes. Because the medial aspect of the amygdala is involved in DAT, imaging such as an MRI could provide insights into behavioural and emotional changes in the person. Be cautious if undergoing the test is problematic for the person.

Cognitive functioning

Cognitive functioning includes memory, reasoning, abstraction, calculation ability and judgment. Refer back to Box 12.1 on page 234 for detailed information on cognitive functioning during the various stages of DAT. People will not respond effectively unless they feel that the information requested is relevant, they see some purpose in the interview and they are interested in the material. Choose testing materials carefully, therefore, and keep the person's endurance in mind at all times. When assessing cognitive functioning, pay particular attention to the following:

Appearance People who appear dishevelled, dirty or unkempt may be experiencing problems with poor memory or a shortened attention span. This diminished ability to perform self-care may not be apparent if the person has a carer who helps with ADLs.

Manner and attitude Some people may exaggerate mannerisms to compensate for a perceived decline in functioning. For example, the person who has compulsive tendencies may become even more set in their ways. An attitude of defensiveness, withdrawal or paranoia may be a response to increasing anxiety about diminished abilities.

Communication Assess communication in the areas of speech, gestures, facial expression and writing. Difficulty in finding words and naming objects may suggest **expressive aphasia**. Difficulty grasping complex concepts may suggest **receptive aphasia**. Assess the person's ability to use gestures and facial expressions to compensate for verbal aphasia. Not using facial expressions and gestures, and speaking in a monotone way, may indicate depression. Also assess the person's written communication and reading and language ability. Older people whose primary language is not English may revert to their native language; therefore, make arrangements for a translator/translation service.

Perception Perception is the person's ability to recognise and integrate sensory information, including the conscious recognition of oneself in relation to the environment. The person with asymmetric brain involvement of DAT may neglect one side of their body. These people may also have difficulty recognising objects (agnosia). The person with perceptual difficulty may distort sensory information, with resulting hallucinations and delusions.

Attention and wakefulness Attention refers to alertness and the ability to attend selectively to stimuli and to direct one's focus. Can the person sustain or pay attention to the interview process, or are they easily distracted? You can assess attention by asking the person to spell a word backwards. Wakeful states range from hyperalertness to stupor. Stupor can be the result of medication intoxication or an acute systemic disease.

Motor activity Lethargy is often a symptom of depression, but it can also be the result of such medications as tranquilisers, antihypertensives, antidepressants and antihistamines. Combinations of medications can also cause lethargy, even when one of the medications alone may not be sedating. Lethargy can be caused by a number of disease processes, such as urinary tract infection, anaemia and meningitis. A shift between hypermotor and hypomotor activity is a sign of delirium. Agitation and physical aggression are occasionally demonstrated.

Mood and affect Depression may accompany earlier stages of dementia. The more serious the dementia, however, the less depressed the person. The person with organic disease of the cerebral area is emotionally labile. Inquire about any changes in eating or sleeping habits, and ask about recent loss of energy and interest in usual activities. If depression is suspected, evaluate the person for risk of suicide (see Chapter 19). Explore thoughts about dying, plans regarding self-harm, or self-neglect to the point of harm or death. Ask questions about suicide in a matter-of-fact manner, without hesitation, and record the findings carefully in your assessment notes.

Orientation Assess awareness of time, place and person in an environment where the person has easy access to the information. Days in hospital are all the same, and there are often no calendars and seasonal cues. Acute disorientation in all spheres is commonly found in people having toxic states and traumatic brain disease. Disorientation to place and person usually indicates a degenerative disorder.

Memory People with dementias have difficulty acquiring recent memory or learning; this symptom may be a key to the early detection of dementia. At present, there is no set of tests that can adequately measure the memory capacity of people with dementia. Most tests measure *episodic memory:* the processing and storage of information, like recalling the events of the day. This type of memory is impaired in most people who have a cognitive disorder, depression, and drug or alcohol intoxication. *Semantic memory,* or knowledge memory, is the ability to synthesise and think about events. It is used in language, abstraction and logical operations. People with DAT have difficulty with semantic memory; however, the person who is depressed does not.

Test episodic memory by asking the person to repeat a series of words or recall a recent event, such as a meal. Test semantic memory by asking the person to develop a scenario, such as describing the events from dinner until bedtime. Episodic memory is also tested in relation to time, and is usually divided into three spheres: recent, remote and past.

Abstract reasoning Proverbs are the most common way of testing abstract reasoning. You might ask, 'What does it mean when we say, "People who live in glass houses shouldn't throw stones"?' or 'What does "A stitch in time saves nine" mean to you?' People with DAT often interpret these proverbs quite literally or concretely; for example, they may reply to your question about the latter proverb with a statement such as 'If you sew a single stitch, you won't have to sew nine.' Be careful, though, as proverbs are culturally- and age-sensitive.

Concentration and focus The most common test of concentration and focus is the serial sevens test: The person subtracts 7 from 100 and then continues to subtract 7 from the answer. This is a difficult process for the person with dementia or delirium. The test measures the person's ability to concentrate and focus thought. However, be aware that it may also be an indication of their educational level.

Judgment The test for judgment can predict whether a person will behave in a socially accepted manner, including the planning and carrying out of activities that require them to discriminate reality from unrealistic situations. You might ask, 'If you needed help during the night, how would you get it?' or 'If you lost your wallet while doing errands, what would you do?'

Nursing care

A discussion of several issues common to those with cognitive disorders follows.

Impaired physical mobility

Gait changes due to neurological involvement are seen in people with a number of the dementias. These include DAT, Huntington's disease, Parkinson's disease and Creutzfeldt–Jakob disease. Restlessness in the person with delirium is reflected in hyperactive behaviour. The person usually alternates between hyperactivity and hypoactivity.

Self-care deficit: bathing/hygiene, dressing/grooming, feeding, toileting

People with delirium are unable to perceive, organise or carry out the activities of daily living (e.g. bathing/hygiene, dressing/grooming, feeding, toileting). They are far too distracted by stimuli and are unable to focus. The person who has a DAT has a distinct problem: apraxia, the loss of ability to perform formerly known skills. In the late stages of all the dementias, total care is a necessity as the person deteriorates.

Readiness for enhanced sleep

Also called *sundowner syndrome,* **sundowning** is commonly understood as confused behaviour when environmental stimulation is low. It can be seen in people with delirium and dementia. The person catnaps during the day and wanders at night. Poor sensory processing can also occur in the person who wanders at night. The person with DAT may not sleep for several days, moving about in a confused state. They become increasingly agitated, disoriented, or even aggressive/paranoid or impulsive and emotional later in the day and at night.

Altered thought processes

Altered thought processes can occur as a variety of experiences. People behave differently depending on their ability to think as a result of these alterations.

Agnosia Agnosia is the failure to recognise familiar objects, and is a progressive problem that eventually renders the person unable to recognise or remember loved ones. Overall, in both delirium and dementia, the person's ability to use information in making judgments may be seriously impaired.

Memory Episodic short-term memory is affected by delirium, dementia and mood disorders. Long-term memory is diminished in the later stages of DAT and acute delirium. See Figure 12.4 ■ for a diagram of how short-term and long-term memory is established.

Orientation Disorientation is seen in people with both dementia and delirium. In the former, it is related to progressive cerebral changes; in the latter, to an acute, usually identifiable, causal agent.

Impaired verbal communication

Confabulation is a common defence used by the person who cannot remember required information and therefore uses fantasy to fill in the memory gaps. Confusion and paranoid ideation require that you interact with the person in a non-threatening manner. Communication: Person with Dementia on the next page describes interactions with this in mind.

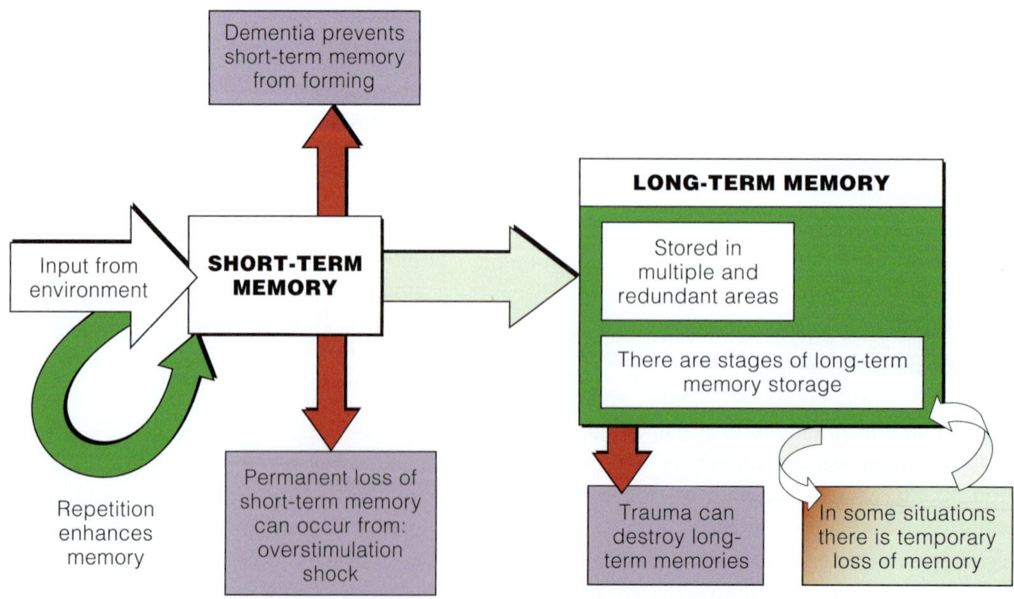

FIGURE 12.4 ■ The path to short-term memory, whether short-term memory is created, and the conversion of short-term to long-term memory.

COMMUNICATION

Person with dementia

Jenni: 'What are you doing here?'

NURSE RESPONSE 1	NURSE RESPONSE 2
NURSE RESPONSE 1: 'Hello, Jenni. My name is Betty, and I would like to talk to you.' *RATIONALE:* This response helps you make contact with Jenni, establish what you are going to do to allay fears, and give an opportunity to interact in a non-threatening manner.	**NURSE RESPONSE 2:** 'I'd like to talk with you, Jenni. Can you tell me if anything is hurting you?' *RATIONALE:* Many people find it easier to talk about physical pain than to articulate complex notions such as feelings and desires.

Aphasia, both receptive and expressive, is one of the hallmarks of DAT. In the late stage of the illness, the person is completely mute. When this occurs, your observations are vital to assess discomfort and pain. Scales that provide descriptors that correspond to how people actually display facial expressions of pain are effective at differentiating intensities of pain (Sheu, Versloot, Nader, Kerr & Craig, 2011).

Risk of self-harm and harm to others

For people with DAT and most of the other dementias, there is a gradual decline in the social acceptability of their behaviour. Overstating distress and making threats are common, especially if this was the previous mode of coping. See Communication: Person with Dementia at Risk for Self-harm for an example of an interaction with a person who is making threats. A high risk for violence is linked with impulsivity and unpredictability. The person may also strike out at others while hallucinating or in a hyperactive phase. These types of behaviours are also seen in people who have a delirium, or who are similarly unpredictable.

The change in role

As a result of decreasing intellectual competence, the person with dementia moves from the role of spouse, parent, employee and community member to that of a dependent person. The role loss and role change are anxiety-provoking, and at times overwhelming for the person, their family and others. Characteristically, the family members experience a period of acute grief after receiving the diagnosis. Assess their level of depression. Feelings of isolation and being overwhelmed are also common. Make sure you provide as much information as they need.

Altered sensory perception

The inability to attend and focus concentration is a hallmark of delirium. Decreased attention is also seen in the later stages of the dementias when the person loses the ability to encode. Delirium alters perception by reducing the person's ability to distinguish and integrate sensory information. As a result, difficulty discriminating reality from hallucinations, dreams, illusions and imagery occurs. In the later stages of dementia, hallucinations and delusions can be experienced, which complicate delivery of care. The person is prone to hallucinations and delusions as a result of a reduced ability to distinguish and integrate sensory information. Communication: Person with Dementia and Hallucinations on the following page shows an interaction with a person who experiences hallucinations.

Self-esteem

During the first stage of DAT and other dementias, the person is acutely aware of cognitive failure. This awareness and the resulting anxiety can be damaging to the self-esteem of a person living in a culture that does not tolerate or provide for dependence. Unfortunately, in many countries there is still stigma surrounding dementia.

Urinary incontinence, bowel incontinence

Incontinence of urine or faeces is usually the result of confusion and difficulty finding or using the bathroom facilities. In the later stages of dementia, the person loses cortical control, but physiological function remains. It is essential to ensure proper hygiene, as poor hygiene will result in infections and skin breakdown.

Nutrition

Poor nutrition and some metabolic disorders can be the direct cause of confusion in the older person. The reverse can also be true; confusion and cerebral change can cause nutritional deficits. Without supervision, many older people are not

COMMUNICATION

Person with dementia at risk for self-harm

Harry: 'I'm going to walk outside and get hit by a truck.'

NURSE RESPONSE 1	NURSE RESPONSE 2
NURSE RESPONSE 1: 'Tell me about why you are so upset.' *RATIONALE:* Harry ventilates feelings in more constructive ways when discussing feeling states with the nurse.	**NURSE RESPONSE 2:** 'Let's take a walk together.' *RATIONALE:* Harry has the opportunity to use physical energy constructively by being distracted with empathic and supportive social interaction.

COMMUNICATION

Person with dementia and hallucinations

Tommy: 'Get those women out of here!'

NURSE RESPONSE 1	NURSE RESPONSE 2
NURSE RESPONSE 1: 'Come with me. We'll go down the hall.' *RATIONALE:* Distracting Tommy from the internal stimuli, which may be transient, calms and addresses the emotional component of his experience.	**NURSE RESPONSE 2:** 'You must be very nervous. Let's get you something to help you feel better.' *RATIONALE:* Tommy may need interventions (nonpharmacological or pharmacological) to control breakthrough symptomatology.

capable of preparing or ingesting adequate amounts of food. During the later stages of DAT, the person may have symptoms of bulimia followed by a total loss of appetite.

Outcome identification

People with these disorders have varying outcomes; delirium in many cases is reversible, while dementia is not. Specific outcomes are often not listed in the nursing care plans. The potential for a return to previous lifestyles remains somewhat intact when disorders are reversible. However, in the deterioration of dementing conditions, carefully scrutinise the expectations for outcomes. Family members and the person need information about the illness and how it will change lifestyle. Maximising quality of life is a worthwhile goal.

Planning and implementation

Nursing interventions for people with cognitive disorders can be divided into two broad groups: interventions for (1) people with dementia and (2) people with delirium. A sample nursing care plan for a person with delirium is presented at the end of this chapter.

With few exceptions, the interventions are similar, although the overall goals are different. The goal is to minimise the loss of self-care capacity. Although functional loss is progressive, at every stage of the illness you must assess and support the person's self-care capacity. Family members must also learn how to work with the person. See Collaborative Care: Family Strategies for suggestions for families. With people who have a delirium, the overall goal for nursing intervention is to support their existing sensory perception until cognitive function can return to previous levels of functioning. Of course, in both conditions, keeping the person safe is the first priority.

Preventing injury

Impaired coordination in dementia means falls become a safety concern. Living areas must be well-lit, and furniture must remain in the same place. Remove any loose rugs, and ensure the person wears properly fitting shoes with a strap that hold the shoe in place and appropriate clothing (e.g. trousers with minimal flares). Assess visual and balance disturbances. Install hand-rails near toilets, showers and tubs. Teach the person and carers how to use walkers and wheelchairs safely. Evaluate the use of medication that could cause postural hypotension. A difference in blood pressures (BP) taken supine and standing, wherein the standing BP is lower than the supine BP, is an indication of postural hypotension. Restlessness and wandering can be dealt with by ensuring a safe environment. Avoid crowds or large open spaces without boundaries.

Hyperactivity in people with delirium can be decreased by controlling environmental stimuli. If this does not help, medications can be used judiciously. Take vital signs one hour before and after the administration of any medication, and observe carefully for signs of stupor. Interrupt prolonged periods of hypoactivity with range-of-motion exercises and frequent turning, and having the person stand up at the bedside, as tolerated. During periods of fluctuating motor behaviour, there is always concern for safety. A staff member should be

COLLABORATIVE CARE

Family strategies

Suggestions for families who have just had a family member diagnosed with DAT

- Have family meetings and discuss strategies to care for the person at the present time and in the future, based on family responsibilities and resources.
- Contact Alzheimer's Australia and request information. Watch videos and read the available material. See https://fightdementia.org.au/
- Attend a support group.
- Make decisions about power of attorney, and the control and distribution of assets.
- Consider developing an advance health directive (AHD). These can be accessed at http://www.publicguardian.qld.gov.au/adult-guardian/health-care-decisions/advance-health-directive (discussed in Chapter 11).
- Become familiar with community resources, such as day-care treatment centers, residential care facilities and respite care for the caregivers.
- Consider purchasing a Medical Alert ID bracelet for the person.

YOUR INTERVENTION STRATEGIES

Strategies for working with the person who wanders

Strategy	Rationale
▪ Stay with the person, or be sure they are in a safe, enclosed area.	▪ People who wander can get hurt. Safety is the first priority.
▪ Maintain a calm demeanour.	▪ People with cognitive disorders pick up on the feelings of others.
▪ Approach the person slowly and give them space. Use touch if they respond positively to it.	▪ The aim is to prevent aggressiveness, fear and anxiety. Each person is different in response to touch, and with specific people.
▪ Determine why the person is wandering. Are they upset? Thirsty? Hungry? Searching for family?	▪ When we understand why the person wanders, we can plan person-centred interventions.
▪ Meet the person's needs. If they are searching, be supportive: 'You are looking for X . . .' 'You must miss X . . .'	▪ Support decreases anxiety, fear and hostility.
▪ Attempt to engage the person in a repetitive activity, such as rolling wool or folding towels.	▪ Repetitive activities use energy and can be diversional.

present at all times; keep the bed lowered and the side-rails up. In DAT, wandering is common, and can be challenging. See Your Intervention Strategies for guidelines for working with the person who wanders.

Maintaining self-care

Allow the person to do as much as possible unassisted. The more the person can effectively control their daily routine, the less anxious they will feel. Remind the person about daily grooming and personal hygiene, and repeat instructions. If the person resists tooth brushing, use other methods for oral hygiene. If the person also resists this, having them eat an apple may help to clean the mouth. If routine procedures are resisted, wait a few minutes and try again. The person often forgets to offer new resistance. The person who is acutely delirious or in the last stages of dementia needs total care.

Sleep

People with dementia and delirium respond poorly to hypnotic medications, which increase confusion and aggravate the disorientation that may be experienced in lowered light. A small warm non-caffeinated drink may produce enough relaxation without side-effects. The most helpful measure may be to allow the person to wander in a safe area until they are tired. If they are disoriented at night, make sure the room is light and without shadows. Possibly leave a radio on to provide more stimulation. Low doses of an anti-anxiety agent may be prescribed. (Use anti-anxiety medications with caution, and re-evaluate them regularly if used on a nightly basis.)

Supporting optimal memory

Gently orient the person. To allay anxiety, do not argue with them about verbal discrepancies. Rather, direct the person towards areas of interest that are familiar and pleasurable. The environment should support whatever memory functions are still intact. If confabulation is used to fill in the memory gap, do not argue; remember that it is an ego-protective mechanism.

Because of their episodic memory loss, the person with DAT does not respond well to reality-orientation. Semantic memory can be triggered by initiating a procedure the person can then complete. In this leading technique, a combination of words and non-verbal cues are used. For instance, while handing the person a toothbrush and pointing towards the mouth with a brushing motion, say, 'Brush your teeth.' Constant repetition in a kind, firm manner is often necessary. Music therapy may also trigger past associations, aid the person's long-term memory, and help someone who is aphasic with social interaction.

Promoting optimal medication management

Medication therapy has been proposed for people in the early stages of DAT to maintain memory and orientation (see Chapter 7). Acetylcholinesterase inhibitors are available to treat DAT, but clinical trials and treatment outcomes for these medications have revealed both positive and negative results. The problems in demonstrating overall efficacy are because everyone is different, and because these medications provide only mild to moderate improvement.

Medication management for people with this group of disorders has a variety of purposes and options.

Orientation

Structure the person's environment to support cognitive functions. Aids (hearing, vision) are often necessary to prevent sensory loss or distortion. Familiar objects from home may also help orient the person. Easily-read clocks, orientation boards, and a consistent daily routine that includes physical activity and socialisation without sensory overload will also help. Verbally orient the person during conversation, but do not quiz the person about discrepancies.

Verbal expression

As communication skills decrease, the person's non-verbal communication becomes more important. People respond physically to the environment, especially if they feel threatened. Use the person's name, approach in clear view, and give simple directions.

Conduct/impulse control

The person may strike out in response to hallucinations or delusions. All measures used to support perception and

YOUR INTERVENTION STRATEGIES Strategies for supporting memory function

Behavioural and psychotherapeutic reminders

- Use large-print calendars or other concrete reminders of what is going on.
- Use objects or wall hangings that mirror the current season or holiday events; pictures that reflect seasonal events and people's actions and behaviours around those events (remember to be culturally sensitive).
- Display family photos in the person's room.
- Discover a person's preferred hobbies and interests to add cues to the environment (e.g. a team photo for a sports fan).

Reminiscence

- People need to talk, even repetitively, about important prior experiences, which encourages the process of resolving feelings about these experiences as well as difficulties in recalling them.
- Encourage discussion of likely social and historical contexts operative during earlier phases of the person's life (e.g. World War II, the moon landing, the Queen's coronation).

Adaptive functioning and cognitive preservation

Evaluate remaining cognitive strengths through:

- observation
- psychological testing
- diagnostic interviewing.

When areas of strength are noted:

- provide opportunities for the person to exercise them
- give positive reinforcements such as praise, a pleasant experience such as listening to music, or a special caring interaction.

When areas of deficit are noted:

- assist the person in coping with deficits (e.g. training and encouragement to use written reminders to compensate for failing memory).
- provide positive reinforcement for using such strategies.

orientation are imperative here, because the person with a cognitive impairment functions best in an environment where stimulation is controlled and sensory overload prevented. All changes, whether environmental or personal, need to be made slowly wherever possible. Approach the person in full view, calling their name, and refrain from touching. Requests should be simple and non-demanding.

SELF-AWARENESS
Triggering semantic memory

The person with DAT experiences episodic memory loss; therefore, interactions may not be retained, and repetition is necessary. Answer the following questions about your skill level at triggering semantic memory.

1. Are your words and non-verbal cues:
   Precise? ☐ Yes ☐ No
   Concise? ☐ Yes ☐ No
   Clear? ☐ Yes ☐ No
2. Constant repetition in a kind, firm manner is necessary. When you have to repeat yourself a number of times, are the following interaction impacts present?

   Is your tone on the third repetition identical to your tone the first time you said this? ☐ Yes ☐ No

   Is your affect kind the fourth time you have repeated yourself? ☐ Yes ☐ No

   Do your movements remain the same even though you have to repeat them? ☐ Yes ☐ No

   Are you consistent? ☐ Yes ☐ No

   If you answered 'Yes', you are using good communication techniques with people who have cognitive impairment, and your interactions are more likely to be successful. If any of these areas has a 'No' response, you may need to improve the connection between your verbal and non-verbal cues, and evaluate your personal reaction (action, emotion, attitude) to the need to repeat basic instructions.

Role performance

To promote functioning in the family, the person must be viewed as an active member. Most people with dementia remain at home until the caregiver can no longer manage the person's needs. The family, especially the main caregiver, requires support throughout this time.

If the person is in residential aged care, the family can be an integral part of the person's daily routine. Family members need extra emotional support as the rewards for maintaining involvement diminish. For the person with dementia, role maintenance involves supporting the person's need to be oriented.

Attention span

Repeat requests as needed. Speak in simple phrases, loud enough to be heard, and reinforce the meaning with gestures. To decrease distractibility and hyperalertness, keep environmental stimulation at a minimum. Make every effort to lower anxiety by moving slowly, speaking clearly and providing new information slowly.

Self-concept/self-esteem

During the early stages of dementia, make every effort to maintain the person's self-esteem as they struggle with their awareness of cognitive loss. Encourage the expression of fears and concerns, and listen attentively. Allow for the verbal expression of anger and sadness.

Manipulate the environment to help the person with a failing memory. Helpful measures include labelling the bathroom and bedroom, posting notes to remind the person to turn off the oven and lock the door, and labelling the contents of drawers. Gently remind the person of forgotten events, and do not confront confabulations. Encourage the family to include the person as a productive member.

Perceptual functioning

A quiet environment with soft music prevents sensory overload. When speaking, stand or sit so that you are in direct view. Use touch with caution. First give a verbal warning before touching the person's shoulder or forearm, and slowly and clearly explain all procedures. Sometimes even a very soothing touch can overexcite the person, who may respond by striking out. Make sure that the person is wearing hearing aids and glasses if necessary.

In responding to hallucinations, simply state that you understand that these sensations can be very powerful and even disturbing. Do not argue or seek elaboration. Take care of the emotional response in your interactions (e.g. if the person is frightened, reassure). Give reassurance that these thoughts will go away. Say, 'We will help you.' Do not leave the person alone or in an isolated room without some stimulation to help them block out the hallucinations, and support reality testing. The room should be well-lit and without shadows or glare. If the person becomes combative, briefly intervene to redirect and prevent harm to themselves or others. Then attempt to distract, reassuring the person, 'You are in a safe place.'

Elimination

A regular toileting schedule helps the person with dementia control incontinence. The person is often unable to let anyone know when they have to use the toilet or have soiled themselves. Use clothing that is easy to remove.

During the early stage of dementia, a toileting routine is essential. It helps the confused person if you place a large sign on the bathroom door labelled 'Toilet'. As the disease progresses, a toilet may no longer be recognised. Resistance to sitting on the toilet may occur. Forcing the person will only produce agitation and combativeness. Distract and try again. If all efforts at maintaining a routine fail, use disposable pants. The use of catheters and external drains is not recommended because of the possibility of infection and their certain removal by a confused person.

Nutrition

Monitor the person's food and fluid intake. Give people who are hyperactive a diet high in protein and carbohydrates in finger-food form. Some people may need double portions. The person who chews constantly needs to be reminded to swallow. Depending on the person's level of perception and motor activity, supervision and assistance at mealtimes may be necessary. Weigh the person routinely, and increase caloric intake as needed. In the final stages of the disease, the person will lose all interest in food, and may receive nasogastric, gastrostomy or intravenous feedings.

Evaluation

Assess both the effectiveness of all interventions and the person's response to them.

Delirium evaluation criteria

The evaluation of nursing care for the person with delirium is based on the premise that the person is capable of returning to their previous level of functioning. During that process, the goal is to help the person maintain optimal levels of sensory perception, participate in activities of daily living and maintain physiological homeostasis.

Dementia evaluation criteria

Dementia entails progressive intellectual, behavioural and physiological deterioration. The goal of nursing care is not to cure, or to return the person to previous levels of functioning, but rather to sustain the person at the optimal level of self-care. Help the family sustain a personally rewarding relationship with their loved one throughout this terminal and difficult process.

CARE COORDINATION

Care coordination of the person with dementia involves developing and organising a program to address symptoms. It must be individual, flexible and responsive to changing needs. There is a great deal of contact with the caregiver(s). Provide regular monitoring and supervise the following:

- regular physical examinations with a primary care provider
- prescription medications
- nutrition
- over-the-counter medications
- finances
- interpersonal relationships.

One of the challenges in managing the care of a person with advanced stages of dementia include how to physically intervene in everyday activities. Nutrition concerns are relevant, especially in how to feed someone who has advanced DAT when other problems are likely and contribute to difficulties.

SELF-AWARENESS
An inventory for nurses who care for people with cognitive disorders

Caring for the person with cognitive disorders can be challenging. The self-awareness information you gather by thoughtfully considering your responses to the following questions will help you to become more successful in working with people who are cognitively impaired and their families.

- How do I feel about working with people who have cognitive disorders?
- What do I like about working with them?
- What frustrates me about working with them?
- What behavioural symptoms (e.g. wandering, agitation, hallucinations, delusions, hostility, eating problems, etc.) do I feel most competent to deal with? Least competent?
- What strategies have I used with people that have been successful? Unsuccessful?
- Who are my favourites? Why? My least favourite? Why?
- What can I do to become more knowledgeable and/or skilled in dealing with people with cognitive disorders?

COLLABORATIVE CARE

Nutrition and feeding

Suggestions for families on effective nutrition and feeding skills with someone with advanced dementia include:

- Recognise that eating problems are not unusual in people with late-stage dementia and, in fact, are quite common.
- Enhancing the quality of life through feeding can be accomplished with involved caregivers.
- Discuss with the treatment team some of the specific nutritional needs.
- Assist family members with oral feeding for as long as possible—this promotes comfort and provides basic contact.
- Take the person's food preferences into account, and remember that the person's tasting and smelling senses may be poor.
- Be aware of the typical problems in feeding at this stage. The person may get distracted, spit out or cheek food, and have swallowing difficulties or poor coordination. Resistance to being fed is often the person's assertion of their last area of control.
- Helpful environmental features include lighting sufficient to contrast and illuminate food and utensils, and avoid overcrowding.
- Maintain appropriate eye contact.

Sources: Chang, C. C., & Roberts, B. L. (2011). Strategies for feeding patients with dementia. *American Journal of Nursing, 111*(4), 36–44; and Lee, T. J., & Kolasa, K. M. (2011). Feeding the person with late-stage Alzheimer's disease. *Nutrition Today, 46*(2), 75–79.

COMMUNITY CARE

Community-based care for the person with dementia could involve appointments in a clinic setting, a day program designed for their current level of difficulties in functioning, medication clinic appointments, a supportive group, or some combination. Frequently, a family member or caregiver is involved, especially due to the need for transportation.

Counselling and face-to-face contacts are a way to decrease the social isolation inherent in a person with dementia. Psychotherapy can be useful to help people with mild to moderate dementia cope with the loss of cognitive functions. The features of counselling or therapy would include:

- empathic listening
- support
- working on coping methods
- providing the person with outlets for distress that might otherwise exacerbate disturbed behaviour (e.g. have them talking over fears rather than acting out behaviourally).

HOME CARE

The most effective treatment for the person with dementia is a balance between stimulation/environmental demand and whatever internal resources remain for the person. The home might need to be modified to meet changing needs. Some modifications are usually necessary so that safe wandering is possible, dangers are minimised through safety devices, and activity can be controlled. A cycle of stimulation and rest is best, so that the person's abilities are engaged but not overwhelmed.

Supportive counselling is frequently helpful when providing home care for people with dementia. You must understand the premorbid personality and developmental history of someone with dementia, because the process of dementia is superimposed on the pre-existing personality. Determine how anxiety affects the person's life and their previous self-view, and how conscious they were of themselves and the impact of their actions on others. Once the person's anxiety is reduced, the tendency towards better functioning will ensue.

The focus of treatment includes carers. Whether the caregivers are relatives, friends or health care providers, they may require explanations of symptoms and help in designing behavioural interventions. Caregivers working with people who have severe levels of dementia may require help in coping with stress, discouragement and a sense of hopelessness.

The concept of respite care is one where carers are able to either have someone come into the environment to care for the person and the carer can exit the situation temporarily, or the person is cared for in a facility with skilled and experienced respite services (Brighton et al., 2016). This allows carers the freedom of movement and action. In either case, the caregiver can have some personal time.

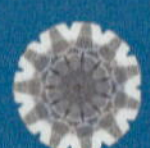

NURSING CARE PLAN: THE PERSON WITH A DELIRIUM

Identifying information

Mr Hennessey is a 50-year-old married man who entered the hospital to have colon surgery. He is a physically fit man in a physically demanding job, typically jogging several miles a week for exercise. This is his first serious physical problem. His wife of 25 years is extremely devoted, and stayed with him following his surgery. While still in the intensive care unit (ICU), Mr Hennessey became disoriented. Staff members were careful to check his electrolyte balances, which were within normal limits. Within two days he began hallucinating. He cried out that the hovering bats he saw in the corners of the room were trying to kill him. He has had other hallucinations and believes that his life is at great risk. When

(continued)

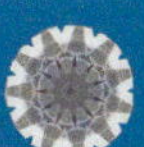

NURSING CARE PLAN: THE PERSON WITH A DELIRIUM (*continued*)

his wife offered him a newspaper, he whispered that she should give him the bucket of pills he had been hiding under his bed. He lashed out at his wife following this exchange, and ripped out his intravenous and nasogastric tube.

History

Mr Hennessey has no prior psychiatric history, nor are there any family members with mental illness. His wife and two grown children, who live nearby, are concerned about his wellbeing. All are attentive to Mr Hennessey, love him, and are willing to help with his care.

Mr Hennessey is a contractor and owns his own business. He and his wife have many friends and activities. He was diagnosed with a colon tumour a month ago and had a colon resection. The pathology report was positive for cancer. Mr Hennessey had been healthy all his life, until he noticed rectal bleeding a month ago. He has had regular physical check-ups and responded immediately when symptoms of a problem arose.

Current mental status

Mr Hennessey is disoriented the majority of time, and he is often aggressive. He has been having frightening visual hallucinations, especially at night. He is delusional that people are trying to hurt him.

Other clinical data

Mr Hennessey is on morphine for pain management.

There is a high risk for violence, related to the confusion and fear inherent in delirium.

Short-term goals	Interventions	Rationales
Mr Hennessey will have decreased symptoms of persecutory delusions.	■ Directly address the fear he is feeling (i.e. 'I understand how frightening this all is, and we will make sure you are safe').	Talking about the feelings is more reassuring, and shifts interactions from argumentation.
	■ Prevent overstimulation and understimulation.	ICUs can be overwhelming in certain sensory areas, while not providing enough cues to the outside world (such as windows).
Mr Hennessey displays considerably less agitation and fear.	■ Orient Mr Hennessey whenever he is confused. ■ Promote relaxation in both active and soothing modes. ■ Move slowly, speak clearly, and explain all procedures. ■ Make sure only one person is speaking to Mr Hennessy at a time. ■ Explain to the family about ICU psychosis and the temporary nature of it.	Decrease the stimuli that can exacerbate symptoms or confusion.

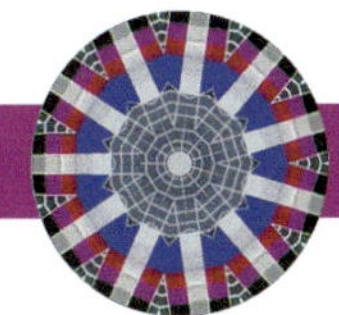

REFERENCES

Alzheimer, A. (1907). Über eine eigenartige Erkraukung der Hirwrinde. *Allegmeine Zeitschrift für Psychiatrie, 64,* 146–148.

Alzheimer's Australia. (2016). Key facts and statistics. Retrieved from https://fightdementia.org.au/national/statistics

American Psychological Association, Task Force to Update the Guidelines for the Evaluation of Dementia and Age-Related Cognitive Decline. (2011). *Guidelines for the evaluation of dementia and age-related cognitive decline.* Adopted by the APA Council of Representatives on 2011, February 18. Retrieved from *www.apa.org/pi/aging/resources/*dementia-guidelines.*pdf*

Andrew, C., Traynor, V., Carmody, J., & Erven, J. (2015). Evaluating the efficacy of the Driving and Dementia Decision Aid (DADD) as a resource for health professionals to support drivers living with a dementia facing decisions who may need to consider driving retirement. In *30th International Conference of Alzheimer's Disease International: Abstract booklet* (pp. 89–89). Perth, Australia: Alzheimer's Disease International.

Blazer, D., Hughes, D. C., & George, L. K. (1987). The epidemiology of depression in an elderly community population. *The Gerontologist, 27,* 281–287.

Brighton, R., Patterson, C., Taylor, E., Moxham, L., Perlman, SD., Sumskis, S., & Heffernan, T. (2016). The effects of respite services on carers of individuals with severe mental illness, *Journal of Psychosocial Nursing, 54*(12), 33–38.

Chang, C. C., & Roberts, B. L. (2011). Strategies for feeding patients with dementia. *American Journal of Nursing, 111*(4), 36–44.

Chung, P., & Khan, F. (2014). Traumatic brain injury (TBI) diagnosis and treatment: A systematic review and update. *Brain Injury, 28*(5–6), 744–745.

Djukic, M., Wedekind, D., Franz, A., Gremke, M., & Nau, R (2015). Frequency of dementia syndromes with a potentially treatable cause in geriatric in-patients: Analysis of a 1-year interval. *European Archives of Psychiatry and Clinical Neuroscience, 265*(5), 429–438.

Eubank, K. J., & Covinsky, K. E. (2014). Delirium severity in the hospitalized patient: time to pay attention. *Annals of Internal Medicine, 160*(8), 574–575.

Gallagher, M., & Long, C. O. (2011). Advanced dementia care: Demystifying behaviors, addressing pain, and maximizing comfort: Research and practice: Partners in care. *Journal of Hospice and Palliative Nursing, 13*(2), 70–78.

Galvin, J. E. (2015). Improving the clinical detection of Lewy body dementia with the Lewy body composite risk score. *Alzheimer's and Dementia: Diagnosis, Assessment and Disease Monitoring, 1*(3), 316–324.

Gannon, P., Khan, M. Z., & Kolson, D. L. (2011). Current understanding of HIV-associated neurocognitive disorders pathogenesis. *Current Opinion in Neurology, 24*(3), 275–283.

Krueger, J.M., Piantino, J., Smith, C. M., Angle, B., Venkatesan, C., & Wainwright, M. S. (2015). A treatable metabolic cause of encephalopathy: Cobalamin C deficiency in an 8-year-old male. *Pediatrics, 135*(1), 202–206.

McKeith, I. G., Galasko, D., Kosaka, K., Perry, E. K., Dickson, D. W., Hansen, L. A., . . . Perry, R. H. (1996). Consensus guidelines for the clinical and pathologic diagnosis of dementia with Lewy bodies (DLB): Report of the consortium on DLB international workshop. *Neurology, 47,* 1113–1124.

Mercello, M., & Starkstein, S. E. (Eds). (2014). *Movement disorders in dementias.* London: Springer.

Noriega, F. J., Vidán, M. T., Sánchez, E., Díaz, A., Serra-Rexach, J. A., Fernández-Avilés, F., & Bueno, H. (2015). Incidence and impact of delirium on clinical and functional outcomes in older patients hospitalized for acute cardiac diseases. *American Hearth Journal, 170*(5), 938–944.

Pan, W., & Kastin, A. J. (2015). Can sleep apnea cause Alzheimer's disease? *Neuroscience and Behavioral Reviews, 47,* 656–669.

Sheu, E., Versloot, J., Nader, R., Kerr, D., & Craig, K. D. (2011). Pain in the elderly: Validity of facial expression components of observational measures. *Clinical Journal of Pain, 27(7), 593–601.* doi: 10.1097/AJP.0b013e31820f52e1

Voyer, P., Richard, S., Doucet, L., & Carmichael, P.-H. (2011). Factors associated with delirium severity among older persons with dementia. *Journal of Neuroscience Nursing, 43*(2), 62–69.

Substance use disorders

RENEE BRIGHTON AND KYLIE SMITH

13

LEARNING OUTCOMES

After completing this chapter, you will be able to:

1. Assess your own feelings about the lived experience of substance use disorders.
2. Explain how the physical, psychological and withdrawal effects of the major categories of substances manifest.
3. Discuss the major theoretical explanations for substance use disorders.
4. Describe the populations at risk for substance use disorders.
5. Identify treatment approaches for the main groups of substances.
6. Implement person-centred strategies when caring for an individual experiencing a substance use disorder to help prevent relapse.
7. Discuss how the presence of both a substance use disorder and a major mental disorder (such as schizophrenia) impacts on the life of the person.
8. Assess your own feelings and attitudes about people with substance use disorders, and how these feelings may impact on your professional practice.
9. Formulate outcome criteria for people living with substance use disorders.
10. Compare and contrast the short-term and long-term nursing intervention strategies for people with substance use disorders.

KEY TERMS

LIVED EXPERIENCE

Living with addiction

Living with addiction is like living in a parallel universe. It entirely changes your perception of 'reality', the things that matter to other people don't matter to you; the things you're meant to care about seem trivial and mundane. It's not just that addiction is all-consuming, which it is, it's also the awareness that you are living closer to death than to life, and this separates you from people. It's safer not to be connected, because you can't trust anyone anyway, and you know you're not really normal, somehow. You forget how to be normal, all you think about is using and everything related to it, fear of hanging out, fear of not having money to score, fear of being caught. Fear is the thing I remember most, fear of what would happen, what I would feel, if I wasn't out of it. That fear over-rides everything else, even the fear of dying.

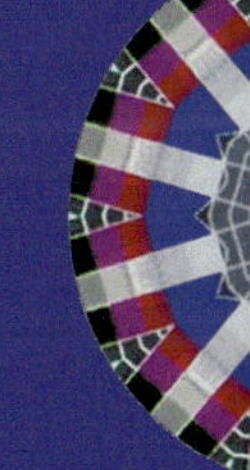

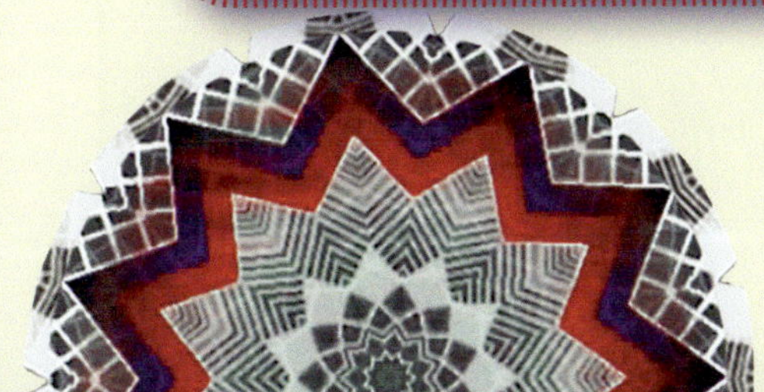

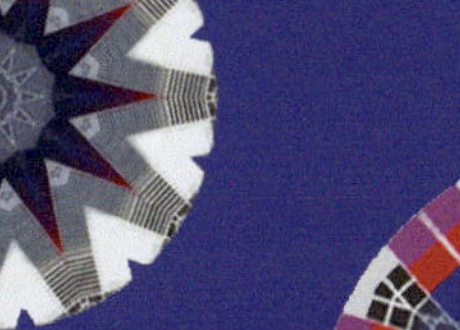

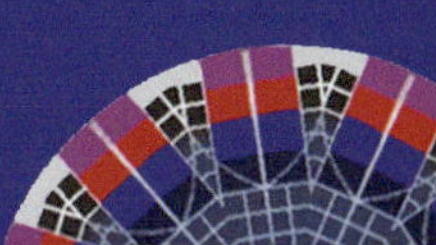

INTRODUCTION

Drug and alcohol use in our society has now reached alarming proportions. As health care professionals, nursing staff are often faced with the complexities of caring for individuals who live with substance use disorders. Drug and alcohol use affects individuals in all parts of society, regardless of the person's race, cultural background, education, religion, gender and age. It is important to recognise that substance use is common, and those who use substances may be affected because of ignorance and the prejudices of other people, including health care staff.

Substance use is a complex public health issue. The use of licit and illicit drugs is widely recognised in Australia as a key health challenge; one that has wide social and economic costs (Australian Institute of Health and Welfare [AIHW], 2011). The use of drugs and alcohol contributes to thousands of deaths, significant illness, disease and injury, social and family disruption, workplace concerns and community safety issues. The draft of the National Drug Strategy (NDS) 2016–2025, which is the seventh iteration of a national policy addressing the use of alcohol, tobacco and other drugs, starting in 1985 as the National Campaign Against Drug Abuse, is now available. It is frequently updated to ensure that it remains current and relevant to contemporary Australian society. The NDS provides a framework for a coordinated, integrated approach to drug and alcohol issues in the Australian community.

Harm minimisation is the key philosophy and basis for government policy in the management of drug- and alcohol-related issues in Australia. The concept is based on the acceptance that drug and alcohol use exists, is likely to continue, and is widespread across all levels of Australian and international communities. Harm minimisation is a way of reducing the impact of drug- and alcohol-related harm to individuals and the community through a range of public health strategies and practices. It encompasses three pillars: *demand reduction* (reduce drugs in the community, support people in their recovery, promote social inclusion), *supply reduction* (reduce supplies of illicit drugs, control and manage supply of legal drugs such as alcohol and tobacco) and *harm reduction* (reduce harms to communities, families and individuals). Nurses are particularly well-placed to identify risks of harm associated with substance use, and can apply a range of harm-minimisation strategies and interventions.

This chapter is a biopsychosocial exploration, applying the nursing process to individuals who live with substance use disorders. The importance of having a knowledge base on this topic, developing person-centred and non-judgmental attitudes, and developing skilled therapeutic interventions are discussed by the peak Australasian drug and alcohol nursing body DANA (Drug and Alcohol Nurses of Australasia). Links to DANA standards and competencies can be found on http://www.danaonline.org/

SUBSTANCE USE DISORDERS

A substance use disorder is described in the 5th edition of the *Diagnostic and statistical manual of mental disorders* (DSM-5) (American Psychiatric Association [APA], 2013) as being a cluster of cognitive, behavioural and physiological symptoms designating that the person continues to use the substance regardless of significant substance-related problems. An important characteristic of substance use disorders is underlying brain changes, often exhibited in behavioural effects, such as repeated relapses and intense substance cravings. All drugs (including alcohol) taken in excess directly activate the brain's reward system. The activation of this reward system is central to challenges arising from substance use—the rewarding feeling people experience as a result of substance use may be so overpowering that they neglect other typical activities in favour of taking the substance. The DSM-5 recognises that people are not equally vulnerable to developing substance use disorders. Certain people experience lower levels of self-control even prior to substance use, which may be reflective of impairment to the inhibitory mechanisms in the brain. This predisposes these individuals to developing problems when exposed to substance use.

Severity

Substance use disorders, as specified in the DSM-5, may range in severity from mild to severe, with severity based on

DIAGNOSTIC FEATURE

DSM-5 criteria (American Psychiatric Association [APA] 2013, pp. 483–484)

The diagnosis of a substance use disorder in the DSM-5 is based on a pathological pattern of behaviours related to the use of the substance. The classification of the different substances this can be applied to will be discussed in more detail later in this chapter, but includes alcohol, opioids, cannabis and tobacco. Substance use disorders in the DSM-5 span a wide variety of behaviours arising from the use of a substance or substances, and cover 11 different criteria.

The first grouping of criterion (Criteria 1–4) is specific to the impaired control over substance use. For example, Criterion 1 specifies the person may take the substance in larger amounts or over a longer period than was initially intended. The person may desire to cut down or discontinue substance use and report multiple attempts to do so (Criterion 2).

The social impairment associated with substance use is specified in the second grouping (Criteria 5–7). For example, the individual may experience recurrent substance use that has resulted in them forsaking major role obligations at work, school or home (Criterion 5). The person may continue substance use despite interpersonal problems caused or exacerbated by substance use (Criterion 6).

The third grouping (Criteria 8–9) relates to the risky use of the substance. This may take the form of recurrent substance use in situations where it is physically hazardous (Criterion 8). The person also may continue to use the substance despite knowing they will experience problems caused by use of the substance (Criterion 9).

The final grouping (Criteria 10–11) is specific to pharmacological criteria. This includes **tolerance** (Criterion 10), which is indicated by the person requiring an increased dose of the substance to achieve the desired effect. Tolerance also refers to the person experiencing reduced effects from the substance when the usual dose is taken. The degree to which tolerance develops varies across individuals and the substances taken, and may involve a variety of central nervous system effects. It is also important to mention that Criterion 11 relates to **withdrawal**. Substance withdrawal will be discussed in more detail later in this chapter.

the number of symptom criteria endorsed. As a guide, a mild substance use disorder is suggested when the person presents with two to three symptoms (criteria), moderate by four to five symptoms, and severe is when the person exhibits six or more symptoms.

ICD-10

While the term 'substance use disorders' is not used by the World Health Organization (WHO) in the *International classification of diseases*, 10th edition (ICD-10) (WHO, 2010), it is important to mention that the terms 'harmful' and 'dependence' are specified in this classification system. This is owing to the ICD-10 being commonly used to classify diagnoses in the Australian health sector.

Harmful use

The **harmful use** of a substance or substances is use that is causing damage to the health of the person. The damage may be physical, such as hepatitis from intravenous substance use, or mental, such as the experience of a mood disorder secondary to the persistent use of alcohol.

Dependence syndrome

A **dependence syndrome** is a cluster of physiological, behavioural and cognitive phenomena in which the use of a substance takes on a much higher priority than other behaviours that once had greater value for the individual. A key descriptive characteristic of the dependence syndrome is the desire (frequently strong, sometimes overpowering) to take the substance or substances. Dependence refers to both physical and psychological elements. Psychological dependence refers to the experience of impaired control over substance use, while physiological or physical dependence refers to tolerance and withdrawal symptoms.

SUBSTANCE INTOXICATION AND WITHDRAWAL

Criteria for **substance intoxication** are included in both the DMS-5 and ICD-10 classification systems. The essential feature in the DSM-5 is the development of a reversible substance-specific syndrome due to the recent use of a substance. The ICD-10 refers to 'acute intoxication', this being a transient condition following the administration of a substance. Both classification systems refer to intoxication in terms of the direct effects of the substance taken on the central nervous system, which result in changes in behaviour

DIAGNOSTIC FEATURE

Substance use disorders, intoxication, tolerance and withdrawal

Substance use disorder: A cluster of cognitive, behavioural and physiological symptoms indicating that the individual continues using the substance despite significant substance-related problems. An important characteristic is the underlying brain circuitry changes.

Intoxication: Reversible or transient condition following the administration of a substance. Attributable to the effects of the substance on the central nervous system that develop during or shortly after the substance is taken.

Tolerance: Indicated by the person requiring an increased dose of the substance to achieve the desired effect. Also relates to the person experiencing reduced effects from the substance when the usual dose is taken.

Withdrawal: A syndrome which develops when the individual's blood or tissue concentrations of a substance decline after prolonged or heavy use. To help relieve the symptoms, the individual is likely to reuse the substance. The features associated with substance withdrawal are directly related to the type of substance taken. Typically, these features are directly opposite to those of acute intoxication.

LIVED EXPERIENCE

Withdrawal

Withdrawal is a much more emotional experience than people realise. It wasn't just the physical symptoms that I feared, although they were bad enough: excruciating headache, cold sweat, bones aching, severe nausea. They were really compounded by a feeling I can only describe as terror—a terror that you feel physically, in your nerve endings. Partly it's the terror of facing reality, of the mess your life has become. If you can get wasted again, then that just doesn't matter, it's like that all disappears. But it's also a terror at what you are going to feel, and that you don't know how to cope with that feeling, that you don't know how to cope in the world at all, and that if you aren't stoned you can't even cope with going to the supermarket and having people look at you. In my case, it was also terror at having to face the things I was running from, the trauma I was trying to hide, and the way that had affected my sense of self. Those are very powerful motivators.

and psychophysiological functioning. Intoxication is highly dependent on the type and dose of the substance, and is influenced by the person's level of tolerance and other physiological and psychological factors. Generally, a substance is taken in order to achieve an anticipated degree of intoxication.

Substance withdrawal is a syndrome which develops when the individual's blood or tissue concentrations of the substance decline after prolonged or heavy use. The person will more than likely reuse the substance in an attempt to alleviate the withdrawal symptoms. Symptoms related to withdrawal vary greatly across the different classifications of substances. Typically, the symptoms seen in a withdrawal syndrome are directly opposite to those seen with intoxication. Withdrawal symptoms specific to the different classification of substances will be discussed in more detail later in the chapter.

THEORIES RELATED TO THE DEVELOPMENT OF SUBSTANCE USE DISORDERS

Many theorists have tried to account for why people use drugs and alcohol, especially when people continue this use despite negative consequences. Some theorists suggest genetic and other biological factors, while others accentuate the influence of personality or social-environmental aspects. While these factors have all been shown to contribute to the development of substance use disorders, no one set of factors can account for the development of all the different types of disorders. No one theory can answer the question of 'why do some people use drugs while others do not?' It is now thought that substance use likely results from complex interactions of biological, psychological and social-environmental processes.

Theories of substance use—disease model

The disease model was first associated with the excessive consumption of alcohol. Records of 'drink madness' can be traced back to ancient Greek and Egyptian times. Physician Benjamin Rush's work in 1784, entitled *Inquiry into the effects of ardent spirits on the human mind and body*, was thought to be the first to medically categorise the signs of acute and chronic 'drunkenness' (White, 2000). Rush introduced medicalised language into the discussion, describing 'persons addicted to ardent spirits', and declaring drunkenness as an 'odious disease'. Rush provided the first recommended treatments for chronic alcohol use.

In the late 18th and early 19th centuries, a cluster of ideas formed from concepts suggested by physicians such as Samuel Woodward, who recommended the creation of special asylums for inebriates, and William Sweetser, who stated that 'drunkenness' affected all major bodily structures. There was clear opinion that the only hope for the addicted person was complete and enduring abstinence from all substance use. This opinion was bolstered by the rapidly expanding knowledge on the physical effects of excessive alcohol consumption. Swedish physician Magnus Huss's landmark study on the physiological effects of alcohol first labelled the group of symptoms people experience, designated by the name *Alcoholismus chronicus*, later abbreviated to 'alcoholism' (White, 2000). These ideas became the building blocks of an emerging disease concept that included biological predisposition, drug toxicity, cravings, pharmacological tolerance, disease progression, inability to refrain from drinking, and loss of control in relation to the quantity of alcohol consumed.

Twelve-step programs

The need for abstinence formed from the disease model led the way to the development of 'twelve-step' programs, such as Alcoholics Anonymous (AA). However, moral theory (see below) is also attributed to the development of AA. AA had its beginnings in Akron, Ohio, in 1935, and was developed by Bill Wilson (a stockbroker) and Dr Robert Smith (a surgeon), both 'alcoholics' (Gross, 2010). The two men learned that by supporting one another, and with spirituality and character development, abstinence and a productive life were achievable. In 1939 the basic textbook, *Alcoholics Anonymous*, was published. This explained the philosophy, methods and core of AA, which is the 12 steps. Steps 1 through to 12 of the program are designed to bring about total acceptance of the 'illness', then offer a permanent solution to 'alcoholism' and addiction (see Box 13.3, which sets out the 12 steps).

Interventions attributable to the disease model

Classic research by Jellinek (1946) during the 1940s to 1960s, described as the 'disease model of alcoholism', revealed that individuals with chronic alcohol use proceed through phases: pre-alcoholic symptomatic phase, prodromal phase, crucial phase and chronic phase. Jellinek recognised 'loss of control' in addictive people, and hypothesised that it may have a biochemical basis. Although the disease model as a purely medical concept fell out of favour in the late 19th century, the language of this model still exists in terms such as 'biological vulnerability', 'tissue tolerance' and 'morbid appetite (cravings)' (White, 2000). Building on this early work, current research examines biochemical differences in people with substance use disorders, such as lower levels of dopamine (DA) neurotransmission, and the increased density of dopaminergic D_2 receptors in the brain.

Based on the development of understanding of neurochemistry, the **pharmacological management** of substance use disorders includes the use of standard and new pharmacological therapies:

1. Acamprosate (Campral) is indicated for the maintenance of alcohol abstinence in people experiencing alcohol dependence but who are abstinent at treatment initiation. This compound alleviates the physiological and psychological distress during the post-acute withdrawal period, making it easier not to drink. Its mechanism of action is not completely understood; the main interaction is believed to be with the glutamate system.
2. Buprenorphine (Subutex) was developed for the treatment of opioid addiction. It is a partial

opioid agonist, and works by reducing withdrawal symptoms and cravings for opioids. Buprenorphine binds tightly to, and dissociates slowly from, endorphin receptors, giving it a slow onset and a long duration of action.

3. Naltrexone (Revia) was developed for the treatment of heroin addiction. It is an opioid receptor antagonist and blocks the normal reaction of the part of the brain that produces the feeling of pleasure when opioids are taken. While the mechanisms behind why it works are not fully understood, naltrexone is also prescribed for blocking the cravings for alcohol and the pleasure derived from drinking it.
4. Disulfiram (Antabuse) inhibits acetaldehyde metabolism. With disulfiram, acetaldehyde, which is highly toxic, accumulates in the bloodstream when alcohol is consumed. This combination of disulfiram and alcohol produces nausea, vomiting, dizziness and other uncomfortable and potentially dangerous symptoms. It is used to discourage alcohol use; however, the severity of the associated adverse effects, the cost of treatment and the extensive planning required for disulfiram therapy has resulted in it rarely being used in Australia.

There is also much research regarding an individual's susceptibility to inheriting vulnerability to addiction. Genetics has been established to contribute significantly to the development of substance use disorders. In recent years, significant progress has been made in identifying susceptibility genes for addictions. Regions on human chromosomes 4, 5, 9–11 and 17 are more likely to harbour susceptibility genes for multiple substances (Li & Burmeister, 2009). Twin studies have been used to demonstrate the genetic influence of substance use disorders. To use alcohol as an example, numerous twin studies for alcohol-related behaviours have shown that heredity for alcohol use disorders ranges from 50 per cent to 70 per cent (Agrawal & Lynskey, 2008).

Changing attitudes to substance use—moral theories

Developed from moral theories were some of the first models used to explain alcohol addiction. During the 17th century, alcohol was generally held in high esteem by society, although becoming inebriated on a regular basis was considered immoral. At this time, people were considered to be separate from Nature in terms of free will. An understanding of personal choice is commonly based in a conception of rationality and the analysis of human behaviour developed by the early classical theorists Cesare Beccaria and Jeremy Bentham (Clark, 2011). Consequently people (freely) choose all behaviour based on their rational intentions. Humans could use free will, and people who drank to excess were seen as 'evil'.

People with alcohol or drug dependence were thus regarded as sinners or criminals. Punishments included whippings and public beatings. 'Public morality' refers to attempts made by the more conservative Christian denominations to enforce moral values through both societal conducts and legislation (Clark, 2011.) Proponents of moral theory saw the individual with substance use as unable or unwilling to 'do the right thing'.

The moral theories began to lose their influence when physicians were seen as having more expertise than theologians regarding human behaviour. Initially, the disease model was integrated with the moral model. In early disease models, substance use was seen as only a problem for those with weak morals. However, the fact that addiction also affected people with strong morals could not be ignored. As such, the disease model of addiction became the more prominent model in the late 18th and early 19th centuries.

Nowadays, health care professionals, families and carers who adhere to moral theory believe that the person experiencing a substance use disorder does not have the moral strength to resist the temptation of the substance of their choice. The moral model is prominent in traditional approaches to recovery. 'She just needs to strengthen her willpower to resist temptation and get on with her life', for example.

The criminal justice system in Australia and in many other countries approaches substance use from a moral perspective. Punishments for substance-related crimes, such as the use of 'illicit' drugs, are intended to motivate people to behave 'better'. However, the notion of drug use being 'illegal' did not emerge in Western societies until the late 19th century.

The consumption of alcohol was once seen in this country as a crime to be punished. The temperance movement in Australia in the 1800s portrayed alcohol as the source of society's degeneration. Temperance societies opposed excessive drinking and encouraged abstinence. They viewed people who drank or used drugs as being closely linked to crime, even when this was not the case. This movement influenced the development of alcohol and drug laws in this country that were thus based not on evidence but on stigma and hegemony.

There exists much debate over the **decriminalisation** of illicit drugs in Australia, with many people arguing that by criminalising the supply and use of drugs, governments around the world have driven drug production and consumption underground. Many feel that decriminalisation in this country would make drug use safer, and that the effects of drug control policy are at least as harmful as the effects of the drugs themselves (Room, 2010). Many are of the opinion that individuals with substance use disorders (health disorders) should not be imprisoned. Importantly, prohibitionist and 'drug war' approaches, historically, have been shown to have little impact on levels of substance use, and even less impact on the levels of harm associated with substance use (Lang, 2004).

Psychological theories

Psychological approaches to the explanation of substance use disorders are often based on concepts common to those of human behaviour. Emphasis is given to the fact that there is impaired control over the use, and the use is continued despite the problems that arise. There are a variety of psychological approaches

LIVED EXPERIENCE

Seeking help

In my experience, if you are a user, and even many years after you have stopped, other people's moralising can be the single biggest barrier to seeking help. It always frustrates me to have health professionals tell me how I just need to stop being so weak and to 'snap out of it'. First, I think this is often hypocritical. Who isn't guilty of some vice, who isn't addicted to something? Secondly, I always wonder why my using exactly is such a problem for society, especially when once upon a time these things weren't illegal. Why are they illegal now? And why are people with addictions seen as morally defective in some way? In my experience, no one enjoys or chooses addiction as a way of life. It is usually always about medicating some other problem, some untreated trauma. I always responded better to people who didn't 'judge' me, who were able to step outside of social norms and deal with me like a person who needs help.

to the explanation of drug and alcohol use, but two main themes emerge—one that emphasises the mechanism of reinforcement, and the other that stresses the influence of personality.

Reinforcement

The history of reinforcement theory in relation to substance use is attributable to the works of behaviourists Pavlov and Watson, and more recently Skinner. Skinner, a psychologist and radical behaviourist, developed his theories in the early to mid-1900s and advanced the theory of operant conditioning, the idea that behaviour is determined by its consequences, be they reinforcements or punishments. This makes it more or less likely that the behaviour will occur again (Gronnerod, Overskeid & Hartmann, 2013). His principles are still incorporated within treatments for substance use disorders. There are thought to be two distinct types of reinforcement: positive and negative.

Positive reinforcement occurs when the person receives pleasurable sensations, and these sensations motivate the individual to repeat the behaviour that caused the pleasure. 'The pleasure mechanism may . . . give rise to a strong fixation on repetitive behaviour' (Bejerot, 1980, p. 253). In relation to drug and alcohol use, this denotes that being intoxicated or 'high' is pleasurable, and what is pleasurable tends to be repeated.

Negative reinforcement occurs when the person behaves in a way to seek relief or avoid pain, thereby being rewarded and 'motivated' to repeat the behaviour that resulted in relief or an alleviation of their pain. In substance use disorders, this can be applied to withdrawal. More of the drug is taken to alleviate the discomfort or pain associated with withdrawal symptoms. According to this theory, the person with a substance use disorder who is withdrawing will experience an extremely strong desire for the substance (Baker, Piper, McCarthy, Majeskie & Fiore, 2004). People will continue taking the substance just to feel 'normal', and not just to achieve a 'high'.

Personality

A number of psychological theories of substance use propose that young people who have behavioural problems early, such as a difficult temperament, or behaviours that are oppositional, aggressive or impulsive, will be at high risk of developing substance use disorders (Midford, 2010). Certain personality characteristics have been shown to influence an individual's decision to use drugs and alcohol to excess, such as impulsivity, low self-esteem, willingness to engage in risk-taking behaviours and neuroticism. The need for sensation-seeking, or the need to seek intense sensations along with a willingness to take risks for the sake of having such experiences, has been found to be a key personality trait in people with substance use (Ersche, Turton, Pradhan, Bullmore & Robbins, 2010). The difficulty with personality theory lies with the debate that these types of personality traits may not actually be vulnerability factors for substance use, but rather that substance use disorders may over time alter a person's personality. Many studies examine the personality traits of those already addicted, thus it is difficult to determine premorbid personality influences.

Sociocultural theories

Sociocultural models of substance use emphasise social forces, role models and adaptive responses to stress in the sociocultural environment. Life's harsh realities come in many forms: the hopelessness and defeat of poverty, the academic and social pressures generated by upper-middle-class families, the adolescent's feeling of impotence and alienation, the peer group pressure to join in and share experiences, the social vacuum of unloving families in which meaningful attachments are dissolved or dissolving.

All of these social conditions and contexts help create and sustain substance use. Another sociocultural aspect is situational—people who develop substance use disorders tend to live in environments where access to drugs is easy and initiation into their use is widespread. People with substance use disorders describe in interviews how they learned to drink or use drugs at school, in social circumstances with their peers, or at home by watching their families. Many of these people experienced some form of violence or assault while growing up. Studies have shown that up to 90 per cent of people who use opioid drugs (namely heroin) have experienced childhood sexual assault. People therefore recognise drugs and alcohol as social lubricants, as an escape, or as a remedy for psychological and physical pain. See Developing Cultural Competence for specific information about culture and substance use.

Family systems theories

A family systems explanation for substance use has gained increasing acceptance among health care professionals. When assessing substance use and the psychological impacts, ask yourself, 'Could the substance dependence be serving a purpose in this family?' It may serve to do any or all of the following:

- shift the family's focus away from other more anxiety-provoking feelings or events
- give them a purpose or a challenge to distract them from other issues
- relieve one family member of a burden, or provide a needed burden to one or several members
- provide a cohesive cause in which all family members can involve themselves.

The family systems perspective includes the phenomenon of co-dependence. **Co-dependency** involves being preoccupied with controlling another person's behaviour. Co-dependency can be seen when a family member both rescues and blames (persecutes) the person with a substance use disorder

Although AA does not openly endorse the family systems theory, it does recognise that alcohol use disorders are family diseases. Al-Anon and Ala-Teen are groups for spouses, parents, friends, co-workers and teenage children of people experiencing alcohol use disorders. The focus is on helping people learn to live and work effectively with their loved ones and colleagues experiencing such disorders.

The underlying process, as the Lived Experience example on the next page illustrates, is that other people assume an enabling role, and this perpetuates the drinking patterns of the person with an alcohol use disorder.

A cycle begins when people who enable cover for the person dependent on a substance—such as by saying that they have a cold, are bruised because of stumbling in the dark, are asleep because of fatigue. Protected by the enabling behaviour, the person with the problem sees that there are no consequences for their bad or antisocial behaviour, and so has no motivation to stop drinking or using drugs. The person who is **enabling**—believing that the person with substance use is coping with family, marital or work problems 'the best way they can'—denies the disorder of addiction. The person with the substance use disorder blames the person who is enabling; the person who is enabling feels guilty and then attempts to control family life and the behaviours of the person by throwing out the alcohol or by taking the car keys. Enabling behaviour was employed to protect, rescue, control and blame, but none of

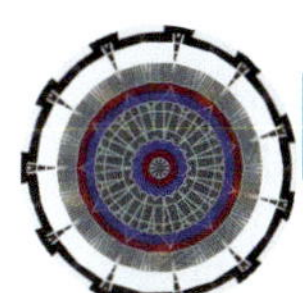

DEVELOPING CULTURAL COMPETENCE

Substance use in specific cultures

Studies clearly show that substance use is present in all cultures; however, which substance people use is often culturally determined. In Western culture, alcohol is the drug of choice. In Muslim countries, marijuana is used because Islam prohibits alcohol use. Opium is used in China and other Eastern countries, while people in India, Africa and South America use native herbs and chemicals. Native Americans use peyote (a cactus button with hallucinogenic properties) and alcohol more than other drugs. South Americans use ayajhuasca (a hallucinogenic herb) in cleansing spiritual hallucinogenic rituals.

Aboriginal and Torres Strait Islander people

The rates of drug and alcohol use by Aboriginal and Torres Strait Islander people are often inaccurately portrayed in the media. For example, compared to non-Indigenous people, a higher proportion of Indigenous people actually *abstain* from alcohol use. Nevertheless, the use of alcohol, tobacco and illicit substances is both the cause and effect of much suffering among Aboriginal and Torres Strait Islander people. It causes serious harm to the physical and psychological health of Indigenous people, but also to the social health of individuals and communities (AIHW, 2009).

The pattern of drug use by Aboriginal and Torres Strait Islander peoples has been shaped by history—dispossessed and alienated from their lands, Australia's first people were controlled by tobacco rations and prohibited from drinking alcohol. This has contributed to the social conditions that they live under today, and has led to excessive use of drugs, which in turn has resulted in poorer living conditions.

Substance use also plays a significant role in the gap between Indigenous and non-Indigenous Australians in terms of life expectancy and health. The rates of smoking—the leading cause of preventable mortality in Australia—among Aboriginal and Torres Strait Islander people remain high, with nearly half of these populations being smokers. Indigenous people living in remote and very remote areas were more likely to smoke and drink at higher levels, but are less likely to use illicit drugs compared with those living in major cities and inner regional areas.

Actions to help with substance use by Aboriginal and Torres Strait Islander communities need to take account of remoteness, traditional practices, access to services, and drugs and safety. They need to be comprehensive, covering physical, spiritual, cultural, emotional and social wellbeing; and be conducted at a local level as well as on a national scale. They need to be culturally valid, involve Aboriginal and Torres Strait Islander people, and be controlled by the community rather than by people from outside (AIHW, 2009). Actions need to take account of mainstream services where alternatives are not available.

For more information on programs aimed to reduce rates of substance use by Aboriginal and Torrres Strait Islander people, please see the Australian Indigenous Health *InfoNet* at http://www.healthinfonet.ecu.edu.au/, and the National Indigenous Drug and Alcohol Committee (NIDC) on http://www.nidac.org.au/

CRITICAL THINKING QUESTIONS

1. Why is it important to know the specific substances someone may use, depending on their culture?
2. What challenges could you anticipate when someone uses these substances for spiritual/cultural reasons?

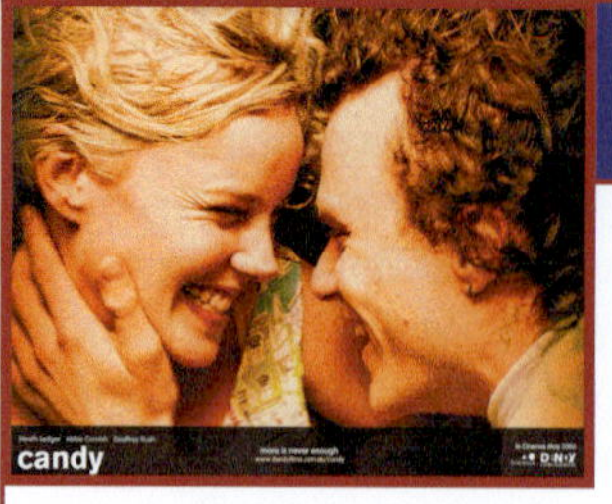

MENTAL HEALTH IN THE MEDIA

Candy

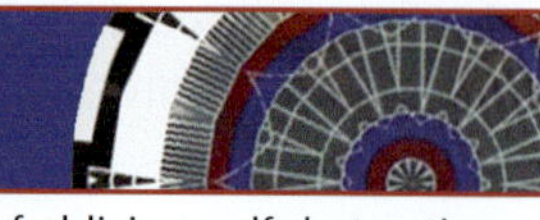

The Australian movie *Candy* depicts the powerful and destructive love between an aspiring poet Dan (Heath Ledger) and the beautiful artist Candy (Abbie Cornish), who is on the brink of success as a painter. When they first meet, Dan uses intravenous heroin regularly, while Candy very occasionally smokes heroin. The enabling behaviours used by Dan result in Candy slowly gravitating to Dan's bohemian lifestyle and his love of injecting heroin. The result is that their relationship alternates between states of oblivion, self-destruction and despair. They steal to get enough money for drugs, Candy prostitutes herself and they hit rock bottom. Candy can't deal with the things that happen to her, and she ends up admitted to a mental health unit. Dan's final visit to the hospital marks his own realisation that he has been dragging Candy down, and he makes the ultimate sacrifice in his love for her to end their marriage in the chance she may have a better life without him, free from addiction. The film is a honest portrayal of addiction and does not hide the devastating effects of heroin use.

LIVED EXPERIENCE

Enabling

Some of the worst enablers I saw among my peers were family members. I wasn't the only addict in my family; my cousin was using as well. My mother completely disowned me (which had its own problems), but I watched my aunt rescue my cousin time after time, and he would say all the right things, and then completely abuse her trust every time. I even told her that he wouldn't stop so long as she kept rescuing him, but how do you explain that to a mother? Her whole life revolved around my cousin's dramas, and her own guilt kept her locked into this cycle of trying to save him—it was more about protecting her own feelings than doing what was right for him.

these behaviours is effective in altering the course of the disorder. Those who enable feel worthless and helpless because they are unsuccessful in helping the person with substance use.

Enabling can also allow someone to stay in a relationship with a person experiencing a substance use disorder (see Mental Health in the Media). This occurs when someone outside the relationship, such as the best friend of the family member, provides a way to continue to ignore or deny the problem. See Box 13.1, How Significant Others Enable, for an example of a relationship involving enabling.

Box 13.1 How significant others enable

Enabling can allow the person with substance use to continue using without immediate consequences; however, enabling can also allow a relationship with the person to continue when this may not be in the best interests of either party. Best friends being supportive in their relationship can have enabling occur when a third party experiences a substance use disorder.

Nell's friend Tish married a gentleman with an alcohol use disorder. Following the honeymoon, Tish called Nell every day to describe how stressed she felt, to talk about her feelings and to receive support. Nell's allowing Tish to vent daily gave Tish the energy to stay in her marriage. Because this took the lid off her stress, Tish did not have to acknowledge the negative aspects of her marriage. Eventually, Nell realised she was enabling Tish, and was actually helping her to avoid recognising that she needed help to deal with her husband's disorder.

Nell explained this process to Tish, along with her decision to refuse to talk with Tish about her husband and his addiction. This decision needed to be reinforced every time Tish brought up the topic. Eventually Tish got 'fed up' with her predicament, sought therapy, and made changes so she could take better care of herself and her husband.

ALCOHOL (ETHANOL, ETOH)

Alcohol is a common, accessible substance that has just as much if not more destructive power as any other substance. According to the World Health Organization, alcohol is one of the most widely used substances in the world, and causes as much, if not more, death and disability as measles, malaria, tobacco or illegal drugs. Alcohol consumption also raises the overall risk of cancer, including cancer of the mouth, throat and oesophagus, breast cancer and bowel cancer. In Australia, one in five people drink at levels that put them at risk of harm, and approximately 3.7 million Australians drink alcohol in risky quantities (AIHW, 2011). Alcohol can be a dangerous, liquid recreational drug that happens to be legal.

The effects of alcohol

Alcohol is a sedative anaesthetic and a central nervous system (CNS) depressant. It depresses physiological (gag, heart rate, breathing rate) and psychological functions. If taken in high doses, alcohol can depress respiration and cause death. Blood alcohol concentration (BAC) refers to the amount of alcohol present in the bloodstream. In all Australian states and territories, a fully licensed driver has to have a BAC reading of under 0.05 per cent when driving. A BAC of 0.05 per cent denotes that there is 0.05 grams of alcohol in every 100 millilitres of blood. Intoxication usually refers to blood alcohol concentrations elevated above 0.05 g/100mL, but this is dependent on many characteristics, such as the weight of the person, their gender and their food intake prior to alcohol consumption.

SELF-AWARENESS

When working as a nurse, interacting with someone who is intoxicated from alcohol requires implementing a set of guidelines, and understanding the processes at work. Because of the increasing incidence of the over-consumption of alcohol and alcohol use disorders, and motor vehicle accidents, assaults and violence attributed to alcohol use, the excessive use of alcohol is now the focus of magazine articles and radio and television programs. Media attention heightens awareness of the devastating effects of excessive alcohol use: depression; loss of self-respect; alienation from family, friends and co-workers; malnutrition; infections; and damaging physiological effects to most body systems. More information on the physiological effects of alcohol use can be found in your medical/surgical nursing textbooks.

Although alcohol use was historically viewed as a moral problem, increased awareness played a part in redefining alcohol use disorders. As research about its biochemical aspects became known, earlier beliefs were challenged. The social stigma attached to alcohol is decreasing, and more people are seeking help. Professionals, laypeople, people with alcohol use disorders and their loved ones are attending workshops and seminars on the use of alcohol; educational recovery programs are reported widely in the media. The latest research related to the treatment of alcohol use disorders and other drugs can be accessed at the website for the National Drug Strategy at http://www.nationaldrugstrategy.gov.au/

Table 13.1 ■ Alcohol and effects on behaviour

BAC	Likely effects
Up to 0.05 g%	Talkative Relaxed More confident
0.05–0.08 g%	Talkative Acts and feels self-confident Judgment and movement impaired Inhibitions reduced
0.08–0.15 g%	Slurred speech Balance and coordination impaired Slowed reflexes Impaired vision Unstable emotions Nausea, vomiting
0.15–0.30 g%	Unsteady on feet, need assistance to walk Apathetic, sleepy Laboured breathing Memory deficits Loss of bladder control Possible loss of consciousness
Over 0.30 g%	Severe respiratory distress Coma Death

BAC = blood alcohol concentration

Alcohol is absorbed in the mouth, stomach and small intestine. Approximately 95 per cent of alcohol is broken down by the liver; the rest is excreted through the lungs, kidneys and skin. Alcohol usually starts to affect the brain within about five minutes of being swallowed. The BAC reaches its peak about 30–45 minutes after the consumption of one standard drink (10 grams of alcohol). Rapid consumption of multiple drinks results in a higher BAC, because the liver has a relatively fixed rate of metabolism regardless of how many drinks are consumed (National Health and Medical Research Council [NHMRC], 2009) It generally takes about one hour for the body to clear one standard drink. However, a person's BAC can continue to rise for a period of time after the last drink is consumed. Table 13.1 ■ compares BAC levels and the behaviours you will observe at various levels of intoxication. Table 13.2 ■ shows standard drink measures.

Adolescents do not have the same behaviours in response to BAC levels as adults. Their neurological and physiological responses vary, so their behaviours vary significantly as a result. We need to know three important differences: no slurred speech, no ataxia and no drowsiness. As a result, a teen may not know they are intoxicated. Because they do not get drowsy, nothing stops them from drinking, so their BAC levels may become toxic.

Table 13.2 ■ 'How much in a standard drink?' (National Health and Medical Research Council, 2011)

How much is in a standard drink?	
Can/Stubbie low-strength beer	= 0.8 standard drink
Can/Stubbie mid-strength beer	= 1 standard drink
Can/Stubbie full-strength beer	= 1.4 standard drinks
100 mL wine (13.5% alcohol)	= 1 standard drink
30 mL nip spirits	= 1 standard drink
Can spirits (approx. 5% alcohol)	= 1.2 to 1.7 standard drinks
Can spirits (approx. 7% alcohol)	= 1.6 to 2.4 standard drinks

History of alcohol use in Australia

Alcohol has always been part of the Anglo-Australian way of life. Rum arrived with the First Fleet in 1788, and was often used as currency in the early days of settlement (Lewis, 1992). In 1974, the drinking age was lowered to 18 from 21, which led to a rise in alcohol consumption by youths and a rise in alcohol-related accidents, mortality and morbidity.

Alcohol and risk of harm

Alcohol plays a complex cultural role in Australian society. Most people drink alcohol, generally for enjoyment, relaxation and sociability (NHMRC, 2009). However, a growing proportion of Australian people live with alcohol use disorders. In Australia, alcohol consumption causes over 5000 deaths per year, and for each death about 19 years of life are prematurely lost.

'**Risk**' is a common word used to describe potential levels of harm to the person from drinking. 'Short-term risk' refers to the risk of accidents and injuries occurring immediately after alcohol consumption, while 'long-term risk' is the risk of developing alcohol-related diseases from regular drinking over a lifetime (NHMRC, 2009). Approximately one-third (35 per cent) of the Australian population drink at levels that puts them at risk of short-term harm, while about 10 per cent of the population drink at levels that puts them at risk of long-term harm. The National Medical and Research Council of Australia (NHMRC) *Australian guidelines to reduce health risks from drinking alcohol* provides evidence to help Australians make informed decisions about their level of alcohol consumption. For more information, see the organisation's website: http://www.nhmrc.gov.au/your-health/alcohol-guidelines.

Regardless of the type of risk, people who drink excessively experience numerous negative physiological and psychological symptoms. See Mental Health in the Media for one of the many stories about alcohol use.

Alcohol withdrawal syndrome

Alcohol withdrawal often includes the symptoms described in the following section.

The term *hangover* is used to describe the unpleasant symptoms of mild alcohol withdrawal occurring approximately four to six hours after alcohol ingestion. These symptoms include the following:

- nausea and vomiting
- gastritis
- headache
- fatigue
- sweating and thirst
- restlessness
- irritability
- the 'shakes'
- vasomotor instability.

The cause of the symptoms is unclear, but they are attributed to dehydration, hypoglycaemia and the accumulation of lactic acid and acetaldehyde in the blood.

Alcohol-related psychosis is a rare condition that refers to hallucinations and delusions reported by people with alcohol use disorders. The hallucinations occur approximately 24 to 48 hours after heavy drinking, and may be vivid and frightening.

Generalised tonic–clonic or withdrawal **seizures** occur in about 5 per cent of people withdrawing from alcohol. They usually occur early, approximately 7 to 24 hours after the last drink. They can be prevented with appropriate nursing assessment of the withdrawal state, and with the administration of medications used in withdrawal, such as diazepam.

Delirium tremens (DTs) is the rare, most severe form of alcohol withdrawal syndrome. It is to be treated as a medical emergency. Symptoms include acute memory disturbances, confusion and disorientation, extreme agitation or restlessness, anorexia, paranoid ideation and hallucinations. The symptoms are described more thoroughly in the section on withdrawal that follows. Generally, the DTs occur two to five days after stopping or significantly reducing alcohol consumption. The usual course is 3 days, but can be up to 14 days. Additional medical illnesses may be present, such as pneumonia, pancreatitis and hepatic decompensation.

The clinical assessment and management of alcohol withdrawal syndromes

Alcohol withdrawal syndrome is composed of a constellation of physiological and behavioural symptoms that occur when the alcohol concentration in the bloodstream drops. Alcohol withdrawal is a syndrome of central nervous system hyperactivity characterised by symptoms that range from mild to severe. The clinical management of alcohol use disorders involves the assessment and management of withdrawal symptoms. Effective management of withdrawal in its early stages can reduce or prevent progression to a complicated withdrawal syndrome. See Table 13.3 ■ for the three main classes of signs and symptoms of alcohol withdrawal.

Assessing withdrawal

Usually withdrawal is brief and resolves after 2 to 3 days without treatment; occasionally, withdrawal may continue for up to 10 days. Withdrawal can occur when the blood alcohol level is decreasing, even if the person is still intoxicated. If alcohol use is suspected, the following questions, known as the *suspicion of alcohol withdrawal*, will assist the nurse to

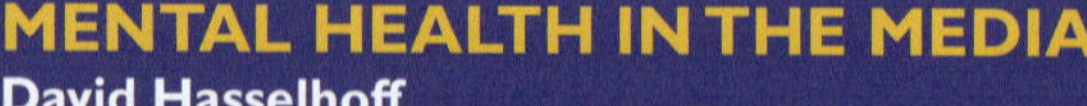

David Hasselhoff

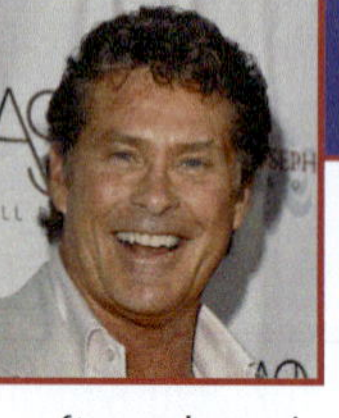

The media exposes us to a variety of situations concerning alcohol. Some are fictional, some are partially autobiographical, and some are real. The fully-fictional or partially fictional depictions often glamorise the situation and minimise the damage and embarrassment. When actor David Hasselhoff was so intoxicated he was crawling around eating a cheeseburger off the floor, he was videotaped. The 2007 home video clip surfaced, showing Hasselhoff apparently in a drunken stupor. He was lying on the floor in a hotel room, shirtless, drunkenly trying to consume a cheeseburger. His then 17-year-old daughter, who shot the video, can be heard saying, 'Tell me you are going to stop, tell me you are going to stop.' The video brought the undeniable reality of alcohol intoxication to light. In 2009, David Hasselhoff was hospitalised with a BAC of 0.39. He has publicly admitted past treatment for alcohol use. In 2010, David was hospitalised for an alcohol-related seizure. In late 2016, he was reportedly alcohol-free, but still 'battling' his addiction.

Photo courtesy © Everett Collection Inc/Alamy.

TABLE 13.3 ■ Main signs and symptoms of alcohol withdrawal

Autonomic overactivity	Gastrointestinal	Cognitive and perceptual changes
Sweating	Anorexia	Anxiety
Tachycardia	Nausea	Vivid dreams
Hypertension	Vomiting	Illusions
Insomnia	Dyspepsia	Hallucinations
Tremor		Delirium
Fever		

Source: NSW Ministry of Health (2009), 'Main signs and symptoms of alcohol withdrawal', *Nursing and midwifery clinical guidelines—identifying and responding to drug and alcohol issues*.

determine whether the person is likely to move into alcohol withdrawal (NSW Health, 2009):

- Does the person have a regular alcohol intake of 80 grams (eight standard drinks—males) or 60 grams (six standard drinks—females) of alcohol or more per day?
- Does the person drink lesser amounts of alcohol than that mentioned above, but drink in conjunction with taking other CNS depressants?
- Are there previous episodes of alcohol withdrawal?
- If hospitalised, is the current admission alcohol-related?
- Evidence of chronic alcohol use, such as:
    - oparotid swelling (swelling in the gland under the ear)
    - ocushingoid face (full/moon-looking face)
    - ofacial telangiectasia (red spots/blood vessels)
    - oeyes reddened or signs of liver disease
    - oascites, jaundice, limb muscle wasting
- Pathology results show raised serum gamma-glutamyltransferase (GGT).
- The person is displaying symptoms such as:
    - oanxiety
    - oagitation
    - otremor
    - osweatiness or early morning retching.

Alcohol Withdrawal Scale (AWS)

The use of a withdrawal scale helps guide the nurse's assessment as to the severity of the withdrawal syndrome. Scales provide a baseline against which changes in withdrawal severity may be measured over time. It is important to note that withdrawal scales *do not* diagnose withdrawal; they are merely guides to the severity of an already diagnosed withdrawal syndrome. The AWS is a widely used scale throughout Australia, and is a seven-item scale that allows a quantitative rating (from 0 to 4) of the following components:

- perspiration
- tremor
- anxiety
- agitation
- axilla temperature
- hallucinations
- orientation.

Practice example

Alcohol withdrawal

Sindi and Alex have just been married and have chosen a cruise for their honeymoon. Towards the end of the cruise, Alex became very sweaty and feverish during dinner, and told Sindi that he thought he had caught the flu. On returning to their cabin, Alex became disoriented, had a seizure and collapsed. The ship's doctor told Sindi that Alex was going experiencing severe alcohol withdrawal. He had stopped drinking just before they went on the cruise, and was now in the fifth day of abstinence from alcohol.

Management of alcohol withdrawal

Nursing pharmacological management for alcohol withdrawal includes the following:

1. Monitoring the person's fluid status. If the person is unable to take fluids by mouth, fluids may be administered intravenously.
2. Administration of benzodiazepines, most commonly diazepam. There are two types of regimens used for hospitalised people: diazepam-loading regimes and fixed-schedule regimes. With loading regimens, high doses of oral diazepam are administered in the early stages of withdrawal (can be up to 80 mg in the first day), and are indicated if the person has a history of severe withdrawal complications (seizures, delirium), presents with an AWS score of 8 or over, and/or presents with severe withdrawal complications. Fixed-schedule is generally indicated once the person reaches an AWS score of 5–7. The regimen involves the regular administration of diazepam, the dose being reduced over the course of four to five days, according to the AWS score. Dosing regimens may vary from setting to setting, depending on the level of support available, the duration of admission and clinician preference.
3. Administration of vitamins, especially thiamine (vitamin B_1), as alcohol interferes with the absorption of B vitamins.

The clinical management of withdrawal from alcohol should include controlling the potentially life-threatening symptoms of withdrawal, and reducing the extreme discomfort. Nursing management also includes supportive care (nutrition and hydration, psychosocial support, withdrawal information), the regular monitoring of vital signs, and the administration of prescribed medications to relieve symptoms (antidiarrhoeals and antiemetics).

Having **blackouts** is frequently confused with 'passing out'. In fact, passing out refers to unconsciousness, whereas a blackout is anterograde amnesia: loss of short-term memories with retention of remote memories. A person can function effectively for several days—talking on the phone, working and shopping—yet have absolutely no memory of doing so. To others, the person may appear normal or 'high'. This is because the cognitive impairment occurs before motor impairment. Interestingly, people with alcohol use disorders appear unconcerned about the blackouts, and eventually learn to cover

YOUR ASSESSMENT APPROACH Stages of alcohol withdrawal

State	Peak time of onset after last drink	Symptoms	Potential duration of symptoms
Tremulousness	24 hours	At rest: slight tremors; during activities: gross and irregular tremors	1 week
		Diaphoresis	3–4 days
		Anorexia, nausea, vomiting	3–4 days
		Increased vital signs	3–4 days
		Sense of agitation and inner shakiness	2 weeks
		Insomnia with nightmares of seemingly real events	2 weeks or longer
Tremors and transitory hallucinosis	24 hours	Tremors plus visual hallucinations of events (e.g., having an accident while driving drunk)	3 days
Alcoholic hallucinosis	24 hours	Cues of tremulousness state plus vivid perse cutory and auditory hallucinations, agitation, increased suicide, preassaultive potential	3 days–2 weeks
Delirium tremens	24–48 hours	Cues of tremulousness state plus delirium, generalised seizures, disorientation for time and place, visual hallucinations, agitation, panic level of anxiety	3–5 days

them up. This appearance of unconcern may, in part, be due to euphoric recall: the person recalls feeling good, but does not recall their behaviour. Reality is distorted. Some people find blackouts very disturbing and seek treatment at that point.

There are two types of blackout: *en bloc* or complete inability to recall a time period, and *fragmentary* where the memory loss is not complete. The faster the person's BAC increases, the more likely there will be a blackout. Women are more susceptible to blackouts due to pharmacokinetics and female body composition (Rose & Grant, 2010). When assessing a person experiencing an alcohol use disorder, it is important to determine whether blackouts are part of the symptoms. See the nursing care plan for alcohol use disorders at the end of this chapter.

Wernicke–Korsakoff syndrome

Wernicke–Korsakoff syndrome is a disturbance of short-term memory that occurs in people who have undertaken long-term, heavy alcohol consumption. It is a neurological disorder caused by thiamine (vitamin B_1) deficiency. If not treated early, this syndrome can result in irreversible and permanent brain damage and memory loss. Wernicke's encephalopathy is usually the first stage of the syndrome.

Wernicke's encephalopathy is a neurological condition associated with excessive alcohol use and subsequent thiamine deficiency. It is characterised by ataxia, sixth cranial nerve palsy, nystagmus and confusion. Wernicke's encephalopathy may clear spontaneously in a few days or weeks, and responds rapidly to large doses of parenteral thiamine in its acute, early stage. If signs and symptoms are treated early enough, the next stage of the syndrome (Korsakoff's) may not develop.

Korsakoff's syndrome most often is preceded by untreated Wernicke's encephalopathy. Korsakoff's involves neural damage, and is generally irreversible even with thiamine administration. The main symptoms include amnesia, severe memory loss, confabulation (invented memories due to memory loss that that are taken as true), lack of insight and apathy.

Fetal alcohol spectrum disorders

Nurses need to be aware of the harmful effects of alcohol on pregnant women and unborn children. **Fetal alcohol spectrum disorders** (FASD) may occur in children of women who engage in alcohol use during pregnancy. FASD is an umbrella term used to describe a range of adverse effects, which include the diagnostic terms 'fetal alcohol syndrome', 'alcohol-related neurodevelopment disorders', 'fetal alcohol effects' and 'alcohol-related birth defects', all of which are attributable to prenatal exposure to alcohol (National Indigenous Drug and Alcohol Committee [NIDAC], 2012). There has been significant debate about the levels of alcohol consumption that can result in fetal harm. It is now generally accepted that large quantities of alcohol consumed (either chronically or intermittently) during pregnancy can cause FASD. However, lower levels of consumption have also been shown to result in harm to the developing fetus (NIDC, 2012). This is why the *Australian guidelines to reduce health risks from drinking alcohol* (NHMRC, 2009) advises that not drinking while pregnant or breastfeeding is the safest option.

FASD results in a range of symptoms and impairments in development, learning and behaviour. Symptoms related to neuropsychological impairment may be present in early childhood, while other symptoms may only be recognised

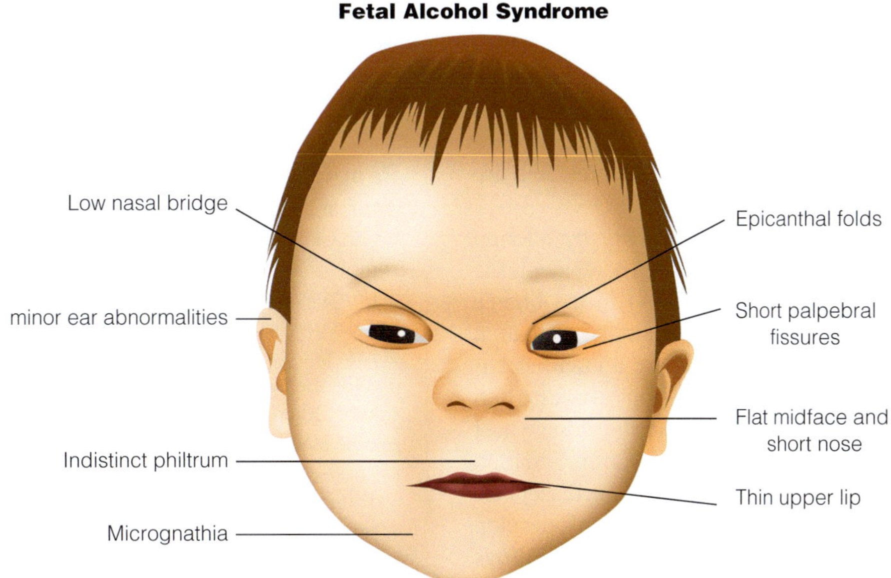

FIGURE 13.1 ■ Facial characteristics that are associated with fetal alcohol exposure. Fetal alcohol spectrum disorder is the result of alcohol consumption during pregnancy, and it can have many severe effects on the child, including physical malformations such as those shown here: narrow forehead, short palpebral fissures, small nose, and long upper lip with deficient philtrum.
Source: *Alcohol Research and Health, 34*(1) http://pubs.niaaa.nih.gov/publications/arh341/4-14.htm

after formal education has commenced. Children displaying characteristic facial abnormalities, such as small eye openings, a smooth philtrum and a thin upper lip, growth retardation and development abnormalities are defined as having fetal alcohol syndrome (FAS). The characteristic physical features of a child with FAS are seen in Figure 13.1 ■.

The prevalence of FASD in Australia is difficult to determine. There is a lack of accurate and current research data across all population groups, as well as confusion between FASD and FAS, as FAS is more clinically recognisable. The first report to estimate the prevalence of FAS in Australia indicated a rate of 0.02 per 1000 for non-Indigenous children, and 2.76 per 1000 for Indigenous children (Bower, Silva, Henderson, Ryan & Rudy, 2000). Other Australian studies have found similar estimates. It is important to note that FASD is not a problem unique to Aboriginal and Torres Strait Islander peoples. The difference in rates reflects under-reporting by non-Indigenous people, as well as other factors, such as socioeconomic status, drinking patterns and differences in diet (NIDC, 2012).

For up-to-date information about FASD, see the link to the National Organisation for Fetal Alcohol Spectrum Disorders (NOFASD) (http://www.nofasd.org.au/).

Suicide and alcohol use

Alcohol is linked to suicidality and self-harm. Alcohol use may lead to suicide through disinhibition, impulsiveness and impaired judgment, but may also be used to ease the distress associated with an act of killing oneself. Increased suicide risk may also be foreshadowed by social withdrawal, breakdown of relationships and social marginalisation, all of which are common in the experience of alcohol use disorders. There is also growing evidence that alcohol increases the risk of highly prevalent mental health disorders, in particular depressive disorders (NHMRC, 2009). It also may affect the efficacy of antidepressant medications. Suicide is thoroughly discussed in Chapter 19.

SEDATIVE-HYPNOTICS

The group of drugs called sedative-hypnotics are prescribed for anxiety, stress and sleep difficulties. There are about 30 different types of benzodiazepines, the most commonly prescribed sedative-hypnotics, available in Australia, including diazepam (Valium), oxazepam (Serepax) and alprazolam (Xanax). Nationally, there are over 7 million annual prescriptions written for benzodiazepines. Benzodiazepines act on the central nervous system, and produce sedation, muscle relaxation and feelings of calm and wellbeing. However, because of these sought-after effects, there is potential for the overuse of these drugs, as in the Practice Example that follows.

Practice example

Elizabeth is 45 years old, and has been depressed and irritable over an impending divorce. Her GP prescribed diazepam 5 mg for sleep and for anxiety (every six hours as needed). Because this dosage was not helping decrease her anxiety as much as she wanted, Elizabeth increased her dosage and began taking 50–100 mg a day over a period of a few weeks. This evening, Elizabeth's estranged husband found her mumbling incoherently. Her speech was slurred, she was bumping into furniture, and she was quite drowsy.

The effects of sedative-hypnotics

Sedative-hypnotics are drugs that cause people to feel euphoric, yet relaxed. They are frequently prescribed to relieve pain, reduce anxiety (sedative effects) and induce sleep (hypnotic effects). Anxiolytic drugs, the benzodiazepines, began to be widely used because of their ability to reduce anxiety without causing significant CNS depression. However, they also have the drawbacks of producing dependence and withdrawal syndromes. Benzodiazepines can cause respiratory depression, but this effect is minimal unless other CNS depressants are taken (such as alcohol or opioids).

These drugs are thought to modify anxiety by altering the balance of neurotransmitters, especially norepinephrine (NE) and gamma-aminobutyric acid (GABA) in the brain's limbic system. The limbic system is involved in the regulation of emotion (see Chapter 6). These drugs have a high risk for overuse and dependence. When the drug stops working and tolerance develops, people tend to increase the dosage just 'to cope'. As the dose increases, effects move from sedation through to hypnosis to stupor. People who take benzodiazepines on a regular basis (whether prescribed or not) may develop tolerance to the sedative effect. In some people, these drugs produce a paradoxical reaction of violence and disinhibited behaviour (NSW Health, 2009). Even the non-benzodiazepines, such as zolpidem (Stillnox), can be used to excess and have dependence issues associated with their use (see Chapter 8).

Patterns of use

Approximately 1.6 per cent of the Australian population uses benzodiazepines recreationally (AIHW, 2009). In party situations, some teenagers and young adults take high doses of benzodiazepines, often in combination with alcohol, to get 'high'. The resultant CNS depression makes this practice especially dangerous. People with amphetamine use disorders may use benzodiazepines to 'come down' from symptoms associated with stimulant use. People with opioid use disorders also may use benzodiazepines when opioids are unavailable, or to increase the effects of the opioid drugs. In Australia, there are two main patterns of benzodiazepine dependence, the most common being low-dose dependency over many years, particularly among women and older people (NSW Health, 2009). High-dose dependence, often in the context of polydrug use as described above, can also occur.

Action

Benzodiazepines are metabolised in phases by the liver. When taken orally, they are initially absorbed and partially metabolised. However, the unmetabolised parts become active metabolites that are stored in the fatty tissues. Consequently, taking these drugs over a period of time results in a cumulative effect, unsuspected dependence and possible **overdose**. Nurses in every area need to be aware of the frequency of substance use and its impact. See What Every Nurse Should Know: People With Substance Use Disorders for further information.

More Australians die from benzodiazepine overdose than from opioid overdose. Many people take alcohol and benzodiazepines together. The use of benzodiazepines in alcohol withdrawal can be confusing for some, and they commence taking diazepam while still intoxicated. While judgment is impaired, they take more pills, thereby unintentionally overdosing. Because alcohol and benzodiazepines are synergistic, an overdose can occur quickly. Benzodiazepines are often used in suicide attempts (see Chapter 19).

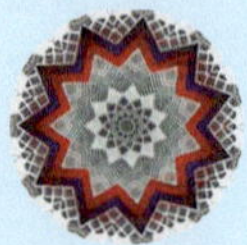

WHAT EVERY NURSE SHOULD KNOW

People with substance use disorders

Drug and alcohol use is commonplace in our society. As health care professionals, nursing staff are often faced with the complexities of caring for individuals who are affected by the use of drugs and alcohol. The focus of nursing practice aims to give equal regard to the physical, psychosocial and cultural wellbeing of all people receiving care. All practice should therefore include a comprehensive substance use assessment, and offer suitable interventions and harm minimisation strategies to all people identified as being at risk of, or experiencing, problems associated with substance use disorders.

Imagine that you are an emergency department nurse. When a person comes in the complaint may be physical or psychiatric in nature, and either of these could be the result of substance use, look for the hallmark signs of substance use. In an emergency situation, you would be able to detect substance-using people because they may not be able to answer key questions like these:

- Have you had any medications, drugs or alcohol today?
- What did you take?
- How much did you take?
- When did you take it?
- What have you taken in the last 24 hours? In the last week?
- Most importantly, how long have you been taking the substance for (duration of use)?

When people are not able to provide the necessary information, you may have to rely on family or friends as data sources, and then corroborate what you learn with the person once they are alert.

Withdrawal

Benzodiazepine withdrawal is unpleasant and can be life-threatening, particularly with abrupt withdrawal from high doses. High-dose benzodiazepine use should not be ceased suddenly; a dose reduction regimen should be used under the management of a GP or an addiction medicine specialist. This is because sudden cessation can result in seizures, hallucinations, coma and death. The onset of withdrawal depends on the half-life of the particular benzodiazepine being used. Withdrawal from short-acting benzodiazepines, such as oxazepam, generally occurs earlier, and is more severe than withdrawal from the longer-acting ones (such as diazepam). Withdrawal symptoms include autonomic hyperactivity (alterations in vital signs and diaphoresis), marked anxiety, agitation, insomnia, depression and seizures. Clinically supervised withdrawal management can prevent a potentially serious emergency during withdrawal.

OPIOIDS

The opioids as a group of substances include heroin and morphine, derived from the poppy plant, and synthetic drugs, such as oxycodone (Oxycontin), codeine and methadone. They all share a common core structure which allows them to interact with the endogenous opioid receptors in the central nervous system.

The effects of opioids

Opioids have analgaesic qualities, and are prescribed after surgery. They are quite potent, and have the ability to remove painful stimuli. Depending on the person, the drugs may produce a euphoric high, but they generally cause people to feel drowsy and out of touch with the world. Postoperative nurses, for example, need to be knowledgeable about the use of opioids because of the potential for tolerance and dependence. However, nurses should never withhold analgaesics when the person is reporting pain. See What Every Nurse Should Know: Pain Medication Use for information on this topic.

Opioids have a depressant effect on the central nervous system. They decrease the spontaneous activity of neurons, which produces drowsiness, mood changes and mental clouding (NSW Health, 2009). They also have features quite distinct from other depressant drugs, such as alcohol and sedative-hypnotics. They are powerful analgaesics and can cause suppression of reflex cough and constipation. However, unlike alcohol, and to some extent sedative-hypnotics, the cessation of opioid use is not likely to be life-threatening. Withdrawal will be discussed further below.

Heroin use by itself is not inherently dangerous. Unless there is an accidental overdose, heroin alone as a substance will not harm the individual. The ancillary issues of possibly contaminated diluting agents, needle cleanliness, and exposure to blood-borne viruses diseases, such as hepatitis C and HIV, along with typically criminal behaviours necessary to support the use, put the individual at great risk.

History of opioid use

Heroin (diacetylmorphine) was first developed in 1874 by the German Bayer Company to treat wounded soldiers and send them back into battle as 'heroes' (hence the name 'hero-in'). Heroin is processed from morphine, a form of opium.

In Australia, the discovery of gold in the 1850s resulted in a huge influx of migrants in search of instant wealth. Many of these people were Chinese men. The smoking of opium was a natural part of the way of life for many Chinese people. In the Chinese camps, which grew in and around towns in regional New South Wales, regular reference was made to opium dens and opium sales. Racism and resentment directed towards Chinese people by Europeans during the 18th and 19th centuries led to the first Australia drug law being passed in 1857, which imposed an import duty on opium. The primary purpose of this law was to discourage the entry of Chinese people to Australia, rather than to restrict the importation of opium itself. In fact, Europeans in Australia at this time were among the world's prime opioid users. Laudanum, a mixture of morphine and alcohol, was regularly taken by upper-class matrons and administered to children to calm them. The first laws restricting opium use were carefully worded to apply only to opium in smokeable form only. Opium use was eventually outlawed in 1905, although heroin was available on prescription until 1953.

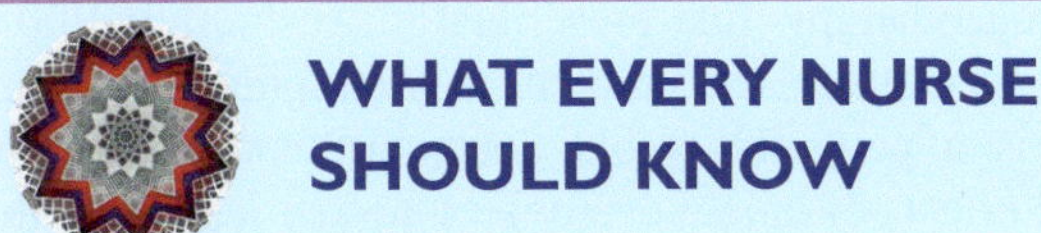

Pain medication use

Imagine you are a postoperative nurse. Following a surgical procedure, it is important to instruct the people in your care on the proper use of pain medications to prevent establishing chronic pain pathways. At the same time, you have to be vigilant not to instruct the person in your care in such a way that promotes inadvertent or deliberate overuse of pain medications. There will be times when people electively choose repeated surgeries so that they have access to pain medications. Under these circumstances, it is important to evaluate the person's intent for surgical interventions, and also tend to the follow-up behaviours after each surgery. Assess for **substance dependence** in the form of prescription pain medication overuse or dependence. Use the assessment skills described in this chapter to ensure healthy recoveries and intervene appropriately.

Current opioid use

The most common opioid drug used recreationally in Australia is heroin, although the use of 'street' morphine (morphine obtained without a prescription) has increased in recent years. Approximately 1.4 per cent of the Australian population use opioids for non-medical reasons (AIHW, 2011).

Although heroin can be smoked or taken orally, many people use this drug intravenously because of the increased bioavailability of the drug with intravenous use. This places people with opioid use disorders at high risk of blood-borne viruses, predominantly hepatitis C. Other problems associated with heroin use include medical and psychological complications, social and family disruption, and violence and drug-related crime. Overdose also is a risk with heroin and other opioid use, as the purity of the drug can vary. People who sell heroin often 'cut' it with other substances, thus increasing the quantity and their own profit. Opioid dependence is a chronic, relapsing disorder that generally requires long-term treatment.

Overdose

Constricted pupils, euphoria, psychomotor retardation, slurred speech and/or drowsiness indicate opioid intoxication.

If a person overdoses, naloxone (Narcan) is given intravenously (IV). It is a fast-acting narcotic antagonist that counteracts respiratory depression. Abdominal cramps, rhinorrhoea and lacrimation may be treated with supportive pharmacotherapies.

Withdrawal

People who use high doses of opioids intravenously are at high risk for severe withdrawal symptoms. Heroin and morphine are relatively short-acting drugs. Withdrawal symptoms are usually evident within 6–24 hours after the last dose, reaching a peak at 24–48 hours. The symptoms generally resolve after 5–10 days. The opioid withdrawal syndrome can be very uncomfortable

LIVED EXPERIENCE

Overdoses were common when I was using heroin. They always seemed to happen in slow motion, including my own. You just knew, straight away, could feel the drug hit the back of your throat and your eyes get heavy straight away. I remember looking at someone as I fell, I didn't have time to speak, I just thought 'Oh no, I can't move my legs', and then I slid off my chair and the last thing I saw was them getting up and reaching out towards me. It's just like falling asleep, but in a matter of seconds; you can't stop it. Even when you are still conscious, it can be hard to keep your head upright, or your eyes open.

I watched other people overdose in front of me—the way the blood drained from their face, pupils dilating really quickly. One person's lips turned blue and we called an ambulance, but you were always worried about the police. The ambos were great, they gave her Narcan on the spot and she came around, but they took her to emergency anyway. I've seen some people get aggressive after Narcan, but I'd rather be alive and in withdrawal than dead and stoned.

and distressing, but not life-threatening unless there is a severe underlying disease. People may have a low tolerance to pain due to the effect of long-term opioid use, and this needs to be acknowledged and treated effectively (NSW Health, 2009). Signs and symptoms are depicted in Table 13.4 ■.

Pharmacotherapy treatment for opioid use disorders

Opioid pharmacotherapy involves replacing the drug of dependence with a legally obtained, longer-lasting opioid that is taken orally. This type of therapy is part of the harm-reduction pillar of harm-minimisation philosophy. Research suggests that pharmacotherapy treatment reduces heroin use and associated criminal behaviour, and improves physical and mental health and social functioning (Chalmers & Ritter, 2009). People seek or are referred to pharmacotherapy treatment (replacement) programs, and a health care professional authorised to provide opioid pharmacotherapy prescribes either buprenorphine, buprenorphine-naloxone or methadone as part of treatment. A comprehensive assessment is undertaken before the person is accepted into a treatment program.

Table 13.4 ■ Symptoms and signs of opioid withdrawal

Symptoms	Signs
Anorexia and nausea	Restlessness
Abdominal pain	Yawning
Hot and cold flushes	Perspiration
Bone, joint and muscle pain	Rhinorrhoea
Insomnia and disturbed sleep	Dilated pupils
Cramps	Piloerection
Intense cravings for opioids	Muscle twitching (particularly restless legs when lying down)
	Vomiting and diarrhoea

This assessment includes undertaking a detailed history of drug use (opioids and other drugs/alcohol), a physical examination (vital signs, pathology), and questions regarding the person's social circumstances and motivations for treatment. People are registered as part of any pharmacotherapy treatment program, and records are kept of the therapies given (counselling, psychosocial support, medications). The person generally attends a 'dosing point' (a specialised treatment clinic, general practitioner or pharmacy) regularly (usually daily or second-daily), and takes a dose of their prescribed medication under the supervision of a registered nurse, pharmacist or other health professional. In Australia, on any one given day, there are approximately 47 000 people receiving pharmacotherapy treatment for opioid use disorders (AIHW, 2013).

Buprenorphine is the drug of choice for a significant amount of people undergoing pharmacotherapy treatment for opioid dependence. It was introduced in Australia in 2000 (under the trade name 'Subutex') for the treatment of opioid use disorders. Buprenorphine is a derivative of the morphine alkaloid, thebaine, and is a partial opioid agonist. Buprenorphine diminishes cravings for heroin and other opioids, and prevents and alleviates opioid withdrawal. This drug has a higher affinity for opioid receptors than full opioid agonists (such as heroin). Buprenorphine can thus block the effects of other opioid agonists in a dose-dependent fashion (AIHW, 2013). Buprenorphine comes in a sublingual tablet that dissolves under the tongue in around five minutes.

Buprenorphine-naloxone (Suboxone) is another commonly used pharmacotherapy, first prescribed in Australia in 2005. This drug contains a 4:1 ratio of buprenorphine:naloxone. Naloxone is a powerful opioid antagonist and is used to reverse the effects of opioid overdose. One key reason for the development of buprenorphine-naloxone was to prevent people from diverting and injecting buprenorphine, as naloxone has no effect when taken sublingually (buprenorphine-naloxone comes in sublingual preparations only). However, if the buprenorphine-naloxone preparation is somehow crushed and injected, the naloxone will result in the opioid being displaced from the receptors, thereby causing immediate and very unpleasant withdrawal effects. This makes it possible for more people to receive 'takeaway' doses so that they can take their medication at home rather than have to present to a dosing point daily or second-daily.

Methadone remains the most commonly prescribed pharmacotherapy in Australia. Methadone was introduced for use in opioid addiction in Australia in 1969. Methadone is a synthetic opioid agonist which comes in the form of oral syrup.

The effects of methadone are therefore similar to that of the other agonists such as morphine and heroin. However, as methadone is taken orally, it has a much longer bioavailability and half-life when compared to other agonists. The aims of a methadone maintenance program are to reduce or eliminate heroin or other opioid use, improve the health and wellbeing of those in treatment, facilitate the social rehabilitation of the person, reduce the spread of blood-borne viruses, reduce the risk of opioid overdose, and reduce the level of involvement in crime associated with opioid use disorders (AIHW, 2013). However, methadone is not without its controversy. There are many critics of methadone treatment programs, mainly centred on the fact that programs are providing a drug of dependence to already drug-dependent people. There is also the view that this drug prolongs opioid dependence by maintaining people on therapy when they may otherwise be drug-free (Robertson & Daniels, 2012). Despite this, methadone treatment programs have been demonstrated to be highly cost-effective and successful interventions for people experiencing opioid use disorders.

Nursing care of the person undertaking a pharmacotherapy treatment program

All nurses need to know about the pharmacotherapy treatments for opioid use. If a person on a program is hospitalised or needs clinical treatment, it can be very dangerous if other opioid drugs are prescribed. For example, if the person taking methadone is given morphine, an overdose can easily occur. If the person is taking buprenorphine-suboxone and they are given opioids, they can experience precipitated withdrawal. Standard doses of pain relief, if the administration of this cannot be avoided, will not likely be effective in someone taking a replacement pharmacotherapy. Advice should be sought from an addiction medicine specialist, a drug and alcohol nurse practitioner, or a staff member belonging to a specialist drug and alcohol program on how to best manage and treat people on pharmacotherapy programs.

PSYCHOSTIMULANTS

Drugs labelled as 'psychostimulants' include a diverse range of CNS stimulants such as amphetamine (speed), cocaine (coke, snow), methamphetamine (crystal meth, speed, ice), methylphenidates (Ritalin), and methylene dioxy-methamphetamine (MDMA—ecstasy). (Note that MDMA is discussed separately later in this chapter.) The following Practice Example shows how the best intentions can lead to dire and unexpected consequences.

Practice example

Amphetamines and weight loss

Laura, a 16-year-old high-school girl, was on a diet so that she could fit into her favourite bikini. Her friend's brother, a pharmacist, gave her some dexamphetamine 'just until you lose the weight'. Laura's mother initially noticed her rather unusual hyperactivity, her euphoria and the fact that she refused dinner. Over a period of a few weeks, Laura's behaviour changed. She appeared suspicious and irritable, and continued to speak and move rapidly, and her grades dropped significantly. Laura was rushed to the hospital after being found unconscious in the girls' changing room at school.

The effects of psychostimulants

In small doses, psychostimulants cause a person to feel energetic and euphoric. A growing number of people take psychostimulants to counteract the effects of sedative-hypnotics and other depressant drugs in a cyclic fashion. Psychostimulants activate the CNS, having a peripheral sympathomimetic action, and are often used for effects such as euphoria, increased sense of wellbeing, increased energy, more confidence or over-confidence, improved cognitive and psychomotor performance, suppression of appetite and insomnia (Kinner & Degenhardt, 2008). See Table 13.5 for the effects of psychostimulants. Psychostimulants can be dangerous because

EVIDENCE-BASED PRACTICE

Kevin tried a lot of drugs as a teenager, but never visualised that he would one day be living with an opioid use disorder. Kevin started using heroin occasionally on weekends, but soon found himself needing this drug every day. After his long-term partner left and his parents refused to see him because of his opioid use, Kevin sought treatment. He was started on a methadone pharmacotherapy program, and was given counselling and psychosocial support as part of this.

Kevin soon learnt that he is fairly characteristic of a person attending opioid replacement treatment; he is in his early forties, male and lives in an urban area. His treatment is managed by his GP. Kevin started attending his local pharmacy daily to take his methadone under the supervision of the pharmacist. After being stable on this program for some time, he was given 'takeaway' doses and able to take his methadone unsupervised at home. Since commencing the program, he has only relapsed back to heroin use twice, and only for short periods of time. Kevin now feels more in control of his life, he has recently met a new partner and started working on his family relationships.

CRITICAL THINKING QUESTIONS

1. What factors do you believe will increase the likelihood that Kevin will remain drug-free?
2. What factors do you believe will decrease this likelihood?
3. How can Kevin's family better help Kevin to stay drug-free?
4. If Kevin needed hospital treatment for another illness, what could you do as a nurse to support Kevin in his recovery?

they alter judgment and obscure feelings. Taken in high doses or intravenously, psychostimulants such as methamphetamine can have dangerous side-effects. Tolerance develops rapidly, and people who use these drugs regularly may experience a toxic, paranoid psychosis. Argumentativeness, delusions, hallucinations, stereotypic compulsive behaviour, increased libido, interpersonal sensitivity, panic and violence may occur (American Psychiatric Association [APA], 2013).

Psychostimulants act by mimicking two of the brain's most important neurotransmitters, dopamine (DA) and norepinephrine (NE). A drug must be able to act on a receptor site or on a number of receptor sites to have an impact. The body may not have a specific amphetamine or cocaine receptor site, so amphetamine and cocaine will take what is called *illegal control* at the existing receptor sites. Dopamine and dopamine receptor sites are intricately involved in the effects substances have on the nervous systems. (The specific ways in which morphine, amphetamine and cocaine are involved in this process are shown in Table 13.5 ■.) Regular use of psychostimulants changes the way a person thinks and behaves, because the brain's cortex is no longer activated during decision-making. This change in the ability of the brain to transport dopamine, to any significant degree (see Figure 13.2 ■), creates the clinical characteristics you see as severe psychiatric symptoms.

History of psychostimulant use

Amphetamines

The use of amphetamine has been documented for centuries in China, where the ma huang plant (*Ephedra vulgaris*) has been used to treat people with asthma (Ransley et al., 2011). The ma huang plant contains ephedrine, which is a CNS stimulant first produced by chemical synthesis in 1887 in Germany. Following this discovery, amphetamines came into medical and recreational use in the 1920s, primarily through the treatment of colds and asthma. In 1932, the Benzedrine Inhaler was introduced as an over-the-counter product, and became a licit substitute for cocaine, which had been declared illegal by the US federal government in 1914 (Ransley et al., 2011). By 1940, 39 disorders had been identified for which Benzedrine—one of the three main kinds of amphetamine—was the recommended treatment, including night blindness, sea sickness and impotence.

Methamphetamine, more potent and easier to make than amphetamine, was discovered in Japan in 1919. The crystalline powder is soluble in water, making it easy to inject. During World War II and the Vietnam War, methamphetamine was widely used by the armed forces to increase alertness, confidence, feelings of increased strength and to suppress appetite. Legally manufactured tablets of both dextroamphetamine (Dexedrine) and methamphetamine (Methedrine) became readily available, and were used by students, truck drivers and athletes. By the 1960s, the market in methamphetamine had changed from being predominantly licit to illicit. The Australian experience of amphetamine use and supply largely followed that of the United States.

TABLE 13.5 ■ Effects of psychostimulants

Immediate effects	Effects at higher doses
Increased alertness	Headaches
Increased energy	Pale skin
Increased confidence	Restlessness
Euphoria	Dizziness
Increased talkativeness	Rapid or irregular heartbeat
Loss of appetite	Paranoia
Insomnia	Anxiety
Increased heart rate and breathing	Panic attacks
Nausea/vomiting	Depression
Headaches	Confusion (feeling 'scattered')
Jaw-clenching	
Hot and cold flushes	
Sweats	

Cocaine

For over 4000 years, coca (*Erythroxylon coca*, the plant from which cocaine is harvested) has been used as a medicine and stimulant in what is now Colombia, Peru and Bolivia. European explorers in the 16th century made note of its existence, and that it was used by South American people to elevate mood, help with digestion and suppress appetite. Coca did not find use in Western medicine until the late 19th century, however, when American drug companies began to explore that part of the world for new medicines. At first considered a safe stimulant and nerve tonic, coca's addictive and destructive properties became apparent within 30 years of its introduction as a pharmaceutical product.

Cocaine was first imported to Australia in the late 1800s. It was used as a local anaesthetic, for treatment for morphine and alcohol addiction, as well as to treat fatigue and depression (Australian Institute of Criminology, 2007). Throughout the 1920s and 1930s, Australia's rates of cocaine consumption were some of the highest in the world. The subsequent ban on selling cocaine without a prescription (during the 1920s) significantly reduced levels of use among the general population.

Current use of psychostimulants

Methamphetamines

Approximately 2.5 per cent of the Australian population uses methamphetamines on a regular basis (AIHW, 2011). Australia has one of the highest rates of amphetamine use in the world, heavily influenced by its proximity to the high production areas of South-East Asia (Lee & Rawson, 2008). In the 1990s, there was a shift away from the manufacture and supply of amphetamine to the more potent methamphetamine. The introduction of methamphetamine increased harms for existing people who used amphetamines, and resulted in an increase in the uptake of smoking methamphetamine among the broader groups of people who used drugs 'recreationally' (Ransley et al., 2011). Methamphetamine is structurally similar to amphetamine, but is more potent with stronger effects. These changes resulted in methamphetamines now being the

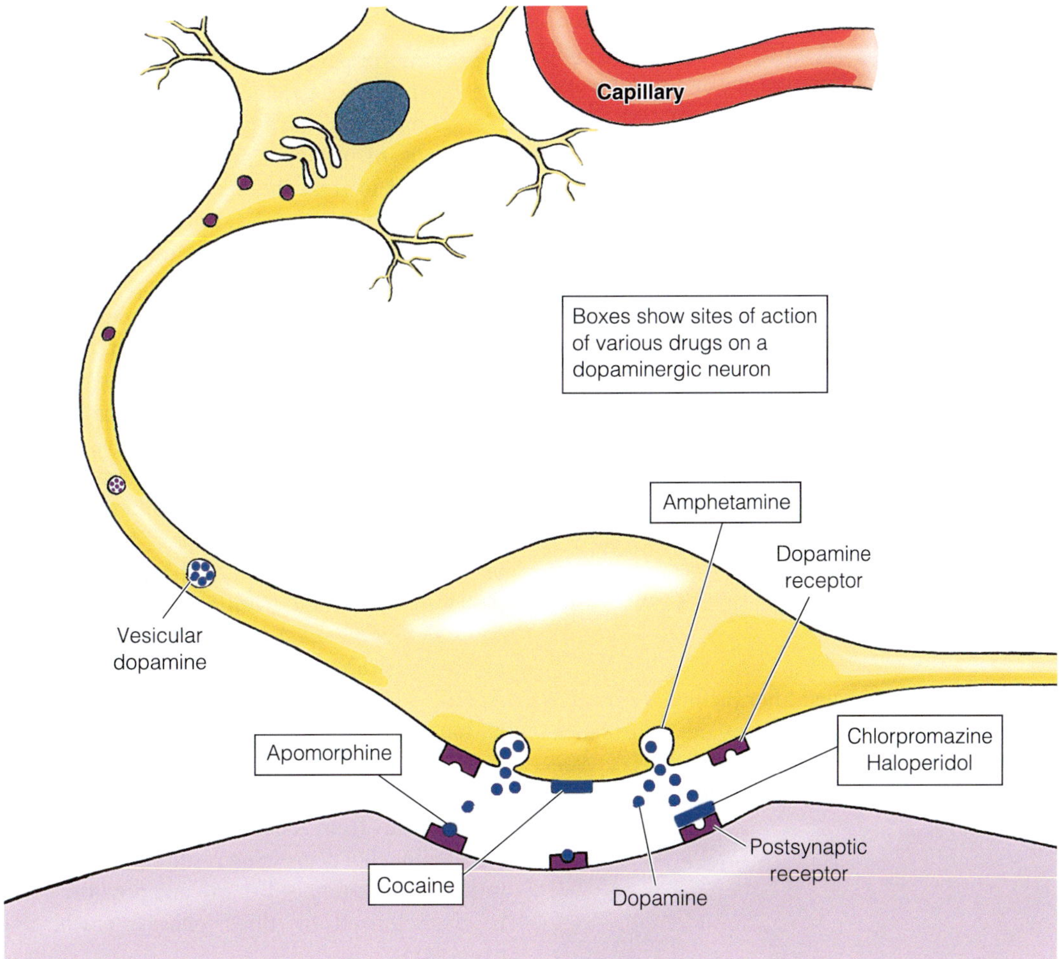

FIGURE 13.2 ■ Action of drugs on dopaminergic neurons. Note how apomorphine can take the place of dopamine in the receptor, and cocaine can perform the blocked reception of a neurotransmitter instead of an antipsychotic.
Source: Smock, T. K. (1999). *Physiological psychology: A neuroscience approach*. Upper Saddle River, NJ: Prentice Hall.

second most common illicit substance used in Australia (cannabis being the first).

Methamphetamines are available in several different forms, with different routes of administration. They can be used intranasally (snorted), smoked, taken orally as a powder or tablet, or used intravenously (IV). They include an oily form known as 'base' and a crystalline form known as 'crystal' or 'ice'. The current appeal of methamphetamines is prominently their relative cheapness, accessibility, flexibility of use, sustained effect on stamina, and feelings of pleasure. Smoking methamphetamine has become particularly associated with young Australians, especially in recreational environments such as nightclubs and dance parties. Its use is generally undertaken by older populations who have established psychostimulant use disorders. However, both routes are associated with an increased risk of dependency.

The harms associated with methamphetamine use are extensive, and include: significant heart disease, liver, kidney and lung damage, malnutrition and anorexia, dehydration, risk of blood-borne viruses (if injected), disorientation, mood swings and confusion. Methamphetamine morphologically changes the corpus callosum and causes skin lesions, perinatal complications, and hypertension (Ransley et al., 2011). The use of methamphetamine is associated with a range of mental health problems that can include anxiety, panic attacks, paranoia, mood swings, mania, hallucinations, aggression, suicidal thoughts and depressed mood. Many of these problems occur during intoxication; consequently, even people who use occasionally are at high risk of harm. People who use methamphetamine are also more likely to have polydrug use disorder than people who use other drugs.

Cocaine

In Australia, cocaine use is most prevalent among the 20–29-year age group. A gram of cocaine costs approximately $300, making this drug unattainable for many people. It also has an extremely short half-life when compared to the other psychostimulants, such as methamphetamine, and the effects diminish after about one hour. This results in people who use cocaine regularly developing very expensive habits. Harms associated with cocaine use include: hypertension and tachycardia, arrhythmias, hyperthermia, anxiety, anorexia, irritability and seizures. Long-term use can result in kidney damage and failure, stroke, drug-induced psychosis, depression and anxiety, and ongoing respiratory problems if snorted. Snorting also damages the mucosal lining of the nose, which can result in nosebleeds, nasal perforation and sinus problems. See the following Practice Example on cocaine use.

The use of crack cocaine, which is produced from treating cocaine with a mild base (usually sodium bicarbonate), is much less available in Australia as it is in other countries, namely the United States and South America. This drug is generally smoked through a glass pipe, and people experience rapid, intense euphoric effects of the drug.

Practice example

Will, a 32-year-old male, was brought to the hospital by his father. He was talkative and jumpy, and his eyes darted around the examination room. He repeatedly wiped his nose with his finger and rubbed the bottom of his face. He acted suspicious, and kept saying someone was after him. His family stated he had a $400-a-day cocaine habit. He began casually snorting a few lines once in a while when he needed a sense of control over his full load of university courses and full-time work. His cocaine use increased to every day, then every few hours.

See Figure 13.3 ■ for before and after pictures of people who use methamphetamine. The changes in appearance demonstrate the severity of the physiological effects. See Figure 13.4 ■ for the ongoing effects of cocaine use.

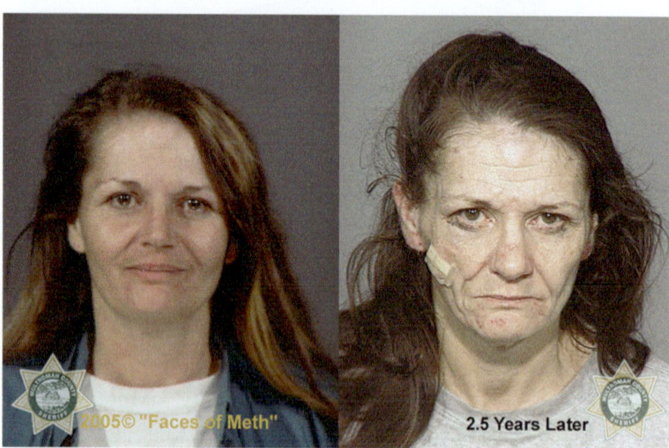

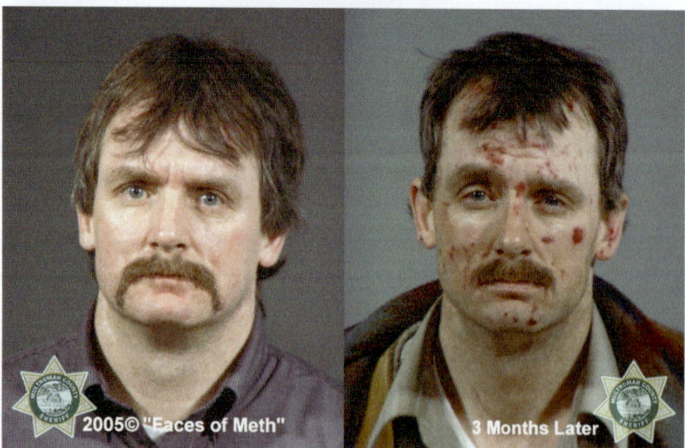

FIGURE 13.3 ■ Weight loss, apparent stress, and opportunistic infections are some of the visible consequences of using methamphetamine.
Photo courtesy of Faces of Meth Program.

Treatments

Treatment for psychostimulant use disorders continues to be a combination of behavioural and psychosocial approaches. No medications have yet proven to be effective in the treatment of psychostimulant use disorders, apart from those used to treat the symptoms (such as antidepressants or antihypertensives). Best practice in treatment involves a clear, mutually accepted treatment plan designed to meet the needs of the individual. Cognitive behavioural therapy (CBT) and contingency management, where the person has a backup plan for each stage of recovery, have been the most successful versions of behavioural and psychosocial treatment (Roll, Rawson, Ling & Shoptaw, 2009). CBT also assists with mental health problems, such as depression and anxiety, which are common among people who use methamphetamines. CBT and other behavioural therapies are discussed further in Chapter 25. For more information on treatments for methamphetamine use disorders, see the report entitled *Treatment approaches for users of methamphetamine: A practical guide for frontline workers* by the Australian government's Department of Health and Ageing (Jenner & Lee, 2008; retrieve from http://www.nationaldrugstrategy.gov.au).

Withdrawal

Withdrawal from cocaine or amphetamines is not life-threatening, but depression resulting from withdrawal can lead to suicidal ideation, self-harm and possibly death. Withdrawal is characterised by three phases: crash, withdrawal and extinction.

The 'crash' phase occurs approximately 12–24 hours after last use for methamphetamines, and within hours for cocaine. Signs and symptoms include exhaustion, fatigue, sleep disturbances, mood disturbances, low cravings and generalised aches and pains.

The 'withdrawal' phase commences around two to four days following last methamphetamine use, one to two days for cocaine. Signs and symptoms include strong cravings, fluctuating mood and energy levels, fatigue, restlessness, anxiety, agitation, vivid dreams, insomnia, muscle tension, poor concentration and attention, disturbances in thought (paranoid ideation, strange beliefs) and perception (hallucinations, misinterpretations).

The 'extinction' phase commences in weeks to months following last methamphetamine and cocaine use. Signs and symptoms include gradual resumption of normal mood with episodic fluctuations in mood and energy levels, alternating between irritability, restlessness, anxiety, agitation, fatigue, lacking energy and anhedonia. Episodic cravings and disturbed sleep are also common.

There are no effective pharmacology therapies identified for psychostimulant withdrawal. However, symptomatic medications may be beneficial, such as benzodiazepines for anxiety, agitation, insomnia and mood changes. Antipsychotic medications are also used when psychotic symptoms are evident.

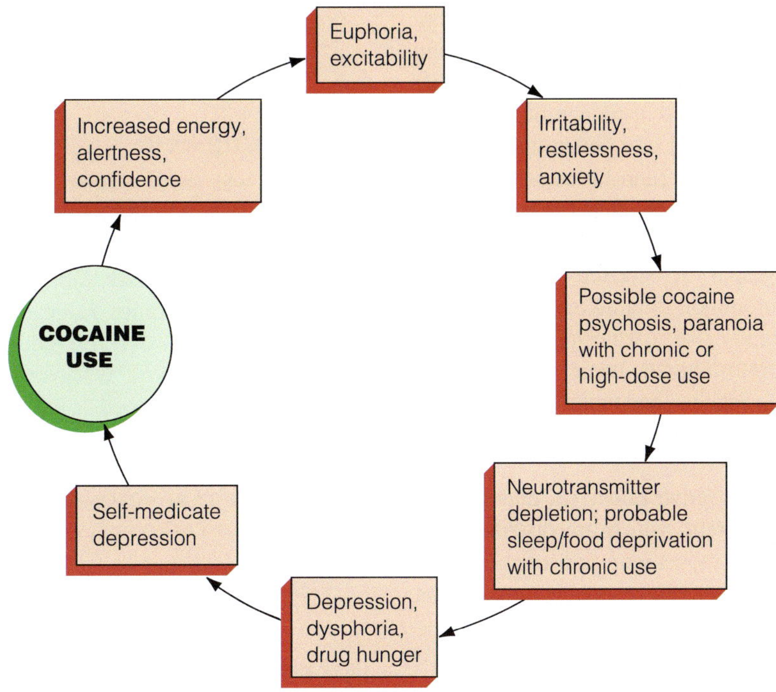

FIGURE 13.4 ■ The cycle of cocaine use.
Source: Reprinted with permission from Mim Landry, Danya International, Silver Spring, MD.

CANNABIS

Cannabis is a generic term used for drugs that are made from any of the genus *Cannabis* plants, including *Cannabis sativa* and *Cannabis indica*. Cannabis-derived drugs are usually produced in three main forms: marijuana (the dried leaves and flowering top of the plants), hashish (cannabis resin) and cannabis oil. Cannabis is not a 'single drug' that induces one single effect. Rather, it consists of over 400 chemical substances. Over 60 of these are cannabinoids, which, when ingested, activate the cannabinoid receptors in the body and produce a variety of effects on movement, appetite, emotion, memory and cognitive functions. The most commonly recognised cannabinoids found in the cannabis plant are Delta-9-Tetrahydrocannabinol (THC). THC is responsible for producing the psychoactive effects of cannabis. It can also be used to produce therapeutic effects that help to reduce pain, nausea and vomiting, and to stimulate appetite (NSW Health, 2009).

THC is found in the sticky yellow resin secreted by the tops and leaves of the ripe plants. Unlike alcohol, which is water-soluble and leaves the body through urine, breath and perspiration, THC is stored in the fatty tissues (especially the brain and reproductive system). Consequently, it can be detected in the body for up to six weeks.

Researchers have found that cannabis produces a significant analgaesic effect, and is modestly effective against the nausea and vomiting associated with chemotherapy. Medicinal applications of both THC and cannabidiol (a derivative) on pain have been examined, showing significant pain relief.

The medical use of cannabis for the treatment of nausea, glaucoma, cachexia, pain and spasticity has been consistently supported by the medical community, but there are legal and ethical risks that are not new and remain problematic (Nelson, 2011). The use of cannabis-based products for medical use is a subject of continuing social, political and medical debate. Specialists in some states of Australia can now prescribe medicinal cannabis for their patients who have exhausted standard treatment options. In New Zealand at the time of writing, ministerial approval is required before cannabis-based products can be prescribed.

History of cannabis use

The medicinal properties of cannabis have been recognised for thousands of years. Physicians in ancient China used it to relieve constipation, loss of appetite, and pain during childbirth. With the development of synthetic drugs in the 20th century, herbal remedies in general fell into disuse.

The first record of common hemp seeds brought to Australia was with the First Fleet, in the hope that hemp would be produced commercially in the new colonies for cloth for the sails of the wind-driven fleet. Until the late 19th century, 'cigares de joy' (cannabis cigarettes) were widely available, these claimed to relieve asthma, bronchitis, hay fever and influenza (Copeland, Gerber, Dillon & Swift, 2006).

Cannabis was not used widely in Australia until the 1970s. From that time, use of cannabis has increased steadily, peaking in the late 1990s. Since 1998, cannabis use has fallen slightly, but still remains the most widely used illicit drug in Australia.

Current use of cannabis

Approximately 10.5 per cent of Australia's population use cannabis on a regular basis (AIHW, 2011). Cannabis use is most prevalent among those aged in their twenties. The majority of people who try cannabis will use it sporadically during adolescence and early adulthood, and cease use once the late twenties is reached. However, there is a proportion of people who will use cannabis for longer and more often, and become dependent on the drug. Although most cannabis users will not go on to use other illicit drugs, such as amphetamines or heroin, most people who use these other drugs will have used cannabis first.

Cannabis can be ingested or smoked. In Australia, smoking cannabis is more common than taking hash. People who smoke cannabis generally use a water-pipe or 'bong', where the drug is packed into a small, metal bowl ('cone') which is lit. The person then inhales the smoke that is filtered through water. Cannabis is also smoked using cigarette papers ('joints'), similar to tobacco.

Cannabis exerts its psychoactive effect via endogenous cannabinoid receptors in the brain, which are distributed in areas that affect the control of movement, appetite, emotion and cognitive functioning. Subjectively, cannabis intoxication can lead to relaxation, enhanced sensory experiences, increased sociability and mirth, and a distorted perception of time (McLaren & Mattick, 2011).

Harms associated with cannabis use include adverse physical, psychological and social outcomes. Long-term cannabis use can result in respiratory problems, such as chronic cough, sputum production, wheezing and bronchitis. Cannabis smoke also contains carcinogens, and it has been found that more tar is inhaled and retained with cannabis when compared to tobacco (McLaren & Mattick, 2011). Cannabis also results in tachycardia, and has been associated with stroke and heart attack. It has also been associated with motor vehicle accidents, as THC compromises reaction times, attention, decision-making, hand–eye coordination and concentration.

Cannabis use has increasingly been associated with psychosis. People who use cannabis are more likely to suffer from psychosis than those who do not use cannabis. Moreover, those who experience psychosis are more likely to use cannabis than those who do not experience psychosis, and cannabis use has been found to make psychotic symptoms worse. Other negative effects of cannabis include anxiety, paranoid ideation, confusion, and impairment of short-term memory and attention. Long-term cannabis use has been associated with both physical and emotional changes.

Cannabis withdrawal

Withdrawal symptoms generally commence on day 1, peaking at days 2–3, returning to baseline after a week or two. These include anger and aggression, decreased appetite and weight loss, irritability, restlessness, stomach pains and cramping, chills, depressed mood, tremors and sleep disturbances. However, there is temporal variation in the profile of specific symptoms, with the late onset of aggression (day 4) and anger (day 6) being particularly significant, with the former often peaking after two weeks of abstinence (NSW Health, 2009).

With pharmacological treatment, not all people will need medications used in withdrawal. Symptomatic relief is needed for some people, generally for those who were using large quantities, such as low-dose benzodiazepines for anxiety and sleep disturbances. There is evidence that small doses of antidepressants such as mirtazapine assist with withdrawal symptoms.

Cannabis use is common in teenage culture. Therefore, nurses who work with teenagers must be knowledgeable about cannabis and its effects. When admitting a teenager to a psychiatric unit or interviewing a teenager as an outpatient, be aware of a variety of indicators of cannabis use. Parents need to be knowledgeable about cannabis use and alert to the following indications that it is being used:

- Cannabis smells like hemp or burning rope.
- Teenagers often burn incense or use perfumed sprays to mask its pungent odour.
- Teenagers may use eyedrops (Murine) so that their eyes will not be red, and they may cough a lot. Conjunctival redness and coughing can occur with cannabis use.
- A teenager who uses cannabis may have smoking paraphernalia—small plastic bags filled with dried leaves and cigarette papers

> **LIVED EXPERIENCE**
>
> **Seeking help**
>
> There was never a worse feeling than going into a service with the intention of trying to get help, even when I felt completely helpless, and having someone roll their eyes or say 'Oh, you again'. (This did happen!) Sometimes you can't articulate the space you are in, how bad you feel. To have someone who has stuck with you, who you know you can turn to without being judged, is invaluable. It really helped me to know that someone was there who wasn't enabling me, but was just waiting for me to find my own way. Then they stepped in and took charge.

HALLUCINOGENS

Hallucinogens (also known as 'psychedelics') include naturally occurring and synthetic compounds. They produce distortions in thoughts, mood and perceptions—typically inducing illusions or hallucinations. They are most commonly used in one-off social contexts, such as dance or rave parties, clubs and pubs, or at home. Hallucinogens cause hallucinations and unusual sensory experiences. Developed in 1938 for scientific research, LSD (lysergic acid diethylamide) became popular in the 1960s when Timothy Leary, a Harvard psychologist, described how it stimulated great insight and increased awareness. In the 1960s and 1970s, the US Army experimented with LSD by giving it without informed consent to unsuspecting army employees. One dramatic and much-publicised event concerned an army officer who leapt to his death from a window after unknowingly

SELF-AWARENESS
Maintaining therapeutic optimism

As with mental illness, people experience personal recovery with or without continued substance use.

- ***Realise that both mental illness and substance use disorders are often long-term, relapsing conditions.*** Understand that progress may be slow and setbacks inevitable, despite your best efforts and those of the person. Appreciate small steps forward and reframe setbacks as learning opportunities.
- ***Understand that even if the person is not currently making much effort towards better management of their disorders, the development of a trusting relationship with you is helping to set the stage for movement toward recovery in the future.*** A positive, person-centred and valued relationship with a mental health professional or with a peer support worker is one of the factors that prompt people with mental health disorders to move toward recovery.
- ***Talk to people who are in recovery.*** Hearing about how these individuals overcame challenges to become happier and more stable will give you more confidence that people who are currently struggling with similar obstacles can also overcome them. You may be able to work with a peer support worker who has a lived experience of recovery from drug and alcohol use disorders.
- ***Don't be afraid to talk to people about spirituality.*** Mental health providers often underestimate how important spiritual concerns are in the lives of people with substance use disorders. Ask people about their spiritual beliefs and practices, and be flexible in helping them find support for their spirituality. Access to these inner resources is especially important when people lack external support.
- ***Find mentors who are successful in working with people with substance use disorders.*** Seek their help in dealing with situations you find difficult or frustrating.
- ***Take good care of your own physical, mental and spiritual health.*** You can role-model healthy behaviour (never underestimate the power of a good example!), and renewing your own energy means you have more to give in your relationships with the people in your care.

LIVED EXPERIENCE
Connection

I always responded better to health professionals who were open and available emotionally. I don't mean they babied me, you don't need that, but they didn't speak down to or belittle me, they didn't make assumptions about me. They were just open and honest and tried to make a real connection.

ingesting LSD. Once the danger of LSD use was publicised, the unethical research became public knowledge. Physician researchers also were interested in experimenting with the uses of LSD in the treatment of a variety of diseases.

The effects of hallucinogens

There are a number of drugs that come into this category. They include lysergic acid diethylamide (LSD), phencyclidine (PCP), psilocybin (magic mushrooms), and dimethyl tryptamine (DMT). They come in a wide variety of forms, from plants to small tabs of printed blotting paper ('trips'). Teenagers today are unacquainted with the LSD horror stories of the 1960s. Today, people use LSD predominantly to get high rather than to expand consciousness. Approximately 1.4 per cent of the Australian population use some form of hallucinogen on a regular basis (AIHW, 2011). Psychological and physical dependence are unlikely, because each experience with a hallucinogen is different. Increased creativity and brilliant personality revelations, presumed effects of the drugs, are short-lived at best. Some people may present to hospital with pronounced mood swings: detachment may alternate with fear, paranoia, distress and panic. It is important that the nurse provide reassurance and supportive care so that the person does not injure themselves or others during a panic attack.

LIVED EXPERIENCE
LSD

LSD was always treated like a bit of a party drug in my circles, but it was one of the most dangerous drugs I ever took. For me, it always seemed to open the gates to underlying fears and anxieties, so I had mostly bad experiences. At first it seems great, colours are the first things that change, everything becomes deeper and more vivid. I've never seen trees quite so green. You feel like you can reach out and touch it, and if you do your skin will change colour, too. Things start to move randomly, become multi-dimensional where before they were flat, so it's quite sensory at first. But then it becomes emotional and a little scary—I was sure I saw people chasing me through the trees, and I became really paranoid and frightened. I couldn't control my body temperature, and words that people said didn't make sense. I remember one time knocking for ages on a door because I couldn't figure out how to turn the handle. Another time I started to pull my skin off because I was sure there was something crawling on me. I had flashbacks for many years afterwards; if I stared at a pattern on a wallpaper, for example, the flowers would start to move, colours change, that kind of thing.

Treatment

The dangers of hallucinogens include 'bad trips' and flashbacks. People who experience *bad trips* may appear psychotic and extremely fearful. Reassuring the person and pointing out reality are helpful; occasionally, tranquilisers or antipsychotics are given. The symptoms usually disappear within 12 hours, but may persist for months. People who are mentally ill or emotionally conflicted are more likely to have bad trips and flashbacks and to require hospitalisation than are ordinary users.

Flashbacks are a spontaneous reliving of the experiences the person felt while under the influence of the drug, although the person is drug-free. The experience may involve perceptual distortions, a variety of physical feelings, and strong emotions such as fear and pleasure. Flashbacks are generally brief, and they occur less frequently over time. Flashbacks may be induced by stress, fatigue, and drug or alcohol ingestion.

SOLVENTS

Solvents—glue, fuels, paints, aerosols, air fresheners, the substance used to re-sole shoes, hairspray, and the propellants in canned whipped cream—can be used by school-age children because they are cheap and easy to obtain.

The effects of inhalants

Solvents are also known as 'inhalants' or 'volatile substances', and are products that vaporise in the air, causing a 'high' feeling when the fumes are inhaled. Inhalants are inexpensive, easily available and often legal. Their use causes euphoria, light-headedness and excitement. Children are the most frequent users. Adults who use inhalants often have a long history of polydrug use.

> **Practice example**
>
> **Inhalant use**
>
> Jack is 13 years old child, is homeless and living on the streets of Sydney. He came to the attention of the clinic because he had been arrested for purse-snatching. On clinical examination, Jack appears giddy, dirty, dishevelled, confused and belligerent. His speech is slurred, he has an unsteady gait, and he smells like glue. His eyes are red and tearing, he is coughing, and he is nauseated. He has avoided attending school and has received no health care.

Patterns of use

Solvents are sniffed or inhaled in a variety of ways, such as from a rag soaked with the inhalant and placed in a plastic bag. Gas is frequently inhaled directly from a tank. Amyl and butyl nitrate (called 'poppers') can be easily concealed and passed around, and paint thinner can be concealed in a soft drink can. This group also includes gases (e.g. nitrous oxide) and highly volatile compounds or mixtures of compounds (petrol, paint—'chroming', glues, aerosol propellants and paint thinners).

Metallic-coloured spraypaints are popular choices, as the propellant—the substance being inhaled—must be more powerful to push out the heavy metal flakes. You will know this is occurring when you see a paper bag concealing the spraypaint and tell-tale gold or silver flecks around the mouth. Use of these inhalants and solvents can cause ventricular fibrillation, decreased cardiac output, serious brain damage and sudden death.

Treatment

Although withdrawal must be managed, as with the other substances covered in this chapter, careful assessment, early identification, education and prevention are particularly critical, because so many people who use inhalants are children and teenagers. Be aware of the programs and resources available, and support legislation to make it more difficult for minors to obtain glue and paint products. For more information on solvent use in Australia, the Drugs Council of Australia has developed a website entitled the *National Inhalants Information Service,* accessed at http://www.inhalantsinfo.org.au/statistics.php

TOBACCO

Tobacco is the major cause of drug-related deaths in Australia. There are over 4000 chemicals in tobacco smoke, many of which are poisonous, and 43 of which have been proven to be carcinogens. These chemicals include nicotine (the addictive component), tar (which causes throat and lung cancer), and carbon monoxide (together with nicotine, it increases the risk of heart disease, atherosclerosis and other circulatory problems). There is no safe level of tobacco consumption (NSW Health, 2009). Populations with psychiatric conditions and substance use disorders have higher rates of smoking, and show a lack of responsiveness to smoking cessation treatments. People with schizophrenia have particularly high rates of smoking. It has been shown that tobacco cravings are increased in those with schizophrenia when compared to the smoking population with no comorbid psychiatric disorders (Potvin et al., 2016). There are interactions between the chemicals in tobacco and the dopamine systems in the brain, which are involved in schizophrenia.

The effects of nicotine and tobacco

Nicotine is a stimulant that acts in the central and peripheral nervous systems at cells that are normally acted upon by the neurotransmitter acetylcholine. In the CNS, nicotine occupies the receptors for acetylcholine in both the dopamine and serotonin neural pathways. This causes the release of both dopamine and norepinephrine. The stimulant nicotine initially increases alertness and cognitive ability, and then has a depressant effect.

Research suggests that dopaminergic processes have a role in regulating the reinforcing effects of nicotine, making cessation of use more difficult. Dopamine blockers can alter smoking behaviour for a limited time, but people compensate for this by smoking more. The usual effect of increased dopamine turnover in the system is the reduction of hunger impulses. Once when someone tries to quit smoking and dopamine is reduced, hunger impulses return and the person may gain weight.

The use of tobacco also interferes with the pharmacological effects of many psychiatric medications, particularly those metabolised by the liver. This results in lower plasma levels of the medications, thus the person needs more medication to achieve the intended results. This effect appears to be due not to nicotine but to the effects of benzopyrenes (tobacco carcinogens).

Although the amount of tobacco consumed by smokers in the general population has fallen somewhat over the past decade, smoking is still of concern to the Australian public. Tobacco smoking is the single most preventable cause of ill health and death in Australia, contributing to more drug-related hospitalisations and deaths than alcohol and illicit drug use combined (AIHW, 2016). Tobacco is associated with cancer, heart disease, emphysema, hypertension and death. Given its negative physiological impact, tobacco use in Australia remains a major public health issue.

Patterns of use

Smoking tobacco is an extremely common addiction, and is seen routinely despite smoke-free environments and restrictions on cigarette access. Approximately 15 per cent of the Australian population smokes, around 2.8 million people (AIHW, 2011). A person's smoking status varies by social characteristics, including education, employment, socioeconomic status, geography and Indigenous status. This is especially true with psychiatric–mental health clients. Their work activities may be dictated by their symptom level, and they frequently experience unemployment.

Typically, people begin smoking at a young age, because of peer pressure, or during times of stress. Use of tobacco products can be interrupted briefly during respiratory illnesses, hospitalisations, pregnancy, and following health care providers' advice on smoking cessation. Return to tobacco use after a brief time is all too common; smokers find it very difficult to quit smoking successfully. Only 10 per cent to 25 per cent of people maintain their smoking abstinence over a long period of time, even if they received pharmacological cessation support, such as nicotine replacement systems and psychopharmacology (Raupach & van Schayck, 2011). Evidence indicates that smoke-free environments only protect people from the force of second-hand smoke, but do not reduce actual smoking. Smokers practise anticipatory smoking (that is, they smoke more before they are going into a smoke-free environment) to ensure their desired level of nicotine is maintained. Smokers also continue to smoke to avoid the symptoms of nicotine withdrawal.

Treatment

The most commonly-used approach for treating nicotine dependence is nicotine replacement therapy (patch, inhaler, lozenge, gum), which reduces craving by maintaining the blood level of nicotine. Support in a variety of forms is also useful in assisting clients with this difficult addiction. Centralised telephone counselling and support services, such as the Quitline, with an emphasis on relapse prevention, have demonstrated long-term abstinence effectiveness. Understanding the mechanisms of behaviour change will enhance your ability to help people transition to healthier behaviours.

POLYDRUG USE

Over the past two decades, Australian people have increasingly used more than one drug at a time. In fact, a person who presents with a single type of drug use is becoming increasingly rare (NSW Health, 2009). Medications, over-the-counter drugs, naturopathic, homoeopathic, legal and illicit drugs all have the potential to interact with each other. This fact complicates diagnosis and treatment, and increases the hazards associated with substance use. The impact of these multiple drugs on one another occurs in a variety of ways, as follows:

- *Synergistic or potentiating effects* are possible where the effects of two or more drugs taken together are greater than the singular effects of each drug.
- *Addictive effects* occur when two drugs that have similar effects are used together.
- *Paradoxical effects* occur if a drug causes a reaction opposite to that expected. Paradoxical effects may occur when only one drug is taken or when several drugs are taken.
- A *pathological reaction* may also result from the ingestion of only one or several drugs; it is an unexpected and dramatic response to the drug. For example, the combination of alcohol and cannabis is especially dangerous, because THC suppresses the nausea that results from an overdose of alcohol. Consequently, the person may continue to drink, risking respiratory depression, coma and death.

Cocaine and alcohol are frequently used together; the cocaine gives the user a brief high, and the alcohol masks the ensuing depression. When the cocaine wears off, the person is intoxicated and unable to drive safely. Prescription drugs and alcohol are also a common combination.

DESIGNER 'PARTY' DRUGS

Designer drugs are also called 'party drugs', 'recreational drugs' and 'club drugs' in Australia. They include ecstasy (3,4-methylenedioxymethamphetamine or MDMA), gamma hydroxybutyrate (GHB), rohypnol (flunitrazepam), ketamine and mephedrone. However, new drugs are emerging at an unprecedented rate as manufacturers use new chemicals to replace those that are banned. The potential harms associated with these new drugs are difficult to quantify. There is very little information about whether the substances are toxic or even carcinogenic.

Methylenedioxymethamphetamine, also called 'ecstasy', 'X' and 'MDMA', is an amphetamine with hallucinogenic properties with effects lasting three to six hours. It is easily and readily accessible. In high doses, MDMA has been associated with malignant hyperthermia and rhabdomyolysis. The effects of ecstasy are caused by stimulating the secretion of serotonin in the brain, as well as inhibiting the reuptake of serotonin and dopamine.

Other drugs are now sold as 'ecstasy', and ecstasy tablets often contain a range of drugs (including amphetamine, various amphetamine derivatives, caffeine, aspirin, paracetamol or ketamine) in addition to, or in place of, MDMA. According to the AIHW (2011), around 3.0 per cent of the Australian population take ecstasy on a regular basis, namely people aged 20–29 years of age.

Flunitrazepam, also known as 'Rohypnol', 'roofies' and the 'date-rape pill', is a fast-acting benzodiazepine that causes anterograde amnesia (memory loss of events occurring while under the influence of the drug) and is tasteless, colourless and odourless. Because it can be used to sexually assault victims when mixed into drinks, it is the modern-day version of a 'Mickey Finn' (alcohol and chloral hydrate).

Another 'date-rape' substance is gamma-hydroxybutyrate (called 'GHB', 'liquid ecstasy', 'grievous bodily harm', 'fantasy' and 'blue nitro'). It produces euphoria, disinhibition and strong sexual urges. GHB was first manufactured and used as a general anaesthetic. It was also widely available in the 1980s as a dietary supplement and bodybuilding product. GHB has since been withdrawn from use in many countries because of unwanted side-effects, such as seizures, drowsiness, agitation, depressed breathing, unconsciousness and even death. It is now considered an illicit drug in Australia.

Ketamine hydrochloride ('special K') is a dissociative anaesthetic drug used by veterinarians and medical professionals. It is also used recreationally because of its hallucinogen properties, and is mostly obtained from the diversion of licit supplies (veterinarians and pharmaceutical companies). Non-medical use is illegal in Australia. The physical effects of ketamine include drowsiness, numbness and nausea. The psychological effects include altered perception, disorientation, hallucinations and a dissociative state. Anxiety, panic attacks, nightmares and 'flashbacks', mania, depression, ongoing disassociation and suicidal ideation are some of the unwanted side-effects.

Mephedrone ('miaow-miaow', 'plant food', 'kitty cat') was originally marketed as a plant fertiliser. It is a synthetically produced cathinone (hence the 'cat' names), a synthetic copy of cathinone found in the khat plant of eastern Africa. Mephedrone produces similar effects to ecstasy and amphetamines. It is one of the newer types of 'synthetic' drugs, with more and more becoming available on the market and sold over the internet.

GROUPS AT RISK FOR SUBSTANCE USE DISORDERS

People in a number of different circumstances can use drugs and alcohol. However, there are those who are at greater risk for substance problems than others.

Teenagers

Although many adolescents experiment with drugs and alcohol for only a brief time, many more who do so develop substance use disorders. Susceptibility to addiction seems to depend on the following variables:

- form and potency of the drug
- dosage
- frequency of use
- pattern of use
- stress
- personality and genetic make-up of the user
- family culture.

People use drugs and alcohol that initially produce good feelings to escape from the stress and strain of life. A teenager who relies on a quick 'fix' (a drug) to ease mental pain does not learn healthy coping skills. If teenagers do not learn healthy coping skills or work through the pains and mood swings associated with living, they will not achieve a necessary developmental stage. Consequently, they remain fixated at a dependent level of development. They enter a dangerous cycle that is unlikely to be interrupted without professional intervention. Drug use, regardless of what drug is used, inevitably affects all areas of a teenager's life: school, work, social and family relationships, and sense of self-worth. (See Chapter 21 for an assessment of teenage drug use.)

Adolescences with substance use disorders manifest more psychopathological conditions than non-using adolescents do. Symptoms include feelings of depression, inadequacy, frustration, helplessness and self-alienation. These teenagers also have ego structure deficiencies and poor impulse control. As you can imagine, once a person starts using a substance instead of doing the personal work to learn how to self-soothe and cope, it predicts continued substance use. The earlier a child begins using a dependence-producing drug, the more likely the child is to use other dependence-producing drugs. Teenagers who use alcohol and drugs are likely to continue to use them in adulthood. Substance use during adolescence has been associated with alterations in brain structure, function and neurocognition, because of the toxic effects of drugs and alcohol on the developing brain. Alcohol, the legal substance, can be dangerous for teenagers, as adolescence may be a period of heightened vulnerability for alcohol's effect on the brain (Clark, Thatcher & Tapert 2008).

People with co-occurring mental health disorders and substance use disorders

There are a number of different ways to refer to people with mental health disorders who also have substance use disorders. *Comorbid mental health and substance use disorders, co-existing disorders* and *dual diagnosis* (referring to both a mental illness and substance use disorder diagnosis), among others, are terms that try to explain the co-existence of two or more demanding and divergent disorders. Co-occurring disorders presents particular challenges in terms of identification, prevention and treatment.

The numerous problems facing people with mental health disorders make them susceptible to both substance use and targeting by drug dealers. Poor coping mechanisms, heightened stress, economic factors, and challenging and demoralising symptoms influence a person's ability to steer clear of the escapism that drugs and alcohol offers. People may also use substances to self-medicate the symptoms of their mental disorder (e.g. the use of alcohol to try to alleviate the symptoms of an anxiety disorder, such as social phobia).

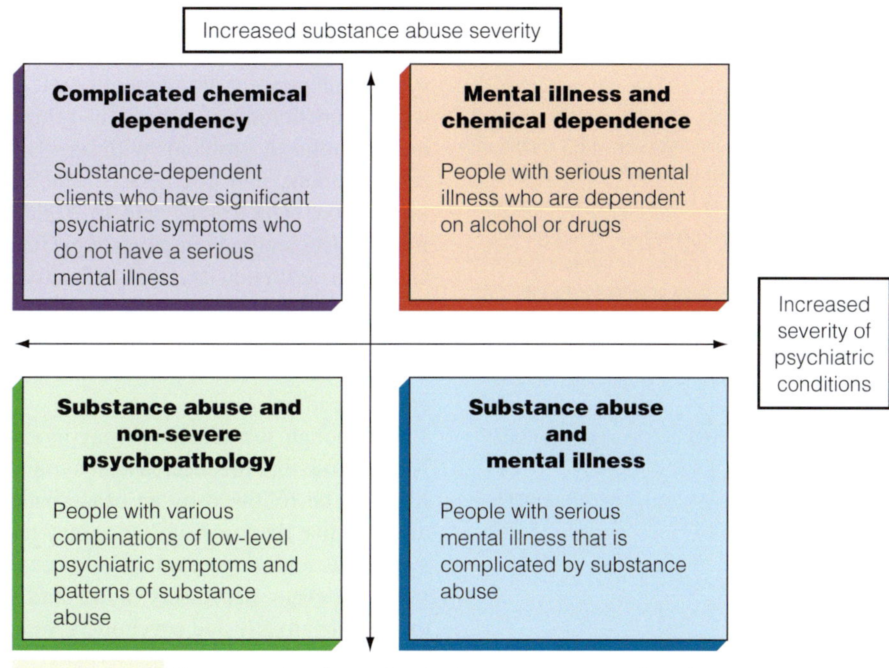

FIGURE 13.5 ■ Characteristics of people who have co-occurring disorders.

It is important to remember in this discussion, as highlighted early in this chapter, that substance use disorders are types of mental health disorders. Both substance use disorders and other mental illnesses are caused by overlapping factors, such as underlying brain deficits, genetic vulnerabilities and/or early exposure to stress or trauma (Croton, 2011). The characteristics of people who have co-occurring disorders are discussed in Figure 13.5 ■.

In an Australia context, in mental health treatment settings, approximately 20 per cent to 75 per cent of people in treatment will have co-occurring substance use. In drug and alcohol treatment settings, approximately 19 per cent to 85 per cent of people receiving treatment will have been diagnosed with a co-occurring mental health disorder (Croton, 2011).

Characteristics of people with co-occurring disorders

The challenges of the problems that these people face impede on their ability to attend appointments and adhere to medication regimens, thereby increasing the likelihood of relapse. The focus of any intervention for people with co-occurring mental health and substance use disorders therefore needs to empower the person to manage their own lives to their full potential. Some people take longer than others to trust practitioners and services. People with co-occurring disorders are more likely to enter into a relationship where they are assisted in identifying and expressing their own needs and can set goals and objectives to achieve them (NSW Health, 2009).

Treatment programs for people with mental health and substance use disorders are best constructed with harm-minimisation perspectives and built-in extensive psychosocial supports. Because this combination creates consequences (see Box 13.2) of which people may not be aware, it is important to educate yourself as a nurse and the people in your care. Staff members with credentials in mental health nursing and substance treatment and rehabilitation work collaboratively with people to manage the numerous chaotic upheavals characteristic of either one of the disorders at any time. Mental health nurses are equipped to deal with people who have co-occurring substance use. The high prevalence of co-occurring disorders in Australia indicates that many mental health nurses have been providing care to people with mental health and substance use disorders within the course of their practice for many years (NSW Health, 2009). The populations that are cared for in both the alcohol and drug and mental health treatment sectors are frequently stigmatised, commonly have chronic, relapsing disorders, and experience illnesses which have a marked impact on behavioural and social functioning. Therefore, both workforces tend to be very effective in dealing with complex presentations.

Box 13.2 Consequences of using substances when living with a serious mental illness

- Increased psychiatric symptoms
- Poor treatment adherence
- Increased need for, and use of, emergency health care services
- Poor response to psychiatric medications
- Unstable clinical course
- Increased frequency and length of hospitalisation
- Chronic threats to health
- Increased risk of tardive dyskinesia
- Behavioural problems
- Suicide
- Homelessness
- Violence

Practice example

Comorbidity

Ian, age 25, was diagnosed with schizophrenia six years ago, when he was a university student. After becoming ill, Ian lost most of his friends, because he was preoccupied with a delusional relationship with a radio talk-show host and spent most of his time alone in his room. He dropped out of university, because his mental disorganisation and frequent psychiatric hospitalisations interfered with his ability to attend classes. Several times he has tried to work, but has not been able to keep a job.

After Ian's most recent hospitalisation, he was moved into a mental health rehabilitation unit and began receiving biweekly injections of a long-acting neuroleptic medication. His delusional symptoms reduced and he started making friends. Several months ago, Ian and two of his male friends from the rehabilitation unit moved into an apartment in a neighbourhood known for its high incidence of opioid use.

Ian's case manager believes Ian is using heroin. He has lost weight, become irritable and paranoid, and has been threatened with eviction for failing to pay his rent. Ian was brought to the emergency department by the police after becoming agitated and threatening the cashier in a service station.

People with co-occurring disorders display a wide range of clinical characteristics and service needs, depending on the nature and severity of their mental health and substance-related disorders (Dickerson & Johnson, 2012).

Gender differences

Because men and women have different rates of substance use disorders and different rates of some psychiatric disorders, gender differences in the range of co-occurring mental health and substance use disorders also exist. Women have a lower prevalence of all types of substance use disorders when compared to men; however, women often have more serious and disabling medical complications from alcohol use disorders.

Women are more likely to have pre-existing mood and/or anxiety disorders than men. They are also reported to link their substance use with specific past traumas, such as physical or sexual abuse, much more often than men do. Women are much less likely to have antisocial personality disorder, which is a significant risk factor for substance use disorders.

Women often have different motivations for entering treatment, such as childcare concerns. Research on women and alcohol makes it clear that treatment programs should be geared to women's needs. Such programs might include women-only groups, lesbian-only groups, female health professionals, meetings with recovered women, and help for families.

Biological, as well as psychological, factors are thought to contribute to the person's use of drugs and alcohol to **self-medicate** (use substances such as drugs and alcohol to address symptoms of mental illness). Some substances of use may stimulate neurotransmitter systems in the brain that have been altered both by the disease and by some of the agents used to treat schizophrenia. Animal studies indicate that addictive agents increase activity in the brain systems dependent on dopamine (DA), a neurotransmitter whose functioning is altered in schizophrenia. In addition, nicotine relieves problems with sensory processing caused by schizophrenia, and counteracts side-effects of psychotropic medication, which may help to explain the extremely high frequency of smoking in this group (Gandhi, Williams, Menza, Galazyhn & Benowitz, 2010). Positive benefits of smoking for those with schizophrenia have also been found, making it very difficult for people to cease tobacco use, as smoking provides people with a purpose and something they feel they can succeed in.

Although substance use may produce symptom relief, it is often true that this decrease in symptoms is short-lived and likely to be followed by an exacerbation of symptoms. It is also true that the same substance may relieve some psychiatric symptoms and worsen others—for example, stimulants may briefly elevate depressed mood and increase energy, but exacerbate anxiety and psychotic symptoms.

Hospitalised people

Nurses working across all clinical areas need to be alert to the possibility that people with physical illnesses may have a substance use disorder and may be in danger of withdrawal. All episodes of care provide an important opportunity or a critical moment for a person to be offered appropriate and easy-to-understand health information and education related to drug and alcohol use, and assessment and evidence-based interventions if a problem is identified. In Australia, access to comprehensive health care is every individual's right. All health professionals need to ensure that their own attitudes, value judgments and personal experiences do not interfere with a person's right to quality care (NSW Health, 2009). If you see symptoms that do not mesh with the condition under treatment, you may want to keep in mind that you may be seeing symptoms of substance withdrawal. Be alert and sensitive if your nursing assessment reveals any of the following:

- debilitation out of proportion to the presenting health problem
- physical findings that do not correlate to the chief complaint
- unsteady gait, slurring of speech, dilated pupils, night sweats, chills, blackouts, tremors, skin tracks, abscesses, nasal septum perforation, or jaundice
- weight loss, poor hygiene and poor nutrition
- symptoms of substance withdrawal syndromes
- failure to attain pain relief with the usual and customary dosage of medication.

Alert the primary health care provider and suggest appropriate laboratory studies (such as liver function tests). A nursing assessment should include questions about the person's drinking habits. If alcohol use disorders are suspected, a helpful, matter-of-fact, but nonjudgmental stance will facilitate the person's acceptance of treatment for possible withdrawal symptoms. Keep in mind when asking about alcohol use that you do not use terminology such as 'standard drink', as many people will not understand what that is. If you want to use this term, you will need to explain this first to the person. It is best not to quantify the amount for the person (i.e. 'Do you drink around three drinks per day?'), as many people will just agree with your estimation or try to go under this amount. If you are finding it difficult to quantify the amount, and you suspect an alcohol use disorder, overestimate the person's use before asking them quantifying questions (i.e. 'How much do you drink daily? Around 10 drinks?'). People will be more likely to come in under your overestimation, and you will then have an accurate answer. However, please be mindful not to use this type of questioning with young people—they may try to match or beat your overestimates!

Older adults

Older adults who are being treated for several chronic illnesses by different health care providers are at risk for drug interactions and/or drug dependence. Alcohol use is also prevalent in older Australian adults. For men and women aged 65 years and over on a day when alcohol was consumed, 40 per cent of all men and 45 per cent of all women had one or two drinks, 23 per cent and 7 per cent had three or four drinks, and 15 per cent and 1 per cent, respectively, had five or more drinks (AIHW, 2011). For this reason, you should obtain a good history from the older person, including a list of all the drugs and alcohol regularly taken, frequency of use, dosage and duration of use. It is often useful to ask the family of an older person to bring all of their drugs to the hospital for review, rather than relying on memory. Frequently, the confusion seen in older people is a direct consequence of drug interactions or malabsorption.

In addition, substance use, especially alcohol use disorders, is less likely to be detected and treated in older adults than in younger people. It often goes unrecognised because the signs of substance use are difficult to distinguish from the changes associated with normal ageing or degenerative brain disease. Therefore, it is likely that problematic drinking behaviours and other substance use are likely to increase with the ageing Australian population. Older adults with alcohol use disorders—those who started drinking at a younger age as well as those who commenced harmful levels of consumption later in life—have reported loneliness, losses, depression and meagre social support networks as antecedents of their alcohol use.

Health care providers

Substance use occurs across all generations, cultures and occupations, including nursing. Many factors place nurses and other health care providers at risk for developing substance use disorders. Nurses in general tend to work under a great deal of stress and have easy access to drugs. Every day, they give people medication to relieve pain. It is an easy leap to self-medication.

Colleagues of substance-dependent health care workers need to be alert to behaviours that suggest a problem. Making ethical decisions can be difficult. That is why when evaluating a health worker and substance use situation, the colleague must review the total picture. They should attempt to talk with the professional who they suspect is having difficulty, before documenting and reporting such behaviour to a supervisor. It is very common for colleagues to cover up for one another. Shielding a drug- or alcohol-dependent health care provider—whatever the professional discipline—puts at risk public safety, the health care provider and the profession. Nurses, however, need to understand that their dependent colleagues experience a health disorder not a moral problem. This understanding empowers us to work together to help one another. Warning signs of behaviour by health care providers that suggest substance use disorders are in Your Assessment Approach.

All states and territories in Australia have employee assistance programs (EAP) for nurses and other health care professionals working in the public sector, and who experience impairment-related issues, such as substance use disorders. We have an obligation to our colleagues and the people in our care to ensure that the health professional voluntarily seeks help, and we should encourage and support them to do so.

YOUR ASSESSMENT APPROACH — Warning signs of health care providers with substance use disorders

Be alert for the following behaviours that suggest a colleague may be experiencing a substance use disorder:

- frequent absenteeism before and after days off
- always working (in order to obtain a supply)
- irritability
- abrupt mood changes
- inappropriate affect
- careless charting and care activities
- problems with the record-keeping of drugs or drug inventory (missing drugs, frequent 'wasting' of drugs, inaccurate records)
- frequent errors in judgment
- alcohol (stale or fresh) on breath
- frequent disappearance from the assigned area
- offering to give medication to people who do not request or do not seem to need it
- frequent night-shift work
- having people who complain of little or no pain relief after the health care provider has administered the medication.

LIVED EXPERIENCE

Peer worker

I worked in a large health service for some time during my using. At first it was quite manageable; I would use once a day or every couple of days, always after work. But it did affect my behaviour and concentration. I was always a little distracted in the afternoons and would rush off. I didn't socialise with my workmates, because they would have known, some of them were drug and alcohol workers! As my tolerance worsened, I would have days off, or be running late, and then eventually using became more important than work. I think the real turning point came when a client of the service looked at me and said 'Oh, you're stoned right now, aren't you?', and here was I trying to tell them why they should go to rehab. They just laughed at me, and I realised I'd crossed the line and lost all credibility and had no right to tell anyone else what they should be doing. I quit my job soon after that.

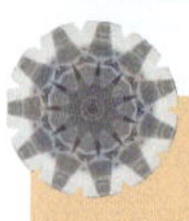

NURSING PROCESS
People with substance use disorders

As substance use becomes more prevalent in society, a greater number of people will be admitted to hospitals and clinics for help with intoxication and withdrawal. Substance use is a health disorder, and not a weakness or flaw. It may be true that some health care providers have negative biases regarding people who use drugs and alcohol, labelling their behaviours as selfish and self-destructive. Some may question whether the person with a substance use disorder has a right to health care resources. A moralistic attitude such as this always alienates the person, and is not scientifically sound. Nurses need to keep in mind that, in the health care setting, drug and alcohol use is always seen as a health issue and not a moral issue.

It is always important for the health care provider to maintain an objective, clinical perspective that does not lapse into personal bias or prejudice, particularly in ways that sabotage the delivery of quality health care to the recipient. Recognising and accepting that substance use disorders are challenging for the person, often with remissions and exacerbations, should keep you from succumbing to the frustration felt by many who care for people who relapse. At stressful times in life, anyone may develop a dependence on drugs or alcohol; however, certain people seem to be predisposed to the disorders. Your expertise in the stages of the nursing process is vital to the care of people with substance use problems. Your focus should be on helping people work toward self-awareness, good health, and good interpersonal relationships so that they can lead productive, fulfilling, happy lives.

Drugs change rapidly, and nurses must keep up with the 'drug scene' to be able to assess and treat substance use. Along with the knowledge acquired from reading, continuing education programs and seminars, nurses need self-knowledge to be good therapists with people who experience substance use disorders. Ongoing critical self-analysis of your own susceptibility to substance use is useful. See Self-awareness for a list of questions to guide this self-analysis.

Assessment

Carry out an accurate assessment of the substances used to anticipate potential toxic and withdrawal effects, and to make nursing care plans as specific and relevant as possible.

SELF-AWARENESS
Your stress response and susceptibility to substance use

Examine who you are when you are stressed, by answering the following questions. Attend to what your answers suggest about your coping mechanisms and your susceptibility to substance use.

Check the substances you choose to use when you seek comfort from stress:

- Food (carbohydrates)
- Food (non-carbohydrates)
- Cigarettes
- Coffee
- Wine
- Beer
- Spirits
- Chocolate
- Tea
- Pain relievers (paracetamol, ibuprofen, other)
- Cannabis
- Recreational drugs

At what rate do you use any of the above?

- More than five times a day
- More than two times a day
- Daily
- Only at work/school
- Only on the weekends
- Only at dinner
- Only at parties
- Monthly
- Occasionally

At what rate would you use these substances if you had the money, time off, no weight concerns, or other release from responsibility?

- More than five times a day
- More than two times a day
- Daily
- Only at work/school
- Only on the weekends
- Only at dinner
- Only at parties
- Monthly
- Occasionally

For example, a person with a methamphetamine use disorder who is malnourished, exhausted and depressed needs immediate diet regulation, rest and gradual involvement in a treatment program. See the nursing care plan for the person with methamphetamine intoxication at the end of this chapter. People with cocaine use are likely to be resistant to treatment, and need active staff intervention and a structured program to involve them in treatment. They should not be left alone or purposefully isolated. It is important that all people over 16 years of age who are hospitalised are assessed for substance use. There is evidence to suggest that alcohol use disorders in Australia are detected in only 25 per cent of hospitalised people who have alcohol use problems (Haber, Lintzeris, Proude & Lopatko, 2009).

Subjective data

As part of the mental status exam and the psychiatric history, conduct a thorough, nonjudgmental substance use assessment. Include the following interview questions:

1. How many packs of cigarettes do you smoke?
2. Do you take any prescription drugs?
3. Do you drink alcohol each day? If yes, do you drink 15 drinks per day? (As mentioned earlier, let the person correct you on your overstatement rather than fear shocking you with the truth.)
4. When was your last drink?
5. When did you last drink more than you wanted to?
6. Do you use drugs?
7. What drugs do you use, how do you use them, and what is their daily cost?

Drug and alcohol use must be qualified and documented in the clinical notes. Key elements of assessment also include: type of drug, route of administration, frequency of use, dose, duration of use, time and date of last amount taken (e.g. grams of alcohol, grams of cannabis, etc.)

Accurate responses to these questions are most likely when they are part of an interview that includes general lifestyle inquiries about smoking, coffee consumption and exercise habits. Experts agree that skilful assessment interviewing of people and their family members remains the best source of data.

Common defence mechanisms Denial, rationalisation and projection are three defence mechanisms common to people with substance use disorders. These defence mechanisms, along with other behaviours—conning, bargaining, feigning illness or an injury—complicate the assessment. Chapter 8 has details of these defence mechanisms.

People with substance use disorders tend to deny that they have a problem or minimise the problem: 'I drink/use drugs every day, but it rarely interferes with my work.' Rationalisation is common: 'I know I shouldn't drink, and I'll stop as soon as I get through this problem. Drinking keeps me calm enough to function.' Projecting the problem onto others is also common: 'You are so uptight that perfectly normal social drinking bothers you for no good reason. It's your issue, not mine.'

A detailed assessment, along with family/co-worker interviews, reveals that the problem is generally worse than the person says.

A person with an alcohol use disorder may think, 'I know I shouldn't hang out with Benny and Paul since we all like to drink/use together, but I like them. I'll just be with them, I won't drink/use.' Later on, the person may think, 'I'll only smoke a couple of cones'; later, 'I'll just smoke a few more, and maybe take some benzos to help me sleep.' This person may tell the nurse, 'I'll be glad to go to group therapy next week; just let me rest for a few days.'

Motivation for treatment Nurses need to consider some important psychosocial issues when people come for treatment. In Australia, people enter treatment programs voluntarily. This situation is best, because they are internally motivated, and therefore have a better chance of success. However, they may be coerced by family, friends, physicians or the police to undergo treatment.

Coerced treatment inevitably causes anger and resentment. People may lash out at others, blaming them (including you, the nurse), and demonstrate resistant or arrogant behaviours. In these difficult situations, you must remain detached and nonjudgmental to avoid both power struggles and taking the role of persecutor or rescuer. At this time, you function as a data gatherer: 'I know you are [uncomfortable/anxious/afraid/angry] now. To help you feel better, I need to ask you some questions about your drug use.' A judgmental question is, 'Don't you know that if you don't get help now you will only get worse?' Such questions prevent rapport and alienate the person.

YOUR ASSESSMENT APPROACH Interview questions for substance use

Your assessment of individuals who may have difficulty with a substance can include general types of questions about their substance use and what kind of feedback they have received from others, if any. The following questions help explore those possibilities:

1. What have you thought about your drinking or substance use?
2. Do you think it is contributing in a negative or a positive way to your life?
3. How would you describe it?
4. What have those who are important to you said to you about your drinking or substance use?
5. Do you agree or disagree with their input?
6. Tell me what happens the next day after you drink or use a substance.
7. Do you notice when you are drinking or using a substance whether you must do certain actions or cannot do others?

The importance of language Knowing the language of the drug world is important in obtaining an accurate nursing assessment of substance use. People with drug use have a language all their own; to understand them and the extent and nature of their habit, you need to be familiar with this language. For example, smoking weed, pot or cones is cannabis use, using ice or crystal is methamphetamine, and pills and pingers are generally ecstasy-type drugs. Often, the person themselves or someone in treatment can teach you this language.

Mental status Changes in mental status findings are seen in substance use disorders, but are not specific to them.

- Confusion, disorientation and agitation are often seen in intoxicated individuals, but can also indicate other problems, such as dementia, head injury or metabolic abnormalities.
- Paranoia is common in psychostimulant use, but can also indicate paranoid schizophrenia.
- Hallucinations can be caused by hallucinogens, withdrawal from alcohol, or psychotic disorders.
- Signs of impaired thinking, such as loose associations, are unlikely to be caused by substance use and are more likely to be due to schizophrenia.

Objective data

In addition to assessing subjective data, you should include a thorough consideration of relevant objective data. An assessment of behavioural changes can cue you to drug use.

Physical findings Less dramatic physical findings may include dry skin, hangnails, malnutrition, ascites, elevated blood pressure, and the smell of alcohol or an inhalant on the person's breath. As alcohol use disorders progress, be alert to signs and symptoms of liver cirrhosis. Your medical/surgical nursing textbooks will have these physical signs and symptoms.

Laboratory tests For years, researchers and clinicians have been searching for an objective biological marker that will reflect problem drinking and make assessment less challenging. Following are common laboratory tests in which elevated values are associated with excessive alcohol intake:

- blood alcohol concentration
- liver function tests
- alanine aminotransferase (ALT)
- aspartate aminotransferase (AST)
- serum gamma-glutamyltransferase (GGT)
- carbohydrate-deficient transferrin (CDT)
- high-density lipoprotein cholesterol (HDLC)
- mean corpuscular volume (MCV)
- uric acid.

Elevated laboratory test values are only one of the alerting factors for alcohol use disorders. No single test or combination of tests alone is appropriate for clinical screening. Confirmation of the excessive use of alcohol in a sensitively conducted assessment interview remains the preferred assessment approach, and is considered a prerequisite for successful intervention. Assessment should include diagnostic interviews, physical examination, investigation of clinical and biological markers, and gathering of collateral information about the person.

Planning and implementation

General hospital care

People who live with substance use disorders and who are suicidal or acutely ill with alcohol withdrawal, heroin overdose, hepatic coma, respiratory depression or cardiac dysrhythmias are often treated in the medical/surgical or intensive care units of a general hospital. See Communication on interacting with an alcohol-intoxicated individual.

Attend to life-threatening physiological symptoms first. In this setting, nurses perform the following tasks:

- monitor vital signs and respiratory and cardiovascular support
- administer prescribed medications
- apply ice packs for fever, such as fever caused by amphetamine intoxication or following cocaine use
- decrease stimulation; provide a darkened, quiet room
- point out reality ('I know you are seeing things, and I know you are frightened. You are in the hospital, and we are caring for you. There are no bugs or monsters here. You are safe and will feel better soon.')
- make sure people receive adequate nutrition and fluids (they are disoriented and generally forget to eat and drink)
- assess changes in level of consciousness
- monitor fluid intake and output
- protect skin integrity
- offer emotional support and encouragement to the person and their family
- refer people to community resources for substance use treatment programs.

COMMUNICATION

Person intoxicated with alcohol

PERSON: 'I'm so sorry I'm such a burden to you. You're such a good nurse, and I never want to be the type of person who . . .'

NURSE RESPONSE 1: 'I'm going to take your vital signs, and then you will have some time to yourself.' *RATIONALE:* This interaction treats the event as a health disorder in which there are physical consequences to the behaviour, as well as set limits on the interaction.	**NURSE RESPONSE 2:** 'We will talk later when you are able to concentrate.' *RATIONALE:* An intoxicated person may not benefit from a detailed discussion.

When the person is out of danger, then the issues associated with their substance use can be addressed.

Specialty care options

Specialty care for withdrawal management (formerly called 'detoxification') is given in inpatient units that are geared specifically for the treatment of substance use. These facilities are equipped with trained personnel and appropriate resources, so that people experiencing acute withdrawal may be admitted. The physical environment is modified to be as therapeutic as possible; for example, rooms that offer a quiet, unstimulating environment that help decrease anxiety and agitation.

The need for inpatient (residential) admission is generally warranted when there is history of a complicated withdrawal syndrome, such as seizure activity or delirium tremens. Withdrawal from alcohol is what most people will be admitted for, as this can be life-threatening. Members of the multi-disciplinary staff are experts in withdrawal management, substance-related education and treatments, including pharmacology for withdrawal. People also receive treatment for co-existing medical and mental health disorders Staff efforts are geared towards stabilisation and enhanced outcomes for the person. Post-withdrawal treatment options, such as ongoing counselling or residential rehabilitation, is organised for when the person has completed the withdrawal management program.

Withdrawal management provides an opportunity for engagement, planning and coordination of post-withdrawal care. It is important to highlight that withdrawal management is only the first step in the person's recovery journey. Note that there are only a few government-funded inpatient withdrawal management units in Australia, as ambulatory care is now considered the best treatment option for people undertaking substance withdrawal (see below). Therefore, people with a history of complicated alcohol withdrawal are admitted to medical wards and other general hospital facilities. Consult liaison nurses specialising in substance use disorders, who are available to help with admissions in metropolitan areas in most Australian states and territories. For more information, see the website for the Australian Drug Information Network (ADIN) at http://www.adin.com.au/help-support-services

Ambulatory care

Ambulatory supportive care (treatment that occurs in the person's home or at a specialised community-based facility) is the preferred way of withdrawal management in Australia. People are more likely to undertake withdrawal management if they do not require inpatient treatment. During ambulatory treatment, the person generally attends their local area health drug and alcohol service, and undergoes monitored withdrawal or reduction in substance use. Supportive pharmacologies are used, and psychosocial support from the multi-disciplinary team is an integral part of these programs. However, the person must first meet with the criteria for ambulatory programs—a history of complicated withdrawal and/or active mental health symptoms such as psychosis or depression generally warrants an inpatient admission. A comprehensive substance use, mental health and psychoscocial assessment is used to determine people's suitability for ambulatory withdrawal.

LIVED EXPERIENCE

Nursing care

While I appreciate the sentiment, it may be the case that actually the thing I most want is for the nurse to take some time to talk to me. Nurses were always the most caring people I ever had to deal with, and you know they are stressed, and as an addict you are used to being told you are a waste of time and space. I think I would have got clean a lot earlier if someone had just taken the time to say 'What's going on with you?'

Residential rehabilitation

Rehabilitation facilities offer residential-based care for people with substance use disorders. These residential centres have a variety of lengths of stay (four weeks to a year or more). People generally need to have undertaken substance withdrawal before attending a residential program. However, some programs do offer withdrawal management (usually non-medicated) as part of their services. Residential rehabilitation programs in Australia are not government-funded, so the person will need to pay a cost (generally minimal) for their stay.

Self-help groups

With self-help groups, people with similar substance use histories help one another. Groups composed of peers share experiences and knowledge of the problem to support and educate one another.

Twelve-step programs In contrast to the previously described treatment programs, 12-step programs such as AA and Narcotics Anonymous (NA) are not specifically treatment programs. They are spiritual programs based on the fellowship among its members. Both are successful self-help groups that meet daily or more often in different parts of large cities, and weekly in smaller towns. Meetings are held in places of worship, schools, community centres and various mental health treatment facilities. Anyone with a desire to stop drinking or taking drugs is welcome. This belief pervades both organisations: 'Once an alcoholic/addict, always an alcoholic/addict.' Members admit they are powerless over drugs/alcohol, live 'one day at a time', recite the serenity prayer, and believe in 'a power greater than man'. Members learn to turn their problems over to 'the God of my understanding'. Their philosophy is revealed in part through their key slogans: 'First things first', 'Easy does it' and 'Let go and let God.' Members of both organisations learn the '12 steps'. The 12 steps of AA are reproduced in Box 13.3. Through AA/NA, people learn to change negative attitudes and behaviours into positive ones. A key concept of AA/NA is that total abstinence is essential to recovery.

As members become sober or drug-free, they begin 'sponsoring' (helping) other substance users. This offering of support is believed to be vital to recovery, as is regular attendance at AA/NA meetings. Twelve-step recovery programs also emphasise spirituality through meditation and prayer, rather than willpower, as the means to recovery.

However, it needs to be recognised that AA's 12 steps were written in the 1930s by and for white Christian males, and so may not be culturally relevant for all people. Adapting the language to a less patriarchal, less traditionally Christian, approach that is spiritual yet culturally relevant to diverse groups of people makes the 12-step principles available to people who might otherwise discount them.

AA and NA, while excellent for some people experiencing substance use disorders, may not be suitable for others. These programs can be difficult for the person with comorbid mental health and substance use disorders. The AA/NA philosophy of complete abstinence from substances has been said to include psychiatric medications. This requirement causes a rift between what people are told by their psychiatric–mental health nurses and the path towards wellness according to AA/NA. Programs work best when they are designed to provide the most effective treatment for the psychobiological underpinnings of mental health disorders and to accommodate the added stress of substances of use.

The harm-minimisation framework that underpins all Australian drug and alcohol policy helps support people with comorbidities, as it focuses on prevention for high-risk groups, such as those with comorbid substance use and mental health disorders. Harm minimisation is not about making moral judgments; it is about supporting and working with people in a respectful way whether their goal be reducing their use or achieving total abstinence.

SMART Recovery SMART Recovery is a voluntary self-help group to assist people in recovering from alcohol and drug use. SMART Recovery is based on cognitive behavioural therapy (CBT) principles. The group helps people to understand, manage and change their thoughts on substance use so as to prevent relapse. The SMART Recovery program comprises of four key points.

1. building and maintaining motivation
2. coping with urges
3. problem-solving
4. lifestyle balance.

Many government-funded drug and alcohol services now run SMART Recovery programs. There are gender-specific and targeted programs available (i.e. women only, or for teens).

Box 13.3 The 12 steps of Alcoholics Anonymous

1. We admitted we were powerless over alcohol—that our lives had become unmanageable.
2. We came to believe that a Power greater than ourselves could restore us to sanity.
3. We made a decision to turn our will and our lives over to the care of God, as we understood Him.
4. We made a searching and fearless moral inventory of ourselves.
5. We admitted to God, to ourselves, and to another human being the exact nature of our wrongs.
6. We were entirely ready to have God remove all these defects of character.
7. We humbly asked Him to remove our shortcomings.
8. We made a list of all people we had harmed, and became willing to make amends to them all.
9. We made direct amends to such people wherever possible, except when to do so would injure them or others.
10. We continued to take personal inventory and when we were wrong, promptly admitted it.
11. We sought through prayer and meditation to improve our conscious contact with God, as we understood Him, praying only for knowledge of His will for us and the power to carry that out.
12. Having had a spiritual awakening as the result of these steps, we tried to carry this message to alcoholics, and to practice these principles in all our affairs.

Source: The 12 Steps are reprinted with permission of Alcoholics Anonymous World Services, Inc. (AAWS). Permission to reprint the 12 Steps does not mean that AAWS has reviewed or approved the contents of this publication, or that AAWS necessarily agrees with the views expressed herein. AA is a program of recovery from alcohol use *only*—use of the 12 Steps in connection with programs and activities which are patterned after AA, but which address other problems, or in any other non-AA context, does not imply otherwise.

Relapse

Relapse is common among people who experience substance use disorders. Clinicians in the field of alcohol use disorders estimate that 60 per cent to 75 per cent of those who complete treatment programs drink again within the first 90 days. Data suggest that only 10 per cent to 20 per cent of people remain abstinent for one year following treatment, and that only 35 per cent of these are abstinent five years later. In fact, recidivism rates are notoriously high across the spectrum of substance use disorders.

Stages of recovery Several common stages of the recovery process are as follows:

1. commitment to recovery and motivation for abstinence
2. initiating change
3. maintaining change.

As a result of a successful initial change, the person experiences perceived control while remaining abstinent.

Stages of relapse The feeling of perceived control continues until the person encounters a high-risk situation involving negative emotional states, interpersonal conflict or social pressure. Collaborative Care includes a checklist of symptoms leading to relapse. The person can avoid relapse by using effective coping responses in the high-risk situation. (See Communication for an example of how you might discuss these issues with a person with a history of substance use but not currently using them.)

COLLABORATIVE CARE

Teaching about relapse

A checklist of symptoms leading to relapse

1. ***Exhaustion.*** Don't allow yourself to become overly tired or to have poor health. Many substance-dependent people are also prone to other addictions, such as being 'workaholics'. Perhaps they are in a hurry to make up for lost time or are overworking to compensate for feelings of guilt or personal inadequacy. Good health and enough rest are essential to recovery. Good feelings of physical wellbeing are associated with a healthy, optimistic mental outlook. Fatigue and feelings of physical illness often induce negative thinking and a pessimistic attitude. You may begin to think a drug or drink would help you return to a positive frame of mind.
2. ***Dishonesty.*** This symptom begins with a pattern of unnecessary little lies and deceits with fellow workers, friends and family. Then come important lies to yourself. This is called *rationalising*—making excuses for not doing what you do not want to do, or for doing what you know you should not do.
3. ***Impatience.*** Things are not happening fast enough; others are not doing what they should or what you want them to.
4. ***Argumentativeness.*** Arguing about small and ridiculous points of view indicates a need to always be right. People with substance dependence need to learn an attitude of acceptance of their disorder and the value of the tools of recovery.
5. ***Depression.*** Unreasonable and unaccountable melancholy and despair may occur from time to time as a *natural part of recovering* from substance dependence. Periods of depression are times when the risk of relapse is very high. Deal with your negative feelings; talk about them.
6. ***Frustration.*** Remember, not everything is going to be just the way you want it.
7. ***Self-pity.*** 'Why do these things happen to me?' 'Why must I be dependent on drugs/alcohol?' 'Nobody appreciates what I'm doing for them.'
8. ***Cockiness.*** 'I've got this problem licked; I have nothing to fear from drugs or grog.' This dangerous attitude may lead to going into situations where friends are drinking and using drugs to prove to others that you don't have a problem. Do this often enough and your defences against relapse will wear down. *Don't test* your recovery. You may lose!
9. ***Complacency.*** It is dangerous to let up on discipline because everything seems to be going so well. Always having a little fear is a good thing when it comes to maintaining abstinence. *More relapses occur when things are going well than when things are going badly.*
10. ***Expecting too much from others.*** 'I've changed—why hasn't everybody else?' It's a plus if they do, but be prepared to deal with disappointment in your expectations of others. They may not trust you yet, or they may be looking for more evidence of your improved physical and mental health. You may be setting yourself up for a lot of frustration and other negative feelings if you expect others to change their lifestyle just because you have.
11. ***Letting up on discipline.*** This attitude may stem from complacency or from boredom. No chemically-dependent person can afford to be bored with their recovery. The cost of relapse is too great. Therefore, continue with faith, meditation, daily inventory and 12-step meeting attendance.
12. ***Wanting too much.*** Do not set goals you cannot reach with normal efforts.
13. ***Forgetting gratitude.*** You may be looking negatively on your life, concentrating on problems that still are not totally corrected. It is important to remember where you started from and how much better life is now.
14. ***'It can't happen to me.'*** This kind of thinking is very dangerous. Almost anything can happen to you, and is all the more likely to happen if you become careless with your recovery. Remember that you have a health disorder and will be in even worse shape if you relapse.
15. ***Omnipotence.*** This is a feeling that results from a combination of many of the attitudes listed here. You may come to believe you have all the answers for yourself and for others. No one can tell you anything new. You may begin to ignore suggestions or advice from others. Relapse is probably imminent unless drastic change takes place.

COMMUNICATION

Person with a history of substance use but not currently using them

PERSON: 'I don't need to spend a lot of time talking to you about this stuff. I'm not going to take it anymore, and you can bet on that.'

NURSE RESPONSE 1: 'I hear that you have no intention to use again, and that's good. I also want to make sure you have every support available to you when that time comes when your resolve gets shaky.'

RATIONALE: This interaction provides direction around the eventual difficulties that face everyone dependent on a substance—temptation and relapse.

NURSE RESPONSE 2: 'We don't have to do a lot of talking, but you have to make the changes in what you do and who you do it with.'

RATIONALE: Clear statements about how the person is responsible for their behaviour and for making necessary changes interfere with urges to shift blame.

LIVED EXPERIENCE

Support systems

There is a fine line between supporting someone and enabling them. It can seem easier for health service people to say 'Well, if you won't change I can't help you', but sometimes people with addiction have no idea how to change. Asking people to take responsibility for themselves can't be done without adequate referral to other support systems. The power of a peer group can be completely overwhelming. If you are going to quit, you need to leave your old friends behind, and that can be the hardest part. I was only able to stop when I was referred to inpatient rehabilitation and found new people like me who were trying to change, too.

If, however, the individual cannot cope successfully, an initial 'lapse' occurs in which they resort to the use of a substance to control stress. The person then feels less able to exert control and develops a tendency to 'give in' to the situation ('It's no use, I can't handle this'). In subsequent high-risk situations, the individual again resorts to substance use to relieve stress. Repeated lapses set the stage for a return to uncontrolled use (relapse).

Relapse prevention Many treatment services incorporate the concept of relapse prevention into their treatment programs. This concept is designed to teach people how to anticipate relapse. By learning skills to use in high-risk situations, people gain confidence and the expectation of being able to cope successfully, thus decreasing the probability of relapse. Strategies include the identification of 'triggers' to substance use (i.e. stressors), stress management advice and short- and long-term goal-setting.

General treatment approaches

A number of general interventions for substance use disorders have been found to be useful are discussed next.

Using confrontation strategies For many years, it was believed that people with substance use disorders needed to 'hit bottom' before they could accept their disorder and request help. Today, evidence shows that intervention can and should occur as soon as the substance use is identified. Nurses are often 'intervention specialists' and leaders in the process.

Evaluation

Evaluating the recovery process requires an evaluation of the person's want to change. Is there evidence that the person is being honest, open and willing to take responsibility for their own actions? Regardless of the substance of use, once a person stops blaming others for their use, treatment has made a positive impact. Another criterion is the amount of substance the person is placing in their body. Has it decreased? Other indications of positive treatment outcome are increased job stability, improvement in interpersonal relationships, and improved problem-solving techniques. Evaluating people for emotional maturity and the ability to make lifestyle changes that include people, places and things are critical for victory over substance dependence. Improvement in these areas is a good indication that the person is well on the road to recovery.

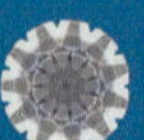

NURSING CARE PLAN: PERSON WITH AN ALCOHOL USE DISORDER

Clinical example—identifying information

John Mills is a 54-year-old married lawyer. He was referred from the residential facility where he has been for the past 28 days.

John states, 'I've had a drinking problem for 35 years. My wife and boss told me if I don't shape up they'll kick me out of my home and my job. I want to feel better. It's been a living hell. But I'm not sure I can stop drinking; I've tried before.' He describes his drinking as a way 'to cope with my problems for most of my life'. He wants to 'stay dry'. Fifteen years ago, his social drinking escalated and he began over-using alcohol on the weekends. He then began drinking throughout the week. He has been drinking daily for most of the past three years. He drank 'enough to keep a buzz on' and occasionally 'enough to pass out'. John's problems with work include tardiness, absenteeism and errors on the job. Marital problems are described as 'she either yells at me or takes care of me'. He gives as examples his wife pouring out his hidden alcohol, and calling his boss to say John had the flu when he was really 'hungover'.

History

John has been in and out of AA groups, and has seen three psychiatrists. He has been hospitalised three times for car accidents and injuries due to drinking (broken leg and ribs, contusions, concussion). After the last general hospital admission, he was admitted to the residential unit for a 28-day alcohol treatment program.

Both of John's parents are deceased, and both had alcohol use disorders. His sister, age 58, is also recovering from an alcohol use disorder (she has been 'dry' for 10 years). The family has never been close. John feels he was 'never allowed to be a normal, active kid'. His sister cared for him when he was young, and functioned as a surrogate mother.

John developed normally, but always 'felt different'. He started a full-time job after graduation. He enjoyed being with his 'drinking buddies' from work, but has never had a close friend on whom he could

(continued)

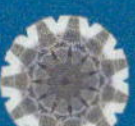

NURSING CARE PLAN: PERSON WITH AN ALCOHOL USE DISORDER (*continued*)

depend. He smokes one pack of cigarettes daily, and uses no other drugs. He spends his spare time watching TV and at the pub with friends.

John has the early signs of liver disease. He is malnourished and has a long history of insomnia.

Current mental status

John is well-groomed, clean and alert. His sensorium is within normal limits; affect appropriate yet apathetic. He appears depressed, and expresses feelings of self-reproach and guilt for his years of drinking and its effect on others. Speech is slow and spontaneous. Motor behaviour, thought content and thought processes are within normal limits. Insight is questionable.

Other clinical data

Multivitamins qd; no indications of suicide or violence potential.

Issue identified: Ineffective coping related to alcohol use.

Expected outcome: John will reduce ineffective and self-destructive coping through alcohol use and regular use of more effective coping styles.

Short-term goal	Interventions	Rationale
Identification of two effective coping mechanisms	■ John inventories those situations that challenge his ability to cope. ■ John recognises the automatic mechanisms involved in habitually responding to stress with alcohol. ■ John rehearses various coping strategies to prepare to select two for regular use. ■ John begins to substitute effective coping for alcohol use when stressed.	Revision of coping styles requires identification of the situations that place him at risk, typical problematic responses, and acknowledgment of the need to learn new coping styles. Rehearsing new behaviours and thoughts; incorporates them into a repertoire.

Issue identified: Insomnia related to alcohol use.

Expected outcome: John will use sleep-inducing strategies nightly and report satisfaction with his quality of sleep.

Short-term goal	Interventions	Rationale
John will sleep a total of 6 hours per night.	■ Assess current pattern and effective strategies. ■ Respond to awakening with sleep hygiene: warm milk, reading, relaxation strategies. ■ Employ effective strategies regularly.	Re-establish a consistently healthy sleep routine.

Issue identified: Imbalanced nutrition: less than body requirements, related to alcohol use.

Expected outcome: John eats three meals every day plus snacks, and takes a multivitamin and thiamine as recommended.

Short-term goal	Interventions	Rationale
John identifies the relationship between alcohol use and malnutrition. John gains weight through a balanced diet.	■ Monitor intake of meals and snacks. ■ Initiate dietary consult. ■ Investigate dietary preferences to maximise John's abilities to expand his intake appropriately. ■ Educate regarding the impact of chronic alcohol ingestion on the digestive tract, metabolism and overall health. ■ Offer frequent food and fluids throughout contacts.	Malnutrition from chronic alcohol use can be addressed with a comprehensive nutrition program. John is more likely to eat food he prefers, as part of a balanced diet. Alcohol impairs the ability of the digestive tract to absorb nutrients.

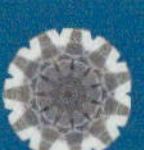

NURSING CARE PLAN: PERSON WITH METHAMPHETAMINE USE INTOXICATION

Clinical example—identifying information

Brianna is a 29-year-old married woman. Her husband brought her to the hospital. Brianna was an advertising executive with a large local firm prior to being recently fired. She has a Master's degree in marketing. She has never sought treatment for drug or alcohol use.

Brianna does not believe she needs to be hospitalised, especially because she needs to find work. She asserts she is extremely creative and productive, and needs 'to get my ideas down on paper before someone steals them as their own'. She is agitated, aggressive, elated, loud and occasionally incoherent during the interview. Her only complaint is increased libido 'that my husband can't keep up with'. Brianna admits to 'working very hard at working very hard', but does not believe she needs treatment right now. She feels she can handle this herself.

She has been using methamphetamine for one year, spending most of her salary on it. For the past five days she has used methamphetamine two to three times a day. Prior to that, her use was once or twice weekly. Brianna explains her recent increase in use as 'helping me work harder and faster to find a job somewhere in this town. I feel more productive.' She is having trouble sitting still, and she is perspiring visibly. Brianna states she has been feeling nauseous for several days. Brianna's husband and one female friend are her main support system.

History

Brianna has no prior psychiatric history. Her parents are both living, and work together in their own business (a retail shoe store). Her younger brother is a college senior. Although close and loving, Brianna's family is 300 kilometres away and they seldom see each other. Brianna's father has a history of alcohol use, but has not touched alcohol for five years.

Brianna is a competitive woman who has always excelled at academic study and at work. She 'likes being number one'. Brianna has few close friends and socialised with acquaintances from work, who have not been accessible to her since she was fired from her job. Smoking cigarettes since age 17, Brianna admits to 'moderate' drinking with occasional weekend alcohol bingeing. She has experimented with a variety of recreational drugs, but states 'meth really works for me'. Brianna describes herself as 'the best kind of hard-driving, career-focused woman', but enjoys reading and tennis when time permits.

Brianna has no current or past medical problems. She states she is in good health, despite 'feeling horrible now'. Her blood pressure is 140/90, and her pulse is 110.

Current mental status

Brianna is attractive, dishevelled, agitated, hyperalert, alternatively compliant and hostile, and occasionally incoherent. Sensorium is impaired. She is oriented to time, place and person. Her judgment is impaired. Her affect is labile, and mood swings are evident. Her motor behaviour is notable for rapid and frequent movements. Her thought content is grandiose. Delusions are present. Brianna reports seeing 'signs' on billboards that are messages to her that she should 'move onward and upward to take over a company'. Thought processes are occasionally incoherent, tangential, with difficulty concentrating and easy distraction. There is limited insight: 'I can take care of myself. I have a great deal of innate skill and knowledge. I know what I'm doing.'

Other clinical data

Brianna is not taking any medications; suicide/violence potential is minimal.

Issue identified: Ineffective coping related to methamphetamine use.
Expected outcome: Brianna will complete a withdrawal management program and will remain free of methamphetamine.

Short-term goal	Interventions	Rationale
Meets with staff and attends group meetings according to schedule without prompting.	▪ Hold individual meetings with Brianna regarding the consequences of drug use in work, home, social and physical arenas.	Improve Brianna's awareness of her behaviours, reduce denial, and educate about the processes involved when experiencing a substance use disorder.
Brianna to approach one staff member when feeling the urge to use methamphetamine.	▪ Convey agreement to assist Brianne on working through her strong desire to return to drug use.	Monitor behaviours that indicate a strong urge to use drugs as an inevitable aspect of her substance use disorder.
Brianna discusses problems created by methamphetamine use.	▪ Assign Brianna to daily individual and group therapy.	
Replaces destructive coping with two effective individual coping options.	▪ Observe every half-hour. When Brianna has a strong urge to use drugs, encourage her to express feelings, educate about cravings and timeframes for resolution.	
	▪ Assist Brianna in recognising the automatic mechanisms involved in turning to methamphetamine.	Revision of coping styles requires learning and practice.
	▪ Encourage Brianna to rehearse various coping strategies and select two for regular use.	
	▪ Explore with Brianna how to substitute effective coping for methamphetamine use.	

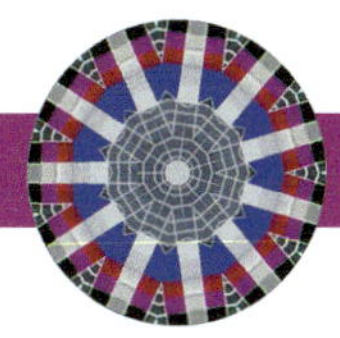

REFERENCES

Agrawal, A., & Lynskey, M. T. (2008). Are there genetic influences on addiction? Evidence from family, adoption and twin studies. *Addiction, 103*(7), 1069–1081.

American Psychiatric Association (APA). (2013). *Diagnostic and statistical manual of mental disorders* (5th ed., DSM-5). Washington, DC: APA Publishing.

Australian Institute of Criminology. (2007). *Australian crime: Facts and figures 2006.* Canberra, Australia: Australian Institute of Criminology.

Australian Institute of Health and Welfare (AIHW). (2009). *Measuring the social and emotional wellbeing of Aboriginal and Torres Strait Islander peoples*. Cat. No. IHW 24, Canberra, Australia: AIHW.

Australian Institute of Health and Welfare (AIHW). (2011). *2010 National Drug Strategy Household Survey report.* Drug Statistics Series No. 25. Cat. No. PHE 145. Canberra, Australia: AIHW.

Australian Institute of Health and Welfare (AIHW). (2013). *National opioid pharmacotherapy statistics annual data collection 2012.* Drug Treatment Series No. 20. Cat. No. HSE 136. Canberra, Australia: AIHW.

Australian Institute of Health and Welfare (AIHW). (2016). *Australian Burden of Disease Study: Impact and causes of illness and death in Australia 2011*. Australian Burden of Disease Study Series No. 3. BOD 4. Canberra, Australia: AIHW.

Baker, T. B., Piper, M. E., McCarthy, D. E., Majeskie, M. R., & Fiore, M. C. (2004). Addiction motivation reformulated: an affective processing model of negative reinforcement. *Psychological Review*, *111*(1), 33.

Bejerot, N. (1980). Addiction to pleasure: A biological and social-psychological theory of addiction. *NIDA Research Monograph*, *30*, 246–255.

Bower, C., Silva D., Henderson, T. R., Ryan, A., & Rudy, E. (2000). Ascertainment of birth defects: The effect on completeness of adding a new source of data. *Journal of Paediatrics and Child Health, 36*, 574–576.

Chalmers, J., & Ritter, A. (2012). Subsidising patient dispensing fees: The cost of injecting equity into the opioid pharmacotherapy maintenance system. *Drug and Alcohol Review, 31*, 911–917.

Clark, J. L. (2011). The evolution of human culture during the later Pleistocene: Using fauna to test models on the emergence and nature of 'modern' human behavior. *Journal of Anthropological Archaeology*, *30*(3), 273–291.

Copeland, J., Gerber, S., Dillon, P., & Swift, W. (2006). *Cannabis: Answers to your questions.* Randwick, Australia: National Drug and Alcohol Research Centre, University of New South Wales.

Croton, G. (2011). *Potential: Australia's evolving responses to co-occurring mental health and substance use disorders.* Submission to Senate Community Affairs Committee—Commonwealth Funding and Administration of Mental Health Services Inquiry. Wangaratta, Australia: Northeast Health Wangaratta.

Dickerson, D. L., & Johnson, C. L. (2012). Mental health and substance abuse characteristics among a clinical sample of urban American Indian/ Alaska Native youths in a large California metropolitan area: A descriptive study. *Community Mental Health Journal, 48(1), 56–62.* doi: 10.1007/ s10597-010-9368-3

Ersche, K. D., Turton, A. J., Pradhan, S., Bullmore, E. T., & Robbins, T. W. (2010). Drug addiction endophenotypes: Impulsive versus sensation-seeking personality traits. *Biological Psychiatry*, *68*(8), 770–773.

Gandhi, K. K., Williams, J. M., Menza, M., Galazyn, M., & Benowitz, N. L. (2010). Higher serum caffeine in smokers with schizophrenia compared to smoking controls. *Drug and Alcohol Dependence, 110*(1–2), 151–155.

Gronnerod, C., Overskeid, G., & Hartmann, E. (2013). Using Skinner's skin: gauging a behaviorist from his Rorschach protocol. *Journal of Personality Assessment, 95*(1), 1–12.

Gross, M. (2010). Alcoholics Anonymous: Still sober after 75 years. *American Journal of Public Health, 100*(12), 2361–2363.

Haber, P., Lintzeris, N., Proude, E., & Lopatko, O. (2009). *Guidelines for the treatment of alcohol problems.* Publications No. P3-5625 (pp. vii–232). Canberra, Australia: Commonwealth Department of Health and Ageing.

Jellinek, E. (1946). *Phases in the drinking history of alcoholics.* New Haven, CT: Hillhouse Press.

Jenner, L., & Lee, N. (2008) *Treatment approaches for users of methamphetamine: A practical guide for frontline workers.* Canberra, Australia: Australian Government Department of Health and Ageing.

Kinner, S. A., & Degenhardt, L. (2008). Crystal methamphetamine smoking among regular ecstasy users in Australia: Increases in use and associations with harm. *Drug and Alcohol Review, 27*(3): 292–300.

Lang, E. (2004). Drugs in society: A social history. In M. Hamilton, T. King, & A. Ritter (Eds.), *Drug use in Australia: Preventing harm* (2nd ed.) (pp. 1–16). Melbourne, Australia: Oxford University Press.

Lee, N. K., &, Rawson, R. A. (2008). A systematic review of cognitive and behavioural therapies for methamphetamine dependence. *Drug and Alcohol Review*, *27*(3), 309–317.

Lewis, M. J. (1992). *A rum state: Alcohol and state policy in Australia, 1788–1988* Canberra, Australia: AGPS Press.

Li, M. D., & Burmeister, M. (2009). New insights into the genetics of addiction. *Nature Reviews Genetics,* 10(4), 225–231.

McLaren, J., & Mattick, R. P. (2011). *Cannabis in Australia: Use, supply, harms, and responses.* Monograph Series No. 57. Canberra, Australia: Australian Government Department of Health and Ageing.

Midford, R. (2010). Drug prevention programmes for young people: where have we been and where should we be going? *Addiction, 105*(10), 1688–1695.

National Health and Medical Research Council (NHMRC). 2009. *Australian guidelines to reduce health risks from drinking*. Canberra, Australia: Commonwealth of Australia.

National Indigenous Drug and Alcohol Committee (NIDAC). 2012. *Addressing fetal alcohol spectrum disorder in Australia.* Canberra, Australia: Australian National Council on Drugs.

Nelson, R. (2011). Cannabis use in long-term care: An emerging issue for nurses. *American Journal of Nursing, 111*(4), 19–20.

NSW Ministry of Health (NSW Health). 2009. *Nursing and Midwifery Clinical guidelines—identifying and responding to drug and alcohol issues*. Retrieved from http://www0.health.nsw.gov.au/policies/gl/2008/ GL2008_001.html

Potvin, S., Lungu, O., Lipp, O., Lalonde, P., Zaharieva, V., Stip, E., . . . Mendrek, A. (2016). Increased ventro-medial prefrontal activations in schizophrenia smokers during cigarette cravings. *Schizophrenia Research*, *173*(1), 30–36.

Ransley, J., Mazerolle, L., Manning, M., McGuffog, I., Drew, J. M., & Webster, J. (2011). *Reducing the methamphetamine problem in Australia: Evaluating innovative partnerships between police, pharmacies and other third parties*. National Drug Law Enforcement Research Fund, Monograph Series No. 39. Canberra, Australia: Commonwealth of Australia.

Raupach, T., & van Schayck, C. P. (2011). Pharmacotherapy for smoking cessation: Current advances and research topics. *CNS Drugs, 25*(5), 371–382.

Robertson, J. R., & Daniels, A. M. (2012). Methadone replacement therapy: tried, tested, effective. *Journal of the Royal College of Physicians of Edinburgh, 42*(2), 133–136.

Roll, J. M., Rawson, R. A., Ling, W., & Shoptaw, S. (2009). *Methamphetamine addiction: From basic science to treatment.* New York, NY: Guilford Press.

Room, R. (2010). The long reaction against the wowser: The prehistory of alcohol deregulation in Australia. *Health Sociology Review*, *19*(2), 151–163.

Rose, M. E., & Grant, J. E. (2010). Alcohol-induced blackout: Phenomenology, biological basis, and gender differences. *Journal of Addictions Medicine, 4*, 61–73.

Smock, T. K. (1999). *Physiological psychology: A neuroscience approach.* New Jersey, NJ: Prentice Hall.

White, W. L. (2000). Addiction as a disease: Birth of a concept. *Counselor*, *1*(1):46–51, 73.

World Health Organization. (2010). *The ICD-10 classification of mental and behavioural disorders: Clinical descriptions and diagnostic guideline* (online). Retrieved from: http://apps.who.int/classifications/icd10/ browse/2010/en#/F10.1

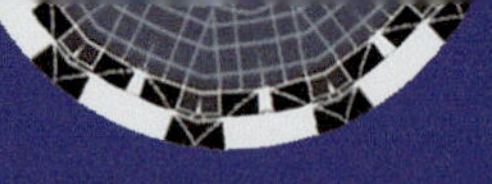

14

Working in collaboration with people living with schizophrenia and other psychotic disorders

MIKE HAZELTON AND SIMON SWINSON

KEY TERMS

LEARNING OUTCOMES

After completing this chapter, you will be able to:

1. Describe the central features of schizophrenia.
2. Distinguish among classical and emerging views of schizophrenia.
3. Compare and contrast the various biopsychosocial theories that address the possible causes of schizophrenia.
4. Explain how psychological and social pressures can influence the course of schizophrenia.
5. Implement recovery-oriented care in working with people living with schizophrenia.
6. Partner with, and provide support to, the families of people living with schizophrenia.
7. Work with people to help them minimise the risk of relapse in schizophrenia.
8. Reflect on the personal characteristics you bring to working with people living with schizophrenia that might affect your ability to provide recovery-focused care.
9. Understand and appreciate the experience of living with schizophrenia.

LIVED EXPERIENCE

Living with schizophrenia has its fair share of ups and downs, traumas and anxieties. But when looked at from the vantage point of age and experience, I do seem to have covered a lot of ground, not so much in linear terms, but rather the sheer bulk of experience that makes me feel good about myself. Even though there have been many disasters, I can still look myself in the face and congratulate myself for having got here. From time to time I perform with a mental health choir named 'Under Construction'; as the name suggests, our lives are constantly 'under construction'.

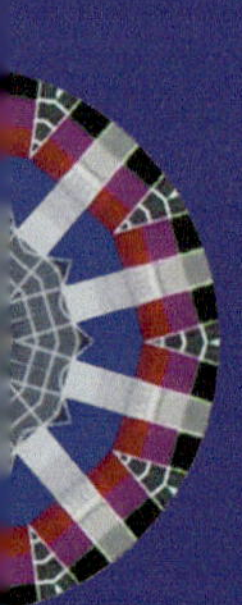

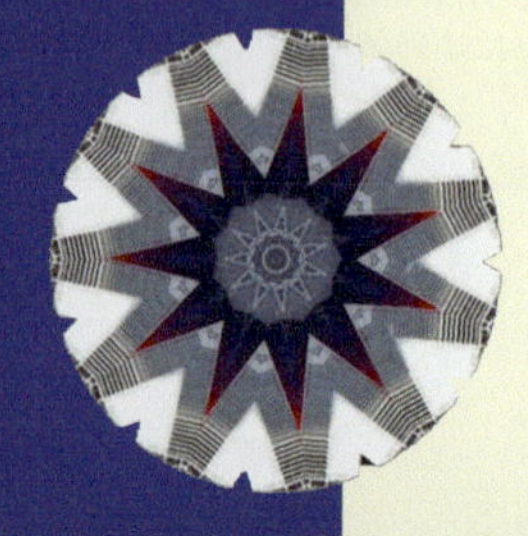

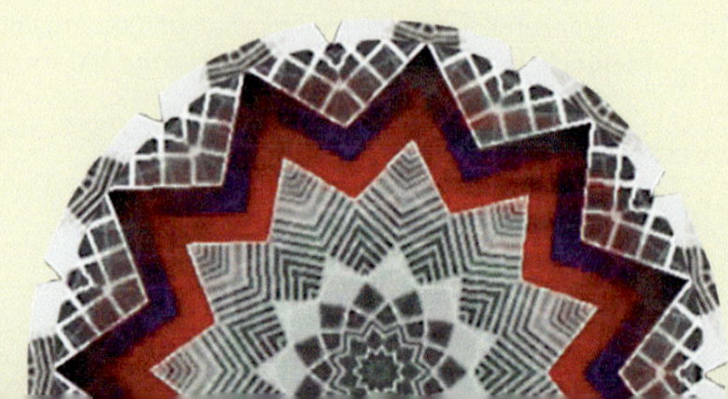

INTRODUCTION

Schizophrenia is a complex disorder with an extremely varied presentation of symptoms. It affects cognitive, emotional and behavioural functioning. According to the Schizophrenia Research Institute, approximately 1 in 100 people in Australia will develop schizophrenia during their lifetime, with similar rates being found in other countries. Schizophrenia spectrum disorders rank among the leading causes of disability in developed countries worldwide, and onset usually occurs between the mid-teens and early thirties. Beyond the considerable emotional cost to families, schizophrenia costs the Australian community more than $2.5 billion per annum in direct health costs and lost productivity (Schizophrenia Research Institute, 2015). The illness is diagnosed most frequently in the early twenties for men and the late twenties for women. The progression of the illness is as variable as its presentation. In some cases, the disease progresses through exacerbations (an increase in the seriousness of the disease marked by a greater intensity in symptoms) and remissions; in other cases, it takes a chronic, more stable course; while in still others, a chronic, progressively deteriorating course evolves. It is important to note, however, that the majority of people living with schizophrenia attain a high level of **recovery** and are satisfied with their lives. Organisations such as the Schizophrenia Research Institute (http://www.schizophreniaresearch.org.au/schizophrenia/about-schizophrenia/), SANE Australia (http://www.sane.org) and The Schizophrenia Fellowship of Australia (http://www.schizophrenia.org.au) maintain up-to-date websites that can be used as resources for you, people living with schizophrenia and their families.

SYMPTOMS OF SCHIZOPHRENIA

The diagnosis of schizophrenia requires not only the presence of distinct symptoms, but also the persistence of those symptoms over time. Symptoms must be present for at least six months, and some symptoms (called *active-phase symptoms*) must be present for at least one month during that time, before schizophrenia can be diagnosed. See the section on the essential features of schizophrenia in the American Psychiatric Association's *Diagnostic and statistical manual of mental disorders* (DSM-5) (American Psychiatric Association [APA], 2013).

The symptoms of schizophrenia are conceptually separated into **positive symptoms**, which represent an excess or distortion of normal functioning, or an aberrant response; and **negative symptoms**, which represent a deficit in functioning.

Positive symptoms

Positive symptoms include the three most pronounced outward signs of the disorder: hallucinations, delusions, and disorganisation in speech and behaviour.

Hallucinations

Hallucinations are the most common perceptual disturbance in schizophrenia. **Hallucinations** are subjective sensory experiences that are not actually caused by external sensory stimuli.

One or more of the five senses are involved in hallucinations. Hallucinations may be auditory (heard), visual (seen), olfactory (smelled), gustatory (tasted) or tactile (touched).

The most common form of hallucination in schizophrenia, at least in Western countries, is hearing voices or sounds that are distinct from the person's own thoughts. If a voice is heard, it (or they) may be friendly or hostile and threatening. It is particularly characteristic of schizophrenia if the person hears two or more voices conversing with each other, or hears a voice that provides continuous comments on the train of thought.

Having auditory hallucinations does not necessarily mean that the individual hears human speech. As you will see later in Table 14.3, several other sounds may be present in hallucinations. It is important that hallucinatory experiences not be confused with *synaesthesia*, which is the experience of having multiple senses involved in a single event. Synaesthesia is not a disease or disorder. Distinguishing between synaesthesia and hallucinations can be accomplished by ensuring that there is no external stimulation to the sensations. Examples of synaesthesia include seeing sounds, seeing colours when in pain and hearing smells.

Hallucinations may also occur in other illnesses besides schizophrenia. Dementia (Chapter 12), substance abuse (Chapter 13), and depression (Chapter 15) are some examples.

DSM ESSENTIAL FEATURES

Schizophrenia

The person presents with some combination of symptoms, including delusions, hallucinations, disorganised speech/behaviour, reduced range of emotion, little speech or low motivation, and has not received treatment for at least a month. Work, social life or self-care are poorly conducted. There is evidence that these symptoms have been present for months. Also, no sustained symptoms of mania or depression are noted, and substance ingestion, a medical problem or developmental disability, do not explain the symptoms.

Through the work of the Hearing Voices Movement, it is becoming evident that many people without mental illness also hear voices, and that this is an unusual but meaningful human experience (Corstens, Longden, McCarthy-Jones, Waddingham & Thomas, 2014). Table 14.1 ■ links hallucinations with commonly associated disease processes. Hallucinations can also be experienced under extreme physiological stress or as side-effects of medications.

TABLE 14.1 ■ Types of hallucinations

Perceptual disturbance	Commonly associated disease process
Auditory	Schizophrenia
Visual	Dementia
Tactile*	Acute alcohol withdrawal
Somatic*	Schizophrenia
Olfactory*	Seizure disorders
Gustatory*	Seizure disorders

*Also called *proprioceptive hallucinations*, associated with infections, heavy metal poisoning or vitamin and mineral toxicities, and tumours.

Delusions

Delusions are mistaken or false beliefs about the self or the environment that are firmly held even in the face of disconfirming evidence. Delusions may take many forms. In *delusions of persecution*, the person may think that others are following them, trying to spy, or to damage, torment or take something of value like a reputation (e.g. 'They have misters in my apartment that spray drugs onto me when I walk around.'). In another common form, *delusions of reference*, the person thinks that public expressions, like a story on the television or a newspaper article, are specifically addressed to them or that the event occurred because of their thoughts or actions (e.g. 'When the newsreader wears navy blue, she is speaking my thoughts to the world.'). ***Folie à deux*** is a delusion shared by two people, who are usually emotionally close to each other. Specific types of delusion are discussed in Table 14.2 ■.

Disordered speech and behaviour

Other positive symptoms represent excesses of language or behaviour. Disorganised speech is the outward sign of disordered thoughts, and may range from less severe forms (the person moves rapidly from one topic to another), to severe forms (the person's speech cannot be logically understood). Positive symptoms include low-level behavioural responses to the environment characterised by such disorganised behaviour as agitated, non-purposeful or random movements, and waxy flexibility (which is discussed and defined later in this chapter). The positive symptoms of schizophrenia are discussed in Table 14.3 ■.

Negative symptoms

Negative symptoms of schizophrenia are less dramatic but just as debilitating as positive symptoms. They are called *negative* symptoms because people are missing something they would normally have if they were not ill. Negative symptoms are also predictors of a poor outcome to treatment (Stanford et al., 2011). Table 14.4 ■ provides examples of negative symptoms of schizophrenia.

Flat affect

People living with schizophrenia often appear to have unemotional or very restricted emotional responses to their experiences. **Flat affect** is defined as the absence or near

TABLE 14.2 ■ Types of delusions

Disturbances in thinking	Definition	Example
Delusions of persecution	Belief that others are hostile or trying to harm the individual	A woman notices a man looking at her and believes that he is trying to follow her.
Delusions of reference	False belief that public events or people are directly related to the individual	A man hears a story on the evening news and believes it is about him.
Somatic delusions	Belief that one's body is altered from normal structure or function	An elderly woman believes that her bowel is filled with cement and refuses to eat.
Thought broadcasting	Belief that one's unspoken thoughts can be heard	A young person believes that everyone around him knows he's attracted to a nurse although he has said nothing.
Delusions of control	Belief that one's actions or thoughts are controlled by an external person or force	A woman believes that her neighbour controls her thoughts by means of his home computer.
Nihilistic delusions	Belief that reality and existence are gone or were never there	A young man states that nothing exists. Makes statements such as 'Everything is lost', 'I have no head, no stomach', 'I cannot die' or 'I will live to eternity.'
Delusions of self-deprecation	Belief that one is not worthy of routine or usual aspects of life	A young mother believes she is ugly and smells like garbage. Severe depression can cause feelings of being unworthy, sinful, ugly or foul-smelling.
Delusions of grandeur	Inflated sense of self-worth and abilities	A woman with mania believes she is 'extraordinarily wealthy and intelligent with a fully evolved value system'.

Table 14.3 ■ Positive symptoms

Positive symptom	Examples	
Hallucinations		
Auditory	Human speech (speaking clearly, mumbling, whispering, singing, yelling, screaming, one voice, several voices, voice speaking to the person, voices speaking to each other, male, female, both, indistinguishable, imitating non-human sounds)	
	Mechanical sounds (clocks, metal clanging, clicking)	
	Music	
	Animal sounds	
	Insect sounds	
	Wind through the trees	
	Grating sounds made by walking on sand	
	Crinkling sound from plastic or aluminum wraps	
	The sound of the earth moving or heaving as during an earthquake	
Visual	Blood	People
	Animals	Movement of large objects
	Distortions of everyday sights	Auras
Olfactory	Green peppers	Blood
	Fumes	Burning materials
	Garlic	Urine or faeces
	Semen	Rotting meat
	Sulfur	
Gustatory	Metallic flavour	Blood
	Urine or faeces	Semen
Tactile	Being pregnant	Giving birth
	Being beaten	Electrocution
	Being raped	Band around head
	Grease on hands	Moving tumours
	Internal movements	
Delusions		
Persecutory	'I cannot leave my unit more than once a month. I have to have this cardboard in my pockets when I go out so the police can't take pictures of me.'	
Referential	'I didn't mean to do it. I was just thinking what would happen if the train derailed. I'm sorry I killed all those people.'	
Somatic	'I am going to be haemorrhaging, bleeding to death through my mouth.' Or: 'I am carrying an alien in my belly. When he is mature he'll drip from my palms like sweat.'	
Religious	'My daughter is the devil, saturated with evil, because her age of ascendancy is 666 (6 June 2006).'	
Substitution	'It looks just like my wife, but it's really a robot.'	
Thought insertion	'These thoughts are being put in my head by the alien conspiracy.' Or: 'When I get angry it's because the police are altering my brain waves.'	
Nihilistic	'Everything is falling apart. My insides are rotting away, and so is everything else.'	
Grandiose	'I made $7 million from a software program I developed, and they're keeping it from me until I tell them my secret programming wizardry.' Or: 'I am not who you think I am. I work midnights at all of the top law firms so I can get all of their work done for them.'	

(continued)

Table 14.3 ■ Positive symptoms (*continued*)

Positive symptom	Examples	
Disorganised speech		
Loose associations	'I take a shot of Haldol every four weeks; it's not weak, it's strong and so is the pill twice a day. I don't care if it does me wonders or not, wonder bread, terrorist. I'm taking it for the hell of it. Bread and soldier. Who cares if it helps me or not. I'm doing phenomenal.'	
Word salad	'Wimple sitting purple which the twilighted cheshire, for then frames of silver ticking bubble and.'	
Clanging	'I want to eat neat treat seat beat.'	
	'I'm fine it's a sign fine whine wine pine dine.'	
Echolalia	The person repeats pieces of what is said or entire phrases: Nurse asks 'How are you today?', and the person states 'You today.' Or the person states 'I love smelling roses. I love smelling roses.'	
Behaviour		
Disorganised	The person walks around aimlessly picking up everything available to them and touching all objects and surfaces.	
Catatonic	Excited catatonia: a person living with schizophrenia in the emergency department is repeatedly assaultive, hyperactive or cannot sit still.	
	Waxy flexibility: The person maintains a rigid position, allows another to move them into new positions and maintains that new position.	
Thinking		
Lack of planning skills	Indecisiveness	Lack of problem-solving skills
Concrete thinking	Blocking	Difficulty initiating tasks

LIVED EXPERIENCE

For me the most disturbing positive symptoms were a combination of delusions and 'voices', where the voices fed off the delusions, modified delusions and created an alternative reality that was self-reinforcing. The main recollection I have is of snakes descending from my ceiling; giant pythons and poisonous snakes. I was preoccupied with snakes at the time; my family manifested the delusions and hallucinations as snakes, and they were waging a kind of psychological warfare against me in the form of snakes. At the same time I had no comprehension of being unwell. While I now think of this as a classic acute psychotic episode, there had been times prior to this in which I had experienced other positive symptoms, such as hearing whispered voices, paranoid delusions and also grandiose delusions, such as believing I was a reborn spiritual warrior.

Table 14.4 ■ Negative symptoms

Negative Symptom	Examples
Flat affect	The person maintains the same emotional tone when told their mother has died as when told it is time to attend programs. 'Okay.'
Apathy	The person has feelings of indifference towards people, events, activities and learning.
Avolition	The person does not get to the job they really wanted because they couldn't get up in time to catch the bus.
Anhedonia	The person apparently derives no pleasure from listening to music when, prior to getting sick, they used to enjoy it.
Alogia	Rather than using a series of sentences or several words, the person, when asked about their day, speaks sparsely in a limited, stilted manner: 'Fine.'

absence of any signs of affective expression, and can include poor eye contact (Black & Andreasen, 2014). To see how flat affect differs from a normal range of affect, imagine someone responding to winning a prize ('This is great! I'm so happy!'). Now imagine that same person with much less emotion in their response and no emotion showing on their face ('Oh.'). The difference between the two responses is the flattening of affect.

Alogia

Brief, empty verbal responses are known as *alogia*. Rather than saying a few sentences in response to a question, a person with alogia will reply with a single word or a very limited number of words. This **poverty of speech** is thought to be symptomatic of diminished thoughts, and is different from a refusal to speak. With alogia, the person does not use many words to express experiences or thoughts.

Avolition

A symptom that is frequently misunderstood by families and the community is **avolition**, an inability to pursue and persist in goal-directed activities. It can also be thought of as not being motivated. You may see evidence of this negative symptom when a person living with schizophrenia fails to keep an appointment or fails to become involved in an easily available activity. The person living with schizophrenia who has avolition is often misinterpreted as being lazy or unwilling to support themselves, rather than displaying a symptom of the illness. This misunderstanding often affects the ability of family members and friends to stay involved in relationships with the person. They may feel frustrated, as if their efforts have been wasted, or feel personally rejected because their suggestions have gone unheeded.

Anhedonia

Anhedonia, the inability to experience pleasure, may pose a challenge as you work with people living with schizophrenia. It is difficult to imagine, and empathise with, someone who cannot seem to enjoy even small aspects of life. It is important to remember that some people who live with schizophrenia cannot enjoy experiences because of a physiological reason over which they have no control.

Recognising the presence of negative symptoms

The negative symptoms of schizophrenia can be difficult to assess, because they are part of our everyday experiences, just more intense and durable. While few of us have experienced true hallucinations, many of us know what it is like to have a day in which our energy levels are very low and we struggle to get things done. Another difficulty in recognising the presence of negative symptoms stems from the fact that people living with schizophrenia often live in difficult situations that may lead to restricted emotional expression and disturbed goal-directed activities.

When asked to identify immediate challenges, participants in the Survey of High Impact Psychosis (SHIP) in Australia identified financial matters, loneliness/isolation, lack of employment and poor physical health ahead of uncontrolled symptoms of mental illness (Carr, Whiteford, Groves, McGorry & Shepherd, 2012). These findings suggest that the priorities of health professionals, such as mental health nurses, and people living with schizophrenia can be quite different. While health professionals are likely to see symptom management as the main priority, people living with schizophrenia may consider loneliness, secure accommodation and financial support as more important. Living alone, in poverty, or in unsettled circumstances—homelessness, for example—can induce feelings of desperation or despair, which may mimic the negative symptoms of schizophrenia. It is thus important to try to separate environmental influences on experience from the disease process, and to note the persistence of the symptoms over time across a variety of circumstances. For example, if a person is living in a boarding house where others around them are likely to steal, that person will not be safe talking excitedly about having received a gift from their parents. If, however, the person is not excited when in their own home in front of their parents and trusted others, the presence of limited verbalisations may be a negative symptom of schizophrenia.

While the media is not typically a reliable source of accurate information about schizophrenia, there have been some reasonably accurate depictions of the experience of psychosis in films; one example is *A Beautiful Mind*. See Mental Health in the Media for details about the plot. You see an authentic representation of what individuals and families struggle with in the depiction of negative symptoms in the movie.

Another important criterion for recognising schizophrenia is detecting an impaired ability to perform and complete social and work obligations. It can be diagnostic of schizophrenia if a person has difficulty performing in one or more areas

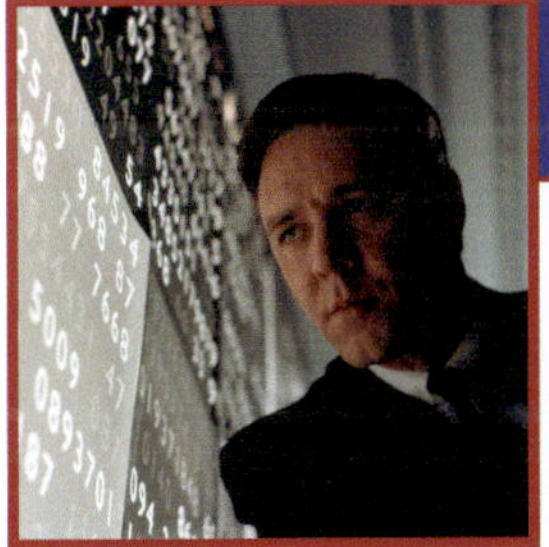

MENTAL HEALTH IN THE MEDIA

A Beautiful Mind

The movie *A Beautiful Mind* is based on the true story of Nobel Prize-winning mathematician and economist John Nash and his life with schizophrenia. The movie begins with his college years at an ivy-league school, and moves through the beginning of his career and the formation of his relationship with his wife. His brilliance and unique perspectives, as well as his quirky behaviours and strongly held views, bring you to the realisation that something else may be shaping his experiences. You find out about his illness when he finds out about his illness. John's best friend and roommate from college and his friend's young niece turn out to be visual hallucinations. Delusions of being involved in special government work greatly influence his behaviour. Antipsychotic medication had not yet been developed when he was diagnosed, so his journey included insulin shock therapy and then, later, the traditional or conventional antipsychotics.

In one scene, John sits and stares while his wife tells him, 'Meaning is all around you, all you have to do is look for it.' Her exasperation is evident. The side-effects of the medications interfere with his relationship with his wife in other ways as well. After he stops taking them, he is once again plunged into symptoms. This movie shines a light on the illness of schizophrenia, how an individual and his family cope, provides hope about the power of caring relationships, and demonstrates how people can take charge of their own recovery. Sadly, John Nash and his wife, Alicia, passed away in 2015.

Photo courtesy of Everett Collection.

LIVED EXPERIENCE

In the 15 years in which I went untreated, I gradually deteriorated into a shell of my former self. I was extremely depressed and anxious, but at the same time also managed to live a very marginal existence. A major problem I struggled with was finding pleasure in anything; I now recognise this as anhedonia. Another problem was avolition—I just could not do anything. For about five years I withdrew into the country and could not work, despite having qualifications and experience in teaching languages at high-school level. Even now I have a tendency to spend too much time watching television and being on my own. I sometimes think of this as being a hangover from the period of untreated psychosis.

of life, including work, school, social relationships, and the maintenance of everyday activities, such as dressing and providing food for themselves.

REMOVAL OF SUBTYPES OF SCHIZOPHRENIA IN DSM-5

In a significant departure from earlier versions of the *Diagnostic and statistical manual of mental disorders*, in DSM-5 the diagnostic criteria for schizophrenia no longer identifies subtypes based on the predominant presenting symptom; for instance, paranoid type, disorganised type, catatonic type, undifferentiated type and residual type. Over time these classical subtypes of schizophrenia were found to be unhelpful clinically, as symptoms often changed from one subtype to another over time, and frequently overlapped in the same person. The elimination of the subtypes from DSM-5 can thus be put down to the heterogeneity of schizophrenia—except for the paranoid and undifferentiated subtypes, other subtypes were rarely used in diagnosing the disorder (Tandon et al., 2013).

SOMATIC TREATMENTS

Prior to the 1950s— a period of time sometimes referred to as the *pre-neuroleptic age*—insulin coma, drug or electrically induced shock treatments, and psychosurgery, including prefrontal lobotomies, were used to treat schizophrenia. The impact of these extreme somatic treatments were thought to make a difference, for a time, in symptomatology, but raised ethical concerns. Initially, it was hoped that these treatments would lead to a cure for schizophrenia, and they seemed to be relatively quick and inexpensive compared to lengthy and costly analytic therapies. This hope was not realised.

Under current mental health legislation in Australia, psychosurgery is regulated to the point of being effectively banned. However, electroconvulsive therapy (ECT) has been improved upon in the past 30 years, and is in widespread use throughout Australia. Effective treatment with minimal risks has been offered mostly for people living with mood disorders.

The introduction of psychoactive drugs in the 1950s provided new alternatives for the treatment of schizophrenia. Psychotropic medications, which influence the thoughts, mood and behaviour of people living with psychotic illness, made previously uncontrolled symptoms more manageable. In the period following the introduction of psychotropic medications, the use of seclusion and restraints declined, as did the duration of hospital stays and the numbers of people detained in state mental hospitals. It ought to be noted, however, that despite concerns raised by policy-makers, consumer and carer representatives and some health professionals, seclusion and restraint remain in widespread use throughout Australia (Gaskin, Elsom & Happell, 2007; National Mental Health Working Group, 2005).

A new optimism arose regarding the possible outcomes of mental illness. Because they controlled to some extent the most difficult symptoms of psychosis, psychotropic medications made psychosocial or behavioural treatments possible for a much greater percentage of people living with mental illness. There is no cure yet for schizophrenia; current thinking and practice focuses more on recovery than cure, stressing the importance of maintaining hope, understanding personal abilities and disabilities, engaging in an active life, exercising autonomy, expressing identity, meaning and purpose in life, and building a positive sense of self (Department of Health, 2010). Importantly, such recovery can be both personal and clinical in nature. Antipsychotic drugs can relieve the more debilitating symptoms of schizophrenia, and make an important contribution towards recovery for many people living with schizophrenia. Unfortunately, these medications are often accompanied by distressing side-effects, such as weight gain, that can contribute to the development of physical illness and thus impede recovery. Refer to Chapters 5, 6 and 7 for more details on the history and the science behind somatic treatments. Ethical and legal aspects of somatic treatments are discussed in Chapter 11.

LIVED EXPERIENCE

For me, medications should not be thought of as 'magic bullets', which is what both my family and I thought initially. My improvement was so slow and gradual that medication proved to be a steadying influence, contributing to the possibility of recovery over time. However, it was still necessary for me to work hard on myself, which has involved years of therapy, especially interpersonal psychotherapy.

RELAPSE

A person living with schizophrenia can be vulnerable to a return of symptoms after a period of stability, however brief or extended, partial or complete. This is called a **relapse**, and the disease itself often has a pattern of relapse and recovery. As a chronic disorder, schizophrenia is characterised by relapses alternating with periods of full or partial remission.

Although antipsychotic medication is effective in reducing relapse rates, 10 per cent to 30 per cent of people relapse within one year after hospital discharge, even if they are receiving maintenance medication (Emsley, Chiliza, Asmal & Lehloenya, 2011). It is important to understand the sense of demoralisation that may accompany such a recurrent and debilitating course, and the need to improve methods for relapse prevention. The following two Practice Examples detail how relapses can occur under certain circumstances.

Practice example

Daryl, a 26-year-old man living with schizophrenia, decided to stop taking his quetiapine (Seroquel) because he didn't think he needed it anymore. Within a few days of stopping the medication, he was unable to leave the house for fear of someone harming him. Although he liked his job at a local supermarket, he refused to go to work for fear that he would be hit by a bus on his way there. He was eventually fired because of poor attendance. The loss of a structured schedule furthered his deterioration, and Daryl relapsed, requiring hospitalisation.

In this instance, a decrease in medication increased Daryl's biological vulnerability, with marked behavioural, and eventually environmental, consequences. His relapse began with a medication issue and could have been prevented.

Practice example

Jeanne, 22, has lived with her divorced mother and younger sister Maura since her release from hospital after her second psychotic episode. She found living alone too frightening, and was more comfortable staying in her old room at home. When Maura began preparing to leave home for university, Jeanne became increasingly anxious, demanding to sleep in Maura's room at night and hiding Maura's belongings. As Maura's departure grew near, Jeanne began actively hallucinating and withdrew to her room, refusing to talk to her mother or sister.

In this case, Jeanne did not have sufficient coping skills to deal with her sister's departure from the household, and her psychosis re-emerged. Jeanne's relapse may have been averted had she been taught more effective coping skills and had the opportunity to practise them. Learning can be unfavourably affected by schizophrenia, as motivation and energy are problems, and even a competent program of teaching cannot remove all of the negative consequences in response to life stress.

OTHER PSYCHOTIC DISORDERS

Psychosis occurs in a number of disorders in addition to schizophrenia. The problems with symptoms can be short-lived, or may extend into significant periods of time with disability.

Schizophreniform disorder

Schizophreniform disorder is part of the schizophrenia spectrum in DSM-5, and is very similar to schizophrenia except the person has not been ill for very long. The main difference is that the symptoms have been experienced for at least one month, and the person has either recovered from the symptoms before six months, or six months have not yet elapsed since the original symptoms began. Under the latter set of circumstances, the diagnosis of schizophreniform disorder is provisional until the six months have elapsed and then a diagnosis is made. A second difference, besides duration, is that the person may show no impairment in social and work functioning.

Schizophreniform disorder may occur just prior to the onset of schizophrenia (i.e. be prodromal to [precede] schizophrenia), yet approximately one-third of people diagnosed with this disorder recover. The other two-thirds go on to develop either schizophrenia or schizoaffective disorder.

Schizoaffective disorder

In **schizoaffective disorder**, two sets of symptoms—psychotic and mood symptoms—are present concurrently in the same period of illness episode: positive symptoms of schizophrenia and symptoms of a mood disorder (either a major depressive or manic disorder; see Chapter 15). Under DSM-5, there is a requirement that a major mood episode be present for the majority of time in which psychotic symptoms are present. Schizoaffective disorder is less common, and has a slightly better prognosis, than schizophrenia, but it has a substantially worse prognosis than mood disorders. Interacting with a person living with schizoaffective disorder may require the same skills you would employ with a person living with schizophrenia. Disorganised speech may be an expression of this type of psychosis. The Communication feature provides examples of therapeutic communication with a client with the clang association form of disorganised speech.

COMMUNICATION

A person with clang associations

PERSON: 'The dining room lining trying to eat forever.'

NURSE RESPONSE 1: 'Jack, are you having a problem getting your food?'	NURSE RESPONSE 2: 'Come with me and let's get you set up.'
RATIONALE: A direct question allows the person experiencing clang associations to answer with a 'yes' or 'no' response, models how the communication can be stated, and labels the situation as a problem.	*RATIONALE:* This response reinforces the appropriateness of the person coming to the nurse with a problem and concretely shows the person how to resolve the problem.

One of the defining characteristics of schizoaffective disorder is when the hallucination or delusion occurs. A person living with schizoaffective disorder is likely to experience hallucinations or delusions regardless of mood state. In other words, if the person were delusional only when they had extreme problems with mood (mania or depression), it is likely the diagnosis would be mood disorder with psychotic features rather than schizoaffective disorder.

Delusional disorder

In DSM-5, **delusional disorder** is diagnosed when a person holds one or more delusions for a period of at least one month. This represents a departure from earlier versions of the DSM in which there was a requirement that such delusions be non-bizarre.

People living with delusional disorders may function quite well in areas of their life not affected by the delusion, yet behave oddly in activities touched by the delusion. Delusional disorders are not common, and arise predominantly during middle and late adulthood.

A type of delusional disorder, the erotomanic type, occurs when people believe that another person is in love with them. Typically no such relationship exists, or is superficial at best. Contacting the person, stalking the person, and displays to impress the imagined lover have involved celebrities, politicians, and the man or woman next door.

Brief psychotic disorder

In DSM-5, brief psychotic disorder is included in the schizophrenia spectrum; at least one of the positive symptoms for schizophrenia must be present (hallucinations, delusions, disorganised speech or behaviour) for at least one day, but for less than one month. Upon remission of these symptoms, the affected person returns to their level of functioning prior to the onset of the illness. This disorder may be brought on by a particular stressful event in the person's life, including childbirth. In other instances, a stressful life event cannot be specifically identified. Brief psychotic disorder is an unusual and seldom-seen phenomenon.

Additional psychotic disorders

Several additional psychotic disorders are specified in the DSM-5, as follows:

- psychotic disorder associated with another medical condition
- substance- or medication-induced psychotic disorder
- psychotic disorder, not elsewhere classified.

Consult the DSM-5 for diagnostic criteria for these disorders. However, in the diagnosis of any psychotic disorder, it is important that alternative explanations are explored, as symptoms may also be caused by an underlying medical disorder or by substance use.

BIOPSYCHOSOCIAL THEORIES

Beliefs about the causes of schizophrenia have changed over the centuries since schizophrenia was equated with early senility. Theories about the treatment for schizophrenia have also undergone change. For example, at one point it was erroneously believed (based on the writings of Sigmund Freud) that people with schizophrenia could not be treated because they were unable to form a therapeutic relationship with a psychoanalyst. At another point, a now-discredited theory pointed to the behaviour of parents, especially mothers, causing schizophrenia in their offspring. It is likely that a number of factors interrelate to cause schizophrenia, and several forces influence the effectiveness of treatment. A multifactorial cause and a varied approach to treatment, responsive to an individual's needs, seem most consistent with current expectations of recovery-focused practice.

Biological theories

It is unlikely that schizophrenia is caused by one specific biological abnormality. Scientists have searched unsuccessfully for a unique biological marker consistently present in people with schizophrenia but absent in healthy people. At the same time, evidence suggests that the disorder is not merely psychological, and that biological alterations are present. The symptoms associated with schizophrenia, such as delusions or hallucinations, are generally only found in healthy people only when they are in a state of metabolic imbalance or suffer from organic diseases. Individuals who have brain tumours, have infections, or have ingested certain drugs, for example, may experience hallucinations. However, the Hearing Voices Movement (HVM), a mental health consumer/survivor movement which has gained in prominence since the 1980s, advocates that hearing voices in the absence of other symptoms of psychosis or underlying health problems is a relatively common if unusual human experience. The main points advocated by the HVM are that hearing voices is a normal part of human experience; that various explanations for hearing voices be acknowledged and respected; that those who hear voices take ownership of their experiences; that hearing voices be understood in relation to social context and personal narratives; that accepting voices is generally more helpful than trying to quell them; and peer support is beneficial in helping people understand and deal with voices (Corstens et al., 2014).

Genetic theories

It is believed that people living with schizophrenia inherit a genetic predisposition to the disease rather than inheriting the disease itself. What supports this theory is the fact that relatives of people with schizophrenia have a greater chance of developing the disease than do members of the general population. While about 1 per cent of the population develops schizophrenia, 10 per cent of the first-degree relatives (parents, siblings, children) of persons living with schizophrenia are diagnosed with the disease during their lifetimes. The risk of developing schizophrenia increases with the closeness of one's relationship to a diagnosed person. Siblings have a greater risk of developing the disease than do half-siblings or grandchildren, and these have a greater risk than more distant relatives, such as cousins.

There is no clear genetic marker for schizophrenia at this time, although research is underway to discover susceptibility genes. The most promising development has been research looking at the large number of genes involved in developing our nervous systems, and the smaller number of genes called *epigenetic regulators*, or genes that can moderate genetic expression (Zahir & Brown, 2011). Because schizophrenia is complex and there are so many forms of the disorder, a single gene is unlikely to be responsible for causing schizophrenia. It has been suggested that schizophrenia may be a collection of disorders rather than a single disease entity.

Research examining the occurrence of schizophrenia in twins indicates that both environmental and genetic factors are important. Rates of concordance (in which both twins either express or do not express the trait) for schizophrenia are consistently higher for monozygotic twins than for dizygotic twins. Interestingly, monozygotic, or identical, twins need not both have schizophrenia, but the chance of both twins having schizophrenia is 25 per cent to 40 per cent. This finding supports the hypothesis of some level of genetic transmission. The fact that both twins are not always affected when they are genetically identical, however, indicates that environment plays a large part in the expression of the illness. If the disease were solely genetically determined, the concordance rates in this group would be close to 100 per cent. (See also pages 105–166 in Chapter 6 for another discussion of genetics in schizophrenia.)

Brain structure abnormalities

As a group, people living with schizophrenia differ in their brain structure from people who do not have schizophrenia. People living with chronic schizophrenia show changes to their frontotemporal cortical grey matter, among other areas. Magnetic resonance imaging (MRI) studies show hippocampal structural differences between people who have schizophrenia and those who do not. When the hippocampus is formed, brain-derived neurotrophic factor (BDNF) is involved. Checking for abnormalities in BDNF may be able to tell us who is at risk for developing schizophrenia. Also, the BDNF increases when clients are on antipsychotic medication (Lee, Lange, Ricken, Hellweg & Lang, 2011).

Altered brain structures may be genetically based, and could represent a marker of vulnerability to schizophrenia that precedes any other symptomatology. How brain structure abnormalities influence the progress of the disease is not well understood and requires further study. An example of PET scan differences between someone who has schizophrenia and someone who does not is seen in Figure 14.1 ■.

Biochemical theories

The biochemical basis of schizophrenia is captured in the **dopamine hypothesis**, which states that schizophrenic symptoms may be related to overactive neuronal activity that is dependent on dopamine (DA). In other words, positive psychotic symptoms are associated with excessive DA transmission.

The hypothesis was supported by numerous studies demonstrating the alleviation of symptoms from treatment with DA blockers, which are medications that decrease DA activity. The traditional antipsychotic medications were shown to be effective because of their ability to antagonise DA receptors; however, this causes undesirable side-effects, such as extrapyramidal symptoms. The relief of positive symptoms with these traditional agents was not complete, and the negative symptoms of the disorder were much less responsive to DA blockers. See Figure 14.2 ■ for a graphic representation of this concept.

Research suggests that the relationships between DA activity and the symptoms of schizophrenia are much more complex than originally hypothesised. It is now known that there are various types of DA receptors, and different types of receptors are concentrated in different regions of the brain.

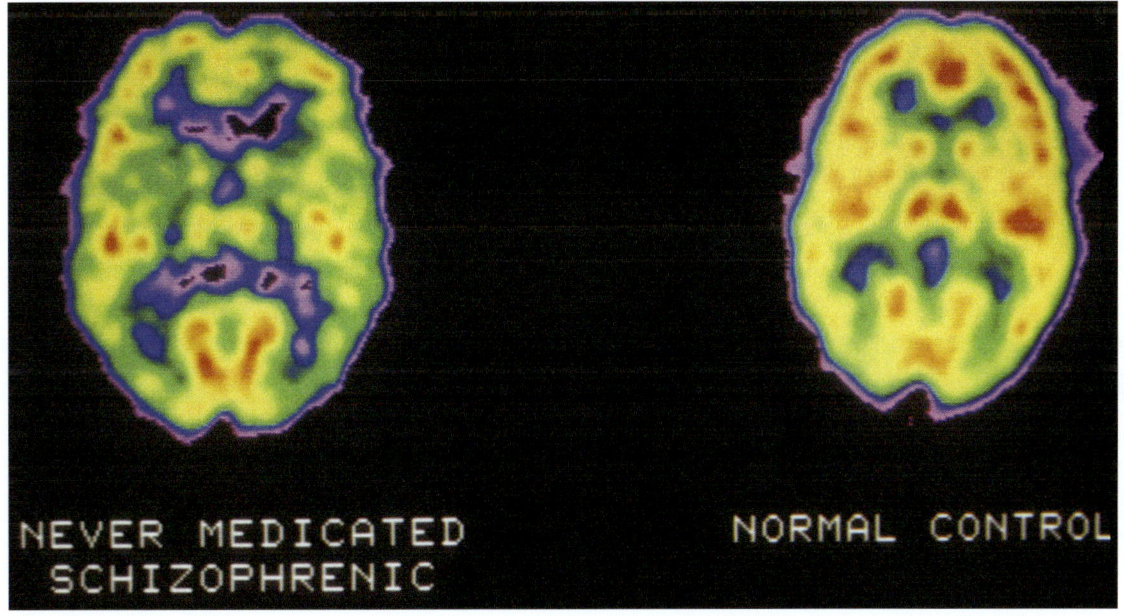

FIGURE 14.1 ■ PET scans measuring regional cerebral blood flow. (a) Areas of lower blood flow and brain activity are seen in the individual with schizophrenia. (b) Areas of normal blood flow and brain activity are visible in the unaffected individual.
Photo courtesy of Merritt/Photolibrary.

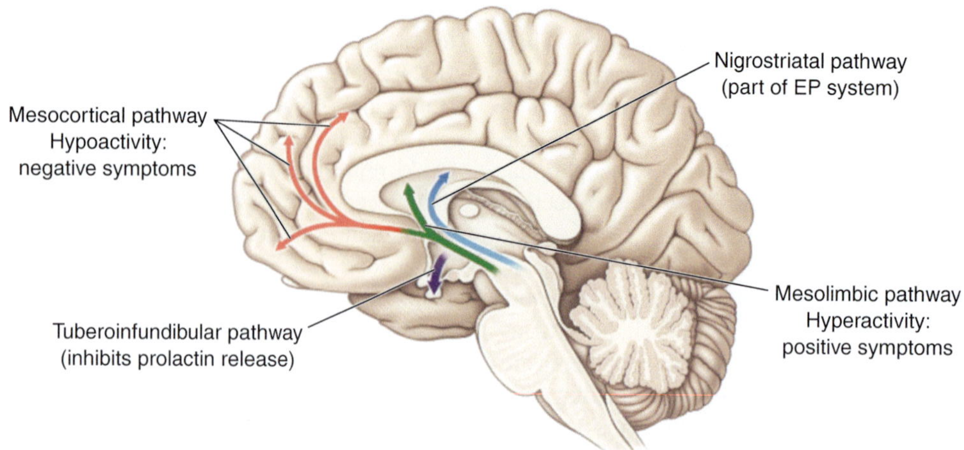

FIGURE 14.2 ■ The dopamine hypothesis of schizophrenia holds that the amount of dopamine in various areas of the brain creates the various symptoms of the disease. Note how too much dopamine in the mesolimbic area (the middle of the limbic system) is thought to cause positive symptoms, while too little dopamine in the mesocortical area (the middle of the cortex of the brain) is thought to cause the negative symptoms of schizophrenia. Antipsychotic medications are designed to address this problem, and attempt to stabilise these excesses and deficits.

The regulation of DA activity continues to be thoroughly studied, because DA dysregulation is recognised as being inherently involved in the pathology of schizophrenia.

Psychological theories

Most psychological theories focus on the processing of information as well as attention and arousal states in schizophrenia.

Information processing

Many people living with schizophrenia have information-processing deficits. Two central types of information processing have been identified, as follows:

1. automatic processing
2. controlled or effortful processing.

Automatic processing occurs when you take in information unintentionally. Automatic processing can occur without your being aware of it, and does not interfere with conscious thought processes that occur at the same time. An example of automatic information processing is being aware of the physical features of a new environment, such as a room being large and spacious as opposed to small and confined.

People living with schizophrenia have difficulty in the skill called *controlled information processing*. Their ability to perform directed, conscious, sequential thinking—for example, making comparisons between two stimuli or organising a set of stimuli—is consistently inferior to that of people who do not have schizophrenia. Someone living with schizophrenia would not be easily able to perform the series of steps necessary to organise a classroom debate. Any level of cognitive dysfunction creates ripple effects in treatment and quality of life. See the Communication feature for an example of an interaction with a person who is unfocused and having a problem processing information.

We do not know whether the inability of a person living with schizophrenia to sustain conscious, directed thought is the primary problem or the result of a primary deficit in automatic thinking. If the primary deficit is in automatic processes, then the person is forced to complete automatic tasks at the conscious level, inhibiting and slowing controlled information processing. Sufficient evidence to resolve this question is not yet available.

Attention and arousal

Attention and arousal are measured by physiological states and alterations, such as galvanic skin response, heart rate,

COMMUNICATION

Unfocused person

PERSON: 'I went to the rugby match and I had great seats and I saw the whole game and I saw all the tries, goals, penalty kicks, scrums, kick-offs, tackles and . . .'

NURSE RESPONSE 1: 'Keith, tell me about this more slowly so I can keep up with you.' *RATIONALE:* This response defines the special skills required for a conversation.	**NURSE RESPONSE 2:** 'How about if I ask you some questions about the game? If you give me a chance to ask questions, I'll have a better idea of what you saw.' *RATIONALE:* This response is structured to be brief and focused, and to direct the person's attention to the speed with which he speaks.

LIVED EXPERIENCE

My experience of knowing many people living with schizophrenia has been that performance levels are often higher than might typically be expected (and health professionals and textbooks imply). For many people recovery is experienced as a struggle to get by; but it is worth the effort!

blood pressure, skin temperature and pupillary response. Physiological studies of attention and arousal in people living with schizophrenia show promise in identifying clinically significant subgroups.

One subgroup exhibits abnormally low response levels to novel, or different, stimuli. This finding suggests that these people are less adept than healthy people at attending to and responding to novel situations. An example of this state can be seen when a person living with schizophrenia does not register that a ball is being thrown to them during a catching game. The ball may even strike them, drop to the ground and roll away before the person looks at it.

A second group of people living with schizophrenia demonstrates a state of hyperarousal evidenced by elevated electrodermal activity, heart rate and blood pressure. Hyperarousal has been noted during both symptomatic and non-symptomatic periods. This group of people demonstrates symptoms of irritability, excitement and anxiety rather than apathy and withdrawal. An example of this state occurs when a person living with schizophrenia angrily and loudly criticises someone for using incorrect grammar in a sentence.

Family theories

Numerous theories implicating family interaction alone as a cause of schizophrenia have been proposed and subsequently not supported. Research has failed to support the theory that dysfunctional family interaction alone causes the illness.

Suggestions have been supported that disordered family communication (the inability to focus on and clearly share an observation or thought) causes schizophrenia only in the presence of a genetic predisposition to the disease. For example, the communication taking place at the dinner table may be chaotic and constant. No one finishes a sentence and nothing is discussed to its logical conclusion. Living with this pattern of family communication during early development is thought to impair the ability of the person living with schizophrenia to perceive the environment and communicate with others about it. People living with schizophrenia are more likely to show symptoms of thought disorder when they are raised by people who have dysfunctional communication.

Individuals living with schizophrenia who are raised by adoptive parents, who themselves showed elevated levels of communication deviance, demonstrate as much thought disorder as those raised in birth families. In contrast, adoptees who were raised by adoptive parents with more functional communication were less likely to show thought disorder. This suggests there is not a 'schizophrenogenic' environment for individuals who do not have a pre-existing genetic liability. These examples support the view that genetic factors alone do not explain the development of schizophrenia, and that interactions with the environment are important. Individuals who live in aversive environments tend to have higher rates of schizophrenia, suggesting there may be a neighbourhood and social context to development of the disease.

The family or the environment's emotional tone can influence the course of schizophrenia over time. Researchers found that individuals living with schizophrenia from families who are highly critical, hostile, overprotective or over-involved tend to relapse more often. Families exhibiting such characteristics have been described as having high **expressed emotion** (EE). There is some evidence that family expressed emotion, life events and biological factors combine with the individual's genetic susceptibility to the disorder to cause schizophrenia. In other words, the disorder is responsive to psychosocial attributes such as the emotional climate of the interpersonal environment (Rylands, McKie, Elliot, Deakin & Tarrier, 2011). Recent research on schizophrenia can be found on the website for the Schizophrenia Research Institute at http://schizophreniaresearch.org.au/schizophrenia/about-schizophrenia/

Humanistic interactional theories

An interactional model of schizophrenia integrates many of the biological and psychosocial theories already discussed. In this view, schizophrenia is due to the interaction of a genetic predisposition or biological vulnerability, stress or change in the environment, and a person's social skills and supports. In an interactional model, the influences are multi-dimensional. A biological vulnerability may inhibit an individual's capacity to cope with even minor stressors, such as the loss of a primary source of support. Similarly, the symptoms of schizophrenia may worsen upon entering an environment that demands coping skills the person living with schizophrenia may not have developed.

A precursor to present-day interactional theories is the enduring interpersonal–psychiatric theory of Harry Stack Sullivan (discussed in detail in Chapter 5). Sullivan, a psychiatrist, emphasised modes of interaction and the role of anxiety as the real focus of psychiatric inquiry in his work with people living with schizophrenia. Hildegard Peplau (a central figure in the development of mental health nursing) based her interpersonal psychiatric nursing approach on the work of Sullivan. However, Peplau had more to say than Sullivan about the social and cultural conditions that influence behaviour. The ideas of Sullivan and Peplau continue to influence our practice with people living with schizophrenia.

Stress–vulnerability model

An interactional model for understanding schizophrenia that has received wide acceptance is the stress–vulnerability model, which suggests that people living with schizophrenia have a genetically based, biologically mediated vulnerability to personal, family and

EVIDENCE-BASED PRACTICE

Assessing the coping skills of a young person living with schizophrenia

Michael is a 16-year-old male who lives with schizophrenia. He is one of the people with whom you work in an outpatient clinic for moderately ill people who have schizophrenia. Your education and experience have taught you that schizophrenia is a complex illness that requires more than medications to address it adequately.

As a teenager, Michael has difficulties with interactions, problem-solving and coping that an older person may not have to the same extent. Older people would have developed those skills prior to getting ill, or had access to psychoeducation and treatment from nurses and other professionals. You note that Michael becomes stressed very easily, and typically retreats into sleeping or wishful thinking to cope. He often feels anxious, fearful and irritable. You notice that, although he will feel better for a brief time after he withdraws to bed or to daydreaming, over time Michael is not learning how to cope, nor is he developing problem-solving approaches.

This situation suggests the need to be active in helping Michael learn new skills. Coping based on problem-solving instead of emotions can lower Michael's stress levels. It is important to remain up-to-date with research on what might be helpful for people living with schizophrenia. The following article might assist in deciding the kind of help you would offer Michael.

Lee, H., & Schepp, K. G. (2011). Ways of coping in adolescents with schizophrenia. *Journal of Psychiatric and Mental Health Nursing, 18*(2), 158–165.

CRITICAL THINKING QUESTIONS

1. Is it possible for Michael to learn new coping skills? Why, or why not?
2. How would you know if Michael is using a problem-solving coping mechanism?

environmental stress. In this model, risk factors and protective factors interact in any of the following three ways:

1. stressors, risk and vulnerability factors combine and potentiate each other
2. as long as stress is not excessive, it enhances competence
3. protective factors modulate or buffer the impact of stressors by improving coping and adaptation.

People living with schizophrenia have a potentially increased vulnerability to stress. High-EE relatives or environments may cause them great stress, resulting in an exacerbation of symptoms and/or a relapse. It is now almost standard practice to aim to reduce high EE and criticism in the environment and relationships of people who live with schizophrenia.

As we know, the stressors a person living with schizophrenia experiences can overwhelm the resources available, and symptoms result. Psychobiological stressors include the stress of living with schizophrenia itself. Altered attention and perception, as well as problems with motivation and energy, create stresses for people living with schizophrenia. Environmental and interpersonal stressors include those we all encounter; however, a person living with schizophrenia is particularly sensitive to them. These include stressful life events, environments that are highly demanding or stimulating, and family or living environments that are highly negative.

It is not unusual for people living with schizophrenia to make statements that point to the validity of the stress–vulnerability concept, especially the protective qualities. As one person said: 'I'm not saying it [an antipsychotic medication] is a perfect solution. It's not. There are painful side-effects. But I know I can count on it when the going gets rough. If things get stressful, it will help me through it.' A second person said: 'I feel raw inside and out when I'm off it [an antipsychotic medication]. Everything bothers me. So it cushions the blows that are my life.'

Resources that moderate stress

Resources that can moderate stress (and are thought to affect the development of symptoms in schizophrenia) include having someone who will recognise symptoms and help manage them, having social support, and taking antipsychotic medication. Social support has proven helpful in moderating stress for general populations, and for people living with schizophrenia in particular. Supportive others who provide empathy, interpersonal contact, financial aid, problem-solving and other forms of support, help to mitigate the difficulties of schizophrenia. Finally, antipsychotic medications moderate some, and sometimes many, symptoms of the disease, and thus some of the stressors induced by the disease.

The capacities to self-monitor the waxing and waning of schizophrenia and to develop coping strategies to influence symptoms at the first sign of trouble show promise in influencing the longer-term course of the illness. It is important for a person living with schizophrenia to learn how to self-monitor symptoms and develop effective coping strategies. This capacity to detect prodromal symptoms and acute symptoms, and institute self-care before symptoms interfere significantly with functioning, is a resource that may work to mediate the stress that occurs in the person, family or environment. Evidence-based Practice, above, shows how some coping mechanisms are better than others.

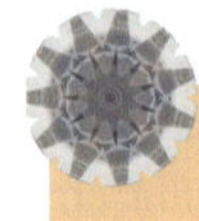

NURSING PROCESS
People living with schizophrenia

For some people, schizophrenia will be experienced as a severe and enduring illness requiring understanding and competent care in many facets of the person's life. In addition to the discussion that follows, a nursing care plan for the person living with schizophrenia is presented at the end of the chapter.

Assessment

Assessing people who live with schizophrenia occurs at individual, family and environmental levels. Be aware of the person's status and of changes in their personal life, family situation and environment, in order to plan care and intervene effectively. In addition, care that addresses multiple levels of the person's life is consistent with the interactional theory of schizophrenia, because it is assumed that changes in any aspect of the person's environment influence all other aspects of the personal environmental balance. The most effective way of collecting and making sense of information on what is troubling a person, and the history of and context to that experience, is in collaboration with the person themselves.

Subjective data

These data describe the person's inner experience of schizophrenia.

Perceptual changes The perceptions of people living with schizophrenia may be either heightened or blunted. These changes may occur in all of the senses, or in just one or two. For example, a person may see colours as brighter than normal, or may be acutely sensitive to sounds. Another may have a heightened sense of touch, and therefore be extremely sensitive to any physical contact.

Illusions occur when the person misperceives or exaggerates stimuli in the external environment. A person living with schizophrenia may mistake a chair for a person, or perceive that the walls of a hallway are closing in. The perceptual changes are sufficient to cause them to mistake the stimulus for something else (see the example of an illusion in Figure 9.1 on page 173). Hallucinations are the most extreme and yet the most common perceptual disturbance in schizophrenia. Auditory hallucinations are the most common form of hallucination. Although hallucinations are a hallmark of schizophrenia, their presence alone does not establish the presence of the disorder. Refer back to Table 14.1 on page 292, which lists the various types of hallucinations.

Assess perceptual disturbances by asking the person about the experience, and by observing for behaviours that indicate that they are frightened or attending to internal stimuli. Ask: 'What are you seeing and hearing?' Note the degree to which this description differs from your perceptions of the environment. People living with schizophrenia may be reluctant to discuss the extreme perceptual disturbance of hallucinations. One of the ways you can introduce the topic is to discuss physical symptoms such as pain or discomfort. Then ask about hearing and vision skills. This can open the way to asking about unusual experiences with hearing and seeing.

A classic sign of auditory hallucinations is placing the hands over the ears when a person is frightened by voices and attempts to block them out. Less obvious signs of hallucinations are inappropriate laughing or smiling, difficulty following a conversation, and difficulty attending to what is happening at the moment. Fleeting, rapid changes of expression that are not precipitated by events in the real world can be another sign. The degree to which a person believes the hallucinatory experience is real, and their ability to verify the reality of the experience by checking with others, have important implications for interventions. It is important to note a person's emotional response to hallucinations. Some people may experience depression or despair about the continued presence of voices; others may be comforted or kept company by their voices. A person's coping strategies, and their effectiveness or ineffectiveness, are also an important aspect of assessment. People living with schizophrenia may also talk to themselves, presumably in answer to the voices they hear. Specific guidelines for assessing hallucinations are given in Your Assessment Approach.

YOUR ASSESSMENT APPROACH

The person who is hallucinating

An effective assessment of hallucinations should identify the following:

- whether the hallucinations are solely auditory or include other senses
- how long the person has experienced the hallucinations, what the initial hallucinations were like, and whether they have changed
- which situations are most likely to trigger hallucinations, and which times of day they occur most frequently
- what the hallucinations are about (Are they just sounds, or voices? If the person hears voices, what do they say?)
- how strongly the person believes in the reality of the hallucinations
- whether the hallucinations command the person to do something and, if so, how potentially destructive the commands are
- whether the person hears other voices contradicting the commands received in the hallucinations
- how the person feels about the hallucinations
- which strategies the person has used to cope with the hallucinations, and how effective those strategies were.

Sleep disturbances Significant sleep disruption may occur with an exacerbation of the symptoms of schizophrenia. Great difficulty getting to sleep (called *extended sleep latency*) may accompany extreme anxiety and concern about delusional and hallucinatory phenomena. The overall circadian cycle may also be disrupted. People living with schizophrenia have a deficit of deeper sleep in stage 4, and reduced rapid-eye-movement (REM) sleep. A careful sleep history looks for other contributing factors—such as obesity-hypoventilation syndrome; in that case, the sleep problem can be minimised by continuous positive air pressure (CPAP).

Objective data

These data are the observable symptoms and manifestations of schizophrenia that you, as a nurse, will assess.

Disturbances in thought and expression People living with schizophrenia find that their thinking is muddled or unclear. Their thoughts are disconnected or disjointed, and the connections between one thought and another are vague. The clarity of the person's communication often reflects the level of thought disorganisation. Such responses may be simply inappropriate to the situation or conversation. The person may have difficulty responding or may stop in midsentence, as if they are stuck, which is a sign of **thought blocking**.

Note the rate and quality of the person's speech. Is it unusually loud, insistent and continuous? Do they wander from topic to topic or have *tangential communication* (communication with only a slight or tenuous connection to the topic)? An example is: 'You want to know how I came here? I came here by bus, but bussing is kissing, I wasn't kissing, but if you keep it simple that is a business tenet for KISS. That was a great group that played on and on but I'm not playing with you.' Does the person bring up minute details that are irrelevant or unimportant to the topic at hand (*circumstantial communication*)? An example is: 'You want to know how I came here? I came here on a blue and yellow bus with a lady bus driver. There were three teenage kids and a blind man with a seeing-eye dog on the bus. It didn't have to make a stop at the railway station.' Are the person's responses slow and hesitant, reflecting difficulty in taking in stimuli and responding to them?

People who live with schizophrenia may also have difficulty thinking abstractly. Their responses may be inappropriate because they interpret words literally rather than abstractly. For example, when told to prepare to have his blood drawn, a young man readied some paper and marking pens. You can assess the person's ability in abstract thinking by asking them the meaning of proverbs, a test requiring them to abstract a general meaning from a specific or metaphysical statement. For example: 'People who live in glass houses shouldn't throw stones.' A person living with schizophrenia is more likely to give a concrete response ('If you throw a stone, the glass will break') rather than abstract response ('Don't criticise someone else if you behave the same way').

Disruptions in emotional responses Tone of voice, rate of speech, content of speech, expressions, postures and body movements indicate emotional tone. Many individuals living with schizophrenia demonstrate inappropriate affect—emotional responses that are inappropriate to the situation. For example, a person may smile or laugh while relating a history of having been abused as a child, or may become angry or anxious when asked to join a group for dinner. The degree to which a person's emotions are inappropriate is a prognostic indicator. People whose emotional response is preserved and generally appropriate have a more favorable prognosis than those who demonstrate inappropriate affect.

A marked decrease in the variation or intensity of emotional expression is called **blunted affect**, and is discussed earlier in this chapter under negative symptoms. The person may express joy, sorrow or anger, but with little intensity.

Motor behaviour changes Disruptions seen in schizophrenia include disorganised behaviour and catatonia. Disorganised behaviour lacks a coherent goal, is aimless or is disruptive. Catatonic behaviour is manifested by unusual body movement or lack of movement. This activity disturbance includes *catatonic excitement* (the person moves excitedly, but not in response to environmental influences), *catatonic posturing* (the person holds bizarre postures for periods of time), and *stupor* (the person holds the body still and is unresponsive to the environment). Another motor concern is body posture and falls. People who live with schizophrenia—especially those who are older—are more likely to be overweight, have extrapyramidal side-effects (from their medication), and have some postural instability. These are risk factors for falling (Koreki et al., 2011) and early death.

Neurological signs Schizophrenia involves neurological deficits in many cases. Assessing for soft and hard neurological signs can help you design appropriate interventions, given the individual person's needs. See Box 14.1 for specifics on these neurological signs.

Changes in role functioning An important factor in predicting the course of schizophrenia is the person's level of functioning before the symptoms of the disorder became pronounced. Assessment should therefore include a complete history of the person's success at completing developmental tasks. The prognosis is best if the person functioned at a high level prior to the onset of psychotic symptoms. Assess how well the person fulfilled role responsibilities in the family, in school, in relation to peers and at work. Obtain a history of the rate of decline in these various roles. The onset of schizophrenia may be relatively acute, or degeneration may be slow.

Drug use People with drug toxicity, intoxication or withdrawal may have behaviour disturbances similar to those seen in people with schizophrenia. They may have auditory or visual hallucinations, and may be confused, illogical and highly anxious. For this reason, it is essential to obtain a

Box 14.1 Neurological soft and hard signs

Neurological soft signs are as follows:

- increased frequency of eye blinking
- difficulty following moving objects (abnormal smooth-pursuit eye movements, called SPEMs)
- impaired fine motor skills
- abnormal motor tone
- mild muscle twitches, choreiform movements (rapid, jerky movements that can cause leaping, jumping or dancing motions), tic-like movements, facial grimaces not related to emotional responses
- not able to recognise objects simply by touch (astereognosis)—the person has to look at the object.
- cannot identify letters or numbers traced out on their skin (agraphesthesia)
- impaired in ability to smoothly alternate and sequence movements, such as alternating palm up and palm down (dysdiadochokinesia).

Neurological hard signs are as follows:

- loss of physical function
- loss of strength
- slowing of reflexes
- impairment in motor and sensory behaviours.

detailed drug history. Assess both long-term and recent use of chemical substances. If the person is not a reliable historian, you may try to interview their family or friends. In addition, both blood and urine should be tested for drugs if you cannot obtain reliable information.

Family health history Part of a thorough and complete assessment is noting any history of mental disorder in the person's family. Of particular interest is a history of schizophrenia or any thought disorder, mood disorders (such as cyclical highs or depressions), or alcoholism in any family member. Note any report that family members had 'nervous breakdowns' or any other colloquial descriptions of mental or emotional disorders.

Family cohesion and emotion In families of people living with schizophrenia, enmeshment (see Chapter 24), combined with a negative emotional tone, is thought to be detrimental to the ill member's wellbeing. However, the presence of acquaintances and family members showing emotional warmth in low expressed emotion (EE) situations can have a protective function.

Much of the assessment of family cohesion and emotion can be carried out unobtrusively. Chapter 24 has specific guidelines for assessment of these and other family dynamics. The nursing staff, in conjunction with the interdisciplinary team, can also arrange formal family assessment interviews (also discussed in Chapter 24). When you are observing interactions, note signs of dysfunction.

Family over-involvement and negativity At present there are no clear-cut clinical determinants of exactly how much over-involvement and negative emotion in families is problematic. Note families who seem excessively bonded emotionally. The inability of family members to maintain emotional, social or physical separateness is a clear sign of this problem. Also assess for the presence of a high level of criticism among family members. Discuss with the treatment team families that seem seriously enmeshed or hypercritical.

Family communication problems Unclear or incomplete communication is frequent in families of people living with schizophrenia. This area requires nursing assessment. Unclear communication may result from continual interaction with the ill family member, or may contribute to the disorder. Clinicians must evaluate how effectively the family communicates to determine the potential need for intervention.

Assess the following aspects of family communication:

- ability to focus on a topic
- ability to discuss a topic in a meaningful way with other family members
- ability to maintain the discussion without wandering from the subject or becoming distracted
- use of language and explanations that are generally understandable (not peculiar to that family alone).

Also note who in the family seems to do the talking, who talks to whom, and whether members talk for, or interrupt, one another. Box 14.2 shows communication problems that commonly occur with the diagnosis of schizophrenia and interfere with interpersonal relationships.

Box 14.2 Problematic communication patterns common in schizophrenia

Blocking

The person has trouble expressing a response or stops in mid-sentence, as if stranded without a thought.

Clang associations

Words that rhyme or sound alike are distributed throughout conversations without necessarily making sense.

Echolalia

Phrases, sentences or entire conversations said to the person are repeated back by them.

Neologisms

Words or meanings are invented by the person. This can include multisyllabic, pseudo-scientific words or simple words.

Perseveration

The person maintains a particular idea regardless of the topic being discussed, or attempts to change the subject.

Word salad

An incoherent medley of words is emitted in conversation as if it was a sensible and articulate phrase.

Family burden Most families of individuals living with schizophrenia report that caring for the ill member places a burden on the family unit. Ask about the challenges the family is facing so that you can determine the information and support needs to be met. See Chapter 24 for examples of common family burdens.

Environment Assess the availability of support and services beyond the bounds of the family, including extended family and friends, as well as community groups and organisations that support people living with schizophrenia. Assess also the availability of mental health services that address the specific mental health needs of people living with schizophrenia.

Responding to the needs of a person living with schizophrenia

Much of the work undertaken by nurses when working with people living with schizophrenia involves helping them with problems with functioning, cognition, emotion regulation, interpersonal processes and perceptions. Increasingly, physical health status is also emerging as a major area of concern (Bradshaw & Pedley, 2012), with recent research, such as the Survey of High Impact Psychosis (SHIP), highlighting the extent of physical illness among people living with schizophrenia and related disorders in Australia. Among other things, the findings of the SHIP study indicated that more than half of those living with a psychotic disorder met the requirements for metabolic syndrome, a group of risk factors that increase the risk of coronary heart disease and other health problems, such as diabetes and stroke (Morgan et al., 2012). All help offered ought to be informed by the principles of recovery-oriented care (Department of Health, 2010).

Impaired communication

Schizophrenia interferes with the ability to communicate, a complex and demanding function.

Verbal People living with schizophrenia may communicate in a disorganised, sometimes incomprehensible fashion. Some people, because their thinking is disorganised, speak very little (alogia, or poverty of speech). Also note that there may be a poverty of content in speech, in that the person converses but actually says very little. Often, people living with schizophrenia communicate in ways that are overly concrete (a sign of an inability to think and communicate abstractly) or overly symbolic (a sign of preoccupation with unreal or delusional material). The symbols are usually difficult to decipher because their meanings are idiosyncratic to that particular individual.

Non-verbal The facial and bodily expressions that accompany the verbal communication of people living with schizophrenia frequently do not match the content of the verbal message. This lack of congruence is primarily due to the blunting of emotions found in schizophrenia. Expected facial expressions—smiles, looks of concern or disgust—may not accompany the person's statements. In addition, clients with motor or behavioural abnormalities—posturing, unusual movements or grimacing—convey a confusing mix of verbal and non-verbal messages.

Self-care deficits

People living with schizophrenia frequently appear indifferent to their personal appearance. They may neglect to bathe, change clothes, or attend to minor grooming tasks, such as combing their hair. Some show little awareness of current fashion styles, and many wear clothing that makes them look out of place. Of greater concern are those who wear clothing that is inappropriate to the current season and weather conditions.

Although lack of attention to grooming might be a simple annoyance to those who must live in close proximity to the person living with schizophrenia, health risks related to prolonged poor hygiene can arise. Assess immediate problems, such as inadequate nutrition, fluid intake and elimination, as well as long-term problems, such as dental caries and increased susceptibility to infections.

Disregard for appearance and hygiene may extend to the person's environment. The person may fail to maintain a clean and safe living space. They may not take good care of personal belongings and may misplace them. Self-care deficiencies may result from consistently disturbed thought and perceptual processes. For example, a person whose chronic hallucinations are only partly relieved by medication may have difficulty concentrating for long periods and paying attention to grooming.

Activity intolerance

The emotional disturbances of ambivalence and apathy, common in schizophrenia spectrum disorders, can result in a lack of interest and inactivity. Inactivity induced by ambivalence is associated with higher levels of emotion. Anxious about choosing one course of action and rejecting another, the person is immobilised. The following Practice Examples describe the experience of intolerance to activity.

LIVED EXPERIENCE

It can be difficult to maintain socially approved levels of self-care when you are prone to severe depression, the medications are making you fat, you live on a limited budget, and have little interest in eating an appropriate diet, and your self-esteem is so low. This, of course, does not mean giving up the battle. Rather, there is a need to develop strategies for regular showering and other personal hygiene practices that overcome reticence or negative feelings and, of course, ongoing negative symptoms.

Practice example

Jim is ambivalent about taking up an opportunity to go out alone from the inpatient unit for the first time. He is undecided about taking the risk of leaving the hospital setting without a staff member, yet yearns for the freedom of walking the streets alone. Indecision leaves him standing, immobilised, by the doorway to the unit.

Extreme ambivalence can manifest itself in even the most automatic of behaviours.

Practice example

Melissa cannot eat because of ambivalence about where to sit or what to eat. She stands in the centre of the dining room, turning first to one chair and then another, unable to choose where to sit so that she can begin eating.

A person who is inactive because of apathy demonstrates little emotional tone. They may spend long hours lying in bed staring into space or listening to music. Often, but not always, apathetic individuals prefer isolation. You might find several people sitting in the same room, engaged in no apparent activities, and interacting with one another only when absolutely necessary.

Social isolation

Extreme anxiety about relating to others often leads people living with schizophrenia to withdraw from interaction and to isolate themselves. Some people tolerate only a few moments of direct communication, whereas others can manage extended periods of contact. Assess the person's tolerance of brief periods of contact with staff and other people using the mental health services. Document patterns of relating and withdrawal, also noting in which activities the person engages when in contact with others, and which activities they undertake when alone.

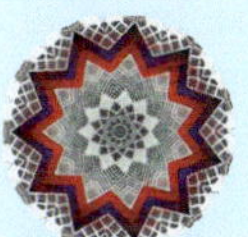

WHAT EVERY NURSE SHOULD KNOW

Primary symptoms of schizophrenia

Imagine you work in a nursing home or residential rehabilitation facility. You need to be familiar with the primary symptoms of schizophrenia—delusions, hallucinations, agitation and general decompensation—in order to competently assess the people with whom you work. There are at least two reasons why being familiar with these symptoms is important:

1. these symptoms are part of an illness process that require treatment
2. the presence of these symptoms can distort or mask the presentation of symptoms of physical illnesses, and severe psychiatric distress can impair healing from medical and surgical procedures and injuries.

When a resident within a nursing home or rehabilitation facility has symptoms that appear to include behavioural and psychiatric features, the nurse should be able to document, classify and report these symptoms correctly, and help ensure the resident receives necessary treatment. Knowing the interventions, pharmacological and nonpharmacological, can speed stabilisation and improve the quality of life the residents experience.

Decisional conflict

Decisional conflict in schizophrenia is probably due to biochemical alterations in the brain that make it difficult for the person to take in, synthesise and respond to information. Decisional conflict may be evident both in the mundane activities of daily life (e.g. selecting one's diet) and in major life decisions. This can be frustrating for caregivers and for people living with schizophrenia. The following Practice Example shows how decisional conflict can remove what is a pleasant aspect of life from the person living with schizophrenia.

Practice example

Murray refuses to take medications, even though not taking them means that he faces the possibility of being discharged from the residential treatment program he likes.

Disturbed sensory perception

Alterations in the five senses (sound, sight, smell, taste, touch) create an altered perception of the world.

Hallucinations Hallucinations are both a clinical diagnostic sign of schizophrenia and a focus for nursing care. You need to know the extent and nature of the person's hallucinations so that you can document the hallucinatory experience. Discuss with the person, if possible, the details of their symptoms. Look for major themes in the content of the hallucinations, particularly whether the hallucinations command the person to take action. *Command hallucinations* such as 'Jump up and down. Jump up and down. Don't look at her, she has cancer and you'll catch it' can be difficult for the person to cope with

LIVED EXPERIENCE

One of my experiences of hallucinations involved believing I had a trusted 'inner' guide from Red Rock in the mid north coast of New South Wales. 'He' was fictitious, but at the time seemed entirely real to me. I have been told it is unusual to hear voices of actual people, but in my experience of command hallucinations I was hearing voices of famous Indigenous Australians, and they were giving me commands to pack up all of my belongings and wait to be picked up by a truck that never came; or to buy train tickets for a journey to inland New South Wales, where I would undergo tribal initiation. At the time this seemed completely real to me, and I acted upon it.

and can affect their behaviour. The person may not be able to withstand pressured commands to say things or perform acts that could include a refusal to remain in a housing situation (which could lead to homelessness), violence or suicide (Kasckow, Felmet & Zisook, 2011).

Illusions Illusions (mistaken perceptions) make the person vulnerable to emotional and physical injury. We all have these experiences from time to time, and they are not part of a pathological process. For example, you may see what you think is water on the road, but another look tells you it is a shadow from a nearby tree. But for someone living with schizophrenia, the level of misperception may vary from day to day and even throughout the day. Misperceptions of the social environment make the person vulnerable to inappropriate responses that may be ridiculed by others. Misperceptions of the physical environment, such as misjudging the speed of an oncoming car, may lead to physical harm.

Disturbed body image

Body image disturbance is common in people living with schizophrenia. People may lose the sense of where their bodies leave off and where inanimate objects begin. They may become dissociated from various body parts and believe, for example, that their arms and legs belong to someone else. They may worry about the normalcy of their sexual organs. People living with schizophrenia often verbalise this altered sense of self directly, saying 'I don't feel like myself' or 'I feel like I am looking at my body from somewhere else in the room.'

Excess fluid volume

Excess fluid intake, or water intoxication, is a physiological state brought on by excessive drinking, characterised by hyponatremia, confusion and disorientation, and progresses to apathy and lethargy. In severe cases, seizures and death may result. This behaviour can lead to irreversible brain damage. Polydipsia appears to be significantly associated with the male gender, smoking, celibacy and psychiatric chronicity. Polydipsia in schizophrenia is a difficult problem to treat, in that behavioural interventions must be balanced against maintaining the person's independence. Acetazolamide (Diamox) and clozapine (Clozaril) are included as effective pharmacological treatments for this population (Takagi, Watanabe, Takefumi, Sakata & Watanabe, 2011). For people considered to be at risk because of frequent drinking, preventive measures include regular measures of urine-specific gravity, and regular weights designed to screen for increases in the body's fluid volume.

Disturbed thought processes

Schizophrenia changes the way thoughts are processed by distorting logic and organisation.

Delusions People living with schizophrenia may express delusional thinking in direct interactions and, to a lesser extent, through behaviours. When asked, many people willingly describe their delusional beliefs in detail. They seldom withhold this information because they believe firmly in the validity of the delusion, no matter how bizarre it seems to others. A person's actions can reflect the fixedness of their beliefs.

Practice example

Jill has the somatic delusion that her body is riddled with holes. She flatly refuses to drink, convinced that the fluid will flow directly out of the holes and soil her dress.

The content of delusions varies: delusions of persecution, reference, and so on (see Table 14.3). Reality-based delusions may seem plausible because they could, under some circumstances, actually occur. Bizarre delusions, more common among people living with schizophrenia, have no possible basis in reality. On the other hand, the false belief that one's husband is having an affair with a neighbour has a possible basis in reality, and is called a *reality-based delusion*. In contrast, the belief that one's thoughts are directed by a television announcer, or that one's unspoken thoughts can be heard by others, are known as *bizarre delusions*.

Delusions often reflect an individual's fears, particularly about personal inadequacies. For example, a man's grandiose delusion that he is the mayor of Melbourne could be a defence against feelings of inferiority. Similarly, persecutory delusions defend against the person's own feelings of aggression. Aggressive feelings are projected onto a person or organisation—for example, the police—whom the person then fears.

Magical thinking Magical thinking is the belief that events can happen simply because one wishes them to. Some people living with schizophrenia claim that they can exert their will to make people take certain actions or make specific events occur, like winning the lottery.

Thought insertion, withdrawal and broadcasting Disturbances of thought in schizophrenia include beliefs that others can put ideas into one's head (*thought insertion*) or take thoughts out of one's head (*thought withdrawal*). In addition, some people living with schizophrenia believe that their thoughts are transmitted to others via radio, television or other similar means. This belief is known as *thought broadcasting*.

Dysfunctional family processes

When a family has a member with a significant illness, regardless of whether it is a mental or physical illness, that family's functioning and dynamics change. The operations of the family must change to accommodate the ill family member, as well as how the rest of the family deals with the illness. The symptoms of the illness may be alien to family members, and they may not know how they should respond. See Collaborative Care: People Living with Schizophrenia and Their Families for guidelines on how to teach families about the negative symptoms of schizophrenia.

COLLABORATIVE CARE

People living with schizophrenia and their families

Teaching about the negative symptoms of schizophrenia

Families and caregivers have a difficult time understanding that the symptoms of an illness include not just those experiences that are unusual and extra, such as hallucinations and delusions, but also those aspects of being human that are missing, such as enjoyment and motivation. It is important to evaluate the family's current level of awareness of negative symptoms and provide up-to-date information.

Suggestions	Rationale
Discuss how not having motivation and not seeming to care about surroundings are part of the illness.	Families may be comforted to know that their loved one is not choosing to behave in this way.
Inform the family members about how these symptoms look and feel to the person living with schizophrenia.	Family members may not understand what it is like for their relative experiencing these symptoms.
Help families identify their responses to the negative symptoms.	Families often misinterpret negative symptoms as laziness or refusing to cooperate, and communicate this to the relative living with schizophrenia. This increases the negativity to which the person is exposed.
Talk about when and how negative symptoms respond to medications.	The timeframe of 18–24 months before negative symptoms respond to atypical antipsychotics may seem a long time to family members, and they will need support so that their expectations are realistic.

Interrupted family processes

Families burdened with the long-term responsibility of caring for a relative living with schizophrenia may suffer disruptions in their household routine, work, social interactions and physical wellbeing. The household may be disrupted by the insistence of the family member living with schizophrenia that the family act on and accommodate delusional beliefs. The family may bend to such expectations, fearing an increase in their family member's anxiety and possible fighting or shouting if they do not comply.

Practice examples

The Walker family built an extra bathroom rather than fight with Tim, their son who lives with schizophrenia, who spends hours in the bath completing elaborate washing rituals.

The Sherman family must eat out several times a week because Suzanne, their daughter who lives with schizophrenia, refuses to allow anyone in the room when she eats.

The family social life may be disrupted. For instance, the family may fear leaving the ill person alone, or they may fear that friends will be embarrassed if they are invited into the home. Some families are willing to be open about the adjustments made to accommodate a loved one living with schizophrenia, whereas others choose to live isolated lives.

Family members' work can suffer because of the emotional strain of living with a relative who is unwell. They must take time off to accompany the person living with schizophrenia to doctors' appointments, make hospital visits, and help during interviews with social agencies or the police. Family health may suffer because of general inattention or because of prolonged stresses within the home.

Supporting recovery

Working with the principles of recovery-oriented practice provides a strong basis for offering help to a person living with schizophrenia. These principles include: acknowledging and valuing the uniqueness of the individual; building and supporting opportunities for real choice; promoting and protecting civil and human rights; respectfulness in dealing with others, and promoting and protecting civil and human rights; engaging in shared decision-making; and evaluating recovery in terms of goals and milestones set by the person with lived experience of mental illness (Department of Health, 2010).

Planning and implementation

Interventions are most effective when they focus on the strengths of a person to maximise functioning. In order to accomplish this, you must attend to the issues that are important to the person with whom you are working. Their perspective is the most valuable tool you have to create competent and meaningful treatment interventions. Box 14.3 discusses issues likely to be important to a person living with schizophrenia.

Practice example

Can culturally adapted interventions make a difference in outcome?

Schizophrenia may present differently and pose many challenges for the people who live with it. The distress experienced during symptom exacerbation motivates the search for treatments that are effective and useful in fulfilling the needs of people living with the disorder. The search for answers has taken a variety of pathways, including the realm of spirituality and cultural sensitivity.

The quality of mental health services available to people living with schizophrenia are greatly enhanced when the relevant content of both psychoeducational and mental health interventions are culturally linked. Think about the last time you spoke with somebody about a problem you were having. If that person had an understanding of both your culture and your value system, such as spirituality, you probably had an easier time explaining your problem. Now think about a time when you spoke with somebody about a problem you were having and that person had no idea what you were talking about. How would you describe that experience? As you can imagine, this happens quite often with people living with schizophrenia when their symptoms are unusual or they are not able to articulate them clearly.

Culture, spirituality and a value system are intricately interwoven. They form the fabric for a system of meaning. Symptom expression, stressors, coping mechanisms and interactions with others arise from this system. Keeping the cultural and spiritual context of a person's experience in mind while interacting around psychiatric symptoms and treatment may reduce their frustration and increase the effectiveness of your communication.

Box 14.3 Important issues for the person living with schizophrenia

People living with schizophrenia have to deal with an illness different from any other disease. The symptoms are unlike anything else, and anosognia (unawareness of the illness) can further complicate their lives. Imagine not knowing you have an illness, and not, therefore, needing help. It makes accepting treatment and staying in treatment particularly challenging. The following are important considerations for developing effective nursing care:

- personal power and efficacy
- interpersonal relationships
- social expectations
- differences between what one hoped for oneself and what one has now
- connecting with people
- personal growth
- stability
- coping with relapses
- expression of spirituality
- understanding the symptoms of the illness.

When planning care in collaboration with any person with a chronic illness, care should be taken to set realistic goals for changing health behaviour. Take particular care when working with people living with schizophrenia, because they can be very sensitive to change and failure. Deterioration in functioning may result from the worsening of symptoms, lack of opportunity and support, or exposure to discrimination and stigma, or a combination of all of these. It is important to focus on the most troublesome areas of personal functioning and set incremental, short-term goals that pave the way for successes in achieving long-term goals. Answering the questions in Self-awareness: Working with People with Schizophrenia will increase your effectiveness in working with a person living with a psychotic illness.

Preventing relapse

Programs for relapse prevention with schizophrenia typically combine standard doses of maintenance antipsychotic medication with psychosocial treatment. Early clinical intervention when low-level symptom worsening occurs is effective in preventing a full relapse in people living with schizophrenia. If they reside with their family, educational and supportive family interventions have an important effect on relapse prevention. Further discussion can be found in Chapter 26.

Promoting effective communication

As with all human communication, people living with schizophrenia communicate in relation to personal experience and social context. It is thus important that close attention be paid to what is being said, and genuine attempts to understand the real and symbolic aspects of the message are important. The person will make their own interpretations of your behaviour. Therefore, one of the most direct and successful ways to demonstrate caring and respect is to attend seriously to the person with whom you are working (this is discussed in depth in Chapter 9).

SELF-AWARENESS
Working with people living with schizophrenia

To increase self-awareness about working with a person living with active psychosis, ask yourself the following questions:

- How do I feel about approaching a person who is experiencing hallucinations?
- How do I feel about talking to someone who is experiencing delusions that frighten them?
- Have I ever encountered someone in public who was experiencing a psychotic episode?
- Do I fear that I might do something that might make things worse for the person living with schizophrenia?
- What kinds of understanding and knowledge do I need to feel comfortable working with people living with schizophrenia?

To increase self-awareness about working with people experiencing difficulty in caring for themselves, ask yourself the following questions:

- Do I react negatively when I think about someone my age who has never worked?
- What goes through my mind when I see someone who is dishevelled, unclean or oddly dressed?
- How can I find a point of connection between myself and someone whose life is so dramatically different from my own?

People living with schizophrenia make valid observations about their environment, needs and concerns. Their observations and sensations make sense to them, although these may be different to what others are experiencing. It is important to note that severe symptoms of schizophrenia, when they occur, are likely to be present during acute episodes of the illness, and are not experienced all or even most of the time. It would be a (stigmatising) misapprehension to always read psychotic symptoms into the thoughts, feelings and behaviours of a person living with schizophrenia. The sensitivity to the environment that can be experienced by someone living with schizophrenia may also clue them into aspects to which others may not have access. Observations may be made about events or situations that are beyond your awareness. For example, a statement about another person's drug use or suicidal threats should be taken seriously. Similarly, complaints about physical symptoms, such as stomach distress, should be taken seriously. It is easy to dismiss the statements of a person living with mental illness, especially if they are experiencing delusions. Doing so, however, is stigmatising and shows a lack of respect for the person.

Promoting adherence with medication regimen

Psychotropic medications play an important part in the treatment of schizophrenia spectrum disorders for many people living with schizophrenia. Although in dispute by some mental health advocates, it is widely held that the newer antipsychotic drugs diminish focal symptoms (hallucinations and delusions) and yet produce fewer and less severe untoward effects. Adherence to treatment, which for schizophrenia means medications, is a complex expectation. You will need to be creative and ever-mindful of the barriers to learning and maintaining behaviours of particular people with whom you are working. The illness itself causes difficulty in adhering to a treatment regimen when a person lacks the ability to recognise the illness. This is called poor insight, and can be compared to the unawareness or lack of insight into neurological deficits following a stroke. It is important to recognise that individuals respond to their illness, their circumstances and their medications in different ways.

The idea of adherence can be expressed through a number of terms, such as treatment adherence, role reliability, collaboration for health behaviours, and cooperation. Interviews and clinical contacts tell us that people are more likely to participate in treatment if they are included and made an integral part of the design of their care. See Box 14.4 for a description of the barriers and challenges to treatment adherence. Consistent adherence in taking medications as prescribed is a problem for many people living with mental illness, although this population is not unique in that regard. People in endocrine, paediatric, antiretroviral and antibiotic situations also struggle with adherence to medications. However, non-adherence is especially problematic for people living with psychosis, because it may lead to an exacerbation of illness, with an increased risk of violence and suicide.

Box 14.4 Challenges to adherence

People living with schizophrenia may stop taking their medications for these reasons:

- difficulties with prescribed psychotropic medications
- severe level of symptomatology
- cognitive difficulties secondary to thought disorder
- motivational problems secondary to negative symptoms
- motivational problems secondary to flight into health (wanting to be 'normal')
- side-effects that are difficult to tolerate
- persistence of positive symptoms (delusions) mitigating against adherence
- financial issues
- misperceptions and misunderstanding of the information presented in medication teaching
- cursory or minimal medication teaching that lacks relevance to all areas of the person's life
- unresolved issues with the treatment providers
- cultural impacts
- misunderstanding the administration instructions
- disorganisation that prevents the person from following the instructions
- uncomfortable side-effects of major tranquilisers
- rejecting treatment in order to avoid being stigmatised as having schizophrenia
- feeling better and believing the medication is no longer necessary
- having difficulty in easy access to pharmacies because of transportation, financial or interpersonal difficulties.

LIVED EXPERIENCE

The points raise above are important and ring true to me. For me, medication has been a life-line to who I want to be. If I were not on medication—and I did go unmedicated with psychotic symptoms for about 15 years—my coping mechanisms, interpersonal relations and general functioning would be massively impacted. However, I would also add that, apart from GPs discussing and largely minimising possible side-effects, I have had little formal education related to the various medications I have been prescribed over the years.

Not taking medications can increase vulnerability to stressors and the risk of more frequent relapse of symptoms. Efforts to educate people about their medications, and to have them practise self-medication prior to discharge, have increased the rate of adherence marginally. A person's attitude towards the medications prescribed also influences their willingness to adhere to the regimen. You must be an active participant in assessing adherence and fostering a positive attitude towards medications. Commonly used antipsychotic medications and side-effects are presented in Chapter 7.

People living with schizophrenia can be ambivalent about taking medications. Maintaining adequate blood levels of therapeutic medications is important for people living with schizophrenia. To help them overcome ambivalence, allow time to think about taking the medications. Set a time limit. If a person admitted to an inpatient unit fails to take the medication, come back later and try again. Two useful strategies are giving reminders of the positive effects of the medication, and framing the action as a way for people to become actively involved in their own recovery. The following Your Intervention Strategies is a compendium for increasing treatment adherence for people living with schizophrenia.

Assisting with grooming and hygiene

Helping with the establishment and maintenance of personal care habits is a complex process. If a person clearly lacks the skills, then teach the skills. If, however, grooming skills have been learned but are not being practised, focus on ways to motivate the person to do so. Intervention begins by negotiating with the person to establish clear expectations about essential grooming habits. The frequency and timing of all aspects of grooming—including bathing, dressing, hair care, oral hygiene, and room care—can be specified in writing if that would be a useful learning device for the person with whom you are working.

Formal training programs for helping people living with severe enduring schizophrenia improve their grooming skills can be applied in inpatient as well as outpatient settings. They systematically help in all steps of personal grooming, including collecting grooming supplies, moving to the grooming area (a bathroom or a bedroom with a sink and mirror), completing each grooming step, completing appropriate dressing, and storing grooming materials. Interventions at each step can progress from simple verbal coaching, to modelling, to gentle physical guidance. It is important to acknowledge the person's efforts during each phase with realistic encouragement and praise. The success of these programs probably depends on daily staff attention to personal training, along with consistent, meaningful rewards. Avoid power struggles regarding the completion of tasks. If initial prompts don't work, leave the person alone for a short period.

Promoting organised behaviour

People whose behaviour is disorganised require guidance and support to make their actions more effective and goal-directed. In working with a person who is disorganised, proceed slowly and remain calm. The person's perception of the environment may be distorted, but your calmness can be a settling influence. Try to direct the person in simple, safe activities. Nursing goals and interventions for a person who is disorganised must focus on manageable steps. A Practice Example of one such intervention follows on page 313.

Promoting social interaction and activity

The efforts of a person living with schizophrenia to withdraw from social contact may stem from real experiences of stigma,

YOUR INTERVENTION STRATEGIES

Increasing medication adherence for people living with schizophrenia

- Involve the person as a partner in medication-based treatment planning decisions.
- Change to another medication with a different neurotransmitter action with lower or different side-effects that may be more tolerable. Atypical antipsychotic medications have a lower side-effect profile, and can increase adherence because they are not so hard to take.
- Teach the person how to report side-effects, such as dry mouth, priapism (persistent, usually painful, erection of the penis). This may require role-playing or assertiveness training.
- Teach the person how to manage the side-effects they experience (sugar-free, hard candy or sugar-free gum helps with dry mouth, and a rubber pillow case liner helps with night-time drooling). This may make it tolerable to continue on the medication.
- Instruct, educate and arrange for reminders well before discharge to maximise both knowledge and adherence. (Knowledge can be the number-one factor determining adherence.)
- Explore options to simplify the medication regimen.
- Match the medication dosing strategy to the person's schedule, preferences, work situation and recreational pursuits.
- Discuss the person's expectations of the medication—are they realistic?
- Take cultural impacts into account during comprehensive treatment planning.
- Use concrete educators. The tried-and-true cognition enhancers are: pamphlets, booklets, handbooks, workbooks, fact or information sheets, cards, videos, audiotapes, posters, magnets, logs, journals and so on.
- Assess the person's perception of control over the treatment regimen.
- Assess the person's self-administration of medications.
- Help the person take action to prevent untoward effects, such as maintaining fluid intake to avoid postural hypotension.
- Teach coping efforts that involve problem-solving, which increases adherence.
- Encourage peer support. Hearing from *peers* how a new medication could help with symptoms, and asking the prescriber to consider it, improves adherence.
- Give hope—it pays to be well. It takes all the small steps to recovery in addition to medications to get better.
- Use repetition—say the same thing over and over, with patience, especially if working with people living with schizophrenia or depression.
- Develop reminders, cues to remembering (visual cues—'when I see this, I need to take my pills', 'when I eat lunch, I take my pills', rubber band on wrist, calendars, to-do lists; auditory cues—alarm clocks or watches).
- Explore the option of using depot medications, which are given weekly, biweekly or monthly; these can contribute to adherence because the person does not have to remember to take pills. The marketing of an atypical antipsychotic in depot form (risperidone, olanzapine) adds to the choices.
- Teach the person to use pill-boxes—they come in many shapes, sizes and organisational styles (multiple daily doses, layers for time of day, Braille markings, timer with a small alarm-clock feature that opens the compartment).
- Keep all of the medications, and the information about them, in one dry, cool place. Use plastic products such as containers and bags—do *not* store in the bathroom or by a dishwasher in the kitchen.
- Involve the family.
- Match the degree of autonomy in treatment to the needs of the individual person with whom you are working.
- Inform the person about sources of possible financial assistance.
- Involve people who are well-established in taking medications in the teaching of others about medication use. Nothing speeds up learning so much as teaching others.

LIVED EXPERIENCE

These strategies seem practical and worthwhile. To me, it sometimes seems to be a question of whether time is available for busy health professionals to work through the information with people who are prescribed the medications. To me, the key is the quality of the working relationship I have been able to develop with the health professional prescribing and/or monitoring the medication I am taking.

LIVED EXPERIENCE

The importance of social interaction cannot be overstated; friendships within and outside the community of people touched by mental illness have been absolutely fundamental to change and adaptation to new circumstances for me. I feel great sorrow that there are mentally ill people who, because of their symptoms (e.g. paranoia), find it really hard to maintain relationships. Having good friends can be as important to recovery as effective medication.

trauma and discrimination, and/or from past relationship failures and fear of rejection. Under such circumstances, a person's internal world may seem less risky, and therefore more attractive than a world that requires interpersonal relating. When making efforts to help a person become less withdrawn, it is important to understand what can sometimes be an overwhelming anxiety about human contact.

Practice example

George is moving quickly yet aimlessly from the refrigerator to the cupboard. He pulls a box of cereal from the cupboard, opens it, and then wanders away. Next he goes to the refrigerator, opens the door, peers in, and closes the door. Rummaging through all his pockets, he locates a comb, combs through his hair, sets the comb on the counter, and wanders back to the cupboard. This effortful yet unproductive behaviour continues for several minutes when the nurse enters.

Nurse: 'George, are you trying to get some cereal for yourself?'

George: 'Sort of. I was going to . . . brush . . . no, comb . . . no, eat something. Yeah, I wanted something to eat.'

Nurse: 'Try to concentrate on one thing. First, put the comb back in your pocket.' (He does so.) 'Now, come over here and get the cereal box. Here's a bowl. Here's a spoon.' (She hands him the utensils.) 'Why don't you sit right here?' (She seats him so that he has his back to the rest of the activity in the room.) 'Can you sit still for a little while?'

George: 'I think so.'

Nurse: 'Pour yourself some cereal. I'll get the milk for you.' (She does so.)

George begins to eat his cereal quietly. The nurse stays with him for a few minutes, and directs him to continue eating each time he becomes distracted by others who come into the room.

After establishing a basic level of trust, the person can be encouraged to try out new behaviours within the relationship. The goal is to set up situations in which success can be experienced; therefore, encourage even small increments of change. If, for example, the person has difficulty initiating conversation, they can be encouraged to practise this skill once a day. Similarly, if the person avoids any activity in the environment because of fear of relating to groups, activities can be arranged that include yourself, the person with whom you are working, and other people who use the service within which you work. Opportunities to should be encouraged, even if that communication contains problematic patterns (refer back to the Communication features on pages 297 and 300).

Promoting social skills and activities

Social skills that are essential to functioning in the environment should be addressed: introducing oneself, starting a conversation, ending a conversation, saying no, asking for assistance and listening. Staff members can model these skills and help in role-playing each skill. Focus discussion on situations in which specific skills might be needed. Motivation to learn a skill is likely to be greater where the applicability of that skill to daily living has been highlighted. Praise and, if available, material rewards can also be used to enhance motivation. Social skills training can also be done in small groups (see Chapter 23).

Schizophrenia can disturb a person's will and capacity to accomplish meaningful activity. People who experience distorted perceptions and thinking expend considerable energy merely taking in and interpreting their immediate worlds. In addition, major tranquilisers, which control the positive symptoms of the disease, can further inhibit active involvement and interest in activities. Be aware of how much work it takes to cope with the symptoms of schizophrenia. Do not assume that periods of quiet or inactivity are due to laziness or lack of interest. Rather, assess each person's need for quiet periods in which to organise their perceptions and thoughts. At the same time, people living with schizophrenia exist within a culture in which action and accomplishment are highly prized and rewarded. They are not immune to the pressure for personal productivity as a measure of personal worth. As with most of us, they are likely to feel better about themselves when they are involved in meaningful activities. Your task is to help in finding activities that are intrinsically rewarding or that bring some social or tangible reward, and can be realistically achieved. See Developing Cultural Competence for ideas about this aspect of psychiatric–mental health nursing.

Learning about the personal interests of the person with whom you are working is a first step. Providing opportunities

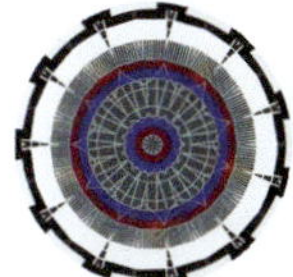

DEVELOPING CULTURAL COMPETENCE

Culture, religion and schizophrenia

In developing your cultural competence with people living with schizophrenia and their families, keep in mind the potent influences culture has on the perception of illness. In a very religious family, a young man who hears a spiritual presence speaking to him and sees its influence around him may be considered blessed or chosen, as opposed to ill or disordered. Therefore, there would be no reason to seek treatment for an experience thought to be special and advantageous. This could continue for a significant period of time, deepening problematic neurochemical processes.

In order to determine whether intervention is necessary, you would need to know the elements of the cultural environment and obtain additional information. An assessment of the young man would include his spiritual and cultural beliefs. You would also consider his overall functioning, because the concept of schizophrenia encompasses more than sensory experiences. If you found him to have poor interaction skills—he does not make sense when speaking—and he has been poorly groomed over a long period of time, you may consider these to be clues to a disorder, and not necessarily related to religious beliefs and practices.

If the family continued to see their son's experience as religious despite evidence of cognitive and emotional dysfunction, psychoeducation might be considered. You might discuss with his family how it would be possible to explore the need for diagnosis and treatment while maintaining the possibility of this being a unique religious experience.

CRITICAL THINKING QUESTIONS

1. Why is it important to know an individual's and family's interpretation of unusual experiences?
2. How might a person's religious and cultural background shape your plan for therapeutic interventions?

for actively engaging in an activity of interest (by providing records, books, craft materials, or access to newspapers and television) is the next intervention. In addition, activities within the therapeutic milieu, such as attending groups and completing unit 'jobs', can provide the external rewards of praise from staff and peers. These activities give confidence, and develop and promote work habits. Success in these activities can lead to success in volunteer or paid work in the community after discharge.

Intervening with hallucinations and delusions

Delusions or hallucinations can be frightening experiences. You can intervene by doing the following:

- reassure people that they are safe
- protect them from physical harm as they respond to their altered perceptions
- validate the feelings they are having in response to their experience
- validate reality
- help the person distinguish what is real from what is a hallucination or a delusion.

Hallucinations are especially frightening if the person has never experienced them before or if their content is threatening or angry. Attempt to alleviate this anxiety by describing your perception of the frightened behaviour and asking the person to discuss what they are experiencing. Make simple reassuring remarks, such as 'I hear what you are telling me. This sounds very frightening. No one means to harm you.' See Your Intervention Strategies for intervention strategies that help a person manage hallucinations.

Provide protection from harm, and give reassurance about safety. A person living with schizophrenia may take impulsive action to escape the frightening experience or to obey voices in the hallucination. Prevent this by doing the following:

- closely observe the person's behaviour during active hallucinations
- use calming techniques and one-to-one interactions to shape and guide the situation
- reduce excess noise and distractions; one person speaks at a time
- intervene quickly by giving additional doses of psychotropic medications and/or taking the person to a quieter location within the unit
- if necessary, put in place safety precautions so that the person is not at risk of engaging in self-harming behaviours.

Make every effort to help the person attend to real rather than internal stimuli, encourage orientation to the real situation, and encourage them to focus on you rather than on the hallucination. 'George, listen to me rather than to the sounds you hear. Remember, you are in the hospital and I am your nurse. I will help you find your shoes. Come with me.' Active involvement in some activity, such as finding shoes, will help in maintaining a focus on real events and perceptions.

General guidelines for working with people experiencing delusions are to avoid arguing with their false beliefs, to focus on the reality-based aspects of their communication, and to protect them from acting on their delusions in a way that might harm themselves or others. It may also be important to teach them that the sharing of delusional content directly with others in community settings, such as the workplace or the social club, may frighten others and lead to stigmatisation. See the following Your Intervention Strategies for suggested nursing interventions that contain or manage delusions.

Promoting congruent emotional responses

Working with people who display blunted or flat affect can be confusing for nurses who are accustomed to reading emotional responses that fall within a more normal range. Be aware that people living with schizophrenia have feelings about events around them, including their interaction with you and other staff members, yet may have difficulty expressing those feelings.

YOUR INTERVENTION STRATEGIES
Helping a person manage hallucinations

- Determine the kind of hallucinations (auditory, visual, etc.).
- Can the symptom be managed with current coping?
- Access resources (advocacy groups, peers, staff, literature) for fresh ideas or better management techniques.
- Discuss options and success rate with professionals.
- Select options for coping with the stimuli:
  - distraction
  - resisting
  - calming
  - treatment (such as medication).
- Practise using an option to cope.
- Use a technique based on the success you have with it.
- Address the emotions evoked by the hallucinations (so that even if the hallucinations are not eradicated by medications, they can be managed).
- Be ready to replace coping styles when they do not work anymore.

LIVED EXPERIENCE

From the perspective of the Hearing Voices Movement, it is worth making the following points: (1) the person hearing the voices experiences them as real; (2) 'hallucinations' as a term is not encouraged; (3) people typically have a relationship with their voices, and that relationship can be as real as anything that exists 'in reality'. Speaking personally, I had primarily positive experiences with voices; they were mainly genial, but often led me astray. However, on one occasion when I realised the primary voice I had been experiencing for about eight months wasn't real, it hurt like losing a good friend.

YOUR INTERVENTION STRATEGIES

Helping a person living with schizophrenia manage delusions

- Determine whether the person can tell the difference between the delusion ('I don't drink the water because it's poisoned') and a personal preference ('I'm not drinking water because I prefer orange juice').
- Work with advocacy groups, peers and professional staff to clearly demarcate what constitutes delusional thinking.
- Suggest options to cope with delusional thoughts:
  - support from others
  - concrete tasks
  - caretaking activities
  - refocusing thoughts
  - determined efforts to steer thinking in another direction.
- Make sure the person understands how important it is to be surrounded by people who reinforce their efforts.
- Encourage the person to self-validate the struggle they are in, and any level of effectiveness they achieve at coping.

Note any lack of congruence between the person's affect and the content of the message. If your relationship with the person is well established, you might comment on the incongruity and explore it with them. ('Malcolm, what you are telling me is sad, but you are laughing. What shall I pay attention to?') Modelling clear, congruent communication is helpful. Little can be done to change the person's anhedonia, yet empathic listening might comfort them.

Ambivalence—the simultaneous experience of contradictory feelings about a person, object or action—can trouble people living with schizophrenia. Ambivalence can become great enough to immobilise a person. The experience of ambivalence makes it difficult to express one emotion or the other, or choose one action over the other. You may be able to partially alleviate the person's unease by identifying aloud the emotions they may be experiencing. ('Lily, I think you might be feeling both very happy to see your father and at the same time very angry.') Naming the conflicting emotions gives the opportunity to talk about them, although many times the person may not be able to do so.

Immobility due to ambivalence is extremely uncomfortable. One way of intervening is to limit the number of choices the indecisive person has to make. For example, a man may be immobilised by his inability to decide whether to go out alone for the first time. You can help by telling him that it seems too soon for him to go out alone, and that, for today, he must be accompanied. Another example is a young woman who is undecided about where to sit. You can remove extra chairs at the table in the dining room so that she has only one choice.

Promoting family understanding and involvement

When a person living with schizophrenia is hospitalised, encourage the family and help them remain involved in the loved one's care. Except for unusual circumstances, share information on the person's status, treatment program and future treatment plans, including discharge plans. Nurses may need to be active advocates for families' rights to information about, and involvement in, the care of their loved one with schizophrenia. Of course, nurses need to comply with the wishes of the person living with schizophrenia and with the laws governing disclosure of information, which are governed by both state/territory and Commonwealth legislation in Australia.

Psychoeducation programs If assessment suggests that family members need information about the disease and treatment, the family can be referred to education programs, through carer organisations such as the Mental Illness Fellowship of Australia (www.mifa.org.au/) or Mental Health Carers ARAFMI Australia (www.arafmiaustralia.asn.au/). Family psychoeducation programs are preferable to direct teaching, because they often combine education with mutual support. In such groups, families can meet others who share their life difficulties. These peers can provide informal support and information to help the family deal with the tasks that lie ahead. You can reinforce the formal teaching that occurs in such programs when you meet with individual families.

Mental Health Carers ARAFMI Australia The families of people living with schizophrenia can access information and support from the national organisation Mental Health Carers ARAFMI Australia, which has incorporated branches in most Australian states and territories. Mental Health Carers ARAFMI Australia serves families through educational programs, local support groups and advocacy work. Most local branch meetings are listed in telephone directories and/or advertised on the internet, or can be contacted through local community mental health services.

The importance of Mental Health Carers ARAFMI Australia and other similar organisations to families is discussed in detail in Chapter 24.

Promoting community contacts

An awareness of a person's community supports and potential treatment programs can guide nurses in preparing plans for discharge. For example, the person's most important peer support group might be those attending a local day treatment

LIVED EXPERIENCE

Families deal in their own ways with information and interventions. In some instances, people will be resistant to being better informed. And in others, families will seek to learn as much as they can. I have seen some families learn about mental illness largely from experience, with little or no exposure to formal access mental health education. I have also seen families pursue information about mental illness and treatments with great eagerness. I would not want to assign value judgements to either of these approaches, as I have seen both work in my own life.

Practice example

The Oldfields were worried about their daughter's failing grades at university for the last semester, and were surprised to learn that she had broken up with her boyfriend. When she came home for the university break, she seemed disinterested and uncommunicative, and wouldn't eat or socialise with the family. Her parents found her burning incense and chanting to herself in the mirror at 3am. In a panic, they took her to the local emergency department. After her admission to hospital, they were shocked to learn that the probable diagnosis was schizophrenia. Furthermore, the psychiatrist wanted their daughter to begin taking medication.

The rapidity of the decline in their daughter's functioning, and the fact that she had hidden many of her symptoms from them, left the Oldfields feeling guilty, sad and disbelieving. They could not fathom how this had happened to their beautiful daughter. A nurse at the psychiatric unit had given them the number of a local ARAFMI group. In their anguish, they called and were able to speak with other parents, who helped them begin to deal with their emotions and directed them to helpful books and online resources that explained schizophrenia and its treatment.

program or clubhouse. If so, several visits prior to discharge will help the transition back to the community.

Working with people to prepare for living in the community after hospital discharge is an important nursing task. Often, there will be opportunities while the person is in hospital to work on developing some of the capabilities required to manage one's life in the community. Opportunities are likely to present to discuss how medications can be managed; what to do if side-effects become difficult to tolerate; how to deal with stressful situations; how deal with boredom to make good use of free time; and how to manage personal hygiene. Nurses work with people living with schizophrenia to help them achieve their highest level of functioning. They document the abilities of the people they are working with to perform various tasks, and make recommendations to the treatment team about existing strengths and areas of functioning that could be further developed.

Evaluation

To complete the nursing process, nurses evaluate how the people with whom they are working respond to the interventions offered. Evaluation criteria are linked to intervention goals, and reflect an understanding of the challenges faced by people living with schizophrenia and their capabilities in meeting such challenges. Crucially, all considerations of evaluation are influenced by the concept of recovery, because living a more meaningful, hopeful and contributing life is a possibility for all people living with schizophrenia.

Communication

The person living with schizophrenia will, with greater regularity, express their thoughts clearly and congruently. They will feel sufficient trust to talk to the nurse about troublesome symptoms or experiences. Because some symptoms may persist even after medications have taken effect, this trust allows the person living with schizophrenia to express what has changed and what is still troublesome.

Self-care

The person living with schizophrenia will consistently appear clean and well-groomed, and will independently manage personal grooming and hygiene. They will have clean and reasonably appropriate clothes, in terms of both fashion and season. Individual styles of dress, which are the person's way of expressing or presenting the self, will be supported by nurses. The means for maintaining self-care after discharge from acute care are identified.

Activity intolerance

The person living with schizophrenia will participate in goal-directed activities with minimal intervention. They will complete any activities they begin. The person will demonstrate a broader range of interest and activities than they did on admission.

Social isolation

The person living with schizophrenia will demonstrate the capacity to interact, at least for brief periods, with nursing staff, with other service users, and in small groups. They will consistently demonstrate socially required interactions, such as greeting and starting a conversation with a stranger, asking for assistance, saying no, and listening to another's conversation. They will be inactive for shorter periods, and will spend more time engaged in interesting or meaningful activity. The person will demonstrate the capacity to function outside the protective environment of acute or sheltered care.

Sensory/perceptual alterations

The person living with schizophrenia will have fewer episodes of attending to internal stimuli. If hallucinations or delusions persist, they will begin to identify stressors or situations that precipitate them. The person will identify and practise personal coping strategies that decrease the hallucinations, delusions or their effects, such as going to a quiet room, engaging in social activities and performing activities that demand concentration.

Thought processes

The person living with schizophrenia will engage in reality-based discussions. If delusions persist, they will not act on delusions in ways that are harmful or detrimental to themselves or others. They will also identify significant others in their current living environment who can help them limit their hallucinations via distraction or social contact.

Emotional responses

The person living with schizophrenia will have increased awareness that their emotional expressions at times do not match their verbal communications. They will monitor others' responses to them, to learn cues about how they are varying their emotional expressions. The person will experience fewer episodes of extreme discomfort due to ambivalence about people, events or actions.

Family functioning

If appropriate, the family of the person living with schizophrenia will be involved in all aspects of care, including assessment, planning and carrying out interventions, inpatient treatment choices, and planning for discharge. Family understanding of the illness trajectory and the person's capacities and limits will improve. Family difficulties in caring for family members living with schizophrenia will be considered in the treatment and discharge planning, and adequate resources will be identified to support family needs. Families will report that their questions surrounding the nature of, treatment for and recovery from schizophrenia have been answered.

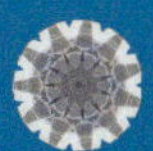

NURSING CARE PLAN: A PERSON LIVING WITH SCHIZOPHRENIA

Identifying information

Jack May is a 24-year-old single male who lives with his mother and receives a Disability Support Pension. He is brought to the emergency department of the local public hospital by his mother. He currently attends a work-transition program for people living with mental illness five days a week, but stopped attending eight days ago.

Jack says that he does not need to be hospitalised and that his mother is the one with the problem. He wants to be left alone to work on his computer projects. He admits that he has been hearing multiple voices in his head for the past week. For the past two weeks, Jack has been increasingly isolated, working on his personal computer in his room. He will not tell anyone what the work is about, but his mother has seen printouts that suggest it is a plan to soundproof and secure his room. When Jack stopped attending his work-transition program a week ago, he said that he had 'more important work' to do at home. He refuses to eat or talk with his mother. His mother believes he has stopped taking his medications. An identifiable stressor is that two weeks ago his mother announced that her boyfriend would be moving into the house in the near future.

History

Four years ago, Jack had a first episode of psychosis towards the end of his first year at university. He was diagnosed with schizophrenia. He was hospitalised for two weeks, stabilised on Risperidone, and discharged home. Persecutory delusions that shift with news events are always present at a low level. He has lived with his mother since diagnosis, attending day treatment and, for most of the past year, a structured work-transition program. He has occasionally attended a local hearing voices group. He has had several short periods of casual work, but has lost these due to unreliable work attendance. He receives medications and follow-up treatment at the community mental health centre.

Jack's mother and father are both living and well. They separated 10 years ago, and divorced five years ago. Jack's father is a high-school teacher and lives interstate, and Jack sees him rarely, but they do communicate by email and social media from time to time. His mother is also a teacher, and is agreeable to having Jack live with her. There are no other children. Jack first met his mother's boyfriend about two years ago, but up until recently had not had much direct involvement with him.

Jack completed high school at the local public high school. He was an above-average student, and was always involved in school and extracurricular activities. Since the first psychotic episode, he has socialised primarily with his mother, and on rare occasions with a few acquaintances from the clubhouse or hearing voices group. He had not smoked while at high school, but for the past four years has smoked a pack of cigarettes a day and drinks beer occasionally. He denies any illicit drug use. Jack has a keen interest in computers. He was undertaking a degree in computer science at university at the time of his first psychotic episode, and subsequently dropped out; he has collected considerable equipment and software. Other pastimes are listening to rock music and watching television.

No notable medical problems.

Current mental status

Jack is a healthy-looking 24-year-old man who is anxious, somewhat guarded, but cooperative in the interview. He is oriented to person, time and place, and demonstrates good memory and recall. Judgment is impaired. His affect is anxious. Speech is rapid, pressured, tangential. He is hyperalert to his environment, and is notably startled by a siren outside. Persecutory delusions about people trying to take over his home and work are present, and he has hallucinations of unrecognisable voices and the voice of his father. He has no command hallucinations. Some loosening of associations is present. Abstractions are concrete and self-referential. His insight is poor; he believes that his mother is 'sick', and that she should not impede him in his important projects.

Other clinical data

There is evidence that Jack may have stopped taking medications approximately two weeks ago. Suicide/violence potential is minimal.

Issue identified: Disturbed thought processes.

Expected outcome: Jack will demonstrate the ability to cope effectively with delusions.

Short-term goals	Interventions	Rationales
Jack is able to function in a variety of settings without intrusive delusional thought content.	■ Allow description of delusional thoughts, and acknowledge emotional impact of same. ■ Focus discussions on Jack's feeling level concerning the delusions, and not the content.	Some contacts can be overwhelming for a person living with schizophrenia and need to be of a manageable length.
	■ Teach Jack how to cope with delusional thinking through engagement in activities for distraction, active self-talk promoting his efforts, support from others, treatment. ■ Reinforce adaptive efforts.	Jack must be taught how to cope with the symptoms of the illness in an effective manner.

(continued)

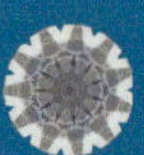

NURSING CARE PLAN: A PERSON LIVING WITH SCHIZOPHRENIA (*continued*)

Issue identified: Anxiety related to delusions.

Expected outcome: Jack will demonstrate decreased anxiety.

Short-term goals	Interventions	Rationales
Jack is able to describe a reduction in his anxiety. Jack participates in his treatment.	■ Make frequent, supportive and brief contacts.	Some contacts can be overwhelming for a person living with schizophrenia and need to be of a manageable length.
	■ Reassure Jack verbally, with a structured routine, and by giving explanations congruent with Jack's ability to understand.	People living with schizophrenia often do not have their feelings acknowledged. Reassurance validates their feelings.
	■ Prompt Jack to interact with others when able, to reduce feelings of isolation and alienation.	You must teach a variety of coping skills to suit various situations.
	■ Provide an array of coping skills Jack may use when anxious.	

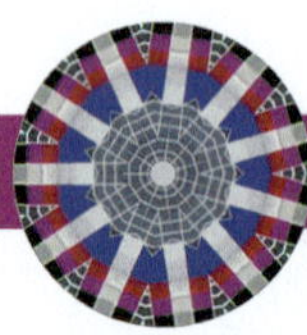

REFERENCES

American Psychiatric Association (APA). (2013). *Diagnostic and statistical manual of mental disorders* (5th ed., Text Revision). Washington, DC: APA Publishing.

Black, D., & Andreasen, N. (2014). *Introductory textbook of psychiatry* (6th ed.). Arlington, VA: American Psychiatric Publishing, p. 624.

Bradshaw, T., & Pedley, R. (2012). Evolving role of the mental health nurse in the physical health care of people with serious mental illness. *International Journal of Mental Health Nursing, 21*, 266–273.

Carr, V., Whiteford, H., Groves, A., McGorry, P., & Shepherd, A. (2012). Policy and service development implications of the second Australian National Survey of High Impact Psychosis (SHIP). *Australian and New Zealand Journal of Psychiatry*, *46*(8), 708–718.

Corstens, D., Longden, E., McCarthy-Jones, S., Waddington, R., & Thomas, N. (2014). Emerging perspectives from the hearing voices movement: Implications for research and practice. *Schizophrenia Bulletin, 40* (Suppl. 4), S285–S294.

Department of Health. (2010). *Principles of recovery oriented mental health practice*. Retrieved from http://www.health.gov.au/internet/publication/publishing.nsf/content/mental-pubs-n-servst10-toc~mental-pubs-n-servst10-pri (Accessed 2015, September 18.)

Emsley, R., Chiliza, B., Asmal, L., & Lehloenya, K. (2011). The concepts of remission and recovery in schizophrenia. *Current Opinion in Psychiatry, 24*, 114–121.

Gaskin, C., Elsom, S., & Happell, B. (2007). Interventions for reducing the use of seclusion in psychiatric facilities. *British Journal of Psychiatry, 191*, 298–303.

Kasckow, J., Felmet, K., & Zisook, S. (2011). Managing suicide risk in patients with schizophrenia. *CNS Drugs, 25*(2), 129–143.

Koreki, A., Tsunoda, K., Suzuki, T., Hirano, J., Watanabe, K., Kashima, H., & Uchida, H. (2011). Clinical and demographic characteristics associated with postural instability in patients with schizophrenia. *Journal of Clinical Psychopharmacology, 31*, 16–21.

Lee, A. H., Lange, C., Ricken, R., Hellweg, R., & Lang, U. E. (2011). Reduced brain-derived neurotrophic factor serum concentrations in acute schizophrenic patients increase during antipsychotic treatment. *Journal of Clinical Psychopharmacology, 31*, 334–336.

Lee, H., & Schepp, K. G. (2011). Ways of coping in adolescents with schizophrenia. *Journal of Psychiatric and Mental Health Nursing, 18*(2), 158–165.

National Mental Health Working Group. (2005). *National safety priorities in mental health: A national plan for reducing harm*. Canberra, Australia: Health Priorities and Suicide Prevention Branch. Department of Health and Ageing, Commonwealth of Australia.

Morgan, V. A., Waterreus, A., Jablensky, A., Mackinnon, A., McGrath, J., Carr, V., . . . Saw, S. (2012). People living with psychotic illness: The second Australian national survey of psychosis. *Australian and New Zealand Journal of Psychiatry 46*(8), 735–752.

Rylands, A. J., McKie, S., Elliott, R., Deakin, J. F., & Tarrier, N. (2011). A functional magnetic resonance imaging paradigm of expressed emotion in schizophrenia. *Journal of Nervous and Mental Disorders, 199*, 25–29.

Schizophrenia Research Institute (2015) About schizophrenia. Retrieved from http://www.schizophreniaresearch.org.au/schizophrenia/about-schizophrenia/ (Accessed 2015, September 17.)

Stanford, A. D., Corcoran, C., Bulow, P., Bellovin-Weiss, S., Malaspina, D., & Lisanby, S. H. (2011). High-frequency prefrontal repetitive transcranial magnetic stimulation for the negative symptoms of schizophrenia: A case series. *Journal of ECT, 27*, 11–17.

Takagi, S., Watanabe, Y., Takefumi, I., Sakata, M., & Watanabe, M. (2011). Treatment of psychogenic polydipsia with acetazolamide: A report of 5 cases. *Clinical Neuropharmacology, 34*(1), 5–7.

Tandon, R., Gaebel, W., Barch, D. M., Bustillo, J., Gur, R. E., Heckers, S., . . . Carpenter, W. (2013). Definition and description of schizophrenia in the DSM-5. *Schizophrenia Research, 150*(1), 3–10.

Zahir, F. R., & Brown, C. J. (2011). Epigenetic impacts on neurodevelopment: Pathophysiological mechanisms and genetic modes of action. *Pediatric Research, 69*(5), 92R–100R.

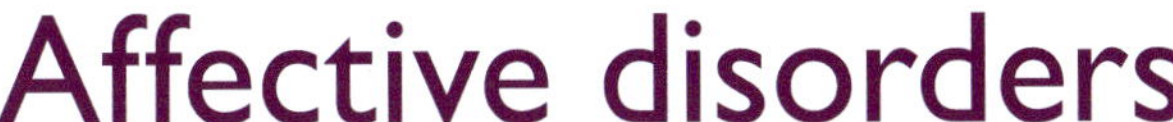

Affective disorders

15

CHRISTOPHER PATTERSON AND DOUGLAS HOLMES

LEARNING OUTCOMES

After completing this chapter, you will be able to:

1. Compare and contrast the similarities and differences between major depressive and bipolar disorders.
2. Describe the elements of the biopsychosocial theories that contribute most to the current understanding of disorders of mood.
3. Explain the principles upon which the various biological therapies for people with disorders of mood are based.
4. Systematically conduct a nursing assessment of a person with a disorder of mood.
5. Implement an understanding of suicide prevention and safety promotion in the plan of care for individuals with disorders of mood.
6. Design a plan of care to reduce negative thinking and promote improved self-esteem.
7. Educate individuals and their families about the biological treatments for disorders of mood, such as antidepressant medications and electroconvulsive therapy.
8. Assess personal feelings, values and attitudes towards people with disorders of mood that may provide challenges to professional practice.

KEY TERMS

affect *320*
anergy or anergia *322*
anhedonia *321*
bereavement *326*
bipolar disorders *323*
cyclothymic disorder *325*
electroconvulsive therapy (ECT) *334*
flight of ideas *324*
grandiosity *324*
grief *326*
hypersomnia *322*
hypomanic episodes *324*
insomnia *322*
learned helplessness *327*
major depressive disorder *321*
manic episodes *324*
psychomotor retardation *322*
tyramine *334*
vegetative symptoms *321*

LIVED EXPERIENCE

Douglas Holmes

The graph highlights the journey I have been on since being born in Bellingen, in Northern New South Wales, in 1949. It highlights when I have submitted tax returns since 1965; I use it when doing mental health presentations to highlight that something was obviously wrong at different points in my life.

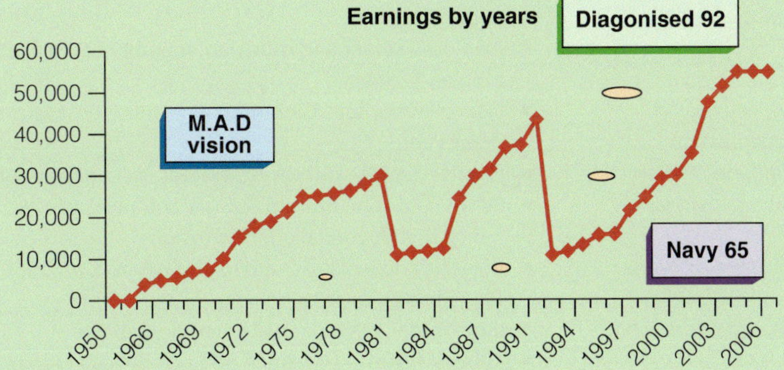

The manic episodes started again during 1991, and I ended up in treatment with the community mental health team in Batemans Bay in June 1992.

(continued)

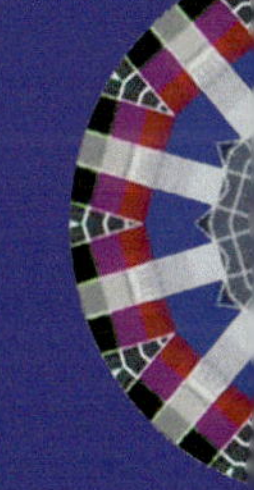

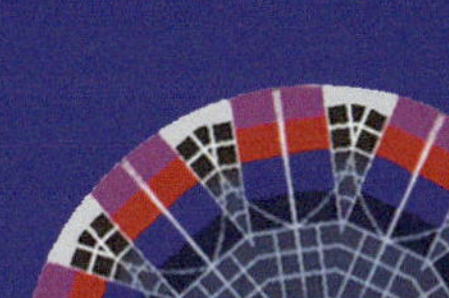

LIVED EXPERIENCE *(continued)*

One of the realities of being in the BAD Club (i.e. being diagnosed with *Bipolar Affective Disorder*—BAD) is that you usually need to have experienced two episodes (one high mania and one low, depressed) to qualify for membership. This concept had never been explained before I experienced my last manic episode in 1992. I had my first interaction with a community health centre in 1965, some 27 years before.

The main things that have helped me cope with being diagnosed with BAD have been:

- having contact with other people who have had similar experiences
- being involved in sharing those experiences with others
- working to make mental health services more responsive to people who have been through this experience
- speaking up to help reduce the stigma associated with the illness
- receiving information about mood disorder.

INTRODUCTION

The disorders discussed in this chapter are a group of psychiatric diagnoses characterised by disturbances in physical, emotional and behavioural response patterns. These patterns of **affect** (mood) range from extreme elation and agitation to extreme depression with a serious potential for suicide. The disorders discussed in this chapter are considered disorders of mood: depressive disorders and bipolar and related disorders. The publication of the DSM-5 (American Psychiatric Association [APA], 2013) saw changes to the classification of disorders of mood. DSM-IV (APA, 2000) classified depressive and bipolar disorders together, as 'Mood Disorders'. However, DSM-5 has identified these affective disorders as requiring their own individual classification, that being 'Depressive Disorders' and 'Bipolar and Related Disorders' (APA, 2013). The 2007 National Survey of Mental Health and Wellbeing (Australian Bureau of Statistics [ABS], 2007) identified 6.2 per cent of Australians as experiencing affective disorders (including depressive episodes, dysthymia or bipolar affective disorders) in the 12 months previous to the study. The prevalence of major depressive disorder in the community, estimated at more than 5 per cent, is of great public

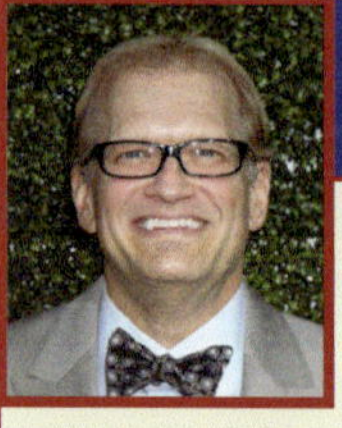

MENTAL HEALTH IN THE MEDIA

Famous people with depressive or bipolar disorders

- Bev Aisbett—writer (*Taming the Black Dog*); depression
- Sheryl Crow—singer and musician ('All I Wanna Do'); depression
- Carrie Fisher—actor; bipolar disorder
- F. Scott Fitzgerald—writer (*The Great Gatsby*); depression
- Sigmund Freud—'father of psychoanalysis'; depression
- P. J. Hogan—movie director (*Muriel's Wedding*); depression
- Billy Joel—singer and musician ('Piano Man', 'Uptown Girl'); depression
- Vivian Leigh—actress (*Gone With the Wind, A Streetcar Named Desire)*; bipolar disorder
- Abraham Lincoln—President of the United States; depression
- Demi Lovato—singer; bipolar disorder
- Gary MacDonald—actor; depression
- Matthew Mitcham—Olympic diver; depression
- Marilyn Monroe—actress (*Some Like It Hot*); depression
- Alanis Morissette—singer and musician ('Jagged little pill'); depression
- Axl Rose—singer and musician, member of Guns n' Roses; bipolar disorder
- Jessica Rowe—television news presenter; postpartum depression
- Charles Schulz—cartoonist, creator of *Peanuts*; depression
- Sting: (Gordon Sumner)—singer and musician ('Roxanne'; 'Every breath you take'); depression
- Magda Szubanski—actor and comedian (*Kath & Kim*; *Dogwoman*); depression
- Ian Thorpe—Olympic swimmer; depression
- Robin Williams—comedian and actor (*Good Morning, Vietnam*; *Dead Poets Society*); depression

Photo courtesy of Helga Esteb/Shutterstock.com.

health significance. Other disorders that occur less frequently than depression, but can be severely incapacitating, include dysthymic disorder and the bipolar disorders. Mental Health in the Media lists just some of the people who have these disorders.

The symptoms related to depressive or bipolar disorders—like poor memory and concentration, fatigue, apathy, indecisiveness and loss of self-confidence in those with depression, and grandiosity and unrealistic overconfidence in those with mania—reduce the capacity to work and maintain the activities of daily living. Some health authorities believe that major depressive disorder is more disabling than many medical disorders, such as chronic lung disease, arthritis and diabetes. It is the leading cause of lost workdays and diminished productivity on the job.

Many people with depressive or bipolar disorders are never seen for treatment in mental health settings because of the following:

1. some people may not realise they have a problem
2. other people do not realise they have a treatable illness
3. physical complaints brought to primary health care providers may be determined to require medical or surgical treatment instead of mental health care
4. health care policy and insurance coverage for mental disorders may be non-existent or meagre
5. stigmatising attitudes in the community may mean that people do not seek help.

Nearly two-thirds of depressed people in Australia go undiagnosed and untreated. As a nurse and a citizen, you are in an excellent position to identify early signs of these disorders in people and initiate action leading to early treatment.

MAJOR DEPRESSIVE DISORDER

A major depressive episode is characterised by a change in several aspects of a person's life and emotional state consistently throughout a two-week period. Of prime importance is the person's mood state. Be aware that people do not always describe their mood as 'depressed'. Instead, they may say they are sad, discouraged or 'down in the dumps', or say that they feel helpless. Or they may complain of having no feelings at all, or of feeling 'blah'. In other cases, vague somatic complaints such as aches and pains are reported, while other people report increased anger, frustration and irritability, with uncharacteristic outbursts over minor matters. It is not difficult to imagine that someone who looks and feels sad or empty is depressed. A diagnosis of depression is more likely to be missed when a person simply seems anxious or irritable. The description of the diagnostic criteria for single-episode and recurrent major depression is found in Diagnostic Features.

Major depressive disorder may consist of a single episode or may recur as recurrent major depression at various points in life. Key facts about major depression are in Box 15.1. When a person experiences a major depressive disorder, activities that previously gave pleasure—such as socialising, hobbies, sports and sexual activities—often are no longer enjoyed. This condition is known as **anhedonia**. Changes in physiological functioning during depression are called **vegetative symptoms**.

DIAGNOSTIC FEATURES
Depressive disorders

Types of depressive disorders include major depressive disorder—a single event or recurrent episodes—and dysthymic disorder. The presence of sad, empty or irritable moods, accompanied by somatic and cognitive changes cause significant distress in social, occupational or other important areas of function. The individual may never have had a manic episode or symptoms of mania. Any of these depressive disorders can vary in relation to the seasons or time of year, and cannot be due to ingesting a substance or from a medical problem or another psychiatric problem.

Major depressive disorder: The various symptoms of a major depressive disorder include a depressed mood and loss of interest or pleasure, changes in appetite and weight, sleep problems, observable restlessness or underactivity, and low energy. Additionally, the person with depression may have difficulty concentrating and have feelings of worthlessness and/or excessive guilt that are inappropriate for the behaviours. Thoughts of suicide or death occur. Symptoms also have to be more than would be expected after the loss of a loved one.

Persistent depressive disorder (Dysthymia): Symptoms of persistent depressive disorder include depressed mood for most of the day, for more days than not, for at least two years, accompanied by some of these symptoms: poor appetite or overeating, sleep problems, low energy, low self-esteem, poor concentration or difficulty making decisions, and hopelessness.

Box 15.1 Key facts about major depression

- The average age of onset is the mid-twenties, although it can begin at any age, and seems to be occurring in much younger people.
- Depression and anxiety are the leading causes of injury and disease burden for males and females aged 15–24 years (Australian Institute of Health and Welfare [AIHW], 2007).
- In any year in Australia, 4.1 per cent of people aged 16–85 will have experienced a depressive episode (Australian Bureau of Statistics [ABS], 2008).
- Major depressive disorder results from both genetic and environmental factors. Gene-environment interaction is hypothesised to be a significant factor in aetiology (Saveanu & Nemeroff, 2012).
- Symptoms usually develop over time. The person may experience anxiety and mild depression for several days, weeks or months before the onset of a full major depressive episode.

Changes in appetite, usually experienced as a reduction or loss of interest in food, are often seen, although increased appetite and cravings are also reported.

Sleep disturbances are common, particularly **insomnia** (the inability to fall asleep or stay asleep, or awakening early in the morning) with depression. An association between depression and the chronic inability to get to sleep or to remain asleep during the usual sleep period was observed at the time of Hippocrates. Two types of insomnia are most often experienced by people experiencing a major depressive episode. *Middle insomnia* refers to waking up during the night and having difficulty falling asleep again. *Terminal insomnia* refers to waking at the end of the night and being unable to return to sleep. The sleep-pattern disturbance may actually precede other symptoms of depression, and likewise may respond to antidepressant medication more rapidly than the depression. Also reported is **hypersomnia**, in which the person sleeps for prolonged night-time periods as well as during the day, but still wakes up tired or fatigued.

Fatigue and decreased energy are characteristic symptoms of depression, a condition known as **anergy or anergia**. Individuals report being tired upon awakening, regardless of how long they have slept. Even the smallest task seems insurmountable, and routine activities require substantial effort and take longer to accomplish. Decreased energy may manifest in **psychomotor retardation**, in which thinking and body movements are noticeably slowed, and speech is slowed or absent. Psychomotor agitation also may occur, where the person cannot sit still, paces, wrings their hands, and picks at the fingernails, skin, clothing, bedclothes or other objects. Psychomotor retardation is a prominent symptom in the Practice Example that follows.

Sleep disturbances secondary to mental health disorders are generally related to mood disorders and anxiety disorders. While recognising that a cyclical relationship is usually involved, it is helpful to try to differentiate primary sleep disorders from those that are secondary to a mental illness. Such differentiation is particularly important for people with depression.

Practice example

Becky is a 26-year-old insurance underwriter who visited a local Family Planning clinic for a yearly checkup and Pap test. During the examination by the nurse, Becky asked whether she might be anaemic because she was 'just exhausted all the time'. Becky revealed that for the past month she had had difficulty getting out of bed in the morning. Getting dressed and ready for work left her feeling drained. She described standing in front of her closet for long periods, unable to decide what to wear. Becky was also having extreme difficulty calling potential clients. Whereas she was normally an assertive salesperson who approached strangers with ease, she now described sitting at her desk for hours, trying to work up the motivation to pick up the phone. Co-workers, including her boss, had commented on her 7-kilogram weight gain, and these comments precipitated several uncharacteristic angry and tearful outbursts at work. Other common symptoms in significantly depressed individuals include guilt or a sense of worthlessness, self-blame, impaired concentration and decision-making ability, even about trivial things, and suicidal ideation.

Differentiating sleep disorder secondary to mental illness from primary sleep disorder is a complex process that requires collaboration between the individual, their family and health professionals. The sequence of onset may provide a clue. Many people with unipolar depressive disorder initially see primary care practitioners or sleep clinics because of insomnia. It may take an intervention known to be effective for one or the other type of disorder to assess the circumstances and clarify the primary diagnosis.

Vigilance is required for potential effects of a mismatched primary diagnosis and intervention. A person experiencing a depressive episode who has been misdiagnosed as having a primary sleep disorder of insomnia may be at risk of suicide if given a usual supply of hypnotic medication; likewise, obstructive sleep apnoea with a modest ingestion of alcohol can be mislabelled as alcohol abuse. As in any area of nursing practice, all components of the nursing process must be carefully and critically utilised.

The characteristics of a major depressive episode are illustrated in Figure 15.1 ■. Individuals with a history of a

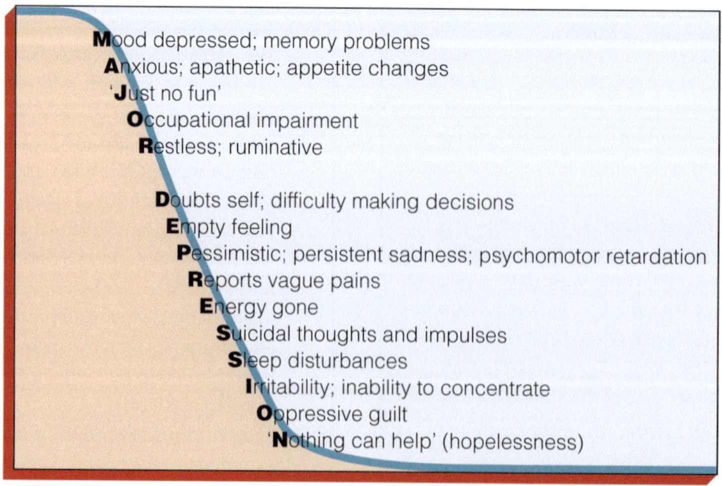

FIGURE 15.1 ■ Characteristics of major depression.

manic or hypomanic episode (discussed later in this chapter) are considered to have a bipolar disorder and are not classified under these categories.

There is a recognised association between depression and cardiovascular disease (CVD) (Hare, Toukhsati, Johansson & Jaarsma, 2014). According to Hare and colleagues (2014), people with CVD have higher rates of depression than the general population, and people with depression are more likely to develop CVD. Stress hormones and mortality concerns following a cardiac event such as a myocardial infarction (MI) could increase a person's vulnerability to depression. Psychopharmacological treatments for depression need to be cardiac-safe (not challenge a person's cardiac functioning) so that people with depression can adhere to treatment. Undela, Parthasarathi and John (2015) conducted a systematic review and meta-analysis of the association between antidepressants and risk of MI. They found an increased risk for MI associated with tricyclic antidepressants (TCAs), but no association between MI and selective serotonin reuptake inhibitors (SSRIs).

PERSISTENT DEPRESSIVE DISORDER (DYSTHYMIA)

The term **persistent depressive disorder** describes chronic depression for the majority of most days for at least two years (one year for children and adolescents). Throughout those two years, no more than two months can be described as symptom-free. The symptoms of persistent depressive disorder, while distressing, tend to be less severe than those in major depressive disorder, with fewer physiological symptoms. The diagnostic criteria for persistent depressive disorder were outlined in Diagnostic Features on page 321. In the DSM-5, persistent depressive disorder represents a consolidation of DSM-IV defined chronic major depression and dysthymic disorder. According to the most recent reported National Survey of Mental Health and Wellbeing of 2007 (ABS, 2008), dysthymic disorder (as per the DSM-IV-TR definition of the time of the study) had prevalence in the adult Australian population of 1.3 per cent. Females were more likely to have dysthymic disorder, with prevalence of 1.5 per cent compared to 1 per cent in males.

Nursing care of a person with persistent depressive disorder is similar to that of a person with major depressive disorder. The Practice Example included here describes this.

BIPOLAR AND RELATED DISORDERS

The **bipolar disorders** are a group of disorders that include manic episodes, hypomanic episodes, major depressive episodes and cyclothymic disorder. A *bipolar I disorder* consists of one or more manic episodes, and the course of illness may be accompanied by major depressive episodes. A *bipolar II disorder* consists of one or more major depressive episodes accompanied by at least one hypomanic episode. The diagnostic criteria for these disorders is outlined in Diagnostic Features.

Bipolar disorders tend to be recurrent, and have the unusual tendency to increase in frequency as the person ages. The majority of people with bipolar I disorder do not have the chance to experience a baseline mood—called euthymic mood—because a major depressive episode may quickly follow. Many people return to normal functioning during

Practice example

Gregory is a 14-year-old boy who was brought to a youth mental health centre by his mother on the suggestion of the guidance counsellor at his school. In a letter to the mother, the counsellor stated that she was concerned because of Gregory's 'persistent pessimistic outlook on life'.

According to Gregory's mother, who was interviewed alone, Gregory has always been a cranky and irritable child. Since starting kindergarten, he has had difficulty relating to other children, and is often left out of activities and social invitations. At home, he stays in his room much of the time, where he plays computer games and writes poetry. He does not do well in school, although testing has shown him to have far above average intelligence. Despite their best efforts, his parents have never been able to interest him in scouting, sports or other activities they deem appropriate for a boy of his age. His parents reported that Gregory's weight, eating habits and sleeping patterns were unchanged.

When Gregory was interviewed, he responded in monosyllables, made poor eye contact with the therapist, and sat slumped in his chair with no facial expression. He stated that he knew his parents were 'disappointed' in him.

DIAGNOSTIC FEATURES
Bipolar disorders

Types of bipolar disorder can include *bipolar I disorder*, *bipolar II disorder* and *cyclothymic disorder*. The symptoms cause significant distress in social, occupational or other important areas of function, and are not caused by taking a substance, for a medical or other mental illness.

Bipolar I disorder: For bipolar I disorder, the criteria for a manic episode must be met. These include an elevated, expansive or irritable mood and persistently increased energy for most days of least one week. Manic episodes may be preceded by or followed by hypomanic or major depressive episodes. The person has a combination of three or more of the following symptoms: inflated self-esteem, reduced sleep, talkative and hard to interrupt, racing thoughts, quick and unusual series of ideas, is distractible, overactive, has an increased focus on goal-directed activities, and takes risks that are not typical for them.

Bipolar II disorder: For bipolar II disorder, the criteria for a current or past hypomanic episode must be met, as well as the criteria for a current or past major depressive episode. The hypomanic episodes of bipolar II disorder include an elevated, expansive or irritable mood and persistently increased energy, for at least four consecutive days. The depressive episodes of bipolar II disorder must meet the criteria of major depressive disorder, lasting at least two weeks. For bipolar II disorder, the person has never had a manic episode.

Cyclothymic disorder: A diagnosis of cyclothymia disorder requires two or more years of numerous periods with both hypomanic and depressive symptoms (meeting fewer criteria than required for an episode major), with no history of meeting the criteria for major depressive, manic hypomanic episodes. These periods of hypomanic and depressive symptoms must have been present for a least half the time, and not be absent for more than two months at a time.

remissions, but approximately 20 per cent to 30 per cent have residual mood symptoms, and as many as 60 per cent have continuing interpersonal and occupational difficulties. Vazquez and colleague's (2015) systemic review of recurrence rates in bipolar disorder was 55.2 per cent in naturalistic studies. In randomised control studies, they found the recurrence rate to be 39.3 per cent for people on mood-stabilising treatments, compared to 60.6 per cent for those receiving a placebo.

Manic and hypomanic episodes

Manic episodes are characterised by an abnormal and persistently elevated, expansive or irritable mood and persistently increased energy for most days of at least one week. This mood significantly impairs social or occupational functioning, and may require hospitalisation. The disturbance in mood must be accompanied by at least three additional symptoms, such as: inflated self-esteem or **grandiosity**, a decreased need for sleep, pressure of speech, **flight of ideas** (rapidly changing, fragmentary thoughts), distractibility, an increased involvement in goal-directed activities or psychomotor agitation, and excessive involvement in activities with a high potential for painful consequences (APA, 2013). Psychotic symptoms, such as delusions or hallucinations, may exist.

Hypomanic episodes are a less extreme form of a manic episode, in that they are not severe enough to markedly impair social or occupational functioning or require hospitalisation. A hypomanic episode is present most of the day, lasting at least four consecutive days. Episodes are characterised by a definite change in functioning, recognisable to those who know the person. Psychotic features are not associated with hypomanic episodes.

The onset of manic episodes is usually in the early twenties, but may begin at any time. It may follow a psychic stressor, such as a recent severe disappointment or embarrassment. The mood of people experiencing a manic episode is euphoric or 'high'. Behaviour is exaggerated and excessive. It may be characterised by overly-enthusiastic involvement in projects of an interpersonal, political, religious or occupational nature.

Practice example

Mr Gery, a 52-year-old engineer, was brought to the emergency department by his two adult sons at 2am. Their mother had called them to help with their father, who had not slept in three days. When they arrived at their parents' home, they found their father working in the backyard on a large landscaping project involving stonework, a waterfall, a fish pond, and extensive plantings of trees, shrubs and flowers.

According to the sons, Mr Gery had had three prior episodes of 'manic behaviour', the first when he was in the Army many years earlier. He was stabilised on lithium carbonate for years, but stopped taking it about a year ago because he felt so good. The current episode began about a week ago, after he was passed over for a promotion at work. He then took a leave of absence from his job to create what he called 'the world's first home-based theme park'. Any attempt by his wife to talk him out of the project was met with anger and renewed resolve. Mr Gery angrily told the admitting nurse, 'I don't know why these boys have brought me here. I need to get back to work! I'm going to get millions for this franchise.'

When someone or something gets in the way or appears to get in the way of the person's goals, they may become irritable. Moods alternate between euphoria and irritability. Increased sexual behaviours are often seen, including flirting, making sexual overtures, having inappropriate sexual relationships, and feeling compelled to seduce and be seduced. Speech is pressured, and racing thoughts or flight of ideas are often present. Grandiosity can reach delusional proportions. People experiencing a manic episode may believe their disturbance in mood is of no concern, even when they are in financial or legal trouble, and may vehemently protest the need for treatment. Characteristics of a manic episode are described in the Practice Example, above, and illustrated in Figure 15.2 ■.

Major depressive episodes

A diagnosis a bipolar I disorder or bipolar II disorder does not always mean that manic or hypomanic episodes are currently present. Major depressive episodes may have occurred in the past. A major depressive episode is not required criteria for a

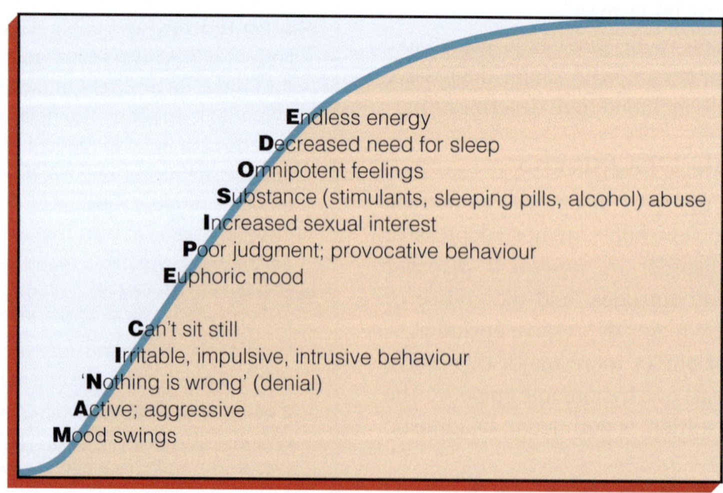

FIGURE 15.2 ■ Characteristics of a manic episode.

diagnosis of bipolar I disorder, but a major depressive episode may precede or follow a manic episode. A current or past major depressive episode is required criteria for bipolar II disorder.

Treatment of major depressive episodes associated with either bipolar I disorder or bipolar II disorder is similar to treatment of major depression disorder, with the exception that the pharmacological treatment may include a mood stabiliser.

The misdiagnosing of bipolar disorders as unipolar depressive disorders can occur due to symptoms being mistaken or not identified (Altamura et al., 2015; Knezevic & Nedic, 2013). This may lead to an incorrect diagnosis, and may result in a person losing years of appropriate treatment.

Mixed features

Mixed features is the term used to identify where symptoms associated with a manic, hypomanic or depressive episodes are present in an episode not usually associated with those symptoms. For example: a manic episode with additional depressive symptoms would be referred to as 'manic episode with mixed features'. The mixed feature specifier may apply to the manic, hypomanic or depressive episodes of bipolar I disorder or bipolar II disorder (APA, 2013). A manic or hypomanic episode with mixed features includes the person meeting the criteria of a manic or hypomanic episode, but with at least three depressive symptoms co-occurring for the majority of the days (APA, 2013). A depressive episode with mixed features includes the person meeting the criteria of a major depressive episode, but with at least three manic/ hypomanic symptoms present. The Practice Example that follows illustrates mixed features (APA, 2013).

Practice example

Mrs Jai is a 32-year-old high-school teacher who was readmitted to the mental health unit two weeks after she was discharged following treatment for a major depressive episode. Her husband described her recent behaviour as extremely unstable, with a strange mix of moods. 'She is driving herself and me crazy, crying and talking about killing herself because her life is so sad and she is so depressed, but every action is so full of energy. She tried to go back to work right after she got out of the hospital the first time, but her boss put her on a leave of absence until the end of the year. He said she made wildly gesticulating movements while describing how miserable she was to some of her students.'

Cyclothymic disorder

When a person has experienced at least two years of 'chronic, fluctuating mood disturbance involving numerous periods of hypomanic symptoms and periods of depressive symptoms', they are diagnosed with **cyclothymic disorder** (APA, 2013, p. 140). They must be free of severe symptoms that qualify for the diagnosis of a manic, hypomanic or major depressive episode. These individuals are often considered to be moody, unpredictable or temperamental. As a result of the mood disturbances, there is significant distress or impairment in social, occupational or other important areas of functioning. Figure 15.3 ■ compares mood in major depressive disorder, bipolar disorders, dysthymic disorders and cyclothymic disorder.

Cyclothymic disorder begins early, usually in adolescence or early adulthood (APA, 2013). It is thought to predispose the person to other bipolar or related disorders. According to the APA (2013), the incidence of cyclothymic disorder is approximately equal between males and females.

AFFECTIVE DISORDERS DUE TO ANOTHER MEDICAL CONDITION

It is widely recognised that affective disorders may be manifestations of physiological conditions such as hepatitis or thyrotoxicosis. Affective disorders may also be induced

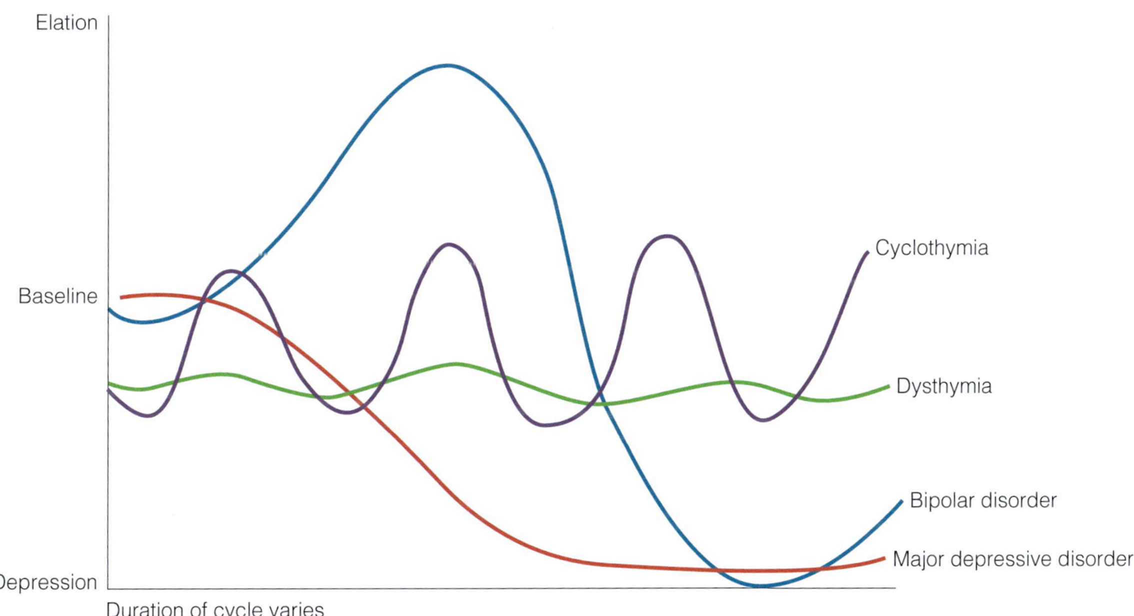

FIGURE 15.3 ■ Comparison of affect (mood) in major depressive disorder, bipolar disorders, dysthymia disorders and cyclothymic disorder.

by: substance abuse, such as cocaine or amphetamines; prescribed medications, such as antihypertensives or oral contraceptives; or toxins, such as lead or carbon monoxide. Affective disorders may also be precipitated by withdrawal from substance intoxication or abuse. Chapter 13 has details on this phenomenon. The general medical condition of consumers should be carefully evaluated before making a diagnosis of specific affective disorder.

EPISODES DURING PREGNANCY OR POSTPARTUM

The majority of women experience the 'baby blues'—transient mood changes, usually depression, that do not impair functioning—in the two-week period after the birth of a baby. However, when the symptoms meet the criteria for any of the depressive disorder or bipolar or related disorder categories discussed earlier in this chapter, and these symptoms occur during the pregnancy or in the four weeks following delivery, the person is diagnosed as having an episode *with peripartum onset* (APA, 2013).

The symptoms the person experiences are no different from the symptoms of other manic, hypomanic or major depressive episodes. An episode with peripartum onset can present with or without psychotic features (APA, 2013). For example, the woman may have delusional thoughts about her baby (the baby is possessed by an evil presence) or command hallucinations (to kill or injure the baby). The following Practice Example describes this.

Practice example

A woman drowned her six children, ages two months through to seven years old, believing that they were evil and that she was saving them from Hell. Each of the six births, all within a period of seven years, was characterised by a major depressive episode with peripartum onset, some with psychotic features that required hospitalisation and psychotropic medications. She had attempted suicide at least twice during a mood episode.

BEREAVEMENT

Bereavement is a term that refers to the state of loss. We all have losses that have to be dealt with, and how we cope affects not only us but also our loved ones. Bereavement is a natural process and not a mental illness. People may have significant difficulties at some point; however, this is usually transient. Bereavement is a process that everyone copes with differently. Although we might wish for a logical and set process, there is no set progression of bereavement or grieving. According to the DSM-5 (APA, 2013), when bereavement and major depressive disorder occur together, the depressive symptoms and functional impairment tend to be more severe, and the prognosis is poorer compared with bereavement that is not accompanied by major depressive disorder.

Grieving

You may notice with people experiencing depression that many episodes of major depressive disorder may be preceded by a significant loss of some kind. **Grief** (the feeling of sadness for a loss) is a multifaceted reaction to loss. It has emotional components as well as physical, cognitive, behavioural, social, spiritual and philosophical dimensions. Caring about someone or something and having a real relationship means putting yourself at risk for intense feelings of grief when the relationship changes or ends. People do not grieve for losses that are unimportant to them. The term 'grief-struck' is appropriate, as many people are shocked by the jarring impact of the loss. Grieving is a personal process that is best supported by understanding and care.

Careful consideration needs to be given to the delineation of normal grief from a major depressive episode (APA, 2013). In distinguishing the experience of grief and major depressive disorder, the DSM-5 (APA, 2013) identifies differences that are likely to exist in a person's affect. The American Psychiatric Association (2013) says:

- In grief, the predominant affect is feelings of emptiness and loss, while in major depressive episodes it is persistent depressed mood and the inability to anticipate happiness or pleasure.
- The dysphoria in grief is likely to decrease in intensity over days to weeks and occurs in waves, the so-called 'pangs of grief'.
- The thought content associated with grief generally features a preoccupation with thoughts and memories of the deceased, rather than the self-critical or pessimistic ruminations seen in major depressive episodes.
- In grief, self-esteem is generally preserved, whereas in major depressive episodes feelings of worthlessness and self-loathing are common.

BIOPSYCHOSOCIAL THEORIES

People with certain personality types or temperaments are more prone than others to develop depressive and elated behaviours. Significant efforts have been devoted to identifying a single psychological factor, trait or mechanism that is unique to the development of mood disorders.

Research exploring the causative factors of mood disorders has focused on reactions to early separation from parents or parental loss, early mother–child relationships, errors in thinking, inherited tendencies, biological factors, and other aspects of human development and experience. To date, no single personality type, biological or psychological trait, or constellation of experiences has been established to account for all forms of mood disorders. Multiple complex factors contribute to the development of mood disorders.

Psychoanalytic theory

The psychoanalytic theory of depression was originally formulated by Freud and later refined by others. It focuses on an unsatisfactory early mother–infant relationship as the primary factor predisposing individuals to later depression. If an infant's needs go unmet, a sense of loss occurs. Unresolved grief over the loss results in anger turned inward and the development of self-hate. The child's ego development is thereby adversely affected, resulting in a weak ego and an overdeveloped, punitive superego.

The psychoanalytic school of thought suggests a different aetiology for bipolar disorder. This theory holds that the mother/primary caregiver derives pleasure from the infant's early dependence, but feels threatened by the child's increasing autonomy as they develop. Independent behaviours are considered 'bad', and the child must suppress their needs in order to sustain parental affection. Ambivalence resulting from the co-existing desires to please the parents and become more autonomous causes resentment and leads to a love–hate relationship with the parenting figures. Again, a weak ego and punitive superego create depression. Mania is seen as the denial of depression taken to the extreme. Contemporary theorists and researchers criticise psychoanalytic theory for its tendency to blame mothers while ignoring biological factors.

Cognitive theory

Cognitive theorists such as Clark and Beck (1999) suggest that depression results from impaired cognition, or distorted thinking processes. People who think negative thoughts evaluate themselves critically and interpret stressful events as having a powerful, global impact on them. They feel guilty, inadequate and hopeless about the future. Recent models of cognitive vulnerability to depression theorise that negative thoughts alone are not sufficient to cause depression unless the individual already suffers from a mildly depressed mood. In these instances, the combination of adverse life events (or the perception of adverse life events) and mildly depressed mood combine to create a downward spiral into depression. The Beck Depression Inventory is a clinical assessment tool. It asks the person to rate themselves on 21 groups of questions designed to detect negative thinking. Cognitive therapy seeks to teach individuals how to stop negative thinking and replace it with more positive self-appraisals. Cognitive therapies are discussed in detail in Chapter 25.

The theory of **learned helplessness** is a cognitive theory that proposes that learning plays an instrumental role in the development of depression. This theory holds that depression is based on the person's belief that they have no control over life situations. This conclusion is drawn from repeated failures, either real or perceived, to control life events and environmental influences. The result is that the person gives up, stops trying to control, becomes dependent on others, and is thereby predisposed to depression (Lazenby, 2011).

Biological theories

Research on the physiological basis for depression has been conducted for more than 60 years, and has generated a variety of hypotheses. Because mental illness such as depressive and bipolar disorders vary widely, it is unlikely that any single biological causative factor can be isolated. This has led to research on how the various biological factors already identified relate to one another, how they affect behaviour, and how they respond to different therapies. In searching for biological changes in depressive and bipolar disorders, it is important to remember that, although a biological abnormality may co-exist with a disorder, it is not necessarily a causative factor. It could be a cause, a co-existing factor or a consequence. Your Assessment Approach lists some abnormal findings on laboratory tests that may indicate the presence of a mood disorder.

YOUR ASSESSMENT APPROACH
Abnormal biological findings in affective disorders

While there are no laboratory studies that definitively diagnose depressive or bipolar disorders, some abnormal findings are noted more often in individuals when symptoms are present than in control subjects. These are as follows:

- sleep abnormalities in 40 per cent to 60 per cent of outpatients and up to 90 per cent of inpatients with major depressive episode and in 25 per cent to 50 per cent of adults with dysthymic disorder; decreased need for sleep and abnormal polysomnographic findings in people with manic episode (sleep abnormalities may precede the onset of a mood disorder and may persist in the absence of other symptoms)
- neurotransmitter and neuropeptide dysregulation in major depressive episode and manic episode
- hormonal disturbances (blunted growth hormone and thyroid-stimulating hormone); elevated urinary free cortisol; dexamethasone nonsuppression of prolactin; elevated plasma cortisol
- brain imaging studies may show increased blood flow in limbic and paralimbic regions, and decreased blood flow in the lateral prefrontal cortex in depression; increased rates of right hemispheric lesions, or bilateral subcortical or preventricular lesions in persons with bipolar disorder
- preventricular vascular changes when depression begins in late life
- urine and blood drug screens may indicate a substance-induced mood disorder.

Gender and age

Women are more prone to major depressive disorders and dysthymic disorders than are men (Slade et al., 2009). This is true across cultures (Kessler & Bromet, 2013). Endocrine and reproductive cycles may play a role, although menopause alone, contrary to popular belief, does not appear to be a risk factor for depression in women. It is also unclear whether peripartum depressions are hormonal in nature, result from the increased stress of motherhood, or represent an interaction of these and other factors. A person's gender is important given the propensity of women to succumb to depression more than men. However, environment and life experiences play a major role in the development of depressive disorders in both sexes. For example, according to the Australian Institute of Health and Welfare (2008), males aged 45–64 years living in rural and remote areas report depression at 1.4 times the rate of men the same age from major cities.

Genetic theories

Numerous studies have concentrated on the role heredity plays in depressive illness. It was noted that the incidence of depression is higher among relatives of depressed individuals than in the general population. Studies of illness rates within and between generations of families, of monozygotic and dizygotic twins, and of the general population, and those using known genetic markers such as blood type or colour blindness, all validate the increased incidence of depression in relatives of depressed individuals.

Studies have demonstrated that bipolar disorder is also increased among first-degree relatives of individuals with that disorder. Studies of identical twins report an 80 per cent concordance rate in bipolar disorder. This means that if one twin has the disorder, there is an 80 per cent chance that the other twin will also develop it.

The role of genetics in the development of major mood disorders is complicated by the familiar question: which plays the more important role—genes or environment? The Nature or nurture debate. People who are biologically related tend to spend time together and influence one another's thinking. They share similar values and beliefs, and are subjected to similar stressors, such as poverty or the death of loved ones. It is therefore difficult to determine the relative influence of genetics, thinking patterns, family relationships and learning in the development of mood disorders.

Depression and the most effective treatments for it can now be tested. Following the US Food and Drug Administration's approval of a test to predict differences in the cytochrome P_{450} (CY_{P450}) gene, clinicians and those experiencing depression in the United States must decide whether using genetic tests to select a specific antidepressant medication from the class known as selective serotonin reuptake inhibitors (SSRIs) might improve the response to treatment for depression. Currently, genetic testing has not been found to predict the most effective treatment, but it can be used to assist those people who may experience adverse reactions related to medications acting on the P_{450} gene (Dubovsky, 2015).

Biochemical theories

Early biochemical studies established that an error in metabolism results in an electrolyte imbalance that seems to play a role in depression. The studies demonstrated that sodium and potassium were transposed in the neurons of depressed individuals. This transposition alters the sensitivity of the neuronal cell membranes. Alterations in the sensitivity of the neuronal receptors are likely to lead to alterations in behaviour. This may account for the efficacy of medications, such as lithium carbonate and antidepressants, in the treatment of mood disorders.

Since then, research has focused on the role of certain chemicals, the neurotransmitters, in the central nervous system. These are chemicals that transmit nervous impulses along neuronal pathways in the limbic area of the brain. Levels of certain monoamine neurotransmitters—norepinephrine, serotonin, epinephrine and dopamine—were found to be deficient in many depressed people. Until the 1980s, scientists believed that major depression resulted from norepinephrine or serotonin deficiencies, and the early antidepressants were formulated accordingly.

The monoamine hypothesis prevailed for years, until it was found insufficient to explain fully the aetiology of a complex disorder such as depression. Deficient levels of monoamine neurotransmitters have not been consistently found in depressed people, and have not been able to relieve symptoms reliably. It is now believed that monoamine deficiencies are only one manifestation of depression. Many pharmacological agents successfully used to treat depression and mania, however, do enhance monoamine activity. For example, the study of the metabolism of serotonin and the discovery of the dysfunction of certain serotonergic neurons in depressed individuals led to the development of the SSRIs and subsequent generations of these useful antidepressants.

Much current biochemical research focuses on the role of psychosocial stress in the pathophysiology of depression. The damaging effects of chronic stress, including its impact on limbic activity, are under extensive study. Research indicates that the underlying biochemical process involves the neurotransmitters dopamine, gamma-aminobutyric acid (GABA), serotonin and norepinephrine (Lin et al., 2011). Interferences with the smooth transmission of impulses from one neuron to another, associated with depressive and manic phases of bipolar disorder, can be explained by the inadequate release of neurotransmitters or faulty storage mechanisms. It is expected that interactive hypotheses of depression—that is, those that take into consideration a variety of biological and psychosocial factors—are most useful when trying to understand these complex disorders.

Biological rhythms

Humans have self-sustained internal physiological cycles that occur every 24 hours. These circadian rhythms, which include body temperature, sleep and appetite, are activated, controlled and integrated by the hypothalamus in the brain. The central controlling pacemaker is commonly known as the *biological clock*.

Diurnal variations in mood, rest and activity cycles, EEG patterns, and neuroendocrine secretions have been clinically demonstrated. No doubt you have experienced these variations yourself. Circadian rhythm dysfunction can explain a number of mood disorder symptoms, such as insomnia, hypersomnia, early morning awakening, and variations in appetite, rest and activity cycles. Animal studies have demonstrated that alcohol and antimanic medications, such as lithium, slow the biological clock, while oestrogen and tricyclic antidepressants accelerate it or restore normal rhythms. The precise role that biological rhythms play in mood disorders is yet to be determined.

The presence of physical problems is thought to play a role in mood disorders. There may be a common factor at work with certain illnesses in which both depression and another physical problem are present, as referred to earlier in this chapter regarding cardiac dysfunction. In order to make a diagnosis of mood disorder, the clinician must rule out infections, chemical imbalances, environmental toxins, alcohol abuse and other biological processes. All of these physical problems may present in such a way as to look like depression.

Psychological factors

Regardless of temperament and personality patterns, people can and do become depressed. Mild depression is widely acknowledged as a part of the human experience. Although most of us have had 'the blues' from time to time, certain people are more prone to developing true depression than others. Individuals thought to be at risk for the development of depressive disorders exhibit certain attitudes and beliefs—such as low self-esteem, lack of personal goals and direction, the tendency to avoid difficult situations rather than facing them directly, dependence and passivity in interpersonal relationships, acting and reacting impulsively, a limited ability to form enduring, mature relationships, and internalisation of blame.

Sociocultural factors

Life events and environmental stress play a role in mental illness, including depressive and bipolar disorders. Whether life events play a primary role or merely contribute to the onset of an inevitable episode of a disorder is unclear. Certain events, such as the death of a loved one, divorce and other losses, are widely recognised as precipitating events for depression. The impact of stress reactions and stress hormones on mood has been established. The unremitting stresses of living in poverty, and society's devaluation of the disadvantaged, also seem to predispose people to developing a depressive disorder.

Predictors of bipolar disorders, for the most part, include stressful life events, increased number of previous bipolar episodes, decreased interval between bipolar episodes, and persistence of the effect of symptoms on functioning. The stressors of pregnancy are excellent examples of life events that can create a psychological vulnerability (Maina, Rosso, Aguglia & Bogetto, 2014).

Having longer periods between episodes is typically associated with active involvement in psychotherapy, adhering to a medication regimen, and having a strong support system. The presence of substance abuse interferes with any semblance of stability, and the prevalence of substance use in this population is notably high.

Culture exerts a powerful influence on how individuals experience and communicate distress. Spiritual or religious concerns such as guilt may predominate and mask some symptoms of an underlying depressive disorder. Some cultures experience depressive episodes largely in somatic terms. Be alert to complaints, such as a weakness in spirit in some Australian Aboriginal populations (Brown et al., 2012). Weakness or 'imbalance' in Asian clients, and body metaphors involving the heart in Middle Eastern people may be culturally determined ways of expressing depression.

Be aware of the unique needs of the person who perceives the meaning and severity of psychiatric symptoms in relation to the norms of their cultural reference group. They include new migrants to Australia, individuals who are still heavily involved in their culture of origin, those who do not speak English, and those whose entire network of social and religious support remains embedded in their culture of origin.

Differences in culture and social status can create problems in diagnosis and treatment. Language differences, for example, create barriers in forming therapeutic relationships in talk therapies and in other treatment settings. Cultural differences in the expression of symptoms make it difficult to determine whether a behaviour is normal or pathological, and the culture itself may dictate or affect the person's attitudes towards and adherence to treatment (Buckner-Brown, Tucker & Rivera, 2011).

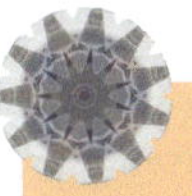

NURSING PROCESS
The person with major depressive disorders

Assessment

Depression is characterised by low mood, and may be related to loss. The loss may be concrete, such as the loss of a loved one or a job, or perceived, such as the loss of a cherished wish or disillusionment with a respected role model.

Subjective data

The person with depressive disorders may express some of the following:

- feelings of sadness
- fatigue
- lack of interest in relationships and activities that were previously pleasurable
- feelings of worthlessness
- impaired concentration
- impaired decision-making ability
- sleep disturbances
- appetite changes; weight loss or weight gain
- excessive sleep.

People will often describe how long it takes them to complete activities that formerly were easily accomplished, such as preparing a meal. Tearfulness and emotional outbursts may also be a part of their description of the problem. They may or may not mention a loss or disappointment that they relate to the feelings.

Somatic concerns Somatic concerns are often the presenting complaint. People experiencing depression may complain of abdominal pains, headaches and vague bodily aches. A problem with sexual functioning or a lack of desire may also be a presenting complaint. Constipation is a common result of the general slowing of metabolism due to inactivity. Some cultures more easily express symptoms of depression through complaints about body function and discomfort. See What Every Nurse Should Know on the next page for information on how you can detect depression evidenced by somatic concerns in other settings.

Suicide assessment Assess all people who describe depressive symptoms for suicide risk. This is best accomplished through direct questioning. Ask about suicidal thinking, history of suicide attempts, and whether the person has a specific suicide plan. This aspect of assessment is often reassuring, not alarming, to people experiencing suicidal ideation. Ask these questions in a direct fashion. You might ask, for example, 'Are you thinking

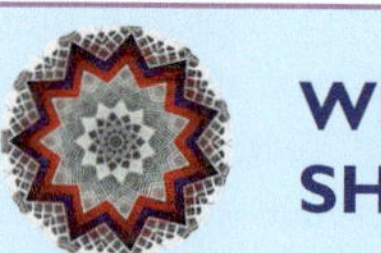

WHAT EVERY NURSE SHOULD KNOW

Physical complaints and depression

Imagine you are a general practice nurse. Frequently, you would note that people feel aches and pains more acutely when they are depressed. The natural reaction to pain is to seek help from one's general practitioner (GP). According to a recent study, depression accounts for 4.3 per cent of all GP encounters; and of all reasons for which clinical treatment is provided by a GP, the most common reason is depression (Britt et al., 2014). However, people with somatic concerns may not recognise these as possible symptoms of depression. The early detection and treatment of depression is important to promote a person's wellbeing (Carey et al., 2014). It is important for people who are experiencing depression to talk to their health care providers about other experiences and symptoms over their lifetime. Be aware that in some cultures people express depression through body systems—headaches, stomach aches, muscle spasms and visual problems, among others. When you assess people from these cultures, consider the possibility that they may be depressed.

People seldom self-diagnose depression. They are much more likely to assume that not enjoying their usual activities, experiencing changes in eating or sleeping habits, and feeling bad in one way or another are caused by a medical problem. Identifying the real cause of distress will ensure effective responses to treatment.

of suicide?', 'Are you thinking of killing yourself?', 'Tell me how you plan to kill yourself', 'Do you have the gun/pills/poison?' It is important to know whether the person has actually planned the suicide, or whether it is a vaguely formed thought. Often, the more organised the plan is, the more concern it generates, particularly if the person has access to a lethal weapon, chemical or other means of suicide. Further discussion of other aspects of suicide will be discussed under the heading Preventing Suicide and Promoting Safety. Suicide lethality assessment is discussed at length in Chapter 19.

Objective data

Depressive disorders are common in the general population. Those with depressive disorders are more likely to be female: 14.5 per cent of women will experience major depressive disorder in their lifetime compared to 8.8 per cent of men (ABS, 2007). Both genders are at significant risk for a depressive episode. People with depression often have had prior episodes of depression and a family history of depression or another disorder, such as anxiety. A history of a recent stressful event and the lack of social support are also common features.

Objective signs The objective signs and symptoms of depression are few. Psychomotor agitation or retardation may be observable if it is profound, or if the nurse is familiar with the person's usual level of functioning. Family members may report observations of a person's agitation or apathy and lack of pleasure in usual activities. They may describe a pattern of social withdrawal and lack of social participation, combined with an intense preoccupation with their own feelings. Be alert to any change in behaviour.

Screening During assessment, many clinicians find it useful to provide a list of symptoms and ask the person to identify the ones they are experiencing. A widely used and highly regarded self-reporting instrument designed to assess mood against a scale is the Kessler Psychological Distress Scale (K10). It is a 10-item questionnaire used to measure psychological distress, based on the frequency of symptoms related to depression and anxiety.

Medical illnesses Other objective information to obtain during the nursing assessment includes concurrent general medical illnesses. Autoimmune, neurological, metabolic, oncological and endocrine disorders often trigger depression. For example, hypothyroidism may be accompanied by depressive symptoms due to the underlying medical disease, while a person with a distressing diagnosis such as cancer may become depressed as a result of the diagnosis, prognosis or disability connected with the disease.

Substance use and abuse Alcohol, which is a CNS depressant, and certain legal and illegal drugs can cause or complicate depression. Obtain a complete list of all of the substances and medications used by the person through matter-of-fact questioning. A few prescription medications have depression as a side-effect; do not overlook these in the complete assessment. Contraceptives, sedatives, reserpine, glucocorticoids and anabolic steroids have all been associated with the development of depression.

Laboratory tests There are currently no laboratory tests specific for depression, but abnormal findings on several tests were discussed earlier in this chapter in Your Assessment Approach on page 327.

Nursing practice

The following sections discuss presentations commonly seen in people experiencing a depressive disorder.

Self-harm behaviour

There are many reasons that a person may partake in self-harm behaviours. These may include the person wanting to punish themselves, distract themselves from painful feelings or anxieties, or feel in control of their body or of others. The person may be experiencing feelings of worthlessness, guilt, repeated failure experiences, helplessness and hopelessness, or be experiencing psychotic thinking. Self-harm behaviours do not necessarily mean that the person is having thoughts of suicide; however, a strong correlation between the two exists (Kerr, Muehlenkamp & Turner, 2010). A person may be partaking in self-harm behaviours to distract themselves from thoughts of suicide. Regardless of setting, whenever a person is at high risk for self-harm behaviour, that becomes *the* priority, and the person's safety becomes the most important aspect of nursing care. In such a scenario, a nurse should remain calm and non-judgmental, avoiding a negative reaction.

Situational low self-esteem or chronic low self-esteem

People expressing a depressed mood often express, either directly or indirectly, negative feelings about themselves and their abilities. Reduced self-esteem may be related to a variety of factors, including feeling abandoned by loved ones, experiencing repeated failures or losses, lacking positive feedback from others, thinking negative thoughts, engaging in negative 'self-talk', or feeling guilty over real or perceived transgressions.

Evidence of low self-esteem may be seen in people who: withdraw from social interaction; have difficulty accepting compliments or positive feedback; are harshly critical of themselves or others; are reluctant to try new activities because of fear of failure; express feelings of inferiority, worthlessness and pessimism about the future; are overly sensitive to criticism; see social slights where none are intended; or set unrealistic goals and engage in grandiose thinking (denial of low self-esteem).

Hopelessness

Individuals who experience hopelessness often believe there is no solution to their problems. They may believe that their own actions cannot significantly influence an outcome, and come to doubt their own abilities and worth.

Evidence of hopelessness is heard in the experience of people as a lack of energy and initiative, as difficulty in engaging in self-care. It may be seen as someone not participating in decision-making, a lack of interest or involvement in activities, and being passive in response to others. People may verbally express a lack of control and doubts about their abilities. They may also be reluctant to express feelings, and exhibit decreased affect.

Social isolation

Low self-esteem and self-doubt lead many people with depression to withdraw socially. Because inadequate social skills and self-absorption create impediments to positive interpersonal relationships, people with low self-esteem are frequently avoided by others. This further reinforces their fears of undesirability and increases their social isolation. Evidence of social isolation and impaired social interaction is seen in behaviours such as spending inordinate amounts of time in bed, lack of verbalisation, lack of eye contact, limited or monosyllabic responses to others' attempts at conversation, a preference for being alone, turning away or closing the eyes, and exhibiting discomfort in the presence of others.

Care planning and implementation

When planning and implementing interventions designed to help people experiencing a depressive disorder, keep the following two general principles in mind:

1. It is impossible to make people with depression feel better by being cheerful. In fact, an overly cheerful attitude tends to make them feel even worse because it trivialises or minimises the impact of their feelings. Try to adopt a more emotionally neutral attitude, while maintaining confidence and hope that they will feel better.
2. Recognise that working with people with depression may eventually lower your own mood and also make you feel 'down'. This is called *emotional contagion.* Stay in touch with your own feelings. If you find yourself feeling down, discuss this with your supervisor or explore options of clinical supervision.

Examine and learn from your interventions by reflecting on your interactions with people with depression. Engage in clinical supervision. One way to reflect on your interactions is the process-recording method. The process-recording method helps you to structure your interaction. A process-recording usually consists of three columns—one for the nurse's statements, one for the person in care, and one that identifies the process or action taking place. A sample process-recording of an interaction between a nurse and a depressed person is given in Box 15.2.

Preventing suicide and promoting safety

There are few times when 'always' and 'never' are applicable. A person's safety, however, *always* takes priority. When the risk for self-harm is high, a number of actions call for immediate intervention. These actions are discussed in the following Your Intervention Strategies. *Be aware that the risk of suicide increases as the severest stage of depression is alleviated, because people then have sufficient energy and cognitive ability to plan and successfully implement a suicide plan, even though they are still deeply depressed.*

Box 15.2 A sample process-recording with a person who is depressed

Person	Nurse	Process
'I don't think I can take this anymore—it's too much for me.'	'You sound so overwhelmed. How long have you felt this way?'	Validating, exploring
'It's been like this for as long as I can remember. It just never ends.'	'How have you handled these feelings over the long time you've had them?'	Opening the topic of person's successes in managing
'I just put one foot in front of the other. It doesn't make it better, though.'	'It does seem to work to some extent. You've made it through this long.'	Reframing the effort as a success
'I guess. I just don't know how I can keep doing it.'	'It can be tiring. Keep in mind you're not alone in this effort. You have people who support you and care about you.'	Validation, reinforcing the social supports in place
'As long as I have some help.'	'There is help you can depend on.'	Reassurance

YOUR INTERVENTION STRATEGIES Preventing inpatient suicide and promoting safety

Check the policy of the health care facility and implement the procedures.

- Evaluate the level of suicide intent regularly, and institute the appropriate level of supervision following unit policy.
- People who are suicidal need to know that the environment is safe for them. Reassure them by removing sharp objects, razors, breakable glass items, mirrors, matches, and straps or belts, and explain why these objects are being removed. Monitor the use of scissors, razors and other potential weapons.
- Nurse the person where they can best be observed.
- Avoid establishing a predictable pattern of observation during the day, and especially at night.
- Be particularly alert during change of shifts and on holidays, or at other times when staffing is limited, and during times of distraction, such as mealtimes and visiting hours.
- Ensure visitors do not bring unsafe items.
- A no-suicide contract, discussed in detail in Chapter 19, is a useful intervention.

Encourage the person to seek staff support when bothered by suicidal thoughts or impulses. Discussing these thoughts and impulses may be sufficient to diminish them and prevent a suicidal crisis from occurring. Avoid discussing suicidal ruminations in repetitious detail, because this may reinforce maladaptive behaviour.

Encourage discussing all feelings. People experiencing suicidal thoughts need to know that all feelings are valid, and that it benefits them to express their emotions, particularly anger and hopelessness, rather than act them out through maladaptive behaviours. Having the feeling is always accepted. Acting on the feeling, however, may be problematic. What counts in the long run is what one decides to do about the feeling. Assist in the transition from inpatient care to home by helping the person identify supportive people in their usual environments to whom they can express feelings candidly without being judged.

Use a calm, hopeful, empathetic and nonjudgmental approach, and teach calming measures, such as stress management and controlled breathing. Provide safe physical outlets for the expression of anger or increasing tension.

Collaborate with the person to identify community resources to which they can turn if suicidal thoughts recur outside the treatment setting. Most communities have access to hotlines like Lifeline (phone = 13 11 14) that are staffed around the clock with trained volunteers who are available to discuss feelings before they reach crisis proportions. Refer to Chapter 19 for specific information on suicide and suicide prevention.

Promoting self-esteem

While low self-esteem is a chronic problem, there are a number of actions that can help reduce negative thinking, thereby promoting improved self-esteem.

- Provide distraction from self-absorption by involving the person in recreational activities and pleasant pastimes. An example is Recovery Camp (Moxham, Liersch-Sumskis, Taylor, Patterson & Brighton, 2015).
- Simple conversations or engagement in activities with staff or peer workers can help interrupt the pattern of negative thoughts.
- Dispel the notion, which people often have, that *when* they feel better they will want to engage in activities. Explain that they must begin doing things *in order* to feel better. Being active promotes a more balanced feeling state. Be sure to acknowledge that it takes self-discipline and energy to do something when one does not really feel like it. Explain this in a respectful manner, being careful not to pressure or challenge the person in an argumentative fashion.
- Recognise accomplishment; do not use flattery or excessive praise. Give positive, matter-of-fact reinforcement, such as 'I notice that you combed your hair', rather than overly enthusiastic compliments, such as 'What a great hairstyle!' Appropriate recognition will increase the likelihood that a person will accept the positive feedback, while insincerity can be perceived as ridicule.
- Help identify personal strengths. It may be useful to write these down. Recognise that it often takes some time for a person with low self-esteem to realise that they have any strengths. Avoid the temptation to point out the characteristics you have noticed. It is far more useful to support their ability to recognise their own positive qualities.
- Be accepting and nonjudgmental of a persons' negative feelings. Be alert for opportunities to interrupt the negative conversational patterns with conversation that focuses on the person's resilience or strengths.
- Teach assertiveness techniques, such as the ability to say 'no' to protect one's own rights while respecting the rights of others. A person with low self-esteem often allows others to take advantage of them. Defining passive, aggressive and assertive behaviour, and giving examples of each, are also helpful when teaching assertiveness. Encourage the person and their family members to practise the new techniques in their relationship with you, so that you can give feedback on how it feels to be the recipient of an assertive communication or action.

Instilling hope

Assisting those who are experiencing depression to develop a positive outlook is a priority nursing intervention. People who feel hopeless tend to form dependent relationships. Be aware of this tendency, and work from the first contact to minimise the likelihood that maladaptive dependence occurs in your nurse–consumer relationship. The list in Self-awareness will give you direction on minimising maladaptive dependence.

COLLABORATIVE CARE

Teaching about aggressive, passive and assertive behaviours

Assertiveness is a learned behaviour. Everyone has assertiveness potential, but we are not born knowing how to be assertive. Children learn patterns of communicating from the adults around them. However, you can unlearn communication patterns if they are not working, and learn new ones. The goal is to help people express themselves without fear of disapproval from others. Being assertive does not guarantee that others will always agree with you, but you do have the satisfaction of giving your opinion.

Definitions

Aggressive behaviour is directed towards getting what one wants without considering the feelings of others. Aggressive communicators want to get their own way at any cost. They want others to 'back off', and use intimidation to convey this message. An example of aggressive behaviour is demanding something of someone and yelling to intimidate them. The outcome of aggressive behaviour is that, although you may get what you want in the short run, others feel discredited and tend to avoid you.

Passive behaviour consists of avoiding conflict at any cost, even at the expense of one's own happiness. An example of passive behaviour is agreeing to go to a movie you do not want to see because your friend pressures you to go. Passive communicators hold their feelings in and allow anger to build up. Anger can come out suddenly in an explosion, or can be expressed in what is known as passive–aggressive behaviour. An example of passive–aggressive behaviour is taking a long time to get ready to go out while your friend is waiting, because you are angry at him for insisting on seeing a movie you do not want to see. The outcome is that the passive person gives up control and is left with resentment, which usually emerges in other ways that damage relationships.

Assertive behaviour consists of expressing one's wishes and opinions, or taking care of oneself, but not at the expense of others. An example of assertive communication is saying, 'I really don't care for violent movies. Let's look at the movie listings and see if there is something that we can both enjoy.' The outcome of assertive behaviour is self-confidence and self-esteem. Consumers and family members can learn about assertiveness in other ways as well. As a psychiatric–mental health nurse, you can help with this type of education.

SELF-AWARENESS

Minimising maladaptive dependence

Be aware that people experiencing a sense of hopelessness may form dependent relationships. Work from the first contact to minimise the likelihood that maladaptive dependence occurs in the therapeutic relationship.

- Emphasising the short-term nature of the relationship is essential.
- If the person singles out one staff member exclusively and refuses to relate to others, this is a clue that undue dependence is developing.
- Avoid giving dependent people the hope that their relationship with the nurse can continue after the end of the therapy.
- Kindly, but firmly, refuse requests for your address or telephone number.
- Remind the person in your care that social contact is not allowed.
- If you find yourself wanting to continue relationships with certain individuals, discuss these feelings with your facilitator or preceptor (if you are a student), or your supervisor or a respected professional peer (if you are a registered nurse). It is essential that you separate your professional and social lives.

Enable personal choices in the planning of care, and encourage consumers to assume self-responsibility. Encouraging those in your care to set their own goals that identify what they hope to achieve reinforces the message of self-determination. Remember that these are the person's goals and you are there to encourage. If you are concerned that a goal may be unattainable, encourage them to consider goals that are more attainable. This will help to reinforce the person's sense of power and achievement. Collaboratively set attainable goals.

Someone who feels hopeless may also need help in identifying how they can gain a sense of control in their relationships and lives. Collaborate with them to identify changes they wish to make, and take steps towards achieving them. Make the steps small and manageable. Accomplishing even small steps leads to a sense of mastery and optimism.

Teach the person coping measures, such as problem-solving techniques, and encourage them to use these when confronting life situations. For example, if the person has difficulty paying the rent, help them identify options, such as moving to a less expensive flat or taking in a flatmate. Explore the pros and cons of each option and their possible consequences. Emphasise confidence in the person's ability to identify, select and carry out problem-solving activities that will result in a greater sense of involvement in their life. Equally important is to help the person identify the aspects of their lives that are not within their control. The ability to accept what *cannot* be changed is just as essential as developing the ability to bring about positive change.

Planning for discharge should begin at admission, and is particularly important with people who may be at risk of maladaptive dependency. Help the person and their significant others identify community resources and support systems. Support groups, therapy groups and social groups can all help a person bring about positive change.

Enhancing socialisation

When considering interventions for promoting social interactions, understand that both the quality and the quantity of a person's social behaviour may be impaired.

COMMUNICATION

Client experiencing major depressive episode

PERSON: 'I am upset and irritated all the time. All I do is yell at my kids and snap at my husband.'

NURSE RESPONSE 1: 'What can you tell me about feeling so upset?'	**NURSE RESPONSE 2:** 'It sounds like you are feeling out of control right now.'
RATIONALE: Open-ended questions elicit the person's perception of the problem and allow them to begin to explore feelings. It accepts the person where they are now without judgment.	*RATIONALE:* This response shows empathy and acceptance. By reflecting the expression of feelings, you validate the accuracy of your understanding and lay the groundwork for further exploration.

Early in the therapeutic relationship, make brief but frequent contacts with the person if they are withdrawn, but without making any demands. Your interest can increase a person's self-worth.

With people who are extremely uncommunicative, simply spending time sitting quietly without any demand for interaction may be helpful. This approach communicates your belief that they are worth the investment of time. If you find it difficult to be comfortable with silence, you may communicate that discomfort to the person. Remember that silence conveys acceptance and is a useful therapeutic communication technique. Using silence therapeutically is discussed in Chapter 9.

When someone expresses feelings or shows emotions, remember to be nonjudgmental. Avoid showing surprise or disapproval. Two examples of how you can do this are outlined in the above Communication feature. Recognise that venting feelings may provide temporary relief, particularly if anger is expressed. If a person is unable to verbalise their feelings, they sometimes can act them out in safe and appropriate ways, such as tearing up an old magazine or beating on a pillow or bed. Provide privacy during these times.

Encourage both verbal and non-verbal expressions of feelings by teaching the person that these are healthy behaviours. This intervention reinforces your acceptance of each person as unique and valuable individuals. Avoid disagreeing with, or otherwise belittling, a person's feelings by using overly cheerful reassurances like 'Now, now, Mrs Liu. You're feeling down right now, but you'll feel better after a good night's sleep.'

Once someone is comfortable interacting with one person, encourage group activities. Although this step may be difficult and frightening for some, you can minimise their discomfort by attending the activities with them at first. If their anxiety becomes too uncomfortable, let them know that they can leave the situation without losing your approval. Give recognition for even small steps, gradually removing yourself and allowing them to stay in groups on their own.

Sometimes people avoid social situations because they lack social skills and self-confidence. Create opportunities for the person to learn social skills and practise them in a protected environment. For example, teach them to read the newspaper or see a movie and select several items of interest to use in making 'small talk'. Demonstrate making small talk, and encourage them to practise with you. Give feedback on their progress. Make sure this is an enjoyable and non-threatening activity.

Individuals who are either extremely passive or too aggressive in their social interactions are often avoided by others. Teaching such people how to use assertive behaviour can improve their interpersonal relationships. Use role-playing to help them become comfortable with these new skills.

Administering medications

Common types of antidepressants that nurses administer to people experiencing a depressive disorder are tricyclic antidepressants (TCAs), monoamine oxidase inhibitors (MAOIs), selective serotonin reuptake inhibitors (SSRIs), serotonin and norepinephrine reuptake inhibitors (SNRIs), and atypical antidepressants such as bupropion. See Chapter 7 for detailed discussions of these medications. The intended action of all antidepressants is to exert positive effects on mood and behaviour. Because some are sedating and others are energising, an individual's symptoms guide the choice of medication. The use of antidepressants during pregnancy may be necessary, and is weighed against both the dangers to the fetus of an untreated, distressed mother and the risk of birth defects. Current clinical practice is to treat the depressive disorder to protect both the mother and the baby.

Antidepressants are generally effective in alleviating most people's symptoms, and are helpful adjuncts to treatment. Because they do nothing to affect any underlying psychosocial conflicts, they should not be used as the single treatment modality for someone with depression, but should be used in conjunction with other therapies and supports. Specific information, such as maintaining a low-tyramine diet (**tyramine** is an amino acid) while on MAOIs, is an educational point that might need to be discussed with the person and their families. People taking MAOIs cannot consume anything (food, drink, medications) containing tyramine, because this can cause a dangerous rise in blood pressure called *hypertensive crisis*. Chapter 7 has additional information about antidepressant therapy and related nursing responsibilities.

Monitoring electroconvulsive therapy

Electroconvulsive therapy (ECT), a treatment procedure during which a small electric current is passed through particular areas of the brain, appears to be useful to individuals

YOUR INTERVENTION STRATEGIES Working with people receiving ECT

- Explain the procedure and answer all questions as fully as possible.
- A separate consent for treatment must be signed, because ECT requires the administration of anaesthesia. While informing the person and obtaining consent forms is legally a medical responsibility, in practice it is often shared by nurses.
- Nil by mouth for at least four hours before treatment.
- Just prior to treatment, request that the person void and remove any contact lenses, jewellery, hairpins and dentures.
- Assess the person's vital signs.
- The anaesthetic preparation usually consists of the following:
  1. Generally, an atropine-like medication, such as glycopyrrolate (Robinul), is given to decrease secretions and block cardiac vagal reflexes during the modified seizure.
  2. A short-acting anaesthetic, such as methohexital sodium (Brevital), is administered intravenously.
  3. Following induction, a skeletal muscle relaxant, such as succinylcholine chloride (Anectine), is administered to prevent injuries during the modified seizure.
  4. The person must be artificially ventilated until the muscle relaxant is fully metabolised, usually in two to three minutes. Oxygen is administered with a rubber bite-block in place. If necessary, oxygen may be administered by positive pressure.
- A controlled electrical current is passed through the brain by means of unilateral or bilateral electrodes placed on the temples. This causes a generalised (or tonic–clonic) seizure, the effects of which are masked by the muscle relaxant. Often the only observable signs of seizure are a fluttering of the eyelids and carpopedal spasms.
- Recovery occurs in the lateral recumbent position to facilitate drainage and prevent aspiration. Upon awakening, the person will be confused and somewhat disoriented. After they are fully recovered and have been reoriented, they may consume food.

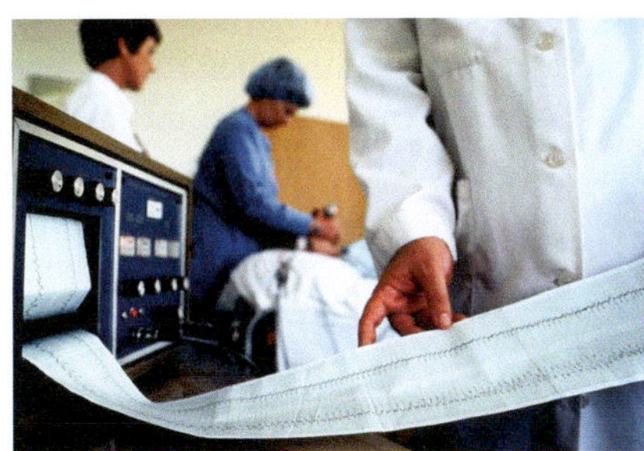

Photo courtesy of Will McIntyre/Photo Researchers, Inc.

with severe depression, acute mania, some psychotic conditions, and those who are acutely suicidal. It is usually given several times a week until a course of 12 treatments is completed. Exactly how ECT works is not well understood. Evidence suggests that it may resynchronise circadian rhythms, like a 'brain defibrillator'; it may act as an anticonvulsant, like carbamazepine; it may restore the equilibrium between cerebral hemispheres; or it may help prioritise function over depressive thoughts. Historically, ECT has been controversial, probably due to its crude beginnings. Current use, known as 'modified ECT', is not the intense physiological event it used to be, because of the use of muscle relaxants and short-acting anaesthetic agents.

ECT causes no tissue damage or neuronal cell loss (structural brain damage). Most people who receive ECT report positive associations with the treatment and general improvement in cognition, in addition to relief from depression for several weeks following ECT. There are very few cautions or contraindications for ECT use. Guidelines for working with people receiving ECT are discussed in Your Intervention Strategies.

During a course of ECT, a transient short-term memory loss is expected. This may be distressing, and reassurance that memory is usually completely restored is required. Because ECT is not curative, ongoing psychotherapy and pharmacotherapy are often continued to prevent *relapse*. This treatment modality is considered the treatment of choice for treatment-resistant depressive disorders. The practical issues of ECT treatment and how the treatment is conducted are described in the following Practice Example.

Practice example

Barry has been depressed for a number of months after having been accused of unfair practices at work. His feelings of guilt and worthlessness are far out of proportion to reality. Although he believes he has a successful defence against these charges, many people at work see it differently. His psychiatrist has tried several different antidepressants with him, but his symptoms continue to worsen. Barry has developed severe depressive symptoms, such as suicidal thinking, psychomotor retardation and weight loss, because he believes that he does not deserve to eat.

Barry's psychiatrist has recommended a course of ECT for his treatment-resistant depression. Barry is concerned because he has heard many rumours about the negative effects of ECT. The psychiatrist has explained that it is a safe and effective treatment about which there are several negative and inaccurate myths. After several discussions, Barry agrees to try ECT. He is given a course of six ECT treatments over two weeks, and experiences a significant improvement in his mood. He is no longer suicidal or delusional, and no longer has psychomotor retardation. It has become possible for him to function more effectively at work, including defending himself against what he declares are unfounded charges. Due to advances in ECT techniques, Barry has had no discomfort during or after any of the ECT treatments. He is relieved that ECT has been an effective treatment for his depression.

Evaluation

Specific behaviours indicate that nursing interventions have been successful. Evaluation criteria answer the question: 'How do we know that the person's condition has improved?'

Impulse control and suicide self-restraint

The risk for self-harming behaviour is lessened when the person reports a decrease in suicidal thoughts and impulses and commits no acts of self-harm. People who are not suicidal can express negative feelings appropriately and avoid high-risk environments or situations. They become more adept at identifying alternative ways of coping with problems, and no longer depend on suicide as their primary coping skill.

Self-esteem

People who have improved self-esteem can verbalise self-acceptance and identify positive self-characteristics. They can speak about increased feelings of self-worth. Behaviours are consistent with increased self-esteem; for example, their posture may be erect, and they may groom and dress themselves with some care. They are more ready to accept a compliment, to express feelings directly and openly, and to communicate assertively with others, including maintaining eye contact. They express some optimism and hope for the future. People demonstrate self-esteem when they evaluate their own strengths realistically, set realistic, attainable goals for themselves, and work towards reaching them.

Hopelessness

People experiencing depression demonstrate progress towards eliminating hopelessness by consistently weighing and choosing among alternatives, and by expressing hope, the will to live, reasons to live, meaning in life, optimism and belief in self or others. They can identify their own personal strengths, show interest in achieving life goals, and demonstrate satisfaction with life conditions, or work to change them.

Social involvement

Improved social involvement is apparent when people communicate and socialise with others. Voluntarily attending group activities is a measure of success. They can initiate interaction with another person appropriately, and assume responsibility for dealing with feelings, including finding others with whom to talk. An individual can identify their own personal characteristics or behaviours that contribute to social isolation, and accept responsibility for them. They report fewer experiences of feeling excluded. For additional information about working with people who have depression, see the nursing care plan at the end of this chapter. A person plans for discharge by establishing or maintaining relationships, a social life, and a support system outside the hospital, and by participating in leisure activities.

CARE COORDINATION

Care coordination with people experiencing depression should always attempt to ensure that the person receives the services they need in a timely, flexible, cost-effective manner. This requires that the care coordinator understands any risk factors and possible complicating factors of major depressive episodes, recognises prodromal/recurrence/relapse symptoms early, anticipates possible complications, and understands effective care coordination outcomes. Depending on their level of expertise, the care coordinator may deliver direct psychotherapeutic interventions like cognitive behavioural therapy (CBT).

WHY I BECAME A MENTAL HEALTH NURSE

Paul Beckett RMN, BSc(Hons) MA

Like many mental health nurses whom I have met through my career, my path into this fascinating and highly rewarding field was a combination of chance and circumstance. I had enrolled in nursing on a spur-of-the-moment whim, and chose paediatrics as my specialty. Towards the end of the initial training, and questioning if I was cut out for paediatrics, I was allocated to a dementia care facility in a local hospital for my mental health clinical practice. I remember being greeted warmly by the staff and encouraged to get to know the people in our care and develop the nurse–client relationships that had been drilled into us in uni, but which were generally discouraged in the majority of clinical areas. I became fascinated with the work of mental health nursing, and knew then that I had found my calling. Twenty years on, I can reflect on many great opportunities and experiences that have resulted from that chance encounter. The most important lesson I have learned, and which I impress on others, is that reflective practice and openness to learning are the key to maintaining passion and engagement.

Risk factors for recurrence or *relapse* of depression include being female, a family history of depression, previous depressive episodes, a lack of family/social support, stressful life events or losses, and substance abuse. Suicide attempts, substance abuse continuance or increase, having a personality disorder, having a co-existing medical or psychiatric condition, resistance to treatment and/or failure to respond to treatment complicate the course of a depressive episode. While recurrence of depressive symptoms is of concern, the length of time it takes to recover from depressive symptoms affects longer-term planning and care coordination. Symptoms of depression must resolve to a certain extent before the person can experience healthier functioning (Sheehan, Harnett-Sheehan, Spann, Thompson & Prakash, 2011). As treatment continues, symptom relief and then functionality proceed. Recognising depressive symptoms and treating them earlier in the process can be an effective tool in reducing the long-term impacts of the illness.

Symptoms that would alert the care coordinator to evaluate a person's need for treatment for major depressive disorder have been discussed in Diagnostic Features on page 321. Care coordination interventions would respond to suicidal thoughts, suicide plans or suicide attempts, prior self-destructive violence, concurrent chronic or severe acute medical problems, prior medication-resistant depression, social withdrawal, and decline in work productivity. Teach the person and their family members to be alert for symptoms that indicate the need for treatment.

People experiencing depression and their families may find the following websites helpful:

- *beyondblue*: http://www,beyondblue.org.au
- SANE Australia: http://www.sane.org/
- National Institute for Mental Health: http://www.nimh.nih.gov/

Desired outcomes include symptom remission, improvement in social, family and occupational functioning, reduced risk of self-harm, and either avoidance of hospitalisation or shortened hospital stay. Individuals who lack financial resources and family, social and employer support, and who resist or respond poorly to treatment, represent greater challenges for goal attainment. The ultimate goal is the earliest possible detection of symptoms, effective symptom reduction, and a rapid return to maximal premorbid functioning.

COMMUNITY-BASED CARE

People with a depressive disorder can be effectively treated in community-based settings such as a general practice, medical centres, private psychiatric or psychology practices, and community mental health clinics, among others. Community-based care involving nurses can also occur in a person's home. Nurses in community settings play a major role in providing coordinated clinical care, recognising and monitoring symptoms of depression, providing screening and assessment, providing therapeutic support and information, managing antidepressant therapy, providing care for physical health, improving links to other health professionals, and educating family members and significant others about depression. Severely depressed and/or suicidal people, however, should be referred to inpatient treatment to ensure their safety. What Every Nurse Should Know presents information on depression for nurses.

Nurses working in general community health settings may not be as educationally prepared as specialist mental health nurses. However, with continuing education focused on the detection and treatment of depression, they can play a valuable role in a person's recovery while enabling them to remain in the community.

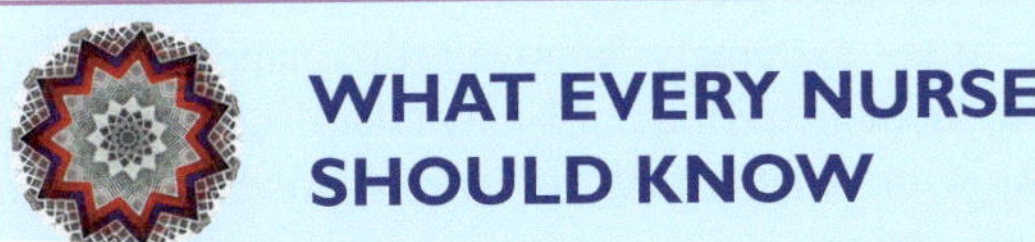

WHAT EVERY NURSE SHOULD KNOW

Grief and depression

Imagine you are a palliative care nurse helping people live the last months of their lives. Depression is thought to be the natural reaction when people have been diagnosed with a terminal illness. When people know that their life is coming to an end, there is sadness and grieving. However, depression is much more than that. Symptoms of depression that last for 14 days or more are not a necessary emotional state. The final months of someone's life, while sad, can be made more comfortable, functional and potentially satisfying when depression is treated. Nurses working in palliative care settings interact with people whose lives will end in a few short months. Spending those months in an emotionally healthy setting is the priority.

Differentiating between normal sadness and grieving and the state called depression is done by a comprehensive assessment and through observations. Statements such as 'I never should have sold the house. That house is where my children grew up and I took all their memories away when I sold it' may represent irrational guilt more than legitimate regret. Similarly, taking more responsibility than is reasonable, interpreting interactions in morbid ways, not being able to enjoy any aspect of their current life, and drastic changes in appetite and sleeping patterns that are not related to their medical condition are all signs of depression. Make arrangements for a psychological consult when you detect depressive symptoms as a palliative care nurse. Consultations of this nature are performed by consultant mental health nurses, psychologists or psychiatrists.

Effective treatment of depressive symptoms, even during the final stages of life, is not only a possibility but a responsibility. Psychotherapy and/or medications can have an impact within a matter of days or weeks, allowing the person to say goodbye and face this transition positively and peacefully.

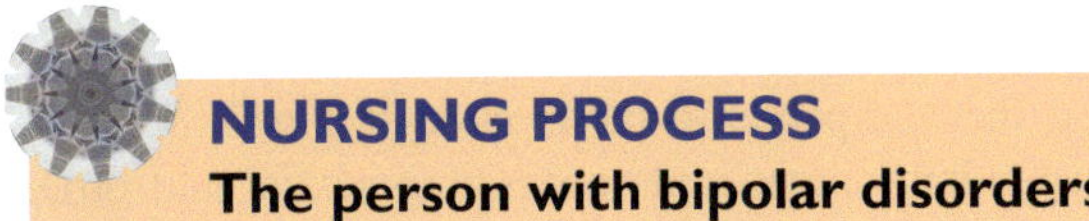

NURSING PROCESS
The person with bipolar disorders

Because the nursing care of people experiencing depressive symptoms is the same whether the diagnosis is major depressive disorder, dysthymic disorder, or depressed episode of a bipolar disorder, this section will focus on hypomania and mania, which constitute the other half of the bipolar continuum of behaviours.

Assessment

The onset of a hypomanic or manic episode may be gradual or dramatic. The affect is euphoric or elated, but can change quickly to irritability or hostility if the person is confronted with limits or is otherwise frustrated. The signs and symptoms range in severity from mild (in hypomania) to extreme (in a frank manic episode).

Subjective data

People who experience mania have changes in their thought processes, sometimes stating that their 'thoughts are racing'. They often experience inflated self-esteem, sometimes to the extent of having delusions of grandeur. Delusions of persecution also may be a feature. They ignore fatigue and hunger, being too involved in activity to focus on physiological sensations. Suffering from an inability to concentrate, they are easily distracted by the slightest stimulus in the environment. They may experience hallucinations. Hypomanic individuals and those early in manic episodes feel wonderful and do not understand why people are upset with their behaviour. See Box 15.3 for all the main symptoms seen in mania.

Box 15.3 Mania symptoms—DIGFAST

Distractable
Insomnia
Grandiose
Flight of ideas
Agitation
Rapid **s**peech
Thoughtlessness (impulsivity)

Objective data

People who are experiencing mania for the first time are most likely to be young people in their twenties, although adolescents are sometimes affected. Although bipolar disorder appears to have little gender specificity, the initial episode is likely to be manic in males and depressive in females (APA, 2013). To date, there is no documented evidence of the effect of race or ethnicity on bipolar disorder.

The hallmark of mania is constant motor activity. During a manic episode, the person will not stop to eat. They do not rest, have disordered sleep patterns, and may go for days without sleep. Bruises and other injuries sometimes result from the constantly agitated behaviour.

Flight of ideas is manifested in manic communications, and pressured speech is an obvious symptom. Family members often report that the person exhibits poor judgment, such as going on spending sprees and committing sexual and other indiscretions that are completely out of character with their usual behaviour. Their appearance may be unusual, such as inappropriate dress and garish make-up or being dishevelled and unkempt. Just as they fail to settle down long enough to eat and sleep, they may also neglect bathing.

Impairment in occupational functioning may result in being dismissed from work or being placed on a leave of absence because the behaviour is disruptive in the workplace. People who have mania cause interpersonal chaos with their manipulative behaviour, testing of limits, and playing off one person against another. If their manipulation attempts fail, they become irritable or hostile, and such behaviour further alienates others. The movie *Michael Clayton* depicts bipolar behaviour and the occupational sequelae.

There are no laboratory findings specific for the diagnosis of mania. Abnormal biological findings were discussed on page 327 earlier in this chapter in Your Assessment Approach. Individuals experiencing manic episodes have been noted to have abnormal cortisol levels as well as abnormalities in their neurotransmitter systems, but it is not known whether these abnormalities are a cause of or result from the disorder.

People who have mania are not usually able to cooperate fully in the assessment process. You will often find it necessary to rely on your own assessment skills and secondary sources, such as family members, to obtain essential assessment data. Family members can often provide detailed information about the onset and progression of symptoms, as well as information about previous episodes, if any.

Nursing practice

Several features are common when caring for people with mania.

Risk for injury

Individuals with mania are at risk for injury, because their usual adaptive and defensive abilities are impaired. Because of their hyperactivity and agitation, they often lose control of their movements and bump into objects, fall and otherwise injure themselves.

Their impulsivity, poor judgement and propensity towards hostile outbursts also place them at risk for injury. Other people are often extremely annoyed by inappropriate or unacceptable social behaviour, and may attack the person who is manic. As with self-harming behaviour, preventing injury becomes a priority.

Disturbed thought processes

People with mania experience disruption of their usual cognitive processes. This may be related to a variety of factors, including:

- biochemical alteration
- genetic predisposition
- sleep deprivation
- a severe blow to self-esteem
- massive denial of depression.

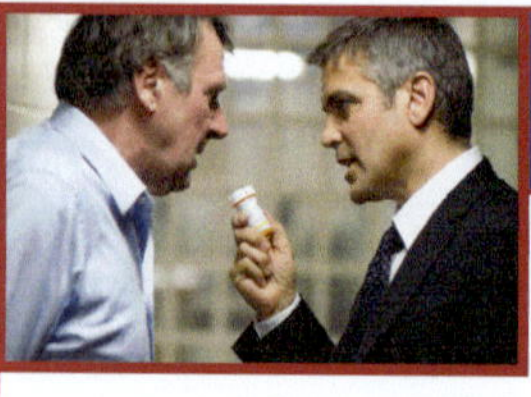

MENTAL HEALTH IN THE MEDIA

Michael Clayton

Michael Clayton is a movie about an attorney, Michael Clayton (played by George Clooney), who fixes problems in law firms caused by the idiosyncratic behaviours of various attorneys. Crimes, sexual misconduct and ethics issues, along with behaviours related to mental disorders, are his usual assignments. One of the attorneys he is asked to extract from an embarrassing situation is a brilliant man who happens to have bipolar disorder. Arthur Edens (played by Tom Wilkinson) has had a bizarre outburst in the middle of a deposition in a class action lawsuit against a conglomerate. Michael arrives to fix the situation for his good friend and colleague. He convinces the authorities to let Arthur out of jail, and brings him back to their hotel where he is successfully sedated. However, Arthur escapes from the hotel in the middle of the night.

The lawyers for the conglomerate obtain Arthur's briefcase and discover that Arthur has documentation detailing the conglomerate's decision to manufacture a chemical they know to be carcinogenic. Public knowledge of this decision would severely disrupt the finances of the conglomerate. In addition, the lawyers know about Arthur's bipolar disorder, his failure to take his medications and his outbursts. They follow Arthur, tap his phone and bug his apartment. The conglomerate's lawyers have Arthur assassinated in a manner designed to resemble suicide, a common occurrence with people who are bipolar and unmedicated.

Michael, saddened by the death of his friend and colleague, is suspicious about the circumstances. He cannot reconcile his friend's beliefs and energies with suicidal intent. Because he searches for and finds Arthur's evidence and plans to publicise it, he is also targeted for assassination. However, the attempt is botched. The movie resolves with Michael recording the admission of murder and attempted murder.

Photo courtesy of CAP/FB Supplied by Capital Pictures/Newscom.

Evidence of altered thought processes are evidenced by difficulty concentrating, short attention spans, distractibility, and have impaired problem-solving abilities. They exhibit unwarranted optimism and poor judgment due to inaccurate interpretations of the environment. Delusional belief systems held by individuals indicate a severe impairment of thought processes, as do hallucinations. Pressured speech, tangentiality and flight of ideas are also evidence of disrupted cognitive operations.

Impaired social interaction

Unlike those with depression who may isolate themselves and avoid social interaction, most people with mania are extremely gregarious and excessively social. Social interactions are often highly dysfunctional, however. Manipulating other people to meet their own wishes and needs is a major impediment to positive social interactions. Egocentrism, impulsiveness, lack of interest in the needs and concerns of others, and an unwillingness to accept responsibility for the effect of their behaviour on others all make those with mania difficult to tolerate. Poor personal hygiene aggravates the situation.

Nurses often have difficulty dealing with the challenging behaviour of people with mania. The Self-awareness feature will help you determine how you may be affected by these behaviours.

Self-care deficit

People who are experiencing a manic episode may have an impaired ability to perform the self-care activities of feeding, bathing, toileting, dressing and grooming. This is related to hyperactivity, the inability to make accurate judgments about personal needs, alterations in thought processes, lack of awareness of personal needs, and fatigue. Self-care deficit is evidenced by inadequate food and fluid intake, an inability or refusal to bathe, a lack of interest in grooming and appropriateness of appearance, and an inability or unwillingness to toilet without assistance.

> **SELF-AWARENESS**
> **Potential reactions to working with people who have mania**
>
> Working with the person who has mania will challenge your maturity, self-control and professionalism. Following are some common reactions you may experience when working with this consumer group. Think about, and discuss with classmates and your educator, how you might handle each of these reactions in order to maintain a therapeutic relationship.
>
> - I feel annoyed by the person's demanding behaviour.
> - I feel outsmarted and outmanoeuvered; I question whether my judgments and actions are appropriate.
> - I develop rescue fantasies in response to a person's flattery, and think I am the only one who understands them.
> - I become defensive and angry when colleagues point out a person's manipulative behaviour.
> - I feel anxious and insecure when a person turns on me, saying, 'I'm not progressing because you're cold and mean.'
> - I have difficulty being objective about people who have manic symptoms.
> - I disagree emphatically with colleagues about how to handle the person's manipulative behaviour; they sit back and watch nurses disagree with each other.
> - I become angry and unsure of my judgment when the person consistently exceeds established limits.
> - I withdraw and avoid people who have mania to prevent feeling embarrassed and experiencing self-doubt.

Sleep deprivation

The sleep pattern of someone in a manic episode is so disrupted that exhaustion and even death can result. Disrupted sleep is related to hyperactivity, agitation and possibly to biochemical alterations. Sleep pattern disturbance includes the inability to fall asleep, roaming or pacing the halls during the night, awakening frequently during the night, and sleeping only for short naps with long periods of hyperactive, restless behaviour in between.

Care planning and implementation

With people who are manic, your demeanour should be calm and relaxed, but firm and matter-of-fact, particularly when communicating limits. Your own behaviour serves as a model, and may be reassuring to people who feel out of control. Building a trusting relationship is important. Therefore, make promises only when you are certain you can keep them.

Promoting the individual's safety

Taking steps to ensure the safety of the individual and others in the environment is a priority.

Providing a safe environment Provide a safe environment for those in a manic episode by reducing environmental stimuli. For inpatients, this means providing a simply furnished private room that has had all unnecessary items removed. It should be in a quiet location to reduce noise stimulation. Low lighting can also be calming to someone experiencing mania.

Because people experiencing mania have difficulty interacting appropriately with others, their participation in group activities might need to be limited until they are less agitated. Group settings can overstimulate people with mania, and their behaviour may antagonise others.

Monitoring activities Scheduling a program of appropriate activity, interspersed with rest periods, helps provide the person an outlet for tension while protecting them from exhaustion. Appropriate activities may include walks, exercising or activities with an allied health professional, such as an art therapist, diversional therapist or occupational therapist. Avoid highly competitive activities that bring out hostility and overtly aggressive behaviours.

Setting limits Set and enforce limits on unsafe or socially inappropriate behaviour when individuals are unable to control their impulses. Calm, matter-of-fact intervention rather than angry scolding is the most effective approach. Individuals may respond to verbal reminders, or you can use their distractibility to redirect them into safer and more appropriate activities. Remember to reward appropriate behaviour with positive reinforcement, such as 'I enjoyed our walk today

EVIDENCE-BASED PRACTICE

Mania and substance abuse

Brent is a large, muscular 22-year-old, who was diagnosed with bipolar disorder two years ago. He was admitted to the acute mental health unit after his parents called the police. He stopped taking lithium last month, and had been up and screaming for three days and nights. Today he shouted obscenities at his mother, pushed his father to the floor, and broke the windows of neighbours' cars parked along the street as he ran from his home. Brent's parents also reported that he uses a variety of substances, although they did not know specifics.

Within an hour of his arrival on the unit, he began breaking light fixtures in the hall and in other consumers' rooms with a broom he had found. Other consumers were visibly distressed and frightened by his behaviour. Your plan for intervention options for the immediate situation, and Brent's long-term care, are based on current research. For example, in your review of studies of psychosocial approaches for improving treatment adherence in people with bipolar disorder who are substance abusers, you consider the possibility that Brent will more quickly and effectively gain self-control of his behaviour if you work with him on specific techniques in private. Decreasing stimulation and setting limits on his free activity both contribute to Brent being able to focus. Less stimuli and brief interactions allow a therapeutic relationship to develop. Once Brent is more stable, psychotherapies and psychoeducation about his diagnosis and treatment can proceed. The success rate of treatment for his disorder, and supports that will help Brent's in his recovery, can be discussed at that time. Involving his family is an integral part of this approach, as is linking Brent with peer support.

You should base your action on more than one study, but the following research was helpful in developing this set of multiple intervention strategies:

Malhi, G. S., Tanious, M., & Berk, M. (2012). Mania: Diagnosis and treatment recommendations. *Current Psychiatry Reports, 14*, 676–686.

CRITICAL THINKING QUESTIONS

1. What elements would you take into consideration when planning to interact with Brent?
2. How can Brent and his family benefit from psychoeducation?
3. What topics would be considered priorities for this family?

because you were able to walk with me rather than running ahead.' See Evidence-based Practice for more information on setting limits and other interventions, and the following Your Intervention Strategies for options in communicating limits.

Administering medications

Mood stabilisers form the basis of medication treatment for bipolar disorders. Lithium is still the optimum choice, with antiepileptic drugs (AEDs) that have mood-stabilising features chosen according to their effectiveness in addressing specific symptoms. Antipsychotic medications also contribute to helping individuals think more clearly, and help manage psychotic thinking (grandiose delusions).

Nursing interventions include providing education about medications, and monitoring for adverse side-effects of mood-stabilising and antipsychotic medications. Side-effects include sedation, agitation, postural hypotension, dizziness, dry mouth and blurry vision (see Chapter 7).

YOUR INTERVENTION STRATEGIES

Setting and enforcing limits

Effective limit-setting requires that all members of the mental health team participate in establishing limits, and determining and enforcing the consequences of exceeding them.

1. Keep the person's dignity in mind at all times. Limit-setting is not a punishment, but a part of ensuring safe care.
2. Establish limits only when and where there is a clear need. Limits must help recovery and growth.
3. Establish reasonable and enforceable consequences for exceeding limits.
4. Explain the limits and consequences in language the person can understand. Explain why the limits are necessary, and encourage the person to express their feelings about them.
5. Enforce the limits consistently. Written care plans help ensure consistency.
6. Evaluate the continued need for limits frequently. Turn control over as soon as the person's behaviour indicates their ability to exercise self-control.

Lithium carbonate Lithium carbonate has been used in the treatment and prevention of acute manic episodes since the 1960s. It is now used in preventing the recurrence of bipolar disorder as well. Toxic symptoms begin appearing at blood levels above 1.5 mEq/L. Because there is such a narrow margin of safety, serum concentrations must be closely monitored. The need for close monitoring means that the person may be hospitalised when lithium therapy is initiated. Before discharge, both the person and their family must learn how to continue lithium therapy safely at home. Read Chapter 7 for nursing considerations for people on lithium carbonate.

Anticonvulsant drugs (AED) as mood stabilisers Agents used in therapy for those with bipolar disorder include the anticonvulsants or AED medications. Individuals may have good responses to any of the mood-stabilising AEDs; however, lamotrigine (Lamictal) or topamirate (Topamax) is generally better for depressive symptoms of bipolar disorder, while sodium valproate (Epilum) or carbamazepine (Tegretol) is effective for mania. These medications cannot be discontinued abruptly, because this may precipitate a seizure.

Additional information about the pharmacotherapy of mood disorders, and the practical issues of psychopharmacology, are found in Chapter 7.

Antipsychotic medications For many years, haloperidol (Haldol) has been added to lithium as part of the treatment of bipolar disorder. Psychotic symptoms, such as grandiose delusions, usually respond fairly rapidly to antipsychotic medications. Hyperactive and agitated behaviour also can be managed well with these medications. The atypical antipsychotics, such as risperidone (Risperdal) and olanzapine (Zyprexa), have proven effective as mood-stabilising medications, and are often given in conjunction with anticonvulsive mood stabilisers. Atypical antipsychotics are used to help manage the symptoms of mania when individuals have started on lithium carbonate therapy, because lithium takes one to three weeks to become effective.

Intervening with delusions and hallucinations

Present reality by spending time with the person. Identify yourself, the time and day, the location and other orienting information as needed. Engage individuals in reality-based, somewhat concrete activities, such as discussing a current event. Consistency is reassuring for the person with altered thought processes. Establish consistency by having a schedule so the person understands what is expected of them. Consistency is also enhanced by assigning the same caregivers to work with the person whenever possible.

When dealing with someone experiencing delusions or hallucinations, communicate your acceptance of their beliefs, while clearly stating that you do not share their perceptions. A statement such as 'I understand that you believe you are the owner of this facility, but I see it differently' conveys acceptance without supporting the delusional thinking. You may also validate a person's emotional response to their perceptions. A statement such as 'I can't imagine how that must feel for you, but I can see that you are upset' again conveys acceptance without supporting false perceptions.

It is non-therapeutic to argue or try to reason with someone experiencing delusions. This may serve to enforce the belief system, and risks impairing the development of therapeutic relationship. Instead, focus on assisting the person with the distress they may be feeling, being sure not to engage in the person's belief system.

When people communicate altered reality perceptions, reflect their statements back to them for validation. For example, 'Are you saying that your husband is trying to poison you?' can help them understand how their perceptions sound to others. You will recognise decreased delusional thinking when they make such statements as, 'I know this sounds bizarre, but . . .' Remember to give positive reinforcement when the person begins to focus on reality.

Enhancing socialisation

Nursing activities are designed to facilitate the individual's ability to interact with others by identifying specific needed behaviour changes and assigning tasks that will improve the person's interactions with others. This may require mediating between the individual and others when the individual exhibits negative behaviour. Nursing actions should encourage and demonstrate honesty and respect for others' rights.

A maladaptive behaviour of people who are manic that significantly impairs social interactions is manipulation, an indirect way of getting their needs met. This may take a simple form, such as borrowing money from other people rather than using their own. Or it may be highly complex, such as playing staff members off against one another.

Setting limits on manipulative and out-of-control behaviour Manipulation meets a need for the individual. It serves the purpose of increasing a person's sense of control and interpersonal power (the mania can be frightening as it spins out of control). Nursing interventions, such as setting limits and promoting security, often enable individuals to curb their manipulative behaviour or give it up entirely. Be aware of your own emotions and behaviours, and provide opportunities for the person with mania to be in control when appropriate. Calm, matter-of-fact limit-enforcement, and the consistent application of consequences, are essential in promoting adaptive behaviours.

Out-of-control and manipulative behaviours require the setting of limits. The Communication feature, below, provides some strategies. All staff members must agree on the established limits and must enforce them consistently. Violations of limits must have established consequences, also

COMMUNICATION

The person with bipolar disorder

FRANCIS: 'I can't go to group today! I'm expecting some top-level government officials to visit. The other nurse told me I didn't have to go.'

NURSE RESPONSE 1: 'I understand, Francis, but it is time for group now, and we expect everyone to attend. Let's walk over together.'

RATIONALE: This response acknowledges the need for the false belief without reinforcing or arguing with it. This response also maintains a consistent, routine schedule wherein this person can feel safe; it clearly articulates what is expected and offers self.

NURSE RESPONSE 2: 'Everyone attends these meetings, Francis. You made some constructive comments last week. Let's go so we can get a good seat.'

RATIONALE: This response sets limits on manipulative behaviour. Calm, matter-of-fact enforcement of rules and expectations without allowing the person to involve you in a dispute with another staff member defuses the manipulative behaviour and provides positive reinforcement of adaptive behavior.

agreed on by all staff. Individuals must know what behaviours are expected, and what consequences will result if they exceed limits. Inconsistent application of consequences will cause failure in the efforts to decrease manipulative behaviour. Your Intervention Strategies on page 340 provides an overview of how to effectively set and enforce limits. (See also Chapter 18.)

Monitoring intake and output, and promoting nutrition

Physical health is compromised when people do not receive sufficient nourishment and fluids for extended periods of time, particularly during periods of hyperactivity. Monitoring intake and output is an important nursing activity. Frequent small snacks that can be eaten 'on the go' are most likely to be consumed by someone who is unable to sit down to eat because of their mania. Ensure that high-calorie finger foods and nutritious liquids are available in the nursing unit until the person is able to attend regular meals.

Promoting self-care

A minimal level of personal hygiene is needed to ensure health, self-esteem and healthy social interactions. Assist people who are unwilling or unable to bathe, brush their teeth, shave, wash their hair, change clothes or use the toilet. Autonomy is desirable, so enable individuals to do as much for themselves as possible with verbal encouragement. Reinforce any attempts at self-care with recognition; for example, 'I see you shaved today, Mr Adams.'

Incontinence of urine or faeces is occasionally seen in people experiencing severe mania. This can be disturbing to family and friends, and may impair the dignity of the individual who is experiencing incontinence. Nurses must remain respectful and empathetic, and provide education to family and friends, as needed.

A more common elimination problem is constipation. People with mania may suppress the urge to defecate and may become severely constipated. The anticholinergic effect of some medications may also exacerbate constipation. Frequent fluid intake and a high-fibre diet can reduce constipation.

Enhancing rest and sleep

People in the manic phase of bipolar disorder appear deceptively energetic when they may actually be nearing the point of exhaustion. Design nursing activities to facilitate regular sleep–wake cycles. Monitor the individual closely for signs of fatigue, and make provisions for rest periods. Promote night-time sleeping by limiting extended daytime naps. Sleep may promote the rapid resolution of first episodes of mania. Prior to bedtime, decrease light and noise, and encourage quiet activities and pre-sleep routines, such as listening to soothing music. Administer medications that do not suppress REM sleep, such as zolpidem tartrate (Ambien), as prescribed.

If individuals experience extended night-time wakefulness, avoid engaging them in long conversations or otherwise stimulating or giving them extra attention during the night. Firmly encourage the person to stay in their darkened rooms with the expectation that they will fall asleep. If they will not stay in their rooms, assign a monotonous, repetitive task, such as folding towels or sorting papers to encourage drowsiness. When they are able to sleep, avoid waking them for non-essential care or activities. Promote sleep cycles of at least 90 minutes.

Evaluation

Specific behaviours indicate that nursing interventions have been successful. Evaluation and outcome criteria answer the question: 'How do we know that the individual's condition has improved?'

Risk for injury

If nursing interventions have been successful in promoting safety, individuals experiencing a manic episode will be free of accidental injuries. They will not engage in agitated or impulsive behaviours that can endanger them. Their social behaviours will no longer irritate or enrage other people, so they will no longer risk attacks from others. The person will be able to describe safe ways of relieving excess tension when it occurs, such as the verbal expression of feelings, writing feelings down in a diary or journal, or other adaptive methods. The person will be able to name their medications, understand the proper dosages, describe any adverse effects, and explain any lab monitoring needed, if any.

Cognitive orientation and reality-based thinking

If nursing interventions have been successful, the person's thinking may be based on reality and they will no longer experience delusional thinking or hallucinations. Successful intervention may also be indicated by delusional thinking or hallucinations continuing, but not causing distress, disruption or harm to the person's life or the lives of others. They will be able to establish trust relationships. Their attention spans will increase. Speech will be less pressured, and will reflect diminished flight of ideas and tangentiality. The individual may be able to recognise and verbalise errors in perception when they occur. Their thought processes and perceptions of environmental stimuli will be accurate, and can be validated by others. They will demonstrate logical, organised thought processes.

Social interaction skills

Improvements in social interaction are evidenced when individuals can recognise and describe which of their interactions are successful and which are not, and acknowledge the effect of their own behaviour on social interactions. They demonstrate behaviours that may increase or improve social interactions. Individuals put significant effort into treatment in order to prevent relapse, and have more appropriate social contacts and interactions. The person acquires or improves skills such as cooperation, sensitivity, genuineness and compromise. The absence of, or dramatic decrease in, the use of manipulation as a method of meeting their own needs will also signal improvement in social interaction. They now accept responsibility for their own behaviour.

Other signs of improved social interaction include non-disruptive participation in activities, re-establishment of a social life, and identification of people with whom they can develop a social and support network.

Intake, output and nutrition

Individuals will demonstrate the ability to establish and maintain adequate nutrition and fluid intake.

Self-care

Individuals who have re-established self-care will demonstrate this ability by performing the activities of daily living autonomously and willingly. This includes adequately bathing and grooming themselves, selecting appropriate clothing and make-up, establishing and maintaining adequate nutrition and fluid intake, and establishing and maintaining patterns of elimination without reminders or assistance.

Rest and sleep

The need for uninterrupted sleep varies from person to person, depending on age, activity level and usual pattern of sleep. Generally, individuals who are able to sleep six or more hours per night without sleeping medication and awaken feeling refreshed will have demonstrated healthy sleep patterns. Being able to fall asleep within 30 minutes or less is another indicator. Recognising fatigue and voluntarily resting or napping appropriately also indicates that a person is attending to their bodily sensations once again.

CARE COORDINATION AND COMMUNITY-BASED CARE

Care coordination and community-based care for people with depressed-phase bipolar disorders were described earlier in the section discussing the care of people experiencing a depressive episode. Individuals in the manic phase of bipolar disorders, however, often require hospitalisation until stabilised on medication or through ECT.

Following discharge, goals for those who have mania are the same as for others—high-quality, cost-effective treatment aimed at returning the person to independent functioning as soon and as much as feasible. Communication with family members, mental health professionals, employers, social workers and others involved in the person's case is essential.

Monitoring the person's lithium level is an important aspect of nursing care for the treatment of mania. Additional psychoeducation for the individual and their family is often required to reinforce information received in the inpatient setting. ECT is increasingly used as an outpatient procedure, again calling on the community nurse's teaching skills and sensitivity to concerns about safety, memory loss and effectiveness.

Care coordinators and community mental health nurses must be alert for 'red flags' that signal exacerbation of a person's manic symptoms. These may include non-adherence with treatment, including refusal to take medications as prescribed, escalating activity levels that may include psychomotor excitement/agitation, spending sprees, shortened attention span, impaired occupational functioning, and grandiosity. Early recognition of red flags and mobilisation of the treatment team can ward off rehospitalisation and enable the person to stay at home while being supported in the community. Be sure that family members are also aware of behaviours that signal exacerbation of the person's symptoms.

Information is available from SANE Australia (https://www.sane.org/). Another resource for bipolar disorders (and depressive disorders) is The Black Dog Institute at http://www.blackdoginstitute.org.au/

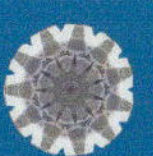

NURSING CARE PLAN: THE PERSON WITH DEPRESSION

Identifying information

Margaret M is a 59-year-old, unmarried legal assistant who was admitted to the mental health unit following a gastric lavage in the emergency department. She had ingested 30 antidepressant tablets in a suicide attempt. Margaret stated that she had been home alone for two days, became increasingly depressed and hopeless, and took the antidepressants that her doctor had prescribed for depression a few weeks ago. She became frightened almost immediately thereafter, was unable to make herself vomit, and called 000. Margaret stated: 'I just don't have anything to look forward to anymore. No one would care if I died.'

History

Margaret is the eldest of seven children from a small remote community. She had to leave school early to stay at home and help with the younger children. At the age of 22, she returned to school and became a legal assistant. She moved to a large city over 400 kilometres from her home town, and built her life around her work. She never married. Because she works long hours in a large metropolitan law firm, she has virtually no social life and, except for a few co-workers, no friends. She stopped going to church recently, stating, 'I just don't fit in anywhere, and I never have.'

Margaret reports that she has been concerned about her impending retirement at age 65 and her elderly mother's declining health. About a month ago, the health of her 86-year-old mother, who still lives in their small town, began to deteriorate. Margaret now fears that she will have to go to care for her mother with whom she has never gotten along. Her siblings are pressuring her to move back home, live with their mother and serve as her caregiver. She fears that, because she has no family of her own and no family ties in the city, she will eventually have to give in to their pressure.

She has no prior history of mental illness and no significant health problems. Vital signs are: temperature, 36.98°C; pulse, 88; respirations, 18; height, 1.6 metres; weight 71 kilograms; blood pressure, 138/78.

(continued)

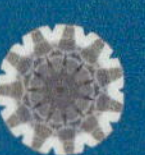

NURSING CARE PLAN: THE PERSON WITH DEPRESSION *(continued)*

Current mental status

Margaret is somewhat dishevelled and weeps occasionally during the interview. She is cooperative with the interviewer, even eager to talk. She reports being 'exhausted' for the past three weeks. She has not slept well, has lost weight, had crying spells, has been irritable with co-workers and had difficulty concentrating at work. She reports having had suicidal thoughts, but did not have a specific plan until the weekend after the firm's senior partner told her to take a few days off to 'get yourself together'. She fears being fired, in which case she will have no reason to resist her siblings' pleas to 'take care of Mum'.

Margaret is alert, responsive and well-oriented. There is no sign of a thought disorder, confusion or impairment. She weeps as she discusses her situation, stating, 'I have always been unattractive, and nobody has ever loved me. If I died, my family would be better off.'

Other clinical data

Margaret reports being in good health, although she is somewhat overweight. She has mild arthritis in her knees, which she treats symptomatically with aspirin. Until she began taking antidepressants, she took no other medicine.

Issue identified: Risk for self-harming behaviour related to recent suicide attempt.
Expected outcome: Able to restrain compulsive or impulsive behaviour. Able to refrain from gestures and attempts at self-harm.

Short-term goals	Interventions	Rationales
Margaret will not harm herself during hospitalisation.	■ Remove all dangerous articles from Margaret's environment.	Margaret's safety is ensured.
	■ Observe Margaret closely, using irregular schedule.	Irregular schedule prevents her from predicting when she will be alone.
	■ Adopt a neutral, matter-of-fact attitude.	A neutral attitude prevents dependency.
	■ Evaluate suicidal intention at every shift, and institute appropriate level of supervision.	Suicidal thoughts and impulses may change rapidly.
	■ Establish a no-suicide contract.	Collaboration promotes self-responsibility.
	■ Encourage Margaret to seek support when bothered by suicidal thoughts or impulses.	Margaret learns to substitute talking it out for acting it out.
	■ Limit repetitive discussion of suicidal ruminations.	Repetition reinforces preoccupation with self-directed violence.
Margaret will demonstrate alternative ways of dealing with stress, such as talking, exercise and relaxation techniques.	■ Assist Margaret to verbalise at least one reason for living.	Identifying reasons for living counteracts negative thinking.
	■ Encourage the expression of feelings in one-to-one and group activities.	Self-expression decreases isolation and elicits peer support.
	■ Assist Margaret to identify and practise alternative ways of dealing with stress.	Margaret's coping behaviours are expanded.
Margaret will identify resources where she can seek help if suicidal thoughts recur following discharge, such as a crisis line, or a church minister.	■ Help Margaret identify community resources and supports.	Margaret becomes more aware of the social supports available to her.
Margaret will verbalise safe uses of antidepressant medication, and describe potential drug–food interactions.	■ Teach Margaret the safe use of anti-depressant medication.	This is information that every person should know.

Issue identified: Self-esteem disturbance related to impaired cognition, fostering negative view of self.
Expected outcome: Self-esteem: personal judgment of self-worth.

Short-term goals	Interventions	Rationales
Margaret will sit and walk erectly, comb hair neatly, and wear clean, appropriate clothes.	■ Help Margaret with hygiene and grooming as needed.	Competent self-care increases feelings of self-worth.

(continued)

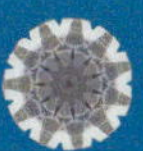

NURSING CARE PLAN: THE PERSON WITH DEPRESSION *(continued)*

Short-term goals	Interventions	Rationales
Margaret will participate in unit activities.	■ Teach Margaret that activity helps decrease depression.	This is information all depressed people should know.
	■ Involve Margaret in simple, non-competitive recreational activities.	Cooperative recreation allows Margaret to experience success.
	■ Increase the complexity of activities as Margaret progresses.	Margaret's growth and self-regard are enhanced by appropriate challenges.
Margaret will verbalise positive aspects of self and increased feelings of self-worth.	■ Set limits on time spent reviewing past failures.	Focusing on personal strengths counteracts negative self-view and increases self-worth.
	■ Help Margaret identify her own personal strengths.	
Margaret will communicate assertively with others; will explain to her siblings that she will not give up her career to come home to care for mother.	■ Teach Margaret assertiveness techniques.	Learning assertiveness validates Margaret's right to take care of herself.
	■ Practise (role-play) Margaret's direct expression of feelings.	Role-playing promotes confidence in asserting herself.
	■ Stay with Margaret during difficult interactions, if desired.	
	■ Give positive recognition when progress is shown.	Encouragement and recognition support healthy behaviours.

Issue identified: Hopelessness related to inability to make and carry out decisions on her own behalf.

Expected outcome: Decision-making: Ability to choose between two or more alternatives.
Hope: Presence of internal state of optimism that is personally satisfying and life-supporting.
Mood equilibrium: Appropriate adjustment of prevailing emotional tone in response to circumstances.
Quality of life: Expresses satisfaction with current life circumstances.

Short-term goals	Interventions	Rationales
Margaret will verbalise feelings about situations over which she has no control; will realise that siblings' expectations do not control her responses.	■ Assist Margaret identify situations over which she has no control.	
	■ Assist Margaret to identify situations over which she can attain control.	A realistic appraisal of her situation allows Margaret to focus on areas in which she can effect change.
Margaret will set realistic goals for herself, and work towards them.	■ Engage Margaret in personal goal-setting.	Setting goals is a crucial step towards self-determination.
	■ Provide options when possible.	Options help Margaret understand the concept of choice.
Margaret will demonstrate a problem-solving system that she has used successfully.	■ Explore problem-solving models with Margaret, and encourage her to select one.	
	■ Practise problem-solving with small daily problems.	Information and practice help build Margaret's confidence.
Margaret will verbalise plans to attain control over life situations; works with siblings to find appropriate caretaker for mother.	■ Role-play possible situations with siblings.	Role-playing increases Margaret's confidence and resourcefulness.
	■ Assist Margaret to prepare for siblings' potential untoward responses.	
	■ Assist Margaret to plan for retirement.	
Margaret expresses some hope for the future.	■ Identify community resources that assist individuals toward fulfilling retirement.	Planning for the future decreases fears of the unknown and introduces new sources of support.
	■ Involve Margaret in identifying enjoyable leisure pastimes.	Positive use of leisure time is promoted.

(continued)

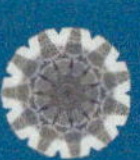

NURSING CARE PLAN: THE PERSON WITH DEPRESSION *(continued)*

Issue identified: Social isolation related to fear of rejection.

Expected outcome: Social interaction skills: Use of effective interaction behaviour.
Social involvement: Social interactions with persons, groups or organisations.
Social support: Perception of availability of reliable assistance from other persons.

Short-term goals	Interventions	Rationales
Margaret will communicate with staff and socialise with others on the unit.	■ Make brief, frequent contacts with Margaret.	Frequent contact demonstrates your availability and interest.
	■ Spend time with Margaret with no demands.	A nonjudgmental approach demonstrates acceptance.
	■ Use a nonjudgmental attitude.	
	■ Encourage Margaret to ventilate verbally or through activity.	Appropriate self-expression decreases internal tension and increases sociability.
Margaret voluntarily attends group activities.	■ Accompany Margaret to group activities initially, withdrawing as tolerated.	Providing support as needed fosters gradual independence.
	■ Teach social skills and assist Margaret to practise them.	Practice increases Margaret's self-confidence in social situations.
Margaret assumes responsibility for dealing with feelings, including seeking others out; identifies key individuals outside hospital and initiates contact to renew relationships; makes concrete plans to go to church again.	■ Teach assertive communication.	Learning assertiveness helps Margaret take care of herself.
	■ Encourage role-playing of phone calls and other contacts, anticipating others' possible responses.	Role-playing decreases social anxiety and builds resourcefulness and flexibility.
	■ Give positive feedback for all signs of progress.	Positive feedback validates Margaret's efforts and reinforces growth.

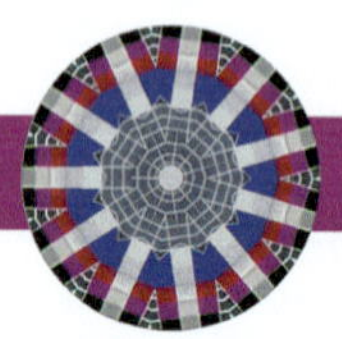

REFERENCES

Altamura, A. C., Buoli, M., Caldiroli, A., Caron, L., Melter, C. C., Dobrea, C., . . . Quarantini, F. Z. (2015). Misdiagnosis, duration of untreated illness (DUI) and outcome in bipolar patients with psychotic symptoms: A naturalistic study. *Journal of Affective Disorders, 182*, 70–75.

American Psychiatric Association (APA). (2000). *Diagnostic and statistical manual of mental disorders* (4th ed.). Washington, DC: APA Publishing.

American Psychiatric Association (APA). (2013). *Diagnostic and statistical manual of mental disorders* (5th ed., Text Revision). Washington, DC: APA Publishing.

Australian Bureau of Statistics (ABS). (2008). *National Survey of Mental Health and Wellbeing: Summary of results, 2007*. Cat No. 4326.0. Canberra, Australia: ABS. Retrieved from http://www.ausstats.abs.gov.au/Ausstats/subscriber.nsf/0/6AE6DA447F985FC2CA2574EA00122BD6/$File/43260_2007.pdf

Australian Institute of Health and Welfare (AIHW). (2007). *Young Australians: Their health and wellbeing 2007*. Cat. No. PHE 87. Canberra, Australia: AIHW.

Australian Institute of Health and Welfare (AIHW). (2008). *Australia's health 2008*. Cat. No. AUS 99. Canberra, Australia: AIHW.

Britt, H., Miller, G. C., Henderson, J., Bayram, C., Harrison, C., Valenti, L., . . . Charles, J. (2014). *General practice activity in Australia 2013–14*. Sydney, Australia: Sydney University Press.

Brown, A., Scales, U., Beever, W., Rickards, B., Rowley, K., & O'Dea, K. (2012). Exploring the expression of depression and distress in aboriginal men in central Australia: A qualitative study. *BMC Psychiatry, 12*, 1–12.

Buckner-Brown, J., Tucker, P., & Rivera, M. (2011). Racial and ethnic approaches to community health. *Family and Community Health, 34*(1S), S12–S22.

Carey, M., Jones, K., Meadows, G., Sanson-Fisher, R., D'Este, C., Inder, K., . . . Russell, G. (2014). Accuracy of general practitioner unassisted detection of depression. *Australian and New Zealand Journal of Psychiatry, 48*, 571–578.

Clark, D. A., & Beck, A. T. (1999). *Scientific foundations of cognitive theory and therapy of depression*. New York, NY: John Wiley & Sons.

Dubovsky, S. L. (2015). The usefulness of genotyping cytochrome P_{450} enzymes in the treatment of depression. *Expert Opinion on Drug Metabolism and Toxicity, 11*, 369–379.

Hare, D. L., Toukhsati, S. R., Johansson, P., & Jaarsma, T. (2014). Depression and cardiovascular disease: a clinical review. *European Heart Review, 35*, 1365–1372.

Kerr, P. L., Muelenkamp, J. J., & Turner, J. M. (2010). Nonsuicidal self-injury: A review of current research for family medicine and primary care physicians. *Journal of the American Board of Family Medicine, 23*, 240–259.

Kessler, R. C., & Bromet, E. J. (2013). The epidemiology of depression across cultures. *Annual Review of Public Health, 34*, 119–138. Retrieved from http://www.ncbi.nlm.nih.gov/pmc/articles/PMC4100461/

Knezevic, V., & Nedic, A. (2013). Influence of misdiagnosis on the course of bipolar disorder. *European Review for Medical and Pharmacological Sciences, 17*, 1542–1545.

Lazenby, R. B. (2011). Depression in the college population: An E-S-A approach to primary prevention. *Nurse Practitioner, 36*(2), 33–39.

Lin, K.-M., Chiu, Y.-F., Tsai, I.-J., Chen, C.-H., Shen, W. W., Liu, S. C., . . . Liu, Y.-L. (2011). ABCB1 gene polymorphisms are associated with the severity of major depressive disorder and its response to escitalopram treatment. *Pharmacogenetics and Genomics, 21*, 163–170.

Maina, G., Rosso, G., Aguglia, A., & Bogetto, F. (2014). Recurrence rates of bipolar disorder during the postpartum period: A study of 276 medication-free Italian women. *Archives of Women's Mental Health, 17*, 367–372.

Malhi, G. S., Tanious, M., & Berk, M. (2012). Mania: Diagnosis and treatment recommendations. *Current Psychiatry Reports, 14*, 676–686.

Moxham, L., Liersch-Sumskis, S., Taylor, E., Patterson, C., & Brighton, R. (2015). Preliminary outcomes of a pilot therapeutic recreation camp for people with a mental illness: Links to recovery. *Therapeutic Recreation Journal, 49*(1), 61–75.

Saveanu, R. V., & Nemeroff, C. B. (2012). Etiology of depression: Genetic and environmental factors. *Psychiatric Clinics of North America, 35*, 51–71.

Sheehan, D. V., Harnett-Sheehan, K., Spann, M. E., Thompson, H. F., & Prakash, A. (2011). Assessing remission in major depressive disorder and generalized anxiety disorder clinical trials with the Discan Metric of the Sheehan Disability Scale. *International Clinical Psychopharmacology, 26*, 75–83.

Slade, T, Johnston, A, Teesson, M., Whiteford, H, Burgess, P, Pirkis, J, & Saw, S. (2009). *The mental health of Australians 2: Report on the 2007 National Survey of Mental Health and Wellbeing*. Canberra, Australia: Department of Health and Ageing.

Undela, K., Parthasarathi, G., & John, S. S. (2015). Impact of antidepressants use on risk of myocardial infarction: A systematic review and meta-analysis. *Indian Journal of Pharmacology, 47*, 256–262.

Vasquez, G. H., Holtman, J. N., Lolich, M., Ketter, T. A., & Baldessarini, R. J. (2015). Recurrence rates in bipolar disorder: Systematic comparison of long-term prospective, naturalistic studies versus randomized controlled trials. *European Neuropsychopharmacology, 25*, 1501–1512.

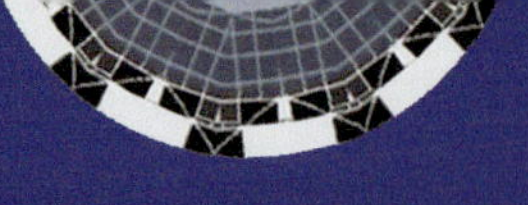

16 Dissociative, somatic symptom and factitious disorders

CHRISTOPHER PATTERSON AND PAULA HANLON

KEY TERMS

LEARNING OUTCOMES

After completing this chapter, you will be able to:

1. Describe theories that aid in the understanding of dissociative, somatic symptom and factitious disorders.
2. Compare and contrast the biopsychosocial characteristics of various dissociative, somatic symptom and factitious disorders.
3. Differentiate among somatic symptom disorders, factitious disorders and malingering.
4. Perform a thorough and comprehensive assessment of individuals with dissociative, somatic symptom and factitious disorders.
5. Incorporate an understanding of therapeutic interventions for the person experiencing selected dissociative, somatic symptom and factitious disorders into their plan of care.
6. Analyse possible personal challenges to professional practice when caring for the person with dissociative, somatic symptom and factitious disorders.

LIVED EXPERIENCE

I am 50 years of age. I have been a consumer worker for almost 18 years (since January 1998) with a community mental health service. I have been a consumer of mental health services since age 12, following a suicide attempt. My first inpatient admission was at age 18. First, the admissions were from alcohol and drug use, then psychiatric admissions. I have been sober and clean ongoing since February 1992. From 1983 until 1992, I was misdiagnosed with the following: schizophrenia, manic depression and borderline personality disorder. I was correctly diagnosed in late 1992 with dissociative identity disorder (DID), when my trauma history and DID symptoms were finally connected.

I worked with a psychologist, who focused on the use of cognitive behaviour therapy and eye movement desensitisation and reprocessing. He also worked closely with the community mental health worker (case manager/care coordinator). Their collaboration was very important to my recovery. I had 15 years (1997–2012) of fairly stable recovery without any major dissociative experiences. I had minor experiences that I was able to maintain. In 2012, I experienced a traumatic relapse, with new memories and trauma surfacing. I have found a psychologist who specialises in DID and therapy, with the occasional inpatient care. I have presented on DID at conferences (the MHS annual conference and the Summer Forum—trauma and impact on healthy lifestyle change), to nursing and occupational therapy students, and to mental health staff. I have written a fact sheet for the NSW Mental Health Association (now called Wayahead), which is available online (https://wayahead.org.au/mental-health-information/fact-sheets/).

INTRODUCTION

The disorders discussed in this chapter cover two separate chapters of the fifth edition of the *Diagnostic and statistical manual of mental disorders* (DSM-5; American Psychiatric Association [APA], 2013): 'Dissociative Disorders'; and 'Somatic Symptom and Related Disorders'. The first section of this chapter will focus on dissociative disorders—disorders characterised by 'a disruption of and/or discontinuity in the normal integration of consciousness, memory, identity, emotion, perception, body representation, motor control, and behavior' (APA, 2013, p. 291). The next section of this chapter will focus on somatic symptom and related disorders, of which factitious disorder is one. Somatic symptom and related disorders are classified by the DSM-5 (APA, 2013, p. 309) as those disorders where prominent somatic symptoms are present, with associated significant distress and impairment.

DISSOCIATIVE DISORDERS

Dissociative disorders have as their common denominator the mechanism of dissociation, in which a person's consciousness, memory, identity, emotion, perception, body representation, motor control and/or behaviour is disrupted (American Psychiatric Association [APA], 2013). Dissociative disorders are complex, and are usually difficult to distinguish from one another; see Diagnostic Features for a comparison of the disorders. In every dissociative disorder, a cluster of related mental events is beyond the person's power of recall, but can return spontaneously to conscious awareness. Dissociative disorders are not attributable to mental illness that has an organic basis, such as dementia. Dissociative disorders are commonly associated with a person experiencing a traumatic event, and symptoms may be influenced by the proximity to this trauma (APA, 2013). People living with dissociative disorders can experience comorbid disorders, such as eating disorders, substance-related and addictive disorders, and other self-injurious behaviours. See Chapter 20 for a discussion of childhood sexual abuse.

DIAGNOSTIC FEATURES
Dissociative disorders

Dissociative amnesia: Inability to recall important personal information, usually of a psychologically traumatic nature; memory loss is too extensive to be caused by simple forgetfulness.

Dissociative fugue: Sudden, unexpected wandering or travel away from home or workplace, accompanied by an inability to remember one's past, confusion about personal identity, or the assumption of a new identity.

Dissociative identity disorder: Presence of two or more distinct personality states or identities; the personality states take control of the person's behaviour; accompanied by an inability to remember personal information; characterised by identity fragmentation.

Depersonalisation/derealisation disorder: Persistent or recurrent feeling of unreality by being detached from one's thoughts or body (depersonalisation) or detached from one's surroundings (derealisation); accompanied by intact reality testing.

Dissociative amnesia

Amnesia is a loss or failure of memory caused by problems in the functioning of the memory areas of the brain. Amnesia can result from concussions, traumatic brain injury, alcohol misuse (Korsakoff's syndrome; see Chapter 13), or disorders of the ageing brain. *Retrograde amnesia* is a loss of memory for events that occurred prior to the onset of the problem. For example, a football player who sustains a head trauma in a game might find that memories of the prior year have been erased. *Anterograde amnesia* is a loss of memory for events that occurred after the onset of the problem. In this instance, the football player may find himself unable to remember people he has met after the injury, or where he parked his car.

Dissociative amnesia differs in its cause; its cause is psychological rather than physical. People with **dissociative amnesia** have one or more episodes of memory loss of important personal information. They are usually unaware of any memory loss. Occasionally, an individual may become suddenly aware that they have a total loss of memory for events that occurred during a period that may range from a few hours to a whole lifetime. In *localised amnesia*, the most common form, a person forgets only specific and related past times, usually surrounding a disturbing event. *Selective amnesia* for some, but not all, of the events is less common. Least common are *generalised amnesia*, which encompasses the person's entire life, and *continuous amnesia*, in which the person cannot recall events up to a specific time, including the present. *Systematised amnesia* is the loss of memory for certain categories of information, such as all memories related to one's occupation, or all memories related to one's family.

Dissociative fugue

A person with **dissociative fugue** wanders, usually far from home and for days, perhaps even weeks or months, at a time. During this period, the person completely forgets their past life and associations, but, unlike people with amnesia, they are unaware of having forgotten anything. The fugue state may be associated with an apparent purpose or confused wandering. People experiencing dissociative fugue are generally reclusive and quiet, so their behaviour rarely attracts attention. During this period, they appear to function unremarkably, but may behave in a manner inconsistent with their usual pattern of functioning. They may assume a completely new and apparently well-integrated identity during the fugue state. Dissociative fugue has been blamed for the 11-day disappearance of the mystery writer, Agatha Christie.

Dissociative identity disorder

Formerly known as multiple personality disorder, **dissociative identity disorder (DID)** is the presence of two or more distinct identities within one individual. Each personality states, called an **alter**, at some time takes full control of the person's behaviour. Each alter has a unique identity, holds different feelings and memories, and performs different functions. The change between alters is called *switching*, and is impacted by extreme anxiety from triggers associated with an early trauma. These triggers can be visual, auditory and/or olfactory—words spoken during abuse, music played, a piece of clothing or items used in the abuse, and physical features of the abuser (hair, smells). Switching can be a singular event for a period of time with one alter maintaining control, or a *revolving door* effect where the primary personality is fighting with numerous alters for that control and the switching can be fast.

Personality states may differ in other ways as well. One alter may have type 2 diabetes or asthma, while the others may not. Some may be right-handed; others left-handed. Allergies and vision may differ. The voice may differ, depending on which alter is in control. Usually, the person's main identity state is unaware of the others' existence.

People living with DID may report periods of memory loss, confusion about reported behaviours and changes in mood, internal voices and conversations, distracted thoughts, physical pain that is not related to diagnosable physical health problems (but is related to an abuse memory), and regular headaches. The alters work as a system, which may or may not be functional. A person may present for treatment when their system is dysfunctional and interfering with their daily life; for example, beginning studies and/or work, intimate or other relationships, family reunions. Treatments can include therapies that support the person to cope with the surfacing memories and the emotional experiences of fear, anger, guilt and shame that create the confusion and anxiety that permeate dissociation. Although medications are not a primary treatment, anxiety medication can be useful to assist in reducing the intensity of the anxiety while developing therapeutic coping mechanisms.

There has been much controversy about dissociative identity disorder (Dorahy et al., 2014). Initially, DID was thought to be a rare condition. However, clinical evidence of the existence of DID abounds, and today it is considered a valid disorder (Dorahy et al., 2014). Refer to the website for the International Society for the Study of Trauma and Dissociation (http://www.isst-d.org).

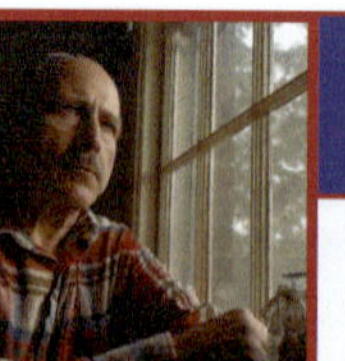

MENTAL HEALTH IN THE MEDIA

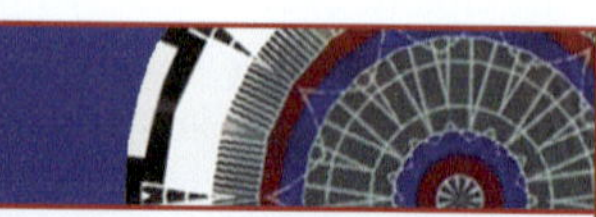

Benjaman Kyle

Known now as Benjaman Kyle, the man in the photograph has been diagnosed as having dissociative amnesia. Benjaman was discovered badly sunburned near a Burger King dumpster in Georgia, USA, on 31 August 2004. He has some memories—of living in Indianapolis as a child, as well as memories of the area around the University of Colorado at Boulder, and recalls having brothers and attending a Catholic school. In late 2004 and 2005, Kyle was diagnosed with schizophrenia and treated in a psychiatric facility. Major worldwide efforts to identify Kyle were unsuccessful for over a decade. Kyle appeared in *National Geographic*, and on CNN and ABC News in the United States, and on Channel 9 in Australia. In 2008, Kyle appeared on the *Dr Phil* show (see https://www.youtube.com/watch?v59nwpvh7E0Mc), but this failed to turn up any useful leads despite 17 million viewers and the efforts of a well-known investigator hired by the show. In 2012, a documentary about Kyle, titled *Finding Benjaman*, was released (see: https://www.youtube.com/watch?v5orn8cCycp1c). In 2015, through a process of DNA profiling, Benjamin Kyle discovered his identity and family.

LIVED EXPERIENCE

Dissociation is a survival mechanism that protected us as a young child being abused and neglected. The disorder helped us to live with each event, and ongoing memories, emotional experiences and interpersonal interactions. The extreme anxiety would trigger the alter that would assist the coping. To progress in the therapy process, we had to understand the alters that were created and their purpose, and develop the skills and confidence to take on these roles without the need for dissociation.

The system of alters needed to be mapped. This involved a lot of painful therapy sessions. The system we have included: a number of child alters, a male who likes train travel, an alter who smokes (we would vomit for hours after she had smoked), an alter who does not experience illness (colds, flu, etc), one who does not need to wear glasses (we would remove them when she was in control), and an alter who would do the housework and be very organised. We also had an alter who was very harmful to the self, and would cut and hit the head against that wall until we were unconscious. Another alter held all sexual knowledge, and would often place us in unsafe and harmful situations.

Depersonalisation/derealisation disorder

The central feature of this disorder is one or more episodes of feeling detached from oneself (depersonalisation) or feeling detached from surroundings (derealisation). The individual feels mechanical. Clive's experience with depersonalisation is recounted in the following Practice Example.

Practice example

Clive feels as if he is living in a dream or a movie. It seems as though he can observe his own life. He explains his experiences by saying, 'I don't feel real anymore. It's like I can watch my life as if it's a TV show. I'm afraid I'm going crazy.'

The feelings experienced by people with depersonalisation are **ego-dystonic**, meaning that they are unacceptable to the person's sense of self, as opposed to **ego-syntonic**, meaning in concert with the person's sense of self. The person has intact reality-testing; in other words, they are not experiencing hallucinations or delusions.

BIOPSYCHOSOCIAL THEORIES

Although biological and genetic factors are being studied as potential aetiological factors, psychosocial theories are used most often to explain dissociative disorders.

Biological and genetic factors

Physiological and neurobiological functions play a significant role in the development of amnesia and dissociative disorders. For example, the neurotransmitter serotonin affects recall of information. The formation and retrieval of memories rely on the intact function of the hippocampus and the limbic system.

- Research suggests that the limbic system may be impaired in individuals who have experienced traumatic experiences in childhood (Sadock & Sadock, 2010).
- One study implicates trauma as an inhibiting factor on the person's ability to process information; there is a disturbance in the cortical visual system (Manning & Manning, 2009).
- Physical illnesses (such as brain tumours, epilepsy and migraine headaches) may lead to symptoms indicative of depersonalisation disorder. Certain drugs (e.g. alcohol, barbiturates, benzodiazepines and hallucinogens) may cause some people to experience depersonalisation symptoms (Sadock & Sadock, 2010).
- One study describes the onset of dissociative disorder after electroconvulsive therapy (ECT), and suggests that ECT may be a risk factor for the occurrence of dissociative episodes (Zaidner et al., 2010).

Psychosocial theories

Pierre Janet (1859–1947) was the first to develop the concept of the 'splitting off', or dissociation, of a part of consciousness. He believed that the individual needed a normal amount of 'mental energy' to maintain integrative mental processes. When the level of energy was high, integration was maintained. When it became low, however, the personality might cease to function as a unit and split or dissociate.

Freud, in contrast, proposed the concept of repression to explain the loss of conscious awareness in dissociation. He then introduced the notion of the dynamic unconscious, a part of the mind in which emotions or ideas that were unacceptable to a person were pushed from awareness. Freud and other early analytic theorists accepted the basic concept of psychological dissociation.

Current explanations of dissociation are based on Freud's dynamic concepts. The repression of ideas that leads to amnesia and other forms of dissociation is conceived of as a way of protecting the individual from emotional pain. External circumstances or internal psychological conflicts are viewed as precipitating factors. A dissociative reaction may be viewed as a flight from crisis or danger—a major psychological route of escape from anxiety. Sometimes, as in states of dissociative fugue and dissociative identity disorder, the dissociated area temporarily assumes direction and control of the entire personality. During such times, the person may appear to be functioning well.

Dissociative identity disorder originates in childhood as a result of chronic trauma, usually child abuse. The trauma may be physical, psychological, or both. The major form of child abuse that contributes to the development of DID is sexual abuse. In attempts to cope with the horror of reality, the child's ego splits through the dissociative process. Each trauma-induced dissociative experience shapes the development of alternate personalities (alters). Chronic abuse leads to a fixation of the dissociated ego splits. Through dissociation, the child may see the abuse as if it were occurring to someone else, as in a movie. This ability to remove the self from the abuse is a mechanism that allows the individual to survive. The development of dissociative identity disorder is illustrated in Figure 16.1 ■.

Dynamic considerations relevant to dissociative disorders include the following. In dissociative amnesia, the pattern is similar to conversion disorder (discussed later in this chapter in the somatic symptom disorders section), except that the individual does not avoid some unpleasant situation by getting sick. Instead, the person does so by forgetting (repressing) certain traumatic events or stresses. In DID, there appears to be a deep-seated conflict between contradictory impulses and beliefs. A resolution is achieved by separating the conflicting parts and developing each into an autonomous personality or alter.

Behavioural theories

Behavioural theorists explain the development of dissociative disorders as learned behaviours. An individual learns that avoidance behaviour provides protection from a painful experience. After repeated experiences, this avoidance pattern is reinforced. Behavioural theory is the framework for many behavioural and cognitive behavioural methods currently used in treating symptoms associated with dissociative disorders.

Humanistic theories

Individuals with dissociative disorders have experienced intense psychological trauma during early childhood. As nurses, we take a holistic approach in dealing with the person, by accepting the fact that the dissociation was used as a defence mechanism that kept the abused child intact.

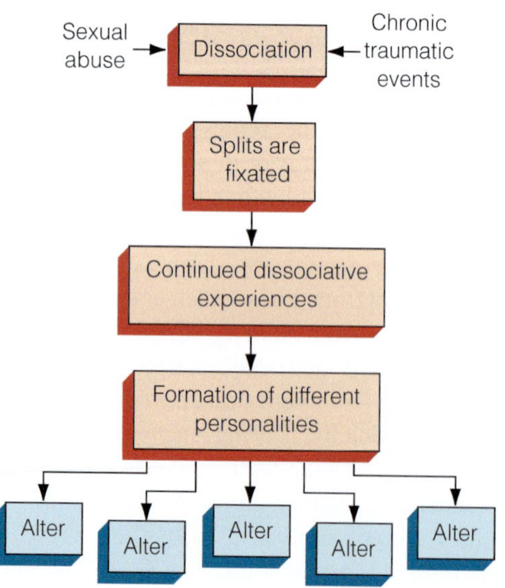

FIGURE 16.1 ■ The development of dissociative identify disorder.
Photo courtesy of Charles Ciccione/Photo Researchers, Inc.

Humanistic theories view people as a composite of life experiences, psychobiological factors and interpersonal interactions. Each person is conceptualised within the context of their culture.

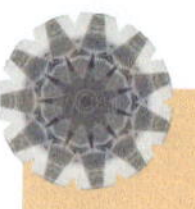

NURSING PROCESS
The person with dissociative disorders

When caring for someone with dissociative symptoms, a systematic approach is required in order to provide holistic, compassionate care. Most people with dissociative disorders are treated in community rather than inpatient settings.

Assessment

It can become extremely challenging when you begin to gather data on an individual with dissociative symptoms. For example, the person's amnesia will likely be problematic when you are collecting a health history. The major areas to focus on during assessment are identity, memory and consciousness. Some other areas to assess are awareness of time, amount of unfinished tasks, goal-setting and inconsistent work attendance (Precin & Precin, 2011). There are a number of measures of dissociation that can be used in assessment. One of the most widely used screening tools (Chu et al., 2011) is the Dissociative Experiences Scale self-report tool (Berstein & Putnam, 1986).

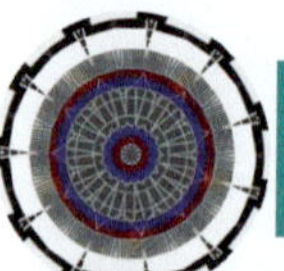

DEVELOPING CULTURAL COMPETENCE

Culture-bound syndromes that can be misdiagnosed as dissociative disorders

Amok A dissociative episode; characterised by a period of brooding followed by a violent outburst; precipitated by a perceived insult; occurs only in males in Malaysia, Laos, Philippines, Papua New Guinea, Polynesia (*cafard* or *cathard*), Puerto Rico (*mal de pelea*) and among the Navajo (*iich'aa*).

Ataque de nervios An episode of distress, usually a result of a stressful event involving the family; common symptoms include uncontrollable shouting, crying, heat in the chest rising to the head, and verbal or physical aggression. Dissociative experiences, such as amnesia about the symptoms, may be experienced. Occurs primarily among Latinos from the Caribbean, but also recognised among many Latin American and Latin Mediterranean groups.

Latah Hypersensitivity to sudden fright, often with dissociative or trancelike behaviour. Other symptoms include echolalia and echopraxia. Primarily occurs in Malaysia and Indonesia; in Malaysia it is more frequent in middle-aged women.

CRITICAL THINKING QUESTIONS

1. Why is it important to understand a person's cultural background?
2. How does cultural knowledge help develop therapeutic interventions?

YOUR ASSESSMENT APPROACH Individual with depersonalisation/derealisation disorder

To determine feelings of unreality, listen for the following:

- 'I just feel weird.'
- 'I'm not myself.'
- 'I feel like I'm floating away.'

To determine altered bodily perceptions, listen for the following:

- 'My body doesn't feel real.'
- 'I looked at my arm and saw that it looked like a piece of wood.'
- 'When I was looking in the mirror, it was like the image was looking back at me.'

To determine impaired behavioural perceptions, listen for the following:

- 'I feel like I'm on automatic pilot.'
- 'I'm walking through life like a zombie.'
- 'I feel like I'm a machine or a robot.'

To determine altered external perceptions, listen for the following:

- 'Everything feels different . . . like I'm in a dream while I'm awake.'
- 'Everyone seems unreal.'

Subjective data

People with dissociative disorders often report a sudden loss of memory of events. The individual may report, for example, that they cannot recall certain important personal events or information. They may not recall important aspects of their own identity, such as their age and where they reside. As you interview them, listen to their pronoun usage. If the person uses 'we' when speaking, this may indicate the presence of alters.

Sometimes amnesia is only partial, and individuals remain conscious of what happened, although they report that they feel no control over it. In cases of complete amnesia, the 'lost' memories can be recovered under certain therapeutic circumstances (e.g. hypnosis), or they may return spontaneously. People who have sustained a loss of their own reality may have adopted a new identity.

If motor behaviour is affected in dissociative disorders, the person or their family may report episodes during which the person physically travelled away from home. In people with DID, the original personality typically is not aware of the existence of alters. However, alters may be aware of the original personality as well as of each other, and may report this awareness to clinicians or peer workers. People with depersonalisation/derealisation disorder may report fears that they are going crazy and experience resulting anxiety. See the above Your Assessment Approach for assessment guidelines for people with **depersonalisation/derealisation disorder**.

Objective data

Conduct a careful assessment of the person's physical condition to rule out the possibility of organic causes, such as a brain tumour. Many of the behaviours of people with dissociative disorders resemble behaviours associated with organic conditions, including post-concussional amnesia and temporal lobe epilepsy. Your observations of the behaviour, character, duration, frequency and context of the dissociative disorder are crucial data. Physical examinations are not continued as part of the long-term intervention program, however, because they reinforce the symptoms and provide secondary gain (defined and discussed later in this chapter in the section on somatic symptom and related disorders). Completeness and accuracy of the initial physical assessment is of the utmost importance.

A psychosocial assessment is conducted to discover the fundamental source of the anxiety as early as possible. Although many episodes of dissociation appear to occur spontaneously, there may be a history of a specific emotional trauma or a situation charged with painful emotions and psychological conflict. Family or friends may provide clues to the person's conflict, so include them in the psychosocial data-gathering. When assessing for the presence of DID, consider the clinical manifestations listed in the Your Assessment Approach feature, below.

Events associated with the trauma can trigger memories that have been repressed; these stimuli can precipitate a switch of alters. When interacting with the person, be alert for evidence of forgetfulness and fluctuations of voice tone, speech and mannerisms. In each interaction, note whether there are uncharacteristic changes in behaviour (Chu et al., 2011). Are there differences in hairstyles, adornment, mannerisms or dress?

To assess for amnesia, ask whether the person has ever had blackouts, blank spells, memory gaps, or has lost time.

YOUR ASSESSMENT APPROACH The person with dissociative identity disorder

To assess for the presence of DID, ask the following:

- Are there blocks of time you are unable to remember?
- Do people call you by another name?
- Do you have physical pain that cannot be explained by health problems?
- Have you ever awakened not knowing your name or where you were at that time?
- Do other people accuse you of being untruthful?
- Have you ever discovered unfamiliar objects, like clothing, in your home, and not known how they got there?
- Do you have headaches? If so, how often? How intense are they?
- How often do you have sleeping problems?
- Do you ever have nightmares?
- As a child, were you hurt or abused by others?

To assess for dissociation, question whether the person ever 'spaces out' or is unable to remember periods of time or events. Ask others who know the person about episodes of uncharacteristic behaviour that the individual does not recall.

Nursing practice

Several features are common with people experiencing dissociative disorders. Dissociation is manifested by disturbances in sensory and thought processes. Dissociative disorders markedly interfere with a person's ability to perform role expectations.

Disturbed sensory perception and disturbed thought processes

The person with dissociative disorders may experience sudden memory loss, disorientation, loss of personal identity and alteration in state of consciousness. The person with dissociative amnesia has a partial or total inability to recall or identify past experiences. In people with depersonalisation/derealisation disorder, feelings of unreality and estrangement can affect their perception of the physical and psychological self and of the world around them. Parts of the body or the entire body may seem foreign, and dizziness, anxiety and distortion of time and space are common.

Role performance

Unexplained disappearances, absences from work, unreliability and unpredictability are common manifestations of dissociative disorders. Thus, the social or occupational functioning of the person is adversely affected. Symptoms of depersonalisation lead to limited or superficial involvement with others, and to withdrawal or disengagement in work or social pursuits. As expected, relationships become highly complicated and disorganised when a person has multiple personalities.

Ineffective coping

In addition to amnesia, a fugue state may occur in the person with dissociative disorders. In this state, people defend against perceived danger by active flight. They may wander away from home and community. Days, weeks or sometimes even years later they may suddenly find themselves in a strange place, not knowing how they got there. There is complete amnesia for the period of the fugue. Individuals experiencing dissociative fugue may adopt a new identity and life pattern.

Care planning and implementation

The role of the treatment team is to identify intervention options and work with the person living with DID to identify their treatment goals. Some people choose to maintain living with DID with system collaboration and co-consciousness, whereas others may opt for integration and eliminating the need for separate alters to cope with life. In choosing intervention strategies with individuals with dissociative disorders, the team must decide whether to alleviate the troublesome symptoms or reintegrate the anxiety-producing conflict. Some teams emphasise the disruptions in day-to-day functioning precipitated by dissociative disorders. These include unexplained disappearances, absences from work, unreliability and unpredictability. The dread associated with them justifies intervention strategies designed to change the disruptive behaviour pattern. Others believe that new problems are created by removing the dissociative symptoms without considering how they help the person control internal anxiety and maintain some balance in external social life.

Although individuals may complain about the difficulties associated with their symptoms, the symptoms often form the basis of relationships with other significant people in their lives. Individuals' roles in social groups are likewise built around their coping styles. Anyone who tries to change these coping styles must offer the person more effective and satisfying ways to handle anxiety and obtain support in their social network. Such a task usually requires long-term psychotherapy. However, behaviour modification strategies can alleviate some of the problematic behaviours. When planning care for a person with DID, remember that trust is a major issue. The basic building blocks of therapy with the dissociative individual are trust, safety and acceptance.

For many individuals, receiving a diagnosis of DID may actually provide a sense of relief. It is possible that for years they have been misdiagnosed and treated incorrectly. However, others may be distressed by the diagnosis: learning the diagnosis may trigger the switching of alters. Thus, a safe, supportive environment is essential when informing the person of the diagnosis. The focus of treatment is to form a therapeutic alliance and work through the issues of each alternate identity.

The goal of integrating the alternate identities into one fused identity is difficult to achieve—but it is feasible. Integration occurs when there is no further need for separateness between the identities. The integration process can be very painful, as memories of previous trauma surface. However, it is important for the person to recall the painful memories in order to work through the unresolved conflicts. Chu and colleagues (2011) state the importance of health professionals remembering that the individual with DID is not a collection of separate people sharing the same body. The person with DID should be seen as a whole person, with the identities sharing responsibility for daily life (Chu et al., 2011).

When planning care for individuals with DID, you must trust them to express their needs. You also need to actively listen to each identity state and provide support, especially when the individual is struggling to accept the realisation that they have DID.

Promoting improved sensory perception and thought processes

Strategies for identifying the underlying source of anxiety include those for recovering unconscious content, such as free association or dream description. At times, more active strategies are used. These may include projective psychometric tests (e.g., Rorschach, Thematic Apperception Test) and hypnosis. These strategies require advanced and specialised training. Strategies that you can use for a person with DID are discussed in Evidence-based Practice.

EVIDENCE-BASED PRACTICE

An eclectic approach to dissociative identity disorder

Sophie is a 34-year-old single female with a history of episodes of which she has no recollection. Family members report that during her blackouts Sophie would spend money uncontrollably, shop-lift, frequent bars and engage in sexually promiscuous behaviour. All of these behaviours are out of character for Sophie. During the past five years, Sophie was involved in six motor vehicle accidents during the blackouts. The family reported that during the blackout episodes, Sophie would dress in a provocative manner and speak in a hostile tone of voice. Sophie has a history of being sexually abused between the ages of 8 and 14 by an uncle. She was also physically abused by her mother for several years.

Your plan for intervention options is based on current research. The primary treatment modality for Sophie is talking therapy. Psychotherapy sessions will focus on desensitising traumatic memories. You have also learned that music therapy may be beneficial in promoting relaxation. Other therapies that will be implemented for Sophie include Gestalt therapy to help give voice to opposing feelings, and hypnosis to assist in reintegrating the alter personalities.

This set of interventions is based on the following literature:

Chu, J. A., Dell, P. F., Van der Hart, O., Cardeña, E., Barach, P. M., Somer, E., . . . Twombly, J. (2011). Guidelines for treating dissociative identity disorder in adults, third revision. *Journal of Trauma and Dissociation, 12*, 115–187.

CRITICAL THINKING QUESTIONS

1. How would you approach a person whose alter personality is in control of behaviour?
2. Why would it be useful to determine the underlying meaning of the person's symptoms?
3. What type of environment should be established for a person exhibiting dissociation?

Supportive insight therapy may be used with the goal of surfacing and integrating traumatic experiences in order to learn new ways of coping with future anxiety. This is especially relevant for those in whom dissociation arises primarily against a background of intrapsychic conflict.

Promoting effective role performance

It is important to work with the person's family in order to help everyone adjust to role performance alterations. Including family members in a therapeutic counselling relationship helps them learn new ways of dealing with the person. Considerable secondary gain is often associated with dissociative behaviour: some individuals may use the illness to escape responsibility and obtain special treatment. Families often need support in learning to avoid reinforcing dissociative behaviour by acting as the source of secondary gain.

Environmental manipulation may be an indicated intervention. For example, it may be necessary to assist the person in problem-solving with the goal of minimising other stressful aspects of the environment. In learning to confront and become desensitised to the underlying conflict, the individual will experience some anxiety and discomfort. This anxiety must be kept within manageable limits. Therefore, obvious stressors should be minimised.

Promoting effective coping

Psychotherapy, environmental manipulation and behaviour modification help the person cope more effectively with any impairments of conduct and impulse, as evidenced by unpredictable and bizarre behaviour. Treatment may prove to be long-term, and progress may be slow. Establishing a supportive therapeutic alliance with the person and their family is crucial in helping everyone understand the periodic occurrence of symptoms, and in supporting improved behaviours. See Communication for the person with depersonalisation/derealisation disorder.

Evaluation

Evaluating the effectiveness of nursing interventions is essential, although it may be difficult with individuals who are experiencing episodes of amnesia. Therefore, you must pay special attention to the person's non-verbal clues and to data obtained from secondary sources.

COMMUNICATION

The person with depersonalisation/derealisation disorder

PERSON: 'I don't feel like myself. In fact, I don't even feel real.'

NURSE RESPONSE 1: 'You sound as if you're afraid when these unreal episodes occur.' *RATIONALE:* This response demonstrates empathy and provides reassurance that it is appropriate to discuss feelings.	**NURSE RESPONSE 2:** 'When you are feeling this way, you look more anxious. We're here to help you learn to cope better with the anxiety.' *RATIONALE:* This response provides feedback on the congruence between the person's feelings and behaviour. It also provides reassurance that methods to decrease the anxiety associated with depersonalisation can occur.

Sensory perception and thought processes

The person will no longer experience sudden memory loss, disorientation, loss of identity or alteration in state of consciousness, or they will experience it less frequently. They will correctly recall and identify past experiences.

Role performance

The person will experience increased satisfaction with family and work relationships. Involvement with others will occur more often and will be more fulfilling. They will attend work or school regularly, without unexplained absences due to dissociative episodes.

Individual coping

The person will no longer exhibit bizarre or unpredictable behaviours, or they will experience them less frequently. For example, incidents of being missing from home without explanation will occur less frequently or not at all.

CARE COORDINATION

Care coordination for people experiencing dissociative disorders usually involves extensive tracking of records for previous hospitalisations, especially for people with DID. The lives of people with DID may often be significantly impacted as a result of the seriousness of the disorder. The care coordinator must maintain ongoing communication with the individual, family members, mental health professionals and other health care providers. Medication management is a major issue for many individuals with dissociative disorders.

COMMUNITY CARE

People with dissociative disorders are not psychotic, and therefore are often managed in the community. Community settings include general practices, medical centres, private psychiatric or psychology practices, and community mental health clinics, among others. However, for those who are hospitalised, discharge goals seem straightforward but present a challenge: to provide quality, cost-effective care that allows the person to return to full functioning as soon as possible. Community care must focus on the person's safety in light of possible continued memory impairments. The individual's ability to live at home is, after all, based on their functional abilities. Some individuals with DID need very close supervision, especially if they rapidly switch alters.

LIVED EXPERIENCE

Therapy and DID

The early trauma prevented us from developing interpersonal communication and social skills. Dissociation was the default in situations that could be happy, sad, angry or fearful. Triggers could include aggression and violence, music, places, food and things that had traumatic memories associated. For example, the violent mother was a matron (director of nursing)—a very strong and powerful woman. For many years any woman in a similar position was perceived as a threat and would trigger dissociation for protection.

The early therapy involved learning to identify the various emotional states, understanding their purpose, how to cope with other people's interactions and how to express these emotions in a balanced and purposeful way. EMDR (eye movement desensitisation reprocessing) was a useful therapy to bring the trauma to the surface to enable us to accept and process the events. The 48 hours following the therapy was the hardest part, as the memory would surface in force, resulting in severe distress, anxiety and depression, heightened fear and strong self-harm thoughts. The psychologist we worked with also worked closely with the community mental health team case manager (care coordinator), so that EMDR sessions would be booked in at times when both would be available to support us during this difficult time. There were nights when we would be sobbing on the floor in the bathroom, holding the pillow so tight to our body to stop us from 'falling apart'. Later, therapy options included dialectical behaviour therapy, which were useful to assisting us to be centred and focused at times when dissociation was problematic.

SOMATIC SYMPTOM AND RELATED DISORDERS

The essential features of somatic symptom and related disorders are physical symptoms suggesting physical disorders for which there is no evidence of organic or physiological causes. **Somatic symptom disorders**, formerly called somatoform disorders, are sometimes confused with physical disorders because the predominant symptoms are physical. These commonly experienced symptoms include fatigue, pain and sensory changes, such as those described in the following Diagnostic Features. Educational information about somatic symptom disorders is available on http://www.psyweb.com.

Somatic symptom disorder

The diagnosis of somatic symptom disorder applies to people who, like Sonya in the Practice Example that follows, have sought medical attention for recurrent and multiple somatic complaints over a duration of several years.

Historically, somatic symptom disorder has been referred to as 'hysteria', 'hysterical reaction' and 'Briquet's syndrome'. This problem usually has a chronic course, and is often accompanied by anxiety and depressed mood. Individuals believe they have been ill for at least six months of their lives, and may report one symptom or a lengthy list of symptoms,

DIAGNOSTIC FEATURES
Somatic symptom and related disorders

Somatic symptom disorder: One or more somatic symptoms that cause significant disruption of daily life for more than six months, with an excessive focus on symptoms or health concerns (APA, 2013).

Conversion disorder (functional neurological symptom disorder): One or more symptoms of altered voluntary motor or sensory function, in the absence of evidence of a medical condition. The symptoms cause significant distress or impairment in social, occupational or other important areas of functioning (APA, 2013).

Illness anxiety disorder: A preoccupation with having or acquiring a serious illness or illnesses that is present for at least six months. A high level of anxiety is present with excessive health-related behaviours. Somatic symptoms are usually not present (APA, 2013).

Factitious disorder: Falsification of medical or psychological signs and symptoms, associated with deception, but in the absence of obvious external rewards (APA, 2013). With *factitious disorder imposed on another*, an individual falsely presents another person with medical or psychological signs and symptoms.

Psychological factors affecting other medical conditions: Significant psychological or behavioural factors adversely affect a medical condition by increasing the risk of suffering, death or disability (APA, 2013).

Practice example

Sonya has appointments with a gastroenterologist, a gynaecologist, a cardiologist and her GP, all in the same month. Now 54 years old, Sonya has had multiple somatic complaints of nausea, bloating, constipation, heart palpitations and dizziness for almost three years. Although several gastrointestinal X-rays, heart studies and physical examinations have not indicated the presence of disease, Sonya is convinced that her disorders are real. She changes GPs regularly.

including blindness, paralysis, convulsions, nausea and other gastrointestinal difficulties. The symptoms may change in the six-month period. These symptoms are not caused intentionally, nor are they faked. The pain experienced by individuals with somatic symptom disorder is real.

Even though it does occur in children, somatic symptom disorder is rarely diagnosed in children and adolescents. With children, complaints are usually associated with a single symptom, and there is rarely worry of a broader illness. The response of parents may influence the level of distress experienced by the child (APA, 2013).

Conversion disorder (functional neurological symptom disorder)

In **conversion disorder**, individuals report impaired physical function, with the symptom not explained by evidence of neurological disease. The loss of functional ability is due to psychological, not biological, problems, identified through inconsistencies in neurological examinations. The symptoms in conversion disorder are not consciously produced. The following Practice Example illustrates this.

Practice example

Ronald is the 17-year-old eldest son of a Baptist minister in a rural community. His father expects his family to be pillars of the community and to serve as wholesome examples for the congregation. Ronald has recently developed a paralysis of his right hand, for which no physical basis has been found. Unknown to others, Ronald has been masturbating almost daily since he was 13 years old. He finds masturbation pleasurable, but feels anxiety and guilt at the same time.

Two mechanisms are thought to explain what a person 'gets' from having a conversion disorder. The first, **primary gain**, helps the person to keep the psychological need or conflict out of conscious awareness. For example, a woman may become blind to avoid acknowledging a traumatic event she has seen. In this instance, the symptom is a partial solution to the underlying conflict (not having to acknowledge witnessing the traumatic event because she has suddenly become sightless). The second mechanism, **secondary gain**, helps the person to avoid a distressing, uncomfortable or repugnant activity while at the same time receiving support from others. For example, a soldier with a paralysed arm could hardly be expected to fire a gun, and is also likely to receive sympathy because of his paralysis. Unlike malingering and factitious disorder, discussed later in the chapter, the symptoms are not deliberately produced to obtain benefits.

Another frequent symptom characteristic of individuals with conversion disorder, although not necessarily present in all instances, is ***la belle indifférence***, an inappropriate lack of concern about a disability. Tom, in the Practice Example that follows, demonstrates *la belle indifférence*.

Practice example

Tom is experiencing a conversion disorder that has led to his inability to walk. Although Tom stated, 'I woke up this morning with no feeling in my legs; for some reason they won't move,' he seems totally unconcerned about his problem despite its severity.

The person is actually calmer as a result of the somatic symptom. This problem usually begins in adolescence or early adulthood, although a conversion disorder may appear at any time of life. Regardless of the time of onset, a conversion disorder can seriously impede normal life activities. Functional impairments may affect the person's ability to function at work, at home or in social situations.

Illness anxiety disorder

Individuals with illness anxiety disorder are preoccupied with the fear or belief that they have a serious disease, which, on physical evaluation, is not present. The preoccupation may be built around any of the following:

- bodily functions (peristalsis, heartbeat)
- minor physical problems (an occasional headache, a slight cough)

- ambiguous, vague physical feelings ('tired ovaries' or 'aching veins').

The unrealistic fear or belief persists for a period of at least six months despite medical reassurance that no illness is present. This fear impairs the person's social and/or occupational functioning.

Practice example

Reading the newspaper and watching the news on television have become anxiety-provoking experiences for Lena, who has become worried about AIDS, avian flu, contaminated spinach and bean sprouts, and even head lice. She attributes any symptom she has—an itch, a runny nose, a loose bowel movement—to any one of a number of possible medical conditions. If her worries have not been relieved by her research on the internet, Lena calls in sick to work and makes an appointment to see her general practitioner.

MALINGERING

Malingering occurs when a person deliberately fakes symptoms in order to benefit. The DSM-5 (APA, 2013) categorises malingering as a condition differentiated from factitious disorder. Malingering is not considered a psychiatric disorder, because it involves deliberate falsification of illness. However, malingering is discussed here because individuals with somatic symptom disorders are sometimes misdiagnosed as faking their conditions. Malingering is consciously motivated and usually results in secondary gain, which may be in the form of extra attention, relief from responsibilities, or financial rewards, as shown in the following Practice Example.

Practice example

Joyce is a police officer. She fakes episodes of back pain in order to avoid street patrol. Whenever she is assigned to this duty, Joyce claims to be in too much pain to work.

Due to the nature of malingering, prevalence estimates are difficult to establish (Bass & Hallingan, 2014). Sullivan, Lange and Dawes (2005) provide the most current Australian estimates of malingering. Their study found that the rates of malingering were variable, dependent on the environment of the individual. Symptom exaggeration or probable symptom exaggeration was reported to involve 17 per cent of criminal cases, 13 per cent of personal injury, 13 per cent of disability or workers' compensation, and 4 per cent of medical or psychiatric cases (Sullivan et al., 2005).

It often occurs in the following situations: personal injury and workers' compensation litigation, and military service and criminal cases. Mental Health in the Media discusses an episode of malingering a mental disorder in order to avoid criminal prosecution. As Chapter 11 discusses, malingering is fairly often linked with legal pleas of guilty by reason of insanity.

FACTITIOUS DISORDERS

The DSM-5 recognises two **factitious disorders**: factitious disorder imposed on self and factitious disorder imposed on another. Malingering and somatic symptom disorders are sometimes mistakenly confused with factitious disorder imposed on self, in which people intentionally produce or feign physical or psychological symptoms (APA, 2013). The major difference between factitious disorder imposed on self and malingering is that a person with a factitious disorder has a psychological need to assume the sick role. Unlike malingering, external incentives for the behaviour are absent. There are numerous difficulties in diagnosing and treating individuals with factitious disorder (Bass & Halligan, 2014; Kradin, 2011). It is also costly when medically unnecessary diagnostic procedures are performed. The course of factitious disorder usually consists of intermittent episodes. If undiagnosed or treated ineffectively, the factitious disorder may become chronic, thereby increasing the risk of danger.

Factitious disorders may occur on a continuum of mild (giving a verbal list of symptoms) to moderate (simulating

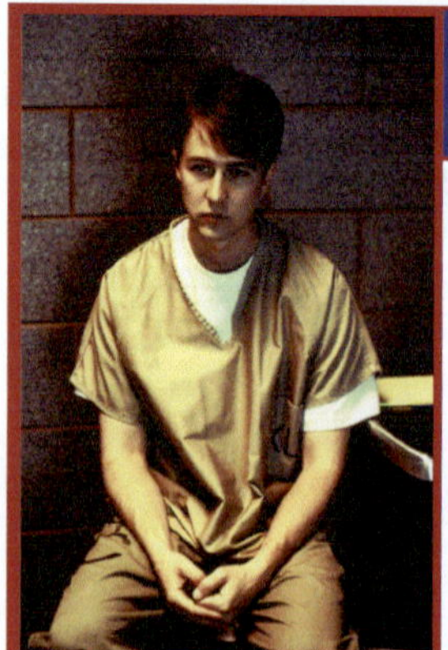

MENTAL HEALTH IN THE MEDIA

Primal Fear

A young, stuttering, timid altar boy, Aaron Stampler (Edward Norton), is accused of the brutal murder of a Catholic priest. A prominent, spotlight-loving defence attorney, Martin Vail (Richard Gere), interested in the publicity the case will bring, volunteers to represent the young man. Despite the considerable evidence against him (Aaron was found running from the archbishop's home covered in blood), he claims not to remember anything about the murder. When Vail discovers more evidence in the archbishop's home, he confronts Aaron and accuses him of lying. In an emotional scene, Aaron breaks down crying, and transforms into the persona of Roy, a violent sociopath. Later, Aaron has no recollection of this event.

In court, Vail arranges a courtroom scene designed to showcase Aaron's vicious alter, Roy. On the basis of Aaron's apparent dissociative identity disorder, the judge dismisses the jury and finds Aaron not guilty by reason of insanity. When Vail returns to Aaron's jail cell to tell him the good news, the no-longer stuttering and no-longer timid Aaron reveals that he has been pretending to have a mental disorder the entire time. As a stunned and disillusioned Vail leaves the jail cell, Aaron taunts him. This film raises the controversial issues of both malingering and dissociative identity disorder.

Photo courtesy of Everett Collection, Inc.

physical symptoms) to severe (inflicting injury). Dermatological manifestations are very common; however, physical symptoms can be intentionally induced for many medical conditions. Thelma, in the Practice Example that follows, exemplifies factitious disorder imposed on self.

Practice example

Thelma has been admitted to the hospital after being seen in a GP surgery with blood in her urine. The admitting doctor has ordered several invasive procedures—catheterisation, blood tests and cystoscopy, among others. The doctor does not know that Thelma has been taking anticoagulants to produce blood in her urine.

People with factitious disorders usually give false medical histories that can be quite elaborate. It can be difficult to detect a factitious disorder, because individuals may use several different names and often seek treatment in several areas to avoid detection or recognition by someone who has encountered them during a previous hospitalisation or GP visit.

The fabricated symptoms—e.g. fever, anaemia, haematuria—are indeed symptoms of 'real' diseases; however, there is no organic reason for the appearance of the symptoms. The individual provides an untruthful account of symptoms and fakes signs of illness in an attempt to receive medical treatment. Uncontrollable lying is the hallmark characteristic of individuals with factitious disorders; stories are fabricated in order to capture the attention of others. Individuals typically describe their symptoms in dramatic terms, yet are vague about the onset and duration of the problems. Individuals with factitious disorders are usually very knowledgeable about medicine. Being knowledgeable, imaginative and sophisticated about medical systems, medical terminology and the routines of treatment facilities allows them to convincingly fake a constellation of symptoms.

Factitious disorders can be severe, chronic and unremitting—involving repeated hospitalisations, travelling between health care providers and health care facilities, and pathological lying of an intriguing and fantastic nature (called *pseudologica fantastica*). Factitious disorder imposed on self used to be referred to as **Munchausen syndrome**. David, in the following Practice Example, is an example of such a person.

Practice example

David is lying on a treatment table in the emergency department. He is in acute pain with a dislocated shoulder. This hospital is located 20 kilometres from the suburb in which David lives. What the medical officer does not know is that David has been to several different GPs in his city and has had multiple prior hospitalisations for factitious symptoms—pain, fevers of undetermined origin, rashes and dizziness. All physical assessments have proved negative. David usually berates the doctor, the nurse or the X-ray technician for being unable to find the cause of his problem, and signs himself out against medical advice. The emergency clinicians do not know that David has dislocated his own shoulder.

As this Practice Example demonstrates, factitious disorder can become a lifelong pattern.

Factitious disorder imposed on another

Factitious disorder imposed on another, previously called **Munchausen's syndrome by proxy**, occurs when parents or caregivers deliberately induce signs of an illness in another, including adults, children and even pets. It is difficult for health care providers to deal with situations in which an individual (usually a parent) deliberately injures the person under their care. In these situations, health care providers should seek clinical supervision or a consultant to help them to cope with their personal responses.

In factitious disorder imposed on another, the individual deliberately injures their victims in order to gain sympathy or attention for themselves. The individual with this syndrome has an insatiable need for attention, even though the person's behaviour is harmful to others. Intentionally producing symptoms in the child (or other victim) is a way to gain attention. The following Practice Example discusses a woman with factitious disorder imposed on another person.

Practice example

A mother has been regularly and deliberately administering large doses of laxatives to her 15-month-old toddler over a period of several months. When the child has episodes of cramping, flatulence and bloody diarrhoea, the mother, appearing to be very concerned, takes her to the emergency department of a local hospital. Diagnostic studies show no medical reason for the toddler's symptoms.

It is wise to suspect the presence of factitious disorder imposed on another if certain indicators are present. These indicators are identified in What Every Nurse Should Know.

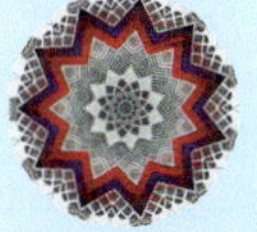

WHAT EVERY NURSE SHOULD KNOW

Factitious disorder imposed on another and child abuse

Imagine that you are a paediatric nurse or a school nurse. Factitious disorder imposed on another is a potentially fatal form of child abuse. Not only is the child's life disrupted, the child is usually subjected to frequent hospitalisations and invasive medical procedures. Therefore, the child's safety is of the utmost concern.

An evaluation by an interdisciplinary team is called for whenever this disorder is suspected. It requires the collection of evidence and the development of a plan to provide appropriate care for the hospitalised child, involve the appropriate authorities (such as child protection services), and obtain help for the child's parent or caretaker. Health care providers should be suspicious of situations in which:

- a child has unexplained, recurrent or rare symptoms
- the parent/caretaker denies knowing the cause of the illness

(continued)

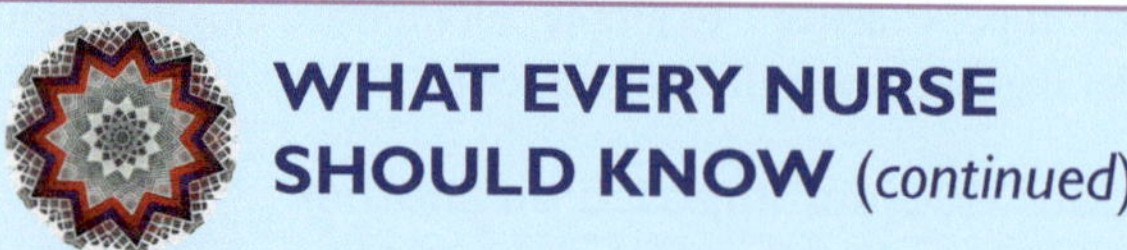

WHAT EVERY NURSE SHOULD KNOW (continued)

- when the parent/caretaker is present, so are the symptoms; however, when the child is separated from the parent/caretaker, the symptoms resolve
- the illness is unresponsive to treatment
- the clinical findings are inconsistent
- there is a history of several hospital visits for treatment.

BIOPSYCHOSOCIAL THEORIES

Biological, genetic and psychosocial theories help to understand somatic symptom disorders. The following section presents research findings about the aetiology of somatic symptom disorders.

Biological factors

In somatic symptom disorders, physical symptoms are present but evidence of physiological disease is not. The symptoms are thought to be linked to psychological factors or emotional conflict. However, there is some evidence that brain abnormalities may lead to altered pain perception (Bourne, 2011; Kregel et al., 2015). Evidence indicates that somatic symptom disorders are associated with increased activity of limbic regions in response to painful stimuli (Browning, Fletcher & Sharpe, 2011). Biochemical imbalances, such as decreased amounts of endorphins and serotonin, may cause some people to experience pain more intensely than those with normal brain chemistry.

Genetic theories

Studies have identified relationships between genetics and somatic symptoms (Klengel et al., 2011; Silber, 2011). A study of somatisation in major depression by Klengal and colleagues (2011) found a strong link between somatisation and a specific genetic variation. There is some evidence to support that some children have a genetic predisposition to somatisation disorders, especially children who exhibit sensitivity to anxiety and trait anxiety (Silber, 2011). There may be a possible genetic predisposition; however, more work is needed to understand the precise genetic contributors and gene-environment interactions (Stein, 2013).

Psychosocial theories

Communication theorists believe that manifestations of somatisation are non-verbal body language intended to communicate a message to significant others. Sometimes the message is as general as 'pay attention to me' or 'take care of me'. At other times the *conversion of anxiety* actually symbolises the nature of the specific underlying conflict. For example, a woman who wants to hit her children may develop a paralysis of her arm. A girl who feels guilty about reading erotic books may become blind. Both experience the primary gain of protection from the anxiety-provoking impulses, and both get secondary gains of attention and sympathy. Such behaviour patterns are most likely to occur among individuals who lack appropriate coping skills.

Many individuals who engage in somatisation were reared in chaotic families. The family dysfunction was usually marital discord, substance abuse and/or personality disorders. For whatever reason, the child received inadequate nurturing. Many adults with somatic symptom disorders experienced physical or sexual abuse as children. The person who deals with anxiety by converting it to physical symptoms usually shows no other psychological symptoms, such as disturbed thoughts or depressed moods.

Pain is associated with a great many disease processes, including some of the organ-specific somatic symptom disorders. Pain can be adaptive or maladaptive, in that it often indicates real danger but sometimes it interferes with functioning. Consciousness, attention, perception and cognition are all necessary for the experience of pain. According to modern theories of pain perception, humans have a control system over pain that operates as a 'gate'. Pain stimuli can be 'allowed in' or 'shut out' from the cerebral cortex, depending essentially on the meaning the person attaches to the stimulus. This underscores the importance of meaning, symbol and affect in the experience of pain sensation. Figure 16.2 ■ shows the basic mechanism for so-called idiopathic pain (pain of unknown origin).

In psychoanalytic concepts, unconscious conflicts are a result of traumatic or frustrating childhood experiences that are reawakened in adult life by a similar stress or frustration. According to this theory, the person cannot express the affect because of feelings of guilt, fear of loss of love, or fear of retribution. The affect is therefore repressed and transformed into physiological correlates, such as pain.

Humanistic theories

It is important to think about the person with somatic symptom disorders in the context of what is happening in their lives. Stress related to relationships and work may be the precipitants for somatic symptoms. There is evidence that psychogenic symptoms associated with conversion disorders are associated with higher rates of childhood trauma and stress (Kaplan et al.,

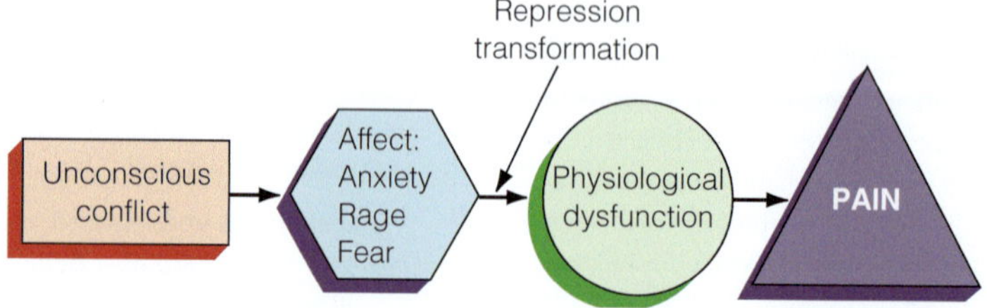

FIGURE 16.2 ■ The mechanism of idiopathic pain.

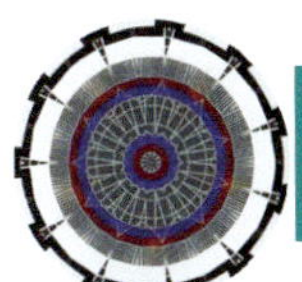

DEVELOPING CULTURAL COMPETENCE

Culture-bound syndromes that can be misdiagnosed as somatic symptom disorders

Bilis and colera (also called *munia*) Occurs in Latino groups. Episodes of extreme anger which can exacerbate existing physical symptoms, including headache, stomach upsets, trembling and loss of consciousness. Chronic fatigue may be a result of these episodes.

Brain fog Term initially used in West Africa for a condition experienced by students; symptoms include impairments in concentration, memory and thinking. Somatic symptoms are headache, blurring of vision, burning in the head and eyes.

Falling-out or blacking out A sudden collapse, which may occur without warning, but is sometimes preceded by feelings of dizziness. Eyes are open, but the individual denies the ability to see; feels powerless to move. Occurs primarily in Caribbean groups.

Shenjing shuairua Characterised by physical and mental fatigue, dizziness, headaches, gastrointestinal problems, sexual dysfunction, other pains, sleep disturbance and memory loss. Occurs in China.

CRITICAL THINKING QUESTIONS

1. Why is it important to know a person's cultural background?
2. How does knowledge of a person's cultural background help to develop therapeutic interventions?

2013). Stressful situations encountered by some children, such as bullying and abuse (either physical or sexual), may be contributory factors (Silber, 2011). Environmental factors may contribute to the development of somatization, in that there is 'a preponderance of these conditions among children of families living in lower socioeconomic strata' (Silber, 2011, p. 63). Research identifies an association between impairments in particular domains of life in adolescence and the development of future somatisation disorders, such as conversion disorder (Keertish & Sharma, 2015).

You must view a person's behaviour within the context of their cultural experience. See Developing Cultural Competence for a listing of culture-bound syndromes that may be misdiagnosed as somatic symptom disorders (APA, 2013).

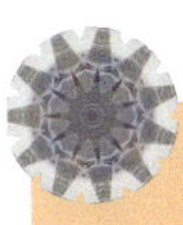

NURSING PROCESS
The person with somatic symptom and related disorders

When you work with individuals experiencing somatic symptom and related disorders, you will be challenged by multiple complex problems, not the least of which stem from your own values and beliefs. Your values and beliefs will influence how well you undertake nursing practice in this area. If you are unaware of your values and beliefs, you are likely to express them non-verbally. Therefore, it is imperative that you increase your self-awareness in order to be more effective when working with the person who has somatoform or factitious disorders. The Self-awareness feature, above, is designed to help you examine your feelings.

SELF-AWARENESS
Exploring your feelings towards the person with somatic symptom and related disorders

Reflect on your feelings when you are caring for individuals with somatic symptom and related disorders. Ask yourself the following questions, and then evaluate the relationship between your answers and your reactions to these individuals.

- How well do you handle frustration?
- How do you respond to the expression of anger, either passive or aggressive, by others?
- How patient are you? Are you able to be satisfied with small successes?
- Can you tell when you are becoming defensive?
- How can you tell if another person is experiencing 'real' pain?

Assessment

Assessment of individuals with somatic symptom and related disorders is often difficult because of the many psychobiological factors involved. Careful and thorough assessment—subjective as well as objective—to rule out the possibility of a physical problem is crucial, as shown in the following Practice Example.

Practice example

Magda was referred for treatment to a local private mental health facility by her GP. She had weakness and numbness of her right arm. When her GP could find no physiological reason for Magda's symptoms, he diagnosed her problem as a conversion disorder and referred her to mental health. The nurse who admitted Magda performed a thorough physical assessment and history-taking. The medical history revealed that Magda had had surgery on her left kidney three months ago. The nurse made the connection between the surgical position (right lateral) necessary to perform Magda's surgery and Magda's symptoms. The numbness and weakness were actually caused by pressure on the brachial plexus in her right arm during surgery. Magda was discharged from the mental health clinic and referred for physical rehabilitation.

In this Practice Example, a complete and accurate assessment of all factors identified the appropriate course of action for Magda and spared her from a potentially stigmatising diagnosis. Some sample questions useful in determining the presence of somatic symptom and related disorders are listed in the following Your Assessment Approach.

YOUR ASSESSMENT APPROACH The person with somatic symptom disorder

The following list provides some sample questions to help determine the presence of somatic symptom disorder:

- Have you ever felt as though you were smothering, or couldn't breathe easily?
- Have you ever had problems swallowing or felt as though you were choking? If so, how long did the episode(s) last?
- Have you ever had burning sensations in your mouth or throat?
- Do you ever experience painful menstrual periods?
- Do you have pain in your joints? If so, how often?
- Have you seen many doctors who have told you that nothing is wrong with you?

Subjective data

Individuals with somatic symptom and related disorders report physical symptoms for which there is no positive evidence of organic or physiological cause. For example, with illness anxiety disorder, the person may return many times to the health service demanding to be re-examined or retested. They believe they are suffering from some major illness that has been undetected. They are not reassured by the lack of physical findings, and may go from GP to GP in an attempt to find someone who will validate their fears. This 'doctor shopping' may lead to fragmented care and misuse of medication. Because the person is usually a poor historian, a complete medical history (including medications taken) is not always obtained. Although individuals with somatic symptom disorder usually describe their condition with colourful, exaggerated language, it can be difficult to obtain specific facts about previous medical and surgical treatments. In conversion disorder, there is loss of, or an alteration in, function.

A nonchalant attitude towards physical problems (*la belle indifférence*) indicates that the symptom is providing primary gain; that is, the anxiety is alleviated through the conversion process. In contrast, persons with somatic symptom disorder or illness anxiety disorder are overly dramatic and emotional when talking about their symptoms and pain. They report the history in vivid detail and colourful language, but often pay more attention to how the symptoms have affected relationships in their lives than to giving a careful description of the nature, character, location, onset and duration of the symptoms.

Careful interviewing frequently reveals a stressful life situation with which the individual is failing to cope, suggesting that the preoccupation with somatic symptom disorder is a way of avoiding underlying conflict. Helping them identify and express feelings is a crucial beginning to psychotherapeutic intervention.

Objective data

Physical examination reveals no organic evidence for symptoms. Likewise, laboratory findings do not substantiate organic or physiological disorder. Despite this, the individual may have undergone many exploratory diagnostic and/or surgical procedures without diagnosis or relief. Family members often report that the person is moody, self-centred or demanding. They feel alienated from the individual, and are frustrated with their chronic preoccupation with physical symptoms.

In a health care setting, these individuals often create scenes that bring them attention without regard for the needs of others. You may find it difficult to be kind, understanding and nonjudgmental with such individuals. If you do not cope with your reactions, you will be unable to effectively work with them. Recognising the person's somatisation as part of the illness will help you to avoid personalising the behaviour. It may help to remind yourself that they do not intentionally produce their symptoms, nor do they understand the effects of their behaviour on others. When you understand the psychopathology of the disorder, you are more likely to have empathy for the individual's coping style. What Every Nurse Should Know will help you apply these understandings in non-psychiatric settings.

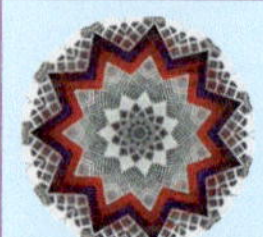

WHAT EVERY NURSE SHOULD KNOW

Somatic symptom and related disorders

Imagine that you are a nurse in a surgical unit.

- Be careful not to rush to judge that 'it's all in their head' when an individual with a somatic symptom or related disorder is admitted. People with somatic symptom or related disorders can be ill or in pain.
- Pain and illness of psychogenic origin is as hurtful as pain of biological origin.
- Be aware that somatic symptom disorder, illness anxiety disorder, conversion disorder and other related disorders are maladaptive responses to stress.
- Remember that unconscious (not deliberate) processes are at work, except for instances of malingering or factitious disorder.
- Be alert for signs of secondary gain, and avoid reinforcing.
- Use a matter-of-fact approach when the individual discusses somatic symptoms.
- Use a calm, patient approach in order to decrease the person's anxiety level.
- Decrease stimuli to promote relaxation.
- Anticipate the individual's needs before somatisation increases.
- Reward appropriate behaviour.

Nursing practice

Individuals with somatic symptom and related disorders experience a multitude of problems. As such, there are likely to be several important focuses for nursing practice. The following section discusses five areas of importance.

Impaired verbal communication

The person with somatic symptom and related disorders has an impaired ability to communicate their needs. Although they may be highly verbal, you need to listen carefully for gaps, over-simplifications, over-dramatisations and over-generalisations in their stories. Somatic symptoms are considered to be non-verbal substitutes for the expression of underlying conflicts.

Role performance and compromised family coping

The manipulative and dependent behaviours of the person with a somatic symptom or related disorder lead to impairments in social, work and family relationships, and to diminished performance in these roles. Friends and relatives eventually tire of the demands and become less available for support. Individuals become emotionally isolated, because their self-absorption makes them unable to respond appropriately to the needs of others.

Work performance may suffer from frequent absences due to imagined illness. Preoccupation with health status uses up creative energy that could otherwise be directed towards work-related activities. When this occurs, the individual usually experiences negative consequences in the workplace.

Ineffective coping

Individuals with somatic symptom and related disorders generally experience anxiety, anger and feelings of helplessness. These may be felt acutely, and they may demonstrate these feelings excessively, as in somatic symptom disorder and illness anxiety disorder. Paradoxically, they may instead show an uncanny lack of feeling, as in the nonchalant reaction to loss of physical function that often occurs in conversion disorder.

Emotions become increasingly restricted with the focus becoming somatic concerns. Individuals no longer experience meaningful emotional connections with other people, activities and events. The range of emotional expression may be limited to making demands, manipulation and symbolic manifestations of anxiety.

Disturbed thought processes and disturbed sensory perception

The person with somatic symptom and related disorders shows selective inattention; that is, they filter out stimuli in response to anxiety. In a further effort to prove their ideas, they distort reality and tend to ramble. Judgment is often impaired and conclusions are not logical. Individuals may also distort memory and show selective memory.

Individuals with somatic symptom and related disorders may have body image disturbances, and often sense that they are weak or vulnerable physically. They perceive sensory data incorrectly; for example, they may perceive abdominal discomfort as cancer rather than indigestion.

Care planning and implementation

In order to intervene effectively, you need to recognise and understand the life problem or adjustment the person is facing. It is also important that you:

- recognise and understand the person's self-perception as an inability to cope
- help the person identify and learn more effective ways of adapting.

These goals may be accomplished by insight-oriented or supportive psychotherapy, behaviour modification, hypnosis, or any of several other psychological, as well as some physical, therapies. No single therapeutic modality has superior effectiveness, and new approaches and techniques are indicated when traditional ones prove inadequate. It is important to recognise that with somatic symptom and related disorders the person is highly resistant to change. Thus, progress can be slow and recovery partial. Specific interventions and rationales are discussed in Your Intervention Strategies.

You may also meet individuals with somatic symptom and related disorders in general health care settings. Refer to What Every Nurse Should Know on the preceding page for specific interventions for non-mental health settings.

YOUR INTERVENTION STRATEGIES The person with somatic symptom disorder

Intervention	Rationale
Establish a trusting relationship.	Promotes psychological safety.
Establish a daily routine.	Decreases anxiety.
Encourage verbalisation of feelings.	Verbalisation is healthier than somatisation.
Assist the individual to relate stress to the onset of physical symptoms.	Pointing out a cause-and-effect relationship helps eliminate triggers.
Encourage writing in a journal.	Increases personal insight.
Limit the time for discussing physical symptoms.	Enables time for problem-solving activities; decreases reinforcement of secondary gain(s).

COMMUNICATION

The person with somatic symptom disorder

PERSON: 'How can they help me get better if they can't even figure out what's wrong with me? I know I'm really sick.'

NURSE RESPONSE 1: 'It sounds as if you are feeling hopeless.' *RATIONALE:* This response focuses on feelings and encourages further exploration. It is also a way to determine any suicidal ideation that may be related to hopelessness.	**NURSE RESPONSE 2:** 'It must be very frustrating for you. All of the examinations and tests show no physical cause for your symptoms.' *RATIONALE:* This response demonstrates empathy while at the same time presenting reality. Reassurance that no organic pathology has been found helps dispute unrealistic beliefs.

Promoting effective communication

After assessing the meaning behind the person's communication patterns, plan intervention strategies, such as encouraging exploration and demonstrating empathy that enhance verbal communication and self-esteem to the point where the individual feels ready to face problems. The Communication feature gives examples of verbal communication strategies.

Establishing a trusting relationship is the key to effective therapy with a person who is somatising. Help them tone down their characteristic extravagances. Express respectful scepticism regarding oversimplifications and over-dramatisations. Group settings provide opportunities to gain feedback about the effect of their behaviour on others.

Promoting improved role performance and family coping

Working with the family is especially important. Collaborative Care discusses educating the family and the individual about the disorder, stressing the importance of avoiding unnecessary surgical or medical procedures.

Encourage independent functioning and reduce the possibility of secondary gain by not focusing on physical symptoms. Assume a matter-of-fact, supportive attitude, with the optimistic expectation that the individual will regain functional abilities in work, family and social roles.

Promoting effective coping

The goal of counselling a person with somatic symptom and related disorders is to help them express their conflicts verbally rather than acting them out through symptomatic behaviours. The aim of long-term (insight) therapy is to promote effective emotional expression by exploring the sources of anxiety. You will likely be challenged to help individuals with somatic symptom and related disorders acknowledge the effects of psychosocial stress on symptoms. Supportive therapy seeks to improve self-esteem, perhaps through measures like expanding the person's interest in their environment.

In general, try to avoid reinforcing symptoms. A well-known psychiatric axiom applies in this general category: *Ignore the symptom but never the person.* Concentrating on the physical symptom by trying to get a paralysed individual to walk or a blind individual to see again is giving the symptom more importance than it merits, thus increasing the secondary gain associated with it. Ultimately, this makes it more difficult for the person to relinquish the symptom.

Promoting improved perception and thought processes

Improve the person's perception and thinking by supporting general measures to reduce anxiety. Maintain a calm, unhurried attitude, listen carefully, and maintain an objective, undistorted view of reality. Avoid a premature challenge to the individual's symptoms and complaints. As the person gradually relinquishes their defences, propose other ways of understanding the condition, such as by suggesting a psychological explanation for a physical complaint.

Evaluation

Consider communication, role performance, coping, perception and thought processes when evaluating individuals with

COLLABORATIVE CARE

Teaching about somatic symptom disorders

- Provide information about the specific disorder.
- Teach about the relationship between stress and physical symptoms.
- Teach relaxation techniques (e.g. progressive muscle relaxation, guided imagery).
- Provide health promotion education (e.g. healthy diet, balance between exercise and rest, healthy sleep patterns).
- Teach the proper use of medications, including target symptoms, side-effects and adverse drug reactions, contraindications, and when to call for help.
- Teach the indicators for emergency treatment.
- Emphasise the need for continued treatment, including follow-up appointments.

EVIDENCE-BASED PRACTICE

Cognitive behavioural techniques for conversion disorder

Alf is a 22-year-old soldier. Even though he voluntarily joined the Army, Alf never told anyone that he believes that killing under any circumstance is murder. After he finished military basic training, he was deployed. When on a routine patrol, Alf's unit was attacked by enemy forces. While aiming his assault rifle at an opposing soldier, Alf suddenly lost his vision. All medical tests show no physical basis for his blindness.

Your plan for intervention options is based on research. You have learned that Alf will likely respond to individual or group cognitive behavioural therapy (CBT) techniques such as those discussed in Chapter 25. Therefore, you teach Alf the techniques of thought stopping and reframing. Using imagery may also be beneficial.

The treatment team also decides to focus on establishing a therapeutic relationship with Alf that includes an open, honest discussion of his disorder. Knowing that somatisation may be triggered by stress, you demonstrate empathy and support to him without reinforcing his symptoms.

These interventions are based on the following research:

Allan, L. A., & Woolfolk, R. L. (2010). Cognitive behavioural therapy for somatoform disorders. *Psychiatric Clinics of North America, 33*(3), 579–593.

Conwill, M., Oakley, L., Evans, K., & Cavanna, A. E. (2014). CBT-based group therapy for nonepileptic attacks and other functional neurological symptoms: A pilot study. *Epilepsy and Behaviour, 34*, 68–72.

CRITICAL THINKING QUESTIONS

1. How would you demonstrate empathy to individuals with a conversion disorder without reinforcing the person's symptoms?
2. In what ways would it be useful to determine the underlying meaning of the individual's symptoms?
3. How would thought stopping and reframing help someone with conversion disorder?

somatic symptom disorder. When evaluating these areas, it is important that you look for evidence of progress. Expect that progress will be gradual, and encourage the individual and family to do the same.

Communication

Individuals will express feelings and conflicts verbally, and will have fewer somatic symptoms. Conversations will 'flow', with fewer monologues and more natural dialogue between the person and you. In other words, the person's communication will become more spontaneous.

Role performance and family coping

They will attend work regularly, without frequent absences due to illness or worry about physical health status. They will be more interested in outside activities, and may begin to engage in socialisation and recreation. Family members and friends will report being more satisfied with their relationship with the person, and will be more willing to interact with them.

Coping

The person will be less demanding, manipulative and attention-seeking in interactions with others. They will appear less anxious, and will talk about topics other than their physical status. They appear less helpless and more able to participate in and make responsible decisions about their health care. For example, they may carry out a plan of treatment without voicing innumerable objections or worries. They will appear more interested and involved in the activities and attitudes of others, and be more aware of the impact of their own behaviour.

Perception and thought processes

Distortion and misinterpretation of reality will happen less frequently. Judgment, insight and memory will improve as a result of reduced defensiveness in perception and cognition. They may report feeling more positive about their bodies, and are more assertive in physical activities because they no longer feel so vulnerable.

CARE COORDINATION

Care coordination with a person who has somatic symptom disorders must focus on occupational functioning, which is usually significantly impaired by the disorder. Provision of job search skills and communication techniques (e.g. how to listen actively to others) will enhance the individual's career opportunities. Rehabilitative agencies can also be called upon to provide specific job-skills training. The care coordinator will often need to refer significant others to services that provide respite care and/or support to family members.

COMMUNITY CARE

Individuals and family members usually need ongoing support for managing in the community. Community mental health centres are very useful in helping individuals obtain medications and adhere to the prescribed therapies. You can also encourage the individual and their family to visit the support service website, Somatoform Australia (http://somatoformaustralia.org/).

Community mental health nurses have a unique opportunity to support individuals and help them maintain independence in their activities of daily living. Home visits are conducted to provide support and education, and to evaluate the person's need for continued treatment. Some tools that are especially useful in the home setting are cognitive behavioural therapy (discussed in Chapter 25) and relaxation skills (discussed in Chapter 8).

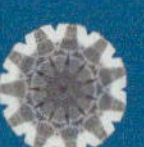

NURSING CARE PLAN: PERSON LIVING WITH DISSOCIATIVE IDENTITY DISORDER

Identifying information

Sally, aged 30 years, is brought to the hospital by her friend, who found her lying on the floor of her home. Sally had cut her wrist and was bleeding moderately. When admitted to the emergency department, Sally states her name is Beth, and she does not understand why she is in the hospital, unless Sally tried to hurt herself again. Beth says that Sally 'is always doing something crazy to herself'. When transferred to the psychiatric unit, Beth admits that she tries to protect Sally from 'terrible things in the world'.

History

Sally experienced sexual abuse from both parents from birth until she was 16, when she ran away from home. She has occasional contact with her younger sister, who lives in another state. She states that she has never been treated for a mental disorder.

Current mental status

Sally is alert and oriented. She answers questions in a vague manner, and has several time lapses with no memory. Her speech is slow but coherent. She acknowledges some problems with short-term memory and the ability to concentrate.

Other clinical data

A thorough nursing assessment identifies the presence of four alter personalities with specific traits and behaviours. Beth is the host personality. Annie is four years old and is looking for 'my daddy'. Sally is 11 years old and experiences all of the pain felt by the others. Bobbie is 17 years old and has the task of protecting the others; Bobbie states she will kill anyone who doesn't do as she wishes.

Issue identified: Risk for self-harm.
Expected outcome: Sally will verbalise a lack of suicidal ideation or plans.

Short-term goals	Interventions	Rationale
Sally will refrain from harming herself.	■ Place on close observation.	Need for continuous monitoring.
	■ Remove all dangerous items from the environment.	Reduces risk of harm by ensuring a safe environment.
	■ Ask Sally to sign a no-suicide contract.	Treats Sally as a partner in treatment by increasing her sense of control. Emphasises seriousness of suicidal thoughts and behaviours.
	■ Ask Bobbie to talk with the nurse if Sally or the others are considering self-harm.	Include the protective part of the system.

Issue identified: Risk for violence directed at others.
Expected outcome: Sally will exhibit control of aggressive behaviour.

Short-term goals	Interventions	Rationale
Sally will verbalise feelings of anger.	■ Teach difference between anger and aggression.	Knowledge increases compliance with expectations.
	■ Encourage Sally to list triggers to anger.	Increases self-knowledge.
	■ Encourage Sally to practise relaxation skills and engage in physical activity.	Provides outlets for the healthy expression of anger.

Issue identified: Disturbed personal identity as evidenced by presence of dissociation (alter states).
Expected outcome: Sally will eventually be able to reintegrate all personality states.

Short-term goals	Interventions	Rationale
Sally will identify two triggers of dissociation.	■ Teach relaxation techniques (i.e. focused breathing, progressive muscle relaxation).	Promotes coping with stress due to recognition of current problems.
	■ Have Sally make a list of warning signs of dissociation.	Conscious awareness helps counter dissociation.
	■ Encourage Sally to write in her journal after each dissociative episode.	Increases self-awareness.

Issue identified: The system of alters.
Expected outcome: The identification and mapping of alters.

Short-term goals	Interventions	Rationale
Mapping the system.	■ Work with Beth, as able, to map her system of alters.	To identify the alters, their reason for being and their function. Promotes trust and safety. Encourages the person's participation.

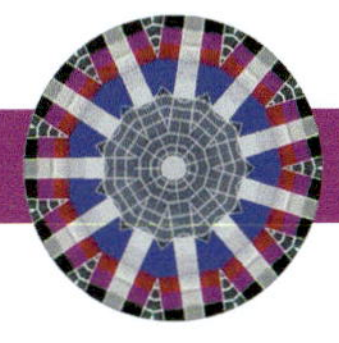

REFERENCES

Allan, L. A., & Woolfolk, R. L. (2010). Cognitive behavioural therapy for somatoform disorders. *Psychiatric Clinics of North America, 33*(3), 579–593.

American Psychiatric Association (APA). (2013). *Diagnostic and statistical manual of mental disorders* (5th ed., Text Revision). Washington, DC: APA Publishing.

Bass, C., & Halligan, P. (2014). Factitious disorders and malingering: Challenges for clinical assessment and management. *The Lancet, 383*, 1422–1432.

Bernstein, E. M., & Putnam, F. W. (1986). Development, reliability, and validity of a dissociation scale. *Journal of Nervous and Mental Disease, 174*, 727–735.

Bourne, E. J. (2011). *The anxiety and relaxation workbook* (5th ed.). Oakland, CA: New Harbinger Publications.

Browning, M., Fletcher, P., & Sharpe, M. (2011). Can neuroimaging help us to understand and classify somatoform disorders? A systematic and critical review. *Psychosomatic Medicine, 73*(2), 173–184.

Chu, J. A., Dell, P. F., Van der Hart, O., Cardeña, E., Barach, P. M., Somer, E., . . . Twombly, J. (2011). Guidelines for treating dissociative identity disorder in adults, third revision. *Journal of Trauma and Dissociation, 12*, 115–187.

Conwill, M., Oakley, L., Evans, K., & Cavanna, A. E. (2014). CBT-based group therapy for nonepileptic attacks and other functional neurological symptoms: A pilot study. *Epilepsy and Behaviour, 34*, 68–72.

Dorahy, M. J., Brand, B. L., Sar, V., Kruger, C., Stavropoulos, P., Martinez-Taboas, A., . . . Middleton, W. (2014). Dissociative identity disorder: An empirical overview. *Australian and New Zealand Journal of Psychiatry, 48*, 402–417. Retrieved from http://anp.sagepub.com/content/48/5/402.full.pdf+html

Kaplan, M. J., Dwivedi, A. K., Privitera, M. D., Isaacs, K., Hughes, C., & Bowman, M. (2013). Comparisons of childhood trauma, alexithymia, and defensive styles in patients with psychogenic non-epileptic seizures vs. epilepsy: Implications for the etiology of conversion disorder. *Journal of Psychosomatic Research, 75*, 142–146.

Keertesh, N., & Sharma, I. (2015). Impairment and classroom environment in adolescents with conversion disorder. *Journal of Indian Association for Child and Adolescent Mental Health, 11*, 99–120.

Klengel, T., Heck, A., Bruckl, T., Hennings, J. M., Menke, A., Czamara, D., . . . Ising, M. (2011). Somatization in major depression—clinical features and genetic associations. *Acta Pscyhiatrica Scandinavica, 124*, 317–328.

Kradin, R. L. (2011). Psychosomatic disorders: The canalization of mind into matter. *Journal of Analytical Psychology, 56*(1), 37–55.

Kregel, J., Meeus, M., Malfliet, A., Dolphens, M., Daneels, L., Nijs, J., & Cagnie, B. (2015). Structural and functional brain abnormalities in chronic low back pain: A systematic review. *Seminars in Arthritis and Rheumatism, 45*, 229–237.

Manning, M. L., & Manning, R. L. (2009). Convergent paradigms for visual neuroscience and dissociative identity disorder. *Journal of Trauma Dissociation, 10*(4), 405–419.

Precin, P. K., & Precin, P. (2011). Return to work: A case of PTSD, dissociative identity disorder, and satanic ritual abuse. *Work, 38*(1), 57–66.

Sadock, B. J., & Sadock, V. A. (2010). *Kaplan and Sadock's pocket handbook of clinical psychiatry* (5th ed.). Philadelphia, PA: Lippincott Williams & Wilkins.

Silber, T. J. (2011). Somatization disorders: Diagnosis, treatment, and prognosis. *Pediatrics in Review, 32*(2), 56–64.

Stein, D. J. (2013). Understanding somatic symptom disorder: The role of translational neuroscience. *Biological Psychiatry, 74*, 637–638.

Sullivan, K., Lange, R. T., & Dawes, S. (2005). Methods of detecting malingering and estimated symptom exaggeration base rates in Australia. *Journal of Forensic Neuropsychology, 4*, 49–70.

Zaidner, E., Sewell, R. A., Murray, E., Schiller, A., Price, B. H., & Cunningham, M. B. (2010). New-onset dissociative disorder after electroconvulsive therapy. *Journal of ECT, 26*(3), 238–241.

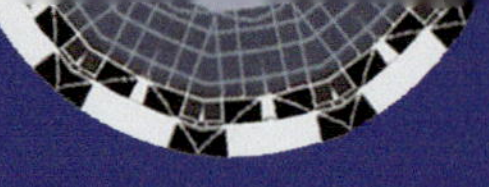

17 Eating disorders

RENEE BRIGHTON AND KATHERINE GILL

KEY TERMS

anorexia nervosa *371*
binge eating *372*
body size *374*
bulimia nervosa *372*
family dynamics *386*
neurotransmitter dysregulation *375*
obsessive rituals *371*
purge *372*
tube feedings *379*

LEARNING OUTCOMES

After completing this chapter, you will be able to:

1. Explain the roles of culture and biology in the development of eating disorders.
2. Compare and contrast the various theories for the causes of eating disorders.
3. Illustrate how psychological and social pressures can influence the course of eating disorders.
4. Assess individual and family problems of individuals with eating disorders.
5. Partner with individuals and their families in both the prevention and the treatment of eating disorders.
6. Formulate intermediate goals in the treatment of those with eating disorders.
7. Create a nursing plan of care for individuals with eating disorders and their families.

LIVED EXPERIENCE

My journey with anorexia has been a long, hard road that left me close to death on a few occasions. At one point I was given two weeks to live. The anorexia began following significant bullying at school. It started with me skipping lunch at school and going to the library to study to avoid the playground bullying. I then went to the library after school to study and skip afternoon tea at home. Very quickly I started to skip and hide all my meals to avoid eating, and I focused all my efforts on study. As my marks improved and my weight went down, I began to feel a sense of achievement that was very reinforcing for the anorexia. This was the start of a 30-year battle with anorexia. The development of my anorexia never had anything to do with body image, cultural ideals or catwalk models.

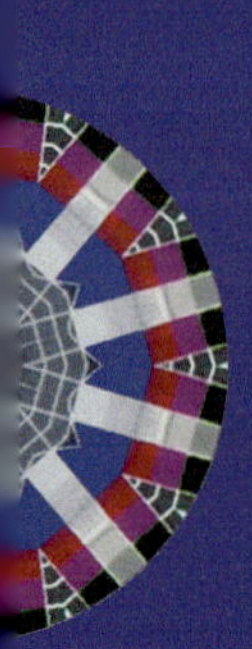

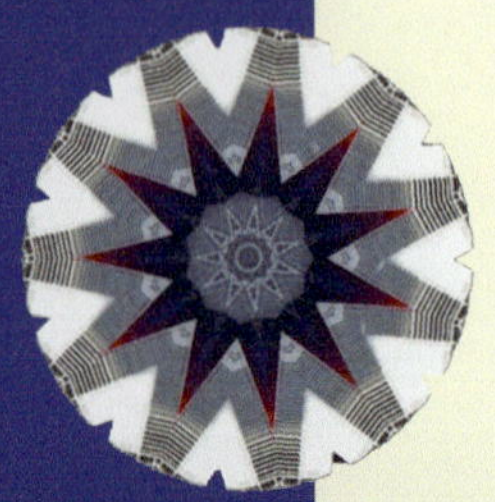

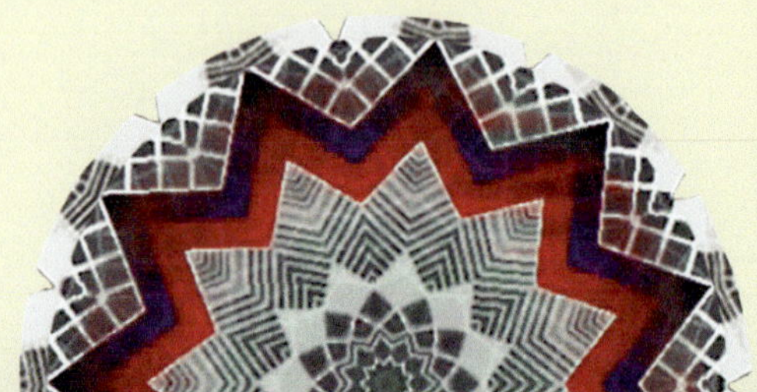

INTRODUCTION

For many, eating symbolises parental nurturing—the love and care that are the prototype of, and basis for, all future intimate relationships. For some, however, eating creates anxiety because of its association with unsatisfactory and unpleasant childhood interactions. Clearly, food and eating have greater individual and cultural meaning and importance than merely sustaining life. Disturbed eating patterns may develop as a means of coping with stress.

Eating disorders can be long-lasting, life-threatening and debilitating conditions. Eating disorders are characterised by disturbances of eating behaviours, and a core psychopathology in relation to food, eating and body image concerns (Hay et al., 2014). The two major eating disorders discussed in this chapter—anorexia nervosa and bulimia nervosa—create biological, psychological and social imbalances that interfere with the individual's functioning. Changes in biochemistry, metabolic rate, emotional state, family relationships and social status brought about by eating disorders can create depression, isolation and sometimes self-destructive behaviour.

Cultural stereotypes contribute to women's preoccupation with their bodies. Attractiveness is determined by how closely a woman's appearance matches the cultural ideal of thinness. Thus, identity and self-esteem are dependent on physical appearance. Being disgusted with one's flesh is the same as having an adversarial relationship with the body—a relationship that often results in eating disorders.

Practice example

A registered nurse who provides nursing support to an élite sports team is aware that a number of girls diet constantly, and several also throw up in the bathroom following lunch. She learns that boys on the team use vomiting as a means of 'making weight'. When the nurse takes her concerns to the head coach on the team to ask his support for an eating disorders educational program, he replies: 'This is a health problem, not an educational problem. We just don't have time for this kind of thing. It's really up to the parents.'

1. In your opinion, what is the responsibility of nurses in educating the public about prevention of eating disorders?
2. What kinds of information do people need in terms of eating and health?
3. What messages have you received that have helped or hindered you in developing healthy eating attitudes and behaviours?

People may starve or binge to make themselves unattractive, or may use food to cope with adverse life experiences. For individuals with a history of traumatic experiences, such as childhood sexual abuse, sexual assault or physical violence, eating disorders can develop as a coping mechanism. The experience of an eating disorder enables the person to avoid the pain, shame or guilt associated with the violation or traumatic experience.

Approximately 90 per cent of women and 25 per cent of men 'diet' at some time in their lives. Over half of teenage girls and one-third of teenage boys use unhealthy weight control behaviours, such as skipping meals, fasting, vomiting and abusing laxatives. Determining the incidence of anorexia and bulimia is difficult because of the secret nature of the illness. Many people will remain undiagnosed for over a decade, and will not present for treatment because of the shame associated with the illness.

It is estimated that the worldwide lifetime prevalence of anorexia nervosa for women is around 1 per cent and 0.5 per cent for men, and bulimia nervosa around 2 per cent in women and 0.5 per cent in men (Hay et al., 2014). Other eating disorders, such as binge-eating disorder (weekly frequency of binge eating and extreme weight-control behaviours) affect around 3 per cent of the population. These estimates may be low, because primary health care providers tend to be accurate in identifying anorexia and bulimia nervosa, but inaccurate in identifying atypical presentations (e.g. eating disorders not otherwise specified) (Allen, Fursland, Watson & Byrne, 2011).

Eating disorders have a high rate of comorbidity with other psychiatric illnesses. The most common comorbidity is depression and anxiety. Borderline personality disorder is also frequently observed, along with histories of childhood trauma. For those with anorexia or bulimia, the most frequently observed disorder is depression. In some cases, depression may be the result of abnormal eating and weight loss, causing starvation in the brain. In other cases, the depression is the primary disorder to which the eating disorder is a response, and yet for another group of people the depression and abnormal eating both are primary disorders.

Post-traumatic stress disorder (PTSD) can co-occur with eating disorders. Engagement in eating disorder behaviours may be a method of coping with the discomforting emotions and experiences correlated with PTSD. Therefore, the chances are great that an individual who has suffered traumatic events will develop an eating disorder as a means of controlling or coping with their circumstances.

There is a high prevalence of several anxiety disorders associated with eating disorders. Social phobias may occur in people with eating disorders, possibly in response to others' awareness of their abnormal eating behaviours and the shame associated with the eating disorder and/or body size and shape. Obsessive–compulsive symptoms are common, especially among people with anorexia. Obsessive–compulsive symptoms often continue even after weight is restored in anorexia. Panic attacks are likely when people with anorexia are prohibited from exercising their usual behaviour patterns. It is unclear whether these are primary disorders or are secondary to the eating disorders (Swanson, Crow, LeGrange, Swendsen & Merikangas, 2011). The following Evidence-based Practice discusses how constructively expressing distress and emotions helps in recovery from anorexia.

EVIDENCE-BASED PRACTICE

Life roles and anorexia nervosa

Suzy, age 45 years, is extremely thin and jogs for several hours every day to maintain her (under) weight. She is 174 centimetres tall, and weighs 55 kilograms. You work with her in an outpatient clinic where she is receiving counselling for marital problems.

Suzy has maintained the same weight since she was 17 years old. Her eating habits have always been tied to her weight. Since she was a teenager, Suzy has added extra distance to her running route, decreased her calorie count, or fasted whenever she was 500 grams over what she considered her ideal weight. The literature reports that adolescence is the peak time for developing eating disorders. Recovery studies will be most helpful to you in understanding and working with Suzy.

As indicated in the following research, many people, through therapy and close relationships, find non-bodily means to express their distress. Events such as committing to a relationship, forming a family, and settling into an identity and occupation all serve to provide a stable platform for overall functioning. Women's drive to be thin tends to decline as they age (conversely, men's drive to be thin tends to increase as they age), but Suzy does not follow that trend. You explore her life roles and what gives her a sense of positive identity (is she a wife, a mother, a daughter, a business executive, a socialite, a student, an athlete, etc.?). Identify the ways in which she expresses a range of negative emotions to determine whether your work with her needs to focus on problematic expression of feelings that may contribute to perpetuating her eating disorder.

You should base action on more than one study, but the following research would be helpful in this situation:

Jenkins, J., & Ogden, J. (2012). Becoming 'whole' again: A qualitative study of women's views of recovering from anorexia nervosa. *European Eating Disorders Review, 20*(1), e23–e31.

CRITICAL THINKING QUESTIONS

1. If Suzy has been maintaining an underweight condition since the age of 17, what are her chances for improvement?
2. What conditions would be necessary for improvement to take place?

Anorexia nervosa and bulimia nervosa are not single diseases but are syndromes with multiple predisposing factors and a variety of characteristics. Although the most obvious symptom is the eating problem, these disorders are not simply a matter of eating too much or too little. It is because of the complex interaction of biological, psychological, developmental, familial and sociocultural factors that certain people develop eating disorders. The focus of Mental Health in the Media, *Superstar: The Karen Carpenter Story,* is on how family dynamics and perception contribute to an eating disorder.

There is no clear-cut distinction between the two disorders, and they have many features in common. However, the traditional division of anorexia and bulimia is still appropriate until more is known about eating disorders. Body weight may be a significant distinguishing characteristic; people with anorexia are underweight, and people with bulimia are at normal or near-normal weight. About 30 per cent of people with bulimia have a history of anorexia. As many as 62 per cent of people with anorexia exhibit bulimic behaviours. Conversion from anorexia to bulimia may be a way of moving from a 'visible' to an 'invisible' eating disorder to deceive family, friends and health care providers. Thus, the two disorders can occur in the same person, or the person can go from one disorder to the other. Low social support during childhood seems to contribute to vulnerabilities to anorexia and bulimia; there are far more similarities than differences between the two diagnoses (Kim, Lim & Treasure, 2011). However, to help you understand the differences, the disorders have been separated in this chapter.

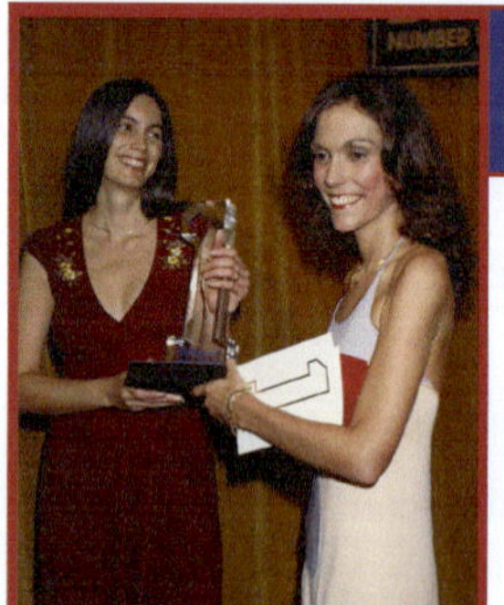

MENTAL HEALTH IN THE MEDIA

Superstar: The Karen Carpenter Story

This documentary investigates the story of Karen Carpenter's life with, and death from, anorexia. Karen's visibility as a popular singer only intensified certain difficulties many women experience in relation to their bodies. The short movie re-enacts her life not with actors but with Barbie dolls, and gives you a feel for a woman pulled apart at the seams by unrealistic expectations. Karen Carpenter's anorexia is a debilitating illness brought on by social, not disease, vectors. Clips of Karen and her brother Richard speaking to Herb Alpert, head of A&M Records, are alternated with black-and-white garish shots of food representing Karen's subjective view of the food she denies herself.

Her family's attempts to cure her anorexia make matters worse. Unable to comprehend the severity of the psychological disorder, Karen's family simply encourage, then force, Karen to eat, deepening the symbolic power of food in her mind. At one point, Richard callously worries that his sister's gaunt frame will ruin their careers, instead of focusing on her withering away. The pace of the film helps us contemplate the sympathetic view of a woman's tragic demise. Although she did not receive psychotherapy, Karen Carpenter began eating normally and was a healthy weight when she died suddenly of cardiac complications brought on by years of starvation.

Photo courtesy of Michael Ochs Archives/Getty Images.

ANOREXIA NERVOSA

Anorexia nervosa is a potentially life-threatening disorder characterised by extreme perfectionism, fear of gaining weight, weight loss, body image disturbances, strenuous exercising, food rituals, and reductions in heart rate, blood pressure, metabolic rate, and the production of oestrogen or testosterone. A well-known pioneer in the treatment of people with eating disorders, Hilde Bruch (1978), called anorexia nervosa 'the relentless pursuit of thinness'. DSM-5 Diagnostic Features defines the eating disorders.

Rigidity and over-control are the hallmarks of anorexia. To control themselves and their environment, these individuals develop rigid rules. Such rigidity often develops into **obsessive rituals**, particularly concerning eating and exercise. Cutting all food into a predetermined size or number of pieces, chewing all food a certain number of times, allowing only certain combinations of foods in a meal, accomplishing a fixed number of exercise routines, and having an inflexible pattern of exercises are rituals common to anorexic people. These rules and rituals help keep anxiety beyond conscious awareness. If the rituals are disrupted, the anxiety becomes intolerable. Paradoxically, all of these efforts to stay in control lead to out-of-control behaviours (Thornton, Dellava, Root, Lichtenstein & Bulik, 2011).

Many people with anorexia are hyperactive, and discover that exercising excessively is a way to increase their weight loss. Solitary running tends to be the exercise of choice, and there are often obsessional qualities to it. For example, people with eating disorders may believe that before they can eat they have to earn calories by exercising. Conversely, if they overeat, people with eating disorders may punish themselves and over-compensate for the calories eaten with excessive exercise. Excessive exercise signifies the triumph of the will over the body, and is an indication of psychopathology (Goodwin, Haycraft, Taranis, & Meyer, 2011).

Young women who experience anorexia often have a desperate need to please others. Their self-worth depends on responses from others rather than on their own self-approval. Thus, their behaviour is often over-compliant; they always try to meet the expectations of others in order to be accepted. They may overachieve in academic and extracurricular activities, but these accomplishments are usually an attempt to please parents rather than a source of self-satisfaction.

The following Lived Experience illustrates over-compliant behaviour and phobia related to weight gain.

DIAGNOSTIC FEATURES
Eating disorders

Anorexia nervosa: There are three essential features of anorexia nervosa: persistent energy intake restriction; intense fear of gaining weight or of becoming fat, or persistent behaviour that interferes with weight gain; and a disturbance in self-perceived weight or shape. The individual maintains a body weight that is below a minimally normal level for their age, sex, developmental trajectory and physical health. People with anorexia often feel hopeless, helpless and ineffective. They may have trauma histories or have experienced being controlled by others. Their refusal to eat may be an attempt to assert themselves and gain some control. As weight is lost, they are rewarded with praise, admiration and envy from their peers, which reinforces the restricted eating pattern.

Bulimia nervosa: There are three essential features of bulimia nervosa: recurrent episodes of binge eating; recurrent inappropriate compensatory behaviours to prevent weight gain; and self-evaluation that is unduly influenced by body shape and weight. To qualify for the diagnosis, the binge eating and inappropriate compensatory behaviours must occur, on average, at least once per week for three months.

LIVED EXPERIENCE

My anorexia was tied up in perfectionism, low self-worth, a reaction to trauma and a way of coping with loneliness. I was extremely fearful of consuming food and calories, and my mind kept telling me to do everything to avoid the intake of nutrition. This led me to hide food, pretend I was eating when I wasn't, and to secretly keep exercising my muscles while I was on medical bedrest in hospital. I was convinced the nurses were the enemies for pushing me to eat. I was isolated from the other patients and punished for not eating. This only exacerbated my feelings of isolation and low self-worth, and I experienced the force-feeding as re-traumatising. I was being held in hospital against my will. My parents didn't want me home until I was 'better', and I felt abandoned; the only friend I had was the voice in my head that would tell me what to do. The nurses seemed to enjoy punishing me, with the behavioural model previously used to get patients with anorexia to eat, which did me more harm than good.

The treatment for anorexia focused on weight gain and food, yet this was the thing I was most fearful of. I was being forced to confront my greatest fears that I had no desire to address at this point in time. What I really needed was for someone to work with me on building a meaningful life, where I didn't need the anorexia and low weight to feel good about myself. I needed help to build supportive connections with understanding people, yet I was isolated from everyone. When I was going through treatment, there were no mobile phones, internet or Facebook; it was just me and the voice in my head. I had to appease the voice in my head by doing 'right' or I had nothing.

BULIMIA NERVOSA

There is a cyclic behavioural pattern in **bulimia nervosa**. It may begin with skipping meals sporadically and overly-strict dieting or fasting. In an effort to refrain from eating, the person may use amphetamines, which can lead to extreme hunger, fatigue and low blood glucose levels. This restriction can lead to a period of **binge eating**, in which the person ingests huge amounts of food (about 14600 kilojoules) within a short time (about one hour). Binges can last up to eight hours, with consumption of around 50000 kilojoules. Binge eating usually occurs when the person is alone and at home, and most frequently during the evening. Many people with bulimia starve themselves throughout the day and come home and plan to only eat a small amount, which gradually develops into a larger binge, whereby the person feels they have lost all control over their eating. The next day the person feels very guilty, ashamed and disgusted with the large intake of food, and will again starve themselves, and so the cycle continues. The cycle may occur once or twice a month for some, and as often as 5 or 10 times a day for others. Although eating binges may involve any kind of food, they usually consist of junk foods, fast foods and high-calorie foods.

Following the binge, the person will attempt to **purge** the body of the ingested food. After excessive eating, many people with bulimia force themselves to vomit. They often also use laxatives and diuretics to further purge their bodies of the food. Some use as many as 50 to 100 laxatives per day. They may resort to syrup of ipecac to induce vomiting. Purging becomes a purification rite and a means of regaining self-control. Some describe it as feeling 'completely fresh and clean again'.

After the purging, the cycle begins all over again, with a return to strict dieting or fasting. Some people with bulimia eat highly nutritious meals when not binge eating/purging, to repair harm done to the body.

Restriction and purging begin as a way to eat and stay thin. Before long, the behaviour becomes a response to stress and a way to cope with negative feelings such as anger, anxiety and depression. For some, it is poor impulse control; for others, it is an expression of rebellion against family members.

People with bulimia may engage in sporadic excessive exercise, but they usually do not develop compulsive exercise routines. They are more likely to take drugs, such as amphetamines, to decrease their appetite, and alcohol to reduce their anxiety. Because their binges are often expensive, costing as much as $100 per day, they may resort to stealing food or money to buy the food. The binge–purge cycle can become so consuming that activities and relationships are disrupted. Many people with bulimia also have problems with excessive alcohol use, and may flip between alcohol use and bulimia as a response to manage stress. To keep the behaviour secret, the person often resorts to excuses and lies. The following Practice Example illustrates the progression of bulimia.

Practice example

Beth is a 17-year-old high school student who had been binge eating and purging with vomiting and the use of over-the-counter diuretics and laxatives for about two years. She was referred to the mental health centre by her school counsellor. Beth stated that her schoolfriends became concerned about her increasing preoccupation with purging, even after eating very small amounts of food. She was spending a lot of time in the girls' restroom; after lengthy bouts of self-induced vomiting following lunch, she was sometimes too exhausted to attend class. Her friends had been 'covering' for her, but had become frightened and went to the school nurse with their concerns.

Beth is of average weight for her height, but admitted that she would be quite heavy if she didn't purge herself of the large amounts of food she consumes in her room at night after her parents have gone to bed. 'I'm so embarrassed. My whole life is totally out of control,' she told the intake worker.

BIOPSYCHOSOCIAL THEORIES

Although many clinical studies have been published, the literature on eating disorders shows no theoretical consensus on aetiology and treatment. Psychoanalytic theory, family systems theory, cognitive behavioural theories, sociocultural theories and biological theories all contribute to an understanding of the development and dynamics of eating disorders. Only by understanding the interrelatedness of the factors in eating disorders can psychiatric nurses take a holistic approach to the care of affected individuals and their families. The interrelationship among these biopsychosocial theories is illustrated in Figure 17.1 ■.

Psychoanalytic theory

Since Freud first identified it as such, eating has been regarded as a critical aspect of psychological growth and development. An infant at the breast is already beginning to internalise a rudimentary understanding about life through the quality of the feeding experience.

Psychoanalytic theory considers eating disorders to be symptomatic of unconscious conflicts. Little attention is paid to biological or cultural factors. Psychoanalytic theory relates eating disorders to regression to pre-puberty and repudiation of developing sexuality. People with anorexia are thought to fear sexual maturity; the anorexia is seen as a rejection of the feminine form and a desperate attempt to regain the contours and dimensions of a pre-pubertal child.

In psychoanalytic thinking, compulsive overeating represents over-compensation for unmet oral needs during infancy. In other words, people eat to compensate for emptiness in their lives. Obesity is also thought to represent a defence against intimacy.

The basic treatment modality in the psychoanalytic model is long-term individual psychotherapy, sometimes accompanied by group therapy. The goal of therapy is the development of insight and subsequent 'working through' of underlying issues to resolve the unconscious conflicts manifested by the eating disorder.

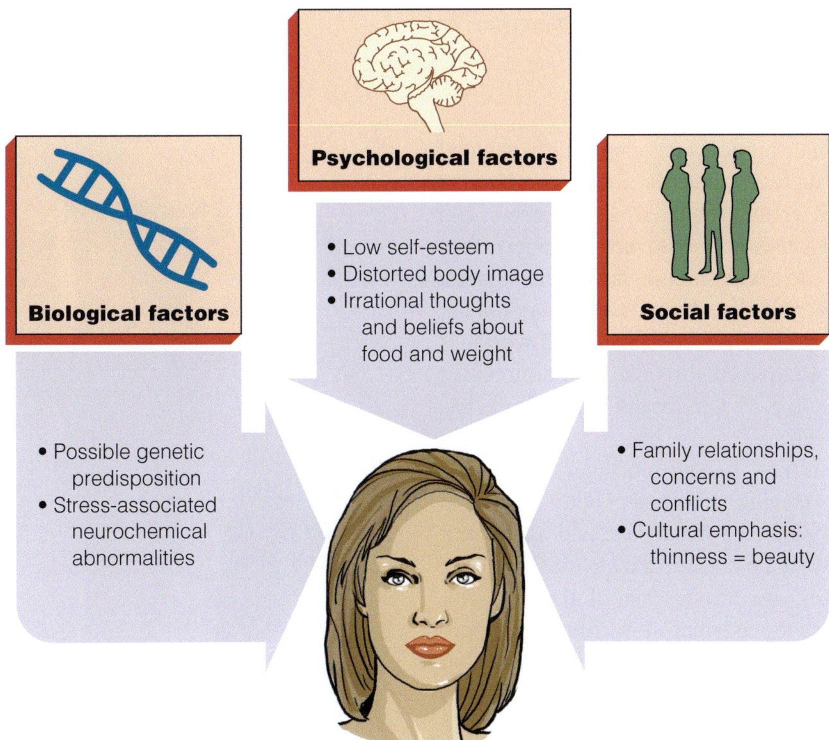

FIGURE 17.1 ■ Biopsychosocial factors in eating disorders. Nurses who understand the interplay among the biopsychosocial factors involved in eating disorders are able to take a holistic approach to nursing care.

Family systems theory

Most family theorists believe family issues are not specific to eating disorders. The family is viewed more as an enabler of the disorder than as a primary causative factor. Some people with eating disorders are survivors of childhood or adolescent sexual abuse, which may or may not have occurred within the family or extended family system.

As the result of anorexia, some families become enmeshed; that is, the boundaries between the members are weak, interactions are intense, dependency on one another is high, and autonomy is minimal. Everybody is involved in each member's concerns, and there is minimal privacy. The enmeshed family system becomes overprotective of the child, and the entire family system becomes preoccupied with food, eating and rituals involving meals. In contrast, current research indicates that families of people with bulimia are less enmeshed than those of people with anorexia. Family members tend to be isolated from one another, and eating behaviour may be an attempt to decrease feelings of loneliness and boredom.

Many families of individuals with eating disorders have difficulty with conflict resolution. An ethical or religious value against disagreements within the family supports the avoidance of conflict. When problems are denied for the sake of family harmony, they cannot be resolved, and growth of the family system is inhibited. The child with anorexia may protect and maintain the family unit. In some family systems, the parents avoid conflict with each other by uniting in a common concern for the child's welfare. In other family systems, the issues of marital conflict are converted into disagreements over how the child with anorexia should be managed. In both systems, the marital problems are camouflaged to prevent the disruption of the family unit.

Many families of people with eating disorders are achievement- and performance-oriented, with high ambition for the success of all family members. The family's focus on professional achievement as well as on food, diet, exercise and weight control may become obsessional.

Cognitive behavioural theories

Cognitive behavioural theories view eating disorders as learned behaviours based on irrational thoughts and beliefs. They focus on changing cognitive and behavioural responses to physiological, psychological and social stimuli. Insight into the nature of the maladaptive behaviour (the eating disorder) is integrated with new and healthier responses to emotional stimuli. Education about the psychology of compulsive behaviour and the physiological effects of starvation and purging behaviours is usually incorporated into the therapy. Other cognitive approaches include the correction of perceptual disturbances of body size, and the elimination of irrational thoughts and beliefs linking weight to self-esteem, such as 'I've gained a couple of kilos; I must run 5 kilometres today and eat nothing' or 'I'd rather be dead than fat.'

Cognitive behavioural therapy has been found to be a successful treatment method for reducing the symptomatology associated with bulimia nervosa, and to result in more rapid treatment than with interpersonal psychotherapy. These approaches are also useful in the treatment of binge-eating disorder (Jenkins & Ogden, 2011; Wilfley, Vannucci & White, 2010).

Sociocultural theory

In Australian society, female attractiveness is strongly equated with thinness. Models, actresses and the media glamourise extreme thinness, which is then equated with success and happiness. The cultural obsession with an extremely thin female body has led to widespread prejudice against overweight people. This prejudice has a significant impact on overall self-esteem and self-acceptance. Self-worth is enhanced for those who are judged attractive, and diminished for those deemed unattractive. Mental Health in the Media has an excellent example of this.

Body size and dieting behaviours can determine popularity with peers. Having a heavier body shape is associated with lower popularity for females, and adolescent males are less popular if they do not fit the male ideal in either direction—that is, if they are heavier and if they are not muscular or fit. When you consider how important peer relationships are at the adolescent stage of development, you can understand how problematic eating behaviours could result from the adolescent's attempts to cope with these pressures. Current examples of 'ideal' body types are presented in Figure 17.2 ■.

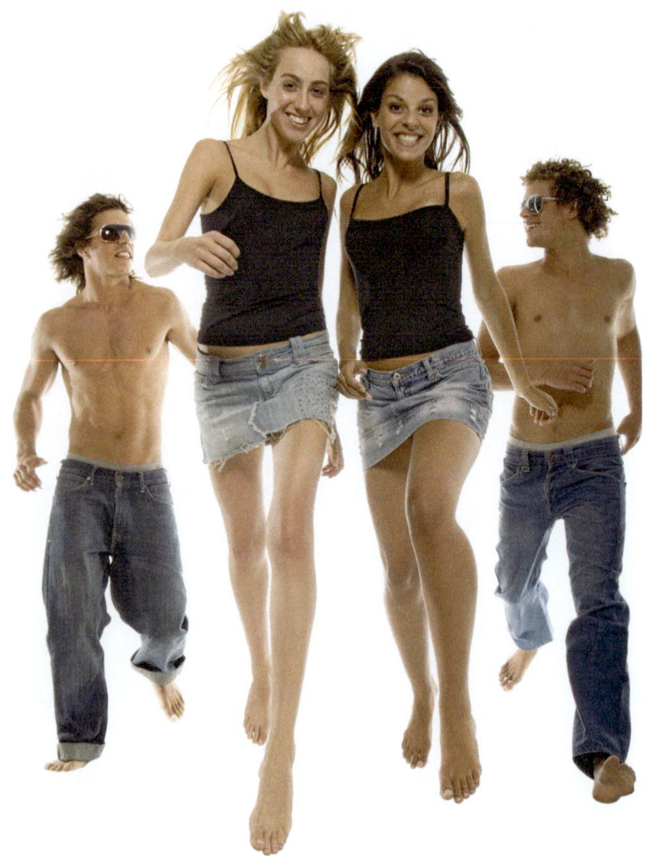

FIGURE 17.2 ■ Advertisements influence our views of attractiveness. The 'ideal' female body is excessively thin. The 'ideal' male body is well-toned with a slim waist and hips.
Photo courtesy of Win Initiative/Digital Vision/Getty Images.

Magazines marketed for adolescent women often present diet and weight control as the solutions for adolescent crises, and contain 90 per cent more articles and advertisements promoting dieting than do magazines read by young men. Frequent exposure to articles about dieting is significantly associated with lower self-esteem, depressed mood and lower levels of body satisfaction. Thus, the body becomes the central focus of existence, and self-esteem becomes dependent on the ability to control weight and food intake. This preoccupation with body image continues throughout women's lives. In fact, dieting and concerns about weight have become so pervasive that they are now the norm for Australian women (Smeets, Jansen & Roefs, 2011).

The ideal of male attractiveness in Australian society has been changing, and has contributed to an increase in eating disorders among men. The ideal male body is becoming more and more difficult for the average boy or man to attain. Little boys are being taught to base their self-esteem on strength and athleticism. Their action toys have washboard abdominal muscles. Men with eating disorders have an overwhelming fear of fatness and a desire to maintain a masculine appearance or shape. It is not uncommon to see males with eating disorders use anabolic steroids to improve muscle tone and build strength (Neri et al., 2011). Men also may be at risk of developing 'reverse-anorexia', where they see themselves as thin and weedy in build, and take anabolic steroids and protein supplements in an attempt to 'bulk up'.

In a sense, anorexia and bulimia could be considered culture-reactive syndromes in the Western world. Developing Cultural Competence discusses this further. Eating disorders are not solely a problem of specific cultural groups, however.

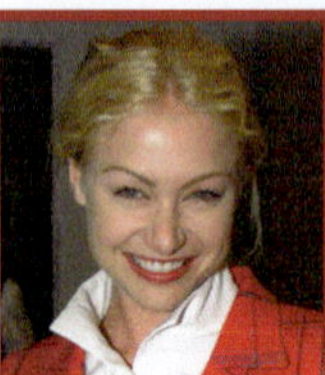

MENTAL HEALTH IN THE MEDIA
Portia de Rossi

Portia de Rossi is an actress who is lucky to be alive. Her memoir, *Unbearable lightness: A story of loss and gain*, deftly describes her years with anorexia and bulimia. She starved herself, over-exercised, and felt guilt and distress for eating a tub of yogurt. Portia limited herself to a total of 150 calories in a day, and at one point weighed 37 kilograms as a 167-centimetre tall woman. Hiding her true self (as a gay woman), and having distorted views of her body ('I just wanted my legs to be straight'), and needing to fit into smaller wardrobe sizes pushed her to protracted behavioural problems with food. Years of treatment taught her how to eat reasonably and restored her to a normal weight that she has since maintained. She is now healthy, has not reverted to bulimic behaviour, and is married to talk-show host Ellen Degeneres.

Photo courtesy © Reuters/CORBIS.

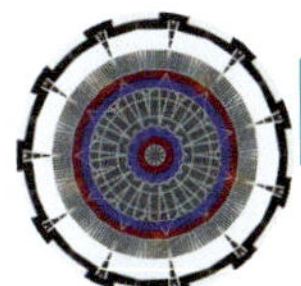

DEVELOPING CULTURAL COMPETENCE

When thin is in

What is considered attractive changes over time and from one culture to another. Attractiveness can also be inconsistent within a culture. Centuries ago, a large woman was considered to be the epitome of beauty, because it indicated that the family had enough money to be well-fed, and enough social status to be spared hard labour. The ideal of attractiveness in Australian society has been fairly consistent for decades—thin—and has contributed to an increase in eating disorders.

Television, magazines, movies and advertisements all define beauty. Women tend to be targeted for messages that, because thin is good, there is no real lower limit on how thin you should be. This, of course, leads to unhealthy and dangerous levels of calorie deprivation and starvation. Men are targeted for being in shape—not too thin, not too heavy—in messages about body building, weight lifting or muscle toning. The 'ideal' male body is one with well-developed muscles on the chest, arms and shoulders, and a slim waist and hips.

Eating disorders tend to occur predominantly in industrialised, developed countries, and less often in traditional societies. For example, Native Canadians (Ojibway-Cree) tend to show a preference for heavier body types than the Euro-Canadian population does. In the Caribbean, the incidence of anorexia among the majority Black population is negligible. African-American women and men in North America are more positive about higher weights in women than are Euro-American women and men. Typically, Asian-American and Latino women were less likely to describe themselves as fat, were less dissatisfied with their body size, and were less likely to diet.

You may see the incidence of eating disorders change, however, as cultures around the world are exposed to each other through media, travel and social media, and become more Westernised. Recently a cultural shift has been noted. In the shift, Asian and Latino women are becoming less satisfied with their bodies because their media, similar to the Anglo media, now promotes thin bodies as ideal for women.

CRITICAL THINKING QUESTIONS

1. How would you initiate a conversation about the culture of ideal beauty with a person in your care?
2. How would you support a person to develop a positive sense of self-worth and identity, to find valued occupations and life roles that provide meaning and purpose in life, so they are less reliant on the eating disorder.

Negative body image and body dissatisfaction lead to problematic eating behaviours. It seems that, culture notwithstanding, negative interactions about body size can create stress and challenges that affect eating behaviours (Rivas, Bersabé, Jiméne & Berrocal, 2010).

Biological theory

Family risk studies show that relatives of people with eating disorders are 5 to 10 times more likely to develop an eating disorder. It appears that in anorexia, the more severe the disorder, the more likely a strong genetic predisposition. Twin studies for eating disorders show that the concordance rate (occurring together) for twins is 55 per cent to 60 per cent. These data suggest that there may be a genetic predisposition (Slane, Burt & Klump, 2011).

Genetic research focuses on behavioural, neurobiological and temperamental variables that may represent core features of these disorders. These features include perfectionism, orderliness, a low tolerance for new situations, low self-esteem and overall high anxiety. If an individual has a high genetic risk, they might develop an eating disorder even if they do not live in a culture that stresses dieting and thinness (Seal, 2011).

Recently, **neurotransmitter dysregulation** has been considered to be a contributing factor in eating disorders, particularly serotonin (5-HT). Being full of food to the point of satisfaction is referred to as *satiety* (Frank, 2013). Normally, a low level of 5-HT decreases a person's satiety, and thereby increases food intake. In contrast, a high level of 5-HT increases satiety, and thereby decreases food intake. Carbohydrates (CHOs) are involved in the synthesis of 5-HT by increasing tryptophan, the precursor of 5-HT. The neurotransmitter hypothesis of bulimia is that recurrent binge episodes may result from a deficiency in 5-HT and low satiety levels (Avena & Bocarsly, 2012). The tendency of people with bulimia to binge on high-CHO foods may be a reflection of the body's adaptive attempt to increase 5-HT levels.

Other neurotransmitters affect eating behaviour. Norepinephrine (NE) and neuropeptide Y (NPY) increase eating behaviour, while dopamine (DA) suppresses food intake (Frank, 2013). DA agonists such as amphetamines and cocaine are appetite suppressants.

Endogenous opioids, such as endorphins, are associated with food intake and mood. Opioids increase food intake and enhance positive mood states; therefore, insufficient levels of endogenous opioids cause decreased food intake and depressed mood. It has been found that underweight people have significantly lower levels of endorphins compared to healthy volunteers (Tortorella et al., 2014). When the person's weight is returned to normal levels, the endorphin level is also within normal limits.

Biological factors, sociocultural factors, and intrapersonal or interpersonal conflicts cannot—and should not—be dealt with separately. The interaction of these factors is extremely important. For example, people experiencing severe obesity may experience shame and helplessness as they attempt to cope with fears of rejection and loss of love. These feelings can lead to compensatory overeating, which in turn can create interpersonal conflict with family members. The person may withdraw from others, thus reinforcing the feelings of rejection and increasing social isolation.

LIVED EXPERIENCE

I became very frightened of the medical profession. I was always scared that if I reached out for help I would be put into hospital and forced to gain weight. I was scared they would take away my control and leave me powerless. No matter how sick I was, I would avoid the medical profession at all costs. After 10 years of avoiding the medical profession, I got to the point where I had become extremely weak and ill, and could no longer study or work.

My day consisted of going to the gym for about four hours in the morning, and then spending the rest of the day in bed. Eventually, I got to the point where I couldn't drive, as I was frequently passing out, due to my dangerously low blood pressure. Once I realised I needed help, and had got to the point where I was ready to get help, a new battle began. I couldn't find anyone who could readily address all my needs. I found that I was too medically unwell for psychiatric treatment, and too mentally unwell for physical health care. I found I was slipping through the gaps in the system. Everywhere I reached out, I found there were closed doors where people and services didn't have the capacity to deal with the complex needs of anorexia and all the other complications I presented with. This made me feel more helpless and abandoned, and I became sicker and sicker, and more and more suicidal while desperately looking for care.

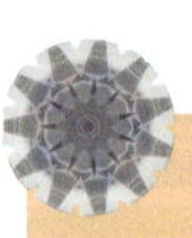

NURSING PROCESS
The person with anorexia nervosa

The following section discusses the specific steps of the nursing process for people with anorexia nervosa. Be aware of your own potential reactions to individuals with eating disorders. Self-aware nurses recognise their own emotional reactions to people with eating disorders, and view those peoples' possible self-absorption as a symptom of the disorder. The Self-awareness feature will help you assess your reactions.

Assessment

When completing assessments with people with dramatic weight loss or gain, you must not lose sight of the fact that both can be caused by physical conditions. Certain illnesses must be ruled out before an eating disorder diagnosis can be made. Wasting conditions, such as advanced cancer, tuberculosis,

SELF-AWARENESS
Possible reactions to working with people with eating disorders

In order to explore your reactions to people with eating disorders, determine which, if any, of the following apply to you.

- You feel exhausted and defeated by the structured demands of the individual's care plan.
- You identify with the individual because of your own personal body image concerns.
- You feel overprotective of the individual, and allow a coalition between yourself and the person to form.
- You feel annoyance and anger toward the individual, and are unnecessarily rough during physical care.
- You have difficulty recognising that the individual's symptoms are as serious as those of a person experiencing psychosis.
- You fail to monitor the individual's mealtime and after-meal behaviours, allowing the individual to continue maladaptive patterns of coping.
- You allow the individual to re-enact power struggles from home, such as those about food, weight and exercising.
- You believe that the individual is deliberately engaging in maladaptive coping behaviours to upset the staff and family.
- You feel repelled by the individual's eating habits or the appearance of their body.
- You feel hopeless and are affected by the individual's despondency.

AIDS, hyperthyroidism and pyloric obstruction, and drug use, must be considered when weight loss is a feature. Rapid weight gain can result from a brain tumour, an endocrine disorder, or as a side-effect of medications.

It is important to note that people with anorexia may not have any significant weight loss. It is imperative for nurses to assess how the person feels about food, weight loss and their self-image. After the presence of an eating disorder is established, you will assess the person using the following subjective and objective data.

Subjective data

People with anorexia nervosa perceive themselves as overweight, no matter how thin they may be. However emaciated their bodies, they can always find some body part they believe is fat. They are preoccupied with thoughts of food, and simultaneously obsessed with rigidly controlling their own intake. They may collect cookbooks, cook prodigious amounts of food, and insist that others eat while not taking a morsel for themselves. They may be fearful of even the slightest weight gain, and view with suspicion anyone who encourages them to eat.

Another preoccupation is with exercise. It is not uncommon for people with anorexia to engage in extremely lengthy sessions of aerobic exercise sessions, or run, bike or walk to excess, even when in an emaciated condition or suffering from severe physical injuries, including fractured bones. They push themselves to greater and greater levels of endurance, and deprive themselves of sleep as a measure of self-control.

People with anorexia frequently deny that they have a weight problem. They insist they have never felt better, and simply wish to be left alone about food. They report feeling strong, powerful and good as a result of self-denial. They report feeling guilty, self-indulgent and weak when they eat. They therefore resist treatment, although they may admit to feeling isolated and lonely, and may even describe themselves as exhausted with the effort it takes to achieve the perfection they seek. They tend to have difficulty accepting nurturing behaviour from others, and therefore have difficulty forming therapeutic alliances. They report a loss of interest in sex, but do not perceive this as a problem.

Objective data

People with anorexia usually experience a weight loss of 25 per cent of their original body weight, but a loss as high as 50 per cent is possible. People with anorexia may also fail to gain weight as a teenager and maintain a low weight to adulthood. Amenorrhoea is extremely common, and is thought to be related to the degree of stress the woman is experiencing, the percentage of body fat lost, and altered hypothalamic function. With low oestrogen levels, these young women are at higher risk for osteopenia leading to osteoporosis. This is a serious medical complication with no known effective treatment.

The person with advanced anorexia is emaciated, with sunken eyes and a skeletal appearance. In very young individuals, growth failure may be present. Lanugo growth (babylike, fine hair) on the face, extremities and trunk may occur. Other physical symptoms include bradycardia, hypotension, arrhythmias, delayed gastric motility, and a hypothyroid-like state manifested by dry skin, listlessness and dry hair that falls out at a higher-than-normal rate. Peripheral oedema may be a feature in advanced starvation. Laboratory tests may reveal leukopenia, anaemia, low serum potassium and elevated blood urea nitrogen (BUN). There may also be low thyroid levels and elevated serum cortisol.

Nursing implications

Once the assessment process is completed, determine appropriate nursing care.

Imbalanced nutrition: less than body requirements

By the time people with anorexia are seen in treatment, their physical condition is often so deteriorated from self-imposed starvation that it becomes the priority for nursing care. Life-threatening malnourishment is seen in 5 per cent to 20 per cent of these people. Death may occur from malnutrition, infection or cardiac abnormalities related to electrolyte imbalances. Intravenous therapy, tube feedings and total parenteral hyperalimentation (TPH) are required in cases of medical emergency.

Another medical emergency that does occur in people with eating disorders is suicidal ideation. Rates of death by suicide among individuals with eating disorders are elevated compared to other mental health disorders, including depression bipolar disorder and schizophrenia (Chesney, Goodwin & Fazel, 2014). The often-relentless thoughts about food and appearance, and the resulting social isolation and disconnection from others, are key risks for suicide.

The person's preoccupation with food, evidenced by reading recipes, discussing food and preparing food for others, is due to suppression and sublimation of their own hunger. Over-exercising creates even more extreme nutritional deficits. In those with anorexia who also purge by vomiting or using laxatives, nutritional status is further endangered, and they are at a significant risk of heart attack.

People in a state of starvation experience hormonal, metabolic and emotional changes. Some of those changes are manifested in amenorrhoea or delay of onset of menses, ketosis, severe vitamin deficiencies, depressed immune response, lethargy, weakness and irritability—conditions that also vitally affect the nursing therapeutic relationship.

Ineffective individual coping

People experiencing anorexia nervosa may demonstrate impairment of adaptive behaviours, such as self-care in activities of daily living. Over time, they may lose cooking skills, or they may never develop basic skills to shop, prepare and cook meals. Due to fatigue, they have difficulty meeting daily demands, and role performance may be affected. Their preoccupation with the pursuit of thinness deprives them of the energy necessary for adaptive behaviour, and distracts them from interest in role fulfilment. The quest for thinness is the entire focus of their lives.

In addition, developmental issues—such as the desire for independence and the longing for dependence—combine with the traditionally adolescent resentment of authority to influence the quality and character of the nursing therapeutic relationship. Family enmeshment and unwillingness to allow the person to separate contribute to self-doubt and the inability to accept responsibility for self.

Disturbed body image

People with anorexia nervosa are unable to make realistic appraisals of their own body size, although they can accurately evaluate the size of others. They drastically underestimate their own bodily needs, even in the face of overwhelming evidence of malnutrition. Profound disturbances in accurate perception of size and intense denial indicate a poor prognosis. The person's body image disturbance is often the source of conflict in family and therapeutic relationships.

Chronic low self-esteem

The person with anorexia may lack of confidence in themselves, and feelings of inferiority are main factors in the disorder. Their self-deprivation and self-denial make them feel powerful and superior to others who cannot muster such profound self-control. The quest for perfection is never-ending, but they can never achieve a level of thinness that is satisfying; there are always a few more kilograms to shed. They often present the picture of helpfulness in contrast to the seemingly more withdrawn people with other mental illnesses.

As a result, newly graduated nurses may have difficulty assessing the severity of the illness accurately.

The low self-esteem of people with anorexia stems from unrealistic expectations by the self and others, complicated by unmet dependency needs. The clinical picture is further complicated because cultural norms of thinness reinforce maladaptive behaviour. The therapeutic nursing relationship is affected by the extreme difficulty these people may have in accepting positive feedback, and by their non-participation in self-care and everyday activities. Their preoccupation with their appearance and with others' perceptions of them may be irritating to other people undergoing treatment. The therapeutic relationship is also affected by the person's need to control versus their need to accept help.

Planning and implementation

When a person meets the criteria for a diagnosis of anorexia nervosa, effective nursing intervention is directed towards ensuring that the person will not die, and helping them to learn more effective ways of coping with the demands of life. A variety of approaches, including behavioural, insight-oriented and cognitive therapies, may be useful; pharmacological therapy may be used also. As a feature of behavioural therapy, a behavioural contract can be very effective. An explanation of how to develop and use behavioural contracts is in Chapter 25.

Symptoms can be extreme and dangerous with this disorder. Protection and improvement may require more intensive and constant treatment. For people who are in advanced stages of the disorder, inpatient treatment is indicated. Box 17.1 lists behavioural characteristics identified by Love and Seaton (1991) and White and Litovitz (1998) that indicate the need for hospitalisation. The suggestions in these classic references are still used today in clinical settings. Recovery from eating disorders is a long process. Individuals with anorexia are ambivalent about treatment, and often terminate treatment early. Symptoms correlated with early termination include higher levels of weight concerns, greater maturity fears and impulsivity. For those who continue treatment, about 40 per cent recover, and the rest experience a chronic course, some with fewer symptoms and some with the same symptoms.

Box 17.1 Criteria for inpatient admission

Inpatient admission is recommended for people with eating disorders who have the following:

- suicidal or severely out-of-control behaviour (self-mutilating; using large amounts of laxatives, emetics and diuretics; using street drugs)
- loss of 25–30 per cent of body weight, resulting in severe emaciation
- cardiac arrhythmias
- fluid and electrolyte imbalances
- the need for more intensive inpatient contacts and therapy if outpatient treatment has proved insufficient
- the need for extensive diagnostic evaluation to rule out comorbidities.

Managing nutrition

To establish adequate eating patterns and fluid and electrolyte balance, assume a calm, matter-of-fact attitude and a positive expectation of the person. Meeting minimal nutritional goals, with the overall goal of gradual weight restoration, is non-negotiable. A person who has been significantly restricting their diet may start with a caloric intake of 5000 to 6200 kJ/day and will increase to around 8400 kJ/day range. Changing the eating pattern to a healthier one (called *graded nutritional therapy*) involves timing, education and reinforcement. Your Intervention Strategies lists guidelines for graded nutritional therapy.

Nursing interventions may include tube feedings or intravenous therapy, which are administered in a nonjudgmental manner. Weighing the person daily, recording

YOUR INTERVENTION STRATEGIES
Guidelines for graded nutritional therapy

Strategy	Rationale
Acknowledge fears of weight gain.	Reassures the person that fears are expected and not unique.
Collaborate with the person and dietician to plan a flexible program for gradual nutrition.	Enlists the person as an active participant in treatment.
Adopt a matter-of-fact, consistent and nonjudgmental attitude.	Conveys your confidence and acceptance of the person.
Collaborate with nutritionists for nutrition supplement options.	Plans the introduction of nutrition because of disruption in the normal flora of the gastrointestinal (GI) tract.
Introduce dietary content slowly.	Gives the person a chance to equilibrate to the psychological impact of eating, as well as allowing the GI tract to accommodate relatively novel items.
Acknowledge that re-introducing food will cause stomach discomfort and pain, but this will dissipate over time.	Helps encourage the person to persist with the re-feeding process.
Support the person during sensations of fullness and bloating; teach that these are normal and transient feelings.	Readjusts the person's GI tract to unaccustomed intake.
Encourage the expression of feelings of loss of control. Acknowledge that this will pass, and the person will not continue gaining weight.	Reassures people, upon resuming adequate intake, that their fear 'losing control' and 'becoming fat' is unfounded in the long-term.
Monitor fluid and electrolyte intake and output, vital signs, body temperature and mood. Prebiotics and probiotics (see your nursing fundamentals texts) will ease the transition.	Provides accurate records that can be acted on if there are changes in the person's vital signs and/or mental state.

intake and output, observing the person during meals, and observing bathroom behaviour may be necessary if you suspect the person is discarding food or inducing vomiting. Weighing should be done 'blinded' (without the person seeing the number on the scale), so as to reduce the person's distress of weight gain. Avoid discussing weight with the person and engaging in conversations about weight. Avoid complimenting the person for gaining weight; always maintain a neutral stance. Avoid discussing food, recipes, restaurants and eating, because these conversations reinforce disorder-related behaviours. Providing a pleasant mealtime environment and adopting realistic expectations of how much the person will eat are critically important aspects of nursing care. People find frequent small meals more acceptable than three large meals. Setting a time-limit of about a half-hour is a good way to forestall mealtime 'marathons'—protracted meals during which the person eats little.

Mandatory **tube feedings**, a controversial intervention, may be the therapeutic regimen in some treatment centres. Although tube feedings will manage a dangerously low weight with perilously disordered electrolytes, tube feedings have a conditioned effect that must be taken into account. (Chapter 25 discusses conditioned responses.) Tube feedings do give a message—that is, taking in calories through food is beneficial to overall health. On the other hand, tube feedings can also deliver the message that the problem is too severe for the person to overcome with voluntary action. This message can be demoralising to the person, and may be further amplified by negative associations with treatment providers because of the unpleasant aspects of the experience. For many people, tube feeding is a necessary part of re-introducing nutrition when the person cannot voluntarily eat.

Education about adequate eating patterns is a necessary part of discharge planning.

Interdisciplinary planning conferences

A target weight is usually chosen by the treatment team in collaboration with a dietician. The target weight for discharge from treatment is usually 90 per cent of the average weight for the person's age and height. Discharge planning can include advice about self-help groups, such as the Butterfly National Support Line and Web Counselling Service. The websites for these self-help groups are included in Collaborative Care.

COLLABORATIVE CARE

Family-based therapies

Friends and family members of people with eating disorders are often at a loss as to how to help. Partnering with family and friends is an important part of family-based therapies. Family-based therapies are often the first line of treatment for children and young adults with eating disorders (Chen et al., 2016):

Family-based therapies are intensive outpatient treatment approaches that put parents at the centre of the person's treatment. Treatment focuses on: (1) weight restoration, (2) restoring control of eating, and (3) returning to normal adolescent development. The main difference between family-based therapies and traditional treatments is that parents are empowered and seen as a key resource in assisting their loved one to recover. There is the belief that the person with the eating disorder is not to blame for any challenging behaviours they may exhibit, but rather that these symptoms are mostly outside of the person's control, thus externalising the illness.

Core to family-based therapies:

- The whole family is involved in treatment, as the family is viewed as the best resource to help bring about recovery.
- In order for attitudes and behaviours to change, everyone must be willing to do things differently. No one is to blame for the development of the eating disorder.
- The person with the disorder must want to make their own change.
- The family must also change to accommodate the person's growth.
- The family must avoid arguments about weight and food, although early on in the process the parents are charged with responsibility of re-feeding their child and containing the eating disorder behaviours.
- The family should express love, appreciation and affection, both verbally and physically.
- The family should work together around the issue of the person's food refusal; each person in the family is assigned a specific role in helping the person.
- When the person is more stable, the family should encourage them to take more control over their eating patterns.

Resources

National

Butterfly National Support Line and Web Counselling Service
Telephone: 1800 334673
Email: support@thebutterflyfoundation.org.au
Website: www.thebutterflyfoundation.org.au/web-counselling

New South Wales

The Butterfly Foundation
Address: 103 Alexander St, Crows Nest, NSW 2065
Support line: 1800 33 4673
Telephone: 02 9412 4499
Fax: 02 8090 8196
Email: support@thebutterflyfoundation.org.au
Website: www.thebutterflyfoundation.org.au
Email: support@thebutterflyfoundation.org.au

Centre for Eating and Dieting Disorders (CEDD)
An academic and service support centre based in Sydney.
Telephone: 02 9515 6040
Fax: 02 9515 6442
Email: info@cedd.org.au
Website: www.cedd.org.au

(*continued*)

COLLABORATIVE CARE (*continued*)

Victoria

Eating Disorders Victoria (EDV)

A non-profit organisation which aims to support those affected by eating disorders and to better inform the community about disordered eating. The EDV helpline operates from Monday to Friday from 9.30am to 5pm.

Telephone: 1300 550 236

Email: help@eatingdisorders.org.au

Website: www.eatingdisorders.org.au

Queensland

Eating Disorders Association Inc Queensland

A non-discriminatory, non-profit organisation. The Eating Disorders Association is funded by the Mental Health Branch of Disability Services Queensland, to provide information, support and referral services for the state of Queensland, Australia.

Telephone: 07 3394 3661

Fax: 07 3394 3663

Email: admin@eda.org.au

Website: www.eda.org.au

Isis The Eating Issues Centre

Isis works with people over 17 with serious eating issues such as anorexia, bulimia and compulsive eating.

Telephone: 07 3848 3377

Fax: 07 3844 6466

Email: info@isis.org.au

Website: www.isis.org.au

Western Australia

Women's Health Works

A non-profit community organisation that provides a range of education, information and support services to women, including self-help groups for people experiencing an eating disorder.

Telephone: 08 9300 1566

Fax: 08 9300 1699

Email: info@womenshealthworks.org.au

Website: www.womenshealthworks.org.au

ARAFMI Mental Health Carers & Friends Association Incorporated

A non-profit community-based organisation that provides information and support for families and friends of people with mental health issues, including family support counselling, support group program advocacy, respite and community education.

Telephone: 08 9427 7100 or 1800 811 747 (rural free call)

South Australia

Centacare: PACE

An organisation that supports individuals living with panic anxiety, obsessive–compulsive and eating disorders, and those who support them. Services include telephone support, face-to-face counselling and referral pathways.

Telephone: 08 8159 1400

Website: www.centacare.org.au/OurServices/HealthWellbeing/

Eating Disorders Association of South Australia (EDASA)

A non-government, not-for-profit incorporated association based in South Australia, providing practical advice, empathic support and guidance for those affected by eating disorders in South Australia.

Email: info@eatingdisorderssa.org.au

Website: www.edasa.org.au

Tasmania

ARAFMI Tasmania

Telephone: 03 6331 4486

Fax: 03 6334 8719

Email: north@arafmitas.org.au

Website: www.arafmitas.org.au

Northern Territory

Top End Mental Health Services (TEMHS)

Telephone: 08 8999 4988

Fax: 08 8999 4999

Website: www.health.nt.gov.au

Facilitating coping

The best way to promote individual coping is by involving people in their own treatment planning. Self-determination fosters adaptive coping mechanisms in the individual's day-to-day hospital experiences; this process carries over to daily life outside the hospital setting.

Although trust may be difficult to establish with people with anorexia, it is the basis for all therapeutic relationships. Being honest, available and matter-of-fact helps establish trust, and encourages people to express their feelings. If necessary, allow the individual to assume a dependent role at first, but, as trust is developed and physical condition improves, encourage them to take more responsibility for themselves. Participating in the planning of care enables the individual to enhance their decision-making capabilities. Provide flexibility in activities of daily living, type and timing of exercise, and choice of occupational and recreational therapy activities. This autonomy increases the person's sense of responsibility.

Giving individuals the opportunity to practise problem-solving may lead to power struggles if the nurse finds themselves disagreeing with a person's choices. Demonstrate positive belief in their ability to regain healthy functioning and a willingness to tolerate 'mistakes'. The treating team must set firm and clear limits, however, to provide the secure environment in which the person is enabled to learn more effective coping behaviours. Another goal is to help people identify ways to feel in control other than by the behaviours associated with their disorder.

Individuals may need to explore their extreme fears of gaining weight before they can relinquish maladaptive behaviours. It is helpful to explore with people their feelings about their family, their role in the family, and their autonomy within the family system.

LIVED EXPERIENCE

Recovery from an eating disorder is hard. People often think that when a person has gained weight, the person is recovered. I find that the weight gain is only a very small part of recovery. For some people, weight gain may mean they are developing another disorder, such as bulimia or binge-eating disorder. A lot of people switch from one disorder to another. People would compliment me on gaining weight and think I was better. In actual fact I was feeling a million times worse, and felt I had gained weight for other people and not for myself. Every time someone complimented me on gaining weight, my head would be telling me off, telling me that I was so fat that people were noticing and that I needed to lose more weight. I felt like a failure for giving in and not being strong enough to keep my weight deathly low.

I would often get suicidal. Sometimes I wanted to starve myself to death. Other times I just wanted to kill myself. The starvation increased my depression. I was so low in energy; I didn't have the strength to keep fighting to live or the strength to keep fighting the eating disorder.

I began to recover when I had a reason to live; when I was able to hold down a valuable and meaningful job, and when I had friends who believed in me. Recovery for me was not about eating and gaining weight; recovery was having a purpose in life, a reason to keep myself alive, and a reason to eat and have the energy to do what I wanted to do.

Many people with eating disorders struggle with self-destructive thoughts, impulse control, emotional regulations and interpersonal skills. Dialectical behaviour therapy is often used to help people with eating disorders manage distressing thoughts without resorting to self-harm and destructive eating disorder behaviours. '*Urge surfing*' is important to address after meals, when people are at their most vulnerable.

Enhancing body image

To help people regain an accurate perception of their body size and nutritional needs, first encourage them to express their feelings about body size. An example is shown in the Communication feature, below. Reframe any misperceptions by using language that emphasises health, strength and evaluation. For example, if the person says 'My thighs are huge', reply 'Your thighs are becoming stronger now that you're gaining weight. Healthy muscles are rounded and firm, like yours.' With practice, people have been shown to replace negative thinking with positive self-talk. Teach and reinforce this skill, and help them practise it. For example, ask the individual to make three positive statements (positive affirmations) about their bodies each day.

You could also use a more structured tool such as the one illustrated in Figure 17.3 ■. In addition, you can access BodyImage, a software program for the assessment of body image disturbance. Any communication about how people perceive their bodies is useful in treatment, because it removes the hidden, shameful aspects of the perception and allows open discussion.

When individuals share feelings honestly, show improvement in accurate perception of body image, or demonstrate healthier eating behaviours, reinforce their efforts through verbal recognition. It is also useful to examine with people the ways in which the fashion and advertising industries support unrealistic cultural norms of excessive thinness incompatible with healthy functioning.

Improving self-esteem

Help people re-examine negative feelings about themselves and identify their positive attributes. Encourage them to record in a diary those thoughts that are difficult to share directly. Be nonjudgmental in your acceptance of negative feelings, and positively reinforce the honest expression of all feelings. Encouragement is particularly important when people experiment with independently made decisions, even when the outcomes are not entirely positive. The individual may need to interpret each experience as worthwhile. Emphasise the feeling of control gained through independent decision-making.

COMMUNICATION

Woman with anorexia nervosa

Woman: [tearfully] 'My doctor says I have to eat and gain weight, but I still have this little fat tummy.'

Nurse response #1: 'Tell me what you are feeling right now.' *RATIONALE:* Asking the woman to focus on her feelings assists her in becoming more self-aware. Obtaining additional subjective data from the woman enables you to better understand her.	**Nurse response #2:** 'It sounds as though you feel caught in the middle of the doctor's expectations and your own.' *RATIONALE:* Nonjudgmental acknowledgment of the woman's conflict shows empathy, and encourages her to clarify the dilemma from her doctor's point of view as well as her own. It avoids directly challenging her distorted perception of her body image.

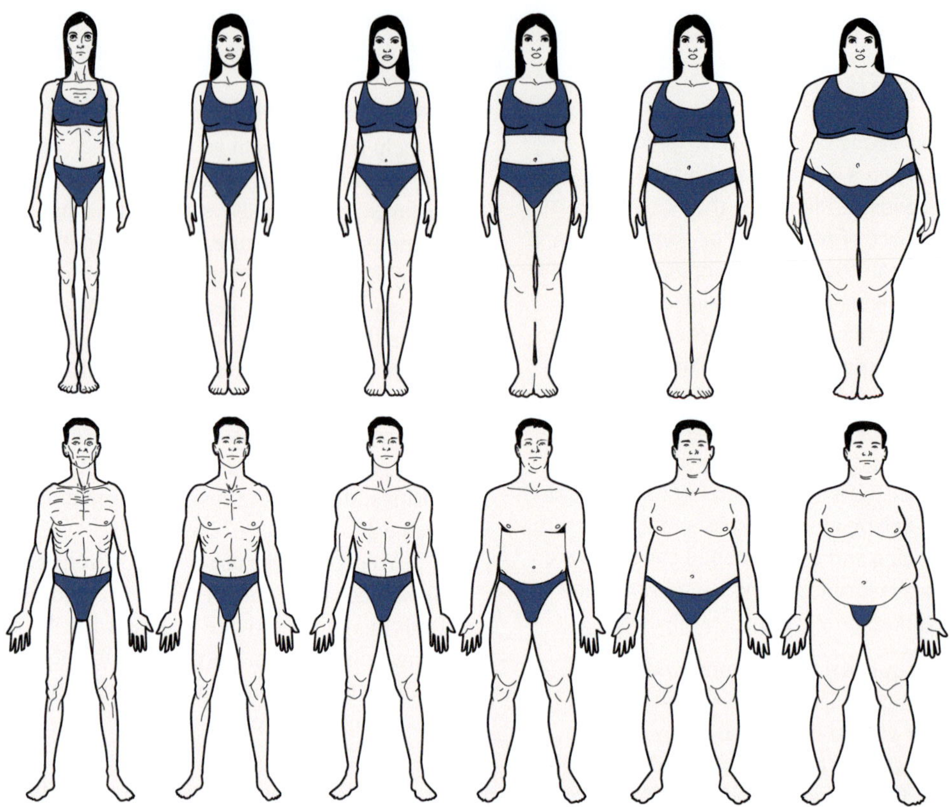

FIGURE 17.3 ■ Assessing body image. A drawing such as this can be used in several ways: (1) People can be asked which image best represents them. This assesses the accuracy of the person's body image. People with anorexia often believe themselves to be larger than they really are. (2) The person can be asked which image best represents the ideal for them. This assesses whether the person has a positive (image is similar to their own body) or a negative (dissimilar image) body image.

Together, you and the individual explore their attempt to achieve perfection by controlling weight. The idea is for the individual to realise that perfection is an unrealistic goal. You are a role model for the person who accepts imperfection yet retains self-esteem. One way to model strong self-esteem is to admit errors willingly. Also model appropriate expressions of anger, and teach people the destructive effects of unexpressed anger.

Evaluation

Evaluation of the effectiveness of nursing interventions with these disorders is an ongoing part of the nursing process.

Nutritional status

The person will regain and maintain at least 90 per cent of the normal weight for their height and age. They will follow eating patterns that demonstrate that they recognise the importance of adequate nutrition. They will regain and maintain normal elimination patterns, vital signs, fluid and electrolyte balance, and muscle tone. Females will have normal menstrual cycles.

Coping

The person will demonstrate effective coping when they participate actively in treatment planning and discharge planning using problem-solving skills. They will demonstrate interest and competence in self-care activities, such as cooking, food preparation, shopping and eating out, as well as sleep, activity, rest and diversional activities. They will accurately identify both maladaptive coping behaviours and adaptive coping behaviours that they can integrate into daily routines. The person will express less anxiety about weight gain, and will verbalise other means of feeling in control of their lives.

Body image

Body image disturbance will be alleviated when the person accurately assesses their own body size and nutritional needs. They will use criteria such as strength and health, rather than appearance alone, to evaluate body size. They will verbalise less preoccupation with body size. They will verbalise positive statements about their own bodies.

Self-esteem

The individual will demonstrate self-esteem when they verbalise their own positive attributes. They will demonstrate less preoccupation with their own appearance, and will focus increasingly on others. They will accept compliments and positive feedback, and show greater interest in activities around them. They will verbalise that perfection is an unrealistic life goal. The person will express anger appropriately, without experiencing incapacitating guilt. They will demonstrate interpersonal relationships substantially free of manipulation. They will work toward success experiences in work, school and/or social groups.

CARE COORDINATION

Care coordinators working with people who have eating disorders must understand the risk factors and possible complications of these disorders. This awareness enables the case manager to recognise symptoms early, mobilise the treatment team and family resources, ensure a smooth transition to inpatient therapy if needed, and ensure adequate follow-up. Failure to respond to treatment occurs in about 50 per cent of cases.

Desired care coordination outcomes include weight gain/loss, normalisation of exercise periods, cessation of binge eating and purging behaviours, and decreased preoccupation with food and body size. Avoidance of hospitalisation, or the briefest possible hospital stay, is a care coordination priority.

The ultimate care coordination goal is early detection of symptoms, effective symptom reduction, and rapid return to maximal premorbid function. Despite the best efforts, about half of individuals with eating disorders progress from acute to chronic illness, which presents them, their families and case managers with lifelong challenges.

COMMUNITY-BASED CARE

Although many, if not most, people with bulimia nervosa and binge-eating disorder can be safely treated in community-based settings, people with advanced anorexia nervosa usually are admitted to an inpatient program. Criteria for hospitalisation are found in Box 17.1 on page 378. Community nurses play a major role in recognising the symptoms of eating disorders. They provide screening, information and support to people with eating disorders and their families, and refer people for specialised treatment. Eating disorders are not self-limiting, and specialised care is required.

Prevention of eating disorders is receiving increased attention as an appropriate and much-needed focus for school-based educational programs. Due to the early onset of body image distortion, education programs as early as primary school should be developed. Eating disorders have become more commonly recognised and, to some extent, normalised. The media have contributed to the idea that the ideal body shape is slimness to the point of extreme thinness. Most recently, the media have called the public's attention to eating-disordered public figures (especially in the entertainment and modelling fields), thus influencing the public's perception of the illness and the community reaction to treatment and relapse.

Nurses in community-based settings can play a valuable role in the education, support and referral of people with eating disorders and their families, often enabling individuals to remain in the community while in treatment.

HOME CARE

Historically, people with eating disorders were isolated from their families during treatment. It was thought that ongoing family conflict would jeopardise their recovery. This approach has been challenged, and attitudes towards community-based care are gradually changing. Having a therapeutic alliance with people with eating disorders and their parents/families is an important aspect of recovery. Many programs have found that increasing family involvement and integration into the treatment program contributes to improved outcomes.

Just as it is important that families are aware of the helpful websites discussed earlier, it is vital for the family to be aware of internet websites that are pro-anorexia and promote treatment sabotage. These websites contain information that promote and support anorexia. Content includes lifestyle descriptions, inspirational photos that serve as motivators for weight loss, and 'tips and tricks' to maintain anorexia. Using the information on these websites disrupts the healing process.

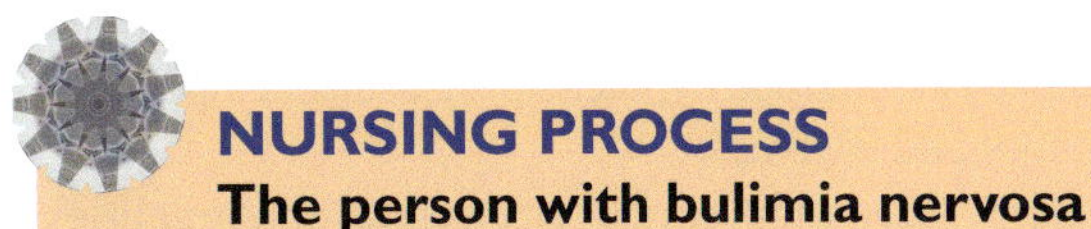

NURSING PROCESS
The person with bulimia nervosa

The following section discusses the nursing process for people with bulimia nervosa. Some individuals with bulimia may also experience anorexia. The nursing process in the previous section (on pages 376–382) covers anorexia.

Assessment

Although the two disorders are described separately, the boundary between anorexia and bulimia is blurred. Many people with bulimia formerly experienced anorexia, while others may become people with anorexia in the future. It is estimated that as many as half of all people with anorexia binge and purge at some time during their illness. During the assessment phase of the nursing process, keep in mind that these two conditions, although distinctly different, often co-exist.

Subjective data

People with bulimia nervosa have feelings of low self-esteem, worthlessness, inadequacy and guilt. They experience shame and embarrassment over their secret binges (eating several tubs of ice cream, buckets of popcorn, or eight or more chocolate bars is not unusual) and subsequent purging activities. This shame may be manifested in self-deprecating remarks. People report feeling out of control, but at the same time they feel an excessive need to control. Unlike people with anorexia, individuals with bulimia nervosa recognise that their eating behaviours are abnormal and bizarre.

Anxiety and unsatisfactory interpersonal relationships are features of this disorder. Anxiety is intensified when others see the person with bulimia as successful and in control, and they often appear so to others. They may be impulsive and cannot delay gratification. Preoccupation with food, weight and dieting is a prominent feature. People with bulimia may report feeling weak and lethargic.

Objective data

Like people with anorexia, those with bulimia tend to be young females. Bulimia first manifests itself later than anorexia, typically during late adolescence or young adulthood. People with bulimia are usually of normal or slightly above-average weight. Appearance does not provide diagnostic clues; hence the term *normal-weight bulimic*. Weight tends to fluctuate, but does not become dangerously low unless anorexia occurs concurrently.

People with bulimia nervosa are more outgoing than those with anorexia, and tend to be more comfortable with sexual relationships. They sometimes manifest impulsive behaviours, such as substance use, shoplifting and self-inflicted injury. In inpatient settings, they may steal others' food and hoard food in their rooms.

Physical signs of bulimia nervosa include hoarseness and oesophagitis, dental enamel erosion, enlarged parotid glands, abrasions or calluses on the knuckles from inducing vomiting, and amenorrhoea in about 40 per cent of cases. The person may also have symptoms of fluid volume deficit: concentrated urine, decreased urine output, hypotension, elevated temperature, poor skin turgor and weakness.

Laboratory tests may reveal electrolyte abnormalities, particularly low serum potassium. Potentially fatal cardiac arrhythmias may result. The overuse of syrup of ipecac, an emetic agent, can create cumulative systemic toxicity affecting the gastrointestinal, neuromuscular and cardiovascular systems, potentially leading to death from cardiotoxicity.

Another concern is the fact that the frequency of bulimia in those with diabetes is increasing, particularly among young women. This is a potentially deadly combination, because binge eating and purging increase the risk for both hypoglycemic episodes and diabetic ketoacidosis (DKA). Closely monitoring blood glucose levels is indicated for these people.

Nursing implications

Anxiety

People with bulimia nervosa experience anxiety: vague, uneasy feelings of moderate to intense severity related to preoccupation with body image. A rise in the individual's anxiety level is usually a forerunner of binge/purge behaviours, and may lead to the purchasing or hoarding of food in preparation for a binge.

Deficient fluid volume

Depletion of body fluids in people with bulimia nervosa is usually related to self-induced vomiting and the excessive use of laxatives and diuretics, combined with decreased fluid intake. Extreme dehydration may lead to changes in electrolyte balance, causing altered mental status. Lethargy and confusion are symptoms of advanced dehydration. Oedema may also be present.

Ineffective individual coping

Binge and purge behaviours are ineffective ways to cope with the stresses of life. Other impulse control problems, such as harmful alcohol use, drug use and shoplifting, are equally ineffective ways to reduce stress. The individual with bulimia's ineffective coping is related to issues such as independence/dependence, identity and self-determination. Ineffective coping is manifested in their preoccupation with body size, poor self-esteem, distorted body image, and excessive overeating followed by purging.

Compromised family coping

The families of people with bulimia nervosa may have distorted perceptions of the problems, and perceive themselves as unable to deal effectively with their loved one's eating disorder. Parents may have difficulty allowing their daughter or son to grow up, and may be overprotective; at the same time, they may have overly high expectations of their offspring. The individual's behaviour may become the family's focus, preventing the fulfilment of essential family roles. If disruption is extreme, the family may not be able to interact effectively with the larger community. Usual problem-solving methods are only partially adequate to deal with the stress of having a family member with bulimia.

Planning and implementation

Several nursing interventions have been somewhat useful in treating those with bulimia nervosa.

Managing medication

Medications, primarily antidepressants, are used to reduce the frequency of disturbed eating behaviours such as binge eating and vomiting. In addition, medications are used to ease the symptoms that may accompany eating disorders, such as depression, anxiety, obsessions or impulse control problems.

Fluoxetine (Prozac), an SSRI, is effective for people with bulimia when given at the higher dose of 50–60 mg per day. Other SSRIs, paroxetine (Paxil) and sertraline (Zoloft), are useful in that they have anti-obsessional and anti-anxiety effects. Typically, the medication is continued until six months following the disappearance of symptoms. In the past, tricyclic antidepressants (TCAs) have been used, but, because these individuals already have a risk for cardiac problems, the side-effect of cardiotoxicity of TCAs is an unnecessary risk.

Reducing anxiety

The goal of nursing interventions with people with bulimia is to help them recognise events that create anxiety and to avoid binge eating and purging in response to anxiety. Initially, being available to the anxious person is useful. Project a calm, reassuring attitude, and provide a quiet, non-stimulating environment. After establishing trust, help the person identify anxiety-producing situations. People experience anxiety as occurring 'out of the blue', and are often unaware that it is related to emotional issues, interpersonal issues, trauma and past abuse. Help them identify previously used coping behaviours to determine whether they might be useful in current situations. How did they handle anxiety before starting to binge and purge? Has positive self-talk or affirmations been beneficial? Box 17.2 shows examples of affirmations. Help those with bulimia identify feelings that precede binge/purge episodes, such as those illustrated in Figure 17.4 ■, and explore healthier ways of dealing with those feelings.

Teach the individual to recognise anxiety early, before it is severe, and to manage increasing anxiety. Energy-consuming activities, such as walking, running and exercising, are useful, but must be used very judiciously if their behaviour includes over-exercising. Individuals with bulimia can benefit from being taught progressive relaxation techniques, dialectical

Box 17.2 Affirmations for those who compulsively overeat

1. I cherish my mind, body and spirit every day in every way.
2. My actions show that I care for myself and for my loved ones.
3. I encourage myself to grow as a kind and loving person.
4. I am honest with other people and true to myself.
5. My body is nourished and satisfied by moderate meals every day.
6. I know that my feelings guide me to my true self—therefore, I tolerate them, welcome them and think about them.
7. I am reliable and trustworthy, to myself and to others.
8. I am lovable as I am, and deserve love and respect.
9. A mild level of anxiety stimulates my creativity.
10. I am honourable to myself by keeping my word to myself.

behaviour therapy and meditation). Administer anti-anxiety medications as ordered, but use caution because of the tendency to habituation. Also review Chapter 8.

Managing fluids and electrolytes

The importance of accurate intake and output records cannot be overstated. Daily consumption of 2000–3000 mL of liquid promotes rehydration. Blinded, accurate daily weights (the person does not see their weight on the scale) are needed, remembering being weighed can be distressful for the person. Always weigh the person at the same time of day (immediately upon arising is preferred) and on the same scale. Assess and document the condition of the skin and oral mucous membranes as well as pulses and blood pressure daily, and monitor laboratory values, particularly urine specific gravity, reporting significant alterations to the physician. Observe the person for at least an hour after meals to prevent purging. To promote comfort in the person with dehydration, give frequent mouth care.

Facilitating coping

People with bulimia nervosa can learn adaptive coping mechanisms to replace the out-of-control, binge/purge cycle. Once you have developed trust, help them plan and practise strategies for dealing effectively with intense feelings and the demands of daily living. It is important for people to identify the situations and patterns of events that precede binge/purge episodes. The following Communication feature provides an example of how you might open up the discussion. People learn to identify, name and express feelings that they formerly perceived only as 'bad'. Once this is accomplished, explore alternative ways for individuals to express those feelings.

Help them to identify times when they are at risk for binge eating and lack impulse control, such as when they are bored, frustrated, angry, lonely or feeling unloved. Teach them ways to nurture themselves during these times other than eating and purging. Suggest taking a warm bath, calling or visiting an old friend, or pursuing a hobby not involving food.

People with bulimia nervosa often perceive feelings of guilt and underlying resentment as overwhelming. They may need to learn effective ways of expressing these feelings and learn assertiveness techniques to diminish guilty interactions in the future. Role-playing with the person helps them practise assertiveness. The worsening of both mood and the symptoms of bulimia during the winter has been reported in eating disorder literature with increasing frequency. Bright white light treatment has proven effective in treating those with bulimia with seasonal mood and symptom patterns. Chapter 15 discusses light treatment.

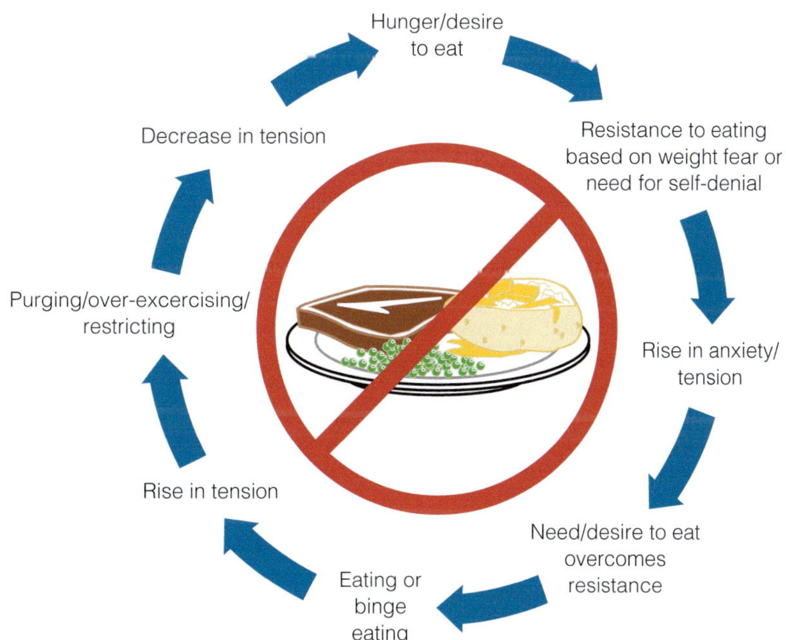

FIGURE 17.4 ■ A disordered eating cycle in bulimia nervosa. A nursing intervention to improve self-awareness and anxiety reduction involves assisting individuals to identify their personal eating cycle, which varies with each individual.

COMMUNICATION

Person with bulimia nervosa

Person: 'Last night I made a tin of brownies and ate the whole lot. Then I had to throw up because I felt so miserable.'

Nurse response #1	Nurse response #2
Nurse response #1: 'Let's talk about what was going on yesterday before you ate the brownies.' *RATIONALE:* Shows empathy for the person. Encourages them to focus on their feelings, and the influence of those feelings on their behaviour, thereby promoting self-awareness.	**Nurse response #2:** 'That sounds uncomfortable. What are the miserable feelings about?' *RATIONALE:* Demonstrates nonjudgmental acceptance. Encourages the person to place events in time sequence. This enables them to connect the cause-and-effect relationship between their experiences, feelings and subsequent behaviour.

People who binge may benefit from a support plan that provides distraction and 'urge surfing' after meals. This may identify what supports and strategies will help a person avoid the post-meal anxiety. Distracting a person after eating can help with the eating disorder thoughts and behaviours after meals.

Involve the person in their discharge planning. Topics covered in discharge planning include the productive use of time, identification of diversional activities not related to food, and participation in support groups. Coordinate care with other nurses who work in specialty areas, such as women's health, and in paediatric settings that also treat the person.

Mobilising the family

Certain **family dynamics** reinforce maladaptive eating behaviours; therefore, families must also develop effective coping mechanisms to support the person's healthier coping behaviours. Assess the family's feelings and perceptions of their loved one's bulimia, listening carefully for what is most stressful and threatening to family members. Correct any misperceptions about the disorder. Encourage family members to explore together their usual coping strategies, and determine whether any previously used strategies can be useful in the present situation.

Help the family identify their strengths and weaknesses. Encourage family members to share their thoughts and feelings with one another and with the person with bulimia, including feelings of guilt, blame and resentment. Teach family members to use 'I' statements, thereby acknowledging their feelings. If the person's disorder impairs family functioning, help the family reorganise roles to reduce stress, and ensure that all family members' needs continue to be met during the person's recovery. Help the family understand that two normal developmental needs of adolescents and young adults are to develop autonomy and to establish identities outside the family. Make appropriate referrals to community resources.

Evaluation

The evaluation process determines the effectiveness of the nursing interventions.

Anxiety

People will demonstrate anxiety control when they verbally identify situations and events that evoke anxiety. They will communicate their needs and negative feelings appropriately. They will identify symptoms that indicate their own anxiety. They will identify ways of structuring the environment to prevent stressful situations that result in feeling out of control. People with bulimia will eliminate binge/purge behaviours and demonstrate the use of anxiety-reduction strategies unrelated to eating. They will verbalise their acceptance of normal body weight without intense anxiety, or will continue healthy eating patterns even though anxiety persists.

Fluid volume

Dryness of oral mucosa and skin will not be evident. Skin turgor will be normal. The person's vital signs and the results of laboratory studies will be within normal limits. Input and output are balanced over 24-hour periods. The person will verbalise their understanding of the relationship between dehydration and self-induced vomiting, and the use of laxatives and diuretics. They will verbalise understanding of the physiological and psychological consequences of dehydration.

Individual coping

The person will demonstrate effective coping when they accurately assess maladaptive coping behaviours. They will demonstrate healthier ways to deal with stress and intense feelings. They will identify times of risk, and verbalise alternative self-nurturing behaviours. They will demonstrate assertive communication techniques. The person will demonstrate self-control in their eating behaviours, gradually maintaining them without supervision. They will verbalise increased self-confidence in their ability to handle the demands of daily life. They will follow through with recommended self-help or support groups and therapy following discharge.

Family coping

Families will verbalise accurate perceptions of their situation. They will verbalise their feelings about having a family member with an eating disorder. They will acknowledge the needs of both the person and the family unit. They will identify useful strategies for coping with the impact of bulimia nervosa on the family. They will use 'I' statements during communication with one another, the individual and the nurse. They will verbalise an understanding of the developmental needs of family members. They will use more flexible problem-solving strategies. The family will reorganise that family roles as necessary. They will identify the community resources available to them and will follow through on referrals.

For additional information about the nursing process with people with bulimia nervosa, see the nursing care plan that follows.

CARE COORDINATION, COMMUNITY-BASED CARE AND HOME CARE

Care coordination, community-based care and home care for people with eating disorders were discussed earlier in this chapter. Refer to page 383.

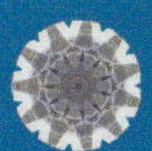

NURSING CARE PLAN: PERSON WITH BULIMIA NERVOSA

Identifying information

Lauren, a 28-year-old married woman, was admitted to the emergency department where she was taken after collapsing during a marathon. She is a social worker who works in a drug and alcohol prevention program.

Lauren reports that she has been training for the marathon for about a year, running at least 35 kilometres a week. She believes that she had to be hospitalised because she did not ingest sufficient carbohydrates and fluids before the race.

Lauren states that she has been binge eating and purging for about three years, ever since she read about ballet dancers' and gymnasts' use of purging for weight control. On a typical day, she arises at 5 am, runs at least 5 kilometres, then gets ready for work. On the way to work, she buys and consumes a dozen doughnuts. She arrives at work before anyone else and vomits in the employees' bathroom. She eats no lunch unless she can be sure of access to a 'good' bathroom, which she describes as one with a single toilet and an outside door that locks. In the evening while preparing dinner, she consumes a can of salted peanuts and four or five glasses of wine. She denies ever getting 'drunk'. After a large dinner she showers, vomiting while the shower is running. Her husband of four years is unaware of her 'problem', but worries about her drinking and wonders how she can eat so much and never gain weight.

History

No prior psychiatric history. Lauren is the eldest of three children and the only female. Her parents, both retired schoolteachers, live in a nearby town. She sees them infrequently because 'they still treat me like I'm a little girl.' She rarely sees her younger brothers, and feels closer to her husband's family. There is no family history of eating disorders or substance use.

As the daughter of two schoolteachers, Lauren was expected to be the top student in her school. She had few friends because she was 'the class geek'. At university, she excelled academically but was a 'social failure'. She states that she can drink an entire bottle of wine, vomit and 'sober up instantly'. She has few friends or interests except running. She describes her job as 'not fulfilling'.

Lauren has no significant health problems. Vital signs are: temperature, 36.8°C; pulse, 68; respirations, 14; height, 170 centimetres; weight, 50 kilograms; blood pressure, 108/68.

Current mental status

Lauren is slim, neatly groomed and cooperative, but reluctant. She is alert and oriented to time, place and person. Her judgment is good and her ability to think abstractly is unimpaired. She is articulate; her affect is appropriate to verbal content; she has no delusions, illusions, hallucinations or other signs of thought disorder. She fidgets in her seat, but makes good eye contact. She expresses embarrassment about hospitalisation and shame about her behaviour. She emphatically does not want her husband or workplace informed of the extent and details of her 'problem'. She maintains that she does not need to be hospitalised and can handle this herself.

Other clinical data

Lauren reports that she has not had a menstrual period in over a year. She takes no medications.

Issue identified: Anxiety-related to low self-esteem.

Expected outcome: Lauren has the ability to control her compulsive or impulsive behaviours, and develop more enhanced coping mechanisms.

Short-term goals	Interventions	Rationales
Lauren will identify at least three sources of anxiety.	■ Adopt a calm, reassuring attitude.	A calm approach conveys safety and confidence.
	■ Provide a quiet, non-stimulating environment.	Reducing stimuli minimises Lauren's anxiety.
	■ Help Lauren recognise the situations and events that create anxiety.	Lauren's self-awareness is enhanced.
	■ Encourage Lauren to identify previously used, successful coping behaviours.	Recognising successful behaviours promotes self-esteem.
	■ Encourage Lauren to identify alternatives to alcohol use, binge eating, and purging in response to anxiety.	Lauren's coping skills are expanded.
	■ Limit over-exercising.	Limits and counteracts unhealthy preoccupations.
	■ Develop a support plan to help Lauren to limit hoarding, vomiting and other compulsive behaviours.	Support plans promote self-responsibility and self-control.

(continued)

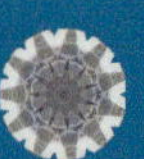

NURSING CARE PLAN: PERSON WITH BULIMIA NERVOSA (*continued*)

Short-term goals	Interventions	Rationales
Lauren will demonstrate the use of relaxation techniques to manage anxiety.	■ Teach progressive relaxation techniques and meditation.	Relaxation techniques improve coping skills.
	■ Assist Lauren to use techniques when feeling tension that would formerly lead to binge eating and purging.	Techniques reinforce and support effective coping.

Issue identified: Deficient fluid volume related to self-induced vomiting and excessive exercising.

Expected outcome: Electrolyte and acid–base balance: balance of electrolytes and non-electrolytes in the intracellular and extracellular compartments of the body.

Short-term goals	Interventions	Rationales
Lauren will drink a minimum of 100 mL of fluids per hour.	■ Teach Lauren the importance of adequate fluid intake.	This is information every person should know.
	■ Offer Lauren her favourite beverages frequently during the day.	Adequate fluid intake maintains hydration.
	■ Blind-weigh Lauren daily to evaluate rehydration.	Hydration status is monitored.
	■ Keep accurate intake and output records.	
	■ Assess skin turgor and condition of mucous membranes daily, and record.	
	■ Encourage frequent mouth care to promote comfort.	Comfort measures promote adherence.
	■ Monitor laboratory values, reporting significant alterations to the physician.	Lab values provide information on electrolyte status.
Lauren will not vomit following meals.	■ Identify supports and activities that will help Lauren distract from the self-impulsive urges to vomit.	Distraction can play a key part in refraining from giving in to disordered thoughts and behaviours.
	■ Provide support for Lauren for at least one hour after meals to prevent purging.	The presence of others provides support and reinforcement.
	■ Give positive recognition when positive behaviours are demonstrated.	Recognising progress reinforces healthy behaviours.

Issue identified: Ineffective individual coping related to feelings of helplessness and lack of control in life situation.

Expected outcome: Development of a sense of control in her everyday activities, ability to self-restrain her compulsive or impulsive behaviours.

Short-term goals	Interventions	Rationales
Lauren will work towards eating regular meals	■ Help Lauren establish a trust relationship with you.	Trust is the basis for a positive therapeutic relationship.
	■ Assist Lauren to plan for and practise dealing with daily demands.	Practice decreases helplessness, promotes self-responsibility and self-control.
	■ Assist Lauren to identify events preceding binge/purge episodes.	Self-awareness is an important step towards self-control.
	■ Encourage Lauren to identify ways of nurturing herself without using food or alcohol.	Concepts of choice, self-determination and self-control are validated for Lauren.
Lauren will identify activities that provide her with meaning and purpose, and will support for emotional growth and empowerment	■ Complete a strengths assessment with Lauren, helping her to identify her strengths and resources for goal setting.	Exploring alternative means of expression increases coping skills, improves impulse control and decreases helplessness.
	■ Help Lauren develop recovery tools, such as learning how to cope in positive ways and effectively managing her emotions.	Recovery tools assist Lauren to identify and practise alternative ways of expressing negative feelings.

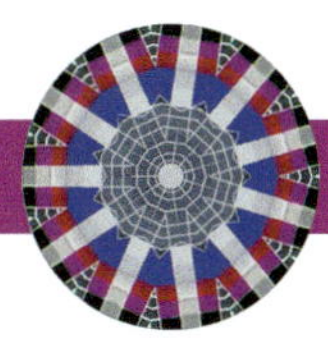

REFERENCES

Allen, K. L., Fursland, A., Watson, H., & Byrne, S. M. (2011). Eating disorder diagnosis in general practice settings: Comparison with structured clinical interview and self-report questionnaires. *Journal of Mental Health, 20*(3), 270–280.

Avena, N. M., & Bocarsly, M. E. (2012). Dysregulation of brain reward systems in eating disorders: Neurochemical information from animal models of binge eating, bulimia nervosa, and anorexia nervosa. *Neuropharmacology, 63*(1), 87–96.

Bruch, H. (1978). *The golden cage: The enigma of anorexia nervosa.* Cambridge, MA: Harvard University Press.

Chen, E. Y., Weissman, J. A., Zeffiro, T. A., Yiu, AQ., Eneva, K. T., Artl, J. M., & Swantek, M. J. (2016). Family-based therapy for young adults with anorexia restores weight. *International Journal of Eating Disorders 49*(7), 701–707.

Chesney, E., Goodwin, G. M., & Fazel, S. (2014). Risks of all-cause and suicide mortality in mental disorders: A meta-review. *World Psychiatry, 13*(2), 153–160.

Frank, G. K., Shott, M. E., Hagman, J. O., & Mittal, V. A. (2013). Alterations in brain structures related to taste reward circuitry in ill and recovered anorexia nervosa and in bulimia nervosa. *American Journal of Psychiatry, 170*(10), 1152–1160.

Goodwin, H., Haycraft, E., Taranis, L., & Meyer, C. (2011). Psychometric evaluation of the compulsive exercise test (CET) in an adolescent population: Links with eating psychopathology. *European Eating Disorders Review, 19*(3), 269–279.

Hay, P., Chinn, D., Forbes, D., Madden, S., Newton, R., Sugenor, L., . . . Ward, W. (2014). Royal Australian and New Zealand College of Psychiatrists clinical practice guidelines for the treatment of eating disorders. *Australian and New Zealand Journal of Psychiatry, 48*(11), 977–1008.

Jenkins, J., & Ogden, J. (2011). Becoming 'whole' again: A qualitative study of women's views of recovering from anorexia nervosa. *European Eating Disorders Review, 20*(1), e23–e31.

Kim, Y. R., Lim, S. J., & Treasure, J. (2011). Different patterns of emotional eating and visuospatial deficits whereas shared risk factors related with social support between anorexia nervosa and bulimia nervosa. *Psychiatry Investigation, 8*(1), 9–14.

Love, C. C., & Seaton, H. (1991). Eating disorders: Highlights of nursing assessment and therapeutics. *Nursing Clinics of North America, 26*(3), 687.

Neri, M., Bello, S., Bonsignore, A., Cantatore, S., Riezzo, I., Turillazzi, E., & Fineschi, V. (2011). Anabolic androgenic steroids abuse and liver toxicity. *Mini Reviews in Medicinal Chemistry, 11*(5), 430–437.

Rivas, T., Bersabé, R., Jiméne, M., & Berrocal, C. (2010). The Eating Attitudes Test (EAT-26): Reliability and validity in Spanish female samples. *Spanish Journal of Psychology, 13*(2), 1044–1056.

Seal, N. (2011). Introduction to genetics and childhood obesity: Relevance to nursing practice. *Biological Research for Nursing, 13*(1), 61–69.

Slane, J. D., Burt, S. A., & Klump, K. L. (2011). Genetic and environmental influences on disordered eating and depressive symptoms. *International Journal of Eating Disorders, 44*(7), 605–611.

Smeets, E., Jansen, A., & Roefs, A. (2011). Bias for the (un)attractive self: On the role of attention in causing body (dis)satisfaction. *Health Psychology, 30*(3), 360–367.

Swanson, S. A., Crow, S. J., LeGrange, D., Swendsen, J., & Merikangas, K. R. (2011). Prevalence and correlates of eating disorders in adolescents: Results from the National Comorbidity Survey Replication Adolescent Supplement. *Archives of General Psychiatry, 68*(7), 714–723.

Thornton, L. M., Dellava, J. E., Root, T. L., Lichtenstein, P., & Bulik, C. M. (2011). Anorexia nervosa and generalized anxiety disorder: Further explorations of the relation between anxiety and body mass index. *Journal of Anxiety Disorders, 25*(5), 727–730.

Tortorella, A., Brambilla, F., Fabrazzo, M., Volpe, U., Monteleone, A. M., Mastromo, D., & Monteleone, P. (2014). Central and peripheral peptides regulating eating behaviour and energy homeostasis in anorexia nervosa and bulimia nervosa: A literature review. *European Eating Disorders Review, 22*(5), 307–320.

White, J. H., & Litovitz, G. (1998). A comparison of inpatient and outpatient women with eating.

Wilfley, D. E., Vannucci, A., & White, E. K. (2010). Early intervention of eating and weight-related problems. *Journal of Clinical Psychology in Medical Settings, 17*(4), 258–300.

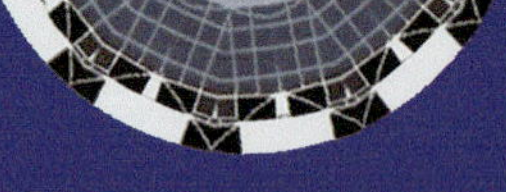

18 Personality disorders

SUSAN SUMSKIS AND ERIN HOWARD-GILLIS

KEY TERMS

antisocial personality disorder *402*
attachment theory *394*
avoidant personality disorder *399*
biopsychosocial theory *392*
borderline personality disorder *398*
dependent personality disorder *395*
lived experience *400*
narcissistic personality disorder *398*
obsessive–compulsive personality disorder *399*
paranoid personality disorder *396*
personality disorder *392*
personality traits *391*
recovery *400*
schizoid personality disorder *396*
schizotypal personality disorder *396*
trauma-informed care *409*
recovery *400*
self-discovery *401*

LEARNING OUTCOMES

After completing this chapter, you will be able to:

1. Understand theories of personality and personality disorder.
2. Understand biopsychosocial theories of disorder.
3. Analyse the role of attachment and trauma in the development of personality disorder.
4. Consider the implications of the classification and diagnosis of personality disorder from both lived experience and professional perspectives.
5. Understand and appreciate the experience of living with a personality disorder.
6. Evaluate trauma informed care, recovery and self-discovery from both the perspective of the person living with a personality disorder and the nurse.
7. Analyse nurses' attitudes to people diagnosed with personality disorder, and the implications for those people.
8. Examine the evidence for the use of medication in the treatment of personality disorder.

LIVED EXPERIENCE

How it feels to receive a diagnosis

When I was diagnosed with borderline personality disorder, I cried—there was a mixture of relief, sadness and anger. After the end of a long-term relationship, I realised that I wanted to get this 'depression' sorted out once and for all. I sat down to browse the internet, and looked around the various Australian mental health resources for answers, when I came across borderline personality disorder (BPD). The more I read, the more I felt that my symptoms fitted with BPD as opposed to major depressive disorder. I saw my GP and asked her whether or not she agreed. My GP turned her computer screen towards me, and there under '*Diagnoses*' was: '*? Borderline personality disorder*'. I looked at her shocked, and asked why she hadn't discussed it with me. Her response was that she wasn't sure how to—that BPD has a lot of stigma attached, and she wasn't sure how I would react. We put together a mental health care plan, and so began the treatment journey.

I felt a huge sense of relief when I was diagnosed, because finally I had some answers—I wasn't inherently 'bad', there was a reason behind my behaviours. At the same time I was sad—no one likes to be told there is something wrong with them, and I was sad that it was largely responsible for the breakdown of many relationships in my life. Then came the anger . . . why was this happening to me?

INTRODUCTION

Through reading this chapter you will understand theories of personality, appreciate the ways in which people can experience disorder within their personality, identify causal pathways, evaluate the classification and diagnosis of personality disorder, and come to understand the highly specialised nature of providing nursing care. You will also develop an appreciation for the challenges and the journey of self-discovery undertaken by people who live with personality disorder.

THEORIES OF PERSONALITY

Box 18.1

A person requests that you, a newly employed nurse on a crisis inpatient unit, bend the rules for her by extending her therapeutic leave for two hours so that she may meet her boyfriend for dinner. When discussing this request with the person, you remind her that decisions about therapeutic leave are made by the entire treatment team. The person then becomes angry and accuses you of 'not being the caring nurse I thought you were'. The person states that she will remember this incident and warn her friends about the uncaring nurses at this facility.

1. What would be wrong with bending the rules a little?
2. Should nurses be flexible and autonomous enough not to require approval from the treatment team? Why, or why not?
3. What purpose could the person's accusations serve?
4. How would you handle this situation with the person? What is your rationale?

Since early Greek times, humans have been interested in personality. Major flaws in personality were of most interest, as opposed to the usual mundane features. Hippocrates initially believed there were four basic temperaments—choleric, melancholic, sanguine and phlegmatic—which were modified in the 2nd century by Galen who associated Hippocrates' choleric temperament with irascible behaviour, melancholic temperament with an inclination towards sadness, sanguine temperament with optimism, and phlegmatic temperament with an apathetic disposition.

In the early 1900s, Kretschmer theorised that normal 'asthenic' (physically thin) individuals are introverted, timid and lack personal warmth, whereas 'phynic' (heavy-set) individuals are gregarious, friendly and independent. In the 1930s, Sigmund Freud observed that we each have an individual character and an individual capacity for adaptation that produces enduring ways of thinking, feeling and behaving, and that these make up our individual personalities. Evidence suggests that an individual's personality emerges through continual interaction between genetically determined constitutional features and experiences in the social environment (Siegel, 1999). Millon (1981, p. 8) provides a useful definition of personality as:

> *. . . a complex pattern of deeply embedded psychological characteristics that are largely unconscious, cannot be eradicated easily and express themselves automatically in almost every facet of functioning. Intrinsic and pervasive, these traits emerge from a complicated matrix of biological dispositions and experiential learnings and now comprise the individual's distinctive pattern of perceiving, feeling, thinking and coping.*

Personality traits have been defined as primary units of personality structure, although there remains a lack of

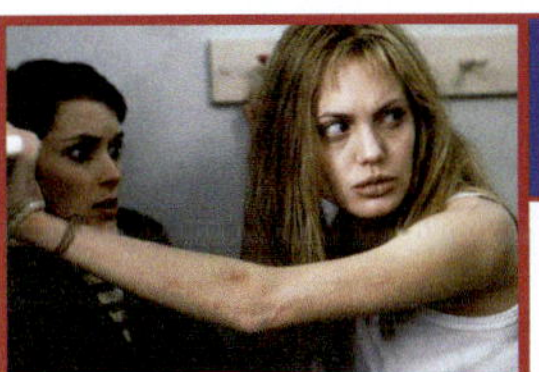

MENTAL HEALTH IN THE MEDIA
Girl Interrupted

This film highlights the experiences of three young women who live with personality disorders and are hospitalised in a mental health hospital. The story is told from the frame of reference of Susanna (Winona Ryder), who was admitted 18 months previously, after a suicide attempt. Susanna has a diagnosis of borderline personality disorder. In addition to having attempted suicide, she self-harms and engages in impulsive sexual behaviour. She experiences depersonalisation several times, and on one occasion bites open the flesh on her hand because she is terrified that she has lost her bones. Although she pushes others away, she is the one who feels abandoned and has low self-esteem.

Lisa (Angelina Jolie) has antisocial personality disorder, and takes pleasure in ordering the other people around. She preys on the others, breaks down their self-esteem and uses their disorders against them. Lisa argues and fights with the staff on a daily basis, and is frequently taken to the seclusion room, kicking and screaming. Lisa has no qualms about hurting herself or others. In fact, she often finds those activities pleasurable, showing no remorse for her actions.

Daisy (Brittany Murphy) has obsessive–compulsive personality disorder. Her focus on orderliness and control is seen most clearly in the way in which she handles food. Her social life and daily routine is hindered by her inability to eat in front of others. Eating involves several rituals—peeling chicken off the bone in a certain order, laying the bones out in an orderly fashion, and saving the carcasses. She counts chicken bones and carcasses over and over. Daisy is aware of her obsessional thoughts and her unusual behaviour, and hides the chicken carcasses so no one will see them.

The personality disorders displayed by the characters in the film are classic and severe enough to warrant hospitalisation, which is not the usual circumstance for people with personality disorders.

Photo courtesy © Columbia/courtesy of Everett Collection.

consensus with regard to the structure (Budge et al., 2013; Leising & Zimmermann, 2011). These primary units are thought to form habitual patterns of thinking, feeling and behaving, which are exhibited in a wide range of social and personal situations. A hierarchical categorisation of personality traits includes several personality schemes, with one such scheme called The Five Factor or The Big Five model of broad personality traits, which are: extroversion, agreeableness, conscientiousness, neuroticism and openness to experience (Markon, Kreuger & Watson, 2005). All five are ways of thinking, feeling and behaving in which differences can be observed. When these differences within traits become maladaptive and inflexible, interfere with daily functioning and cause distress, they constitute a **personality disorder** (American Psychiatric Association [APA], 2013).

THEORIES OF DISORDER

Personality disorders originate in childhood or adolescence, and significantly affect the important development tasks of learning to regulate emotions, developing a conscience, learning to control impulses and developing an individual identity (Skodol, 2008). Personality disorders involve pervasive restructuring of an individual's defensive style, which amounts to a total character restructure and development of 'character armour'. This restructure can result in chronic attitudes and chronic modes of reaction which are evident within four domains: identity, self-direction, empathy and intimacy. Freud believed that personality can change right through into adulthood, and research has since demonstrated that environmental influences are largely responsible for these changes; therefore, even 'chronic' modes of reaction can be altered (Rutter, 2006).

Disorder of personality greatly affects the ability to form and sustain stable interpersonal relationships. A common defensive style is to attribute problems in interpersonal relationships wrongly to others, which causes others to suffer (Tyrer, Reed & Crawford, 2015). This defence has consequences within interpersonal health care relationships, particularly when problems are blamed on individual members of the health care team. To maintain therapeutic effectiveness in this type of situation, nurses need to develop their own interpersonal boundaries (see Chapters 2 and 6). Attributing problems wrongly to others has also contributed to nurses' use of pejorative terms, such as referring to people as 'PDs'. This has been found to lead to therapeutic pessimism and diagnostic hopelessness and exclusion from services through beliefs that people so diagnosed are difficult to help and are untreatable (Tyrer et al., 2015).

THEORIES OF CAUSATION

Biopsychosocial theory

Kuo and Linehan (2009) believe that a combination of being born highly sensitive or more sensitive than most others, combined with an invalidating childhood environment, affects development of emotional responses and leads to problems regulating emotions in adulthood. Linehan's theory is particularly useful for understanding borderline personality disorder, and for linking an individual's biological nature with the way in which they regulate their emotions. Figure 18.1 ■ provides a representation of **biopsychosocial theory**.

Biopsychosocial theory

Sensitive biological predisposition (Nature)
+
Invalidating environment (Nurture)
=
Pervasive dysfunction of emotional regulation systems

FIGURE 18.1 ■ Biopsychosocial theory (Linehan, 1993).

Biopsychosocial theory seeks to validate the individual by identifying the impact of childhood experience and environmental effects on the person's development in childhood. It also asks the individual to accept these experiences, and to learn new skills to facilitate change to improve their future experience.

In an invalidating environment, the individual's inner emotional experiences are not confirmed as being real; for example, expressions of distress may be discounted or denied by parents or caregivers, and the person may be punished and consequently feel shame for feeling distress. If this is an enduring pattern of childhood development, the person is unable to accurately label and modulate their emotions, and therefore does not learn to manage or tolerate distress. Later on, it is no longer necessary for others to invalidate the person's emotions: the person has learned how to self-invalidate and then follow up with feelings of shame, self-criticism and self-punishment (Linehan & Wilks, 2015). Self-invalidation, shame and punishment become a vicious cycle. When others in the environment, including nurses, respond in a critical way to evidence of this cycle, the pattern of invalidation is continued.

SELF-AWARENESS

Shame and punishment

Can you think of a time when you felt punished for a negative emotion (shame, upset, crying, tantrum, acting out)? What emotional response did you develop within yourself to be able to handle this?

An effective nursing response is to accept the individual's sensitive nature, consider the consequences of childhood experience, validate the individual's emotional experience, and facilitate the development of coping skills in a variety of contexts. To validate means to authenticate the person's current experience, either verbally or non-verbally. Validation focuses on listening to what the person is saying, observing non-verbal cues, and responding verbally and physically where appropriate. Examples include nodding your head and perhaps holding someone's hand. Restating what the person had said, and then naming their feelings; for example, 'you are furious about this' is also validating. Conveying hope through normalising feelings—for example, 'it's normal, most people would feel this way'—is also effective. Validation is an extremely important nursing skill, and is best employed to assist an individual to calm down and to help them accurately recognise and label the emotions they are feeling, and to develop non-judgmental self-evaluation (Koerner & Linehan, 2003).

Attachment theory

Each individual's attachment experiences are important to consider in the context of the development of personality disorder. Attachment patterns evolve from a complex array of influences, including genetics, parenting and environmental and social cues. Disorder of an individual's personality is most keenly felt and experienced within social situations. Social behaviour is largely influenced by an individual's mental models of social relationships, and these models are constructed during attachment experiences in infancy (Fonagy, 2003).

Family is the primary agent of socialisation, and attachment experiences with primary caregivers play an important role in each infant learning to bond with others and with the infant's own regulation of emotions (Maccoby, 2000). Attachment to primary caregivers is the earliest experience of causal motivation, and leads to the construction of a representation of self, and a set of intentions aimed at ensuring social collaboration. A self-representation is how we would describe ourselves if someone were to say to us 'tell me about yourself'. Attachment in adulthood, while ever-evolving, seeks to protect the individual's self-representation from the impingements that social encounters create. Severe personality disorder arises when psychological attachment is distorted or dysfunctional, such as through neglect or maltreatment, and cannot fulfil its biological function of preserving self-representations (Fonagy, 2003).

Infants possess an inborn brain-based attachment system which enables them to improve their chances of survival through seeking attachment with caregivers (Meyer & Pilkonis, 2005; Siegel, 1999). The parental biological function of the attachment system is protection of the child (Cassidy, 2008). Attachments are usually formed by around six months of age (Masten & O'Dougherty Wright, 2010), and may form the central foundation for the development of memory, narrative, emotion, representations, states of mind and interpersonal skills (Meyer & Pilkonis, 2005). The way in which an infant attaches to caregivers leads to specific organisational changes in the brain, and is linked with regulation of emotions and behaviour. The quality of attachment relationships between an infant and their primary carer influences later relationships with friends, romantic partners and their own children (Masten & O'Dougherty Wright, 2010). Attachment is a developmental process, and therefore people are able to continue to grow and change despite early attachment problems. Secure attachments convey resilience, whereas insecure attachments convey risk. Insecure attachment creates a risk for later psychological and social dysfunction.

Theories of attachment are useful for understanding people's behaviour in health care situations. Several theories have been created; among them, Ainsworth and colleagues (1978) provide four patterns of attachment which can shed light on behaviour in the context of personality disorder. The four attachment categories are: *secure, anxious/avoidant, anxious/resistant* and *disorganised/disoriented* (Ainsworth, 1985). In situations signalling threat or danger, or in situations of injury, illness, fatigue or excessive distance from the caregiver, infants exhibit attachment behaviour in order to gain the comforting and protective presence of the caregiver (Meyer & Pilkonis, 2005). Attachment behaviour includes smiling, vocalising, crying, approaching and following.

Infants with a *secure* attachment type will separate to explore their environment, will seek reattachment when stressed, and will calm down once reattached (Ainsworth et al., 1978). Securely attached parents are 'tuned in', and are available and responsive to the infant's needs (Cassidy, 2008; Siegel, 1999). Secure attachment is linked with emotionally resilient infants who are able to be restabilised in the face of stress (Fonagy, 1999). Under stress, an adult with this style of attachment might seek out supportive people to help them deal with the stressor and restabilise their emotions.

Infants with an *anxious/avoidant* attachment type over-regulate their affect by avoiding stressful situations. Infants with *anxious* attachment feel stressed when separated, and are not easily calmed down with reattachment (Cassidy, 2008). Parents may be under-involved, erratic or inconsistent with their attention, or may lack parenting skills. Infants with *avoidant* attachment are not stressed with separation, and avoid or ignore the caregiver's return, as the parenting style may be characterised by neglect or maltreatment. Avoidant parents may be consistently cold or rejecting of the infant, may use overstimulated ways of interacting, and may reject close body contact. Avoidant attachment styles are linked with later personality maladjustment. Avoidantly attached children are experienced as controlling and are often disliked by their peers, and as adults they tend to have more stormy, conflict-ridden relationships (Meyer & Pilkonis, 2005). Under stress, an adult with this style of attachment may find it difficult to settle themselves down, even with support at hand.

Anxious/resistant attached infants have a low threshold for threat, under-regulate their emotions, and become more distressed while also showing frustration with caregiver responses, and often do not calm down in the presence of the primary caregiver. Under stress, an adult with this style of attachment may exhibit high levels of emotional arousal, and may become angry with those who care for them or who are seeking to help them.

Children who have attached in a *disorganised/disoriented* pattern exhibit purposeless behaviour, such as freezing, handclapping and head-banging, and deficits in attention, even in the presence of the caregiver. They become detached when overwhelmed, and have difficulty regulating impulses, and this has been recognised as a risk factor for later development of post-traumatic stress disorder. Under stress, an adult with this style of attachment may be a challenge to reach therapeutically, may detach and may self-harm, and would benefit from assistance to reorganise/reorientate their emotions.

> *The pathway followed by each developing individual and the extent to which he or she becomes resilient to stressful life events is determined to a very significant extent by the pattern of* ***attachment*** *he or she develops during the early years (Bowlby, 1988, p. 171–172).*

SELF-AWARENESS

Attachment style

1. Can you recognise your own attachment style?
2. How do you think your style might affect your attachment and communication style within your nursing practice?

Attachment theory is a useful background for understanding behaviour within social settings and in relationships with health care professionals. Threats to personal security, such as during a crisis, activate an individual's attachment system, which is aimed at achieving safety and security, and also triggers their corresponding emotional response styles.

Early infant–caregiver interaction patterns form beliefs and expectations around the individual's worthiness, and the likelihood of others providing empathy, help and nurturance (Meyer & Pilkonis, 2005). People who feel secure and have positive ideas of themselves are not easily compromised by receiving inadequate external validation. People with negative ideas about themselves feel highly anxious about being rejected, and rely on other's approval for their self-worth. Importantly, these processes are automatic, without volitional intent, and therefore individuals may not see the connection between how they are approached and how they respond. Individuals cannot reinvent their attachment in response to critical situations. Intentional psychological therapeutic intervention is helpful for examining and working with attachment styles, and the process of change can take many years. This has implications for nursing care and nurses' ability to provide validation for people in the face of their attachment history and, in particular, their low self-esteem. It is important not to view it as *attention-seeking*, and thus also neglect or reject the person and respond coldly or without empathy.

Trauma

> *Individual* ***trauma*** *results from an event, series of events, or set of circumstances that is experienced by an individual as physically or emotionally harmful or life-threatening and that has lasting adverse effects on the individual's functioning and mental, physical, social, emotional, or spiritual well-being* (Substance Abuse and Mental Health Services Administration, 2014, p. 7)

LIVED EXPERIENCE

Living with a personality disorder

Living with a personality disorder can be challenging and difficult. At times I know my reactions to certain situations are a result of the disorder, yet I cannot control my behaviour—most commonly in the domain of my relationships with others, particularly those close to me.

If I get a sense of abandonment or rejection, I may act out to push that person away before that can happen. In one sense I feel relieved that I have avoided the abandonment or rejection, but I have also achieved what I was wanting to avoid—losing or damaging my relationship with that person. I might push someone away by starting an argument or saying hurtful things—at the same time, in my head, I am willing myself to stop. At the time, it can feel like being on a runaway train where the brakes are failing.

Childhood maltreatment is an important risk factor for personality disorder (Afifi et al., 2011; Hengartner et al., 2015). Attachment style is also severely shaped by childhood maltreatment. Emotional abuse is most perversely and detrimentally associated with the personality traits of extroversion, openness, conscientiousness and agreeableness. Emotional abuse and neglect, physical abuse and neglect, and sexual abuse in childhood are significantly related to neuroticism.

The association between childhood trauma and negative mental health outcomes is strong (Afifi et al., 2011; Ball & Links, 2009). Traumatic experiences such as child sexual abuse, child psychological or physical neglect, parental violence, witnessing intimate partner violence and other types of childhood maltreatment are associated with adverse development across multiple areas of adult functioning, particularly those affected in personality disorder: identity, self-direction, empathy and intimacy (APA, 2013; Godbout & Briere, 2012; Goodman & Yehuda, 2002; Schore, 2003; van der Kolk, 2003). Multiple traumas, cumulative trauma and higher frequency, severity and chronicity of abuse are factors associated with diagnosis of personality disorder (Bandelow et al., 2005). A large US study of adverse childhood experiences (ACE) (Felitti et al., 1998) found that the majority of people who are given a diagnosis of personality disorder are understood to have histories of enduring trauma, of which over two-thirds was physical abuse, sexual abuse or witnessing serious domestic violence (Anda et al., 2006). A study of 21 000 Australians revealed that over 13 per cent of those surveyed reported having been abused in childhood, either physically or sexually, or both (Draper et al., 2008). The Australian Institute of Health and Welfare (Commonwealth of Australia, 2009) identified childhood abuse rates as 23 per cent physical,

29 per cent neglect, 38 per cent emotional, and 10 per cent sexual. Importantly, not all people affected seek psychological help; however, statistics show that two out of every three people presenting at emergency departments and inpatient or outpatient mental health services have experienced trauma (Bateman, Henderson & Kezelman, 2013).

Experiences such as these can lead to a massive disturbance in emotion regulation, interpersonal difficulties, self-integration difficulties, impulse control difficulties, and dissociation when under stress. More than one in three women (35.6 per cent) and more than one in four men (28.5 per cent) in the United States have experienced rape, physical violence and/or stalking by an intimate partner. Furthermore, the ACE study found that one in six men have experienced emotional trauma, 80 per cent of people in psychiatric hospitals have experienced physical or sexual abuse, 66 per cent of people in substance abuse treatment report childhood abuse or neglect, and 90 per cent of women with alcoholism were sexually abused or suffered severe violence from parents (Anda et al., 2006). In Britain, 46.4 per cent of people were found to have experienced at least one ACE, and 8.3 per cent had experienced four or more (Hughes, Lowey, Quigg & Bellis, 2016). A study identifying the prevalence of Australian children's exposure to potential family life difficulties found that chronic health conditions, both physical and mental, are likely indicators of underlying childhood emotional trauma.

Trauma-informed nursing practice is required to ensure physical, psychological and emotional safety within health care settings for people who have experienced trauma. See the trauma-informed care discussion in the nursing care section within this chapter for more on this topic.

CLASSIFICATION AND DIAGNOSIS

Through our personality, we react to the environment, and our individual personality characteristics will be most evident when we are under severe stress or challenge (Rutter, 2006). When our personal pattern of responding in stress or to challenge is determined to be 'maladaptive', we may be given a diagnosis of personality disorder.

Classification of disorders of personality began with Schneider in 1923 (Tyrer et al., 2015), and his nine types of personality are still evident within today's diagnostic classifications. Schneider's work was based on his clinical observations rather than research, and many of contemporary researchers consider modern personality classifications to be unvalidated. The words used to label disorders of personality are also problematic because they impart stigma; for example, diagnostic labels such as antisocial, narcissistic and schizotypal personality disorder. People who are diagnosed are often not aware that they have a disorder of personality, as the symptoms are not as obvious as those for other mental disorders. While classification and diagnosis fall outside of the scope of practice of nurses, it is useful to know that the assessment of personality is largely subjective, and is open to argument and disagreement. In accordance with the person-centred principles of nursing care, people should never be referred to by their diagnosis.

Diagnosis of personality disorders is problematic due to there being no clear threshold between types and degrees of personality dysfunction within the diagnostic system (Tyrer et al., 2015; Widiger, 2015), which causes overlapping diagnoses and diagnostic disagreement (Bateman, Gunderson & Mulder, 2015; Tyrer et al., 2015). Therefore, personality disorder is best understood as a single dimension or continuum, ranging from normal personality at one end through to severe personality disorder at the other. Personality disorders are currently diagnosed using criteria within the 5th edition of the *Diagnostic and statistical manual of mental disorders* (DSM-5) (APA, 2013) or the International Classification of Diseases 10th Revision (ICD-10) (World Health Organization, 1992).

Currently, there are 10 distinct disorder types: paranoid personality disorder, schizoid personality disorder, schizotypal personality disorder, antisocial personality disorder, borderline personality disorder, histrionic personality, narcissistic personality disorder, avoidant personality disorder, **dependent personality disorder** and obsessive–compulsive personality disorder (APA, 2013).

Diagnosis is made from matching an individual's symptoms or presentation to a personality disorder category (Shedler et al., 2010). There are three major categories of personality disorder, called *clusters*: Cluster A, odd–eccentric; Cluster B, dramatic–emotional; and Cluster C, anxious–fearful (APA, 2013). Even though there are differences among the three clusters, the following three traits are common within all three clusters:

- lack of insight and understanding of the impact of their behaviour on other people
- responding to feeling threatened by trying to change the environment rather than looking to change themselves and the way they perceive the environment
- unwillingness to accept the consequences of their own behaviour, and a tendency to project blame onto others.

The essential characteristics of personality disorders are chronicity, pervasiveness and maladaptation. The essential features of these disorders include significant distress or impairment in at least two of the following areas of functioning:

- cognition
- affect
- interpersonal relationships
- impulse control.

These behaviour patterns must be evident by early adulthood, and not be a result of other mental disorders or substance abuse (APA, 2013). It is important to distinguish the behaviour that defines personality disorder from responses that may emerge as a result of specific situational stressors or transient mental states. Therefore, it is necessary to conduct more than one interview with the person over a period of time. While individuals with personality disorder display enduring, inflexible and pervasive maladaptive behaviour in a broad variety of personal, occupational and social situations, they may not view their lifestyles as problematic. Typically, they do not seek professional help unless they are extremely anxious and/or in crisis.

The individual with a personality disorder can become trapped within the same dysfunctional pattern of maladaptive ways of responding across every dimension of life. In a desperate bid to try to gain some form of control over outcomes, the person may be experienced by others as manipulative. This is a highly damaging term once entered into an episode of care, and it is instead more helpful to understand and focus on the underlying issues to be addressed. In crisis, a person with a disorder of personality will be acutely focused on having their needs met, and may be seen by others as narcissistic. Again, this is another highly damaging term, which tends to influence clinician attitudes and distracts from solving the real issues at hand. Impulsive actions are also characteristic of personality disorder, and may be employed as a means of escape from a situation that has become unsolvable or intolerable. It is helpful to remember that the person is escaping from intolerable emotions within themselves in contrast to a deliberate desire to escape from the care they may currently be receiving. Box 18.2 provides the criteria for diagnosis of personality disorder according to the DSM-5.

Box 18.2 Criteria for diagnosis of personality disorder (APA, 2013)

Diagnosis of personality disorder is made after careful consideration of six criteria:

1. The person's own experiences and their resulting behaviour are different to what is evident in their surrounding culture. They view themselves, others and events differently. They appear to have little control over their impulses. As a result, interpersonal relationships are affected because the person's responses are often very intense, highly changeable or inappropriate.
2. The person's way of relating and behaving is fixed.
3. The person experiences major distress which impacts on their life in important areas.
4. The person describes these experiences as having been consistent, including during developmental phases.
5. These phenomena are not caused by another mental disorder.
6. These phenomena are not caused by other internal or external factors, such as illness, injury or substance use.

PERSONALITY DISORDER CLASSIFICATION

Cluster A personality disorders: odd–eccentric

Cluster A consists of the paranoid, schizoid and schizotypal personality disorders. The major features of these disorders are pervasive distrust, social detachment, and subsequent challenges in social and occupational functioning. People with odd–eccentric personality disorders have the most cognitive challenges, as well as the most peculiar behaviour and ineffective defensive styles, of people who experience disorder within personality. Table 18.1 ■ provides the diagnostic criteria,

Table 18.1 ■ DSM essential features—Cluster A personality disorders: odd–eccentric

Diagnostic criteria	Prevalence	Development and experience
Paranoid personality disorder: A pattern of distrust and suspiciousness such that others' motives are interpreted as malevolent: suspecting that others are exploiting, harming or deceiving them; doubting the loyalty of others; reluctant to confide in others; reading hidden meanings into remarks; holding grudges; anger reactions.	Internationally, between 2 per cent and 3 per cent of the general population. More common in men than women. Higher in prison populations. Improvement in behaviour over time. Higher rates of suicide, substance misuse and aggression. Comorbidity with other mental disorders is high (Khalifa et al., 2010).	Childhood and adolescence onset. Appearing odd or eccentric. Distorted private reality. Watchful, on guard, unable to relax. Social isolation to reduce anxiety. Distrust of others' motives, making claims against others leading to discrimination. MOVIE: Humphrey Bogart's character in *The Caine Mutiny*.
Schizoid personality disorder: Pervasive pattern of detachment from social relationships and a restricted range of emotional expression; engaging in solitary activities; lacks close friends; lacks enjoyment of activities; seems indifferent to praise or criticism; emotionally cold or indifferent with flat affect.	Two international surveys identified prevalence between 3.1 per cent and 4.9 per cent (APA, 2013). Schizoid personality diagnosis are said to have poor diagnostic validity. Major difference with schizotypal, below, is flat affect in contrast to anxious affect and magical thinking (Triebwasser, Chemerinski, Roussos, & Siever, 2012).	Childhood and adolescence onset. Is not common in clinical settings due to it not being a medical condition. Individuals adopt a stance in which they withdraw into themselves (Triebwasser et al., 2012). Rosa (2015) argues that there is an inhibition of aggression that gives rise to pervasive defensive postures and creates a struggle with the individual's inborn need to connect. Hess (2016) finds that clinical curiosity is threatening and will be rejected with withdrawal. People date infrequently and often don't marry. MOVIE: Ralph Fiennes's character in *The English Patient*.
Schizotypal personality disorder: A pattern of acute discomfort with, and reduced capacity for, close relationships; cognitive or perceptual distortions (depersonalisation, derealisation) and eccentricities of behaviour. May experience ideas of reference, magical thinking, illusions, and odd patterns of speech and behaviour; excessive social anxiety.	Prevalence estimates vary from 0.6 per cent in Norway to 3.9 per cent in the United States (APA, 2013).	Late adolescence onset thought to be preceded by language development delay, social difficulties, poor academic performance, motor difficulties, magical thinking, bizarre fantasies (Jones et al., 2015). Milder schizophrenia symptoms with individuals having ability to attenuate symptoms (Chemerinski, Triebwasser, Roussos & Siever, 2013). Most often seek treatment for anxiety and depression. Culturally competent assessment required, particularly around beliefs and rituals (APA, 2013). MOVIE: Robert de Niro's character in *Taxi Driver*.

prevalence rates and other information for Cluster A personality disorders.

Cluster B personality disorders: dramatic–emotional

People with antisocial, borderline, histrionic and narcissistic personality disorders can be characterised as dramatic, emotional and erratic. Individuals with these disorders are often in conflict with society through their impulsive behaviour. Impulsive people view the world as a discontinuous, fragmented collection of opportunities, frustrations and affective experiences. They may live mainly in the present moment and not formulate long-range plans. They may act without critical evaluation of consequences. Because they live very much in the present moment, the focus of their intellectual and emotional goals is to achieve satisfaction in the moment. A low level of impulse control, and difficulties with delaying gratification, often result in both verbal and non-verbal outbursts of anger, which may be self-directed or other-directed. Indeed, people with dramatic–emotional personality disorders may experience rapid escalation to distressing levels of anxiety. As interpersonal difficulties increase, they often rely on others to have their needs met or to find a way out of anxious situations. Table 18.2 ■ provides the diagnostic criteria, prevalence rates and other information for Cluster B personality disorders.

Practice example

Paranoid personality disorder

Jim, a 39-year-old engineer, has suspected that his employer is withholding significant data from him pertaining to an important job assignment. Jim began to question others about the reliability and integrity of his boss. He went to the factory one Sunday morning without permission. A security guard found him going through his employer's computer. His employer confronted him the following day, and sent him to the employee assistance program nurse. During the nurse's assessment, Jim states: 'I knew my boss was dishonest from the start. He could never give me a straight answer to my questions. As soon as I was almost onto what he was hiding, he set me up to look bad and maybe lose my job.'

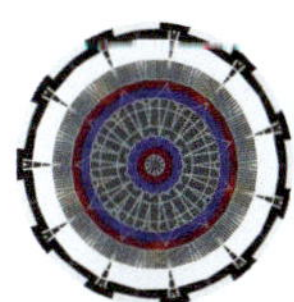

DEVELOPING CULTURAL COMPETENCE

Assessing people with schizoid and schizotypal personalities

Culture determines the meaning of behaviour. When assessing people with schizoid and schizotypal mannerisms, it is important to first consider the person's ethnicity, cultural milieu and spiritual beliefs. Within many cultures, phenomena such as speaking in tongues and psychic experiences are natural and not pathological. Multicultural assessment is necessary to gain a deeper understanding of the context of the person's beliefs and behaviour.

CRITICAL THINKING QUESTIONS

1. When would such experiences as speaking in tongues or being guided by a guardian angel be considered cultural and not pathological?
2. What does it indicate if a person from another culture does not ask questions when you offer the opportunity?

Practice example

Borderline personality disorder

Katie, age 29 years, has been admitted to hospital in a state of crisis, with deep cuts to her arms following the break-up of a relationship. Katie appears to be unable to stabilise her emotions, and becomes distressed very quickly. Katie tells you that she cuts herself to relieve the tension and distress, and that it wasn't an attempt to kill herself.

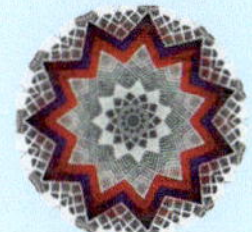

WHAT EVERY NURSE SHOULD KNOW

Person with borderline personality disorder

Imagine that you are a nurse working in a medical/surgical setting and you have care of a woman who has visible scars of cuts up both of her arms. This means that you are dealing with a person who has experienced trauma and *may* have borderline personality disorder. Take note of the following:

- Anxiety and high levels of arousal are expected responses within the hospital setting. The person may be making frequent requests in a bid to reduce anxiety or arousal levels.
- Delivering care according to the principles and practices of trauma-informed care is essential.
- Meet their needs wherever possible, and provide a reasonable explanation as to why other needs are not able to be met.
- Teach them relaxation techniques and encourage their use.
- De-escalate yourself first, remain calm, remain reasonable, *do not judge* the person.
- *Do not* participate in discussions with your colleagues about the 'unreasonableness' of the person's requests.
- Do use practices such as trimvirate team nursing to maintain professional caregiving.
- Maintain peer support and clinical supervision throughout the period of care.

Practice example

Narcissistic personality disorder

Michael has been admitted to the surgical ward for a knee replacement. Michael and his wife have frequent arguments during visits, because Michael does not believe that his wife treats him the way he should be treated. He expects her to put his needs above her own, and to attend to him at the hospital whenever he requires it. Michael is displaying the same attitude towards nurses. When his needs aren't being immediately met, he feels rejected and shouts at nurses or refuses to talk to them. Michael's wife has advised him that she will no longer visit him at the hospital because she is embarrassed by the way he is speaking to her in front of others, and is also embarrassed about the way he is treating the nurses. He tells her in front of everyone 'you will regret doing that to me'.

TABLE 18.2 ■ Essential features—Cluster B personality disorders: dramatic–emotional

Diagnostic criteria	Prevalence	Development and experience
Antisocial personality disorder: Pervasive pattern of disregard for and violation of the rights of others. Characterised by social rule-breaking, offending, deceitfulness, impulsivity, irresponsibility and aggressiveness. Shows reckless disregard for the safety of self and others. May also involve alcohol and illicit drug misuse, anxiety, depression, unemployment, homelessness and relationship difficulties.	Prevalence is higher in adverse socio-economic circumstances. Rates in the general population are between 0.2 per cent and 3.3 per cent, while they are greater than 70 per cent in forensic settings (APA, 2013).	Begins in childhood and continues into adulthood (APA, 2013). Cannot be diagnosed before 18 years of age. Remits as people age. Only half of people who meet diagnostic criteria commit criminal offences (Hatchett, 2015). Considerable comorbidity with other psychiatric diagnoses, and a high rate of rejection by health services (Duggan, 2009). Distressing for the individual and their families and friends; e.g. marital problems and unemployment. Positive outcomes shown to substance misuse treatment (Gibbon, 2010). Clinicians with poor boundaries struggle with the rule-breaking, egocentricity, deceitfulness and disregard for others' feelings of people with this diagnosis (Duggan, 2009). MOVIE: Anne Hathaway's character in *Rachel Getting Married*.
Borderline personality disorder: Characterised by a pattern of unstable relationships, disturbance to affect and disturbance to self-image, with marked impulsivity. Intense fear of abandonment; identity disturbance; impulsivity; chronic feelings of emptiness; intense anger and/or rage. Transient stress-related paranoid ideation or dissociative symptoms. Recurrent suicidal behaviour, gestures and self-mutilating behaviour.	Prevalence ranges from 2 per cent to 5 per cent in Australia, with 75 per cent being female. A strong correlation between childhood sexual trauma and borderline personality has been found (MacIntosh, Godbout & Dubash, 2015); however, trauma experiences are not part of the diagnostic criteria.	Chronic instability in early adulthood. Often engaged with health services. Very sensitive to environmental circumstances, inappropriate anger when fearing abandonment, low tolerance for being alone. Can switch between idealising and devaluing clinicians. Dramatic shifts to sudden disillusionment, with intense anger often played out upon the self. High need for care-givers with strong boundaries and good validation skills. MOVIE: Angelina Jolie's character in *Girl Interrupted*.
Histrionic personality disorder: Pattern of attention-seeking and excessive emotionality; a need to be the centre of attention; uses physical appearance and provocative behaviour to draw attention to self; exaggerated expression; easily suggestive.	Prevalence of 1.84 per cent internationally (APA, 2013). More frequently diagnosed in females. Original term 'hystera' related to 'womb', and belief that women would get angry, hysterical and diseased when unable to bear children. Later converted to 'wandering womb' and 'wicked womb' (Novais, Araújo & Godinho, 2015).	Features mostly within relationships with role identification with 'victim' or 'princess' (Novais et al., 2015). Impaired friendships due to high attention needs. Crave novelty, stimulation and to be the centre of attention. Only diagnosed as a disorder when traits become maladaptive. MOVIE: Vivien Leigh's character in *Gone With the Wind*.
Narcissistic personality disorder: A pervasive pattern of grandiosity (in fantasy or behaviour), need for admiration, and lack of empathy. Characterised by a grandiose sense of self-importance and a belief that one is 'special'. Preoccupied with fantasies of success, power and brilliance; a strong sense of entitlement and a need for admiration. Exploits others, is envious and lacks empathy.	Prevalence 6.2 per cent, with rates greater for men (7.7 per cent) than women (4.8 per cent) (Stinson et al., 2008). High comorbidities with substance use, mood, anxiety and other personality disorders (Stinson et al., 2008). More disability associated with males.	Traits common in normal adolescence, but most individuals do not go on to be diagnosed with the disorder. Those diagnosed devalue others while overvaluing self. May devalue the credentials of those who disappoint them. Clinicians require strong boundaries, the ability to not take things personally, and the ability to validate others. The therapeutic key is in understanding rather than reacting (Romano, 2004). MOVIE: Natalie Portman's character in *Black Swan*.

Cluster C personality disorders: anxious–fearful

Individuals who experience disorder within their personality that is primarily anxious or fearful may be diagnosed with avoidant, dependent or obsessive–compulsive personality disorder. Anxious–fearful people generally experience both social and occupational challenges as a result of their restricted affect, non-assertiveness, difficulty with expressing feelings, unrealistic expectations of others, ineffective decision-making and problem-solving. The lifestyle of the anxious–fearful person is characterised by intense emotional repression and behaviour that is socially isolating and self-defeating. The behaviour of anxious–fearful personalities tends to overlap, and common diagnostic features are described in Table 18.3 ■, along with prevalence rates and other information for Cluster C personality disorders.

TABLE 18.3 ■ Essential features—Cluster C personality disorders: anxious–fearful

Diagnostic criteria	Prevalence	Development and experience
Avoidant personality disorder: Pervasive pattern of social inhibition, feelings of inadequacy, and hypersensitivity to negative evaluation. Avoidance of activities due to fear of criticism or rejection; unwillingness to establish interpersonal relationships; self-perception of inadequacy; reluctance to try new things because of fear of embarrassment.	Prevalence estimates from available studies suggest 2.4 per cent.	Begins in infancy or early childhood as shyness and avoidance (APA, 2013) and remits with increasing age. Link found between avoidant personality disorder depression and anxiety symptoms, childhood maltreatment, parental overprotection and childhood teasing (Hageman, Francis, Field & Carr, 2015). MOVIE: Anthony Hopkin's character in *The Remains of the Day*.
Dependent personality disorder: Pervasive and excessive need to be taken care of, resulting in submissive, clinging behaviour; fears of separation/abandonment; needs others to assume responsibility for major decisions; fears disapproval; lacks self-confidence; feels helpless when alone; exaggerated fears of being unable to care for self.	Prevalence 0.6 per cent, although 14 per cent comorbidity with other personality disorders (Faith, 2009). Should not be diagnosed in children or adolescents due to dependence being developmentally appropriate. Diagnosed more frequently in females (APA, 2013).	Fear of abandonment, fear of losing support or approval. Care seeking is high, as is the need to be seen to be deserving of care. Individuals with this diagnosis have great difficulty expressing disagreement. This feature when combined with the need for close relationships can keep dependent people trapped in abusive relationships. MOVIE: Jennifer Jason Leigh's character in *Single White Female*.
Obsessive–compulsive personality disorder: Preoccupation with orderliness, perfectionism and control. Focusing on details to the extent that the major point of the activity is lost. Perfectionism interferes with task completion. Excessive devotion to work; overly conscientious, scrupulous and inflexible; hoards money and worthless objects; reluctant to delegate tasks due to need for control. Demonstrates rigidity and stubbornness.	Prevalence between 2.1 per cent and 7.9 per cent. Thought to be one of the most prevalent personality disorders. More common in males than females.	May have difficulties prioritising or making decisions. May become angry or upset when unable to control their environment. Anxiety is common in social situations. MOVIE: Jack Nicholson's character in *As Good As It Gets*.

Practice example

Avoidant personality disorder

Michael Jackson lived as a virtual recluse at his Neverland property. Michael wore masks and disguises when going out in public, and also required his children to do the same. Michael didn't enjoy attention in the way that many stars of his calibre do. He built an amusement park on his property so that he could enjoy himself without having to encounter the public. People who knew Michael often stated that he was painfully shy. Michael once stated: 'People think they know me, but they don't. Not really. Actually, I am one of the loneliest people on this Earth. I cry sometimes, because it hurts. It does. To be honest, I guess you could say that it hurts to be me.'

Practice example

Obsessive–compulsive personality disorder

Bryce explained, 'I have all of my clothes hanging in the closet according to the day of the week, including my shoes, socks and underwear. So I know that if it's a Tuesday after a long weekend with a Monday holiday, I need to bypass the clothing on the hanger marked "Monday" and wear the clothing on the hanger marked "Tuesday".'

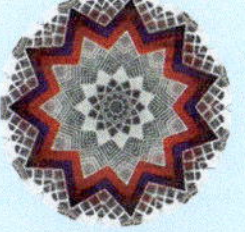

WHAT EVERY NURSE SHOULD KNOW

Person with dependent personality disorder

Imagine that you are a maternal/child health nurse:

- Be alert for signs of depression in new mothers.
- Assess the woman's history for indicators of domestic abuse—conduct a domestic violence screen.
- Women who are excessively dependent may have difficulty in assuming care for a newborn.
- Be attuned to your own feelings of helplessness to ensure that apathy does not interfere with your ability to deliver quality care.
- Avoid the tendency to rescue the dependent person; this will only reinforce helplessness.
- Encourage the woman to do things for herself and her infant; don't do them for her.
- Validate the woman's taking of personal responsibility.

Other personality disorders

Personality change due to another medical condition

This is a personality disturbance due to the direct effects of a medical condition (e.g. frontal lobe lesion). Varying types include labile type, disinhibited type, aggressive type, apathetic type, paranoid type, other type, combined type or unspecified type.

Other specified personality disorder

This is where the individual's personality pattern meets the general criteria for a personality disorder and traits of several different personality disorders are present, but criteria for a specific personality disorder are not met, or meets the general criteria however traits don't meet specific diagnoses, e.g. passive–aggressive personality disorder.

Personality disorder not otherwise specified

A diagnosis of personality disorder not otherwise specified (PD-NOS) may be given to people who do not meet five criteria for diagnosis under another specific personality disorder, but do meet the required criteria of five for a diagnosis to be given. Regardless of the number of criteria that are met, the person will experience psychosocial function and other dimensions of personality consistent with personality disorder diagnosis; however, the difference is in severity of symptoms (Coccaro, Nayyer & McCloskey, 2012). The person may exhibit characteristics of a disorder that are not included in the existing classification system; for example, depressive and passive–aggressive personality disorder.

EPIDEMIOLOGY

Personality disorders are among the most common disorders experienced by people who are mentally distressed (Skodol et al., 2005), and are believed to affect 10–12 per cent of the general population internationally (Torgersen, 2005; Dixon-Gordon, Whalen, Layden & Chapman, 2015) and 6.5 per cent in Australia (Lewin, Slade, Andrews, Carr & Hornabrook, 2005). Very few epidemiological studies have been conducted in the area of personality disorders, particularly in the Australian context. Personality disorders were previously believed to be enduring and relatively stable from childhood into adult life (APA, 2013); however, there is now a reasonable expectation that people can recover, with fewer than 50 per cent of people diagnosed retaining the diagnosis over time (Skodol, Johnson, Cohen, Sneed & Crawford, 2007).

Having a Cluster A personality disorder (odd–eccentric cluster) can lead to lower education and achievement levels, greater partner conflict, childbearing in the adolescent years (Chen et al.) and comorbid mood, eating and anxiety disorders. Cluster B (dramatic–erratic–emotional) traits lead to difficulties with intimacy and relationship conflict (Crawford, Cohen, Johnson, Sneed & Brook, 2004), substance misuse and anxiety, mood and eating disorders, and more challenged daily functioning than other personality disorders (Zanarini, Frankenburg, Hennen, Reich, & Silk, 2006). Cluster C (anxious–fearful) is linked with difficulties or lack of desire to form relationships, and conflict once in a relationship, and also mood and anxiety disorders (Johnson, Cohen, Kasen & Brook, 2006). PD-NOS is linked with educational failure and interpersonal difficulties. People who experience borderline personality disorder are more likely to experience other comorbid mental disorders, greater mental disability and negative impact on role functioning (Jackson & Burgess, 2004). High levels of trait expression in adolescence across Clusters A and B are associated with violence towards others, in Cluster C with suicide, and borderline personality disorder with self-harm. A large longitudinal study of personality disorder outcomes found that 12 per cent of study participants attempted suicide within the six-year study period, and 44 per cent of those made multiple attempts (Yen et al., 2005), suggesting that a diagnosis of personality disorder represents a significant risk for suicide, when compared to the general population.

Experiencing a personality disorder also strongly increases the likelihood of having three or more co-occurring long-standing illnesses, such as depression, asthma, other chest problems, rheumatism or arthritis, migraines and back problems (Fok et al., 2014, Skodol, Geier, Grant & Hasin, 2014). The suicide rate and therefore suicide risk are also higher (Skodol et al., 2005), and are associated with premature mortality (Tyrer et al., 2015).

RECOVERY AND SELF-DISCOVERY

Contrary to traditionally held beliefs, the majority of people recover from personality disorder, and many more experience significant decline in trait expression as they age (Johnson et al., 2000; Lenzenweger, Lane, Loranger & Kessler, 2007; Skodol et al., 2014; Zanarini, Frankenburg, Reich & Fitzmaurice, 2010). Four large-scale longitudinal studies of the course of personality disorders have identified that personality disorder trait expression decreased by 48 per cent between ages 14 and 22. In the first six years of follow-up on longitudinal studies, over 60 per cent experienced a 12-month remission. Those who still express traits in their thirties experience greater challenges with daily functioning, and those who develop a disorder in their thirties also experience significant challenges (Skodol et al., 2007). Longitudinal studies use the term 'remission', and explain a state of remission as meeting two or fewer personality disorder criteria for either 2 consecutive months or 12 consecutive months, depending on the study (Skodol et al., 2005, Zanarini, Frankenburg, Hennen, Reich & Silk, 2005).

Borderline personality disorder has been shown to improve over a 10-year period with 88 per cent of people diagnosed entering 'remission' and only 6 per cent of those experiencing another episode. In recovery terms, this equates to an 82 per cent recovery rate. Cluster A personality disorders are equated with 55 per cent remission rates, and cluster C, 33 per cent (Grilo et al., 2004). Schizotypal personality disorder has the lowest relapse rate, and avoidant personality disorder has the highest. There is no diagnostic exit door from any mental illness diagnosis once given, including personality disorders, and people who do recover are unable to have their psychiatric 'label' or the resulting stigma removed, even though they have recovered.

Recovery in the wider context of mental illness is well explored, and has its origins within the mental health service consumer and survivor movements. Two useful models to guide understanding of the experience of personal recovery have been developed within Australia. First, Glover (2012), a person with **lived experience**, identified five recovery processes as encompassing: passive to active sense of self, hopelessness to hope, other's control to self-control, alienation to discovery, and disconnectedness to connectedness. Secondly, Andresen, Oades and Caputi (Andresen et al., 2011; Andresen et al., 2003) identified four processes: finding and maintaining hope, re-establishing a positive identity, building a meaningful life, and taking responsibility and control. Within Australian policy, the wider definition of recovery from mental illness, such as that proposed by Andresen et al.'s model (2011) and Glover's model (2012), has been adopted thus far for personality disorder (National Health and Medical Research Council [NHMRC], 2012).

There is argument within published literature that these broader definitions of recovery from mental illness are not the best fit for understanding recovery from personality disorders (Gillard et al., 2015; Turner, Lovell & Brooker, 2011). There is a paucity of lived experience literature on recovery from personality disorder, and due to this the unique experiences and challenges of personality disorder are not embedded within current models of recovery. An example is that the social interventions typically delivered within recovery programs can be experienced as challenging, and can lead to social exclusion, alienation and isolation rather than inclusion for people with personality disorder (Castillo, Ramon & Morant, 2013; Gillard et al., 2015).

Some early definitions for recovery within the context of personality disorder are emerging. One idea is that recovery from personality disorder involves a journey of self-discovery rather than recovery of something. Personality disorder involves an intense struggle between internally and externally experienced worlds, with a consequent need to discover a self that can safely co-exist in both worlds. A metaphor for the struggle between external and internal worlds is that of falling through a trapdoor.

> *. . . it can change instantly how I'm feeling . . . I could be fine one minute and the next minute I would just go down, straight down . . . you're walking along sometimes, a trapdoor opens and you just fall through the trapdoor and you can't get back up again . . .* (Gillard et al., 2015, p. 5)

The subsequent intense internal emotional state may lead to the need to isolate or to act out these emotions with volatility or self-harm. Remaining linked to the external world through contact with a nonjudgmental and supportive person helps.

A preferred term for recovery from personality disorder is '**self-discovery**' which includes uncovering latent potential and tapping into undeveloped talents and abilities through an ongoing process of growth and self-actualisation (Turner et al., 2011). Recognition of the need for personal reconciliation of the internal and external selves is necessary within any definition of recovery from personality disorder (Siddiqui, 2014). Figure 18.2 ■ illustrates how the internal and external worlds are intersected by the process of recovery and discovery of a sense of self that co-exists in both worlds.

The Haven Hierarchy of Progress represents key steps in the journey of recovery, self-discovery and growth with personality disorder (Castillo et al., 2013; see Figure 18.3 ■).

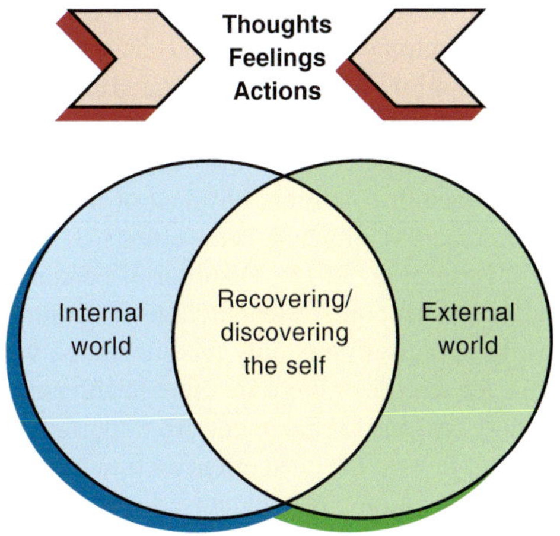

FIGURE 18.2 ■ Reconciliation of internal and external worlds through self-discovery.

Transitional recovery
Achievements
Hopes, dreams and goals
Containing experiences and developing skills
Learning the boundaries
A sense of belonging and community
Feeling cared for
A sense of safety and building trust

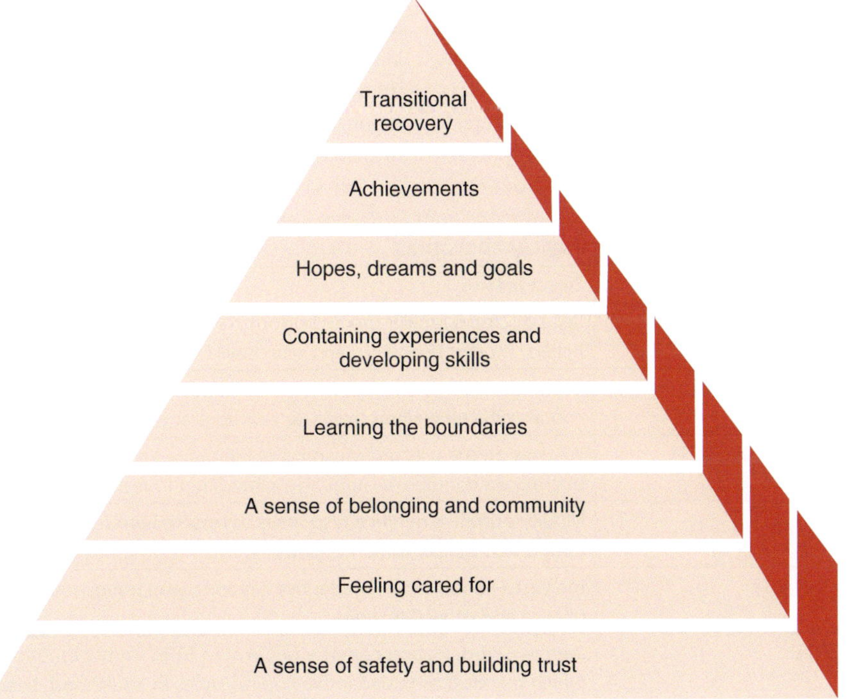

FIGURE 18.3 ■ The Haven Hierarchy of Progress represents key steps in the journey of recovery, self-discovery and growth with personality disorder (Castillo et al., 2013).

The first step starts most essentially with building a sense of safety and trust, and is related to reorganising insecure attachment into secure attachment, as discussed earlier in this chapter. Feeling cared for implies acceptance and leads to a developing a sense of belonging in community. Connecting with community is challenging, as it involves both internal and external selves, intense vulnerability and the need to develop healthy boundaries. Later processes include learning to contain emotional experiences, develop skills to cope, unleash hopes, dreams and goals, and experience achievement and transitional recovery (Castillo et al., 2013).

TREATMENT

Personality disorder is not a discrete illness to be treated. It is a cluster of ways of responding in the social world which tends to complicate situations rather than lead easily to solutions.

Because disorder of personality is related to an individual's lifetime emotional and social development, anyone can be affected. Therefore, personality disorder may be comorbid with any other health condition, physical or mental, and will be encountered across all health care settings (Dixon-Gordon et al., 2015; Tyrer et al., 2015). Disorder of personality has a negative effect on the course and outcome of comorbid health conditions. Hospitalisation is only recommended when there is a high risk for suicide or there are other health concerns that are the primary reasons for treatment. An important reason for this is that people who have experienced trauma are exposed to the risk of becoming re-traumatised within health care settings through the actions of health care professionals.

Psychological therapies

Psychological interventions are regarded to be most effective treatment for personality disorders (Stoffers et al., 2010). Interventions may be delivered by psychologists or nurses, may be on a one-to-one basis over a lengthy period of time, or may be within groups. Nurses are more likely to be involved with group work rather than one-on-one intensive psychotherapy. Therapies used include psychodynamic psychotherapy (all personality disorder diagnoses), cognitive behaviour therapy (CBT) (all diagnoses), dialectical behaviour therapy (DBT) (mainly borderline personality disorder), acceptance and commitment therapy (ACT) (all diagnoses), client-centred therapy, transference-focused therapy (TFT), mentalisation-based treatment (MBT), schema-focused therapy (SFT), and systems training for emotional predictability and problem-solving (STEPPS). Most of these treatments are effective when delivered as longer-term 6 to 12 months outpatient or community therapy. Short-term hospital treatment is effective for gaining emotional stability in a crisis situation or for commencing medication to reduce anxiety or arousal; however, it is generally not long enough to achieve psychological change.

Treatment recommendations for **antisocial personality disorder** include domestic violence groups, boot camps, therapeutic communities, mental health courts and substance abuse programs (Hatchett, 2015), which have shown some improvements in physical aggression and other beneficial outcomes. Table 18.4 ■ provides descriptions of the psychological therapies used in the treatment of personality disorder.

Cognitive behaviour therapy (CBT) and dialectical behaviour therapy (DBT) are widely used in the treatment of personality disorder. CBT encompasses more than 70 techniques aimed at encouraging the person to examine the beliefs underpinning their situational responses, and to learn new ways of understanding and responding (O'Donohue, Fisher & Hayes, 2003). DBT is based on the assumption that the individual's life is currently unbearable. DBT encourages the belief that the person is doing the best that they can, that they want to improve; however at the same time, they need to do better, try harder and be more motivated to change. DBT theory believes that individuals may not have caused their own problems, but they have to solve them anyway through learning new behaviour in all relevant contexts (Linehan and Wilks, 2015). The goal of DBT is to help the person improve interpersonal relationships, tolerate distress and regulate emotional responses. See Chapter 25 for more detailed information on DBT.

TABLE 18.4 ■ Personality disorder psychological therapies

Therapeutic model	Description
Cognitive behaviour therapy (CBT)	Self-directed learning process through which people identify and evaluate their core beliefs, modify behaviour and gain new experiences.
Dialectical behaviour therapy (DBT)	Behaviour change through using mindfulness, role-play and rehearsal to tolerate distress, contain difficult feelings, regulate emotions and learn successful interpersonal behaviour.
Acceptance and commitment therapy (ACT)	Focuses on the use and meaning of language and the ways in which language shapes the human condition. Language is modified to reduce psychological suffering.
Transference-focused therapy (TFT)	Modify primitive defence responses to resolve identity diffusion and achieve an integrated representation of self.
Mentalisation-based therapy (MBT)	Increases an individual's reflective capacity, and builds recognition and understanding of own and others' feelings.
Schema-focused therapy (SFT)	Identify self-defeating core themes arising from unmet emotional needs in childhood which manifest as maladaptive coping styles in adulthood. Learn to get needs met.
Systems training for emotional predictability and problem-solving (STEPPS)	Group-based education which combines CBT and skills training. Used to supplement ongoing treatment.

LIVED EXPERIENCE

The value of therapy

DBT changed my life. I learned skills that were missing from my life. DBT taught me mindfulness, emotion regulation, distress tolerance and interpersonal effectiveness.

Prior to DBT, I was admitted to psychiatric emergency care on almost a monthly basis, and self-harm was a regular occurrence. After completing 12 months of DBT in an outpatient setting, I average one to two visits a year, and very rarely self-harm. People around me noticed the changes in my behaviour even during DBT; in particular, with managing my emotions and coping with distress.

Medication

Prescribing medication (unless it is a standing order) remains outside of the scope of practice of registered nurses (RN); however, nurse practitioners in Australia do have prescribing rights for a wide range of psychotropic medications, including those used to treat the distressing consequences of personality disorder. The registered nurse standards for practice requires nurses to adhere to legal requirements for medications (Nursing and Midwifery Board of Australia [NMBA], 2010), and psychotropic medications are routinely administered by registered nurses in all health care settings, including as prn medications. Nurses are required to understand the different psychotropic medication classes, and to educate and empower individuals receiving the medication, as well as to monitor and respond to therapeutic effects, overdose effects, unwanted adverse effects and life-threatening syndromes that can result from psychotropic medication administration. Within specific mental health care settings and as determined under each state and territory's *Mental Health Act*, medication may be administered by nurses without consent and against the will of the person receiving the medication, particularly if the person is highly aroused and the risk for harm is present. Therefore it is essential that registered nurses understand the legal and practice imperatives around the various *Mental Health Acts* which guide practice in each jurisdiction.

Antidepressants, antipsychotics, mood stabilisers and anti-anxiety medications may all be prescribed to help modulate mood, manage emotions and reduce the symptoms of hyperarousal that are associated with personality disorder (Vollm et al., 2014). The Cochrane Collaboration commissioned systematic reviews of research on pharmacological interventions for Cluster A, B and C personality disorders. Borderline and antisocial personality disorders were the only conditions with sufficient research evidence to produce a pharmacological treatment protocol. Insufficient research has been conducted on medication use for obsessive–compulsive, paranoid, narcissistic, schizotypal, schizoid, histrionic and avoidant personality disorders (Ahmed et al., 2014; Alex, 2014; Farooq et al., 2014a; Farooq et al., 2014b; Stoffers et al., 2014a; Stoffers et al., 2014b; Vollm et al., 2014).

Twenty-eight trials involving 1742 people examined first-generation antipsychotics, second-generation antipsychotics, mood stabilisers, antidepressants and dietary supplementation (omega-3 fatty acid) usage in the treatment of symptoms of borderline personality disorder (Stoffers et al., 2010). First-generation antipsychotics and antidepressants showed only marginal effects. The use of second-generation antipsychotics, mood stabilisers and omega-3 fatty acids is supported; however, the long-term use of these drugs has not been studied. Olanzapine is possibly associated with an increase in self-harming behaviour, significant weight gain and sedation. Topiramate is associated with a significant decrease in body weight.

Eight trials involving 274 people examined eight different medications used for the treatment of symptoms of antisocial personality disorder, and found that only three demonstrated effectiveness compared to placebo (Khalifa et al., 2010). Nortriptyline is associated with a reduction in the number of drinking days for alcohol-dependent men. Nortriptyline and bromocriptine contributed to a reduction in anxiety according to one scale, and phenytoin is associated with reduction in the frequency and intensity of aggressive acts in male prisoners with impulsive aggression (Alex, 2014).

The person who is diagnosed with the types of personality disorders that contribute to psychological distress are often heavily medicated, if not over-medicated, in an attempt to manage anxiety, impulsivity and mood disturbance (Paris, 2015). The nurse's role in medication administration includes understanding and reflecting upon the experience of psychotropic medication from the perspective of those who are prescribed it, and considering the issues related to effective therapeutic alliance and the administration of medications within nursing practice. Nurses need to have open dialogue with those in their care about potential and actual adverse effects, and strongly advocate for review when people feel that adverse effects are impacting on important life responsibilities and experiences. Nurses are also responsible for educating on the therapeutic and adverse effects of medications, appropriately assessing and monitoring progress, valuing the person as an expert on their own experience, and being able to advocate for review when required.

NURSING CARE

Traditionally, nurses do not find the challenging nature of the features of personality disorder a comfortable or attractive work experience, although nurses who choose to commit themselves to excellence within this area find the work rewarding and fulfilling. There is a high need for continuing professional education and development, and a commitment to being therapeutic and effective. The ability to not take things personally is uppermost when working with people who have their own reasons to suspect authority and to choose to either seek treatment or reject treatment (Duggan, 2009). Treatment seekers are often also labelled as attention-seekers by nurses when they choose not to accept or don't respond to the help that is offered. Treatment rejecters can be regarded as not valid recipients of care. Consumer-generated evidence shows that nurses are capable of re-traumatising individuals with personality disorders in their care through practices of invalidation, shaming and dismissal of their right and need for care.

Self-awareness is the first step in developing therapeutic approaches to people with any personality disorder. By examining your own responses and feelings, you will be better able to prevent countertransference from occurring (refer Chapter 6). The Self-awareness feature, at right, will direct you towards reflection. Education on therapeutic approaches for personality disorder such as DBT will ensure that you are therapeutically effective in this area of practice.

Arousal of feelings of anger, powerlessness, a sense of having been 'conned', disappointment, and even guilt and shame is common among nurses (Filer, 2005). Nurses are often unaware of their own underlying beliefs, which may be countertherapeutic. By using introspection and clinical supervision, you can become more aware of the emergence of your own beliefs and the impact of your feelings and behaviour on others.

SELF-AWARENESS

Explore your thoughts and feelings towards people with personality disorder

Your answers to the following questions will help you assess your reactions:

- Can you detect your early physiological and emotional responses to stress?
- How great is your need to rescue or 'save' people from unhealthy situations?
- How do you know when you are becoming defensive?
- How do you respond when you become angry with a person in your care?
- What do you do when you feel helpless to effect change?
- What do you do when you feel guilty about being unable to help a person in your care?
- What is your behavioural response when you feel that you have been 'used'?

Nurses have been found to lack a clear understanding of personality disorder, and this can result in negative attitudes, reactive responses such as rejection, and greater social distance

LIVED EXPERIENCE

Experience of receiving nursing care

I sometimes find that when I present to an emergency department with mental health issues, such as self-harm or suicidal ideation, nursing staff treat me as though I have an intellectual disability. This may include speaking to me very slowly, speaking loudly or as though I don't understand what they are saying. I have also had one nurse speak to another nurse about me, as though I don't understand their conversation. I, like many people with mental illness, have no intellectual impairment—in fact, I hold postgraduate qualifications. I appreciate when nurses speak to me like any other patient.

People who have self-harmed also feel that they are treated like they are not deserving of emergency care because the injury is self-inflicted. The injury is often a result of mental distress, and I feel the physical injury is as valid as any other. It is sad and also dangerous that many of my friends with personality disorders are too scared to attend an emergency department with self-harm—many injuries I have seen should have had medical attention.

When I attended an emergency department a few years ago with self-inflicted burns on my arms, I was assessed by the mental health team. The team decided that I was okay to go home, but that I needed to see one of the medical doctors to have the burns examined first. I approached the triage nurse to ask if I could sit away from the waiting room, as I was still teary and it was drawing unwanted attention. The nurse stood up and said quite loudly and aggressively, 'If you don't want to wait, you can go and see your GP tomorrow.' I was extremely embarrassed. I was okay with waiting; I just wanted to know if it was possible to sit elsewhere. I felt as though the burns on my arm didn't deserve medical attention—and now being even more distressed, I left the emergency department. The burns on my arm developed an infection over the next few days. The risk of infection could have been minimised if I had seen the doctor, and would most likely have been given prophylactic antibiotics and wound care.

When I more recently presented to an emergency department in distress, the triage nurse came and spoke to me while I was waiting to see the psychiatrist. The nurse said that she couldn't offer me any medication before I saw the doctor, but asked if I would like a bag full of ice cubes to hold. This is one of the DBT skills I have been taught to handle intense emotions. I accepted the offer. I don't know whether the intensity of the cold ice in my hand brought my distress down, or the fact that the nurse had acknowledged my distress and offered very practical assistance.

WHY I CHOOSE TO WORK IN MENTAL HEALTH

Sue Sumskis, BN (Hons), PhD, RN, CMHN, FACMHN

Very early on in my mental health nursing career, I chose personality disorder as a practice specialty. When I encountered a person who was having an emotional crisis or who self-harmed in health care settings, I felt therapeutically ineffective and I knew I needed education and skills. I read extensively and went on a study tour to investigate international practices. I came to understand that, more often than not, I was dealing with deeply traumatised individuals, and I came to accept that every individual was doing the best they could with what resources they currently had. The day I discovered dialectical behaviour therapy (DBT) I felt that the windows had been thrown open and the light of improved practice came flooding in. DBT gave me the understanding and the tools I needed to be an effective nurse in this context. Interestingly, studies have shown that it isn't particular therapies that are effective, but rather the therapist's belief in the therapeutic model. I encourage every nurse to align themselves with a therapeutic model that represents a good fit with their practice style. Your nursing practice will thereafter be characterised by rewarding and fulfilling therapeutic relationships.

than other diagnoses (Markham and Trower, 2003). A majority of nurses do not cope well with the key features of personality disorder, in particular instability of interpersonal relationships, which impacts on the development of a therapeutic relationship (McGrath and Dowling, 2012). Poor preparedness to deal with challenging behaviour can lead to the re-traumatisation of admitted individuals. Despite experiences of negativity with some nurses, the therapeutic relationship is still regarded to be the most important support (Fallon, 2003).

Therapeutic challenges

Most therapeutic guidelines recommend that multi-disciplinary and multi-agency networks be established around each individual. Within nursing settings, team nursing with a strong peer-review structure supporting that nursing effort is recommended. Box 18.3 provides key principles for working with people who experience disorder of personality.

To be effective in the therapeutic relationship, nurses need to possess well-developed personal boundaries (Winship, 2010), and strive to maintain practice within the zone of helpfulness rather than being over-involved or under-involved (NMBA, 2010). Studies of nurses' attitudes to caring for people with personality disorders have revealed low levels of empathy and greater social distance than with other mental disorders (Winship, 2010). These attitudes are also found in nursing students (Weight & Kendal, 2013). Key diagnostic features of emotional instability, poor impulse control and deliberate self-harm can lead to some nurses developing beliefs that the person is dangerous (Filer, 2005; Markham, 2003; Winship, 2010). Lack of diagnostic understanding may lead to stigmatisation and exclusion from services (Lamph, 2011). Nurses' responses then feed into the person's poor self-image, chronic feelings of emptiness and fear of being abandoned (Eastwick & Grant, 2005). Early theorists and researchers in the area drew attention to the link between the negative reactions of staff and the increasing malfunctioning and suicidal behaviour of people diagnosed with personality disorders (Adler, 1973; Friedman, 1969; Gunderson, 1984). Box 18.4 provides key principles for responding to a person who is in crisis.

Box 18.3 Key principles for working with people with personality disorders

- Demonstrate **empathy**.
- **Listen** to the person's current experience.
- **Validate** the person's current emotional state.
- **Take the person's experience seriously**, noting verbal and non-verbal communications.
- Maintain a **nonjudgmental** approach.
- Stay **calm**.
- Remain **respectful**.
- Remain **caring**.
- Engage in **open communication**.
- **Be human**, and be prepared to acknowledge both the serious and the funny side of life where appropriate.
- Foster **trust** to allow strong emotions to be freely expressed.
- Be **clear, consistent and reliable**.
- Remember aspects of challenging behaviour have **survival value** given past experiences.
- Convey **encouragement** and **hope** about the person's capacity for change, while validating their current emotional experience.

Source: Grenyer et al., 2015.

Assessment

When assessing people who experience personality disorder, ensure that your words and actions are congruent—that is, be sure that your non-verbal behaviour matches what you say. You must maintain professional distance by using empathy. Specific questions you can ask consumers and their families are outlined in the following Your Assessment Approach.

Box 18.4 Intervention strategies for responding to a person in crisis (Grenyer et al., 2015)

1. Remain calm, supportive and nonjudgmental.
2. Avoid expressing shock or anger.
3. Stay focused on what is happening in the here and now. Avoid discussions about the person's childhood history or relationship problems, as these can 'unravel' the person and are better addressed in ongoing treatment.
4. Express empathy and concern.
5. Explain clearly the role of all staff involved, including how, when and what each will be doing to support the person.
6. Conduct a risk assessment. Remember the level of risk changes over time, so it is important to conduct a risk assessment *every time* the person presents in crisis.
7. Make a follow-up appointment and/or refer the person to an appropriate service.
8. After the crisis, ensure that the follow-up appointment and referral was successful.

YOUR ASSESSMENT APPROACH

People with dramatic–emotional personality disorders and their families

Use the following statements with the person:

- How often do you notice rapid mood changes?
- Tell me about one time you lost your temper.
- Describe how you get along with others.
- Give me an example of what happens when things do not go as you wish they would.
- How do you describe your ability to make decisions?
- Describe what you do when you feel bored.
- What important lessons did you learn from your last mistake?
- Tell me about one time you felt depressed.

Use these statements with the person's significant others:

- Do you often feel that the person takes advantage of you?
- Explain how the person expresses feelings of concern for others.
- What does the person do when they become angry?
- Is the person able to postpone getting what they want?
- Describe the person's judgment.
- Is the person able to share attention with others, or do they need to be the centre of attention?

COMMUNICATION

Person with paranoid personality disorder

PERSON: 'What did you mean by that remark? People are always making fun of me.'

NURSE RESPONSE 1: 'That remark was not meant for you, Jarrod. It was directed at everyone in the group.'

RATIONALE: This response provides a simple explanation without being argumentative or overly detailed in explanation. It also reinforces reality for the person.

NURSE RESPONSE 2: 'Do you feel that others may be picking on you?'

RATIONALE: This question encourages the person to verbalise feelings of mistrust. It is stated in a nonjudgmental manner while maintaining appropriate eye contact, which is a behaviour that promotes trust.

YOUR INTERVENTION STRATEGIES Guidelines for people with paranoid personality disorder

Nursing intervention	Rationale
Respect personal space.	Promotes a sense of security.
Respect the person's preferences as much as is reasonable.	Increases self-esteem.
Give feedback to the person based on observed non-verbal cues of responsiveness, such as eye movement, posturing and voice tones.	Improves interpersonal effectiveness.
Provide the person with a daily schedule of activities, and inform the person of any changes.	Activity schedules will diminish anxiety about social interactions, and may help ensure participation.
Use role-playing to help the person identify feelings, thoughts and responses brought on by stressful situations.	Rehearsing social behaviour in a safe environment provides immediate feedback and time for altering responses.
Encourage the person to evaluate how their behaviour led to the current crisis.	Points out cause-and-effect aspects of interaction.
Use an objective, matter-of-fact approach.	The nurse is a reliable person who gives respect without argument.
Use concrete, specific words rather than global abstractions.	Keeps the intended message clear by decreasing ambiguity.
Respond to suspicious ideas by focusing on feelings: 'It must be distressing.', 'You see him as vindictive.'	Communicates empathy.
Conduct brief one-to-one sessions daily (avoid lengthy sessions).	Shortened sessions decrease fear and anxiety.
Help the person to identify adaptive diversionary activities (leisure, recreation) in one-to-one sessions and in groups.	Participation in groups may increase the person's support system.

Self-harm may be carried out by people diagnosed with borderline personality disorder. Nurses may believe that people have control over self-harm decisions or states of emotional arousal, and may withdraw empathy (Forsyth, 2007; Winship, 2010). Holding a belief that individuals have control over self-harm leads to nurse-imposed labels such as 'attention-seeking' and 'manipulative' (Filer, 2005). Self-harm is not about nurses and is not aimed at services. The majority of self-harm is carried out in private, and is not brought to the attention of health services. Self-harm is not necessarily connected with a desire to end life, but rather is a means of coping with distress. This does not mean that self-harm won't lead to suicide. Self-harm is a complex phenomenon, and readers are encouraged to explore this area further through current literature and research, and also through therapeutic relationships with people as experts on their own experience. Box 18.5 provides insight into the role of self-harm.

Health services will have their own policies and procedures for managing self-harm in inpatient settings; however, it is essential that nurses maintain strong links with best practice in this area, as informed by current evidence and professional guidelines. Box 18.6 provides an effective strategy for helping.

Box 18.5 The role of self-harm

Self-harm is often:

- used to help manage overwhelming and intense emotions or to provide relief from negative or painful emotions
- used to provide immediate relief from emotional distress
- associated with high levels of impulsivity
- performed in secret and presented in crisis
- performed after a triggering event, such as separation, an experience of rejection, loss or failure or when the person feels alone
- accompanied by endorphins, which means some people don't feel pain followed by shame and remorse.

Source: Grenyer et al., 2015.

Box 18.6 Intervention strategies for people who use self-harm

- Show **C**oncern.
- Convey **A**cceptance of the fact that, although you don't approve of self-injury, you do understand that it is helping the person to cope in the best way they currently know how.
- Show **R**espect for their courage and determination to survive.
- Communicate **E**mpathy by listening without becoming judge and jury; by trying to put yourself in their shoes in an effort to understand what it feels like to be in those shoes; by being there for them, and by trusting them to find solutions that feel right for them.

Source: Sutton, 2005.

No-self-injury contracts are generally created to meet the needs of service providers rather than individuals living with cyclical self-harm patterns. Contracts need to be mutually agreed upon and be used very cautiously. Breaking the contract can lead to feelings of shame and further self-harm, and undermine the valuable therapeutic relationship (Sutton, 2005).

People diagnosed with personality disorders are commonly accused by staff of carrying out a behaviour known as 'splitting', which results from an individual believing that a nurse has been disloyal to the nurse–client relationship in some way (McNee, Donoghue & Coppola, 2014; Winship, 2010). The individual becomes dismissive of their primary care nurse and seeks out other staff who will agree to their point of view. The result is two staff members who are at odds with each other, and who are being portrayed in the roles of good nurse and bad nurse. When this happens, nurses often feel devalued, used and unable to help (Woollaston & Hixenbaugh, 2008). Planned, consistent teamwork is important for dealing with the inevitable challenges of this diagnostic group, and includes structured nursing care, within consistent boundaries, clear communication, nursing peer support, training and supervision (McNee et al., 2014; Wehbe-Alamah & Wolgamott, 2014; Winship, 2010). Triumvirate care is a teamwork approach which involves three nurses alternating roles to share care, with built-in clinical supervision between peer nurses and reflection in practice (Swift, 2009).

Care planning requires a collaborative approach, and individualised care plans are essential. Care plans identify both short- and long-term goals, identify situations that trigger distress or risk, identify self-management strategies that reduce distress and risk, strategies that have been helpful in the past, things that make the situation worse, emergency contacts and others who can help (Grenyer et al., 2015). The Project Air Strategy for Personality Disorders has been developed to engage community, families, carers, consumers and health and drug and alcohol services and agencies in better support and treatment for people with personality disorders. The Nursing Care Plan on the next page shows an example of a care plan adapted from Project Air resources.

Partnering with families

Whenever possible, include family members or significant others in some aspects of treatment. Families and significant others can be taught in every setting, both inpatient and outpatient. Inclusion of families recognises them as experts in the person's situation, and helps to improve and increase the support necessary for people to function more independently. Education guidelines for teaching families and carers about personality disorders are listed in Collaborative Care on the next page. Chapter 24 discusses a wide range of family interventions.

People receiving care should be able to identify and verbalise their fears and some specific areas in which change is indicated. The following are among the factors that influence the likelihood of successful change:

- the severity of the person's emotional deprivation
- the rigidity of the person's personality structure

- the person's ego strengths
- the person's motivation to change
- the nurse's skill and commitment
- social support systems in the person's family or milieu that favour the desired change.

People who live with personality disorder report experiencing re-traumatisation within health care settings, particularly through practices such as seclusion and restraint, and they often need to recover from the effects of the system in which they are treated (Bonney and Stickley, 2008).

NURSING CARE PLAN

Sample care plan adapted from Project Air Personality Disorders Strategy

Name: **Clinician name:**

My main therapeutic goals and problems I am working on

(1) In the short-term

(2) In the long-term

My crisis survival strategies

Warning signs that trigger me to feel unsafe, distressed or in crisis

Things I can do when I feel unsafe, distressed or in crisis that won't harm me

Thinks I have tried before that did not work or made the situation worse

Places and people I can contact in a crisis

Lifeline 13 11 13 **Emergency 000** **Mental health crisis team**

My support people (partner, family, friends, psychologist, nurse social worker, GP)

NAME	CONTACT DETAILS	ROLE IN MY CARE	OK TO CONTACT?

COLLABORATIVE CARE

Teaching about personality disorders

- Provide information about the specific disorder.
- Help the person learn to verbally express their needs instead of acting out.
- Provide social skills training (negotiation, cooking, money management), as needed.
- Teach problem-solving techniques, including goal-setting, identifying alternative responses and evaluating consequences.
- Teach stress-reduction techniques (e.g. guided imagery, relaxation).
- Provide instruction in cognitive behavioural techniques (e.g. thought stopping).
- Teach the person, their family members and carers about the proper use of medications, including target symptoms, side-effects and adverse medication reactions, contraindications and when to call for help.
- Practise and/or role-play newly acquired skills (e.g. assertiveness).
- Teach the person and family members/carers about indicators for emergency treatment.
- Emphasise the importance of follow-up care as indicated.

This is particularly true for people who experience personality disorder. Current treatment recommendations are that hospitalisation is used only as a brief, last resort when the person is in crisis and the risk for harm is higher than less restrictive alternatives could accommodate (Grenyer et al., 2015). Most treatment, intervention, recovery and self-discovery occur in the community. Nurses must strive to maintain optimism for care outcomes and for each individual's discovery prospects.

Trauma-informed care

The majority of people served by public mental health and substance abuse service systems are survivors of trauma (see the discussion in the trauma section of this chapter). Coercive practices in hospitals, such as seclusion and restraint, have been shown to re-traumatise people and to trigger memories of previous abuse (Substance Abuse and Mental Health Services Administration [SAMHSA], 2014). Seclusion and restraint is reported to feel like punishment, and the use of force by staff feels like harm rather than protection from harm (Ashcraft & Anthony, 2008; Azeem, Aujla, Rammerth, Binsfeld & Jones, 2011; Borckardt et al., 2011).

To avoid these coercive practices, advance directives, safety plans and de-escalation preferences are used within systems of care that are trauma-informed and which use 'universal precautions'. Universal precautions encompass the belief that we do not know what adverse experiences have happened to people in the past that may be impacting on their behaviour today. By seeking to understand what happened, rather than judging the person, we can avoid re-traumatising them. Every contact with a person will either contribute to a safe, trusting and healing environment, or detract from a safe and trusting environment. We all play a role in assisting the person to heal and make progress in their lives. **Trauma-informed care** places the person at the centre of treatment, includes and empowers family, prioritises wellness and self-management, maintains transparency to outsiders, and minimises power and control (SAMHSA, 2014).

Trauma-informed nursing care involves person-centred care that is respectful, uses calm tones of voice, quiet body language, helpful and hopeful attitudes, and objective, neutral language. It avoids actions that are demeaning, disrespectful, dominating, coercive or controlling. Disruptive behaviour is responded to with empathy, active listening skills, and engaging the person in finding solutions.

Studies of the brains of people who have experienced trauma have identified an automatic learned response of high alert or 'fight or flight' as protection against remembered traumatic experiences.

Triggers can lead to flashbacks, which are recurring memories, feelings and thoughts which bring traumatic stress from the past into the present (Fallot, McHugo, Harris & Xie, 2011). Box 18.7 lists some trauma triggers. A thorough understanding of the profound neurological, biological, psychological and social effects of trauma and violence on the individual is required. Woodland (2011), a person with lived experience, suggests what helps and what hurts in Box 18.8.

Box 18.7 Trauma triggers

Potential trauma triggers (SAMHSA, 2014) are shown below.

- Loud or abrupt noises
- Having to repeat one's story multiple times to multiple people
- Smells
- Filling out forms
- Tone of voice
- Removal of or denial of privileges
- Glaring lights
- Colors
- Waiting for long periods of time to receive services
- Anniversary dates
- Aggressive behaviour
- Signage
- Impatience
- Disorder/chaotic environments
- Not being listening to or being heard
- Lack of choice or options
- Small spaces
- Not being believed
- Crowds
- Darkness

Box 18.8 What helps and what hurts (Woodland, 2011)

What hurts?

When they don't/didn't listen

When they used coercive practices in exchange for my cooperation

When they treated me the same way every time I had a re-admission

When I am excluded from the process

When the different service systems I was in, didn't talk to each other

When I was not treated with respect and dignity

What helps?

When I was shown respect and dignity

When a rapport was establish with my helpers

When they shared the power with me

When they showed me how to, instead of telling me

When I was given choices and alternatives

SELF-AWARENESS
Working with traumatised people

- Why should nurses avoid bringing up traumatic memories?
- How can nurses talk with people about a range of trauma reactions and endeavour to minimise feelings of fear or shame, and to increase self-understanding?
- How can nurses address the emotional stress that can arise when working with individuals who have had traumatic experiences?
- What training would you require to develop the knowledge and skills to work sensitively and effectively with trauma survivors?

People with a history of trauma present across all sectors of the health service, and may in fact never present within mental health services (SAMHSA, 2014). Trauma-informed care emphasises physical, psychological and emotional safety for the people in our care. The nurse–consumer relationship is critical to the quality and effectiveness of care (Muskett, 2014). Nurses using trauma-informed practice empower people to rebuild a sense of control and become masters of their own destiny.

CONCLUSION

Personality is defined as a complex pattern of deeply embedded, unconscious psychological characteristics that express themselves automatically. Personality traits are ways of thinking, feeling and behaving that can be classified within five factors: extroversion, agreeableness, conscientiousness, neuroticism and openness to experience. Maladaption within these traits constitutes disorder of personality, and is identified through chronic attitudes and modes of reaction within an individual's identity, self-direction and capacity for empathy and intimacy. Biological, psychological and social influences all play a role in the development of personality disorder. Being born with a sensitive nature, experiencing problematic attachment to early caregivers and childhood trauma are strong contributors.

Diagnosis of personality disorder is problematic due to a lack of diagnostic agreement caused by no clear threshold between types and degrees of personality dysfunction within the diagnostic system. Receiving a diagnosis of personality disorder is stigmatising, and contact with health services can lead to invalidation, re-traumatisation, therapeutic pessimism and hopelessness. Effective nursing care is trauma-informed and is based on specialist education, teamwork, professional boundaries, self-awareness, reflection, peer support and clinical supervision.

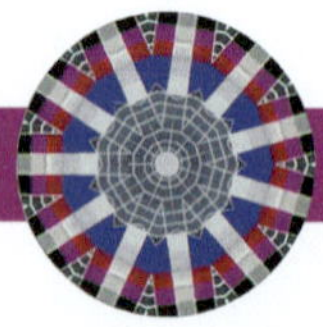

REFERENCES

Adler, G. (1973). Hospital treatment of borderline patients. *American Journal of Psychiatry, 130*, 32–36.

Afifi, T., Mather, A., Boman, J., Fleisher, W., Enns, M., Macmillan, H., & Sareen, J. (2011). Childhood adversity and personality disorders: Results from a nationally representative population-based study. *Journal of Psychiatric Research, 45,* 814–822.

Ahmed, U., Gibbon, S., Jones, H., Huband, N., Ferriter, M., Vollm, B., . . . Duggan, C. (2014). Pharmacological interventions for avoidant personality disorder (Protocol). *The Cochrane Collaboration of Systematic Reviews*.

Ainsworth, M. (1985). Attachments across the lifespan. *Bulletin of the New York Academy of Medicine, 61*, 792–812.

Ainsworth, M., Blehar, M., Waters, E., & Wall, S. (1978). *Pattern of attachment: Psychological study of the strange situation.* Hillsdale, NJ, Erlbaum.

Alex, R. (2014). Pharmacological interventions for obsessive–compulsive personality disorder. *Cochrane Database of Systematic Reviews*.

American Psychiatric Association. (2013). *Diagnostic and statistical manual of mental disorders* (5th edn.) Washington, DC: APA Publishing.

Anda, R. F., Felitti, V. J., Bremner, J. D., Walker, J. D., Whitfield, C., Perry, B. D., . . . & Giles, W. H. (2006). The enduring effects of abuse and related adverse experiences in childhood. *European Archives of Psychiatry and Clinical Neuroscience, 256*, 174–186.

Andresen, R., Oades, L., & Caputi, P. (2003). The experience of recovery from schizophrenia: towards an empirically validated stage model. *Australian and New Zealand Journal of Psychiatry, 37*, 586–594.

Andresen, R., Oades, L. G., & Caputi, P. (2011). *Psychological recovery: Beyond mental illness.* Chichester, England: Wiley & Sons.

Ashcraft, L., & Anthony, W. (2008). Eliminating seclusion and restraint in recovery-oriented crisis services. *Psychiatric Services, 59*, 1198–1202.

Azeem, M. W., Aujla, A., Rammerth, M., Binsfeld, G., & Jones, R. B. (2011). Effectiveness of six core strategies based on trauma informed care in reducing seclusions and restraints at a child and adolescent psychiatric hospital. *Journal of Child and Adolescent Psychiatric Nursing, 24*, 11–15.

Ball, J., & Links, P. (2009). Borderline personality disorder and childhood trauma: Evidence for a causal relationship. *Current Psychiatry Reports, 11*, 63–68.

Bandelow, B., Krause, J., Wedekind, D., Broocks, A., Hajak, G., & Rüther, E. (2005). Early traumatic life events, parental attitudes, family history, and birth risk factors in patients with borderline personality disorder and healthy controls. *Psychiatry Research, 134*, 169–179.

Bateman, A., Gunderson, J., & Mulder, R. (2015). Treatment of personality disorder. *The Lancet, 385*, 735–743.

Bateman, J., Henderson, C., & Kezelman, C. (2013). Trauma-informed care and practice: Towards a cultural shift in policy reform across mental health and human services in Australia, A National Strategic Direction, position paper and recommendations of the National Trauma-Informed Care and Practice Advisory Working Group. Lilyfield, Australia: Mental Health Coordinating Council (MHCC).

Bonney, S., & Stickley, T. (2008). Recovery and mental health: A review of the British literature. *Journal of Psychiatric and Mental Health Nursing, 15*, 140–153.

Borckardt, J., Madan, A., Grubaugh, A., Danielson, C., Pelic, C., Hardesty, S., . . . Frueh, C. (2011). Systematic investigation of initiatives to reduce seclusion and restraint in a state psychiatric hospital. *Psychiatric Services, 62*, 477–483.

Bowlby, J. (1988). *A secure base: Parent–child attachment and healthy human development.* London, England: Routledge.

Budge, S., Moore, J., Del Re, A., Wampold, B., Baardseth, T., & Nienhuis, J. (2013). The effectiveness of evidence-based treatments for personality disorders when comparing treatment-as-usual and bona fide treatments. *Clinical Psychology Review, 33*, 1057–1066.

Cassidy, J. (2008). The nature of the child's ties. In J. Cassidy & P. Shaver (Eds.), *Handbook of attachment: Theory, research, and clinical applications* (2nd ed.) (pp. 3–20). New York, NY: Guilford Press.

Castillo, H., Ramon, S., & Morant, N. (2013). A recovery journey for people with personality disorder. *International Journal of Social Psychiatry, 59*, 264–273.

Chemerinski, E., Triebwasser, J., Roussos, P., & Siever, L. J. (2013). Schizotypal personality disorder. *Journal of Personality Disorders, 27*, 652–679.

Chen, H. A., Cohen, P., Johnson, J. G., Kasen, S., Sneed, J. R., & Crawford, T. N. (2004). Adolescent personality disorders and conflict with romantic partners during the transition to adulthood. *Journal of Personality Disorders, 18*, 505–525.

Coccaro, E. F., Nayyer, H., & McCloskey, M. S. (2012). Personality disorder-not otherwise specified evidence of validity and consideration for DSM-5. *Comprehensive Psychiatry, 53,* 907–914.

Commonwealth of Australia. (2009). *Mental health services in Australia.* Canberra, Australia: Australian Institute of Health and Welfare (AIHW).

Crawford, T. N., Cohen, P., Johnson, J. G., Sneed, J. R., & Brook, J. S. (2004). The course and psychosocial correlates of personality disorder symptoms in adolescence: Erikson's developmental theory revisited. *Journal of Youth and Adolescence, 33*, 373–387.

Dixon-Gordon, K. L., Whalen, D. J., Layden, B. K., & Chapman, A. L. (2015). A systematic review of personality disorders and health outcomes. *Canadian Psychology, 56*, 168–190.

Draper, B., Pfaff, J. J., Pirkis, J., Snowdon, J., Lautenschlager, N. T., Wilson, I., & Almeida, O. P. (2008). Long-term effects of childhood abuse on the quality of life and health of older people: Results from the Depression and Early Prevention of Suicide in General Practice Project. *Journal of the American Geriatrics Society, 56*, 262–271.

Duggan, C. (2009). A treatment guideline for people with antisocial personality disorder: Overcoming attitudinal barriers and evidential limitations. *Criminal Behaviour and Mental Health, 19*, 219–223.

Eastwick, Z., & Grant, A. (2005). The treatment of people with 'borderline personality disorder': A cause for concern? *Mental Health Practice, 8*, 38–40.

Faith, C. (2009). Dependent personaltiy disorder: A review of etiology and treatment. *Graduate Journal of Counseling Psychology, 1*, 1–10.

Fallon, P. (2003). Travelling through the system: The lived experience of people with borderline personality disorder in contact with psychiatric services. *Journal of Psychiatric and Mental Health Nursing, 10*, 393–400.

Fallot, R. D., McHugo, G. J., Harris, M., & Xie, H. (2011). The trauma recovery and empowerment model: A quasi-experimental effectiveness study. *Journal of Dual Diagnosis, 7*, 74–89.

Farooq, S., Vollm, B., Husain, N., Huband, N., Stoffers, J., Gibbon, S., . . . Lieb, K. (2014a). Pharmacological interventions for schizotypal personality disorder (Protocol). *The Cochrane Collaboration of Systematic Reviews.*

Farooq, S., Vollm, B., Stoffers, J., Gibbon, S., Duggan, C., Ferriter, M., . . . Lieb, K. (2014b). Pharmacological interventions for schizoid personality disorer (Protocol). *The Cochrane Collaboration of Systematic Reviews.*

Felitti, V., Anda, R., Nordenberg, D., Williamson, D., Spitz, A., Edwards, V., . . . Marks, J. (1998). Relationship of childhood abuse and household dysfunction to many of the leading causes of death in adults: The Adverse Childhood Experiences (ACE) Study. *American Journal of Preventive Medicine, 14*, 245–258.

Filer, N. (2005). Borderline personality disorder: Attitudes of mental health nurses. *Mental Health Practice, 9*, 34–36.

Fok, M., Hotpof, M., Stewart, R., Hatch, S., Hayes, R., & Moran, P. (2014). Personality disorder and self-rated health: A population based cross-sectional survey. *Journal of Personality Disorders, 28*, 319–333.

Fonagy, P. (1999). Attachment, the development of the self, and its pathology in personality disorders. In J. Derkesen, C. Maffei, & H. Groen (Eds.), *Treatment of personality disorders* (pp. 53–68). New York, NY: Kluwer Acadenim/Plenum Publishers.

Fonagy, P. (2003). The development of psychopathology from infancy to adulthood: The mysterious unfolding of disturbance in time. *Infant Mental Health Journal, 24*, 212.

Forsyth, A. (2007). The effects of diagnosis and non compliance attributions on therapeutic alliance in adult psychiatric settings. *Journal of Psychiatric and Mental Health Nursing, 14*, 33–40.

Friedman, H. (1969). Some problems of inpatient management with borderline patients. *American Journal of Psychiatry, 126*, 299–304.

Gibbon, S. (2010). Psychological interventions for antisocial personality disorder. *Cochrane Database of Systematic Reviews.*

Gillard, S., Turner, K., & Neffgen, M. (2015). Understanding recovery in the context of lived experience of personality disorders: a collaborative, qualitative research study. *BMC Psychiatry, 15*, 183.

Glover, H. (2012). Recovery, lifelong learning, empowerment and social inclusion: Is a new paradigm emerging? In P. Ryan, S. Ramon, & T. Greacen (Eds.), *Empowerment, lifelong learning and recovery in mental health: Towards a new paradigm* (pp. 15–35). New York, NY: Palgrave Macmillan.

Godbout, N., & Briere, J. (2012). Psychological responses to trauma. In C. R. Figley (Ed.), *Encyclopedia of trauma* (pp. 485–489). Thousand Oaks, CA: Sage.

Goodman, M., & Yehuda, R. (2002). The relationship between psychological trauma and borderline personality disorder. *Psychiatric Annals, 32*, 337–345.

Grenyer, B., Jenner, B., Jarman, H., Carter, P., Bailey, R., & Lewis, K. (2015). *Treatment guidelines for personality disorders.* Wollongong, Australia: University of Wollongong.

Grilo, C. M., Sanislow, C. A., Gunderson, J. G., Pagano, M. E., Yen, S., Zanarini, M. C., . . . McGlashan, T. H. (2004). Two-year stability and change of schizotypal, borderline, avoidant, and obsessive–compulsive personality disorders. *Journal of Consulting and Clinical Psychology, 72*, 767–775.

Gunderson, J. (1984). *Borderline personality disorder.* Washington, DC: American Psychiatric Press.

Hageman, T. K., Francis, A. J. P., Field, A. M., & Carr, S. N. (2015). Links between childhood experiences and avoidant personality disorder symptomatology. *International Journal of Psychology and Psychological Therapy, 15*, 101–116.

Hatchett, G. T. (2015). Treatment guidelines for clients with antisocial personality disorder. *Journal of Mental Health Counseling, 37*, 15–27.

Hengartner, M. P., Cohen, L. J., Rodgers, S., Müller, M., Rössler, W., & Ajdacic-Gross, V. (2015). Association between childhood maltreatment and normal adult personality traits: Exploration of an understudied field. *Journal of Personality Disorders, 29*, 1–14.

Hess, N. (2016). On making emotional contact with a schizoid patient. *British Journal of Psychotherapy, 32*, 53–64.

Hughes, K., Lowey, H., Quigg, Z., & Bellis, M. (2016). Relationships between adverse childhood experiences and adult mental well-being: Results from an English national household survey. *BMC Public Health, 16*, 222.

Jackson, J., & Burgess, P. (2004). Personality disorders in the community: Results from the Australian National Survey of Mental Health and Well-Being Part II. *Social Psychiatry and Psychiatric Epidemiology, 39*, 765–776.

Johnson, J., Cohen, P., Kasen, S., & Brook, J. (2006). Personality disorder traits evident by early adulthood and risk for eating and weight problems during middle adulthood. *International Journal of Eating Disorders, 39*, 184–192.

Johnson, J., Cohen, P., Kasen, S., Skodol, A., Hamagami, F., & Brook, J. (2000). Age-related change in personality disorder trait levels between early adolescence and adulthood: A community-based longitudinal investigation. *Acta Psychiatrica Scandinavica, 102*, 265–275.

Jones, H., Testa, R., Ross, N., Seal, M., Pantelis, C., & Tonge, B. (2015). The Melbourne Assessment of Schizotypy in Kids: A useful measure of childhood schizotypal personality disorder. *BioMed Research International, 2015*, 1–10.

Khalifa, N., Duggan, C., Stoffers, J., Huband, N., Völlm, B. A., Ferriter, M., & Lieb, K. (2010). Pharmacological interventions for antisocial personality disorder. *Cochrane Database of Systematic Reviews.*

Koerner, K., & Linehan, M. M. (2003). Validation principles and strategies. In W. T. O'Donohue, J. E. Fisher, & S. C. Hayes (Eds.) *Cognitive behaviour therapy: Applying emipirically supported techniques in your practice* (pp. 229–237). New Jersey, NJ: Wiley & Sons.

Kuo, J. R., & Linehan, M. M. (2009). Disentangling emotion processes in borderline personality disorder: Physiological and self-reported assessment of biological vulnerability, baseline intensity, and reactivity to emotionally evocative stimuli. *Journal of Abnormal Psychology, 118*, 531–544.

Lamph, G. (2011). Raising awareness of borderline personality disorder and self-injury. *Nursing Standard, 26*, 35–40.

Leising, D., & Zimmermann, J. (2011). An integrative conceptual framework for assessing personality and personality pathology. *Review of General Psychology, 15*, 317–330.

Lenzenweger, M., Lane, M., Loranger, A., & Kessler, R. (2007). DSM–IV personality disorders in the National Comorbidity Survey Replication. *Biological Psychiatry, 62*, 533–564.

Lewin, T. J., Slade, T., Andrews, G., Carr, V. J., & Hornabrook, C. W. (2005). Assessing personality disorders in a national mental health survey. *Social Psychiatry and Psychiatric Epidemiology, 40*, 87–98.

Linehan, M. (1993). *Cognitive-behavioral treatment of borderline personality disorder.* New York, NY: Guilford Press.

Linehan, M. M., & Wilks, C. R. (2015). The course and evolution of dialectical behavior therapy. *American Journal of Psychotherapy, 69*, 97.

Maccoby, E. (2000). Parenting and its effects on children: On reading and misreading behaviour genetics. *Annual Review of Psychology, 51*, 1–27.

MacIntosh, H. B., Godbout, N., & Dubash, N. (2015). Borderline personality disorder: Disorder of trauma or personality, a review of the empirical literature. *Canadian Psychology, 56*, 227–241.

Markham, D. (2003). Attitudes towards patients with a diagnosis of 'borderline personality disorder': Social rejection and dangerousness. *Journal of Mental Health, 12*, 595–612.

Markham, D., & Trower, P. (2003). The effects of the psychiatric label 'borderline personality disorder' on nursing staff's perceptions and causal attributions for challenging behaviours. *British Journal of Clinical Psychology, 42*, 243–256.

Markon, K. E., Krueger, R. F., & Watson, D. (2005). Delineating the structure of normal and abnormal personality: An integrative hierarchical approach. *Journal of Personality and Social Psychology, 88*, 139–157.

Masten, A., & O'Dougherty Wright, M. (2010). Resilience of the lifespan: Developmental perspectives on resistance, recovery and transformation. In J. Reich, A. Zautra, & J. Hall (Eds.), *Handbook of adult resilience* (pp. 213–237). New York, NY: Guilford Press.

McGrath, B., & Dowling, M. (2012). Exploring registered psychiatric nurses' responses towards service users with a diagnosis of borderline personality disorder. *Nursing Research and Practice, 2012*, 1–10.

McNee, L., Donoghue, C., & Coppola, A.-M. (2014). A team approach to borderline personality disorder. *Mental Health Practice, 17*, 33–35.

Meyer, B., & Pilkonis, P. (2005). An attachment model of personality disorders. In M. Lenzenweger & J. Clarkin (Eds.), *Major theories of personality disorder* (pp. 231–281). New York, NY: Guilford Press.

Millon, T. (1981). *Disorders of personality: DSM-III Axis II*. New York, NY: Wiley.

Muskett, C. (2014). Trauma-informed care in inpatient mental health settings: A review of the literature. *International Journal of Mental Health Nursing, 23*, 51–59.

National Health and Medical Research Council (NHMRC). (2012). *Clinical practice guideline for the management of borderline personality disorder*. Melbourne, Australia: NHMRC.

National Institute for Mental Health (NIMH). (2003). *Breaking the cycle of rejection: The personality pisorder capabilities framework*. London, England: NIMH, Department of Health.

National Institute of Health and Clinical Excellence (NICE). (2009). *Borderline personality disorder: Treatment and management*. NICE Clinical Guideline 78. London, England: NICE. Retrieved from www.nice.org.uk/CG78

Novais, F., Araújo, A. M., & Godinho, P. (2015). Historical roots of histrionic personality disorder. *Frontiers in Psychology, 6*, 1643. doi: 10.3389/fpsyg.2015.01463.

Nursing and Midwifery Board of Australia (NMBA). (2010). *A nurse's guide to professional boundaries*. Sydney, Australia: NMBA.

O'Donohue, W., Fisher, J., & Hayes, S. (2003). *Cognitive behaviour therapy: Applying empirically supported techniques in your practice*. Hoboken, NJ: Wiley & Sons.

Paris, J. (2015). Why patients with severe personality disorders are overmedicated. *Journal of Clinical Psychiatry, 76*(4), e521.

Romano, D. M. C. (2004). A self-psychology approach to narcissistic personality disorder: A nursing reflection. *Perspectives in Psychiatric Care, 40*, 20–28.

Rosa, M. H. (2015). Love at a distance: Aggression and hatred in a schizoid personality. *Psychoanalytic Review, 102*, 503–530.

Rutter, M. (2006). *Genes and behaviour: Nature–nurture interplay explained*. Malden, MA: Blackwell Publishing.

Schore, A. (2003). Early relational trauma, disorganised attachment and the development of a predisposition to violence. In M. Solomon & D. Siegel (Eds.), *Healing trauma: Attachment, mind, body and brain* (pp. 107–167). New York, NY: WW Norton & Co.

Shedler, J., Beck, A., Fonagy, P., Gabbard, G., Gunderson, J., Kernberg, O., . . . Westen, D. (2010). Personality disorders in DSM-V. *American Journal of Psychiatry, 167*, 1026–1028.

Siddiqui, S. (2014). *Recovery in people with a diagnosis of borderline personality disorder*. (Unpublished Diploma of Clinical Psychology thesis, University of Manchester, Manchester).

Siegel, D. (1999). *The developing mind: How relationships and the brain interact to shape who we are*. New York, NY: Guilford Press.

Skodol, A., Geier, T., Grant, B., & Hasin, D. (2014). Personality disorders and the persistence of anxiety disorders in a nationally representative sample. *Depression and Anxiety, 31*, 721–728.

Skodol, A., Johnson, J., Cohen, P., Sneed, J., & Crawford, T. (2007). Personality disorder and impaired functioning from adolescence to adulthood. *British Journal of Psychiatry, 190*, 415–420.

Skodol, A. E. (2008). Part IV—outcome: Longitudinal course and outcome of personality disorders. *Psychiatric Clinics of North America, 31*, 495–503.

Skodol, A. E., Gunderson, J. G., Shea, M. T., McGlashan, T. H., Morey, L. C., Sanislow, C. A., . . . Stout, R. L. (2005). The Collaborative Longitudinal Personality Disorders Study (CLPS): Overview and implications. *Journal of Personality Disorders, 19*, 487–504.

Stinson, F. S., Dawson, D. A., Goldstein, R. B., Chou, S. P., Huang, B., Smith, S. M., . . . Grant, B. F. (2008). Prevalence, correlates, disability, and comorbidity of DSM-IV Narcissistic personality disorder: Results from the Wave 2 National Epidemiologic Survey on Alcohol and Related Conditions. *Journal of Clinical Psychiatry, 69*, 1033–1045.

Stoffers, J., Ferriter, M., Vollm, B., Gibbon, S., Jones, H., Duggan, C., & Lieb, K. (2014a). Pharmacological interventions for people with histrionic personality disorder (Protocol). *The Cochrane Collaboration of Systematic Reviews*.

Stoffers, J., Ferriter, M., Vollm, B., Gibbon, S., Jones, H., Duggan, C., & Lieb, K. (2014b). Pharmacological interventions for people with narcissistic personality disorder (Protocol). *The Cochrane Collaboration of Systematic Reviews*.

Stoffers, J., Vollm, B., Rucker, G., Timmer, A., Huband, N., & Lieb, K. (2010). Pharmacological interventions for borderline personality disorder (Review). *The Cochrane Collaboration*.

Substance Abuse and Mental Health Services Administration (SAMHSA). (2014). *SAMHSA's concept of trauma and guidance for a trauma-informed approach*. Rockville, MD: SAMHSA.

Sutton, J. (2005). *Healing the hurt within: Understand self-injury and self harm, and heal the emotional wounds,* Oxford, England: How To Books.

Swift, E. (2009). The efficacy of treatments for borderline personality disorder. *Mental Health Practice, 13*, 30–33.

Torgersen, S. (2005). Epidemiology. In J. Oldham, A. Skodel, & D. Bender (Eds.), *American Psychiatric Publishing textbook of personality disorders* (pp. 129–141). Arlington, VA: American Psychiatric Publishing.

Triebwasser, J., Chemerinski, E., Roussos, P., & Siever, L. J. (2012). Schizoid personality disorder. *Journal of Personality Disorders, 26*, 919–926.

Turner, K., Lovell, K., & Brooker, A. (2011). '. . . and they all lived happily ever after': 'Recovery' or discovery of the self in personality disorder? *Psychodynamic Practice, 17*, 341–346.

Tyrer, P., Reed, G., & Crawford, M. (2015). Classification, assessment, prevalence, and effect of personality disorder. *The Lancet, 385*, 717–726.

van der Kolk, B. (2003). Post traumatic stress disorder and the nature of trauma. In M. Solomon & D. Siegel (Eds.), *Healing trauma: Attachment, mind, body, and brain* (pp. 168–196). New York, NY: WW Norton.

Vollm, B., Farooq, S., Jones, H., Ferriter, M., Gibbon, S., Stoffers, J., . . . Lieb, K. (2014). Pharmacological interventions for paranoid personality disorder (Protocol). *The Cochrane Collaboration of Systematic Reviews*.

Wehbe-Alamah, H., & Wolgamott, S. (2014). Uncovering the mask of borderline personality disorder: Knowledge to empower primary care providers. *Journal of the American Association of Nurse Practitioners, 26*, 292–300.

Weight, E. J., & Kendal, S. (2013). Staff attitudes towards inpatients with borderline personality disorder. *Mental Health Practice, 17*, 34–38.

Widiger, T. (2015). Assessment of DSM-5 personality disorder. *Journal of Personality Assessment, 97*, 456–466.

Winship, G. (2010). Attitudes and perceptions of mental health nurses towards borderline personality disorder clients in acute mental health setings: A review of the literature. *Journal of Psychiatric and Mental Health Nursing, 17*, 657–662.

Woodland, M. (2011). *Doomed to be nothing: Destined to be something,* Morningside, MD: Unlock Publishing House.

Woollaston, K., & Hixenbaugh, P. (2008). Destructive whirlwind: Nurses' perceptions of patients diagnosed with borderline personality disorder. *Journal of Psychiatric and Mental Health Nursing, 15*, 703–709.

World Health Organization (WHO). (1992). *International classification of diseases, 10th revision, mental and behavioural disorders*. Geneva, Switzerland: WHO.

Yen, S., Pagano, M. E., Shea, T. M., Grilo, C. M., Gunderson, J. G., Skodol, A. E., . . . Bender, D. S. (2005). Recent life events preceding suicide attempts in a personality disorder sample: Findings from the Collaborative Longitudinal Personality Disorders Study. *Journal of Consulting and Clinical Psychology, 73*, 99–105.

Zanarini, M. C., Frankenburg, F. R., Hennen, J., Reich, D. B., & Silk, K. R. (2005). The McLean Study of Adult Development (MSAD): Overview and implications of the first six years of prospective follow-up. *Journal of Personality Disorders, 19*, 505–523.

Zanarini, M. C., Frankenburg, F. R., Hennen, J., Reich, D. B., & Silk, K. R. (2006). Prediction of the 10-year course of borderline personality disorder. *American Journal of Psychiatry, 163*, 827–832.

Zanarini, M., Frankenburg, F., Reich, D., & Fitzmaurice, G. (2010). Time to attainment of recovery from borderline personality disorder and stability of recovery: A 10-year prospective follow-up study. *American Journal of Psychiatry, 167*, 663–667.

People at risk for suicide and self-harming behaviour

19

MIKE HAZELTON AND CARRIE MILLER

LEARNING OUTCOMES

After completing this chapter, you will be able to:

1. Identify the social, demographic and clinical variables and lived experience that influence suicidal or self-harming behaviour.
2. Compare and contrast the similarities and differences in suicide rates among various demographic groups.
3. Discuss the sociocultural, interpersonal and biological theories and lived experience that enhance our understanding of suicide and self-harming behaviour.
4. Formulate a lethality assessment.
5. Distinguish between the crucial components of basic suicide precautions and maximum suicide precautions.
6. Develop intervention strategies to prevent suicide that can and should be implemented in any health care setting.
7. Integrate family members into the plan of care for the person who is suicidal or self-harming.
8. Develop intervention strategies that may be helpful to survivors of suicide.

KEY TERMS

LIVED EXPERIENCE

I was at my lowest point during one hospital admission. I remember sitting on the floor of my room, my face buried in a cotton blanket that was wet and heavy with every tear I had ever needed to cry. A nurse came in and just sat quietly next to me while my heart broke. He gave me space to exhaust my sadness, and then he said something remarkable: 'This may not make sense to you now, but I know things will get better. I know you will recover.' It was a powerful moment. I had never heard the language of recovery—it had never been spoken in any of my previous treatment. For a mental health professional to hold the hope for someone's recovery when they are too broken to hold it for themselves—that is the essence of transformative practice. I now realise that was the beginning of my recovery journey.

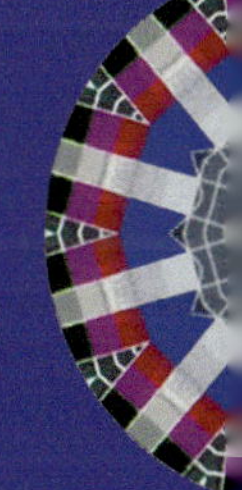

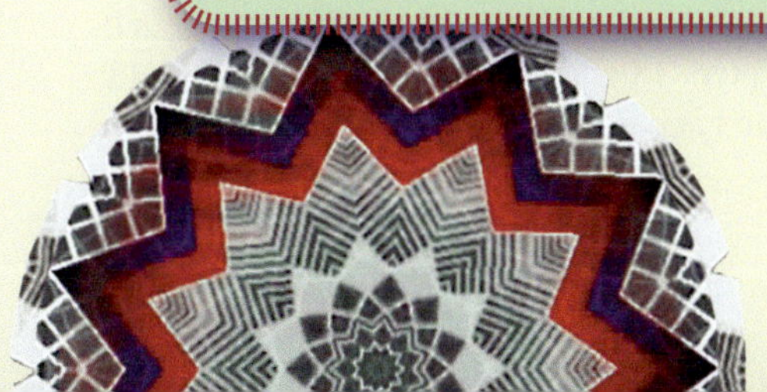

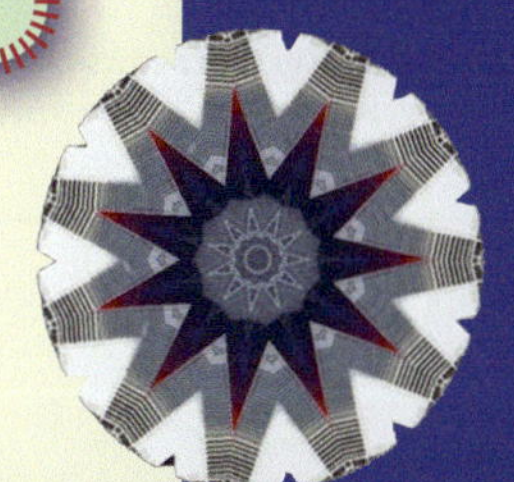

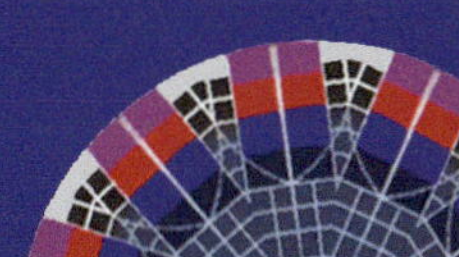

INTRODUCTION

Behaviour in which a person attempts to self-harm or take their own life has been a part of the human experience since time began. **Self-harming behaviours** and suicidal behaviours are maladaptive measures a person uses to restore inner equilibrium when overwhelmed or unable to cope with stressful life events. Distressed and unable to see that they have other options, people attempt to harm or kill themselves thinking that they can take away unbearable emotional pain. Did you know that **suicide**, the wilful act of ending one's own life, is the 14th leading cause of death among Australians, and that over 2800 people kill themselves a year? That is more than seven suicides every day. In Australia, almost 90 per cent of people who complete suicide are living with a mental illness.

Suicide ranks differently as the cause of death for different age groups. There are a number of health problems that cause death in the oldest age group; therefore, suicide might erroneously appear to be of less concern. However, the risk for suicide is high for this group, especially older males.

There are gender and method differences to suicide as well. In any one year about 75 per cent of completed suicides will be by males. The most common causes of death by suicide are hanging, poisoning and firearms, respectively. The rate of suicide has consistently remained much lower for females. In 2014, the age-standardised suicide rate for Australia was 12 per 100 000. In the same year, the age-standardised suicide rate for males was 18.4 per 100 000, while the corresponding rate for females was 5.9 per 100 000.

Stigma and ignorance about mental illness, depression and suicide may embarrass, shame and silence individuals who want to speak with others about their pain. People in distress may believe that others, including nurses and other health care providers, will label them 'crazy' if they speak of suicide. In fact, discussions of suicide do arouse intense and complicated emotions in others.

Suicide is a major public health problem in Australia and in many countries around the globe. Suicide affects all age groups, genders, cultures, religions and socioeconomic classes. It is thus important to be aware that any person receiving care in a health care, occupational or community setting may, given the right circumstances, contemplate suicide. Box 19.1 shows facts about suicide.

As psychiatric–mental health nurses, we frequently find ourselves face-to-face with people who are suicidal or engage in self-harming behaviour. Few people with whom you will work will elicit such intense feelings of anxiety and helplessness. Individuals who are suicidal may cause you to question your abilities to help others and preserve life. Thus, it is critically important to be prepared for all the emotional reactions—fear, anxiety, anger and so on—that a person who is suicidal may evoke in you. Unless you understand them, these reactions may interfere with your ability to establish rapport. This chapter will help you to understand more clearly people who are suicidal or engage in self-harm, so that you can be more comfortable in assessing their needs and providing help.

Box 19.1 Suicide facts

- Every day, more than seven lives are lost to suicide.
- Suicide is now the 14th leading cause of death in Australia for all age groups, and the leading cause of death in the 25 to 44 age group.
- There are more than 2800 deaths from suicide in Australia each year.
- More people kill themselves each year than are murdered; in 2014, the suicide rate was 12 per 100 000 while the homicide victimisation rate was 1.8 per 100 000.
- In the month prior to their suicide, a high percentage of older suicide victims had visited a primary care provider; many had a depressive illness that was not detected.
- More men than women die by suicide; the gender ratio is three males to every one female.
- Over 70 per cent of deaths from suicide are in adult men aged 25–65.
- Many suicidal people never seek professional care.

Source: Australian Bureau of Statistics (2016). *3303.0 – Causes of death, Australia 2014*. Retrieved from www.abs.gov.au/ausstats/abs@.nsf/mf/3303.0

SELF-HARMING BEHAVIOUR

In addition to suicide, other typical self-harming behaviours and acts include, but are not limited to, nail biting, hair pulling, self-mutilation such as scratching or cutting one's wrist or another part of the body, smoking cigarettes, driving recklessly, gambling, drinking alcohol, using drugs, and sexually risky behaviour. **Enduring self-harming behaviour** is behaviour that harms the self, is habitual, and generally poses a low level of lethality. In general, these behaviours range from relatively innocuous acts at one end of the continuum, such as overeating and gambling, to more lethal ones at the other, such as driving recklessly. Such self-harming behaviours can injure one's health and sometimes hasten one's death.

A completed suicide is the most violent self-harming behaviour. It is important to understand that not all individuals who self-harm go on to kill themselves. People who are suicidal may manifest several of the behaviours listed in Box 19.2. Another type of self-harming behaviour is self-mutilation; see Chapters 18 and 20 for information related to specific diagnoses and age groups.

LIVED EXPERIENCE

I would lash out, deeply scratching my wrists with a knife, hitting my head against a wall, dropping heavy objects on my feet. When I was a passenger in a car I would fantasise about grabbing the wheel and causing an accident so I could hurt myself. Once I hit myself in the face with a hammer, hoping that I would be offered plastic surgery and that would fix how ugly I was, inside and out. For me, self-harm was a concrete expression of a deep and abiding self-hatred; it was an externalisation of internal pain and suffering.

I have a history of child sexual abuse, and was very sexually disinhibited from an early age. This risky behaviour was fuelled by my mania and my substance abuse. I repeatedly put myself in very vulnerable situations, I didn't know how to keep myself safe; I hated myself so much I didn't want to. As a result, I experienced sexual assault several times as an adult. I realise now I was unconsciously putting myself in vulnerable situations to try to gain some mastery over the original sexual trauma, but this risk-taking would just end up in further victimisation.

Box 19.2 Continuum of suicidal behaviour

- **Suicidal ideation:** Having thoughts of harming or killing oneself.
- **Suicide threat:** A threat that is more serious than a casual statement of suicidal intent, and that is accompanied by other behaviour changes. These may include mood swings, temper outbursts, a decline in school or work performance, personality changes, sudden or gradual withdrawal from friends, and other significant changes in attitude.
- **Suicide attempt:** A non-fatal, self-inflicted destructive act with explicit or inferred intent to die. The attempt may be thwarted by another person or by circumstances, it may be planned to avoid serious injury, or it may be one in which the outcome depends on the circumstances and is not under the individual's control. For example, someone who takes a heavy overdose of sleeping tablets may or may not be discovered in time.
- **Suicide:** A fatal, self-inflicted destructive act with an explicit or inferred intent to die.

Ethics and suicide

Do people have the right to kill themselves, and can or should nurses intervene when people try to kill themselves? The traditional belief is that mental health professionals should do everything possible to prevent suicide. You should know that, ethical concerns aside, you may be prosecuted under Australian law that makes it a crime to aid or abet a suicide

LIVED EXPERIENCE

I have thought about killing myself since I was nine. It became a card up my sleeve if everything got too much, and so in that way suicidal thinking brought some relief to my suffering. It was like an escape valve on the pressure cooker of my thoughts and feelings. When things got too intense, I could soothe myself with the idea that 'I can always kill myself'.

under any circumstance, even when a terminally ill person decides to end their life. Questions about a person's right to suicide and society's right to control suicide are still being debated, and there is currently much public debate surrounding so-called 'assisted suicide'. Engaging in the process of ethical reasoning presented in Chapter 11 will help you in your search for a personal position.

Meaning and motivation in suicide

Suicide is not a random act. Whether carried out impulsively or after painstaking consideration, the act has both a message

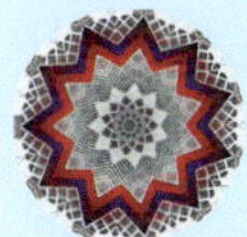

WHAT EVERY NURSE SHOULD KNOW

Suicidal ideation in primary care

Imagine you are a nurse working in a primary care setting, such as a general practice surgery. It is not unusual in primary care settings to see people with suicidal ideation or at high risk for suicide. It is also not unusual for primary care providers to fail to recognise those at high risk for suicide. Suicide risk is increased in both physical and mental illness, especially when both are present. It is important to remember that there is also a strong association between depression, risk for suicide and chronic medical illness. The possibility of suicide risk should be considered in all people with chronic illness, including those with solely physical symptoms.

Although there are more effective medications available to primary care practitioners to treat depression, suicide rates have remained unacceptably high and may be under-reported if unexplained deaths are considered. In instances where uncertainty surrounds a person's death, a psychological autopsy may be performed. A **psychological autopsy** is an assessment tool that reviews the circumstances and events that preceded an individual's completed suicide. Reviews of psychological autopsies and other similar methods have revealed that a high percentage of suicide victims have a comorbid mental disorder (such as mood disorders and/or substance use disorders) and, furthermore, that they were under-treated, despite contact with mental health or other health care services. Recognising this association, screening for it, and providing treatment is a primary care imperative and may prevent unnecessary tragedies.

and a purpose. In general, unless it was an accidental overdose or involved substances of abuse, the purpose or reason for suicide was to escape or end an intolerable situation, crisis or relationship, such as:

- a terminal (especially painful) illness (refer to What Every Nurse Should Know on page 415)
- being a burden to others
- an untenable family situation
- an untenable personal situation
- punishment or exposure of socially, personally or professionally unacceptable behaviour.

Needing to end intolerable situations is the motivation in the clinical examples of the five people discussed in the following example.

Practice example

Howard's lung cancer has metastasised to his bones; any exertion causes spontaneous fractures, and he is in constant pain. He has asked friends, family and health care workers to help him escape his illness by ending his life.

Joan, a widow, fell three times last year and is now in a nursing home. She decided on suicide so that she would no longer be a burden to her family. Joan has not eaten in seven days.

Jeremy, age seven, attempted to run into the path of a car. He had heard his mother say many times, 'If it weren't for you, Daddy and I would never have broken up.' Jeremy believed that if he were dead, his parents would reunite, thus solving what he believes to be an untenable family situation.

Serena, age 33, had been admitted for the third time to a mental health inpatient unit because of thoughts of suicide. Carl, her husband, has broken the last two appointments with a relationships counsellor, and went on a fishing trip with his mates when she came into the hospital this time. Serena believes that she is unlovable and will attempt to leave the hospital tonight to finally stop the pain.

Richard, 22, killed himself on the third anniversary of the death by stabbing of his older brother, Christopher.

Many people who self-harm have long-term difficulties communicating their needs to others. Some people cannot express their needs or feelings; or, when they do, they do not obtain the results they had hoped for. For them, self-mutilation or suicide becomes a clear and direct, if violent, form of communication. The message inherent in suicide tends to be complex and complicated, and may be aimed at a specific person, usually a significant other. Interrupting a suicide plan or suicidal thoughts requires hearing, understanding and responding appropriately to messages of pain, loneliness and hopelessness. Communication has an example of communicating with a person who is suicidal.

BIOPSYCHOSOCIAL THEORIES

Suicide and self-harming behaviour are still not well understood by the public or by the scientific community. In fact, many people's understanding of suicide has been influenced by misconceptions. Some of these myths, and the corresponding explanatory facts that negate them, are discussed in Box 19.3.

Suicide is a complex phenomenon, and there is no single explanation for its complicated process; however, sociocultural, interpersonal and intrapsychic, cognitive and biological theories can contribute to our understanding of suicide. In addition to the section that follows, careful study of Chapters 16 and 18 will help you to understand the behaviours discussed in this chapter.

Sociocultural theory

Sociocultural theories about suicide propose that the social and cultural contexts in which people live influence their expressions of suicidality. The following clinical examples describe two possible social and cultural contexts for suicide:

- experiencing a precipitous deterioration in one's relationship with society (such as the loss of a job or a close friend)
- considering self-inflicted death as honourable.

Practice example

Emma, who is without family or friends, had decided that life was not worth living after retiring from her job with the Commonwealth Government. She came to believe that no one would even know or care if she succeeded in killing herself.

In the Gaza Strip, a suicide bomber detonated explosives strapped to his body as he rode his bicycle into an Israeli checkpoint, killing himself and three soldiers and wounding several Israeli civilians. Those who claimed responsibility for the attack indicated their belief that the suicide bomber's death was an honorable one, and that he is rewarded in Heaven.

COMMUNICATION

A person who attempts suicide

PERSON WHO IS SUICIDAL: 'I just had to do it. I just can't take this pain another day.'

NURSE RESPONSE #1: 'I'm wondering how you felt when you tried to kill yourself.' *RATIONALE:* Gathering more data will help you to understand the person better. You can help the person consider triggers and behaviours if you first encourage them to identify and describe the feelings and emotions around the event.	**NURSE RESPONSE #2:** 'Let's talk about what led up to your trying to kill yourself.' *RATIONALE:* While this response validates the behaviour as real, it also asks the person to begin examining what may have caused an overload or an inability to cope.

Box 19.3 Suicide myths versus suicide facts

- ***MYTH: A suicide threat is just a bid for attention and should not be taken seriously.*** *FACT: All suicidal behaviour should be taken seriously; a bid for attention may be a cry for help.*
- ***MYTH: It is harmful for a person to talk about suicidal thoughts. The person's attention should be diverted when this occurs.*** *FACT: Of prime importance in helping a person who is suicidal is talking with that person in order to assess the extent and lethality of their suicide plan.*
- ***MYTH: Only people who are psychotic kill themselves.*** *FACT: The majority of completed suicides are carried out by people who are not psychotic.*
- ***MYTH: People who talk about suicide won't do it.*** *FACT: Most people do talk about their suicide intention before making a suicide attempt.*
- ***MYTH: A nice home, good job or an intact family prevents suicide.*** *FACT: People of all social and economic backgrounds kill themselves.*
- ***MYTH: A failed suicide attempt should be treated as manipulative behaviour.*** *FACT: Failed attempts are more likely evidence of a person's ambivalence towards suicide.*
- ***MYTH: People who kill themselves are always depressed.*** *FACT: People who kill themselves are not always depressed, although depression is common. People can also be terminally ill, enduring chronic pain, psychotic, agitated, organically impaired or have personality disorders.*
- ***MYTH: Suicide is more common in the winter months.*** *FACT: While the available data are inconclusive, there is some evidence to indicate that suicides peak during spring in Australia.*
- ***MYTH: There is no connection between alcohol or drug use and suicide.*** *FACT: Alcohol, drugs and suicide are often closely connected. A person who kills themselves may have become depressed, impulsive and suicidal after using alcohol or other drugs.*
- ***MYTH: Once suicidal, always suicidal.*** *FACT: Suicide attempts are often made during particularly stressful times in people's lives. If the suicide attempt is managed properly, people can and do go on with their lives without recurrent thoughts of suicide.*
- ***MYTH: Suicidal people rarely seek medical help.*** *FACT: According to studies, a high percentage of people who are suicidal sought help within the six months that preceded the suicide.*

The suicide rate for Indigenous Australians is almost twice that for their non-Indigenous counterparts. In a survey conducted in 2012, about 12 per cent of Indigenous people reported feeling depressed or having depression, compared to 9.6 per cent for all Australians. In the same year, the suicide rate for Indigenous youth aged 15 to 18 (34 per 100000) was five times that of the corresponding non-Indigenous age group (7 per 100000) (Australian Institute of Health and Welfare, 2015).

Age and gender

Similarities and differences exist in suicide rates among people of different ages. Suicide is a leading cause of death in Australian youth. For those aged 14–24, it is the leading cause of death, with young males being twice as likely as their female counterparts to die by suicide. What has become clear in recent decades is that depressed young people need treatment. There has been much debate regarding the role of selective serotonin reuptake inhibitors (SSRIs) in the treatment of moderate to severe depression and suicide in young people. Current Australian clinical guidelines recommend the use of a stepped-care approach, starting with a psychological intervention such as cognitive behavioural therapy (CBT). Further, it is recommended that the SSRI fluoxetine be used in moderate to severe depression only when psychological treatments have not been effective or have been refused, and a close therapeutic relationship has been established with the young person to enable ongoing close monitoring of treatment response and side-effects. A summary of the issues involved in the use of SSRI antidepressant medication to treat depression in young people can be accessed at: https://headspace.org.au/assests/Uploads/Resource-library/health-professionals/ssri-v2-pdf.pdf

Alcohol and substance use

Alcohol consumption is thought to significantly increase the risk of suicide in both young males and young females. Alcohol use among young people has been consistently associated with increased suicidal behaviour. The explanations include the psychologically depressive impact of alcohol, alcohol's disinhibiting effects, impulsivity heightened by alcohol, as well as the individual's high level of arousal and aggression (including past suicidal behaviour) (Dubovsky, 2010). Alcohol use and subsequent suicidal ideation and suicide attempts among pre-teens suggests that efforts to delay and reduce early alcohol use may reduce suicide attempts. Regardless of age, alcohol is a risk factor for completed suicides (Vijayakumar, Kumar & Vijayakumar, 2011). Table 13.1 on page 259 in Chapter 13 on blood alcohol level (BAL) demonstrates alcohol's effect on the human physiology and on subsequent behaviour.

Substances of abuse also increase the risk of suicide. When an individual is intoxicated, rational thought and judgment are impaired and impulsivity is heightened, to the point where, if the person has difficulty resolving a dilemma, suicide may seem the best course of action.

Ethnicity

In general, there are commonalities in all cultures: suicides occur when people are stressed, have poor resilience or poor coping skills, use substances, and have symptoms of depression. Between 2001 and 2010, in Australia 74.9 per cent of all suicides were by people born in Australia. A further 7.4 per cent of suicides in the same time period were by people born in Europe, and 7.1 per cent and 3.8 per cent were by people born in the United Kingdom and Asia, respectively. Between 2004 and 2008, the age-standardised suicide rates by country of birth were: New Zealand, 13.5 per 100000; Australia, 11.6 per 100000; Asia, 5.3 per 100000; Africa and the Middle East, 5.9 per 100000.

LIVED EXPERIENCE

My abuse of drugs and alcohol was always more extreme than that of the people around me, even as a teenager. I would take drugs to the point of overdose, and I would drink to oblivion. I think of my drinking and drug-taking as a kind of suicide-by-instalment plan. For many years I existed in a twilight zone between life and death, not wanting to die, but not knowing how to live with so much unresolved suffering. The substance abuse was a vicious cycle of dangerous and embarrassing behaviour during blackouts, followed by intense feelings of shame and remorse about my actions that inevitably led me back to more using. At first, substances were really helpful in medicating my feelings and dampening down my obsessive negative thoughts, but ultimately they became the primary source of my problems.

Interpersonal and intrapsychic theory

The notion that suicide is an expression of interpersonal and intrapsychic as well as societal conflict is a significant contribution that psychiatry and psychology have made to our understanding of suicide. The following examples describe some possible interpersonal and intrapsychic contexts for suicide:

- having no close relationships with others
- having no personal freedoms and no hope of getting them.

Practice example

Daniel thought that suicide was the best way to solve his problems, after he lost his job with the closure of a local coalmine and his girlfriend of 10 years precipitously broke off their engagement, left the area and married someone else.

Jamie, who is the victim of family violence, believes that it doesn't make any sense to go on living. She has no close friends or relatives. Her husband will not allow her to drive, go shopping or go to work. She is unable to see an alternative, and decides that a life regulated to this extent is not worth living.

According to well-regarded authorities, such as the American clinical psychologist Edwin Schneidman (1996), suicide can often be understood as a dyadic event between two unhappy people, motivated by real or perceived rejection, abandonment, guilt, revenge or pity. Suicide can be better understood if viewed in the context of the relationship between two people: the suicidal person and the significant other. Broadly defined, the significant other can be a spouse, child, boss, landlord, friend, nurse or other health care worker.

Suicidal people very often communicate their intent to significant others before the fact or attempt, although the meaning of the message may not be clear until after the attempt or death. Schneidman found a clear communication of intent in 80 per cent of the cases studied. A suicide threat or suicide attempt can arouse feelings of sympathy, anger, hostility, anxiety or desire for connectedness on the part of a significant other, thus altering the current relationship to meet the need of the suicidal person. Although there is no one cause associated with suicide, there are a number of interpersonal and intrapsychic elements that are commonly associated with it. The list in Box 19.4 summarises common characteristics based on Schneidman's work (1996).

Biological theory

A number of biological and medical markers have been studied in relation to the possible biological foundation of suicidal behaviour. The most promising biological markers to date appear to be decreased central serotonergic function, reduced serum cholesterol levels, decreased platelet 5-HT, low cerebrospinal fluid 5-HIAA, and hypothalamic–pituitary–adrenocortical axis (HPA axis) dysfunction. These biological markers are discussed next.

Neurotransmitter receptor hypothesis

The neurotransmitter receptor hypothesis of depression (see Chapters 7 and 16) holds that errors in the receptors for the specific neurotransmitter serotonin are critical in

Box 19.4 Characteristics most closely associated with suicide

1. The common purpose of suicide is to seek a solution to what appears to be an otherwise insoluble problem.
2. The common goal of suicide is cessation of consciousness or oblivion.
3. The common stimulus in suicide is unbearable psychological pain that may arise from any number of sources.
4. The common stressor in suicide is frustrated psychological needs that often result from family turmoil and occupational and interpersonal difficulties.
5. The common emotion in suicide is a pervasive sense of hopelessness coupled with helplessness.
6. The common cognitive state in suicide is ambivalence—desiring to die, but wishing there were another way out of the dilemma.
7. The common perceptual state in suicide is constriction of thought (tunnel vision) that prevents effective problem-solving.
8. The common action in suicide is escape from intolerable circumstances.
9. The common interpersonal act in suicide is communication of intention (estimated to be 80 per cent in completed suicides).
10. The common pattern in suicide is consistency of lifelong styles; suicidal people generally employ the same coping styles they have used throughout their lives.

the development of depression and suicide. Lower levels of serotonin (called *serotogenic hypofunction*) are associated with suicide and serious suicide attempts. There is evidence that the serotonergic system is partly under genetic control. As yet unknown genetic factors—thought to be independent of the factors responsible for the heritability of major psychiatric conditions associated with suicide—may contribute to the risk for suicidal behaviour.

Normally, serotonin is released from one nerve cell, received by the next nerve cell, and then reabsorbed back into the first nerve cell. Many factors influence how much serotonin is passed from the first cell to the second cell, and how much is reabsorbed back into the first cell. Transmission can be influenced by:

1. the number of receptors
2. the ability of the receptors to function properly
3. whether the body produces monoamine oxidase, which catabolises serotonin (as well as norepinephrine and dopamine).

Whatever the exact mechanism may be when serotonin and serotonin metabolic activity are reduced, more violent lethal suicides and attempted suicides seem to occur in these circumstances. Thus, while psychiatrists continue to debate the relationship between serotonin, depression and suicide, it has been suggested that enhancing serotonin function may reduce suicide risk.

Genetics

A family history of suicide is a recognised marker for the increased risk of suicide, suggesting that in addition to other influences there may be a genetic trait that predisposes some people to suicidal behaviour. Various studies provide evidence for a genetic component in suicidal behaviour (von Borczyskowski, Lindblad, Vinnerljung, Reintjes & Hjern, 2011). Genetic studies at the molecular level have concentrated on the genes of the serotonergic system, because there is evidence, as discussed earlier, that serotonergic neurotransmission is implicated in suicidal behaviour.

Cognitive theory

Suicidologists have speculated about the cognitive style (method of thought processing) of people who complete or attempt suicide. Although there is no single suicidal logic, some cognitive styles are thought to predispose to suicidal behaviour. *Dichotomous thinking* (the belief that there is only an either/or choice) is commonly seen in the person who is suicidal. The person falls into an imminently suicidal state when death seems to be the only escape. The thought processing of people who are suicidal is generally constricted; that is, people who are suicidal have great difficulty considering alternatives to their current dilemma. *Constriction in thought* generally results in the belief that there are only two choices: a 'magical' solution or death.

People who are considering suicide are often divided within themselves. They have two conflicting desires at the same time (**ambivalence**): to live and to die. Any attempt to understand the thinking of someone who is acutely suicidal requires consideration of the concept of ambivalence. Ambivalence accounts for the fact that a person who is suicidal often takes lethal or near-lethal action but leaves open the possibility for rescue, allowing for the possibility of intervention. Failing to intervene and provide life choices increases the person's desperation, and death becomes the more focused choice.

The effectiveness of cognitive behavioural therapy (CBT) in moderating suicide risk in people with significant mental disorders (major depressive disorder, for example) is an important research topic. For instance, it has been found (Curry et al., 2011) that CBT can contribute to recovery in young people with major depressive symptoms. The effectiveness of CBT was sustained at follow-up. Further research is indicated to substantiate these findings and determine how and why CBT works.

SUICIDE PREVENTION

Suicide, a serious public health problem, is often preventable. Krysinska et al. (2016) reviewed the evidence for strategies to reduce the suicide rate in Australia. They concluded that, while there is currently insufficient evidence supporting the effectiveness of specific suicide prevention strategies, those that were most likely to contribute to a reduction in suicide deaths were psychological interventions and well-coordinated aftercare.

Risk factors and protective factors

A combination of individual, interpersonal, community and societal factors contribute to the risk of suicide, as well as to the protective factors for suicide. Risk factors are the characteristics that are associated with suicide. They may or may not be direct causes. Protective factors serve as buffers from suicidal thoughts and behaviour. Both are equally important, and both need more extensive and rigorous research.

Identifying people at risk allows us to engage them in effective treatments, support the presence of protective factors and improve clinical practices. Risk factors and protective factors for suicide are discussed in Box 19.5.

National Suicide Prevention Strategy

The National Suicide Prevention Strategy (NSPS) provides a framework to guide suicide prevention in Australia; it emphasises promotion, prevention and early intervention initiatives. Renewed in late 2015, the NSPS involves:

- a systems-based approach to suicide prevention, operating at the regional level led by the recently established Primary Health Networks, in partnership with local health care providers in both the public and private sectors
- a focus on suicide prevention in Aboriginal and Torres Strait Islander communities.

The NSPS also involves the Living Is For Everyone (LIFE) framework. Information on NSPS and the LIFE framework can be accessed at: www.health.gov.au/internet/main/publishing.nsf/Content/mental-nsps

Box 19.5 Risk factors and protective factors for suicide

Risk factors

- Family history of suicide
- Family history of child maltreatment
- Previous suicide attempt(s)
- History of mental disorders, particularly depression
- History of alcohol and substance abuse
- Feelings of hopelessness
- Impulsive or aggressive tendencies
- Cultural and religious beliefs (e.g. suicide is a noble resolution of a personal dilemma)
- Local epidemics of suicide (suicide clusters)
- Isolation (feeling cut off from other people)
- Barriers to accessing mental health treatment
- Loss (relational, social, work or financial)
- Physical illness
- Easy access to lethal methods
- Unwillingness to seek help because of the stigma attached to mental health and substance abuse disorders or to suicidal thoughts

Protective factors

- Effective clinical care for mental, physical and substance abuse disorders
- Easy access to a variety of clinical and aftercare interventions and support for seeking help
- Family and community support
- Support from ongoing medical and mental health care relationships
- Skills in problem-solving, conflict resolution, and the non-violent management of disputes
- Cultural and religious beliefs that discourage suicide and support the instinct for self-preservation

Source: Adapted from: Centers for Disease Control. (2009). *Injury prevention and control: Suicide prevention* (retrieved from http://www.cdc.gov/ViolencePrevention/suicide/index.html); and Australian Government Department of Health and Ageing (2008). A framework for prevention of suicide in Australia (retrieved from *http://wwwlivingisforeveryone.com.au/uploads/docs/LIFE_framework-web.pdf*)

Suicide helplines

A number of suicide and crisis helplines are available for around-the-clock access in the states and territories and throughout Australia. These include:

- Beyondblue Support Service 1300 22 4636 (24 hours/7 days a week professional support)
- Suicide Call Back Service 1300 659 467 (24 hours/7 days a week professional phone counselling)
- Lifeline 13 11 14 (24 hour/7 days a week phone counselling)
- Suicide Line (Victoria) 1300 651 251 (24 hours/7 days a week professional anonymous support across Victoria)
- Kids Help Line 1800 55 1800 (24 hours/7 days a week professional phone counselling)
- Mensline 1300 789 987 (24 hours/7 days a week professional phone counselling and referral)
- Veterans Line 1800 011 046 (after-hours professional telephone crisis counselling for veterans and their families).

NURSING SELF-AWARENESS

When working with a person who is suicidal, it is imperative that you are aware of, and monitor your own reactions to, this potentially life-threatening situation, because your reactions may interfere with your ability to accurately assess the situation and offer help. The person who is suicidal presents a significant challenge and will call on all of your resources. You must be able to ask the right questions and make the right decisions, as well as manage your own fears and anxieties. Working with a person who not only may not want your assistance but wants deliberately to harm or kill themselves is a very complicated process.

You must be compassionate enough to be able to form an effective link with a person who is suicidal. The goal is to encourage and support the person to see you as an ally, yet maintain enough perspective to avoid being overwhelmed by the person's pain. The person with whom you are working will also bring many feelings into the interaction. Whether the feeling is anger, fear, anxiety, irritability or hostility, it is important to remember that all emotions need to be tolerated, worked through and evaluated.

Our attitudes towards people who are suicidal have many sources. In addition to the direct experience of people in distress, societal, familial and ethical issues, as well as historical antecedents, influence what we think and how we feel about suicide and self-destructive behaviour, euthanasia, abortion rights, the right to kill oneself, and the responsibility to prevent suicide. We can get caught up in the dilemma of how much responsibility to take for the person who self-harms and for how long. (Ethical issues about suicide are discussed in Chapter 11.)

All nurses must be competent not only to assess but also to intervene effectively with a person who is suicidal. This is not easy. People who are suicidal or self-harming seemingly defeat our best efforts by choosing death over life, or by engaging in self-harm. Although it is our responsibility to promote and maintain life, we cannot force the person to stay alive. Instead, we encourage people to examine and understand how it is that they have reached this point, and to expand their repertoire of coping methods.

Your attitudes when working with people who are suicidal or self-harming may include a variety of feelings—frustration and anger among them. Before working with someone who is suicidal or self-harming, it is critically important to assess any personal feelings, experiences, conflicts and memories that may either impede or facilitate your effectiveness. People report a more positive experience in treatment when we have a greater understanding of their experiences of self-harm (McHale & Felton, 2010). The inventory in the Self-awareness feature will help you to explore your own attitudes.

SELF-AWARENESS
An attitude inventory for working with people who are suicidal

To increase self-awareness about managing your own anxiety when working with people who are suicidal, ask yourself the following questions:

- What kinds of things frighten me?
- How do I feel about asking for someone else's help with a person with whom I am working if I am unsure of myself or uncomfortable?
- Are people who are suicidal asking me to take responsibility for their behaviour?
- Are people who are suicidal able to assume responsibility for their own behaviour?

To increase self-awareness of your own feelings about people who are suicidal or self-harm, ask yourself the following questions:

- How do I feel about people who deliberately harm themselves?
- How do I understand self-harming behaviour?
- Do I believe that people who are suicidal or who self-harm are capable of change?
- Do I believe that people ultimately have the responsibility for their own lives?
- Can a person who is mentally ill choose suicide as a reasonable course?

To increase self-awareness about your own anger, ask yourself the following questions:

- What kinds of things make me angry?
- How do I deal with my own anger? Do I tend to ignore it or hide it?
- How do I react to others when they are angry?
- How do I feel about people who don't change immediately?
- How do I deal with people who appear to do illogical things?
- How do I feel when people don't change their behaviour when I have asked them to or when I talk to them about it?

To increase self-awareness about your own feeling of control, ask yourself the following questions:

- In what areas of my life and my work do I feel the need to take control?
- How do I feel when interventions do not go the way I would like them to?
- How do I handle control issues with the people with whom I am working?
- How do I feel about control issues with the people with whom I am working?
- How do I feel about my lack of control over others?

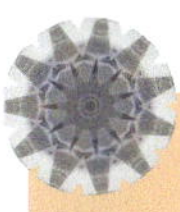

NURSING PROCESS
The person who is suicidal or self-harming

Working effectively with a person who is suicidal or self-harming requires understanding the meaning the behaviour has for the person, performing a **lethality assessment**, keeping the person safe, and helping enlarge their repertoire of adaptive coping behaviours. An example of how this can be done in clinical practice is given in Evidence-based Practice.

Review these other chapters for information on suicide in specific populations: young people, Chapter 21; older people, Chapter 22; people who abuse substances, Chapter 13; and people with mood disorders, Chapter 16.

EVIDENCE-BASED PRACTICE

Finding alternatives to suicide

Marie, a 19-year-old university student majoring in the performing arts, has been admitted to the inpatient unit after a heavy night of drinking alcohol that culminated in a suicide attempt. Marie's boyfriend has just dropped out of the university they attend and returned to his hometown in another part of the country. In the three months prior to this admission, Marie experienced a major injury to her knee. The injury was severe enough to threaten her career plan of being a dancer. Marie's family reports that she became increasingly despondent, saying she had nothing left to live for. They are also concerned that she seems to be reverting to the drinking problem she had in high school.

While in the unit, Marie has been unwilling to attend group therapy, saying that she 'can't think of what to say', that her 'head is messed up', and that she 'doesn't want to be around others'. Her diagnosis is major depression, and she has commenced taking antidepressant medications. As her psychiatric–mental health nurse, you formulate a nursing care plan that addresses the following considerations.

1. Marie is depressed and is working through multiple losses. In order to be able to find alternatives to suicide, she will need to think and process her feelings in a less rigid fashion.
2. Providing a less-demanding but secure environment will allow time to demonstrate to Marie that she has the flexibility to develop new coping skills and behaviours in response to her losses.
3. Cognitive behavioural therapy can help Marie learn to identify and respond more appropriately to circumstances that elicit maladaptive responses (alcohol abuse, depression).
4. Helping Marie to express feelings and perceptions will increase her self-awareness and her ability to plan methods for meeting her needs in the future. Validating Marie's perceptions provides reassurance and can decrease her anxiety.

(continued)

EVIDENCE-BASED PRACTICE *(continued)*

5. Marie's hospitalisation is likely to be short-term. The likelihood of suicide attempts is elevated in the month after starting treatment, when Marie will be back at university. Referrals to her general practitioner and to the local community mental health team and drug and alcohol service will be important in supporting Marie in the community. The range of services likely to be available in the university, and also online sources of information and support such as beyondblue, can also be discussed with Marie and her family.
6. A peer support worker may be able to share their journey of recovery with Marie, and give her hope that there is future to look forward to.

The interventions for Marie are based on the following research:

Curry, J., Silva, S., Rohde, P., Ginsburg, G., Kratochvil, C., Simons, A., . . . March, J. et al. (2011). Recovery and recurrence following treatment for adolescent major depression. *Archives of General Psychiatry, 68*(3), 263–269.

Seo, H.-J., Jung, Y.-E., Kim, T.-S., Kim, J.-B., Lee, M.-S., Kim, J.-M., . . . Jun, T.-Y. (2011). Distinctive clinical characteristics and suicidal tendencies of patients with anxious depression. *Journal of Nervous and Mental Disease, 199*(1), 42–48.

Krysinska, K., Batterham, P., Tye, M., Shand, F., Calear, A., Cockayne, N., & Christensen, H. (2016). Best strategies for reducing the suicide rate in Australia, *Australian and New Zealand Journal of Psychiatry, 50*(2), 115–118.

See also the recently released Royal Australian and New Zealand College of Psychiatrists clinical practice guideline for the management of deliberate self-harm (Carter et al. (2016)).

CRITICAL THINKING QUESTIONS

1. If Marie needs to become less rigid in her thinking and more flexible in her coping skills, how might a structured program such as cognitive behavioural therapy help her?
2. Is a short-term hospitalisation such as Marie's appropriate for someone at increased risk for suicide? Should Marie remain hospitalised until the threat of suicide is over? Why, or why not?
3. What types of strategies are likely to be most effective in reducing the suicide rate in Australia?

Assessment

A thorough assessment should include a self-assessment by the nurse, the identification of clues or cries for help, and an accurate lethality assessment. Because assessment of suicide risk involves a degree of clinical judgment, you should seek advice and support from more experienced professional colleagues if you are a beginning practitioner.

Clues or cries for help

People intent on suicide often give either verbal or non-verbal clues of their plans or ideas. A high percentage of people who kill themselves may signal their need for help by making a social contact or by approaching a health professional. Unfortunately, the cry for help is not always clear until after the event (Dimirci, Dogan, Erkol & Gunaydin, 2009). Because people do want help, you should ask questions about depression and suicide. It is thus important to be alert to patterns that may at first seem coincidental, as in the following example.

Practice example

You are working as a mental health nurse in a suburban general practice when Dulio, a 21-year-old man, presents to see the general practitioner (GP). Although he has described chronic 'aches and pains' and 'not feeling well', a physical exam revealed no physical problems. In the course of the consultation, Dulio talks about how life is just not worth living, and the GP asks you to see him. In his meeting with you, Dulio discloses a recent history of driving recklessly and that he had recently broken up with his girlfriend. Dulio then admits that his reckless driving had a suicidal intent.

The cry for help may be indirect or subtle. Examples of what a person might say are: 'I have had it; I just can't take it anymore', 'There's no reason to go on', 'Sometimes I think I'd be better off dead', 'I won't be seeing you anymore', 'Take care of my dog and cat', 'Too bad I won't get to see my little brother grow up' and 'Will you be sorry when I'm gone?' Sometimes the behaviour of people intent on suicide provides the clue. They may do the following:

- give away prized possessions
- make out or change a will
- take out, or add to, an insurance policy
- cancel all social engagements
- be despondent or behave in unusual ways
- be unable to sleep
- feel hopeless
- have trouble concentrating at school or on the job
- suddenly lose interest in friends, organisations and activities
- have a sudden, unexplained recovery from a depression
- plan their funeral
- cry for no apparent reason.

It is important to be alert to both clear and veiled communications about suicide. Once clues have been identified, the next step is to perform an accurate lethality assessment. You should always perform an assessment for suicide whenever you suspect suicidal thought or intent.

Suicide risk assessment

A suicide risk assessment is an attempt to predict the likelihood of suicide. A careful assessment is essential in formulating

LIVED EXPERIENCE

There is a strange calm that comes with the absence of a desire to live. After months of unbearable anxiety and depression, I experienced a moment of clarity: I could relieve myself of suffering. I had thought about killing myself quite often, but this time it was different. It was like I had been looking into a badly focused kaleidoscope where the images were blurred and distant, and that I had discovered how to adjust the lens so that everything became crystal-clear. I never considered it as ending my life, it was just ending the pain.

a plan for helping a person who is suicidal. An assessment of risk factors is essential in order to determine if there is a need for hospitalisation, or the extent of watchful precautions to take when a person is hospitalised. Carrying out a suicide risk assessment requires direct communication with the person about their intent. Your Assessment Approach outlines aspects of a suicide risk assessment.

YOUR ASSESSMENT APPROACH
Suicide risk assessment

Danger to self	Typical indicators
No predictable risk of immediate suicide	No suicidal ideation or history of attempts; satisfactory social support network; in close contact with significant others
Low risk of immediate suicide	Has considered suicide with less lethal method; no history of attempts or recent serious loss; satisfactory support network; no alcohol problems; basically wants to live
Moderate risk of immediate suicide	Has considered suicide with highly lethal method but has no specific plan or threats; or has plan with less lethal method; history of less lethal attempts; tumultuous family history; reliance on drugs or medications for stress relief; is weighing the odds between life and death
High risk of imminent suicide	Current highly lethal plan with obtainable means; history of previous attempts; unable to communicate with close friends; drinking problem; feels depressed and wants to die
Very high risk of imminent suicide	Current highly lethal plan with obtainable means; history of highly lethal attempts; cut off from resources; depressed and uses alcohol to excess; threatened with a serious loss (unemployment, divorce, failure in school)

Another component of assessing suicide risk is a consideration of the lethality of the proposed suicide method. Box 19.6 compares the lethality of various suicide methods. There are some gender differences in suicide methods. Women tend to use less violent methods—drugs and carbon monoxide poisoning—while men tend to use more violent methods—firearms and hanging. In 2014, the most frequent method of suicide was hanging, strangulation and suffocation (53 per cent), followed by poisoning by drugs (15.4 per cent), poisoning by other methods (e.g. alcohol and motor vehicle exhaust) (6.6 per cent), and firearms (6.2 per cent) (Australian Bureau of Statistics, 2016).

Box 19.6 Lethality of suicide methods

Less lethal methods

- Wrist-cutting
- House gas
- Non-prescription medications (excluding aspirin and paracetamol)
- Tranquilisers

Highly lethal methods

- Firearms
- Jumping
- Hanging
- Drowning
- Carbon monoxide poisoning
- Barbiturates and prescribed sleeping pills
- High doses of aspirin and paracetamol
- Car crash
- Antidepressants (tricyclic and monoamine oxidase inhibitor classes)

It is critical that you evaluate the person's ability and intent to act on an urge or plan. Beyond inquiring into the existence of a plan for suicidal action, ask questions and pay particular attention to whether the person has already taken steps to implement such a plan. For example, has the person already stockpiled medication, written a suicide note, obtained (or have access to) knives or guns, spoken to others about purchasing a gun, written a will, given away valued objects or recently purchased insurance? Also obtain information about prior suicide attempts, as well as the person's history of violence and impulsiveness, alcohol and drug use, and family history of suicide or violence.

Assessment of suicide risk is not easily accomplished. One barrier is the fear inexperienced nurses have of asking inappropriate or possibly harmful questions. It is important that you understand that *it is not possible to 'cause' a person's suicide by assessing feelings and thoughts*. Inquiring about suicidal thoughts may alleviate a person's anxiety about considering suicide, not 'give them the idea'.

These are some suggestions for questions that you might ask:

- 'How bad are things for you?'
- 'How down do you get?'
- 'Are you worried about yourself?'
- 'Do you ever think of harming yourself when you're down?'

Then proceed with questioning the person gently, but directly asking questions such as:

- 'Have you ever thought of taking your own life?'
- 'Have you ever been so sad that you wanted to end it all, maybe by dying?'
- 'How long have you been feeling that way?'
- 'How are you thinking of hurting/harming yourself?'

Do not use euphemisms—be direct and clear in your communication.

The person who asks you to promise not to tell anyone about a suicide plan poses a serious assessment problem. Never promise to keep clinical information of any kind a secret, and explain to the person that information is shared with the treatment team. You will probably need to discuss the issue of confidentiality further and explore the dynamics of the therapeutic relationship.

A comprehensive assessment, including risk and lethality assessments, will help in decisions regarding which interventions are indicated for the person. For example, a careful assessment of level of risk and lethality can prevent unnecessary hospitalisations. Hospitalisations in and of themselves can create a crisis. However, when the suicide plan is lethal and there are inadequate supports to safely maintain the person in the community, hospitalisation will need to be considered.

Responding to the needs of a person who is suicidal or self-harming

Much of the work undertaken by nurses when working with people who are suicidal or engage in self-harm involves:

- assessment of the (degree and immediacy of) risk of suicide or self-harm
- mitigation of the risk of suicide or self-harm
- support for the feelings of powerlessness and hopelessness
- assistance to improve ineffective individual coping
- help in improving low self-esteem

In the course of such work, nurses may also become involved in helping a person to better manage anxiety, improve verbal communication, work through losses experienced, deal more effectively with distressing thoughts, and address family-related issues and pressures.

Identification of outcomes

The following are outcome criteria when working with the person who is suicidal or self-harming:

- acknowledge self-harm thoughts
- admit to the use of self-harm behaviour if it occurs
- be able to identify personal triggers
- learn to properly identify and tolerate uncomfortable feelings
- choose alternatives that are not harmful
- attempt to identify stressors
- engage with interventions designed to reduce suicidal thoughts and control behaviour.

Planning and implementation

The interventions outlined in the following section are based on the belief that mental health care professionals should do everything reasonably possible to prevent a suicide. The descriptions of all clinical interventions strive for the ideal outcome; however, it is important to recognise that ideal circumstances are not always available, and therefore ideal outcomes do not always result.

General guidelines for any setting

The priority task is to work with the person to stop the constricted processing of suicidal thinking long enough to enable the person and family members to consider alternatives to suicide. The nature of the interventions is in large part determined by the setting in which you encounter the person who is suicidal. It is important to be familiar with and work according to state and local policies and procedures. The following list of interventions and suggestions offers general guidelines that are applicable in most settings.

- Take any threat seriously. Evaluate the threat carefully before dismissing it.
- Talk about suicide openly and directly. Remember, asking about it will not put the notion into the person's head.
- Implement suicide precautions (discussed in greater detail later in this chapter).
- Search the person's room, especially if suicidal thoughts or a suicide attempt occur after admission.
- Decide (with the person and other members of the treatment team) if a no-self-harm/no-suicide contract will be used (a sample contract is in the following Your Intervention Strategies).
- Locate the person in an area that is accessible for easy observation. Select a room that is near the nurses' station.
- Be careful not to encourage staff behaviours that convey a false sense of security to the person or staff.
- Develop a plan of care in collaboration with the person who is suicidal or self-harming. Discuss all important problems, prioritise them, and list several approaches to each problem. Write down this plan, noting who is responsible for which actions.
- Do not make unrealistic promises such as 'Don't worry, I won't let you kill yourself.' Remain honest but hopeful. Making unrealistic promises diminishes your credibility with the person with whom you are working.
- Encourage the person to continue daily activities and self-care as much as possible. Assign tasks for the person that are distracting but not taxing.

- Decide with the person which family members and friends are to be contacted and by whom.
- Be prepared to deal with family members who may be worried, confused or angry. Strive to remain neutral, and do not make assumptions about the family's behaviour.
- Expect that the person will likely be experiencing shame, and work to help them towards self-acceptance.
- Remove the person from immediate danger by removing medication or other harmful objects in their possession, or by moving the person to a physically safe environment.
- Address the person's obvious immediate distress. Does the person need a bath, clean clothing, food, sleep?
- Find out what, in the person's view, is the most pressing need. This may be seeing a friend or family member, or arranging for someone to pick up the children after school.
- Assume a nonjudgmental, caring attitude that does not engender self-pity in the person.
- Ask why the person chose to attempt suicide at this particular moment. The person's answer may shed light on the meaning that suicide has for them, and may provide information that can lead to other helpful interventions.
- Provide for the person's safety through close observation and careful monitoring (see the section on safety for the person who is suicidal).
- Review the safety of the environment (see the later section on safety in the therapeutic environment).
- Evaluate the person's need for medication.
- Evaluate the plan developed in collaboration with the person, and arrange for appropriate follow-up.
- Monitor your personal feelings about the person, and decide how they may be influencing your clinical work.
- Work with other team members to evaluate the issues fully. If available, seek the services of a peer support worker. You do not always have all of the pieces of the puzzle.
- Perform a physical examination. (One woman had cut herself severely prior to coming to the hospital, but this injury was not discovered until the physical examination was performed.)
- Recognise that people can and do hang or strangle themselves with shoelaces, brassiere straps, pantyhose, dressing-gown belts, craft materials and so on. Remain alert: sharp objects such as razor blades may be found in pages of books; matches are relatively easy to hide; pills may be hidden in plastic wrap in a cake box; light bulbs can be broken and used to cut oneself, as can wire from spiral notebooks. People are also able to drown in a bathtub, throw themselves through a plate-glass window, set themselves on fire, or drink cleaning solutions such as bleach.

General guidelines for the emergency department

Attempted suicide or suicidal ideation is one of the most common mental health-related reasons for presentation to an emergency department (Weiland, Cotter, Jelinek & Phillips, 2014).

YOUR INTERVENTION STRATEGIES

How to develop no-self-harm/no-suicide contracts

No-self-harm/no-suicide contracts are sometimes used when working with people who are suicidal or self-harming. You may see them being used in hospital or outpatient settings as a means of providing additional support to people who are likely to harm themselves.

- Perform a thorough assessment before developing a no-suicide contract.
- Establish a relationship with the person prior to initiating the contract.
- Specify in the contract the intervals for re-evaluation. In outpatient settings, the interval may be one week; the inpatient interval may range from several times every day, to every one to three days, to weekly.
- Encourage the person to contribute to writing out the contract if at all possible. If the person is unwilling to do so, other options include having the contract audiotaped.
- Have both nurse and person sign the contract and date it.
- Use the contract as a way of connecting with, and staying connected with, the person.
- It is important to note that the contract *does not guarantee the person's safety*; clinical judgement should always be prioritised over a contract.

People who are acutely suicidal may agree to the contract even though they have no intention of adhering to it.

Sample no self-harm/no-suicide contract

I, Cathy Smith, will not harm myself in any way. If I feel as though I am going to lose control, I will tell the staff (inform my nurse, call the crisis number, call my primary health care professional, etc.).

I will not bring, nor will I ask others to bring, harmful articles or substances onto the unit.

This contract lasts until _________ (date), and is renewable at that time.

Signed (and dated)

______________________________, Consumer

______________________________, Nurse

In the emergency department, the main goal of treatment is to save the person's life. Although the emergency staff may be excellent at technical interventions, they may voice or feel frustration with the person who presents frequently, especially if the attempt is not life-threatening. The person needs a professional, non-punitive approach, and a smooth transition to other caregivers or agencies. One-to-one observation and a psychiatric evaluation by an experienced clinician is the standard of care. Leaving the person alone or with access to harmful objects is obviously a hazard to be avoided in a busy emergency department.

Suicide precautions

It is important to maintain the person's safety in the least restrictive manner possible (the right to treatment in the least restrictive setting is discussed in Chapter 11). The length of time **suicide precautions** are in place is of concern to the person as well as the staff. While precautions address the person's safety needs, they do not constitute treatment. On an inpatient unit, times of highest risk for suicide are evenings, nights and weekends. Two factors account for this: during these periods, the unit program tends to be less structured, and fewer staff members are available.

Suicide protocols Most psychiatric inpatient units have developed a set of protocols or guidelines for observing, monitoring and restricting the behaviour of people who are suicidal. These systems of observation have between three and six levels, will almost certainly require an order by a psychiatrist or other medical practitioner, and are usually put into effect by nurses. These protocols are often labelled to reflect the rationale for their use. They may be known as *constant observation*, *special observation* or *close observation*. At the higher levels of observation, the nurse may be required to be within arms-reach of the person at all times; or within direct sight and in the same room at all times; or must be able to sight the person at regular intervals (e.g. every 15 minutes). Examine sample protocols in Your Intervention Strategies.

It is of critical importance that all staff members be familiar with the system being used, and understand the rationale for its use. Maintaining and observing people on these protocols is an important nursing responsibility.

Reserve restrictive status for managing the safety of people who are suicidal or self-harming. Restrictions can confound therapeutic management, and their use simply to restrict the free movement of other people on the unit diminishes their effectiveness. In general, privileges and other components of unit restriction are better dealt with by other measures, such as privilege systems. If there is doubt about the appropriate safety status, the person should remain on a more restrictive status until the treatment team decides

YOUR INTERVENTION STRATEGIES Sample protocols for suicide precautions

Note that these are sample protocols. It is important to be familiar with the policies and procedures of the state/territory health department jurisdiction and specific mental health facility within which you are working. An example of a policy directive from one state jurisdiction in Australia, NSW Health, is *PD2016_007 Clinical care of people who may be suicidal*. This document can be accessed at www0.health.nsw.gov.au/policies/pd/2016/PD2016_007.html (accessed on 28 September 2016).

Basic suicide precautions

Basic suicide precautions are usually ordered by an admitting doctor in consultation with the senior nurse. In circumstances in which a person's clinical condition requires a reconsideration of the suicide/self-harm precautions protocol, this should be raised with medical staff as soon as possible. It is important to note that such protocols involve more than a mere location check. Regular precautionary observations should also include opportunities to engage with and support the person who is suicidal.

- The person is to remain in the room with the door open unless accompanied by a staff or family member. The person may use the bathroom alone.
- Check the person's whereabouts and safety every 15 to 30 minutes, depending on the level of risk. Document safety checks.
- Stay with the person while all medications are taken.
- Look through the person's belongings for potentially harmful objects. Make the search in the person's presence, and ask for their assistance while doing so.
- Check all articles brought in by visitors.
- Allow the person to have a regular access to meals, but be sure to check whether the glass or any utensils are missing when meals are finished.
- Allow visitors and telephone calls unless the person wishes otherwise.
- Check that visitors do not leave potentially dangerous objects in the person's room.
- Maintain the protocol until it is ceased by the treating doctor (usually a consultant psychiatrist).
- Inform the person of the reasons for, and details of, precautionary measures. The nurse and the treating doctor should both provide this explanation and document it in the person's clinical notes.

Maximum suicide precautions

Maximum suicide precautions require a medical order by the treating doctor (usually a consultant psychiatrist).

- Provide one-to-one nursing supervision (sometimes referred to as *constant* or *special* observation). You must be in close proximity to the person and have a direct line of sight at *all* times. When the person uses the bathroom, they must be accompanied by a nurse. A staff member should sit next to the person's bed at night.
- The person should not leave the unit for tests or procedures; if this becomes necessary, they must be escorted by a nurse in close proximity at all times.
- Allow visitors and telephone calls unless the person wishes otherwise. Maintain one-to-one supervision during visits.
- Look through the person's belongings in their presence, and remove any potentially harmful objects, such as medications, matches, belts, shoelaces, pantyhose, brassieres, razors, tweezers, mirrors or other glass objects (such as light bulbs), wire and craft materials.
- If suicide precautions are initiated after the person has been on the unit for any length of time, make a complete search of the room.
- Check that visitors do not leave potentially harmful objects in the person's room.
- Serve the person's meals in their room, ensuring that the tray contains no glass and no metal eating utensils.
- Prior to instituting these measures, explain to the person what you will be doing and why. The treating doctor should also discuss the necessity of maximum suicide precautions with the person. The explanations should be documented in the person's clinical notes.
- These measures should be maintained until ceased or modified by the treating doctor (usually a consultant psychiatrist).

what measures are appropriate. If there is any doubt or concern about moving a person to a different status, it is best to retain the more restrictive status until the clinical direction of treatment is clarified.

Signs of clinical improvement Once you have recognised that a person is at risk of suicide or self-harm and you have implemented a safety plan, you should begin the therapeutic work of addressing depression, psychosis and precipitating factors. The treatment focus shifts as the person begins to show signs of clinical improvement.

The following signs may indicate clinical improvement and signal the need to review or change treatment plans, grant privileges or plan discharges:

- verbalising a range of options other than suicide
- making long-term plans or discussing future events
- verbalising hope
- responding to antidepressant and/or antipsychotic medications
- wanting to reconnect with, or moving towards reconnecting with, family or significant others
- showing more energy
- sleeping better
- feeling less hopeless
- demonstrating a wider range of affective responses to situations that occur on the unit.

Removing suicide precautions While changes to a suicide precautions protocol should be authorised by medical staff, it is best that they occur gradually, rather than all at once. A realistic plan is to change one or two variables at a time, while observing, monitoring and documenting the person's responses. As the treatment team begins to move the person off special status, it is important for all team members to keep communicating openly about the person's progress (Addo et al., 2010). As the person begins to improve, the risk of suicide may increase temporarily (especially if the person has increased energy and ability finally to act on the suicidal ideation). The following times are critical and call for careful evaluation:

- *When the decision is made to move the person off suicide precaution status.* If a person has come to depend on the around-the-clock safety, comfort and nurturance provided by a staff member, they may experience the discontinuing of suicide precaution status as a loss. Gradual removal from suicide precaution status, and careful monitoring of its impact on the person, is indicated in these cases.
- *When the decision is made to increase access to 'sharps' (dangerous objects).* This increased access may make it possible for a person to act on a suicidal impulse. Assess the person carefully before granting this access.
- *During the initial weeks following commencement of antidepressant medication.* At this time, the person may have increased energy but their depression has not been resolved.
- *When the decision is made to allow leave.* Carefully evaluate decisions to allow the person to leave the unit. Where is the person going, and with whom? What timeframe is being considered, and why? Perform a careful assessment both before and after the person goes on leave. Additional searches may be needed at these times.
- *Prior to discharge and while formulating the discharge plan.* Remember that while a person is an inpatient, they will have staff available at a moment's notice. This is not the case once the person is discharged. It is crucial to evaluate the 'holding environment' in the community. Refer the person to resources in the community, and schedule a follow-up appointment at the time of discharge. Family and significant others should participate in discharge planning. It is generally not a good idea to discharge a person (especially one who lacks immediate family support and must rely on agencies or health care practitioners in the community) on a Friday, over a long weekend, or when the primary care provider will be on holiday or otherwise unavailable.

Monitoring the safety of the therapeutic environment

It is important that the safety of the therapeutic environment be evaluated periodically. Does it meet the needs of the current population of consumers, and is the level of restrictions consistent with the milieu philosophy? Here are specific questions to consider:

- Are areas free of glass or sharps?
- Are hazardous objects and areas kept locked?
- Are wardrobe handles or shower rods of the breakaway type?
- Are craft items safe?
- How many people are being treated on the unit? What is the population of people on the unit like now? How many people are in a high-risk group (severe depression, acute schizophrenia)?
- If the therapeutic environment is temporarily deemed to be unsafe—that is, if there are objects (such as razors, glass, drugs) on the unit that can harm others—is there also a need to conduct a thorough 'health-and-welfare search' in order to completely examine all areas of the unit for other potential hazards?

It is also very important to educate the person's family and visitors about safety measures and their rationale. Taking this step helps ensure that family members and other visitors do not bring unsafe objects on the unit. Visitors must understand visit limits and unit policies in relation to leave passes. It is also necessary to explain the need for searches. Families and friends who repeatedly violate the safety measures of the unit may require additional attention, and their visiting privileges may have to be restricted.

Documenting behaviour and treatment

Documentation is essential for those working with people who are suicidal or self-harming on an inpatient unit. Documentation helps all staff members understand the rationale for changes, and comply with ethical and legal requirements. In general, follow organisational rules about documentation. The following should also be documented:

- all team reviews of the status of people in care, and the names of the team members involved
- any decision to remove the person from a more restrictive status to a less restrictive one
- the rationale for any changes in the treatment approach, especially changes in the level of restriction
- statements made by people who are suicidal about self-harm or denial of self-harm
- responses of people who are suicidal to changes, passes, family, visitors
- all telephone calls or interactions with family members
- all searches carried out, and the reason for them.

Working with families

Including family members in the plan of care for the person who is suicidal or self-harming is extremely important. Hospitalisations for suicidal ideation or a suicide attempt may be brief, and may be terminated before the antidepressant medication has had a chance to work. There are two important strategies that families need to be aware of:

1. how to prevent suicide
2. how to help their loved one avoid acting on suicidal thoughts when those thoughts occur.

Guidelines for families in preventing suicide are given in the Collaborative Care feature on helping families prevent suicide. You can also suggest some helpful phone numbers and websites to family members, such as beyondblue Support Service (1300 22 4636; www.beyondblue.org.au/get-support), Suicide Call Back Service (1300 659 467; www.suicidecallbackservice.org.au), Lifeline 24-Hour Counselling and Crisis Support Service (13 11 14; www.lifeline.org.au) and Suicide Prevention Australia (www.suicidepreventionaust.org/).

Evaluation

Suicide, like all crisis situations, calls for ongoing evaluation of the plan made by the nurse and the person who is suicidal. Because events often occur rapidly, you may need to change the initial care plans almost daily. In addition to evaluating individual care plans, services and staff members who work with people who are suicidal need to evaluate their overall approach and philosophy periodically.

CARE COORDINATION

Care coordinators can ensure that planned therapeutic linkages occur once the person has been discharged. Linkages might be established with community health nurses, community mental health nurses, or nurses working in primary care settings such as general practice surgeries.

Make sure that people who have been discharged and their families have all the telephone numbers they need—suicide/crisis helplines, community mental health team, general practitioner. Care coordinators can also find other appropriate resources in the community to meet an individual person's needs. At the time of discharge, a person should also have the time and date of their follow-up appointment.

COMMUNITY-BASED CARE

The treatment team needs to have a realistic approach when planning the care of a person who is suicidal. It is usually not possible to meet all of the therapeutic goals in an inpatient setting. People who are suicidal are often discharged well before antidepressant medication is at full therapeutic response (see Chapter 7 for a discussion of antidepressant medications). It is thus important that careful monitoring is provided in the community, and the person should be encouraged to maintain contact with a mental health professional in a mental health facility, private practice or community mental health centre. A good case manager will have provided helpline and crisis

COLLABORATIVE CARE

Helping families prevent suicide

If family members strongly believe that someone is close to a suicidal act, or the person has indicated that they are close to acting on a suicidal impulse, teaching them these steps can help prevent suicide.

- **Take the person seriously.** Stay calm, listen, but don't under-react. Express concern.
- **Listen attentively.** Maintain eye contact. Use body language to show concern, such as moving close to the person or holding their hand, if appropriate.
- **Do not promise secrecy.** You may need to speak to the person's health care professional in order to protect the person from themselves. Don't make promises that would endanger your loved one's life.
- **Ask direct questions.** Find out whether the person has a specific plan for suicide. If you can, determine what method of suicide the person is considering.
- **Offer reassurance.** Stress that suicide is a permanent solution to a temporary problem. Remind the person that help is available and that things will get better.
- **Involve other people.** Don't try to handle the crisis alone or jeopardise your own health or safety. Call a crisis or suicide support line if necessary. Contact the suicidal person's mental health professional, a crisis intervention team, a suicide helpline, a hospital emergency department, or others who are trained to help.
- **If possible, do not leave the person alone.** Make sure that arrangements are made for your loved one to be in professional hands as quickly and safely as possible.

service telephone numbers to the person with whom they are working.

Day programs, where available, can be options. These activities structure and focus the day, so the person can learn adaptive coping mechanisms, socialise as tolerated, and develop goals in a safe environment.

HOME CARE

In addition to helping family members learn how to be gatekeepers to prevent suicide (such as in the preceding Collaborative Care: Helping Families Prevent Suicide), the person who is suicidal and their family should have a suicide crisis plan in place that will help the person avoid acting on suicidal impulses. Parents and friends can be instrumental in preventing suicide. Most symptoms of depression and hopelessness are universally recognised by parents and friends, although friends tend to be better able to recognise symptoms of substance abuse, which increase the risk for suicidal behaviour. The Collaborative Care: Helping an Individual Develop a Family Suicide Crisis Plan emphasises a role for people who are suicidal in developing a family suicide crisis plan.

SURVIVORS OF SUICIDE

The act of suicide can have long-lasting ramifications for the survivors. Nurses who are working with the families or staff who have worked with the deceased must be alert to the potential after-effects of the death (staff reactions are described later in the chapter).

Farberow (1992), a suicidologist who studied the effects of suicide on survivors, identified these emotional experiences of survivors of suicide that remain relevant today:

- strong feelings of loss accompanied by sorrow and mourning
- anger at being made to feel responsible for the behaviour of the suicidal person
- feelings of separation because their help was refused
- anxiety, guilt, shame or embarrassment because the person killed themselves
- relief that the nagging, insistent demands of the suicidal person have ceased
- feelings of desertion
- the arousal of impulses towards suicide
- anger caused by the belief that the suicide represents a rejection of social and moral responsibilities.

Many survivors do not seek assistance from mental health care professionals. They may be angry and believe that mental health care professionals 'should have prevented this'. Those who work with survivors, including nurses, must be prepared for this reaction. In Australia, a number of organisations provide information and support for survivors of suicide. These include Lifeline (www.lifeline.org.au) and Survivors of Suicide (SOS) (www.survivorsofsuicide.com.au).

Family and friends who are survivors

Families and friends may not receive the same degree of support as bereaved people whose loved ones have died because of illness or accident. People in the support network (including other family members or friends) may be uncomfortable and embarrassed, and may stay away rather than help. If there is shame associated with suicide, that shame may be directed towards the survivors of suicide. Comments may be made about the family not being sufficiently attentive, or that they should have prevented the suicide. Options for establishing an alternative network of support exist with support groups such as Survivors of Suicide Bereavement Support Association (SOSBSA) (www.SOSBSA.org.au), which operates a helpline (1300 767 022).

Sometimes, suicide is denied or concealed by family members, who wish to avoid feelings of shame or avoid being blamed for the death. This secrecy may further impede grief work, because survivors cannot resolve the loss unless they discuss it openly. Suicide exacerbates dysfunctional

COLLABORATIVE CARE

Helping an individual develop a family suicide crisis plan

For most people, thinking about killing themselves is temporary. It is important that when suicidal ideas occur to people that they have a crisis plan in place. This plan will help them avoid acting on suicidal thoughts when those thoughts occur. Teach the person with whom you are working that their plan should contain the following elements:

- **Tell those you trust about your condition.** It is important for the people close to you to be totally familiar with your condition before it becomes a crisis. Discuss your plan with family and friends so that they can respond quickly and effectively if you need their help.
- **Recognise the earliest warning signs of a suicidal episode.** Learn to be sensitive to subtle warnings of illness. This is a time to take care of yourself with the utmost care. Try not to become angry or disgusted with yourself.
- **Avoid drugs and alcohol.** Most deaths by suicide are the result of sudden, uncontrolled impulses. Because drugs and alcohol contribute to such impulses, it is very important to avoid them. Drugs and alcohol also interfere with the effectiveness of medications prescribed for depression.
- **Don't despair if your suicidal thinking recurs.** Suicidal thinking may be a signal of neurochemical imbalance. Call for help.
- **Contact your mental health provider, primary care provider or family doctor.** Have these phone numbers with you, along with a backup number such as an emergency department or a suicide crisis helpline.
- **Set your telephone speed-dial feature with emergency numbers.** Having these numbers available will get you help sooner if you are feeling desperate.

family dynamics, such as scapegoating or blaming other family members. If grief is not allowed to proceed, mental health problems ensue for the survivors. Personal growth can arise from healing after a suicide loss (Feigelman, Jordan & Gorman, 2009).

Besides making the usual preparations after death, which are stressful enough in themselves, families must deal with police investigations, the media and insurance companies. This can precipitate extreme stress, especially if only limited support is available.

Families and significant others who survive a suicide may need health professional intervention, but it is especially warranted for the following:

- families who lack support from usual sources
- dysfunctional families who react by blaming, scape-goating or covering up the death as an accident
- children whose parent has killed themselves
- young people exposed to the suicide of a friend.

Outreach services should be made available to these groups. A typical plan might include contacting the family immediately after the suicide and periodically until the first anniversary of the death, and arranging for staff or a staff representative to attend services, if appropriate. Consider connecting the family to a bereavement support group. Families (first-degree relatives, spouses and significant others of someone who has killed themselves) may experience a significant reduction in maladaptive grief reactions and perceptions of blame in cognitive behavioural counselling programs. Psychoeducational services and family interventions may also be helpful. Families who need assistance towards the positive resolution of grief can be encouraged and supported to contact Compassionate Friends Australia at www.thecompassionatefriends.org.au

Children and young people who experience the suicide of a parent

Children who experience loss as the result of suicide by a parent require urgent intervention to deal with the trauma. It is important to be particularly sensitive with these children, because they often have problems with grieving. A child who loses a parent is also at greater risk for suicide and depression.

Young people who are exposed to the suicide of a friend are at high risk for development of major depression. You should carefully screen, observe and treat for depressive symptoms. A close relationship with the victim, visual exposure to the victim at the scene of death, having a conversation with the victim the day of the suicide, and both a personal and a family history of depression are all predictive of the development of depression subsequent to the suicide.

Suicide clusters

Suicide clusters—an excessive number of suicides occurring in close temporal or geographical proximity to each other—is a phenomenon of great concern to those who work with young people. Internationally, clustering is often seen to be more prevalent in young people located in institutional settings, such as correctional centres or mental health facilities. An Australian study identified 258 suicides out of 10 176 suicides between 2004 and 2008 that were classified as being within a suicide cluster. Data from that research indicated that death was more likely to occur within a suicide cluster if the person was Indigenous, living in a rural area, or living in the northern part of Australia (especially Northern Territory, Queensland or Western Australia). While these findings suggest that geographical factors ought to be considered in developing a better understanding of suicide clustering, more research is required to clarify the importance of other factors, such as age, gender and employment status (Cheung, Spittal, Williamson, Tung & Pirkis, 2014).

Staff survivors of suicide by a person in treatment

Staff members are also survivors of suicide by a person in treatment. Suicide during a course of treatment has sometimes been considered as an 'occupational hazard'.

The reactions of staff members can be as varied as the roles they perform with the people with whom they work. For example, the exact memories and reactions will vary with a nurse who finds a person hanging and administers first aid, a therapist who saw a person for their last session, and a psychiatrist who was the last health professional to evaluate a person. All are likely to experience the suicide as a traumatic event.

Support for staff members is critical after suicide by a person in treatment. Typical reactions to the suicide of a person in treatment may include sadness, anger, denial and

LIVED EXPERIENCE

I'm not sure I will ever be 'recovered', but I am in the process of recovery now. I rarely think of suicide and I haven't self-harmed in more than 15 years. I have definitely had temporary setbacks, but I no longer see these as undermining the permanent gains I have made. What has been vital in this process is having people—friends, family, colleagues and mental health professionals—in my life who speak the language of recovery, who don't look at me as an illness but as someone who sometimes experiences mental distress as a result of trauma. I now view mental health conditions like mine as legitimate responses to what's happened to someone rather than as something maladaptive. When you understand mental 'illness' as a sane response to insane circumstances, you empower people to understand that they are just trying to survive what's happened to them, and that's a very powerful shift in how people like me think of themselves. I see myself as a survivor, and that has given me the sense of agency required for change that was constantly being undermined by the 'system' when I was just a diagnosis.

shame. Some may have the erroneous belief that if you are 'a good enough' nurse or therapist, you will be able to effectively prevent all suicides. Ethical concerns may be the focus of guilt if the person requested, and was refused, an assisted suicide (Levene & Parker, 2011). Staff members may lack confidence and be unable to function. This would be a good time for nurses to review their reasons for becoming nurses in the first place. Thoughts of reconsidering what they do or where they work are common. The range of other common reactions among nurses, doctors and other health care professionals range from refusing to admit people who are suicidal to their caseloads or units, to recognising what the particular problems were and how they might manage them better in the future. Clinicians who have lost a person to suicide may consider discussing their reactions to this in clinical supervision (or less formally with a trusted professional colleague), or seeking support via an employee assistance program (or similar) within their workplace.

Staff members with little health professional training or experience may suffer more than those who have previously encountered illness and death. These workers may need extra attention.

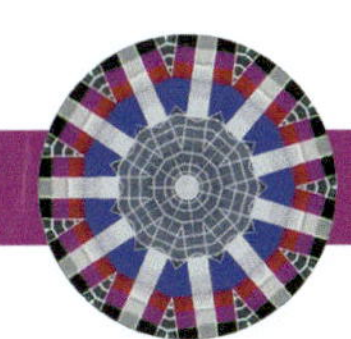

REFERENCES

Addo, M. A., McKie, A., Kettles, A. M., Gibb, J., Gass, J., & Yule, M. (2010). Are nurses empowered to make decisions about levels of patient observation in mental health? *Nursing Times, 106*(9), 26–28.

Australian Bureau of Statistics (ABS). (2016). *3303.0—Causes of death, Australia, 2014*. Canberra: ABS. Retrieved from www.abs.gov.au/ausstats/abs@.nsf/mf/3303.0 (Accessed 2016, August 23.)

Australian Institute of Health and Welfare (AIHW). (2015). *The health and welfare of Australia's Aboriginal and Torres Strait Islander peoples 2015*. Cat. No. IHW 147. Canberra, Australia: AIHW.

Carter, G., Page, A., Large, M., Hetrick, S., Milner, A., Bendit, N., . . . Christensen, H. (2016). Royal Australian and New Zealand College of Psychiatrists clinical practice guideline for the management of deliberate self-harm. *Australian and New Zealand Journal of Psychiatry, 50*(10), 939–1000.

Cheung, Y. T. D., Spittal, M., Williamson, M., Tung, S., & Pirkis, J. (2014). Predictors of suicides occurring within suicide clusters in Australia, 2004–2008. *Social Science and Medicine, 118*, 135–142.

Curry, J., Silva, S., Rohde, P., Ginsburg, G., Kratochvil, C., Simons, A., . . . March, J. (2011). Recovery and recurrence following treatment for adolescent major depression. *Archives of General Psychiatry, 68*(3), 263–269.

Dimirci, S., Dogan, K. H., Erkol, Z., & Gunaydin, G. (2009). Unusual suicide note written on the body: Two case reports. *American Journal of Forensic Medicine and Pathology, 30*(3), 276–279.

Dubovsky, S. (2010, January 4). Suicide—New data on causes and cures. *Journal Watch Psychiatry*. Retrieved from http://psychiatry.jwatch.org/cgi/content/full/2010/104/7

Farberow, N. L. (1992). The Los Angeles Survivors After Suicide program: An evaluation. *Crisis, 13*, 23–24.

Feigelman, W., Jordan, J. R., & Gorman, B. S. (2009). Personal growth after a suicide loss: Cross-sectional findings suggest growth after loss may be associated with better mental health among survivors. *Omega Journal of Death and Dying, 59*(3), 181–202.

Krysinska, K., Batterham, P., Tye, M., Shand, F., Calear, A., Cockayne, N., & Christensen, H. (2016). Best strategies for reducing the suicide rate in Australia. *Australian and New Zealand Journal of Psychiatry, 50*(2), 115–118.

Levene, I., & Parker, M. (2011). Prevalence of depression in granted and refused requests for euthanasia and assisted suicide: A systematic review. *Journal of Medical Ethics, 37*, 205–211.

McHale, J., & Felton, A. (2010). Self-harm: What's the problem? A literature review of the factors affecting attitudes towards self-harm. *Journal of Psychiatric and Mental Health Nursing, 17*(8), 732–740.

Seo, H.-J., Jung, Y.-E., Kim, T.-S., Kim, J.-B., Lee, M.-S., Kim, J.-M., . . . Jun, T.-Y. (2011). Distinctive clinical characteristics and suicidal tendencies of patients with anxious depression. *Journal of Nervous and Mental Disease, 199*(1), 42–48.

Schneidman, E. S. (1996). *The suicidal mind*. New York, NY: Oxford University Press.

Vijayakumar, L., Kumar, M. S., & Vijayakumar, V. (2011). Substance use and suicide. *Current Opinion in Psychiatry, 24*(3), 197–202.

von Borczyskowski, A., Lindblad, F., Vinnerljung, B., Reintjes, R., & Hjern, A. (2011). Familial factors and suicide: An adoption study in a Swedish National Cohort. *Psychological Medicine, 41*(4), 749–758.

Weiland, T., Cotter, A., Jelinek, G., & Phillips, G. (2014). Suicide risk assessment in Australian emergency departments: Assessing clinicians' disposition decisions, *Psychiatry Journal*, Article ID 943574, 1–8. doi.org/10.1155/2014/943574

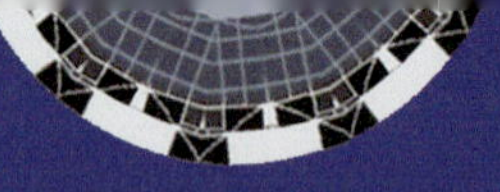

20 Family violence

ELLEN SINCLAIR AND MIKE HAZELTON

KEY TERMS

neglect *435*
physical abuse *433*
psychological abuse *433*
sexual abuse *444*
shaken baby syndrome *435*
stalking *437*

LEARNING OUTCOMES

After completing this chapter, you will be able to:

1. Describe the biopsychosocial causes of family physical abuse and family sexual abuse.
2. Discuss the short-term and long-term effects on victims of family violence.
3. Distinguish who is at greatest risk for family physical and sexual abuse.
4. Integrate the main principles for treating victims of violence into a treatment plan.
5. Explain why spiritual recovery is important for persons who have been victims of violence.
6. Incorporate into your nursing role the specific advocacy actions you would take to reduce family violence.
7. Formulate a plan for managing personal feelings and attitudes that may affect professional practice when caring for victims of violence.

LIVED EXPERIENCE

Recovery from family violence

I experienced physical, emotional, and spiritual abuse in the relationship. I can testify that complete recovery is achievable and attainable, but it requires a lot of hard work. You cannot handle the situation in isolation; you need friends, family and counsellors to pull you through. It takes a lot of courage and strength to walk through it. You will have setbacks along the way; provided you keep heading in the right direction that is all that counts.

Submission to the Royal Commission into Family Violence (State of Victoria, 2016b, p. 39)

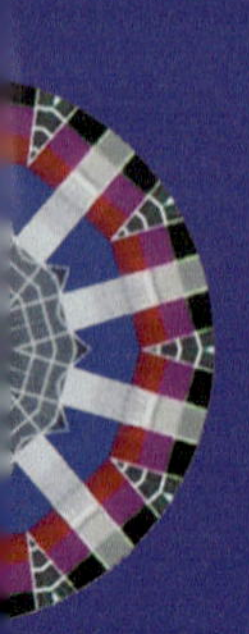

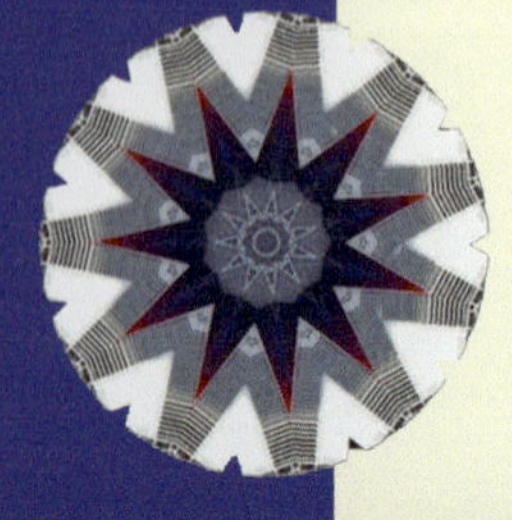

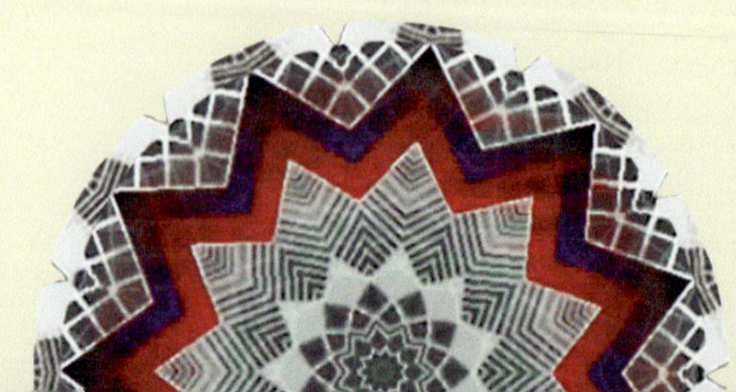

INTRODUCTION

The topic of this chapter—family violence—is a particular type of violence. There are various ways of defining violence. One of the more common definitions is that used by the World Health Organization (WHO):

> The intentional use of physical force or power, threatened or actual, against oneself, another person, or against a group or community, that either results in or has a high likelihood of resulting in injury, death, psychological harm, maldevelopment or deprivation. (Krug, Dahlberg, Mercy, Zwi, & Lorenzo, 2002, p. 5)

This definition addresses acts of omission such as neglect, as well as the more explicit violent acts of commission such as homicide. The definition also stresses intentionality, to differentiate between purposeful violence relating to injury and unintentional incidents such as injury resulting from road traffic accidents. The WHO definition (Krug et al., 2002) also identifies various types of violence based on the characteristics of those who commit the violence: self-directed violence, interpersonal violence and collective violence (Krug et al., 2002). Family violence fits within the category interpersonal violence.

Violence that occurs as physical or sexual abuse within the family is a serious health problem that confronts nurses in every clinical setting both in Australia and internationally. The victims of violence are seen in the community, in paediatric units, in intensive care units, in medical/surgical units, in maternal care settings, in ambulatory care facilities, in geriatric units, and in psychiatric–mental health settings.

Nurses can become involved in assessing and providing appropriate interventions for the emotional and physical consequences of violence and abuse. Depending on the circumstances, nurses may be called upon to give evidence in the prosecution of a perpetrator. Nurses working in the community may become involved in and/or refer victims to support groups and agencies. Increasing public awareness of family violence, through formal and informal teaching activities, can also be an important part of the work of nurses. The nursing profession is thus an important stakeholder in both the prevention of family violence and the treatment of the victims.

It is important to develop a knowledge base and be able to identify factors that contribute to domestic violence in order to assume this preventive role. Such roles may involve taking up opportunities for providing public education and advocating for changes in public policy. This knowledge, along with an increased awareness of the extent of the problem, can play an important role in the early and accurate detection of family violence. When family violence involving children or minors is detected, nurses must comply with Australian state and territory mandatory reporting requirements. Beyond such legally mandated requirements, nurses may bring concerns regarding possible or actual family violence to the attention of other members of the health care team.

FAMILY VIOLENCE: PHYSICAL ABUSE

Domestic violence—violence within the family—occurs at all levels of society. The myth is that violence occurs only among the poor and under-educated; the reality is that violence also occurs among the middle and upper classes, as well as the professional élite. In the past, these problems among wealthy or prominent people were kept hidden from the general public. With an increase in national concern, however, more publicity is being given to cases of domestic violence at all socioeconomic levels.

In this text, the word *family* refers to any one of these three categories of people who are:

- related by birth, adoption or marriage
- in an intimate relationship
- in a domestic relationship; that is, sharing the same household.

Although the image of the family is often one of happiness and harmony, this ideal is often in conflict with the underlying reality of domestic violence. The home is the most frequent place for violence of all types. **Physical abuse** is the non-accidental use of physical force that results in bodily injury, pain or impairment. **Psychological abuse** takes the form of verbal assaults, threats, humiliation and/or harassment. Women and children are more likely to be assaulted, raped and killed by people who claim to love them than they are by strangers. Perpetrators of family violence do to others in their homes what they would not dare do anyplace else. While there is little or no tolerance for violence in schools, at work or on the streets, different standards often seem to apply within the privacy of the family. Family members often appear to believe they are entitled to strike other family members. Mental Health in the Media on the next page discusses a disturbing example of family violence, both psychological and physical.

The incidence of domestic violence is difficult to estimate, and rates are almost certainly underestimates. Moreover, while it is not clear whether the incidence of such violence is increasing, the reporting of it certainly is. Within the limitations of data collection and reporting, a number of trends are nonetheless clear. The most common type of family violence is intimate partner violence, which is mainly perpetrated by men against women, and a large proportion of occurrences are 'hidden'. For instance, a survey of personal safety conducted by the Australian Bureau of Statistics (2013) found that of people who have experienced violence by a current partner 66 per cent (n = 237 100) were women and 34 per cent (n = 119 600) were men. Further, 25.6 per cent of the female respondents and 54.1 per cent of the male respondents reported never having told anyone about violence by a current partner, with even higher percentages (women: 39 per cent; men: 70.3 per cent) indicating having never sought advice or support of any kind. If under-reporting of family

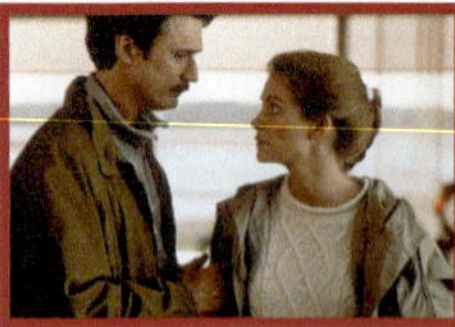

MENTAL HEALTH IN THE MEDIA

Sleeping with the Enemy

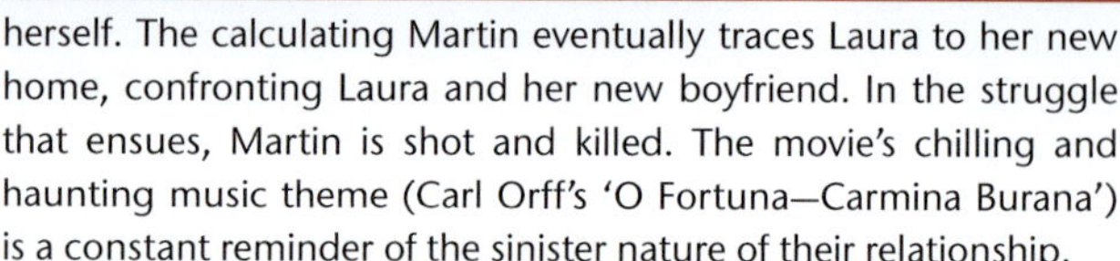

This psychological thriller stars Julia Roberts as the battered and psychologically abused Laura Barney, who is married to an abusing, controlling man with very definite obsessions and compulsions. Laura has been attempting to abide by her husband's compulsive rituals and demands since their marriage. However, when Martin physically assaults her as punishment for what he perceives as flirting with another man, Laura develops a complicated plan in which she fakes her own death in a storm at sea near her Cape Cod home. In her desperation, she flees to Cedar Falls, Iowa, adopts a different identity, and attempts to create a new life for herself. The calculating Martin eventually traces Laura to her new home, confronting Laura and her new boyfriend. In the struggle that ensues, Martin is shot and killed. The movie's chilling and haunting music theme (Carl Orff's 'O Fortuna—Carmina Burana') is a constant reminder of the sinister nature of their relationship.

Despite not having received the most positive of reviews from movie critics, the movie has been remade four times in India, once in Pakistan, and appears to have inspired similar movies in several other countries around the world. This leads one to believe that the movie touches upon a universally important topic.

Photo courtesy © United Archives GmbH/Alamy.

violence is an issue, the information that is collected is also often incomplete and unreliable; demographic data can be recorded inconsistently within and between organisations, and the scope of services is often difficult to determine (State of Victoria, 2016a, p. 48). A good source of information on family violence is the Royal Commission into Family Violence, which delivered its final report to the Victorian government in March 2016 (State of Victoria, 2016a; 2016b). The full report can be accessed at: www.rcfv.com.au.

Family violence is a violent crime against which the victim has the right to be protected, and for which the perpetrator can be arrested and prosecuted. While requirements vary across jurisdictions in all the states and territories of Australia, nurses are required by law to report suspected incidents of child abuse, and there are penalties for failing to do so. In addition, failure to report suspected child abuse or other forms of violence, such as elder abuse, are contrary to the standards and values espoused in codes of ethics and professional conduct for the nursing profession in Australia and internationally (Nursing and Midwifery Board of Australia, 2013). The far-reaching impacts of violence on a child's life are explored in Evidence-based Practice.

Sibling abuse

A form of domestic violence that is very common but not necessarily acknowledged occurs between siblings. Many people assume that it is natural and even appropriate for children to use physical force with one another. Parents may say, 'It's a

EVIDENCE-BASED PRACTICE

Childhood violence and its effects on dating relationships

In your role as a mental health practice nurse working in a suburban general practice, you come into contact with adolescents experiencing interpersonal relationship difficulties, some of which relate to dating. The young people you see are unsure how best to handle strong feelings and impulsivity, and some are involved in physical violence and abuse. In several instances, there are hints of having been exposed to abuse and violence at a much younger age. In thinking about how violence might become 'normalised' through exposure during childhood, you wonder whether there might be ways of predicting and possibly preventing, continuing relationship violence.

Your review of the literature found that adolescents in violent dating relationships had experienced sexual abuse (14 per cent), inter-parental violence (12 per cent), and parent mental illness (11 per cent) during their childhood. Childhood adversity predisposes people to physical dating violence, and almost half of the adolescents in one study were involved in dating violence. The prevalence of violence in young children's lives is fairly high, as are the negative effects on subsequent relationships. In your role as a mental health practice nurse, you can talk with young people about better ways to communicate, help guide them through challenges without resorting to violence, and promote effective coping and conflict resolution.

You should base action on more than one study, but the following article provides a good starting point from which to develop appropriate interventions:

Miller, E., Breslau, J., Chung, W. J., Green, J. G., McLaughlin, K. A. & Kessler, R. C. (2011). Adverse childhood experiences and risk of physical violence in adolescent dating relationships. *Journal of Epidemiology and Community Health, 65*(11), 1006–1013.

CRITICAL THINKING QUESTIONS

1. Whom would you identify as important to contact in order to initiate an effort to reduce dating violence?
2. Why would it be useful to identify the major role models in a child's life?
3. How would an increased awareness of childhood violence make a difference?
4. Why would involving adults in reducing childhood violence likely be helpful?
5. What would be the purpose of talking about violence as if it were not normal?

good chance for him to learn how to defend himself', 'She had a right to hit him; he was teasing her' and 'Kids will be kids.' With these attitudes, children learn that physical force is an appropriate method of resolving conflict among themselves. Children who are hit by their parents are much more likely to exhibit violence against siblings than children whose parents do not hit them. Hitting children increases the probability that they will be violent. Two particular areas of concern in Australia in recent years have been sibling sexual abuse and abuse of a sibling with disabilities. Both of these types of sibling abuse are poorly understood and often missed by health professionals and other human service workers, with family sensitivities and social taboos likely being important contributors to this 'hiddenness'. Nonetheless, sibling sexual abuse is the most prevalent form of sexual abuse (Australian Institute of Family Studies, 2012). Most adults in a position to know about violent confrontations and relationships (parents, police, medically trained personnel) have a very low awareness of sibling and peer violence (Finkelhor, Ormrod, Turner & Hamby, 2011). Identifying child and adolescent victims of sibling abuse is an important aspect of the work of nurses.

Child abuse

Child abuse (sometimes referred to as 'child maltreatment') is seen by the WHO as a serious public health concern worldwide (Krug et al., 2002). Child abuse includes various forms of physical and/or emotional ill-treatment, neglect, negligence and sexual abuse. Also included are forms of commercial exploitation which endanger a child's health, development and dignity. Exposure to intimate partner violence may also be considered a form of child abuse (WHO, 2014). In Australia, a large number of children are exposed to some form of maltreatment, with girls being more at risk than boys. Children who live at home with an abusive parent are at high risk of abuse. Younger parents are more likely to engage in physical abuse against children than older parents, and such abuse may be construed as 'discipline'. For many children, hitting and other forms of violence—punching, grabbing, slapping—begins when they are very young, and may continue until they leave home. Adolescents are more at risk of being attacked physically, sometimes with weapons. Men and women are equally likely to abuse young children, while adolescents who abuse others are more likely to be male.

Acts of violence against children range from a light slap, to a severe beating, to homicide. In some families or cultures, hitting or spanking children is condoned, and even approved as being necessary and good for the child. Many parents, however, do not realise the underlying messages they are giving the child by hitting:

- If you are small and weak, you deserve to be hit.
- People who love you hit you.
- It is appropriate to hit people you love.
- Violence is appropriate if the end result is good.
- Violence is an appropriate method of resolving conflict.

Generally, violence against children can compromise the child's physical and mental health (Lyden, 2011). Research shows that violence against children affects the type of, quality of, and assumptions made in later relationships (Miller et al., 2011).

Shaken baby syndrome

Shaken baby syndrome is a type of inflicted traumatic brain injury (ITBI). In Australia, ITBI is the leading cause of death and disability in children who have been abused. Similar to other forms of child abuse, shaken baby syndrome is under-reported and frequently overlooked. It involves the vigorous shaking of a baby held by the extremities or shoulders, which causes whiplash-induced intracranial and intraocular bleeding. The younger the victim, the greater the likelihood of permanent brain damage and death; consequently, infants are most at risk. Not recognising the danger of their actions, many parents shake rather than hit the child, mistakenly believing that this is less violent.

Child neglect

Neglect is the most frequently reported type of child maltreatment. It differs from abuse in that it is an act of omission that results in harm. Neglect includes lack of adequate *physical care* (including not medicating as prescribed), nutrition and shelter. It also includes unsanitary conditions that often contribute to health and developmental problems. Lack of human contact and nurturance is considered *emotional neglect*.

Homicide of child

In Australia in the period 2010–2012, about 12 per cent ($n = 61$) of all homicides were of children and young people under 18 years of age. During the same period, there were 34 filicides (death of a child or infant under the age of one where the perpetrator was a parent or step-parent) (Bryant & Cussen, 2015). Compared to adults, children are less likely to be become victims of homicide. However, when death occurs in children, it is five times more likely to be due to homicide than is the case for adults (Crime and Misconduct Commission Queensland, 2013). It is thought that many of these deaths are the result of battering in response to colic in the infant and toilet-training difficulties in the toddler. A small percentage of children are killed because they are unwanted, as the result of mercy killings, at the hands of a mentally ill parent, or in retaliation when one parent kills the child to inflict hurt on the other parent.

Internationally, it has been estimated that each year there are about 41 000 homicide deaths of children, with the rate of violence-related child deaths in low-income countries being almost double that in high-income countries. Among economically developed countries, Australia has a relatively low rate of child death resulting from maltreatment. At 0.8 per 100 000 children, Australia's rate is higher than that of Spain, Greece and Italy, and lower than that of New Zealand and the United States (Australian Institute of Family Studies, 2016).

In the context of mental illness, the killing of a child by their parent is referred to as *filicide*. In Australia and comparable countries, filicide is largely perpetrated by mothers. The most common forms of mental illness associated with filicide are mood disorders, schizophrenia and related disorders, and comorbidity is also often present. Mothers living with mental illness who kill their children tend to be older, married, use more violent methods of killing and are less likely to conceal the offence (Crime and Misconduct Commission Queensland, 2013).

The murder of a son or daughter by a biological father is often accompanied by marital discord, suicide and the murder of a wife by her husband. Murders of children by step-parents often involve ongoing abuse and death by beating. Moreover, if parents also have biological offspring, their stepchildren are at increased risk of ongoing abuse and neglect prior to death.

Homicide of parent

Parricide—the killing of a custodial or non-custodial parent or step-parent—is uncommon in Australia. In the period 2008–09 and 2009–10, 510 homicides were recorded in Australia, of which 20 involved the homicide of a parent. This accounts for 11 per cent of the 185 domestic homicides recorded for the period. The gender of parricide victims was 55 per cent ($n = 11$) male and 45 per cent ($n = 9$) female, and their average age was 61.4 years. Parricide offenders and victims tend to be non-Indigenous males, with the perpetrators acting alone.

The literature on parricide suggests three main types of offenders—severely abused children who are pushed to their limits; children living with severe mental illness; and children who are dangerously antisocial—with severely abused children being the most common. The most frequent situation—90 per cent of cases—is one in which the teen has been severely abused and/or the mother is a victim of abuse. The adolescent's attempts to get help have failed, and the family situation becomes increasingly intolerable prior to the murder. A critical factor is the easy availability of knives and other sharp instruments (44 per cent) or firearms (23 per cent) in the home. The other 10 per cent of cases involve either severely mentally ill children who experience hallucinations and delusions, or dangerously antisocial children who have extreme conduct problems (Mousos & Rushworth, 2003).

Partner abuse—heterosexual

Although no socioeconomic class, ethnic group, religion or age group is immune to family violence, most victims are women. If the abused are mothers of dependent children, their children are also likely to be victims. Female partner abuse in heterosexual relationships is the most widespread form of family violence in Australia. It is thought that 1 in 5 women and 1 in 20 men are physically abused by their partners. More than half of the women who are abused have experienced more than one incident. About one-half of men and one-quarter of women who have experienced current partner violence have never told anyone about it. The intensity and frequency of attacks tend to escalate over time. If verbal and emotional assaults were included, the numbers would be much higher. Violence is the single largest cause of injury to women in Australia, accounting for a significant proportion of emergency department presentations.

Typically, the first acts of partner violence occur in dating relationships. Physical abuse occurs among as many as 30 per cent to 50 per cent of adolescent and tertiary education students who are dating. Sadly, many victims and offenders interpret violence as a sign of love. Common reasons teens and young adults give for the violence is betrayal and jealousy.

It is important to also be aware of female abuse of heterosexual males. Men who find themselves in this situation are generally not recognised as 'real' victims, and when they do tell others, they are criticised for not standing up for themselves or for not fighting back. This may account for under-reporting by male victims; admitting the occurrence could be considered a sign of weakness or a cause for embarrassment.

Partner abuse—homosexual

Until very recently, the existence of physical abuse in lesbian and gay relationships had been downplayed or even denied. This denial has been supported by the myths that women are not violent people, and that men can defend themselves. In reality, violence does occur in some gay and lesbian families, for the same reasons as in heterosexual families: to demonstrate, achieve and maintain power and control over one's partner (Wang, 2011). In addition to physical or emotional abuse, the violent partner may use homophobic control—the threat of telling ('outing') family, friends, neighbours or employers about the victim's sexual orientation.

In the Australia, family violence is a significant health problem for gay men, along with substance abuse and AIDS. It is estimated that the level of family violence in same-sex relationships is similar to that of opposite-sex relationships. Men rarely talk about being victims for fear of being considered weak if they admit that their partners are hurting them. Violence in same-sex relationships suggests that violence is not a gender issue but rather a power issue.

Homophobia and hatred of homosexuals in Australia contribute to the difficulties of battered lesbians and gays. Traditionally, they have been cut off from the usual support systems available to heterosexual victims, such as specialised counselling services and shelters, although this is gradually changing. Gays and lesbians who live in rural areas or come from some ethnic minority group backgrounds can be even more isolated than their urban-dwelling counterparts. Because the legal status of same-sex partnerships is still being determined under Australian law, access to the legal system can be uncertain. Being victimised by one's lover can be less frightening than being victimised by the legal system. Fear of being identified as gay or losing custody of children adds to the silence about the violence. However, members of lesbian and gay communities are increasingly advocating for and supporting victims.

Elder abuse

The extent of elder abuse in Australia is difficult to determine due to under-reporting. However, the Royal Commission into Family Violence (State of Victoria, 2016b, p. 59) has suggested that up to 1 in 20 older people can experience elder abuse, and for about half of those the mistreatment is in the form of financial abuse. Elder abuse is any deliberate action or negligence that harms an older adult. Some older adults may be exposed to physical abuse or have their basic physical needs neglected and suffer from dehydration, malnutrition and over-sedation. They may be deprived of necessities such as glasses, hearing aids and walkers. Emotional neglect can mean leaving a person alone for long periods of time or failing to provide social contact. Some older people are subjected to psychological abuse. Remarks such as 'One of these days I am going to poison your food and you won't know when' and 'I am the only thing standing between you and a nursing home' are considered to be instances of psychological abuse.

Families may violate an older person's rights by refusing appropriate medical treatment, forcing isolation or unreasonable confinement, denying privacy, providing an unsafe environment, or demanding involuntary servitude. Some older people are financially exploited through theft or the misuse of property or funds. Others are beaten and even sexually abused or raped.

The perpetrator of elder abuse may be a spouse, child, grandchild, niece, nephew, some other relative, or an unrelated caretaker. The abuse is most likely to be inflicted by a person with whom the victim lives. A number of factors contribute to the abuse of older adults. Perpetrators may have personal problems, such as a lack of support in caring for the older family member, alcohol or drug addiction, or a family history of violence. Family factors include unresolved previous conflicts and power struggles. The perpetrator may be retaliating for previous abuse suffered at the hands of the older person. Older people may be resistant to intervention because they fear that losing a caregiver will mean having to be put in an institution.

Emotional abuse

Although the focus of violence in this chapter is on physical abuse, it is important to note that emotional abuse can be equally damaging. Words can hit as hard as a fist, and the damage to self-esteem can last a lifetime. Emotional abuse involves one person's shaming, embarrassing, ridiculing or insulting another, either in private or in public. It may include destruction of personal property or the killing of pets in an effort to frighten or control the victim. Such statements as 'You can't do anything right', 'You're ugly and stupid—no one else would want you' and 'I wish you had never been born' are devastating to one's self-esteem.

Abuse of pregnant women

Pregnancy is a time of increased risk for abuse. It has been suggested that there are more incidents of violence during pregnancy than of hypertension, gestational diabetes or placenta previa, all of which are screened for regularly (Mitra, Manning & Lu, 2011). A 2015 survey estimated that about 400 000 women aged 15 and above have experienced violence by a co-habiting partner during pregnancy (State of Victoria, 2016b, p. 51). A past history of abuse is one of the strongest predictors of abuse during pregnancy. Non-pregnant women are usually beaten in the face and chest. But pregnant women tend to be beaten in the abdomen, which can lead to miscarriage, placenta abruptio, fetal loss, premature labour, fetal fractures, pelvic fractures, rupture of the uterus and haemorrhage.

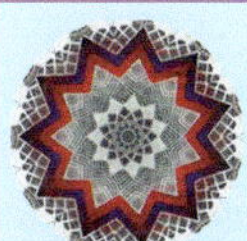

WHAT EVERY NURSE SHOULD KNOW

Assessing for emotional and physical abuse during pregnancy

Jill, a midwife, is having the first prenatal meeting with an expectant woman. In the course of the meeting, Jill explains that she is going to ask questions related to emotional and physical abuse throughout the woman's pregnancy because pregnancy is a time of increased risk for abuse. Jill will try to determine whether there is a prior history of physical or emotional abuse in the current relationship. In so doing, it will be important to avoid making assumptions based on cultural myths (upper-class women are not abused; lesbian women do not abuse their partners; women could leave abusive situations if they choose to; and so on). In addition to assessing for physical injuries, at each prenatal visit the following questions will be asked:

- Do you feel valued as a person by your partner?
- Do you feel safe in your home?
- Are you isolated from others for long periods of time?
- Have you been hurt in any way since your last visit here?

Battering during pregnancy is associated with severity of abuse. The man who beats his pregnant partner is an extremely violent and dangerous man. Battering during pregnancy is also a risk factor for the eventual homicide of the female partner.

The timing of the first prenatal visit is often related to abuse status. Abused women are twice as likely to delay prenatal care until the third trimester. Many abused women report that the abuser forced them to avoid prenatal care by denying them access to transportation. What Every Nurse Should Know outlines specific questions to be asked and cues to be incorporated into an assessment of a pregnant woman.

Physical abuse during pregnancy may be related to ambivalent feelings about the pregnancy, competition for attention with the developing fetus, the increased vulnerability of the woman, increased economic pressures, and decreased sexual availability. Unfortunately, the abuse of pregnant women is often overlooked by health care professionals, even when the victim appears in the emergency department with bruises, cuts, broken bones and abdominal injuries.

Stalking

The term 'stalking' has entered the Australian vocabulary, and all states and territories have stalking legislation. While legal definitions differ across jurisdictions in Australia, **stalking** can be broadly understood as the act of following, viewing, communicating with, or moving threateningly towards another person. Property damage and assault may accompany stalking. Victims often feel trapped in an environment filled with anxiety, stress and fear that often results in their having to make drastic changes in how they live their lives. An important aspect of the Australian stalking legislation is the expectation that offenders intend to cause harm.

Domestic stalking occurs when a former partner, spouse or family member threatens or harasses a person. The stalker often makes it clear that the victim is their 'property'. The stalker is usually motivated by a desire to continue the relationship, which can evolve into an attitude of 'If I can't have them, no one can.' In some cases the stalker is angry and retaliating against the victim, whom they perceive as rejecting them. Frequently, there is a history of domestic violence, and the stalking may end in a violent attack on, or killing of, the victim.

Cycle of violence

Domestic violence is the deliberate and systematic pattern of abuse used to gain control over the victim. The behaviour is always intentional. Perpetrators choose to be violent and give themselves permission to be violent. Perpetrators are not out of control, as is commonly assumed. They may be enraged or cool and calculating, but in either case they have made a choice. The victim cannot 'make them do it'. Generally, perpetrators of domestic violence can appear to be law-abiding citizens; they are dangerous only to their loved ones.

To the victim, domestic violence often happens without warning and without a build-up of tension. A pattern of violence usually develops. The first incident may be precipitated by frustration or stress. If the victim immediately refuses to accept the violence and seeks outside help, there are often no further episodes. If the victim submits to the violence, then physical force, without the stimulus of frustration or stress, becomes a way of relating, and the pattern becomes resistant to change. A typical cycle occurs when conflict escalates into a violent episode, after which the perpetrator begs for the victim's forgiveness. The victim stays in the system because of the perpetrator's promises to reform. With the next episode of conflict, the cycle of violence begins again and becomes part of the family dynamics.

Violent people are often jealous and possessive. They view other family members in terms of property and ownership. Abusers use violence in an attempt to prove to themselves and to others that they are superior and in control. Their use of physical force temporarily eases their sense of inadequacy and compensates for a lack of internal resources.

The abuser is the most powerful person in the life of the abused. The abuser's purpose is to control the victim, while simultaneously demanding respect, gratitude and love. Power over the victim is established by repetitive emotional abuse that instils terror and helplessness. Threats of serious harm or threats against other family members keep the victim in a constant state of fear.

In order to have complete domination, the abuser isolates the victim. Often the victim is forced to give up work, friends and family. The abuser may stalk the victim, eavesdrop, intercept letters and phone calls, and manage access to financial resources. Control and scrutiny of the victim's body and bodily functions, finances and transportation further destroy their sense of autonomy. The victim is shamed and demoralised when told what to eat, when to sleep, what to wear, when to go to the bathroom, and so on. For a victim who has been deprived long enough, the hope of a meal, a bath or a kind word can be a powerful reward. This ongoing abusive behaviour is punctuated by unpredictable outbursts of physical violence. Such domestic captivity, along with traumatic bonding to the abuser, often goes unrecognised. It is also important to recognise that some abusers may adopt only one or two of these behaviours.

Victims can be further immobilised by feelings of anxiety and depression. Feelings of self-blame may be expressed in such statements as 'If I hadn't talked back to my mother, she wouldn't have hit me' and 'If I were a better wife, he wouldn't beat me.' Guilt can contribute to depression, which further immobilises victims and keeps them from leaving or seeking help for the family system.

Fear contributes to victims' inability to leave abusive relationships. Often threatened with violence and even death at the idea of leaving, they live in fear of physical reprisal. Fearing loneliness, some victims may believe that being in

Box 20.1 Lived experiences of physical and sexual abuse

The most distressing thing I lost was me, my [self-worth]. [I] Couldn't think straight. I couldn't write out a shopping list: I couldn't concentrate. I was always worried that I may do or say the wrong thing. It is so hard to describe to you the mental torment, always questioning yourself. Never being able to comprehend that this person who is supposed to love me can hurt you so badly. (State of Victoria, 2016b, p. 19)

I was isolated; he controlled all the money, tracked my phone calls, checked my mobile phone frequently and had a key-tracking program on my computer, banning me from going to certain websites. (State of Victoria, 2016b, p. 29)

And I am so glad I left him. But I am still scared when he threatens me at my door at handovers. I am still scared he won't return my children to me safe and well. I am still married to him because he won't sign the divorce papers. I still feel trapped by him. I can't afford the legal fees to protect my rights in court. I am trapped by the system. (State of Victoria, 2016b, p. 22)

I didn't think I was in domestic violence. I didn't feel I was entitled to it because he did not bash me. I thought there were women out there who needed help more. It's the perception of domestic violence; it's the image of a woman beaten bloody. So, I didn't feel like I deserved the help. (State of Victoria, 2016b, p. 25)

Even now at [redacted] years of age I am distressed to write this. The sense of powerlessness and being different has never left me. I will often feel all wrong and have to leave. I cannot join in conversations as I do not have a shared experience with others. I am deeply ashamed and try so hard to remember how it started; perhaps I am somehow to blame. I can remember when I started to menstruate and he said we now had to be very careful. I still have this sense we are somehow in partnership. (State of Victoria, 2016b, p. 35)

My experience as both a victim/survivor as well as being in a family where sexual violence and abuse has occurred has been difficult not only due to the impacts of the abuse itself but also because of the isolation myself and members of my family felt after the abuse. As victims of the abuse both directly and indirectly we have been made to feel ashamed, labelled, and lost. (State of Victoria, 2016b, p. 35) a bad relationship is better than being alone, and leaving the relationship would not necessarily ensure the end of the abuse. They may become dependent and believe they are incapable of 'making it on my own'. The abuser is often most dangerous when threatened or faced with separation. Box 20.1 (page 438) provides first-hand accounts of exposure to family violence taken from submissions to the Royal Commission into Family Violence (State of Victoria, 2016b).

Practice example

Sandy, age 20, met Ron at work. When they first started seeing each other, Ron often bought Sandy small gifts and commented on how Sandy was the nicest women he had ever met. He told Sandy he'd never really been in love until he met her. Sandy believed him, quickly fell in love and moved in with Ron. Several months later she called her parents from work and begged them to come and get her. Sandy told them that she wanted to leave the relationship with Ron, but didn't know how to get out of it. Ron had taken over Sandy's life, even controlling the use of the car that her parents had helped her buy. He followed her everywhere and rarely let her out of his sight.

Sandy insisted on returning to the apartment that night to get her car, telling her parents that Ron was not a violent person. However, Ron brutally beat her for having called her parents. Sandy moved back home and began trying to put her life back together. Even so, Ron continued to make harassing phone calls and to send text messages to Sandy. Because she had moved out so quickly, there were still financial matters she and Ron needed to resolve, so Sandy agreed to meet with him one evening. At that meeting they argued over who would pay the outstanding bills, and Ron lost his temper and physically attacked Sandy; she was taken to the local emergency department. Ron was arrested by the police and charged with assault.

For a partial list of the reasons why people remain in abusive relationships, see Box 20.2.

Fear also contributes to the inability to leave a partner in an abusive gay or lesbian relationship. Because many couples share close friends within the same community, victims may fear shaming their partners. They may also fear that friends will either deny the problem or take the abuser's side. Homophobia may also contribute to the victim's reluctance to seek help. Calling the police may result in ridicule or offhand responses from the officers. Victims may not seek help from family members to avoid reinforcing negative stereotypes about homosexuality, which might exacerbate the family's homophobia.

Box 20.2 Why do they stay? Why do they go back?

Fear: Victims may be afraid of physical reprisal if they resist, of being found and beaten again, and of their children being hurt. Those who attempt to leave risk suffering worse violence and even death.

Learned helplessness: Victims may believe that they have no choices and no control; they have come to believe that violence is an acceptable way of life.

Traumatic bonding: Victims may stay loyal in the relationship, hoping and searching for meaning in the indifference and abuse. Traumatic bonding results from alternating good and bad treatment; the victim has no sense of autonomy and puts energy into keeping the relationship intact.

Emotional dependence: Victims may be convinced that they are weak, inferior and do not deserve better treatment; they are insecure about their potential autonomy.

Financial dependence: Victims may not have a source of income; if the abuser is arrested, the abuser may lose their job and then the family will have no income. Victims have been taught that they must be submissive in exchange for financial support.

Guilt and/or shame: Victims may have been convinced that they provoked the abuse. They feel guilt over the failure of the relationship or shame for remaining in the relationship despite the abuse. They may feel pressured by family, religious or cultural values against divorce or separation.

Isolation: Victims may have few, if any, friends; little support from family; and/or no car, phone or mail.

Children: Victims may believe two parents are better than one. They may be threatened with loss of custody; the abuser may threaten to harm or kidnap the children.

Hope: Victims may hope that if they change in the way the abuser wants them to, the abuse will stop. They hope the abuser will keep their promise to stop the assaults.

BIOPSYCHOSOCIAL THEORIES

Domestic violence is easier to describe than to explain. There is no single cause of this type of violence. It results from an interaction of neurobiological, personality, situational and societal factors that have an impact on families.

Neurobiological theory

Neurobiological theorists propose that genes and neurotransmitters may contribute to causing violent behaviour. Although a genetic predisposition may make certain behaviours more likely, it does not make them inevitable. Serotonin (5-HT) plays an important role in mood and aggressive behaviour. 5-HT calms us through inhibitory control over aggression. Abnormally low levels of 5-HT result in a lack of control, loss of temper and explosive rage.

Childhood abuse and neglect lead to permanent alterations in the parts of the central nervous system that are known to be stress-responsive. Corticotropin-releasing factor (CRF) is a major regulator of the endocrine, autonomic, immune and behavioural stress responses. It is thought that stress early in life results in the sensitisation of the brain to even mild stressors in adulthood, thus contributing to mood and anxiety disorders long after the abuse or neglect has stopped. As a result, changes in the way CRF performs its function make it more difficult for the adult to cope with stress.

Intrapersonal theory

Intrapersonal theory suggests that the cause of violence lies in the personality of the abuser. It is thought that people who are violent are less able to control their impulsive expressions of anger and hostility. A high proportion of male abusers grew up in homes in which they were abused or observed their mothers being abused. With these family dynamics, the child sees the father as frightening and intimidating, and sees the mother as helpless and non-protective. This early emotional deprivation contributes to the formation of an adult who has an excessive need for nurturing and support. The individual comes to adult relationships with unrealistic demands for time and attention. As the relationship develops, the person discourages their partner's relationships with other people because of their own low self-esteem and fear of abandonment.

Social learning theory

Social learning theory proposes that violence is a learned behaviour, and people are conditioned to respond aggressively and violently. Children learn about violence from observing it, from being victims, and/or from behaving violently themselves. If the use of violence is rewarded by a gain in power, the behaviour is reinforced. If there is immediate negative reinforcement within the family, a decrease in violent behaviour will result. Learning to abuse is the first step in the battering process, but it does not necessarily lead vulnerable individuals to abuse. The social environment affects how the potentially abusive person behaves. The person must have the *opportunity to abuse* without suffering negative consequences. They have the perception that they can 'get away with it'. Although learning may have occurred and an opportunity is present, the potentially abusive person makes a *conscious choice* to abuse. The batterer is solely responsible for the violence.

In addition to family models, the media provide many models of violence to which children are exposed. Some movies and television shows demonstrate that 'good' people use force to achieve 'good' ends. Many of the stories make no attempt to justify the use of force for 'good' ends; they simply present endless, senseless acts of cruelty by one human being upon another—violence without consequences. In recent decades the introduction and widespread use of electronic games has contributed significantly to the 'normalisation' of violence. With these types of family and media examples, children may develop values that tolerate, and even accept as normal, everyday violence between people.

Gender bias theory

The sexist structure of the family and society is an important factor in domestic violence. It is a common belief that men have the right to keep women subordinate through power and privilege (Duran, Moya & Megias, 2010). If there is nothing to contradict this ethos within the family system, then reaching the goal of maintaining female subordination will be accomplished using any means possible. Family violence is a way to promote that goal, because it uses the power assumed to be automatically granted a male in that family system. Victims are sometimes labelled as co-dependent in the abusive relationship, but such labelling is just another way of blaming the victim for the abuse.

The economic system can contribute to the entrapment of women, who are often forced to choose between poverty and abuse. It is often difficult for women to find advocates and solutions within the male-dominated legal, religious, mental health and medical systems. Society effectively sanctions male violence by neglecting female victims. The ultimate outcome of the cycle of abuse from which women cannot extricate themselves is that they become a built-in, ready target. Statistics validate this outcome by documenting that women are being murdered on a regular basis, not by strangers, but by husbands and lovers.

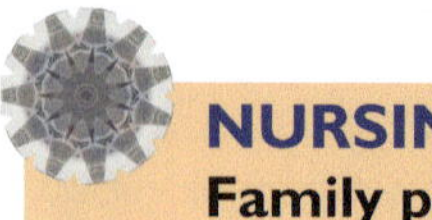

NURSING PROCESS
Family physical abuse

Addressing abuse that occurs within the family system requires an approach that is sensitive and effective.

Assessment

Nurses in all clinical settings should routinely assess for evidence of family violence. Considering how extensive this problem is, it is important to ask one or two introductory questions of every person presenting to a health service. In assessing a child, the following questions can be asked: 'Mums and dads try to help their children learn how to behave well. What happens to you when you do something wrong?' or 'What is the worst punishment you have ever received?' In assessing adults, the approach can begin with: 'One of the sources of stress in our lives is family disagreement. Could you describe how disagreements affect you? What happens when you disagree?' If the responses to these questions are indicative of violence, a more in-depth assessment should be conducted. Guidelines for assessment are given in Your Assessment Approach nursing history tool.

Problem identification

The main aim is to identify the existence of family violence. Priority must be given to critical and serious physical injuries. It is important to consider the severity and potential fatality of the situation, as well as the needs of dependent children and the legal issues surrounding the case. The following should be considered when data is being analysed:

- How might ineffective family coping patterns relate to family violence?
- How might ineffective coping relate to being a victim of violence?
- How might ineffective parenting relate to the physical and emotional abuse of children?
- How might victim feelings of powerlessness relate to the perceived dependence on the abuser?
- How might low self-esteem relate to feeling guilty and responsible for being a victim?
- How might social isolation relate to shame about family violence?

Outcomes of intervention

Achievement of the following outcomes indicates the success of interventions. The victims have:

YOUR ASSESSMENT APPROACH Nursing history tool for assessing victims of family violence

Behavioural assessment

- Tell me about how people communicate within your family.
- What types of things cause conflict within your family?
- How is conflict managed or resolved?
- Who in your family loses control of themselves when angry?
- Have you received verbal threats of harm?
- Have you ever been threatened with a weapon, such as a knife or firearm?
- What happens to you when a family member has violent outbursts? Are you slapped? Hit? Punched? Thrown? Shoved? Kicked? Burned? Beaten up?
- Who in your family has needed emergency medical treatment?
- In what ways have you attempted to stop the violence?
- Have you attempted to leave the situation in the past?
- What happened when you attempted to leave?
- Describe the use of alcohol in your family.
- Describe the use of drugs in your family.

Affective assessment

- Who do you think is responsible for the use of physical force within your family?
- In what way is this (these) person(s) responsible?
- How much guilt are you experiencing at this time?
- Tell me about your fears. Do they concern a lack of security? Financial problems? Childcare problems? Living apart from your spouse? Further physical injury?
- What factors contribute to your feeling of helplessness to leave or stop the abuse?
- How hopeless do you feel about your situation?
- How would you describe your level of depression?

Cognitive assessment

- Describe your strengths and abilities as a person.
- If you were describing yourself to a stranger, what would you say?
- What are your beliefs about keeping your family together?
- Tell me about your reasons for remaining in this situation. Promises of reform? Material rewards?
- Do you believe or hope the violence will not recur?
- What are your expectations of how children should behave?
- What rights do parents have with their children?
- What rights do spouses have with each other?
- What are the rules about physical force within your family?

Sociocultural assessment

- How did your parents relate to each other?
- Who enforced discipline when you were a child?
- What type of discipline was used when you were a child?
- What was/is your relationship like with your mother?
- What was/is your relationship like with your father?
- How did you get along with your siblings?
- In your present family, who is the head of the household?
- How are decisions made in your family?
- How are household jobs assigned in your family?
- Describe recent and current stresses on your family. Unemployment? Financial problems? Illness? New family members? Deaths or separations? Child-rearing problems? Change in job status? Increase in conflict? Change in residence?
- To whom can you turn for support in times of stress?
- Describe your social life.
- What types of contact have you had with the legal system? Telephoned the police? Obtained an apprehended violence order? Obtained a lawyer? Been involved in court cases? Protective services?

- recognised that they are not to blame for the violence of others
- ended the denial and minimisation of family violence
- demonstrated an awareness of their own strengths, skills and competence
- re-established a sense of power over their lives
- verbalised their right to express their own needs and to satisfy them
- established social networks to decrease isolation and secrecy.

Planning and implementation

Most victims of family violence would like it to end, but they may not know how to seek the help they need. It is important that health professionals are nonjudgmental in their interactions with all family members. Initially, people who are the victims of family violence may be unwilling to trust others because of family shame and fear of being judged for remaining in the violent relationship. It is vital that the values of others not be imposed through, for instance, the offering of quick and easy solutions to what are very complicated problems of domestic violence. Both Self-awareness and Collaborative Care will help to debunk myths about family violence and develop understanding of personal feelings and attitudes.

SELF-AWARENESS
Working with victims of family violence

Take some time to think about and consider your reactions to the following questions:

- Is Australian culture violent compared to other cultures?
- The foundation of colonial Australia was characterised by violence. How might this have influenced the values and behaviour of present-day Australians?
- Do you think there is a difference between spanking a child and beating a child?
- Do you think the stalking laws are decreasing the level of violence in Australia?
- What are your views on gun control?

The treatment of families experiencing violence requires a multi-disciplinary approach, with a broad range of interventions. Nurses, social workers, medical practitioners,

COLLABORATIVE CARE

Teaching about family violence

Myths and facts

- ***MYTH: Family violence is rare.*** *FACT: Every year over 3 million women in Australia experience violence by a known person. The most likely type of known perpetrator is a previous partner.*
- ***MYTH: Most violent people are mentally ill.*** *FACT: The available evidence does not support this view; indeed, people with mental illness are more likely to be the victims of violence. The vast majority of violent men are not suffering from mental illness. Most abusers are respectable men able to exercise self-control; they come from all occupations and social classes. Violence usually only occurs in their relationship with their partner and children.*
- ***MYTH: Violence is a trivial matter.*** *FACT: In Australia, violence is the biggest cause of injury or death among women aged 18 to 45. One-third of Australian women will be subjected to physical or sexual violence in their lifetime.*
- ***MYTH: Family violence is confined to people in lower socioeconomic groups.*** *FACT: Family violence and abuse occurs in all income groups, professions, geographical locations and ethnicities.*
- ***MYTH: Family violence is a private matter.*** *FACT: Family violence is increasingly being seen as a serious public concern. Physical assault in the home is a serious crime, and Australian homicide data indicate that for about a third of victims the primary offender is a family member.*
- ***MYTH: Family violence is usually a one-off, isolated incident.*** *FACT: Family violence is a pattern of behaviour that includes the repeated use of various tactics designed to dominate and control a family member. Threats, intimidation, isolation, economic and financial control, emotional and sexual abuse and physical violence can all be used to control another person.*
- ***MYTH: Abused women like being hit; otherwise, they would leave.*** *FACT: There are many reasons why abused women may not leave. These include fear for herself, her children and her pets. Practical barriers to separating from an abusive partner may include a lack of money or uncertain housing options. The most dangerous time for a woman who is being abused is when she tries to leave.*

family therapists, vocational trainers, police, child protection officers, and lawyers must coordinate to intervene effectively in a situation of family violence.

In the initial contact with family members, it is important to ensure their physical safety as much as possible. It is critical to assess the level of danger for the victim; homicide may be a possibility if previous threats have been made. It is also important to assess the level of danger for the abuser. The severity and duration of the violence are the factors that contribute most directly to victims killing their abusers in self-defence. In cases in which the level of danger is high, the involvement of police and family services staff is important; child protection placement or removal to a shelter are likely to be required.

Providing psychoeducation

Interventions can be provided to improve communication. Families experiencing violence often have poor communication skills. Teaching content should focus on active listening with feedback (see Chapter 9), clear and direct communication, and communication that does not attack the personhood of others.

Family dynamics surrounding disagreements can be identified and explored; this may involve discussing how disagreements are inevitable. Consideration can also be given to the use of the democratic process in conflict resolution and decision-making. It is best to practise with simple, unemotional family problems at first.

Family members can be helped to identify methods to manage anger appropriately. All family members must assume responsibility for their own behaviour. They can practise talking about angry feelings as they occur. This can be expressed through the use of relaxation, physical exercise, and striking safe, inanimate objects (such as a pillow, a couch or a punching bag). The family should be guided in establishing limits, and defining consequences if violence recurs. It should be emphasised that violence within the family will not be tolerated.

Parents who are physically abusive can be helped to develop and improve their parenting skills. The beginning point is the recognition of current positive parenting skills to increase self-worth and help engagement in the learning process. It is important that parents be supported to understand that the use of violence is often a desperate attempt to cope with their children. Acknowledging that parents care about their children will increase the likelihood of their active participation in the treatment process.

Because family violence is often trans-generational, there should be opportunities for the parents to discuss how they were punished as children. Parents can be taught about the normal growth and development of children. Unrealistic demands for children to comply beyond their developmental ability often result in violence. An early consideration in the problem-solving process is helping parents identify specific problems they experience with raising children. They can then go on to identify solutions, other than physical force, that are age-appropriate for their children. They will likely need support in implementing, practising and evaluating these new skills.

Empowering survivors

One of the primary goals of intervention is the empowerment of victims. The process of violence removes all power and control from the victim, resulting in low self-esteem, anxiety, depression and somatic problems. The following principles are basic to the empowerment of victims:

- A commitment to the belief that women and men are inherently equal.
- An egalitarian approach to the therapeutic relationship: the person who has been exposed to violence is viewed as an equal partner, rather than as a helpless recipient of interventions.
- An emphasis on the victim's strengths and abilities.
- Respect for the victim's ability to understand their own experiences.
- An emphasis on altering destructive roles and expectations within the family system.
- A willingness to state clear value positions about family violence

Through this approach, people who are the victims of family violence can become aware that they have choices in, and control over, their lives. Sensitivity should be exercised in discussions regarding an adult victim leaving a partner. Notwithstanding the significant challenges in doing so, health professionals must be willing to support people who are the victims of family violence in their pain, rather than telling them what to do about their problems. For the most positive adaptive outcome, it is important that adult victims work towards becoming their own rescuers and take charge of their own safety and protection plan. If they need help with this process, they can be taught to ask for it directly. This is not meant to imply any form of abandonment of victims. Rather, health professionals should stand by, support and cheerlead the positive choices and decisions made by the person.

Adult victims of family violence can be helped to begin identifying ways in which they are dependent on their abusers. High levels of dependence make it difficult for victims to leave abusers without intense support. Help can be given to identify intrapersonal and interpersonal strengths to decrease a victim's feelings of powerlessness. From there, attention can shift to identifying those aspects of life that are under their control. Assertiveness training can be offered to help in the development of new skills for relating to others in the future (see Chapters 4 and 25). If the person receiving help is still in the abusive relationship, they can be cautioned that assertive behaviour may escalate the violence.

Treating the abuser

Most abusers do not seek treatment unless it is court-ordered or there are custody issues involved. It is frustrating to intervene with abusers who deny the reality of, or responsibility for, the violence. Group therapy for abusers is sometimes helpful. The group setting can be more effective than individual therapy, because interactions with a number of people may more successfully address the anger and control problems. The responsibility for aggression is always placed on the aggressor. Issues regarding the patriarchal and power views of relationships are discussed in greater depth. Participants are asked to specify their abusive behaviours, identify the intentions behind those behaviours, and examine the effects of the abuse on their victims. Abusers learn that anger can be controlled and that violence is always a *choice*.

Evaluation

Nurses in acute care settings may not have the opportunity for long-term evaluation of the family system. Short-term evaluation focuses on the following:

1. the identification of family violence
2. the family's ability to recognise that a problem exists
3. the willingness of the family to accept assistance by following through with referrals
4. the removal of the victim from a volatile situation.

Nurses in long-term settings or within the community have an opportunity to evaluate the effectiveness of the multi-disciplinary treatment plan over an extended period of time. When violence no longer exists within the family system, the plan has succeeded. Involvement in the process of family growth and adaptation can be a source of professional satisfaction.

All nurses should evaluate their professional obligations and practice in counteracting those aspects of society that foster family violence. Family violence is a mental health problem of national and international importance, and nurses can be leaders in helping prevent it in future generations. Primary prevention includes interventions of parent education, health education in schools, referral for appropriate child or elder care, establishment of support groups, and education of fellow nurses about the problem of family violence. It also includes community education about the pervasive effects of media violence on individuals and society.

Secondary prevention of family violence includes working with children who are victims or who have seen their mothers beaten, and making referrals for multi-disciplinary intervention. Nurses must be community advocates in supporting hotlines, crisis centres and shelters for victims of domestic violence. On the political level, nurses and nursing professional organisations must make their voices heard with regard to policies and laws affecting children, women and older people. Questions to guide the evaluation of nursing practice and the extent of advocacy activities include the following:

- Have I assessed each person for possible abuse?
- What actions have I taken to decrease violence in the media?
- Have I considered the issue of gun control?
- Have I confronted the use of physical punishment within families?
- Have I written to legislators to protest the lack of funding for programs designed to help children, women and older people?
- Have I spoken out on the need to increase the number of counsellors, lawyers, nurses and medical practitioners who share the same ethnic background as the individuals and families they serve?

CARE COORDINATION

The goal of care coordination for the victims of family violence is to focus on the immediate problems. Intervention is directed towards developing rapport with the victim, clarifying the presenting problems, and enhancing the victim's existing problem-solving ability. The safety of the victim(s) is of primary importance. Once safety is ensured, interventions include the following:

- identification of effective and ineffective coping skills
- emphasis on victim's strengths and abilities
- development of problem-solving skills and new coping behaviours
- identification of available support systems
- group therapy with other victims and survivors of domestic violence
- evaluation of the effectiveness of new coping strategies (Burriss, Breland-Noble, Webster & Soto, 2011).

Care coordination of the victims of family violence raises a number of issues. Developing an expanded understanding of the context of problems encountered is critical if the help offered to a victim is to be effective (Graham-Bermann, Sularz & Howell, 2011).

COMMUNITY-BASED CARE

Prevention of child abuse is a community function that involves the identification of risk factors and crisis intervention. Risk factors include the following:

- parents who were abused as children
- adult relationship dysfunction
- poor self-esteem
- social isolation
- unrealistic expectations of children's abilities
- having a child with special needs.

Interventions are geared towards improving adult–adult relationships as well as adult–child relationships. Helping families connect with other families decreases their sense of isolation. Parenting classes help families develop realistic expectations of their children according to developmental levels. It is very important that families with special-needs children be referred to sources of appropriate support.

Prevention of elder abuse involves supporting older persons and their caretakers in identifying and expanding social support networks. Community resources may be able to help with the activities of daily living (ADLs), transportation, financial advice, and assistance with personal problems. Caretakers can be assisted in exploring their feelings about the older people in their care; they can be supported in identifying the factors that are disturbing to them and that may contribute to neglect or abuse. The caretakers' ability to meet their loved one's needs should be determined, and appropriate education provided. This can include information and contact details on community resources, such as government departments and non-government organisations that may be able to offer assistance and support.

Australia has strict gun control laws that were introduced in the mid-1990s following the mass killings at Port Arthur in Tasmania. The legislation resulted in the strict regulation of military-styled automatic and semi-automatic firearms, and heavy penalties exist for violations. While gun control measures have reduced the number of firearms in the community, they have not removed the threat altogether. The availability of firearms in circumstances of family violence is very likely to prompt police concern and action.

HOME CARE

Nurses providing support to women living at home can help with the development of a 'safety plan' or an 'escape plan' to use when their safety is threatened. They should plan a quick, safe exit from their home, and have a safe place to go to once they do leave. The plan should be straightforward and complete, and it must be taught to their children. As part of the plan, it can be suggested that they have all of their important documents (such as birth certificates and court orders), some money, a list of important phone numbers, and a couple of days' clothing gathered in one secure location. They should have a second set of car keys so that they can leave quickly if the need arises.

FAMILY VIOLENCE: SEXUAL ABUSE

Childhood sexual abuse is a major health problem in the Australia. The majority of cases are probably unreported. What is known is that children are most vulnerable between the ages of 8 and 12; that the average age is between 8 and 9 years; about two-thirds of the victims are 10 years of age or younger; and one in three girls and one in six boys will be sexually abused in some way before the age of 18. **Sexual abuse** is defined as inappropriate sexual behaviour, instigated by a perpetrator, for the purpose of the perpetrator's sexual pleasure or economic gain through child prostitution or pornography. Behaviour ranges from exhibitionism, peeping, explicit sexual talk, touching, caressing, masturbation, oral sex, vaginal sex and anal sex, to forcing children to engage in sex with one another or with animals.

Health care professionals, as well as families, have used denial to cope with ambiguous evidence of the cultural taboos of incest and sex with children. The following Self-awareness feature can be used to help understand your own feelings and attitudes. In order to respond appropriately to cues that signal sexual abuse, it is necessary to understand the characteristics and dynamics of the families involved. A note of caution, however: with the recent increased publicity about the prevalence of child sexual abuse, there is a real danger of jumping to conclusions; any hint or accusation of sexual abuse may be interpreted as absolute proof of guilt. Rumours and false accusations can destroy individuals and families. It is thus very important that any assessment be carefully conducted and balance maintained between the extremes of denial and assumption of guilt (Everson & Sandoval, 2011).

SELF-AWARENESS
Working with victims of child sexual abuse

Take some time to think about and consider your reactions to the following questions:

- Do you think the rate of child sexual abuse is increasing, or is there just better reporting?
- Do you think sex education can decrease the rate of sexual abuse?
- Which situation do you think is more devastating in child sexual abuse—when force is used or when no force is used?
- Does the fact that many perpetrators were sexually abused as children excuse their behaviour? What if the perpetrator is only 11 years old?
- Far fewer women than men are accused of sexually abusing their children. How might you explain this?
- What needs to be done to decrease the incidence of child sexual abuse?

Sexually abused children and adult survivors of childhood sexual abuse (hereafter called *adult survivors*) are crying out for help. A few cry out loudly in protest, but many cry inwardly in silence. In Australia, it is thought that as many as one in three girls and one in six boys are sexually abused before the age of 18. Many of these are single, isolated incidents. Boys are more frequently molested outside the family system than are girls. Adolescent males who sexually abuse tend to have been sexually abused as children, and were exposed to trauma and pornography at young ages (Burton, Duty & Leibowitz, 2011).

Sexual abuse occurs in all ethnic, religious, economic and cultural subgroups. Affinity systems—immediate family, relatives, friends, neighbours, clergy, sporting and youth leaders—account for a high proportion of the abusers. Male perpetrators are involved in up to 90 per cent of reported cases. Although father–daughter incest is more likely to be reported, it is believed that sibling incest is more widespread. Some siblings turn to each other for emotional nurturance and acceptance. In other instances, a sibling uses coercion or violence to perpetrate the abuse.

Types of offenders

Some offenders prefer girls; others prefer boys; and some abuse both, so long as the victim is a child. Some are interested in adolescents or pre-teens, some in toddlers, and some in infants. Some offenders do not abuse until they are adults, but more than half start in their teens.

Juvenile offenders

Many, if not the majority of, cases involving juvenile offenders go unreported. Family members often want to protect and shield the young offender. Sometimes the behaviour is rationalised as adolescent male experimentation. Many juvenile offenders were sexually abused as children, and they gradually develop offending behaviours as they reach adolescence. A high proportion of the remainder show fairly high rates of other delinquent behaviours, and many are diagnosed, or if assessed would be diagnosed, with conduct disorder. Those offenders who were child victims tend to begin abusing at a younger age, to have more victims, and to have male victims when compared with non-abused teen sex offenders. Juvenile offenders may seek victims within or outside the family system. The type of sexual offence often parallels the offender's own experiences of abuse.

Male offenders

Research focusing on fathers who abuse their daughters has identified the following five types of incestuous fathers (Greenberg, Firestone, Nunes, Bradford & Curry, 2005; Schetky, 1999):

1. *Sexually preoccupied abusers* have a conscious and often obsessive sexual interest in their daughters. Many of them regard their daughters as sex objects, in some cases as early as at birth. Stepfathers were more sexually aroused by their stepdaughters than biological fathers, although this was the only difference between the two groups.
2. *Adolescent regressors* become sexually interested in their pubescent daughters. These men sound and act like adolescents around their daughters.
3. *Self-gratifiers* are not sexually attracted to their daughters *per se*, and during the abuse they fantasise about someone else. In effect, they are simply using their daughters' bodies.
4. *Emotional dependants* see themselves as failures, and feel lonely and depressed. They see their daughters as romantic figures in their lives.
5. *Angry retaliators* abuse out of anger, either at the daughter or at the mother. This type of offender is most likely to have a criminal history of assault and rape.

Female offenders

Although female perpetrators commit far fewer cases of sexual abuse, they are now more likely to be reported than once would have been the case. The most common types of sexual abuse by women are fondling, oral sex and group sex.

Female offenders fall into the following four major types:

1. *Teacher–lovers* are older women who teach children about lovemaking.
2. *Experimenter–exploiters* are often girls who have had no sex education growing up. Babysitting is often an opportunity to explore younger children. Many of the girls in this group do not even realise what they are doing or that it is inappropriate.
3. *Predisposers* usually come from a family with a long history of physical and sexual abuse. These families have been dysfunctional over many generations.
4. *Women coerced by males* abuse children because men have forced them to abuse. Usually, they have been victims as children and are easily manipulated and intimidated.

There is agreement that there is often sexual abuse in the female perpetrator's history (Tsopelas, Spyridoula & Athanosios, 2011; McCloskey & Raphael, 2005).

Abusive behaviour patterns

Typically, adult perpetrators initiate sexual behaviour in a manipulative or coercive manner. Often, the adult misrepresents the abuse as a game or 'fun' activity. The behaviour usually follows a progression of sexual activity, from exposure and fondling to oral, vaginal and/or anal sex. Secrecy is imposed on the child by persuasion or threat. The abuser may make threatening statements such as those in Box 20.3. Secrecy and silence are used by abusers to escape accountability. When secrecy fails and the child victims or adult survivors begin to talk to others about the abuse, the perpetrators usually attack the credibility of the victims and try to make sure no one will listen to them. Other perpetrators acknowledge the abuse but minimise the impact, while some use the defence mechanism of projection and blame the child for the abuse.

Child victims

Children know that adults have absolute power over them, so they obey. When they have been threatened with abandonment or harm, they frequently choose to protect others. When asked 'Why didn't you tell sooner?', the answers invariably are 'I didn't know who to tell', 'I was scared' and/or 'I did tell, and no one believed me.'

Children often feel responsible for the adult's behaviour, and ashamed that they have not been able to stop the abuse. Secrecy and guilt keep these children isolated, causing them to feel alienated from their peers. They may act out sexually by initiating oral or genital sex with other children or adults. The feeling of powerlessness is extremely potent, because what the victim says and does makes no difference. If the abuser has an adult partner who does not protect the child, the child may receive the message that this behaviour is normal. When the child's repressed rage comes to the surface, it may be directed against the self in self-defeating and self-destructive ways, such as substance abuse, high-risk sexual behaviour and suicide (Champion, 2011; Denton, Newton & Vandeven, 2011).

Adolescent victims may run away from home to escape an intolerable situation. Because they have learned, at home, that sexual behaviour is rewarded by affection, love and attention, some turn to prostitution. Others are forced into prostitution as a way to support themselves while living on the streets.

Some child victims use denial to cope with the trauma. Acknowledging the abuse would mean acknowledging that the world is dangerous and that those who are supposed to protect and nurture failed instead and caused harm. Other victims minimise the impact, saying things like 'It's not so bad; it only happens once a month' or 'It's all right, because it stopped when I was 11 years old.' The following Practice Example illustrates the impact of child sexual abuse on one child victim.

Box 20.3 Typical threatening statements by sexual abusers

To obtain secrecy and silence

- 'If you tell, you'll be sent away.'
- 'If you tell, I won't love you anymore.'
- 'If you tell, I will hurt you.'
- 'If you tell, I'll do the same thing to your little brother.'

To attack the victim's credibility

- 'It never happened, she's lying.'
- 'He's exaggerating some innocent touching.'

To acknowledge the abuse while minimising the impact

- 'Better for her to learn about sex from her father than from some horny teenager.'
- 'She didn't really mind; in fact, we have a very close relationship.'
- 'Even if it did happen, it's time to forget the past and move on.'

To use the defence mechanism of projection and blame the child

- 'She's a very provocative child, and she seduced me.'
- 'If he hadn't enjoyed it so much, I wouldn't have kept doing it.'

Practice example

Sonja describes her current sexual life as one of promiscuity, and relates this to being sexually molested from age four through to age seven by her grandfather.

This is her description of the abuse: 'Whenever I was alone with him in the car, he would fondle me and expose his penis to me. He would tell me I could touch it, it would be all right.

'So much of the time I tried to block everything out—it's hard for me to recall exactly what happened. Some of the things I remember clearly. I remember Grandad's chair in the lounge room. When we were alone he would make me sit on his lap in that chair, and he would stick his fingers in me. This happened many times. One time he parked in an isolated area and played with me and made me touch him and kiss his penis. He tried to coax me to have intercourse. He told me it wouldn't hurt. But I cried and he masturbated into his handkerchief instead. He made me promise never to tell anyone.

'He always bought me gifts or gave me money. I remember the day he died. I came home from school and when my mum told me, I cried. But deep down I was glad. I was finally safe from him; I hated him for hurting me and making me tell lies all the time.'

Frequently, dissociation is the victim's main defence mechanism. The mind is 'separated' from the body so that the victim is not emotionally present during the sexual attack. Dissociation is evident in statements such as 'I put myself in the wall, where he couldn't reach all of me' and 'When he would come into my room, I would close my eyes and go to my favourite place. Only my body stayed on the bed; the rest of me wasn't there.'

Adult survivors

Adult survivors may come to believe that they were to blame for the abuse and should have been able to resist the adult.

This self-blame may contribute to depression, anxiety, panic attacks and low self-esteem. They feel worthless and different from other people. For some, anger is the only emotion experienced and expressed; all other feelings are repressed. Many adult survivors continue to hate their perpetrators, as well as the non-abusing significant adults who did not protect them. Studies have reported a high incidence of painful life events among people who hear voices; in many cases the traumatic experience involved childhood sexual abuse (Andrew, Gray & Snowden, 2008).

Sexual difficulties

Adult survivors may believe that they are only sex objects, to be used and abused by others. Some have a very strong aversion to sex and are filled with terror in sexual situations. Some are sexually inhibited, and experience discomfort with sexual thoughts, feelings and behaviours. Some engage in compulsive sexual behaviour, perhaps as an unconscious way to validate their shame and guilt, or as a way to feel powerful. Many adult survivors go through a period of celibacy as they try to manage fear, anger and distrust.

Confusion about sexuality is very common among male survivors. Sexual victimisation of a male by a male carries a hidden implication that the victim is less than a man. Heterosexual survivors fear that the abuse has made, or will make, them homosexual. Intense homophobia and/or hypermasculine behaviour may be an effort to disprove their fears. Gay survivors worry that their sexual preference may have caused the abuse. It is important to remember that childhood sexual abuse is not related to adult sexual orientation.

Self-mutilation

Some adult survivors engage in *self-mutilation*; this may involve cutting, slashing or burning themselves. It is important to understand the meaning of such behaviour. For some, the pain of self-mutilation proves their existence and reassures them that they are alive and real. Self-mutilation may be a plea for nurturance, because they come to the emergency department seeking care. Others nurture themselves by cleaning up the wounds after self-mutilation. For those who dissociate, self-mutilation may be a way to stop the dissociation, to focus on the here-and-now with physical pain. Others self-mutilate as a form of self-punishment and a way to decrease guilt feelings. And finally, some self-mutilate as a way to reduce emotional pain through the feeling of physical pain. It is important to understand the function of the behaviour in order to replace it with healthier behaviours that satisfy the same need.

Memory of sexual abuse

Research has shown that many memories of past events are not reports but reconstructions. It is the difference between remembering facts and remembering events. What is remembered is the overall impression rather than the specific details. The details we add when we reconstruct our experience depend on our personality traits and cognitive styles. We may also create pseudo-memories of events that never actually occurred, especially after being told of such 'events' by trusted individuals. Reports of remembered child abuse in adults, therefore, should ideally be corroborated by other people.

BIOPSYCHOSOCIAL THEORIES

There is no single cause of childhood sexual abuse. Rather, the abuse results from a combination of personality, family and cultural factors.

Intrapersonal theory

There are many types of perpetrators of sexual abuse of children. Some traits are contradictory, and there is no agreement on a composite personality. Certain characteristics apply to many people, not just abusers. The descriptions that follow are guidelines for assessment, not proof that the person actually committed sexual abuse:

1. Perpetrators usually have low self-esteem and feel more secure in interactions with children than with adults.
2. Some were emotionally deprived as children, and thus have a great need for constant, unconditional love, which is more easily obtained from children than from adults.
3. Some perpetrators are described as lacking impulse control and the ability to experience feelings of guilt.
4. Some are described as rigid and over-controlled, while others are dominant and aggressive.

If perpetrators were sexually abused themselves as children, they may have learned to associate all feelings of love with sexual behaviour. Most people who were sexually abused as children do not go on to sexually abuse others. Some victimised children, however, develop offending behaviour in late childhood, adolescence or adulthood. It is likely that there are a number of factors involved in why some abuse and others do not. The world of abuse is comprised only of victims (powerless) and perpetrators (powerful). Victims become perpetrators in an unconscious attempt to master the trauma of their own experiences and retrieve power. The move from victim to offender may also result when anger and hostility concerning the past are externalised and projected onto new victims.

Family systems theory

Family sexual abuse most typically occurs in families that have difficulty with structure, cohesion, adaptability and communication.

Family structure is usually hierarchical according to age, roles and distribution of power. Typically, the adults, who are older, assume the parental roles and are the most influential. The structure of incestuous families, however, is often quite different as the result of dysfunctional boundary patterns. An adult may move 'down' in the structure or a child may move 'up' in terms of roles and influence (boundaries). If the father moves downward, he assumes a childlike role and is cared for and nurtured like a child in the family. In this position, the father assumes little parental responsibility. He may then turn to the daughter as a 'peer' for sexual and emotional gratification.

As another example, the daughter may move upward and replace the mother in the hierarchy. The mother does not usually move downward, but rather moves out of the structure by distancing herself emotionally or physically from the family. As the daughter assumes the parental role and responsibilities, the father may turn to her for fulfillment of his emotional and sexual needs.

Families that are enmeshed—that is, the members are immersed in and absorbed by one another—may be at risk for sexual abuse. In addition, incestuous families tend to be either rigid or chaotic in their adaptability. Rigid family systems have strict rules and stereotyped gender-role expectations, with minimal emotional interaction. Children have no power or authority, even over their own bodies. They are not allowed to question or protest inappropriate sexual behaviour. In contrast, chaotic family systems have either no rules or are constantly changing the rules. Within the chaotic system, there may be no assigned roles or no rules regarding appropriate sexual behaviour, which may contribute to the incidence of sexual abuse. Enmeshed and rigid family structures and family dynamics are discussed in Chapter 24.

Communication patterns within the family system may contribute to the occurrence of sexual abuse. Incest depends on keeping the secret within the family. In family systems that avoid conflict, accusations of sexual abuse are not tolerated. Peace, and therefore silence, must be kept at all costs.

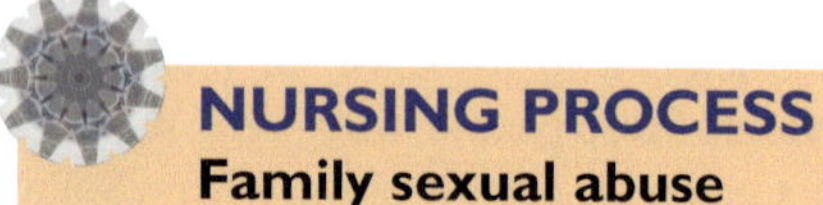

NURSING PROCESS
Family sexual abuse

A nursing care plan for an adult survivor of childhood sexual abuse is provided at the end of the chapter.

Assessment

It is important that the reality of childhood sexual abuse is acknowledged. Nurses who deny the existence of the problem will miss the cues and fail to complete a detailed assessment. If you are knowledgeable about the incidence and characteristics of the problem, you will be alert for cues that demand nursing assessment. Guidelines for assessment are given in Your Assessment Approach.

When assessing children, it is important to remember that some will exhibit most of the symptoms presented in this chapter, others will exhibit only some, and still others will exhibit none. It should also be noted that these same behavioural, affective and cognitive characteristics may be symptoms of other emotional problems. Once it has been discovered that one child in a family is a victim of sexual abuse, the possibility that other siblings, both boys and girls, have also been abused should be considered. Entire families may be sexually abused before someone 'tells'.

It is important to appreciate the power of secrecy and how difficult it is for adult survivors to disclose such information, especially for men, who are expected to be anything other than victimised. Routine questions on nursing histories may provide an opportunity for survivors to share their pain and obtain treatment as adults. See Your Assessment Approach on page 450 on conducting a physical assessment of a sexual abuse victim; the topics included may be easier for the survivor to discuss than details of the actual abuse.

It is important for the health professional to take responsibility for initiating the topic. Shame and confusion may keep the adult survivor from doing so. Avoiding the topic may contribute to pathology by supporting the person's denial of reality. Failure to initiate a discussion of sexual abuse sends a message that such abuse does not occur or does not matter. Now that childhood sexual abuse has been identified as a major health problem, nurses in every clinical setting must be alert for cues from both individuals and families.

When working with adult survivors, it is important to continuously assess the person's comfort level with the physical setting. Closed doors increase anxiety in some people, while others may request that doors never remain open. Some people are uncomfortable in a room with a couch or a bed rather than chairs. How close you sit can be an issue; even normally appropriate physical contact, such as a handshake, may increase anxiety. Permission should always be sought before touching a person who is the victim of sexual abuse. Always ask permission before touching a person you are working with.

Problem identification

Based on assessment data, problem statements are formulated for the individual child victim, the family members and/or the adult survivor. Problems for the child victim may include:

- ineffective coping related to being a victim of sexual abuse
- powerlessness related to being helpless to stop the abuse
- trauma related to being a victim of sexual abuse
- social isolation related to keeping sexual abuse secret.

Problems for families experiencing sexual abuse may include:

- poor family coping related to a child being sexually abused
- poor family coping related to an enmeshed family system that is either rigid or chaotic
- ineffective parenting related to being a perpetrator of sexual abuse
- dysfunctional family process related to disruption when abuse is discovered.

Problems for adult survivors of childhood sexual abuse may include:

- trauma related to being an adult survivor
- distress related to issues about fairness and justice in life
- low self-esteem related to self-blame for the abuse
- denial related to amnesia for childhood events
- social isolation related to difficulty in forming intimate relationships, mistrust of others
- sexual dysfunction related to the trauma of abuse.

YOUR ASSESSMENT APPROACH Nursing history tool for the assessment of individuals and families for family sexual abuse

Behavioural assessment

Individual child

- Have there been any signs of regressive behaviour in the child?
- Is the child having sleeping problems?
- Is the child exhibiting clinging behaviour to the parents or others?
- Does the child have friendships with other children?
- Has there been any sexual acting-out on the part of the child?
- Has the child ever run away or threatened to run away?
- Has the child ever attempted suicide?

Perpetrator

- Describe how discipline is handled in the family.
- Do you see yourself as the dominant person in the family?
- At what age do you believe parents should give up control of their children?
- How many adult friends do you have?
- Describe your relationships with these friends.
- Describe your relationship with your partner.
- What kinds of sexual difficulties are you and your partner experiencing?
- When you were young, who was the closest family member with whom you had any sexual activity?

Family system

- Describe who has responsibility (mother, father, both parents, or children) in the following areas of home management:
  - Caring for the younger children
  - Cooking
  - Cleaning
  - Paying bills
  - Shopping
  - Outside home maintenance
  - Budget planning
  - Decisions about leisure time
  - Supervising children's homework
  - Taking children to activities
  - Putting children to bed
- Who are the best communicators in the family?
- Who talks to whom the most?
- Who is unable to talk to whom very much?
- How are secrets kept from one another within the family?
- How are secrets prevented from leaking outside the family?

Affective assessment

Individual child

- How helpless does the child feel about changing any of the family's problems?
- Does the child feel responsible for family problems?
- Does the child get enough love within the family?
- Is the child more loved than the other children in the family?
- Ask about the fears the child may have if any family secrets are told:
  - Fear of not being believed
  - Fear of being blamed for the problems
  - Fear that your parents will not love you
  - Fear that you will be moved to a foster home
  - Fear that your parents will be taken away
  - Fear of physical abuse

Perpetrator

- Who loves you most within the family?
- Who is able to give you unconditional support and affection?
- Do you see yourself as responsible for family problems?
- How does fear of failure affect your life?

Family system

- Describe the emotional relationships among family members.
- Does everybody know each family member's business?
- How is privacy protected within the family?
- Do you have any fears of the family unit disintegrating?
- What will happen if the family is separated?

Cognitive assessment

Individual child

- Tell me about your nightmares.
- How would you describe the family's problems?
- What effect do these problems have on you?
- What effect do these problems have on the rest of the family?
- Who do you believe is responsible for these problems?

Perpetrator

- Describe what kind of a person you are.
- What are your personal strengths?
- What are your personal limitations?
- Describe how you handle new situations.
- Do you enjoy changing situations?

Family system

- Who sets the family rules?
- Tell me about the most important family rules.
- How do rules get changed within the family?
- What are the expectations of the males in the family?
- What are the expectations of the females in the family?

Sociocultural assessment

- What significant events have occurred for your family in the past year?
- What support systems do you have outside the family?
- How often do you visit with friends?
- Who are the problem drinkers in the family?
- How is the issue of drugs managed within the family?

Outcomes of intervention

Once outcomes have been determined, a collaborative approach is used to identify goals for change. Goals are specific behavioural measures by which progress towards healing can be evaluated. The following are examples of some of the goals appropriate to people who have experienced childhood sexual abuse:

- remains safe and free from harm
- utilises a variety of therapies to express feelings about the sexual abuse

YOUR ASSESSMENT APPROACH
Physical assessment of the sexual abuse victim

A head-to-toe physical assessment with emphasis on the following should be completed:

- weight and nutritional status
- throat irritation
- gag reflex
- episodes of vomiting
- abdominal pain near diaphragm
- smears of the mouth, throat, vagina and rectum for sexually transmitted infections
- genital irritation or trauma
- rectal irritation or trauma
- chronic vaginal infections
- chronic urinary tract infections
- pregnancy

- verbalises improved self-esteem
- manages negative emotions in an appropriate manner
- verbalises a feeling of connectedness to significant others
- verbalises improvement in sexual functioning
- utilises community resources.

Planning and implementation

The first priority of care with child victims is to ensure the safety of the child. Nurses are subject to mandatory reporting of suspected child sexual abuse in all state and territory jurisdictions in Australia.

When families are enmeshed and either rigid or chaotic, family members will need help to move to a more moderate position between the extremes. In such cases, families may need to be taught basic problem-solving techniques. With a rigid family, the purpose of problem-solving is to help family members to increase the flexibility of roles and rules. With a chaotic family, problem-solving may concentrate on ways to organise appropriate roles and formulate consistent rules. Resources to creatively and effectively intervene in cases dealing with domestic violence can be sought (Hassija & Gray, 2011).

Working with children

It is important to facilitate the child's ability to talk and to think about the abuse with decreasing anxiety. A safe and predictable environment in which the child feels supported should be created. It should also be made clear to the child that you understand that talking about the abuse is difficult.

Interventions should aim to encourage affective release in a supportive environment. Child victims must be able to experience a range of emotions. Play therapy helps these children play out traumatic themes, fears and distorted beliefs. It is a non-threatening way to process the thoughts and feelings associated with the abuse, both symbolically and directly. Art therapy provides an opportunity to express feelings for which there are no words. Therapeutic stories present the traumatic issues of abuse, link the victims' feelings and behaviour, and describe new coping methods. Journal writing can help children over the age of 10 to cope with intrusive thoughts and feelings. They may choose to bring their journal into the one-to-one sessions with their therapist.

Empowering survivors

Because the process of sexual abuse is disempowering, it is important to empower survivors. The focus on traumatic stress therapy treats the trauma while acknowledging the process and result of victimisation. Developmental therapy focuses on the 'gaps' in the personality that occurred during the abusive process, such as trust issues, identity issues and relationship issues. Loss therapy focuses on helping the survivors identify and grieve over the things they have lost during their childhood sexual abuse, such as innocence, trust, nurturing and memories.

In working with adult survivors, it should be remembered that they have been robbed of a sense of power and feel detached from others. Recovery includes restoring power and control. It is important to avoid becoming a 'rescuer', as that might send the message that the person with whom you are working is not capable of acting for themselves. The role of the nurse sets up a collaborative relationship, unlike the powerful authority relationship that occurred with the abuser. The most helpful approach is being an ally, partner and supporter as the person struggles through the healing process. Instances can be pointed out in which the person has taken control of their life; they can be supported to identify situations in which they are able to make self-respecting choices.

Supporting spiritual recovery

To recover from sexual abuse, survivors must place responsibility for the abuse where it belongs—100 per cent with the offender. If they fail to do this, they will continue to be paralysed by self-blame and guilt. For this reason, it is essential that the person's need for spiritual healing be supported. Strategies for doing so set out in the following Practice Example.

Practice example

Supporting spiritual recovery from sexual abuse

For many victims, betrayal by abusing adults can be experienced as a spiritual issue. It is thus important that a person's need for spiritual healing be acknowledged. Victims and survivors may be consumed with spiritual questions such as 'Why did it happen to me?', 'What's wrong with me?' and 'Am I an evil person?' When people are sexually abused, they are likely to question their understanding of, and relationship to, God. Questions may arise such as 'What's wrong with God?' and 'Why didn't God stop it?' It is not unusual for survivors to be angry with God and hold God responsible for the abuse. The sexual abuse may also have been perpetrated by a trusted member of a religious organisation, such as a priest. This anger may in turn trigger fear and guilt for hating a divine entity.

Spirituality includes a sense of connectedness to others. Survivors face the long journey of developing trusting relationships. The adult self needs to reach out and care for the hurt inner child by breaking down the walls that have isolated that child. Experiencing the rage and grief are part of the survivor working towards self-forgiveness and more complete healing. For many survivors, experiencing human contact and the warmth of a therapeutic relationship may be the beginnings of re-establishing trust in other humans. As part of a collaborative process, people who have been subjected to sexual abuse may be referred to religious counsellors who understand the emotional issues surrounding sexual abuse and who are sensitive to the need of survivors to work slowly through their spiritual struggles.

Increasing self-esteem

Interventions designed to increase self-esteem can be employed. Adult survivors have a continuous internal monologue of negative statements such as 'You're weak, stupid, incompetent, unlovable and unattractive.' Negative statements become self-administered abuse, and keep the survivor weak and powerless. People can be helped to become aware of the frequency and intensity of these negative thoughts; they can be taught to consciously replace negative thoughts with positive ones. While this is often difficult at first, it becomes easier with practice.

Reducing anxiety

Because adult survivors are often anxious, interventions to reduce anxiety are also necessary. Helping people to learn progressive relaxation and controlled breathing can reduce the likelihood of full-blown panic attacks. Teaching the process, and talking an individual through the stages of relaxation, you can support them in reducing anxiety by themselves. When the person is relaxed, they can be guided through imagining a scene in which they feel safe and comfortable. Anytime they need to, the person can return to this safe scene where they are in total control. Daily practice increases the effectiveness of these techniques (see Chapters 8 and 25).

Facilitating healing

Art therapy can be used to help adults in the healing process. Making group murals to express both individual progress and a sense of unity among survivors can be very effective. Music therapy, combined with movement or dance, may be a way for people to experience very early memories. Another often-used technique is journal writing, which can also include poetry, songs and plays.

Group therapy allows survivors to share their feelings and experiences with others who believe their stories. The group setting fosters mutual understanding, and decreases the sense of isolation. Many adult survivors find self-help groups to be very supportive in the process of healing (see Chapter 23).

Evaluation

Nurses in acute care settings may not have the opportunity for long-term evaluation. Short-term evaluation focuses mainly on identifying child victims and adult survivors, and referring them to appropriate sources of professional help.

Nurses in long-term or community settings can evaluate the effectiveness of the treatment plan over an extended period. Questions to guide the evaluation of the child victim and family include the following:

- Has the child remained safe from further harm?
- Has the child returned to functioning at an appropriate developmental level?
- Is the child able to express feelings either verbally or through play or art therapy?
- Is the child verbalising decreasing feelings of guilt and/or responsibility?
- Is the child developing peer friendships?
- Has the family structure become more flexible?
- Is communication more open within the family?

Nurses have an opportunity to influence the care of adult survivors of childhood sexual abuse. It can be explained to others that the survivor's behaviour is a post-trauma response that makes sense as an adaptation to trauma and to a possibly dysfunctional family. This may be especially important when working with people in relation to personality disorders. It is also important to be watchful for, and intervene in, circumstances in which staff members recreate the dynamics of the abusive relationship by assuming a position of power and control.

Questions to guide the evaluation of adult survivors include the following:

- Has the person remained safe from further harm in adult relationships?
- Is the person able to talk about the childhood trauma? If not, is art therapy, music therapy, movement therapy, or journal writing effective in facilitating expression?
- Is the person able to identify situations in which they have been able, or hope to be able, to make self-respecting choices?
- Is the person verbalising increased spiritual comfort regarding the trauma?
- Is the person verbalising less self-blame?
- Is the person verbalising improved self-image?
- Is there evidence that the person is able to develop trusting and respectful relationships with adults?

Although, as a culture, we say that we protect our children, in reality we often fall short of this value. In the past we have not invested sufficient time, caring and money in the prevention of childhood sexual abuse. As recent inquiries such as the Royal Commission into Family Violence (State of Victoria, 2016a; 2016b) have indicated, current approaches to treatment and also the social control of sexual abuse are not yet effective enough to assure the long-term safety of children. Nurses can and must play an active part of the battle to stop childhood sexual abuse.

CARE COORDINATION

Care coordination in these cases of child sexual abuse is very likely to involve protective services for the child/children and partner/cohabitants. Protective services for children will likely implement one of the following approaches if the abuse is occurring within the family system:

1. Separating the abuser from the family. The non-abusing parent must protect the child from any contact with the abuser.
2. When the non-abusing parent is unable to protect the child, both the child and the abuser are removed from the home. This option maximises the child's safety and decreases the child's feelings of responsibility.
3. In cases in which families have not used physical violence, there is no substance abuse, and there is someone who can ensure the child's safety, the family may be allowed to remain intact while participating in intensive therapy.

4. In some instances, the child may be removed from the family when that is the safest option. Unfortunately, this decision may place additional guilt on the child.

COMMUNITY-BASED CARE AND HOME CARE

A community issue that touches the lives of women, in particular, is how women are treated by men in the workplace. If the environment is one that tacitly supports keeping women subordinate, then those women are being discriminated against. Sexual harassment of women in the workplace and in schools has always existed as a hidden crime. Only recently has it been more fully recognised for what it is—discrimination against, and violation of, the victim. It is part of the continuum of sexual violence, which also includes childhood sexual abuse and rape. Girls and boys and women and men must be taught that they do not have to tolerate harassing behaviours. These behaviours include the following:

- staring or leering
- being unnecessarily familiar, such as deliberately brushing against a person or touching them
- making suggestive comments or jokes
- making insults or taunts of a sexual nature
- indulging in intrusive questions or statements about a person's private life
- displaying posters, magazines or screen-savers of a sexual nature
- sending sexually explicit emails or text messages
- making inappropriate advances on social networking sites
- accessing sexually explicit internet sites
- making requests for sex or repeated unwanted requests to go out on dates
- behaving in ways that may also be considered an offence under criminal law, such as physical assault, indecent exposure, sexual assault, stalking or obscene communications.

Sexual harassment can lead to severe stress in the victims. Many experience depression, isolation, feelings of powerlessness, helplessness, fear, restlessness, inability to concentrate, somatic complaints, sexual problems, and loss of self-esteem. At its most severe, harassment resembles the other sexual traumas of child sexual abuse and may result in post-traumatic stress disorder. In Australia, the Human Rights and Equal Opportunity Commission (HREOC) is the government body responsible for receiving complaints under the *Sex Discrimination Act 1984*. This legislation makes it unlawful for a person to sexually harass another person in a number of areas, including employment, education, the provision of goods and services, and accommodation. About one in five complaints received by the HREOC under the *Sex Discrimination Act 1984* relates to sexual harassment.

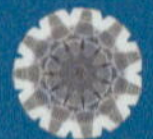

NURSING CARE PLAN: AN ADULT SURVIVOR OF CHILDHOOD SEXUAL ABUSE

Identifying information

Jill is 35 years old and, with her husband John, co-owns and operates a local newsagent business. The couple have been married for 15 years, and have three children aged 14, 12 and 7.

Jill was sexually abused by her grandfather from a very young age until she was about 11 or 12. She states that she told her mother about the abuse when she was 9 or 10, but that her mother just ignored it. Her mother now denies that Jill told her about the abuse when it was occurring. Jill has tried to ignore her abuse history, until several months ago when she saw a television program about incest. She has periods when she is filled with rage at her parents and grandfather.

History

No prior psychiatric history.

Jill is the third child of five in an intact family. She describes her mother as 'strict . . . she would threaten by saying "wait until your dad comes home".' When asked about her father, Jill states, 'He wasn't around . . . he was working . . . he was always distant.' She describes the family communication as 'dysfunctional; only certain people talked to certain other people. For example, none of us kids could talk directly to Dad. We always had to go through Mum.'

Jill describes herself as a 'homebody'; she works in the newsagency several days a week while the children are at school, and says 'the shop is my chance to get out of the house each week.' In the past, she went out with her husband regularly, but says she never really enjoyed doing so. Since having children, Jill's life has increasingly involved parenting, home duties and the newsagency. She states that she has never had close friends and her only friend is her husband, but she also feels intimidated by him. She has a very close relationship with her children.

Jill has no current or past medical problems. She states that she is in good health except for feeling 'down a lot of the time'.

Current mental status

Jill is oriented to person, place and time. Her affect appears dysphoric, irritable and constricted in range. At times she is filled with rage, saying, 'I am mad . . . Mad at the world in general, and at having to deal with all of this.' She states that during her entire life she has spent much of her energy in 'not thinking', 'not imagining' and 'not remembering' the abuse. She has attempted to keep a sense of distance from her inner emotional life. After viewing the television program on incest, she now experiences 'painful, bitter, brooding thoughts about the abuse'. Jill is an anxious and angry woman with extremely low self-esteem and intense feelings of inadequacy. She views herself as unable to function in an autonomous, self-directed and self-reliant fashion, and sees the world as untrustworthy, betraying and often cruel.

Unable to rely on her own resources or depend on the support of others, Jill feels a sense of bitter futility and resignation.

(continued)

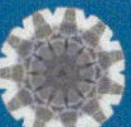

NURSING CARE PLAN: AN ADULT SURVIVOR OF CHILDHOOD SEXUAL ABUSE *(continued)*

She identifies herself as a victim who is inevitably betrayed and disappointed. Many of her dynamics are consistent with those of adult survivors of sexual abuse. She feels intense rage at her parents for being unsupportive, unprotective, and unable to provide her with a sense of safety and security in herself and in the world around her. This contributes to Jill's fear of autonomy, and to the conflict between her need to depend on others and her intense mistrust of the sincerity and commitment that others can offer. There is no evidence of psychotic illness or of a manifest thought disturbance.

Other clinical data

Jill states that she would like more emotional support from her husband. Her husband states that he has been unable to give it to her lately because he is often irritated at the messy and disorganised state of the house. She thinks he is being controlling and uncaring. He has offered to hire a cleaner, but Jill sees that as another failure on her part.

Issue identified: Trauma related to being an adult survivor of incest.
Expected outcome: Jill will resolve associated anger and anxiety.

Goals	Interventions	Rationales
Jill discharges her anger appropriately.	▪ Discuss feelings of guilt. Repeat often that children are never responsible for the incest, but rather that her grandfather is totally responsible.	Jill needs to place the responsibility for this abuse where it belongs.
	▪ Discuss her feelings of anger towards the grandfather and her parents for not protecting her as a child.	Survivors of abuse frequently take blame for the incest.
	▪ Connect feelings of low self-esteem to feelings of guilt and anger.	Jill's current interactions with others are based on what she learned from these experiences as a child.
	▪ Recommend journal-keeping for recording feelings, thoughts and memories.	
	▪ Help Jill identify and grieve over things lost in childhood, such as innocence and trust.	
Jill uses relaxation exercises.	▪ Teach anxiety-reducing techniques, such as muscle relaxation, deep breathing and physical exercise.	Handling stress and taking care of herself were not taught to her as a child by the adults who raised her.

Issue identified: Social isolation related to withdrawal and a decreased desire to interact with others.
Expected outcome: Jill will increase interactions with people outside her family.

Goals	Interventions	Rationales
Jill will be able to initiate relationships outside the family.	▪ Help Jill identify the benefits of social interactions.	Jill may not know that she could feel better when she is in regular contact with other people.
	▪ Help Jill identify a variety of available supportive people.	
	▪ Give Jill positive feedback when she expresses an interest in, or engages in, interactions with others.	Jill will respond to positive feedback and be likely to continue to discover others by answering where, how and when questions on social interactions.
	▪ Provide assertiveness training.	Jill's ability to say 'no' comfortably through assertiveness training will increase her comfort in relationships with others.
Jill will seek out and accept support and help from a self-help group.	▪ Provide information on self-help groups for adult survivors where Jill can share with others and establish trusting relationships.	Self-help groups provide the opportunity to realise that one is not alone.

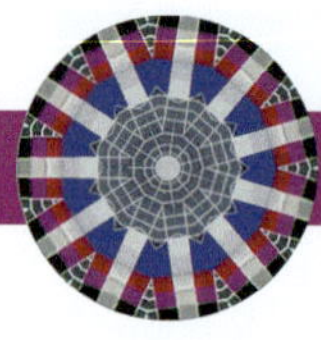

REFERENCES

Andrew, E., Gray, N., & Snowden, R. (2008). The relationship between trauma and beliefs about hearing voices: A study of psychiatric and non-psychiatric voice-hearers. *Psychological Medicine, 38* (10), 1409–1417.

Australian Bureau of Statistics (ABS). (2013). *Personal safety, Australia, 2012*. Cat. No. 4906.0. Canberra, Australia: ABS, Table 23, Table 24.

Australian Institute of Family Studies. (2012). *Sibling sexual abuse*. ACSSA Research Summary No. 3. Retrieved from https://aifs.gov.au/publicationsd/sibling-sexual-abuse/introduction (Accessed 2016, June 2.)

Australian Institute of Family Studies. (2016). *Child deaths from abuse and neglect*. CFCA Resource Sheet May 2016. Retrieved from https://aifs.gov.au/cfca/publications/child-deaths-abuse-and-neglect (Accessed 2016, June 3.)

Bryant, W., & Cussen, T. (2015). *Homicide in Australia: 2010–2011 National Homicide Monitoring Program Report.* Monitoring Report 23. Canberra, Australia: Australian Institute of Criminology. Retrieved from aic.gov.au/publications/current%20series/mr/21-40.html (Accessed 2016, June 3.)

Burriss, F. A., Breland-Noble, A. M., Webster, J. L., & Soto, J. A. (2011). Juvenile mental health courts for adjudicated youth: Role implications for child and adolescent psychiatric mental health nurses. *Journal of Child and Adolescent Psychiatric Nursing, 24*(2), 114–121.

Burton, D. L., Duty, K. J., & Leibowitz, G. S. (2011). Differences between sexually victimized and nonsexually victimized male adolescent sexual abusers: Developmental antecedents and behavioral comparisons. *Journal of Child Sexual Abuse, 20*(1), 77–93.

Champion, J. D. (2011). Context of sexual risk behavior among abused ethnic minority adolescent women. *International Nursing Review, 58*(1), 61–67.

Crime and Misconduct Commission Queensland. (2013). *Vulnerable victims: Child homicide by parents*. Research and Issues Paper No. 10 (June 2013). Fortitude Valley, Australia: Crime and Misconduct Commission.

Denton, J., Newton, A. W., & Vandeven, A. M. (2011). Update on child maltreatment: Toward refining the evidence base. *Current Opinion in Pediatrics, 23*, 240–248.

Duran, M., Moya, M., & Megias, J. L. (2010). It's his right, it's her duty: Benevolent sexism and the justification of traditional sexual roles. *Journal of Sex Research, 14*, 1–9.

Everson, M. D., & Sandoval, J. M. (2011). Forensic child sexual abuse evaluations: Assessing subjectivity and bias in professional judgments. *Child Abuse and Neglect, 35*(4), 287–298.

Finkelhor, D., Ormrod, R., Turner, H., & Hamby, S. (2011). School, police, and medical authority involvement with children who have experienced victimization. *Archives of Pediatrics and Adolescent Medicine, 165*(1), 9–15.

Graham-Bermann, S., Sularz, A. R., & Howell, K. H. (2011). Additional adverse events among women exposed to intimate partner violence: Frequency and impact. *Psychology of Violence, 1*(2), 136–149.

Greenberg, D. M., Firestone, P., Nunes, K. L., Bradford, J. M., & Curry, S. (2005). Biological fathers and stepfathers who molest their daughters: Psychological, phallometric, and criminal features. *Sexual Abuse: A Journal of Research and Treatment, 17*(1), 39–46.

Hassija, C., & Gray, M. J. (2011). The effectiveness and feasibility of videoconferencing technology to provide evidence-based treatment to rural domestic violence and sexual assault populations. *Telemedicine Journal and E-Health, 17*(4), 309–315.

Krug, E. G., Dahlberg, L. L., Mercy, J. A., Zwi, A. B., & Lorenzo, R. (2002). *World report on violence and health.* Geneva, Switzerland: World Health Organization.

Lyden, C. (2011). Uncovering child abuse. *Nursing, 41*, 1–5.

McCloskey, K. A., & Raphael, D. N. (2005). Adult perpetrator gender asymmetries in child sexual assault victim selection. *Journal of Child Sexual Abuse, 14*(4), 1–24.

Miller, E., Breslau, J., Chung, W. J., Green, J. G., McLaughlin, K. A., & Kessler, R. C. (2011). Adverse childhood experiences and risk of physical violence in adolescent dating relationships. *Journal of Epidemiology and Community Health, 65*(11), 1006–1013.

Mitra, M., Manning, S. E., & Lu, E. (2011). Physical abuse around the time of pregnancy among women with disabilities. *Maternal and Child Health Journal, 16*(4), 802–806.

Mousos, J., & Rushworth, C. (2003). *Family homicide in Australia*. Trends and Issues Paper No. 255. Canberra, Australia: Australian Institute of Criminology.

Nursing and Midwifery Board of Australia. (2013). Code of professional conduct for nurses in Australia. Retrieved from www.nursingmidwiferyboard.gov.au/Codes-Guidelines-Statements/Professional-standards.aspx

Schetky, K. H. (1999). Sexual victimization of children. In J. A. Shaw (Ed.), *Sexual aggression* (pp. 107–128). Washington, DC: American Psychiatric Press.

State of Victoria. (2016a). *Royal Commission into Family Violence: Summary and recommendations.* Parliamentary Paper No. 132 (2014-16). Melbourne: Victorian Government Printer.

State of Victoria. (2016b). *Royal Commission into Family Violence: Report and recommendations*, Vol. 1, Parliamentary Paper 132 (2014-2016). Melbourne: Victorian Government Printer.

Tsopelas, C., Spyridoula, T., & Athanosios, D. (2011). Review on female sexual offenders: Findings about profile and personality. *International Journal of Law and Psychiatry, 34*(2), 122–126.

Wang, Y. W. (2011). Voices from the margin: A case study of a rural lesbian's experience with woman-to-woman sexual violence. *Journal of Lesbian Studies, 15*(2), 166–175.

World Health Organization. (2014). *Child maltreatment*. Fact Sheet No. 150. Retrieved from www.who.int/mediacentre/factsheet/fs150/en/ (Accessed 2016, June 2.)

The mental health of younger people

21

ELLEN SINCLAIR, ISABELLA SWINSON AND MIKE HAZELTON

LEARNING OUTCOMES

After completing this chapter, you will be able to:

1. Compare and contrast the biopsychosocial theories important to understanding young people.
2. Incorporate relevant biological and developmental information in the assessment of young people.
3. Illustrate how a humanistic–interactionist perspective contributes to a comprehensive assessment of problems experienced by young people.
4. Design intervention strategies for young people who act out.
5. Formulate strategies for working with young people who are angry or hostile, test the staff, scapegoat others, engage in problematic sexual behaviours, or abuse substances.
6. Construct a therapeutic contract for use with a young person in treatment.
7. Analyse personal feelings and attitudes or unresolved issues about adolescence that may affect your professional practice with young people.
8. Understand and appreciate the lived experience of young people with mental illness and their families.

KEY TERMS

LIVED EXPERIENCE

For me it has been a recovery journey. I don't think recovery ever really ends. It is a process of learning that everyone has to go through at some stage, not only those who experience mental illness. So, for me recovery is a normal part of life. My first experience of mental ill health was in late childhood, but I don't think it was picked up as such at the time. In many instances it probably looks like a normal part of growing up, but is actually the early indications of mental illness. At 16 years of age a suicide attempt led to a long-term psychiatric hospitalisation, first in adult inpatient units in another country, then for a period of time in a small adolescent inpatient unit. By age 17 I had returned to Australia with my family, and became an inpatient within specialist child and adolescent/youth mental health services in Victoria. I think it would be fair to say that many of the

(*continued*)

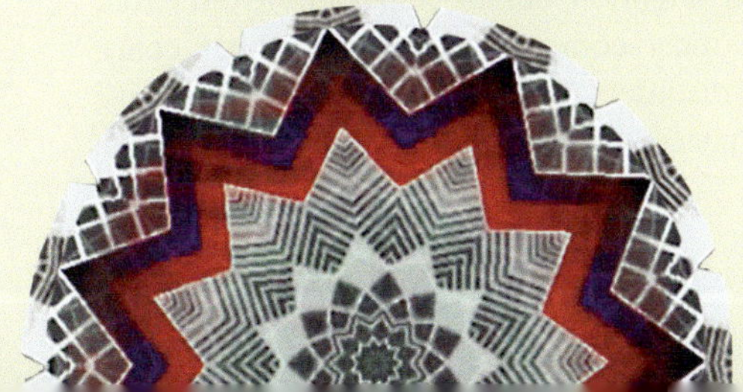

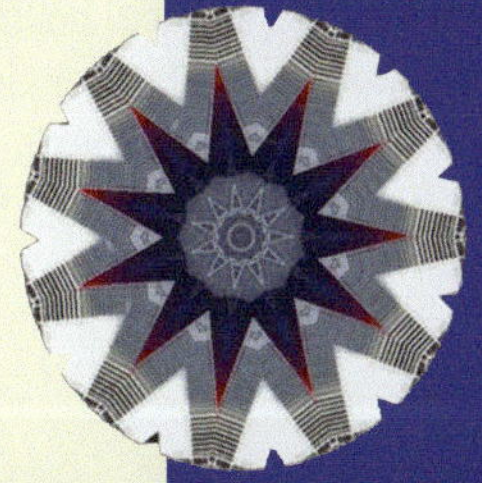

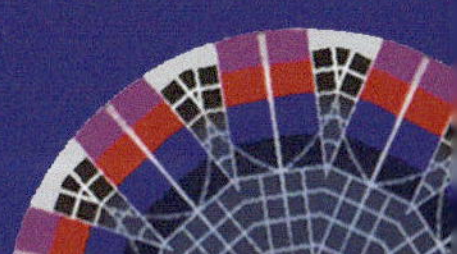

LIVED EXPERIENCE *(continued)*

health professionals I saw in the early stages of being unwell did not hold out much hope for my recovery. The people who did stick by me were my family. One of the points I would make to health professionals and students is that it is critically important that you work with an expectation that people can and will recover from the illness they are experiencing. I can't stress this enough.

INTRODUCTION

What is adolescence? Some sources define it simply as the time of physical and psychosocial development between the ages of 12 and 20. Others have described it as a period of 'normal psychosis'. Still others see it as a perplexing subculture that is not consistent with the beliefs and values of our society. It is not necessary to accept the latter two definitions verbatim to understand their implications. Most people recognise the immense stress that occurs during adolescence, and the importance to a young person's future of managing that stress.

Trying to understand young people can be a challenge for older adults. If you think of your own experiences and reactions during that tumultuous time, it may help you better appreciate the dilemmas that must be faced during this stage of life. Nurses who choose to work with young people find considerable rewards from the challenge. Whether the nurse functions as a generalist, a clinical nurse specialist or a nurse practitioner, today's health care settings integrate professional capabilities, skills and roles to intervene with younger people. The goal is to help the young person to achieve optimal social, emotional, cognitive and physical development. Young people are emotionally and economically dependent on several systems (family, school, community and institution), and nurses work closely with them all to identify relevant changes in the developmental process.

The Australian Youth Affairs Coalition (AYAC) is the peak body representing over 4 million Australians aged 12–25. The Australian government funded AYAC up until July 2014. Since that time AYAC has continued to operate with limited resources. In representing young people, AYAC has sought to facilitate debate on key issues affecting young Australians (information about AYAC can be accessed at www.ayac.org.au). Currently, youth health policy is organised and operated at the state/territory jurisdictional level in Australia. An example of one such policy is the New South Wales government's *Youth Health Policy 2011–2016: Healthy bodies, healthy minds, vibrant futures*. This policy can be accessed at www.health.nsw.gov.au/policies/pd/2010/pdf/_073.pdf

YOUNG PEOPLE AND MENTAL ILLNESS

There is a broad range of mental disorders affecting people in their teenage years. Approximately one in four young Australians meet criteria for a mental disorder, with the potential for severe impairment at different stages during their lifetime. Mental disorders common in adults often first emerge in childhood and adolescence. This highlights the need for an increased focus on prevention and early intervention during adolescence. Such concerns have led to youth mental health policy initiatives throughout Australia, the most prominent of which is the establishment of more than 90 headspace centres nationally. Established as a foundation supporting youth mental health and wellbeing nationally, headspace provides early intervention services to young people aged 12 to 25, in areas such as mental health, physical health, work and study support, and the use of alcohol and other drugs. The services offered by headspace focus especially on supporting young people experiencing high-prevalence disorders such as depression and anxiety. The range of services includes counselling on a walk-in basis, support for schools that have been affected by suicide, and online and telephone counselling for young people experiencing a mental illness and their families. More information on the purpose and services offered by headspace can be accessed at www.headspace.org.au

The findings of the Second Australian Child and Adolescent Survey of Mental Health and Wellbeing (Lawrence et al., 2015; Lawrence et al., 2016) indicated that almost one in seven (13.9 per cent) 4- to 17-year-olds would satisfy diagnostic criteria for a mental disorder in the 12 months prior to the survey (equivalent to 560 000 Australian children and teenagers). Males were more likely to have experienced a mental health problem than females (16.3 per cent compared to 11.5 per cent), with attention deficit hyperactivity disorder (ADHD) being the most common disorder (7.4 per cent), followed by anxiety disorders (6.9 per cent), major depressive disorder (MDD) (2.8 per cent) and conduct disorder (2.1 per cent).

Just under one-third of all 4- to 17-year-olds with a disorder had two or more mental disorders in the 12 months prior to the survey, and in about one in seven (14.7 per cent) of these the disorder was assessed as being severe.

BIOPSYCHOSOCIAL THEORIES

A sound theoretical knowledge base can help in differentiating between what are considered to be 'normal' and 'abnormal', or usual and unusual, behaviours during the adolescent stage of life. When conducting a comprehensive assessment, the focus should be on the psychological development of the individual and the evolution of the young person as a biopsychosocial being. The first task can be approached using an understanding of developmental theory, and the second with an appreciation of biological and humanistic–interactionist theories.

Biological theory

Mental health nursing requires you to integrate a biological focus into your practice, to accommodate both the changing needs of the young person and an expanding biological knowledge base. An appreciation of hormonal changes, growth spurts, stress, immune function, chronic illness, depression and other mental disorders can help you evaluate the needs of young people from a more effective and comprehensive perspective.

Neurobiology and biochemistry

In recent decades, research has been conducted using neuroimaging, magnetic resonance imaging (MRI), and spectroscopy in order to better delineate the anatomical, functional and biochemical imbalances of mood disorders and other behaviours in children and teenagers. As a result, there is now data suggesting that young people who are depressed without a comorbid psychiatric disorder exhibit an abnormally hyperactive amygdala compared to healthy controls (Arnold, Hanna & Rosenberg, 2010). In addition, neuroscientists have identified structural brain changes in correlation with emotional neglect and other early life stress experiences (Frodl, 2010). Researchers recognise that this developmental phase, with its risky behaviours, makes this population even more vulnerable to neurobiological problems, such as substance dependence and abuse (Rutherford, Mayes & Potenza, 2010).

Advancements in molecular biology and biochemistry allow investigations of gene expressions in specific neuronal systems of the brain. Applying advances such as these to common and important health issues for young people—for example—metabolic functioning, indicates the interconnection of systems. Neurobiological systems and specific neuropeptides and hormones are as important as behavioural and familial habits in abnormal body weight regulation. It is now known that neurochemical and humoural substances are related to the traits of overeating, weight gain and eating disorders. These discoveries are important in themselves for clinical treatment. In addition, knowledge regarding the biochemical and physiological aetiology for these physical conditions could help positively influence the tendency within the community to discriminate against people who live with such conditions. Realising that biochemical and neuronal systems are contributing to these medical conditions could alleviate some of the prejudice endured by young people with eating disorders, through exposure to peer taunts such as 'All he has to do is push himself away from the table' or 'Doesn't she know that's disgusting?'

Chronic illness

Also important is the effect of chronic illness on the young person's mental health. Asthma, head injury, diabetes, epilepsy and many of the less common chronic physical diseases can contribute to depression. Equally at risk for depression are young people with various learning disabilities or specific neuropsychiatric illnesses, such as attention deficit/hyperactivity disorders (ADD/ADHD), disruptive behaviour disorders, tic disorders, eating disorders, anxiety disorders (including obsessive–compulsive disorder [OCD] and post-traumatic stress disorder [PTSD]), and schizophrenia.

The proportion of overweight and obese children and adolescents in Australia has increased over time, from 21 per cent in 1995 to 25 per cent in 2007/2008. Within this same timeframe, the obesity rate for 5- to 17-year-olds increased from 5 per cent to 8 per cent (Australian Bureau of Statistics [ABS], 2009). In addition to the more publicised comorbid medical conditions associated with excessive weight (such as diabetes, cardiac abnormalities, hypertension and metabolic syndrome), there is the psychological impact of depression and peer discrimination that burden young people who are overweight or obese. Health professionals who work with young people need to be aware of the stressors inherent in living with a chronic illness. See the following two What Every Nurse Should Know features, which provide some of this information for a variety of settings.

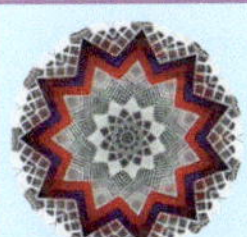

WHAT EVERY NURSE SHOULD KNOW

Allaying the stress of parents and family members of young people

Imagine you are a nurse who works mainly with children and teenagers. In the paediatric acute care or critical care arenas where young people are treated, emotions and fears can run high. Parents and family members frequently feel guilt, anger and helplessness as they watch their adolescent loved ones undergoing invasive procedures. You can help allay their fears as well as obtain much-needed assessment data by talking with them about their stress. Consider comments such as 'This must be very stressful for you. The diagnosis of diabetes must have come as a shock. This is beyond the usual day-to-day stresses and strains. How do you usually cope?' Such questions can yield adaptive measures, and they can draw on or reveal maladaptive measures, such as physical abuse.

LIVED EXPERIENCE

I think it is really important for health professionals to understand and acknowledge that the families of young people living with mental illness are also suffering, probably every bit as much as the young person themselves. In my case, this was true for both my parents and grandparents, and also my younger sister. I am not sure that many nurses and doctors really appreciate the extent of the suffering of the families, which can make it even more distressing when they are told to back off by well-meaning but insensitive health professionals. I recall my mother being told by a doctor that she was a 'helicopter mum'; this term was meant to imply that my mother 'hovered' above me constantly, intruding into my life in every way. I should stress that this was not my view: for me, Mum's support was the most important thing holding me together at that time.

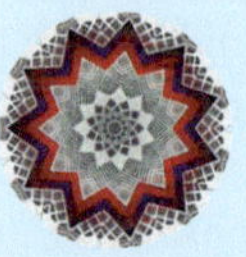

WHAT EVERY NURSE SHOULD KNOW

Helping young people cope with the stress of a cancer diagnosis

Imagine you are working on an oncology ward. Between 1983 and 1993, the incidence of cancer in teenagers and young adults (15 to 29 years of age) increased by 1.5 per cent, but has remained unchanged since that time. Between 1987 and 2007, cancer mortality in 15- to 29-year-olds has decreased steadily (by 1–2 per cent per year). Since 2004, survival rates have been relatively high and continue to improve (Australian Institute of Health and Welfare [AIHW], 2011a). Considerations for physical, cognitive, emotional, social and spiritual strategies are key to helping young people and their families cope during such stressful times. It is also important that you familiarise yourself with evidence-based standards for end-of-life care in circumstances where you may be called upon to assist a young person and their family and friends to prepare for the process of dying. Tending to the physical symptoms of distress (such as dyspnoea, fatigue and nutritional concerns) can provide opportunities for you to help with the psychological and spiritual distress as well.

Psychopharmacology

The value and safety of using psychotropic drugs in the treatment of children and young people—especially in primary care—is controversial. While people living with various mental disorders may benefit from medication, there are serious concerns among mental health professionals regarding the number of prescriptions written for young people in primary care settings without a comprehensive psychological evaluation of symptoms and without sufficient studies of the efficacy and adverse effects of the drugs (Morrato et al., 2010). Of equal concern is the practice of prescribing drugs without offering the benefit of evidence-based, effective and safe treatments, including psychotherapy. There is much evidence suggesting that cognitive behavioural therapy (CBT) and other psychological interventions offer alternative treatments for depression in younger people and adults, especially when considering the implications of receiving unmonitored medications from primary care providers (Naylor et al., 2010). Nurses in various settings can be helpful to young people and their parents by making them aware of the risks as well as the benefits of pharmacological agents, and helping them to make informed decisions about their usage. Up-to-date guides to effective treatments for depression and anxiety in young people can be accessed from beyondblue (www.beyondblue.org.au/get-support/resources).

Developmental theory

An understanding of developmental theory can help in identifying variations in adolescent growth and development processes, and can be a guide in the selection of appropriate interventions. The theories of Freud and Erikson provide considerable insight into the challenges faced by young

LIVED EXPERIENCE

In my mid-teenage years I was commenced on antipsychotic medication for psychotic symptoms. I was treated with a number of atypical antipsychotics, which in each case were accompanied by quite distressing side-effects. For instance, at 16 years of age and with no sexual experience at all, I began producing breast milk while taking a particular antipsychotic medication. When this medication was replaced, the new drug caused significant anxiety. Yet another medication that was tried caused me to put on 30 kilos of weight in three to four months. A number of these medications left me feeling like a 'zombie' for much of the time; these side-effects were occurring alongside the positive psychotic symptoms I was experiencing. Antipsychotic medications do have benefits, but more attention needs to be paid to managing the side-effects more sensitively and effectively. Fortunately, I was able to cease taking antipsychotics some years ago, and now take just one SSRI antidepressant, which I find to be very helpful. For me, medication is an important part of recovery, but needs to be balanced with many other considerations. Medication is not likely to be helpful if it is the only part of the treatment plan.

people in attaining adulthood. These developmental theories are discussed in Chapter 5.

The development of a young person's sense of identity may entail a preoccupation with self-image. It also entails a connection between future role and past experiences. In the search for a new sense of sameness and continuity, many teenagers must repeat the crisis resolutions of earlier years to integrate these past elements and establish the lasting ideals of a final identity. According to Erikson, these crisis periods or stages are reviews of the young person's sense of trust, autonomy, initiative and industry, in that order.

Equally important for a young individual's development is cognition. Piaget's research revealed three stages of cognitive development. The third stage, called *formal operations,* develops between ages 12 and 14, and results in the ability to conceptualise on an adult level. The young person has the capacity to think abstractly, to be self-reflective and to adopt a multi-dimensional perspective on problems.

Humanistic–interactionist theory

As a mental health nurse, you not only need knowledge about psychobiology and developmental theories, you must also integrate humanistic–interactionist principles into your assessments and interventions to develop a trusting, caring interpersonal relationship with the young people with whom you will work. The adolescent developmental period is a time when identity, values and goals are in a state of flux. The immediate situation and the developmental stage are taken into account along with the social, ethnic and cultural factors, family influences and psychodynamic conflicts. To accomplish this, you can explore the meaning of the identified problem or behaviour. See Your Assessment Approach for a list of questions to explore the problem experienced by the young person.

YOUR ASSESSMENT APPROACH
Exploring the meaning of a young person's identified problem or behaviour

Addressing the following questions will help in determining the meaning of a young person's behaviour:

- What meaning does this behaviour or problem hold for the young person?
- What message are they conveying through this behaviour?
- What impact does this problem have on the young person in this developmental stage? Is this a usual or unusual problem or behaviour for the young person's peer group?
- How have resulting changes, if any, affected the young person and their relationships with others?
- What goals does the young person have for the immediate and distant future?
- What personal strengths does the young person have to help deal with this problem?
- What considerations have you and the young person given to other developmental, familial, biological or sociocultural factors involved?

It is insufficient to base nursing interventions solely on adolescent behaviours without a more comprehensive evaluation of the other factors. You may find the following Practice Example to be useful as you gain an increased understanding of young people and what is most important to them.

Practice example

Grappling with life's meaning and purpose during adolescence

Many adults with years of life experience may feel 'settled' with their spiritual beliefs and regular practices, their attitudes about health and healing, and their perspective on optimal living and a peaceful death. For many, turning to their spiritual, religious or philosophical resources is both a proactive and reactive strategy, particularly when faced with an acute stressor, a chronic illness or a life-threatening diagnosis. For young people, life may have offered little such experience or at least few 'hard facts' in dealing with life's challenges. Whereas you may turn to meditation, ritual, yoga or prayer for support during times of stress or illness, the person in their teen years is still grappling with life's meaning and purpose.

If asked, it may be appropriate to offer your beliefs or practices to the wondering teen, but otherwise the best thing you can do in your health provider role is to serve as a positive role model. Rather than imposing your own beliefs or practices on the developing teenager, the most helpful stance you can take is to be objective and receptive to the teen's explorations and experimentation. You can help the curious teen to ponder the interconnectedness of the body with the mind and spirit with some well-considered questions.

You can work to increase the young person's appreciation for physical reactions when emotionally upset. The emotionally distraught teenager can be asked 'Where in your body are you feeling stressed right now?', and then, after a response that could range from a curt reply to a veritable inventory of bodily sensations, the young person can be helped to remember times past when they felt this way. You can ask: 'What worked at that time to improve the upset feelings?' You might encourage deep breathing or progressive muscle relaxation as an immediate means to relaxing the body and to lessening the focus on the emotions. This will improve the teen's sense of confidence in having greater self-control over an upsetting event or situation, at least in the moment before trying to be more rational in designing a plan for intervention.

The young person can be supported to increase their cognitive understanding of events or realisation of emotional stressors that can contribute to physical complaints. Medical sources of pain or discomfort can be ruled out before inviting the teen to consider: 'What was happening just before you realised that your stomach was upset?' To recall an upsetting text message may open a flood of emotional responses from the teen, lessening the need for somatic symptoms and yielding the opportunity for some rational problem-solving.

The teenager can be helped to increase their awareness of positive experiences, daily practices, regular rituals or helpful spiritual resources that have given them support in their daily lives or with unusually threatening events. Try to discover who the young person is before a crisis hits. Explore with them what has given solace and support in the past, and respect their answers. The young individual may have found friendship at a local youth group, or found comfort in talking to a member of the clergy. On the other hand, the teen may tell you that listening to favourite music, immersing oneself in particular television programs, or using social media is as helpful as 'talking it out' with you or another authority figure. You can learn more by allowing the young person to educate you than by believing that you must have all of the answers to teach them at a time of need.

Only by considering all aspects of the young person as a biopsychosocial being can you truly understand the meanings of such behaviours to the individual and intervene effectively.

THE ROLE OF THE NURSE

Nurses working in most areas of health care will come into contract with young people in the course of their work. In many cases, mental health will be an important focus of that work. The goal is to identify distressing or problem-causing behaviour during this difficult period of development, and help maintain the health and wellbeing of the young people with whom you are working. In recent decades, studies have determined that there is a high prevalence of mental illness among Australian youth, but many of those affected do not seek any form of professional help (Jorm, 2015). This combination of high unmet need and poor service access affects up to 1 million young Australians on the threshold of adulthood (McGorry, Hamilton, Goldstone & Rickwood, 2016). Many times these mental health problems are identified in primary care and community health settings. Early intervention for young people with depression and other mental health issues promotes better outcomes (Asarnow & Albright, 2010).

Whether dealing with adolescent stress or with the challenge of a mental disorder, parents and families can experience the gamut of emotions, from feeling mildly frustrated to feeling overwhelmed with the unpredictability of their young family member's behaviours. Collaborative treatment helps families understand why young people behave so differently from adults. Dealing with impulsivity, problem-solving and decision-making can be more productive and less stressful with some guidance.

In outpatient settings

The rapidly changing landscape of mental health service delivery in Australia means that nurses working in most areas of health care are increasingly being called upon to work with children, youth and adults living with mental illness. While psychiatric–mental health nurses provide specialist knowledge and skills in mental health care, all nurses are expected to have acquired and to maintain a high level of mental health literacy.

Nurses working in community and primary care services

Nurses working in community health and other primary care services (e.g. school nurses, nurses working with general practitioners) have many opportunities to observe young people engaging in normal activities in schools, community groups and community health centres. The nurse who knows how to work with young people experiencing common problems will also be adept at identifying obstacles to the effective resolution of emotional problems, and at suggesting treatment. There are many opportunities to counsel young people about solutions to the problems that confront them daily, such as teen pregnancy and substance abuse, and to advise parents, school and community service staff members on their encounters with teens.

> **LIVED EXPERIENCE**
>
> I have had many very positive experiences with nurses, and looking back on it nurses have played an important role in my recovery. To give one example from a time when I was experiencing quite severe psychotic symptoms, I believed 'bugs' were crawling through my skin. One particular nurse used to come and sit with me; he would gently hold my hands so I could not damage my skin by scratching, and would talk about different things to distract me. This helped enormously; apart from limiting the physical damage I would have done scratching my arms, he provided a great deal of emotional support and just plain caring. People can always tell when nurses care; this nurse did, and it made a difference.

As a multicultural nation, there is a steady increase in the number of young people from ethnic minority backgrounds in Australia. The importance of designing culturally sensitive interventions related to a range of health needs is well recognised by policy-makers and practitioners. Key areas of concern include stress management, violence reduction, reproductive health needs, unplanned pregnancies, substance misuse and harm minimisation. One organisation that has been established to provide support services, training and consultancy, and knowledge and advocacy for young people of diverse backgrounds, is the Centre for Multicultural Youth (CMY). Organisations such as the CMY provide a resource for nurses working with young people and their families in any area of health care. The CMY has produced a Good Practice Guide on Youth Work in the Family Context, which can be accessed at: cmy.net.au/sites/default/files/publication/Youth%20work%20family%20context%202011.pdfs

Within the school School is one of the most influential experiences in a young person's life outside the home. Teenage people spend more waking time in school activities than in any other activity, and many of their successes, problems and conflicts are played out in the school setting.

The role of the school nurse includes early recognition of and support for troubled young people at school. Mental health promotion is a key aspect of such work. The closeness of the relationship between the nurse and the young person, and the comprehensive and holistic nature of nursing assessments, may be helpful in exploring areas of conflict in a distressed or disruptive student. Health promotion and early intervention are key aspects of the role of the school nurse. Box 21.1 outlines problems in the school setting that might warrant early intervention.

The Australian Institute of Health and Welfare (AIHW) reports regularly on the health and wellbeing of young people

Box 21.1 Student problems in the school setting that call for early intervention

- Antisocial behaviours such as stealing, setting fires, bullying others
- Avoidance behaviour
- Chronic illness
- Depression
- Disruptive classroom behaviour
- Substance abuse
- Excessive daydreaming
- Hypochondriasis
- Learning difficulties
- Poor school performance or a dramatic shift in school performance
- Temper tantrums

in Australia. The 2011 report (AIHW, 2011b) considered a range of health concerns for young people, including:

- injuries
- tobacco use
- alcohol and other substance use
- sexually transmitted diseases and the use of contraceptives
- unhealthy dietary behaviours
- physical inactivity.

The key trends reported in the AIHW report (2011b) are set out in Box 21.2.

In various health care settings, the work undertaken by nurses will involve contact with the families of young people. Being a parent of a teenager can be challenging for parents. As the child grows into adulthood, with all its perplexing questions and problems, parents normally worry about the child's safety and wellbeing. They may feel rejected because they are no longer needed in the same way. Because many parents of relatively normal young people share this plight, they can usually find receptive listeners who will give them comfort and support.

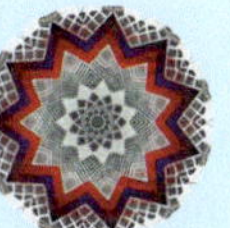

WHAT EVERY NURSE SHOULD KNOW

Teen pregnancy

Nurses working in various health care locations will come into contact with young women who are pregnant. While teen pregnancy has been identified as an ongoing issue by the Australian Institute of Health and Welfare, teen fertility rates in Australia declined from 55.5 per 1000 births in 1971 to 14.6 per 1000 births in 2013. The decision to become a parent involves various personal, social and cultural considerations, and the nature of both parenting and families has changed significantly in recent decades. Raising children now involves a diversity of arrangements, including single parenting and same-sex parenting. In some cases the family may be supportive, in other circumstances less so.

Abortion and adoption are other possibilities to be considered by the pregnant teen and possibly her family. In most parts of Australia, abortions are performed in private clinics, and the associated costs are high and increasing. Abortion laws vary across state and territory jurisdictions in Australia, and nurses should be familiar with the legal issues pertaining to their specialty areas in order to fully address the health and psychological needs of the young women with whom they are working (and if appropriate their partners and families). Organisations such as Children by Choice (www.childrenbychoice.org.au), which is based in Queensland, provide reproduction-choice-related counselling, information and referral for women.

The problems faced by parents of young people living with mental illness are more complicated. Many of these parents may have a strong sense of failure because their children did not turn out 'right'. They may experience guilt, frustration and helplessness if their child is admitted to hospital. They may also feel confused and resentful if offered advice, especially if it is presented in a non-collaborative manner. All such experiences and feelings are likely to be intensified by stigma.

Box 21.2 The health and wellbeing of young Australians

Areas of improvement

- Youth mortality rates are declining (largely due to declining injury rates).
- Asthma prevalence and hospitalisations are declining.
- Cancer survival rates are increasing.
- Tobacco smoking and substance use have declined since 1998 (48 per cent decline for each).
- Most sexually-active Year 10 and 12 students use contraception.

Areas of concern

- Indigenous young people have poorer outcomes in many areas (e.g. death rates over twice as high).
- Incidence of insulin-dependent diabetes is increasing (41 per cent increase since 2001).
- Sexually transmitted disease notifications have increased four-fold (mostly related to *Chlamydia* notifications).
- High death rates for road transport accidents and suicide, particularly for males.
- Over one-third of young people are overweight or obese, and less than half meet physical activity guidelines.
- Most young people (95 per cent) do not consume the recommended amounts of fruit and vegetables.
- High proportions of young people are drinking alcohol at risky or high-risk levels for short-term harm (30 per cent) and long-term harm (12 per cent), and using illicit substances (19 per cent).
- Teenage birth rate compares unfavourably with other OECD countries (22nd out of 26 countries), and is five times as high among young Indigenous women. (AIHW, 2011b)

Unlike the parents of other young people, these parents may have no one in whom to confide, either because they lack the support and understanding of others, or because their own self-reproach prevents them from seeking out confidantes.

Meetings with family members may be indicated if the young person's role in the family seems to compound the problems presented in the school or agency setting. An important part of the problem-solving process is organising initial interviews with parents and family members. The information gathered during these meetings can be used to determine whether the problems stem from difficulties posed by the larger system (the family) and, if so, whether a family intervention is indicated (refer to Chapter 24).

It is important that compassion and understanding be shown for the parents' dilemma without blaming them or their offspring. Parents will be more receptive to family meetings and to exploring their part in the young person's problems if they sense that the health care team will be respectful and support them. Stress and psychological symptoms evidenced by parents can serve as markers for emotional or behavioural problems in young family members.

Any tendency by staff to feel self-righteous or superior to the young person's parents is an obstacle to effective treatment. Such feelings are readily communicated to parents, and can only validate their fear of blame and increase their reluctance to participate in the treatment with their loved one. At the same time, it is important to resist any temptation to over-identify with the parents—this inadvertently perpetuates the family system's problems. The young person and the family need a neutral party who can play an objective, knowledgeable and supportive role in helping them change. The young person's chances for resolving the underlying conflicts and maintaining a healthy life are much more difficult if the family system remains unchanged.

Parents, school and agency staff must understand the objectives and goals of treatment to appreciate the progress the young person has made, and avoid reinforcing the previously maladaptive behaviour. The following Practice Example illustrates the problems that arise when parents and school authorities, particularly those who must deal directly with behavioural problems in the classroom, lack psychological sophistication.

The siblings of a young person living with mental illness may experience many different feelings. Sometimes they share in the parents' guilt and shame. Sometimes, however, they are pleased and relieved when the 'troublemaker' is out of the family and hospitalised. The same understanding given to the parents should be extended to the siblings, helping them to see how each member of the family contributes to the problem. If the troubled young person is hospitalised, another member of the family, usually a sibling, may assume the role of the 'bad' or 'sick' person in the family, because the identified 'bad' person is no longer at home. It is important to be aware of this possibility. In many instances the main responsibilities of non-mental health specialist nurses will be to undertake an initial assessment of the family's needs and refer the family to an appropriate service.

In addressing the needs of a young person living with mental illness, it may be necessary to consider various types of intervention. In some cases, an informal discussion is all that is warranted. In other cases, problems may be identified that require considerable attention. For problems that do not threaten the safety of the young person or the family, sometimes a period of unsuccessful treatment is necessary to determine that outpatient therapy is ineffective and that hospitalisation is indicated. Before making such a recommendation, you need to establish a trusting relationship with the young person and their parents. The national depression and anxiety initiative beyondblue maintains an up-to-date website that families can access for information on youth mental health and sources of support; beyondblue can be accessed at www.beyondblue.org.au. Batyr is another organisation that provides support for young people experiencing mental health problems. Batyr can be accessed at http://www.batyr.com.au/

Practice example

Josh, a 13-year-old boy, was brought into the general practice surgery in which you work as a practice mental health nurse, because he had become increasing introverted and isolated. At school, Josh made little contact with either his peers or his teachers, and rarely spoke unless addressed directly. After he had spent three months seeing you and a registered psychologist, Josh started seeking out his form teacher of his own accord to talk about his depression and the problems he had been having in his family. Both the form teacher and Josh's family believed this to be an indication that his difficulties had worsened; his family complained to the general practitioner about what they saw as the failure of his treatment. Not only had Josh's parents and the form teacher misunderstood the goals of treatment and the behaviours expected to come with change, they were also uncomfortable with the changes in behaviour and with the implications of these changes for their relationships with him.

LIVED EXPERIENCE

One of the things I have come to realise is the extent to which my having been unwell affected my younger sister. At the time my being unwell resulted in our family having to move back to Australia from overseas. For my sister this meant the loss of friends, changing schools, and many other unexpected and unwelcome life changes. I now understand the distress this must have caused her; she blamed me for much of this without realising the extent to which I was unwell. I suspect that most young people in similar circumstances would react in much the same way. We have worked through this in recent years, and now have a shared understanding of what happened and why it was necessary. I could not ask for a better support.

In the inpatient setting

Admission into an inpatient facility may be indicated under the following circumstances:

- if the young person is unable to control impulsivity
- if the degree of destructive or antisocial behaviour escalates beyond normal limits
- if the young person cannot form meaningful, stable relationships within the everyday environment (as in the case of family dysfunction).

The existence of any of these conditions warrants counselling or professional treatment. A combination of two or more is likely to make treatment on an outpatient basis very difficult and indicate a possible need for hospital treatment.

A young person experiencing the symptoms of mental illness may be admitted to hospital for the following reasons:

- to provide additional structure within which to handle the physically and psychologically challenging elements of the young person's behaviour
- to remove the young person from the stresses of a disrupted family environment
- to offer opportunities for supporting existing ego strengths and promoting whatever ability the young person has for forming relationships.

However, it is important to note that, while the criteria for admission of a young person to a mental health inpatient facility (whether it be a specialist child and adolescent mental health service, or an adult mental health service) can vary within and between jurisdictions in Australia, a number of key principles apply. These include:

- care should be provided in the least restrictive alternative, and take account of safety considerations
- care should be provided as close as possible to home and social support networks
- care should be developmentally and clinically appropriate.

An example of an Australian policy governing the hospitalisation of children and adolescents for mental health reasons—NSW Health Policy PD2011-016 Children and Adolescents with Mental Health Problems Requiring Inpatient Care—can be accessed from http://www1.health.nsw.gov.au/policies/pd/2011/pdf/PD2011_016.pdf (last accessed on 2016, September 26).

Your Intervention Strategies on the following page will help you in supporting parents to be more effective.

Hospitalisation is sometimes sought for young people because their ideas are strange or threatening to their families, or because the responsible authorities seek to punish what is seen to be unacceptable behaviour. The results can be disastrous. It is thus important to make accurate assessments and to implement early treatment when indicated. Nurses can play a crucial role in making assessments, undertaking appropriate interventions, and educating parents, teachers and school officials to recognise these needs.

LIVED EXPERIENCE

I have spent a great deal of time in both adolescent and adult mental health inpatient services, both in Australia and overseas. Overall, this was a terrifying experience: I was already anxious when admitted to hospital and experiencing psychotic symptoms, and found myself in close proximity to other people who frightened me; was experiencing symptoms I didn't understand; was not sure of what was happening to me; and had decided that I wasn't going to get better. As time went on I started to think of the unit as 'home'; I spent more than six months as an inpatient, and then had a series of re-admissions. Given the amount of time I was on the unit, it did start to feel like home, and I found the nurses very caring. So over time and with increased familiarity, being admitted seemed much more comfortable, but by then the outside world had become frightening.

Registered nurses in a general hospital setting

Young people with emotional problems may have symptoms of physical illness, and as a result may be admitted to a general hospital setting for evaluation and treatment. Registered nurses in medical and surgical units may thus have opportunities to work with and reach out to young people living with mental illness.

Psychiatric–mental health nurses in a general hospital setting

Psychiatric–mental health nurses working in a psychiatric inpatient unit of a general hospital may be consulted by other nursing staff about young people with mental illness who have been admitted to general medical or surgical units. Some general hospitals have advanced-practice registered nurses who are clinical nurse consultants or nurse practitioners in consultation/liaison mental health nursing roles in acute care areas such as emergency departments.

Registered nurses in a psychiatric setting

Psychiatric–mental health nurses working in inpatient settings also have numerous opportunities to observe and assess the family dynamics among the young person's family members and to possibly intervene. Nurses involved in working with families can perceive maladaptive ways of relating and take direct steps to work towards change. However, it is crucial that such work is undertaken within the structured format of an intervention plan that has been developed by the treatment team.

Because inpatient nursing entails around-the-clock care, the nurse has the responsibility to maintain the therapeutic

YOUR INTERVENTION STRATEGIES **Encouraging more effective parenting behaviours**

Parent behaviour

- Initiates loud verbal arguments during visits with the young person.

Interventions

- Stop the immediate behaviour, pointing out the disruptiveness to the unit.
- Bring the disruptive parental behaviour to the attention of the treatment team to enable interventions to be offered to resolve differences and learn more adaptive ways of relating.
- Suggest to the treatment team that the family be contacted for one or more of the following:
  - staff will monitor visits
  - family will bring up potentially volatile topics only within the structure of family meetings, and not on the unit during visits
  - staff will intervene if arguments ensue on the unit
  - staff may limit visiting time on the unit.

Parent behaviour

- History of physical violence against the young person.

Interventions

- Monitor parent visits with the young person on the unit.
- Limit or deny leave with parents until progress is demonstrated.
- Depending on the parent's level of self-control, refuse visiting privileges with the young person until progress is seen in family relating.

Parent behaviour

- Unable to set limits with the young person during visits (is adversely influenced by manipulative attempts, tolerates verbal abuse, etc).

Interventions

- Intervene if demands or behaviour could lead to physical harm, unit rule-breaking or other negative results.
- Bring the problem to the attention of the treatment team.
- Role-model appropriate and effective limit-setting with the young person, if necessary.
- Offer to discuss the situation with the parents and the young person, if desirable in the immediate situation.
- Offer emotional support to the parent who needs to talk.

Parent behaviour

- Limited interaction with the young person during unit visits.

Interventions

- Initiate discussion between the young person and family members related to visit and treatment goals.
- Communicate observations to the treatment team.
- Initiate discussion with the parents to allow exploration of the difficulty, if desired.
- Suggest that family members and the young person discuss the problem in family meetings.
- Plan outings or special-occasion celebrations to include family, if appropriate.

environment. The role of the nurse working in any inpatient setting includes the following:

- maintaining physical and psychological safety of the unit
- setting verbal and physical limits on the behaviour of the young people admitted to the unit
- establishing meaningful one-to-one relationships with the young people admitted to the unit
- identifying strengths and promoting more adaptive coping skills in the young people admitted to the unit
- role-modeling socially acceptable behaviours
- participating in group interventions and other structured activities.

The importance of milieu

Many authors have described the importance of the therapeutic environment, indicating the strong influence of the treatment environment on the treatment outcome. (For a more detailed discussion, see Chapter 9.) Because of the importance young people place on peer acceptance, their overwhelming uncertainties and fears, and their ever-changing behaviours and attitudes about identity, their chances for success in inpatient treatment are increased by a peer group setting. Much has been written about the value of the therapeutic environment in dealing with the problems experienced by young people, including substance abuse and similar destructive activities. Without the social interaction and living–learning situations provided by the peer group, psychotherapy may be ineffective.

Of course the nature of the psychotherapy, the treatment modalities and intervention strategies will be largely determined by the theoretical base of the treatment setting and the training of the staff. Specifically, most youth mental health units use behavioural management principles as the basis for work with young people. Units that specialise in treating specific disorders or problems use relevant treatment modalities that studies have shown to be effective. As one example, the use of CBT has been used to treat young people with depression, anxiety, PTSD and eating disorders. Another example is dialectical behaviour therapy (DBT), which has been used successfully in individual and group therapy with young people with chronic suicidal thoughts or self-harm behaviours. See Chapter 25 for a more complete discussion of cognitive behavioural interventions.

The therapeutic environment can provide valuable experiences for the following reasons:

- Young people more readily hear and accept limits from peers than from adults.

- Young people more readily respond to feedback, both negative and positive, from peers than from adults.
- Shared goals and objectives facilitate group processes and the development of cohesion among young group members.
- Group interaction allows for the expression of appropriate feelings, and identification with peers with similar feelings.
- Group interaction provides opportunities for learning how to develop relationships with others.
- Group structure allows for the testing of new, more adaptive behaviours.
- Young people receive feedback from the peer group, and have the opportunity to give feedback in a supportive environment.
- The group format provides an opportunity to work out specific issues of conflict with adult group leaders while receiving the support and understanding of peers.

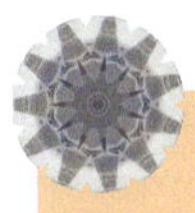

NURSING PROCESS
Young people

Young people present behaviours and problems unique to their developmental stage. Without knowledge and understanding about potentially difficult areas, nurses may respond with confusion, anger and even hostility, which may cause feelings of frustration and failure for both themselves and the young people with whom they are working. The following pages contain numerous examples of either typical behaviours expected of the 'normal' young person or problem behaviours that may provide the impetus for referral to a treatment setting, or both. In many situations, the focus will be on the issues encountered in working with young people. That information is provided in the assessment section. Situations that represent an identified problem necessitating treatment are discussed under planning and implementation.

Assessment

It is important to keep in mind that over the course of normal development, children and teenagers may experience symptoms of anxiety, dysphoria, oppositionality or conduct disorder. On the other hand, there are factors that can contribute to missed or inaccurate diagnoses in the assessment of a young person:

- symptom overlap, which can blur diagnostic boundaries
- effects of normal development on symptom presentation
- high rates of comorbidity in youth with mental illness
- perception of informants (i.e. parents/guardians, teachers or other family members).

Moreover, two other factors that can minimise the effectiveness and comprehensive nature of an adequate assessment in the young person are:

- the impact of managed care, with its emphasis on brevity of contact in inpatient and outpatient settings
- the emphasis in some clinical training on rigid adherence to DSM criteria without the exploration of developmental stages, risk and protective factors, current stressors, temperament, cultural issues and/or family dynamics.

Accurate and comprehensive assessments are more likely to be obtained by viewing the young person as a biopsychosocial being. Only by integrating knowledge from biology, psychology, humanistic–interactionist theory and a young person's lived experience are you likely to begin to understand what a particular behaviour might mean to them. If you can remember your own experiences as a youth—the conflicts and uncertainty, as well as the elation and the triumphs—you will better appreciate the turmoil. It is equally important that you discover who the young person is as an individual.

The meanings of behaviour, values and actions can vary from person to person, and may not reflect the meanings or values that you hold. For example, the person who has trouble with competitive feelings may be reluctant to accept an invitation to play a game of Trivial Pursuit. And because young people are developmentally between childhood and adulthood, they frequently have the feelings and choices of adulthood without an adult's abilities in verbal discourse and impulse control. As a result, young people may 'act out' feelings and decisions non-verbally, in a childlike way. This is particularly true of the young person who is having difficulty regulating their emotions. In settings where tension and anxiety are typically high, such as the emergency department of a hospital, the high emotionality of a young person can be potentiated. See What Every Nurse Should Know about working with young people when they are upset.

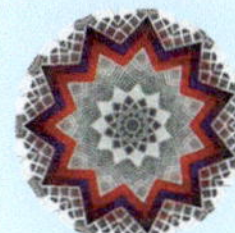

WHAT EVERY NURSE SHOULD KNOW

Working with young people who are upset

Imagine you are a nurse working in an emergency department (ED). If the hospital is often a frightening place for adults, you can imagine what the ED is like for a young person. Young people come to the ED seeking help, as family members of a person seeking help, or as friends of a person seeking help. In fact, if there is an injury or accident at the local school, a group of teens may show up to support their injured or sick schoolmate. Whether seeking help themselves, or supporting another person seeking help, young people may behave dramatically and exaggerate the nature of a problem. You may find it helpful to deal with the upset young person by suggesting deep-breathing or de-escalation techniques. Having teens focus on their breathing can provide a focus for their anxiety, allow them to concentrate, and increase their oxygen level. When they are able to 'hear' what you have to say, you should then ask them questions with simple answers, while also encouraging positive expectations. An example might be: 'Have you felt this way before?' If the answer is yes, ask: 'What did you do to help yourself at that time?'

Acting out

The concept of acting out is complex. The term has been used to describe a variety of behaviours, ranging from antisocial, destructive acts to unconscious impulses expressed in action rather than in symbolic words or symptoms. Acting out may include destructive actions and seemingly undefinable behaviours. The term describes a re-creation of the person's life experiences, relationships with significant others, and resulting unresolved conflicts.

These are all components of what might be thought of as the person's *life script*, which unfolds as they relate, react and behave in accustomed ways. Through observation of, and interaction with, the person, you can uncover the meanings that various behaviours and actions hold for the individual. For example, the child who has assumed the 'black sheep' role in the family seeks to re-create that familiar role with others outside the home, particularly in the inpatient setting. The following Practice Example illustrates one young woman's relationship with her parents as replayed with the staff on an inpatient unit.

Practice example

Xanthe is 14 years old. She has been on the unit for six days. She is an attractive, engaging young person, who has been friendly with both staff and people admitted to the unit. Xanthe has been on the periphery of several rule-breaking incidents, but has not been directly involved. She has begun to establish close ties with Jim, a nurse, and engages in frequent lengthy discussions with him about her innermost feelings and fears. One evening she candidly talks to him about the callous way in which she was treated by one of the female nurses, in regard to a gynaecological problem. Xanthe says with undisguised fear and embarrassment that she is afraid the situation will repeat itself. She expresses great respect for Jim's knowledge and style, and asks him to attend to any subsequent problems himself so that she does not have to interact with the other nurse again.

The implications for treatment are many. The most important factors for Jim to consider are what meaning Xanthe's behaviour has for her and what would be the most therapeutically effective way to deal with the situation. The presenting problems and the expectation that Xanthe will act out previous conflicts and life scripts have provided Jim with information on which to consider options for intervention. The attempt to manipulate and win over the nurse, and the need for nurses to examine their own behaviour and motivations, are discussed in detail later in this chapter.

Practice example

In the previous Practice Example, Jim recognises that Xanthe may be unconsciously acting out her life script by re-creating her relationships with her parents with Jim and one of the female nurses on the unit. Jim remembers that Xanthe's home situation is chaotic. Xanthe's mother and father frequently fight over who is the better parent. Jim surmises that Xanthe also plays a part in these fights. Jim recognises the 'pull' from Xanthe to feel that only he can adequately handle the situation. The present situation seems to indicate that he is about to be pitted against the female nurse, just as Xanthe perhaps plays one parent against the other. Jim responds by reiterating his concern for her dilemma, and suggesting that Xanthe speak with the female nurse about the situation that is causing her concern.

In this example, it is possible that Xanthe is attempting to re-create her home situation, using two of the nurses to re-enact the roles of her parents. Had Jim been drawn into playing the father's role in the script, he would have re-created the family's conflict on the unit. The ideal solution is for staff to interrupt this pathological process by substituting a healthier way of resolving the problem. Thus, Jim does not react with compliance or with anger to Xanthe's attempts. Instead, he recognises the significance of her behaviour and deals with the situation in a concerned yet healthy way, suggesting a resolution to the immediate problem that demonstrates respect for both Xanthe and the female nurse's abilities to resolve the conflict.

Such situations are commonplace when working with young people. They require nursing staff to evaluate the person's psychodynamics and psychopathology, as well as their own inner feelings and behaviour. For these reasons, it is imperative to identify transference and countertransference issues, and to discuss them with your clinical supervisor. Transference and countertransference are discussed in Chapter 9, but these situations are not limited to the inpatient setting. This fact alone obliges you to be alert in observing and assessing verbal and non-verbal communication, and to understand your own feelings and behaviour in order to make accurate assessments and appropriate interventions. In this way, you will be most effective when working with young people. An illustration of how research can help shape interventions to maximise resilience in a young person who is acting out a self-destructive life script is in the following Evidence-based Practice.

Communication

Communication with young people can be challenging. To become proficient in this area, you must accept and understand the following:

- Young people tend to act out feelings and conflicts rather than verbalise them.
- Young people have an unconventional language of their own.
- Young people, especially those that are distressed, may use profanity frequently.
- Many clues can be obtained simply by observing a young person's behaviour, dress or environment.

If you learn the verbal and non-verbal communication skills discussed in Chapter 9, you can use them comfortably and naturally in communicating with young people.

Non-verbal cues Young people may give many non-verbal cues to their specific emotional struggles, underlying confusion or transitory moods. A glance around their rooms or a brief study of their dress may tell you more than what several

EVIDENCE-BASED PRACTICE

Maximising resilience

Danny is a slightly underweight 15-year-old boy who was admitted to the local child and adolescent unit after treatment in the emergency department for an 'accidental' overdose of his insulin. After admitting to his parents that he had intentionally drawn up too much insulin in a suicide attempt 'to get what's coming anyway', he was admitted to the unit for observation and treatment.

Your initial assessment revealed that Danny's depression and guilt seem to have evolved over time, as he endured the loss of several relatives close to him, who died following complications from diabetes. He fears for himself, and also feels guilty for 'surviving' the illness that has taken his loved ones. Talking to him and his family about his diabetes reveals a similarly fatalistic attitude among his family members.

Your consideration of options for intervention is based on current research results. For example, in your review of studies of building resilience in young people, you noted that optimism is a trait that contributes to resilience, and has been identified as the most influential adolescent cognitive factor to moderate the effects of life stressors. Danny's parents commented that they had always regarded him as the 'most positive' of their three children. Prior to puberty (his female cousin with diabetes died at age 12), he had been active in all sports and was 'a cool kid in every way'. You recall that the design and delivery of an intervention to maximise resilience in young people requires gender-specific strategies that are attractive, engaging and easily accessible. You ask his parents to bring in pictures of Danny when he was active in sports. You encourage him to talk about his exploits, and remind him about his physical abilities and competitive nature. You encourage him to be conscientious about managing his diabetes, while inviting him to envision his goals for the future after high school. You incorporate these values and resiliency-building interventions in the nursing care plan and in all treatment team meetings.

Furthermore, your readings and experiences have yielded information regarding the financial and staffing limits of community and school resources. As a result, you understand that local resources may tend to be problem-focused and disease-oriented, because they do not have the funds or time to provide preventive or creative activities. You expect to put a plan in motion that will use pre-existing resources as well as connect Danny with new supports, perhaps even identifying a program or resource to enhance Danny's school and social environments.

With the help of one of the social workers, you set up a 'surprise' visit from a local sports celebrity, an adult who has managed his diabetes since childhood. Danny is thrilled to meet him, but, more importantly, is surprised to learn of his lifelong diabetes self-management and to see first-hand the positive results of his efforts. Over the next few weeks of his treatment, Danny demonstrates renewed optimism and displays a new-found autonomy and self-assurance in his diabetes self-management skills. Moreover, he agrees to explore serving as a mentor to younger kids in a local diabetes camp who might feel the way he 'used to'.

This set of multiple intervention strategies is based on the following research:

Macgowan, M. J., & Engle, B. (2010). Evidence for optimism: Behavior therapies and motivational interviewing in adolescent substance abuse treatment. *Child and Adolescent Psychiatric Clinics of North America, 19*(3), 527–545.

Yancey, A. K., Grant, D., Kurosky, S., Kravitz-Wirtz, N., & Mistry, R. (2010, August 26). Role modeling, risk, and resilience in California adolescents. *Journal of Adolescent Health Online.* Retrieved from http://www.jahonline.org/article/S1054-139X(10)00227-2/-fulltext

CRITICAL THINKING QUESTIONS

1. How would knowing how a young person has coped with earlier problems in life help you to design strategies for intervention?
2. Would an increased awareness of ways to be resilient make a difference in a young person's life? How?
3. Why would involving others in Danny's goal of increased resilience be helpful?
4. Of what value are reminders of earlier active times in Danny's life? Would they be discouraging rather than encouraging?

direct questions would elicit. Sometimes the cues are obvious. A young person who wears a coat around the unit may be planning to run away. Other less obvious behaviours, which are often outside the young person's conscious awareness or control, can also yield vital information. A sudden escalation of horseplay among the boys around bedtime is an example. You might speculate on whether this behaviour is an expression of anxiety related to sexual identity and fears of homosexual feelings. Interactionist theory holds that the adolescent boy's new-found sexual feelings and changing body image provide unfamiliar ways of relating to members of his own gender. As a result, he regresses to pre-adolescent behaviour, which served him well in handling close feelings then, but now proves inappropriate. In this instance, firm limit-setting is in order. Avoid interpreting the behaviour or paying undue attention to the specifics. (Testing and limit-setting are discussed later in the chapter.)

Slang and obscenities Young people may create a language all their own. This takes some understanding and acceptance. In seeking their identity, young people establish a form of communication unique to the group. To gain acceptance into this world, the adult must accept the need of young people to use ambiguous (to the adult) yet specific (to young people) terms to express themselves. In many cases, it may be necessary for you to communicate with young people by using their slang.

This slang often includes obscene and profane words. This is particularly true of young people who are distressed, who have an especially difficult time expressing anger and fear appropriately. The words they use may reveal the nature

COMMUNICATION

The person using swearing or obscenities

YOUNG PERSON: 'Hey, jerk. When is dinner served around this hell hole?' [Other young people on the unit are snickering in the background.]

NURSE RESPONSE 1: [with an exaggerated look of surprise] 'Matt, you're new to the unit. I will give you information about the unit and about mealtimes, but you need to understand something first. Swearing is not an acceptable way to get to know anyone here. I expect you to treat me with respect, as I will you. Now I'll show you your room and you can put your things away.' [The nurse then proceeds with Matt to a less public space, where he talks with him without the other young people for an audience.]

RATIONALE: A person who is newly admitted may be attempting to over-compensate for his anxiety and fears as 'the new kid' with bravado and intimidation. Giving information may allay his anxiety while verbally setting limits on his provocative behaviour, avoiding escalation and the need for physical controls.

NURSE RESPONSE 2: [with an obvious look of surprise] 'Matt, you need to learn about the unit. That includes information about acceptable behaviours as well as mealtimes. Let that be the last time you address me or anyone else here in that way. If you have trouble controlling your behaviour, we can assist you in taking a time out until you're able to control yourself and are ready to be with the rest of the group. Ellen and I will show you to your room, and you can ask us any other questions there.' [The two nurses escort Matt to his room, soliciting information as they evaluate his reactions and degree of control.]

RATIONALE: The young person was newly admitted to the unit. Immediate limit-setting and spelling out of consequences may deter further provocative behaviour to assert domination over staff and intimidate others on the unit.

of the emotional conflict. For example, a young teenage male grappling with his sexual identity and aggressive feelings may resort to sexually graphic words when he feels anxious or afraid. You may sometimes find it productive to use similar words to give explanations or to clarify communication. Understandably, some nurses have difficulty tolerating profane or sexually graphic language. However, you must evaluate the person's underlying reasons for using such language, to help them understand their feelings. Only then can you encourage them to use more appropriate means of expression. If a young person senses that the reason you want them to speak more appropriately is only to make you, the nurse, feel more comfortable, the end result will not be satisfactory. Communication: The Person Using Swearing or Obscenities further demonstrates two examples of this. See, also, Stone, McMillan and Hazelton (2015) for a review of swearing and cursing in health settings.

The young person living with mental illness often has symptoms of disturbed communication, which can affect all realms of daily living, particularly in relationships with peers, family members and non-parental authority figures. Giving information is one way you can help decrease communication deficits and facilitate relationships with others. Other nursing behaviours are outlined in the planning and implementation section.

Confidentiality An emerging body of research underscores the importance of discussing confidentiality with a young person. There will be health concerns, thoughts and feelings that the young person will want to keep private. Assurances of confidentiality will increase the likelihood that they will disclose sensitive personal information to you. Confidentiality, however, cannot be unconditional, in that some information, such as sexual abuse, must be reported by law, and other information, such as a suicide plan, must be discussed with the rest of the treatment team and significant others. In discussing confidentiality with the young person, one way of clarifying this dilemma might be to simply state: 'What you and I discuss is confidential. However, you need to know that *if it means harm to you or to someone else* [emphasise these words], it will be important for me to talk it over with other members of the treatment team, who will likely want to discuss it with your parents. If that happens, I will first discuss it with you to determine the best way to present our concerns to others.'

Anger and hostility

Expressions of anger and hostility are common on a youth mental health unit. Anger expressed verbally usually takes the form of swearing. How effectively you deal with expressions of anger and hostility depends on how effectively you handle your own angry or hostile feelings. You will compromise your effectiveness as a nurse if you are uncomfortable with expressions of anger or hostility, or view anger and hostility as negative or to be avoided at all costs.

Nurse's self-assessment A subject that is rarely considered is anger felt and expressed by the nurse towards the person for whom they are caring. The general focus on the person's need for understanding and good care seems to make it unacceptable to display negative feelings towards the person receiving treatment. In the nursing care of young people, however, a constant all-giving and all-accepting attitude by the nurse, particularly during times of testing, would be not only non-therapeutic but also illogical and dishonest, and young people need honest feedback. Provocative behaviour can sometimes be used to test a nurse's response or to evoke an angry reaction. Pretending that you are not angry in such a situation is as undesirable for treatment as it would be to pretend that you are fond of the young person when you are not.

Being honest about your feelings is a prime prerequisite in establishing and maintaining meaningful and productive relationships with young people. This does not mean that you should vent all your thoughts or impulses. Be aware of your reactions, and use good judgment in handling them. This is also an opportunity to model adult modes of anger expression. The questions in Self-awareness: A Self-awareness Inventory for Working With Young People will help you assess your own ways of dealing with anger.

Anxiety and resistance

All young people are likely to feel anxious as they experience change and inner turmoil in adapting to a new identity. The anxiety evidenced by distressed young people in treatment can indicate many other things. The changes required are much more threatening to young people living with mental illness.

> **SELF-AWARENESS**
>
> **A self-awareness inventory for working with young people**
>
> To increase self-awareness about your own way of dealing with anger, ask yourself these questions:
>
> - What kinds of things make me angry?
> - How do I deal with my anger? Do I tend to ignore or hide it, or do I show that I am angry?
> - Do I sometimes use swearing or act out my feelings in a physical way? How do I feel about others who do this?
> - What do I think about how I handle anger? Am I proud of the way I handle anger?
> - How do I react to others when they are angry?
>
> To increase self-awareness about your tendency to be seduced or manipulated, ask yourself these questions:
>
> - Is this person's friendliness compromising the professional role boundaries between us and 'personalising' our relationship?
> - Do I feel compelled to respond in a personal rather than a therapeutic way, possibly revealing information about my own life and lifestyle?
> - Do I feel uncomfortable with the person's flattering comments or probing questions?
> - Do I tend to forget that this person is a consumer of the service I work in?
> - Is the person encouraging me to keep secrets from other staff or to 'side' with the them against other staff?
>
> To increase self-awareness about your own sexual attitudes and feelings, ask yourself these questions:
>
> - How would I describe my youth as it related to my developing sexuality?
> - What do I remember about the development and changes in my body?
> - How did I feel about these changes?
> - How would I describe my teenage relationships with members of my own sex?
> - How would I describe my teenage relationships with members of the opposite sex?
> - What events stand out in my mind when I recall my sexual experiences during my teen years?
> - How have these past relationships, events and feelings influenced me today?

If treatment is to be successful, people must look at the meaning of their behaviour and must change many of their earlier interactional patterns. This can be frightening. For example, it may be more comfortable to play the role of the 'bad seed' or 'bad kid', with its known pitfalls and expectations, than to attempt a change that entails many uncertainties and unknowns.

Young people may feel threatened and anxious when the nurse does not act according to their expectations, because they must then find other ways of handling the situation. They must also deal with the anxiety. This anxiety may be channelled into a game of 'cops and robbers', as the young person once again assumes a familiar role and maintains the negative or unhealthy image. The anxiety caused by unfamiliar roles is dissipated by further testing and acting out. This should not be taken as an indication that therapy is not working. It may indicate that the young person needs to move ahead more slowly with insightful discoveries, and needs your support to do so.

It is important to keep in mind that 'opening up' in a trusting way does not hold the same positive promise that it might for you. Young people who have been rejected or have experienced loss following close relationships in the past will likely be wary of your expressions of interest or concern, and will be cautious about repeating such experiences. They may respond to you with testing behaviours, anger and mistrust, or outright rejection. Those who expect rejection gain some control over the relationship if they reject others before being rejected themselves.

Nurse's self-assessment Sometimes nurses find it difficult to allow young people to grapple with their anxieties and fears. At other times, you may not recognise the behaviour as a symptom of anxiety or depression. The following Practice Example demonstrates the value of a comprehensive assessment, of exploring all possible reasons for a young person's resistance to your efforts, before implementing action.

> **Practice example**
>
> Kate was the quietest and most aloof person admitted to the unit. She had isolated herself from the others during the week that followed admission, and avoided conversing with staff members outside meetings. One evening she seemed unusually receptive to the new nurse, Ellie, who was able to interest her in a sewing project. Ellie, who was a new graduate, felt pleased that Kate had responded warmly to her during their time together. The next day, Kate did not speak to Ellie and seemed to avoid her at all costs. Later, Ellie noticed that the dress Kate had been sewing had been torn into shreds and stuffed into the wastepaper basket. Ellie took this personally. She felt deeply hurt and rejected.
>
> In her discussion with her supervisor, Ellie expressed her disappointment and anger. Her supervisor observed that, although the good time and feelings that Ellie and Kate had shared the evening before were genuine, Kate had not experienced many such times before with her parents or other adults. She suggested that Kate was possibly angry with Ellie for pointing out what she, Kate, had missed out on in the past. The supervisor suggested that Ellie be patient with Kate. Perhaps later Ellie could re-establish the bond, and they would be able to talk about what had happened.

Fortunately, Ellie did not act on her angry feelings. Had she done so, she might have impulsively assessed Kate's behaviour as 'hopeless', interpreting her anxiety and resistance as an inability to trust, or she may have begun to relate to Kate in a vindictive way, withdrawing her care. Instead, she sought advice. Ellie's supervisor recognised that Ellie wanted to do well and needed positive feedback. She also realised that Ellie did not understand the nature of giving to young people who are emotionally volatile and distressed. Had Ellie not sought advice, she might have acted on her angry feelings, further alienating Kate and causing herself more anger and frustration. Without an understanding of Kate's actions, Ellie would have continued to expect kindness in return for kindness and would have been keenly disappointed.

Non-therapeutic enticement

In working with young people, nurses may be enticed into relating in a non-therapeutic way. Various factors can contribute to the problem:

- the intimate nature of the nurse's involvement with the young person
- the narcissism that is sometimes evident in this age group
- the nurse's all-accepting attitude in working with the young person.

Narcissism in this age group may be caused by the child's withdrawal from the parents and their value system. This withdrawal leads to a general self-centredness, over-evaluation of the self, heightened self-perception, a decreased ability for reality testing, and extreme self-absorption. The result is that the people to whom the young people turn become all-important and perfect in their eyes. Nurses may be strongly tempted to respond accordingly.

Nurse's self-awareness The dangers inherent in this situation are not simply the two possible extremes: total submission to temptation, resulting in an inappropriate relationship with the person; or strong denial of temptation by maintaining a rigid, unapproachable stance that makes it impossible to establish a meaningful, trusting relationship. Neither of these extremes is unknown. The questions in Self-awareness: A Self-awareness Inventory for Working With Young People on page 469 will help you assess how you deal with problems of non-therapeutic enticement and how you deal with your own attitudes and feelings.

It can be tempting to respond to the young person's idealised view, to be the 'rescuer' who succeeds with this 'difficult person' where everyone else has failed, to feel superior to the imperfect parents, the harassed school teacher, or other members of the staff on the unit. However, such temptations should be reflected upon and resisted. Complications will very likely develop that at best will temporarily compromise your effectiveness, and at worst will render the treatment program ineffective. Xanthe's example of acting out demonstrates this. Jim, the evening nurse, could have been enticed by Xanthe to collude with her against the day nurse, had he not been keenly aware of that possibility.

Nurses who work intensively with young people often face situations in which their own unresolved feelings are aroused. You must choose whether to act on these impulses or to explore their origin. Of course, one is not always conscious of these unresolved feelings. It would be unrealistic to expect you to be totally aware of the meaning of your behaviour at any given moment. Nonetheless, the skilled clinician is usually acquainted with the issues or conflicts that have caused problems in the past. In doubtful cases, the knowledgeable nurse will seek consultation from a clinician. The clinician can help you assess the situation and understand what part you may have played in initiating it. Nurses who wish to explore their personal conflicts further may then seek counselling or therapy.

Nursing staff would benefit from establishing one or more of the following to provide a consistent format for assessing and evaluating ongoing situations with the young people with whom they work:

- each nurse's own ongoing supervision with a preceptor or clinical supervisor
- a regularly scheduled meeting (perhaps monthly) for all nursing staff to discuss difficult situations and conflicting feelings
- staff meetings (perhaps weekly) in which all disciplines identify interpersonal obstacles and plan interventions towards more optimal treatment.

Sexual behaviour of the young person

The biological changes that occur in late childhood and early adolescence are rapid and pervasive. It is important that the young person's experimentation and attitude in sexual matters not be underestimated. Likewise, evaluate your own attitudes and feelings about sexual issues as they relate to past experiences and current activities. Conflicts in such matters or resentments left over from the past may affect your decisions or interactions with young people regarding sexual matters. Again, while it is not necessary for you to resolve all of these issues, it is highly desirable to be aware of areas of conflict that might make it difficult to view a situation objectively or to set rational limits.

Until young people master their anxieties and fears about their sexual identity and gain control over sexual urges, they will exhibit a variety of behaviours and attitudes that may confuse or trouble you. In recent decades, rates of pregnancy and live births have declined among youth, and there has been an increase in the use of more effective contraceptive methods. At the same time, the rate of sexually transmitted diseases has increased among young Australians—especially chlamydia.

Heterosexuality Heterosexual activity is normal and desirable during adolescence. However, nurses working with either normal or troubled young people will sometimes see them engage in sexual activities that do not seem healthy or growth-producing. For example, the young teenage girl who appears to be seeking punishment rather than true pleasure in her sexual exploits may display them in an overt, exhibitionistic way in a place where a particularly moralistic person will discover her and give her the reprimands she desires. She may be testing a parent's values in an attempt to resolve her own inner conflicts.

Young people in an inpatient treatment setting where sexual intercourse is prohibited may engage in sexual

COMMUNICATION

The young person with sexual acting-out behaviour

YOUNG PERSON: [Laurie and Bill are discovered together in a linen room on the unit.] 'Hey, a little privacy, if you don't mind!'

NURSE RESPONSE 1: 'Laurie, Bill, not cool, guys. What's going on? You knew I was coming in here to get more towels. Laurie, does this have to do with your weekend leave tomorrow? Let's talk about this in the office. C'mon.' [She escorts the two young people to the office to talk.]

RATIONALE: Both young people have been on the unit for some time and are familiar with the rules and expectations. The nurse believes that the behaviour is a display of Laurie's anxiety about her impending weekend leave, and may be an attempt to sabotage that arrangement. Rather than addressing the rules as the focus for their discussion, the nurse talks with them about the underlying meaning of their behaviour.

NURSE RESPONSE 2: 'That is enough. Stop what you are doing now, and we are going to talk about appropriate behaviour on the unit.'

RATIONALE: This intervention is particularly appropriate if the young people have repeated this inappropriate behaviour.

intercourse where you or another staff member will be sure to discover them. The experience may reinforce their image of sexual behaviour as 'bad' behaviour. Or it may simply provide a means of acting out their defiance of the rules, thereby earning the familiar 'bad kid' label. The incident involving Laurie and Bill, the two young people admitted to an inpatient unit in the above Communication, is an example of this situation.

Homosexuality Homosexuality is the persistent sexual and emotional attraction to someone of the same gender. It is part of the range of sexual expression, and has existed throughout history and across cultures. Pre-adolescents usually choose a member of the same gender with whom to experience intimate or loving feelings. This does not necessarily mean that a sexual relationship will ensue, although it sometimes does. Homosexual activity may continue into the adolescent years. Many gay, lesbian and bisexual individuals first become aware of their sexual thoughts and feelings during their teen years, and may have their first experiences at this time. Recent changes in society's attitude towards sexuality, including homosexual issues, have helped gay, lesbian and bisexual youth feel more comfortable with their sexual orientation. On the other hand, much more needs to be accomplished. Although the scientific basis of homosexuality and bisexuality is not clear, there is agreement that sexual orientation is not a mental disorder. Nor is it a matter of choice. Individuals are no more able to 'choose' whether or not to be homosexual than to be heterosexual.

LIVED EXPERIENCE

I spent so much of my teenaged years in inpatient care that I hadn't had a chance to be a normal teenager, and this included the kinds of experiences through which a young person develops an understanding of who they are emotionally, sexually, attitudinally. This resulted in me putting myself into a number of risky situations that ended badly—I was sexually assaulted. I put this down to my lack of experience as a normal teenager at the time. This is important for health professionals to understand: that young people with mental health issues may try to play 'catch-up' with what they think are normal behaviours, including sexual expression and the use of alcohol and other substances, and they are really poorly prepared to do so. At about 17 or 18 years of age I felt very inadequate; that I was not normal for my age. I desperately wanted to be normal without really knowing what that was, and it got me into trouble.

Like their heterosexual counterparts, gay, lesbian and bisexual teens have many concerns, including: feeling different from their peers; fearing ridicule, rejection or harassment by others; worrying about a negative response from their families or loved ones; and worrying about sexually transmitted diseases, including HIV infection. Moreover, they have an additional fear of discrimination due to their sexual orientation when seeking employment, applying to university, or joining clubs or sports activities. They can become socially isolated, withdraw from friends and activities, have trouble concentrating, develop low self-esteem, become depressed and feel suicidal. Counselling may be helpful for teens who are uncomfortable with their homosexuality or who are unable to express it. Regardless of setting or sexual orientation, young people do have a choice about how and where to express their sexual feelings, just as they do their other emotions.

Generally speaking, however, many young people view homosexual feelings as a threat to the development of their identity. As a result, they may ward off such feelings by engaging in sexual activity with a member of the opposite sex. This is particularly true for boys. It is normal for an adolescent boy to be afraid of feelings of passivity, and to label these feelings as homosexual. Some boys may have been brought up to identify with physical displays of strength or aggressive displays of power. If that is the case, an incident where he feels threatened or powerless would produce feelings of sexual impotence, a feeling of dependence or weakness, and a greater fear of homosexuality. The adolescent boy in treatment may act out these feelings, or he may attempt to reaffirm his masculinity with inappropriate displays of aggression or destructive behaviour. Likewise, the adolescent girl who feels a need to ward off intense feelings for female peers may engage in sexual activity with numerous male partners for similar reasons.

Nurses who work with young people may encounter any of these situations, and they must attempt to understand the meaning that homosexual behaviour has for the teenaged person. The young people may need to explore their feelings and anxieties openly. Open discussion with an understanding yet knowledgeable professional may help resolve many of the concerns and conflicts inherent in adolescent sexual behaviour. It is important to remain objective and nonjudgmental with these young people, allowing them to deal with the feelings of anger or depression that may result from addressing the conflict.

Although homosexual behaviour during adolescence does not predict adult sexual preference, some young people make a lasting identification as homosexual during these years. These young people will not experience conflicts about homosexual relationships or need to flaunt them or act out with the staff in an angry or hostile way. In these cases, however, it may be necessary to deal with your own negative feelings about homosexuality, if any exist. It is important for you to consider what young people's relationships mean to them and to respect them.

Pregnancy Teen pregnancy may reflect social and family expectations and unconscious motivations. Some teenage girls are quite pleased to be pregnant, and suffer no emotional consequences from motherhood. In general, however, a conscious, deliberate decision to become pregnant at this age may reflect a wish to escape a difficult family situation, to express hostility towards parents, or to act out a life script in which the daughter is seen as 'bad'. The adolescent girl who did not receive adequate nurturing as a child could be acting out dependency needs by giving her baby the love and caring she herself did not receive. In so doing, she feels loved and cared for in turn.

It is important to be sensitive to motivational factors in dealing with young people who are emotionally troubled. Interpersonal relationships can be used to help adolescent girls understand their needs and motivations to become pregnant. It is also important to educate young people of both genders about sex and birth control. Highs schools now recognise this need and include birth control education as part of the formal curriculum. Too often parents and professionals alike deny the young person's sexual activity until an unwanted pregnancy occurs.

Dietary problems and eating disorders

The eating habits and food preferences of troubled young people can reveal a great deal about the nature of their inner distress. A comparison between the person's diet and that of a normal, healthy teen may show little difference in variety but probably a great difference in quantity.

Young people who have been deprived of early nurturing tend to eat more than others, and probably place a higher value on mealtimes and on receiving their 'share' of the food. You may notice that young people consume more milk than usual during periods of stress or anxiety. In general, girls want to follow food fads or unreasonable dietary regimens to become slim and attractive. This usually provides an opportunity to engage in health teaching about nutrition and exercise, and to express a cooperative interest in their developing feminine identity. (Eating disorders are discussed in Chapter 17.)

Depression and suicide

Both depression and suicide are thought to be under-reported among young people. The Diagnostic Features box highlights the criteria necessary for a diagnosis of adolescent depression. For young people between the ages of 15 and 24, suicide is the leading cause of death, followed by motor vehicle accidents. In 2014, 92 males aged 15 to 19, and 174 males aged 20 to 24, died by suicide. In the same year, the number of deaths by suicide for females aged 15 to 19 and 20 to 24 was 38 and 58, respectively. Risk factors for youth suicide include antisocial behaviour, poor family cohesion, parents who live with mental illness, poor academic performance, depression and substance abuse. However, youth deaths from suicide are only part of the problem. It has been reported that more young people survive suicide attempts than actually die. It is thought that about 5 per cent of young people engage in self-harming behaviour, with females being more likely to do so than males. Between one-third and one-half of teenagers experience thoughts of suicide at some time. The presence of self-injurious behaviour should always trigger a suicide assessment. (See Chapter 19 for a more detailed discussion of suicide.)

DIAGNOSTIC FEATURES
Adolescent depression

Depression: Core symptoms are the same for children and young people as adults, although the prominence of symptoms may change with age. Somatic complaints, irritability and social withdrawal are particularly common in children and younger teens, whereas psychomotor retardation, hypersomnia and delusions are less common in pre-puberty than in adolescence and adulthood. In young people, depression is frequently associated with disruptive behaviour, attention deficit disorders, anxiety disorders, substance-related disorders and eating disorders. Rather than a depressed mood during depression, a young person may display an irritable mood. In addition to depressed and/or irritable mood, there may also be: a lack of interest or pleasure in activities during most of the day, weight change of more than 5 per cent in a month, psychomotor changes, loss of energy, concentration difficulties, feeling worthless, inappropriate guilt and durable thoughts of suicide. With young people, it is important to consider problematic sleep patterns (insomnia or hypersomnia nearly every day) as a sleep change.

Substance use and abuse

Australian reports have consistently indicated that alcohol and cannabis are the substances most likely to be used by young people in Australia. While the proportion of young people (aged 14 to 17) who choose not to drink has risen from 63.6 per cent in 2010 to 72.3 per cent in 2013, underage drinking remains a significant problem. The average age at which young Australians have their first drink is 15.7, with friends or acquaintances being the most likely suppliers of alcohol. About 17 per cent of 15- to 18-year-olds report having had sex when they were intoxicated, and alcohol contributes to the three leading causes of death among young Australians: injury, homicide and suicide. With the exception of cannabis, reported levels of illicit substance use by young people are low, and in most cases gradually declining. The average age of first cannabis use among young people is 16.7, with just under 15 per cent of 12- to 17-year-olds having tried that drug at some point in their life (Australian Drug Foundation, 2016).

Young people give many reasons for using drugs: to experiment, to get high, to 'get inside my head', to have fun, to understand more about life. They may also use drugs to cope with feelings of worthlessness or loneliness, or to avoid uncomfortable feelings, as in the following Practice Example.

Practice example

Cindy is a 15-year-old Year 9 high-school student who has been abusing drugs since age 12. According to Cindy, her three-year history of substance abuse has involved regular marijuana use one to two times a week, the occasional use of diazepam (which she sneaks from her mother's 5 mg tablet prescription medication), and LSD on two occasions.

Cindy describes herself as 'a bit of a loner' who has few friends and keeps to herself at home and at school. She leaves the house each morning for school before the others are awake, 'to avoid the hassles with my mother and sisters'. She describes one female classmate to whom she feels close, but states that their time together is usually brief and often involves smoking marijuana in the morning just before school. Cindy has recently been suspended from school as a result of the school principal's discovery of Cindy and her friend smoking marijuana behind the canteen block.

Cindy is lonely and depressed, and has extreme feelings of worthlessness. She characterises herself as 'bored', 'bad' and 'hopeless'. Cindy says that when she uses drugs, she does not feel as bad.

Although there may be concern in the general public regarding whether drugs are harmful, the fact remains that using drugs—or at least experimenting with them—is acceptable to many young people.

Assessing drug abuse How can you determine when drug *use* becomes drug *abuse*? Generally, the young person who abuses drugs or alcohol exhibits at least one of these following characteristics:

- The young person's performance at school or work increasingly deteriorates.
- The young person is frequently caught high or in the act of getting high by parents or other authority figures.
- The young person increasingly resorts to alcohol or drugs in times of stress or boredom.
- The young person has seriously deficient interpersonal relationships, and can relate only when under the influence of drugs or alcohol.
- The young person may lose interest in interpersonal relationships altogether, preferring to be high alone rather than to be with others.

Nurses are most effective when they can determine what the particular drug or high does for the young person. A boy with a poor self-image and low-esteem may say that it makes him 'feel like a man'. A particularly shy or introverted girl may say that it makes her 'outgoing and friendly'. You may discover that being high helps rid troubled young people of angry or depressed feelings. Indeed, in the treatment setting, you may see young people resorting to smoking cannabis or using other substances to escape uncomfortable feelings. Your Assessment Approach highlights some of the behavioural changes that may be observed in young people using drugs.

Responding to the needs of a young person living with mental illness

Assessing the mental health needs of a young person requires more than considering the criteria for a DSM diagnosis. For example, look back at Cindy, the 15-year-old girl with a three-year history of substance abuse. Limiting your assessment to a DSM diagnosis alone might yield a substance use disorder, a cannabis (marijuana) use disorder, or a substance-induced mood disorder. While this tells you something about her drug history, it does not reveal any specifics, such as current stressors, temperament, or cultural, social or family dynamics that might contribute to or even underlie her drug abuse.

YOUR ASSESSMENT APPROACH

Behavioural changes associated with teenage drug abuse

- Unexplained periods or reactions of moodiness, depression, anxiety, irritability, oversensitivity or hostility
- Strongly inappropriate over-reaction to mild criticism or simple requests
- Lessening in warmth towards family; avoids interaction and communication with parents, withdraws from family activities
- Preoccupation with self, less concern for the feelings of others
- Loss of interest in previously important hobbies, sports, activities
- Loss of motivation and enthusiasm
- Lethargy, lack of energy and vitality
- Loss of ability to self-discipline and assume responsibility
- Need for instant gratification
- Change in values, ideals, beliefs
- Changes in friends; unwillingness to introduce friends
- Secretive phone calls or other electronic communications
- Unexplained absences from home
- Disappearance of money or items of value from home; handling of money becomes secretive
- Desire for increased sensory stimuli

Specifically, your assessments (and interventions) become more comprehensive and universally informative with an exploration of any or all of the following: difficulties in coping; a family that does not function effectively; low self-esteem; frequent feelings of hopelessness; strengths that can be built upon. It is important to establish a more comprehensive picture of the young person's difficulties and strengths, and to be collaborative and goal-oriented in assessing and planning care.

In many treatment settings, mental health care professionals are reluctant to give a DSM diagnosis during a young person's formative years to avoid labelling them (possibly erroneously). Such labelling may result in inadequate treatment, self-fulfilling prophecy, or both, in subsequent mental health care contacts. For a more thorough discussion of DSM diagnoses with people living with mental illness, see Chapter 10.

Identifying outcomes

The determination of outcomes and interventions will depend primarily on your individualised assessment and the young person's stated goals. As a result, the goals and interventions that are decided upon in collaboration with the young person are more likely to be effective.

With 15-year-old Cindy, for example, an expected outcome that she will no longer use drugs after discharge might be unrealistic. Expected outcomes that would yield more success, yet demonstrate improvement, might be one or all of the following:

- approaches a nurse to discuss the temptation to use drugs
- attends and participates in family meetings
- verbalises negative feelings
- correlates negative feelings with the temptation to use drugs
- demonstrates alternative ways of dealing with stressful situations, such as talking to others, becoming involved in peer group activities, or using 'quiet time' in anticipation of family meetings.

Successful treatment with young people may translate into their use of new skills in many instances, but not 100 per cent of the time. Young people will take some time to 'try out' new behaviours and mechanisms for coping. It is important to acknowledge that the person may take two steps forward and one step backward as progress is made. Moreover, as stressful situations arise, there may be an inclination to resort to previous and maladaptive patterns of behaviour. In Cindy's situation, she may resist attending a difficult family meeting, or may even bolt from the room when confronted with her behaviours or feelings. Either behaviour alone does not mean that she is not showing progress or improvement.

Likewise, correlating interventions to support these expected outcomes might include one or all of the following:

- establishing a no-drug contract with the young person
- adopting a neutral, matter-of-fact attitude when discussing drug usage
- encouraging the young person to seek out a nurse when feeling tempted to use drugs
- drawing a parallel for the young person between drug usage and sad or angry feelings
- encouraging the young person to talk about their feelings in individual therapy, group meetings and family meetings.

Planning and implementation

Nurses in numerous roles and diverse settings are in prime positions to recognise and intervene early with troubling symptoms and behaviours.

Prevention plans

By preventing certain circumstances in the early stages of life—such as smoking or drug use as coping mechanisms—health improvements are more probable at later stages. The progression from primary prevention (education/self-care) to secondary prevention (early problem recognition and treatment) to tertiary prevention (more complicated and serious forms of illness and risky behaviours) includes services that become increasingly more technological, expensive and exclusive.

Establishing a contract with a young person

Contracts can be particularly useful with young people. Teenagers can feel powerless in a treatment setting, especially when referred to treatment by parents or other authority figures. Moreover, with this increased sense of involvement in their treatment and control over their own behaviour, young people become collaborators in, rather than objects of, the treatment plan.

With most young people, a written contract can be considered for these reasons:

- the goals and expectations are less easily forgotten
- the process seems more formal and 'serious'
- the young person has more responsibility as a collaborator, indicating an increased awareness of responsibility and choice of behaviour
- there is less room for misinterpretation and manipulation.

Contracts may be helpful as part of an overall treatment plan in situations of substance abuse, eating disorders, suicidal behaviour, and impulsive or manipulative behaviours. Whether verbal or written, the contract can be simply stated to promote clarity, consistency and cooperation. Here is an example:

- I will not take drugs or bring drugs onto the unit.
- I will not call or accept calls from my drug friends while in the treatment program.
- I will go directly to my therapy appointment and return immediately to the unit.
- I will not harm myself or others. If I feel like hurting myself, others or property, I will tell the staff.

If written, the contract can be signed by the young person, dated and co-signed by you. The contract can be renegotiated at regular intervals (hourly, daily or weekly), depending on the goals, the severity of the symptoms, and the degree of adherence with the agreement. The form of the contract is less important than the way you and the young person jointly set the goals and expectations, carry out the contract, set limits and renegotiate changes, and evaluate the final outcome. However, it is important to recognise that contracts do not guarantee outcomes with respect to adherence to treatment plans or safety concerns. Chapter 19 illustrates no-suicide contracts, and discusses the issues surrounding them.

Moderating anger and hostility

Depending on the degree to which the young person is experiencing and expressing anger and hostility, a variety of interventions can be considered. These range from observing and assessing the young person's behaviour to preventing someone from attempting destructive action.

Choosing an appropriate intervention In some situations, a troubled young person's ability to express anger directly to another person can be a sign of success in treatment. The choice of interventions also depends on your own experiences with these feelings, your knowledge and understanding of this person's life experiences with anger, and the external limits imposed by the mental health agency.

You can attempt to discover what meaning anger and hostility have for the young person by asking the following questions:

- How has this person handled anger in the past?
- Does the person have a history of aggression towards objects or people?
- If so, what were the consequences of this behaviour?
- What does this person describe feeling after such a reaction?
- What kinds of things make this person angry? Which of these would be most likely to occur on the unit or in this setting?

This Practice Example illustrates a situation in which you might choose to observe and assess rather than intervene in response to a person's anger and hostility.

Practice example

Steve had expressed great interest in building a model aircraft. He saved up his money and took a long time to choose 'just the right one' at the hobby shop. After spending most of the afternoon constructing and painting it, he was interrupted by a phone call from his mother. She told him that she would not be able to attend the family meeting that week, giving a number of reasons. This was the third time that she had missed a family meeting. Each time, she gave questionable reasons for being unable to attend.

Steve was disappointed and angry. He slammed down the receiver, started swearing loudly in response to the nurse's questions, and ran into his room. There, he destroyed the plane by throwing it against the wall.

In this example, Steve was not hurting himself or another. Although he did destroy property, the model belonged to him, and he was free to do with it as he chose. The nurse resisted any impulse to stop Steve from damaging his model aircraft. Because it was of significant value to him, he later regretted having taken out his anger on it. However, the situation provided Steve with an opportunity to explore his actions, and he later asked the nurse why he would destroy something that he valued so much after his mother had disappointed and angered him. The parallel between this situation and hurting himself with drugs right after he had argued with his mother seemed only too apparent.

Anger directed towards the nurse Incidents in which the nurse bears the brunt of a young person's anger or hostility do not offer obvious solutions. Troubled young people may not think twice about addressing a female nurse as 'slag' and coupling such a greeting with a request for a favour. Young people direct insults and hostile remarks at nurses for many reasons, most of which have little to do with the nurses as people, but a lot to do with nurses as adults or authority figures.

In choosing interventions, it is important to consider the meaning behind the young person's behaviour, your own relationship with them, your immediate feelings, and the desired result. For example, if the young person insults you the first time you meet, you may interpret this as a form of testing, and may choose to respond immediately with a bewildered look at this unwarranted display of hostility. Later, you may approach the young person, expressing a naïve curiosity as to the origin of the hostile feelings: 'Hey, I don't understand what happened between us a few minutes ago. We just met, and you're insulting me. What's that all about?' This simple question conveys two messages. First, it indicates to the person that you are not accustomed to being addressed this way. Second, it indicates that you are more interested in the motivation for the remark than in curtailing its use.

If the young person resorts to name-calling only when angry or under stress, you may decide to ignore the words and deal only with the feelings involved. For example, if a young person has angrily left an ongoing family meeting and then insults you, it seems reasonable to assume that the anger is displaced. It is probably a result of overwhelming feelings experienced during the meeting. You may elect simply to say, 'I know you're not angry at me right now. It seems like the meeting was pretty rough, though. Do you want to talk about why you don't want to be in there now?' In neither situation is the name-calling intended as a personal affront. However, the way you handle it determines both the outcome of the immediate situation and your chances of furthering your relationship with the young person.

The young person's reactions The reaction to your intervention largely determines its effectiveness. For example, with Steve, the boy who destroyed his model plane, the nurse's goal was to help Steve understand the impulsive reaction that destroyed something he loved, and to encourage a more appropriate and direct expression of anger at his mother. He was able to do this as well as draw a parallel between anger at his mother and his drug abuse, which hurt himself. If the nurse's goal had been simply to stop the destruction of his property, Steve could have felt even greater anger and frustration, and he might have turned his aggression towards himself, the nurse or the environment. Certainly if Steve had escalated his destructive behaviour, turning his aggression towards himself or others, then direct limit-setting would have been indicated.

In first-time encounters with any young person new to the setting, do not be surprised or dismayed about less-than-optimal success with interventions. It may take some time and trial and error to assess the person's behaviours and choose the most effective interventions.

Moderate testing and setting limits

As young people attempt to adjust to the upheaval in their emotional lives and begin to release themselves from parental figures, a good deal of testing is to be expected. This is normal. However, the meaning that testing holds for an emotionally troubled young person can be a more complicated matter.

Young people who lack early nurturing may have difficulty with interpersonal relationships. In many cases, parents were emotionally unable to provide adequate parenting. In other cases, they chose not to impose their values on their children. In either case, the children never developed the internalised values that reduce conflict and avert crisis during adolescence. This may cause identity diffusion (the failure to maintain a cohesive self-concept), which in turn results in emptiness, a lack of basic trust, and difficulties with intimacy on any level.

In the treatment setting, young people who have had such experiences may test by making limitless and absolute demands. Although such reactions to imposed limits may be accompanied by cries of injustice, they may imply a wish for limits as an indication of caring, as indicated in the Practice Example that follows.

Practice example

Alison had been on the unit for only two days. During that time she had seen several older teens run away from the unit, commonly known as 'absconding' or 'absent without leave (AWOL)', and had witnessed the staff members' attempts to encourage those remaining on the ward to deal with whatever feelings they were experiencing. Towards the end of her second evening, Alison abruptly jumped up from a conversation with a nurse and ran towards an open door. The surprised nurse immediately followed, running down the stairs after her. A smiling Alison was waiting at the bottom step when the nurse arrived, breathless and confused, asking why Alison had run away. Alison quickly answered, 'I just wanted to see if you cared enough to come after me.'

In this situation, no further action was necessary.

Sometimes the young person may use annoying or destructive behaviour to test you. At these times, setting firm limits without further interpretation or exploration may be indicated. In other instances, such behaviour may be a reaction to some real threat or to an uncomfortable situation.

Practice example

Mandy was quietly playing pool by herself when she noticed her care coordinator talking to a new female who had recently been admitted to the unit. Mandy's volatile nature gave rise to jealousy and rage, and she began to hit the billiard balls off the table, making a lot of noise and startling everyone around her.

The nurse who had been observing her witnessed the change in her behaviour, and understood that it as a reaction to sharing her care coordinator's attention with the young person recently admitted to the unit. Without questioning Mandy's apparent anger, she stepped up to the table and challenged her to a game, which Mandy immediately accepted. Because Mandy prided herself on her pool-playing ability, she quickly channelled her energy and competitive feelings into the game and won. She then sought out her care coordinator and happily announced her victory.

Had the nurse not understood what had triggered Mandy's outburst, she might have become angry with her for making a noise, and set limits on her privilege to play pool. This would likely have produced a helpless and even angrier Mandy, whose destructive behaviour may have escalated. Because of the nurse's perceptive action, Mandy was able to save face by winning at pool, and was not forced into a situation that would have made her feel more helpless.

Think about what other interventions might have been equally effective with Mandy. In your relationships with young people in care, you might find yourself inclined to respond with myriad, seemingly unrelated, interventions. With a combination of increased clinical experience, a personalised assessment of the young person and the immediate situation, and knowledge of current practice studies, you will be most effective in your interventions.

Reducing scapegoating

Scapegoating—a process by which an individual or group of individuals is identified as different from others and becomes the object of the group's fears, frustrations or anger—is common in many groups, but particularly in adolescent groups. It occurs in three stages:

1. Frustration generates aggression.
2. The aggression is then displaced onto other people.
3. A process of blaming, projecting and stereotyping follows. This displaced aggression is rationalised and finally justified, because the identified scapegoat is 'different' in some real way.

The members of a group tend to attack the scapegoat because they are afraid to attack the person, group or institution on whom their feelings are actually focused. Young people readily identify peers who are 'different', and project onto them their own fears and insecurities about their changing images. The person identified as the scapegoat is the object of much teasing and many hostile remarks.

It is worth considering whether attempting to merely rescue the scapegoat is the best approach, because this may augment the anger and frustration of the others on the unit and encourage an escalation of the hostility. Set limits on the behaviour, and then ask the group to focus on what is going on, to acknowledge the anxiety or other uncomfortable feeling that preceded the scapegoating incident. If possible, anticipate the occurrence of scapegoating in times of stress, and try to circumvent the process before it gets out of control.

Also be aware that identified scapegoats may share some responsibility for their predicament by presenting themselves to others in a different or provocative stance. In some instances, the scapegoat is accustomed to this role or has an inner need to be punished, and the scapegoat meets the group's urgent need to punish as well. You can be valuable to these young people by helping them explore whatever function this role serves for them.

Reducing bullying

A discussion of scapegoating would be incomplete without some information on bullying. Teasing and bullying are a major concern among youth. As a child or teenager, you may have been the object or the instigator of such behaviour. Prior to the electronic age, such behaviours took the form of verbal taunts or physical challenges, and typically were limited to the school or social group setting, events known only to you or perhaps your family or closest circle of friends. Such behaviours were generally perceived by parents and authorities as unfortunate but typical expressions of youthful insecurities and part of growing up. However, in more recent times, with internet access, the prevalence of mobile phones, the advent of online social networks, and the capability of communicating with literally hundreds of others in your peer group with the touch of a key, the term *bullying* has taken on a more dramatic meaning that has sometimes resulted in tragic outcomes. Increasingly, the bullying of children and young people, especially via electronic media—**cyberbullying**—is being seen as a significant modifiable risk factor for mental illness (Scott, Moore, Sly & Norman, 2014). Cyberbullying is discussed in Developing Cultural Competence.

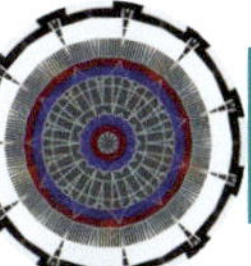

DEVELOPING CULTURAL COMPETENCE

Preventing and dealing with cyberbullying

Cyberbullying may include harassing emails, provocative mobile phone messages or images, and aggressive behaviours communicated through online social networks. Notably, victims of cyberbullying report higher rates of depression than cyberbullies or non-cyber victims. Unlike traditional bullying, which usually involves a face-to-face confrontation, cyber victims may not see or identify their harasser and, as a result, may be more likely to feel isolated, dehumanised or helpless at the time of the attack (Kozlowska & Durheim, 2014; Scott et al., 2014; Wang, Nansel & Iannotti, 2010). See Collaborative Care for information that you can use in helping young people and their parents with incidents of cyberbullying.

CRITICAL THINKING QUESTIONS

1. Why do you need to keep up-to-date with electronic media issues with young people?
2. In what ways might cyberbullying affect the mental health of a young person?
3. Are you familiar with recent news items regarding cyberbullying? Why, or why not?

COLLABORATIVE CARE

Preventing and dealing with cyberbullying

Parents and their teens can be encouraged to design rules for disclosure as well as rules of privacy and confidentiality with all electronic communications. Teens will be more likely to initiate conversation and engage with their parents if they can take part in developing the 'rules of the game'. Visit the websites that your young person frequents. You may join a social networking site to see first-hand the activities of your child and the social connections they have made. Know that such technology is not a passing fad. Moreover, many such websites and online activities can be very helpful to the student in obtaining information and in making beneficial connections with peers with similar interests.

You can suggest to parents that they talk regularly with their child about their online activities. You can offer 'what to say' suggestions to the parent that show sensitivity but also convey concern: 'I'm aware of stories of cyberbullying. I want to trust you, and hope that you will tell me if you are the victim of cyberbullying, stalking or any other illegal or troublesome online behaviour. I will not take away your [specify technology] if you confide in me a problem that you are having.'

Explain to the parent the importance of allowing the young person to respond, and to take part in a dialogue with them before rushing to give limits or warnings: 'My concern for your safety may over-ride my concern for your privacy, and I may need to look at your online communications if I think you are in danger.'

With incidents of cyberbullying, you can help victims and their parents with the following suggestions:

1. Encourage them to not respond directly to the cyberbully.
2. Do not erase the messages or images. They may be needed by the authorities. Save them in a way that avoids subjecting the teen to them again and again.
3. Try to identify the sender. Even if cyberbullies are anonymous, there may be a way to identify them through their internet service provider, website or mobile phone company.
4. If the behaviour/threat is criminal, contact your local police and ask them to investigate. While laws may vary across state and territory jurisdictions, in general the following constitute criminal activity:
    a. obscene or harassing phone calls or text messages
    b. threats of violence
    c. harassment, stalking or hate crimes

(continued)

COLLABORATIVE CARE (*continued*)

  d. child pornography
  e. sexual exploitation
  f. extortion
  g. taking a photo of someone in a place where that person expects to have privacy.

5. Contact the school. If the cyberbullying is coming through the school's internet system, the administrators have an obligation to intervene.
6. Even if the behaviour is happening off-grounds, the school authorities may be able to identify and resolve the cyberbullying, or at least be watchful for an escalation of the aggressive behaviour, as with physical or verbal bullying within the school.
7. Talk with the young person and the family to see whether professional counselling is needed to help deal with the stress and upset of cyberbullying. As with traditional forms of bullying, electronic aggression has been associated with emotional distress in general, and conduct problems at school. Moreover, depression is a major concern for the cyber-victim.
8. As a preventive measure or post-event intervention, consider working with parents and community groups to present a seminar on electronic aggression, develop a zero-tolerance policy for cyberbullying, and encourage a collaborative relationship among all parties.

Because society has become more sophisticated about technology and there are a great number of social media outlets, the opportunity to express emotions electronically is more accessible. It is important to consider the environment of a communicating young person. The following experiences are quite common:

- insecurity
- inexperience managing strong emotions
- communication difficulties
- anger
- fear of the unknown or unfamiliar
- anxiety
- impulsivity
- hostility and resentment.

Once a powerful feeling is felt by a young person who does not have competent skills to deal with it, the path of least resistance is often to resolve the situation with the comfortable and easily manoeuvered cyberspace option.

Managing sexual behaviours

With self-awareness and an understanding of your feelings and attitudes about sexual issues, you can more readily plan interventions to deal with the sexual behaviours of the young person with whom you are working.

Masturbation Masturbation is a normal sexual activity for people of all ages, from the beginning of sexual awareness to senescence. If you have a relatively healthy attitude towards masturbation, you are not likely to run into problems unless the young person masturbates in inappropriate places or uses masturbation to express hostility.

You may be confronted with a teenage boy who fondles his genitals when he is anxious or feels threatened. Understanding his behaviour as an indication of anxiety, you may elect to ignore the gesture and explore the nature of his anxiety with him. At other times, the boy may make a masturbatory gesture to convey contempt or hostility. In this case, it would be ineffective to feign indifference in response.

Your reaction depends on all of the previously mentioned factors, such as the therapeutic relationship you have with the young person and the behaviour that preceded the gesture. Generally, however, it is wise to comment on the gesture—for example, by mentioning it as an attempt to 'make me uncomfortable'—and then to allow the young person the opportunity to express his feelings verbally. It is unlikely that this intervention will produce a tumultuous outpouring of feeling resulting in immediate resolution. However, it does allow you to acknowledge both the young person's and your own feelings, perhaps paving the way for a more appropriate exchange in the future.

Heterosexual behaviour Young people may sometimes use sexual behaviour as a means of acting out other conflicts, and as a testing ground for the nursing staff's feelings and attitudes. The Practice Example of Barbara and Laurie illustrates both issues.

Practice example

This was the third time Barbara, a nurse, had gone into Laurie's room to check on two young people in care, Laurie and Bill, who were an identified couple on the unit. Although there was a rule against people admitted to the unit having sexual intercourse with each other, Laurie and Bill had been discovered in the act each evening Barbara was on duty. Barbara found these discoveries disconcerting. She wondered if she was the only staff member who checked on people on the unit, because no one else had reported any sexual activity. She decided to bring up the subject at the next treatment planning meeting to find a more effective way to deal with the situation.

Imagine Barbara's surprise when her peers suggested that Barbara was actually partly responsible for Laurie and Bill's acting out. It seemed that her frequent checking on people conveyed her expectation that they were 'up to something'. Barbara acknowledged that she expected that sort of behaviour and was quite afraid of discovering Laurie and Bill in the act of intercourse.

The team helped Barbara see that her own expectations were being met. Laurie and Bill were doing exactly what she expected them to do—maybe even wanted them to do. Laurie and Bill were following their scripts of being 'bad' and expressing their hostility towards Barbara. When Barbara heard how other staff members spent time with the couple to encourage them in indirect ways to join the larger group activities, she realised how obvious her anxiety and unconscious messages actually were. She then began to question her own attitudes about sexual matters, and to explore why she feared discovering the couple engaged in sexual intercourse.

In this example, Laurie and Bill used sexual behaviours to act out their own underlying feelings. Had Barbara's assessment been limited to each immediate situation, she would have focused only on the couple's unacceptable behaviour and would not have been open to the implications their behaviour had for her. By seeking out information and feedback from her peers, she made a discovery about herself, and realised that it was more effective to anticipate and possibly circumvent such behaviours than to intervene after the fact. Had Barbara not asked for feedback, the problem would have continued, with a likely increase in the sexual behaviours and in Barbara's frustration. The situation would then have required intervention by an astute supervisor or an empathic colleague.

Homosexuality In situations in which homosexual activity is an expected developmental step or a lifestyle without expressions of anger or hostility towards parents or staff, little or no intervention may be indicated. As mentioned in the assessment section, it is as important for the nurse to understand and provide emotional support for the young person who is homosexual or bisexual as for the young person who is heterosexual and dealing with sexual identity and other developmental issues. Moreover, it is important that young people be supported to decide when, and to whom, to disclose their sexual orientation.

Counselling directed specifically at insisting that the counsellor's sexual orientation be considered the norm, when it is not, may be traumatic and cause lasting harm for an unwilling young person. Professionals and laypersons alike can obtain understanding and support from organisations such as Parents, Family and Friends of Lesbians and Gays Australia (www.pflagaustralia.org.au).

The term *metrosexual* is sometimes used in young adult references. The term, a combination of the words 'metro' meaning *urban* and 'sexual', has nothing to do with the man's sexuality as much as his lifestyle choice. The term *metrosexual* refers to the urban lifestyle of a man who typically spends a great deal of time and money on his appearance and lifestyle. While his fastidious grooming, beauty treatments (which can include nail care and facials), and fashionable clothes might stereotypically be identified with a homosexual lifestyle, he is heterosexual. The term was introduced in 1994 by Mark Simpson, a British journalist, who explores male and female roles and lifestyles in his writings and in the popular media (Hagood, 2010).

On the other hand, when homosexual behaviour is used to act out feelings of impotence, or aggressive behaviour is used to counteract feelings of intimacy, limits must be imposed. Try to anticipate this behaviour and provide other ways for the young person to work with the anxiety. As one example, with a male needing to demonstrate his masculinity, perhaps you could organise a game of football or tennis, if he is fairly proficient at these skills, or engage him in some other activity in which he excels. With a female who fears intimate feelings, anticipate and circumvent a similar display of acting out, perhaps with a group activity where intimate or competitive feelings can be channelled in a more socially appropriate way. The point is to re-establish the young person's feeling of competence and control. Without these interventions, feelings of impotence will escalate to the point where the young person will act them out in a negative way. The young person who uses homosexuality to express defiance towards authority figures will flaunt homosexual activities and consistently incur the anger, embarrassment, or both, of staff and others in care alike.

Reducing substance abuse

You will benefit from self-awareness and an understanding of the feelings that working with people who abuse substances can evoke. For example, the nurse who feels angry and punitive with the person who abuses drugs, or who over-identifies with and finds adventure in drug stories, will struggle to establish a therapeutic relationship with the person. Feelings of disdain or envy can compromise nursing care and, indeed, may make treatment ineffective. Only by viewing substance abuse as a symptom of a broader illness can you be effective in dealing with young people.

Cultural and generational factors are important in understanding the young person's choice of drug as well. You may wonder why the current teen population had not learned lessons from your generation or previous generations. **Generational forgetting** occurs as a result of older drugs being rediscovered by a newer generation of young people. Such drugs make a comeback from previous years when they fell from popularity, because the adverse consequences are unknown or forgotten by the next generation. Such drug examples that were popular in the 1960s and saw a resurgence in the 1990s were LSD, methamphetamine, heroin, cocaine and crack (Johnston, O'Malley, Bachman & Schulenberg, 2010). Nurses who have contact with young people, especially in school or community settings, should familiarise themselves with the general effects of various drugs and the first-aid treatment for each (see Chapter 13).

Interventions are determined to be effective or ineffective by the use of subjective and objective behavioural criteria, as described in the section on identifying outcomes on page 474. These criteria should reflect the individualised plan of care and the goals agreed upon by you and the young person with whom you are working. Only then can you expect to see the benefits of the interventions and experience the satisfaction that can come from working with young people.

Evaluation

Evaluating interventions for young people can be tricky for numerous reasons:

- The young person may need to test the limit one more time following an intervention to avoid appearing 'too compliant' or to 'save face' with the group.
- Although it is important to set limits, it is equally important to be flexible. To set a limit and immediately 'draw the line' with the next infraction is to invite the young person to step over that line to test its seriousness.
- This is a slow process. Do not make quick judgments if immediate results are not obtained.

- The behaviours that brought the young person to psychiatric treatment will continue long after treatment and interventions have begun. Despite a well-designed care plan and behavioural contract, the young person may resort to previous maladaptive ways, immature and impulsive acts, or destructive behaviours in the face of change, particularly if this change represents improvement or growth (such as an increase in privileges or an impending discharge). The nurse who thinks this means that the interventions are not effective may feel hopeless about progress, and convey that hopelessness to the young person and the rest of the treatment team.
- Using a behavioural contract without understanding the underlying reasons or factors contributing to the young person's problems will result in a superficial approach with an equally superficial evaluation.

If the young person had the desire or the impulse control simply to 'act right' after being given the rules and consequences, then they would be doing so, and psychiatric treatment would not have been necessary. The young person needs the structure and consistency of a care plan and a behavioural contract without the rigidity that can be imposed by a 'now or never' approach with absolute consequences.

You can make a more adequate evaluation if you are aware of the social context and the meaning of the behaviour to the young person. For example, you may be wrong in determining that an indicator of increased self-esteem for a young female would be to stop dyeing her hair purple. Dyeing one's hair an unusual colour may have been an indication of low self-esteem during *your* youth, but for the young person in question that may or may not be the case. For that young woman and her peer group, purple hair may be a well-defined cultural symbol.

CARE COORDINATION, COMMUNITY-BASED CARE AND PRIMARY CARE

Mental health nurses who work with young people need to be able to function as care coordinators and to work in community-based and primary care settings. The skills required in these roles include the following:

- assessing troubled young people and dysfunctional families wherever you encounter them
- educating professional colleagues, community organisations and parents about the importance of preventive attention and the resources available to help teens and their families
- preventing youth violence and drug abuse if possible
- advocating for online treatment (e-mental health) models where indicated
- refining therapeutic skills to work with young people and their families
- teaching about sensitive health topics, such as drug use, STDs, unwanted pregnancy and the consequences of violence
- advocating for social policies and programs that help keep families out of poverty, a major risk factor for young people.

Mental health nurses are most likely to encounter troubled young people in community-based settings such as schools, emergency rooms, general practice surgeries, on university campuses, detoxification programs, STD clinics, and other outpatient settings that provide programs for angry, abused, neglected or otherwise troubled teenagers. The earlier section in this chapter on mental health nursing roles in outpatient settings addresses in detail the skills needed when working with young people presenting with these problems.

Of particular interest to mental health nurses who are committed to advocating for young people who are troubled or in trouble are opportunities to effect change at the state, territory and national level. It is known that, despite treatment advances and improved early identification, most youth living with mental illnesses do not receive treatment. Some of the barriers to treatment include a shortage of child/adolescent psychiatrists and psychiatric mental health nurses, a lack of adequate coverage of mental health services within health care systems, a lack of research funding, and a lack of community mental health services. As the peak professional organisation representing psychiatric–mental health nurses in this country, the Australian College of Mental Health Nurses (www.acmhn.org) plays an important role in advocating for improvements in mental health policy and practice, including child and youth mental health.

On a global scale, youth of all nations should be recognised for the hope they bring to the health and vitality of their countries. The World Health Organization (WHO) states that child and youth mental health is a necessary priority for the healthy development of societies. In particular, child and youth mental health is central to the future development of low-income countries throughout the world (WHO, 2016). Developing Cultural Competence details serious challenges faced by the youth of other nations—challenges that impact on not only low-income countries, but on Australia and other developed countries as well. The accompanying critical thinking questions might challenge you and your professional peers to be dissatisfied with the status quo in your clinical setting, your local health district, your neighbourhood or your state/territory.

Discussion among your colleagues might prompt you to make changes to improve the quality of care provided to teens of minority groups or immigrant populations within your local areas in particular. You might want to access numerous WHO publications that are available free online from the WHO library database in numerous languages.

Many nurses, and especially mental health nurses, are in prime positions to influence the movement towards proactive partnerships among schools, families and the community in enhancing the health and ensuring the future of young Australians. Moreover, with an increased appreciation and knowledge of the challenges facing young people on a global scale, we can hope to improve the quality of life in our multicultural communities, the mental health of youth throughout the world, and the future of human societies.

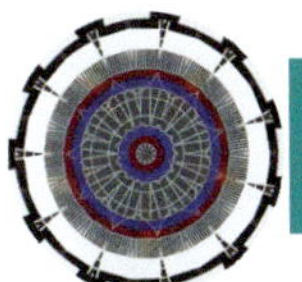

DEVELOPING CULTURAL COMPETENCE

Cultural and societal obstacles to displaced and disenfranchised youth

In low-income countries, such as sub-Saharan Africa, the health and societal challenges of AIDS orphans, AIDS-infected youth, displaced populations of child combatants, reintegrated child soldiers, and youth marginalised because of lack of economic opportunity are all jeopardising the future of these nations. Furthermore, the voluntary and forced migration from Africa and other parts of the world affected by internal conflict brings to the shores of Australia and elsewhere youth who struggle to integrate into these new societies because of mental health and health-related problems (WHO, 2016). Seeking health care from you in your clinical setting may be a daunting challenge for any young person for the usual developmental reasons, but for these displaced and disenfranchised youth, cultural and societal reasons pose added obstacles as well. Moreover, the stigma associated with certain medical problems, such as HIV infection and mental health disorders, particularly in ethnic minority groups and/or immigrant populations, cannot be overestimated.

CRITICAL THINKING QUESTIONS

1. How youth-friendly is your hospital, health centre or other practice setting? Do you have literature available to prompt a discussion with young people about awkward or embarrassing topics?
2. What are your attitudes and biases related to teens with a different cultural background from yours?
3. How might the unknown practices or unfamiliar customs of a different race, religion or ethnic group affect the assessment and care given to a minority member teen at your clinical setting?
4. What actions can you take on your local, regional or state/territorial level that might impact on a multicultural teen population?

LIVED EXPERIENCE

For me, youth mental health is different to adult mental health. It comes with its own set of difficulties and challenges. In growing up—through childhood, to adolescence, to young adulthood—young people have much to go through anyway, and the experience of mental illness makes this so much more difficult. One of the things that has really helped me is having a peer worker; I have had ongoing contact with a particular peer worker since I was 18 and I am now 22. We still chat from time to time, and she is very important to me. I should also say that during the times when I have made very strong therapeutic connections with nurses, it was when they were prepared to share aspects of themselves with me; though not quite in the way in which a peer worker might (I understand there are limits to the extent of self-disclosure a health professional might offer). Really, what I am saying is that it is beneficial when nurses and other health professionals allow themselves to be seen as real people rather than just authority figures. In my experience, nurses who were able to do this effectively were very good professional helpers.

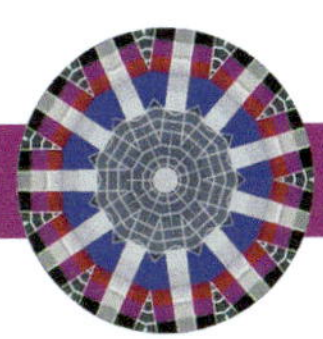

REFERENCES

Arnold, P. D., Hanna, G. L., & Rosenberg, D. R. (2010). Imaging the amygdala: Changing the face of gene discovery in child psychiatry. *Journal of the American Academy of Child and Adolescent Psychiatry, 49*(1), 7–0.

Asarnow, J. R., & Albright, A. (2010). Care management increases the use of primary and medical care services by people with severe mental illness in community mental health settings. *Evidence-Based Nursing, 2010*(4), 128–129.

Australian Bureau of Statistics (ABS). (2009). *Children who are overweight or obese*. ABS Social Trends 4102.0. Retrieved from www.abs.gov.au/AUSSTATS/abs@nsf/Lookup/4102.0Main1features2-Sep12009 (Accessed 2016, July 6.)

Australian Drug Foundation. (2016). *Facts and resources about alcohol and other drugs*. Retrieved form www.druginfo.adf.org/topics/quick-styatistics#alcohol (Accessed 2016, July 14.)

Australian Institute of Health and Welfare (AIHW). (2011a). *Cancer in adolescents and young adults in Australia.* Cancer Series No. 62. Cat. No. CAN 59. Canberra, Australia: AIHW.

Australian Institute of Health and Welfare (AIHW). (2011b). *Young Australians: Their health and wellbeing 2011.* Cat. No. PHE 140. Canberra, Australia: AIHW.

Frodl, T. (2010). Childhood stress, serotonin transporter gene and brain structures in major depression. *Neuropsychopharmacology, 35*(6), 1383–1390.

Hagood, C. (2010, April 13). Wo-metrosexuality and the city: My chat with Mark Simpson. *Huffington Post.* Retrieved from http://www.huffingtonpost.com/caroline-hagood/metrosexuality-and-the-ci_b_535333.html

Johnston, L. D., O'Malley, P. M., Bachman, J. G., & Schulenberg, J. E. (2010). *Monitoring the future, a continuing study of American youth. National results on adolescent drug use: Overview of key findings, 2009.* NIH Publication No. 10-7583. Bethesda, MD: National Institute on Drug Abuse.

Jorm, A. (2015). How effective are 'headspace' youth mental health services? *Australian and New Zealand Journal of Psychiatry, 49*(10), 861–862.

Kozlowska, K., & Durheim, E. (2014). Is bulling a modifiable risk factor for mental illness? *Australian and New Zealand Journal of Psychiatry, 48*(3), 288–289.

Lawrence, D., Hafekost, J., Johnson, S., Saw, S., Buckingham, W., Sawyer, S., . . . Zubrick, S. (2016). Key findings from the second Australian Child and Adolescent Survey of Mental Health and Wellbeing. *Australian and New Zealand Journal of Psychiatry, 50*(9), 876–886.

Lawrence, D., Johnson, S., Hafekost, J., Boterhoven De Haan, K., Sawyer, M., Ainley, J., & Zubrick, S. R. (2015). *The mental health of children and adolescents. Report on the Second Australian Child and Adolescent Survey of Mental Health and Wellbeing*. Canberra, Australia: Department of Health.

Macgowan, M. J., & Engle, B. (2010). Evidence for optimism: Behavior therapies and motivational interviewing in adolescent substance abuse treatment. *Child and Adolescent Psychiatric Clinics of North America, 19*(3), 527–545.

McGorry, P., Hamilton, M., Goldstone, S., & Rickwood, D. (2016). Response to Jorm: headspace—A national and international innovation with lessons for redesign of mental health care in Australia. *Australian and New Zealand Journal of Psychiatry, 50*(1), 9–10.

Morrato, E. H., Nicol, G. E., Maahs, D., Druss, B. G., Hartung, D. M., Valuck, R. J., . . . Newcomer, J. (2010). Metabolic screening in children receiving antipsychotic drug treatment. *Archives of Pediatric and Adolescent Medicine, 164*(4), 344–351.

Naylor, E. V., Antonuccio, D. O., Litt, M., Johnson, G. E., Spogen, D. R., Williams, R., . . . Higgins, D. L. (2010). Bibliotherapy as a treatment for depression in primary care. *Journal of Clinical Psychology in Medical Settings, 17*(3), 258–271. Retrieved from http://www.springerlink.com/content/93qr8335907n37k5/

Rutherford, H. J. V., Mayes, L. C., & Potenza, M. N. (2010). Neurobiology of adolescent substance use disorders: Implications for prevention and treatment. *Child and Adolescent Psychiatric Clinics of North America, 19*(3), 479–492. Retrieved from http://www.ncbi.nlm.nih.gov/pubmed/20682216

Scott, J., Moore, S., Sly, P., & Norman, R. (2014). Bullying in children and adolescents: A modifiable risk factor for mental illness. *Australian and New Zealand Journal of Psychiatry, 48*(3), 209–212.

Stone, T., McMillan, M., & Hazelton, M. (2015). Back to swear one: A review of English language literature on swearing and cursing in Western health settings. *Aggression and Violent Behaviour, 25*, 65–74.

Wang, J., Nansel, T. R., & Iannotti, R. J. (2010, September 22). Cyber and traditional bullying: Differential association with depression. *Journal of Adolescent Health Online*. Retrieved from http://www.jahonline.org/article/S1054-139X(10)00343-5/pdf

World Health Organization. (2016). *Adolescents: Health risks and solutions.* Fact Sheet No. 345. Retrieved from http://www.who.int/mediacentre/factsheets/ fs345/en/ (Accessed 2016, July 15.)

Yancey, A. K., Grant, D., Kurosky, S., Kravitz-Wirtz, N., & Mistry, R. (2010, August 26). Role modeling, risk, and resilience in California adolescents. *Journal of Adolescent Health Online.* Retrieved from http://www.jahonline.org/article/S1054-139X(10)00227-2/fulltext

Older people

22

BRYAN MCMINN AND AMTUL SHAH

LEARNING OUTCOMES

After completing this chapter, you will be able to:

1. Identify the age-related demographic projections that have implications for planning future mental health services for older people.
2. Analyse personal biases, feelings and attitudes that may be experienced in professional practice when caring for older people who suffer from mental disorders.
3. Discuss the major theories of ageing and the ideas associated with each one.
4. Differentiate the normal physical and psychosocial changes that accompany ageing from mental disorders affecting older people.
5. Synthesise the key components of a recovery-focused biopsychosocial assessment into the plan of care for an older person.
6. Develop treatment plans, including cognitive therapies, reminiscence therapy, life review, reality orientation, validation and socialisation enhancement for older people.

KEY TERMS

LIVED EXPERIENCE

I worked in the public service for 28 years before asking for a retirement package, as I was diagnosed with mental illness after having been a diabetic for 11 years and having coronary artery disease diagnosed six months previously.

The next year I moved to another city after over 30 years. My husband and I lived between these two cities for 14 years. Initially, he used to travel six hours each way once a fortnight just for the weekend, and both boys and I visited him during school holidays, etc. Later on, my husband and I started travelling between the two cities alternate fortnights.

The next year my mother died of a stroke after having been in a coma for more than a year. My father had been dead for some 25 years prior, having died in a car accident. A 17-year-old sister had died from a burst appendix two years before my father's death. Over 30 years ago I had my first baby (a boy), who was diagnosed with acute myeloid leukemia at three months of age. For the following 13½ months, we lived between the two cities, and life became very traumatic for both my husband and I. I suffered from lack of sleep so much that, even after the baby's death at 18 months of age, I became an insomniac, and to this day I can only sleep three to four hours

(continued)

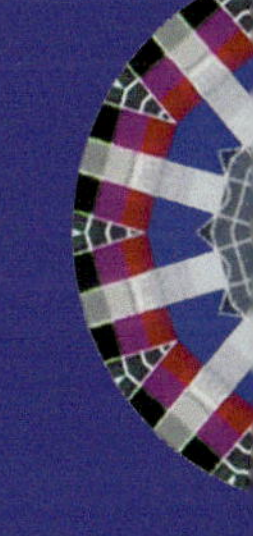

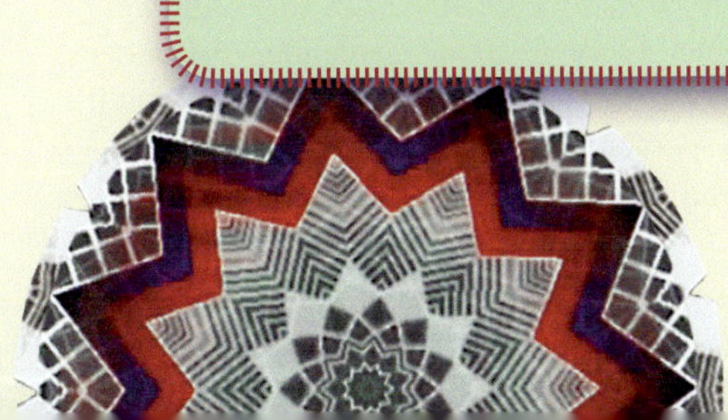

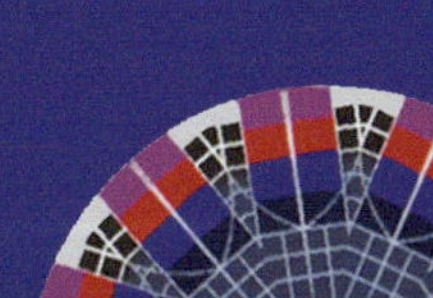

LIVED EXPERIENCE *(continued)*

at night. None of the sleeping tablets, relaxation techniques and other remedies have ever helped with the insomnia.

I was first admitted to hospital after a psychotic episode as a result of leaving my old home for good. I had gone into a deep depression because of leaving my job, the shock of Mother's death, selling my dream home, leaving all my friends and other networks, but most of all because my baby was buried there.

CRITICAL THINKING QUESTIONS

1. What are some background and triggering factors contributing to her first admission?
2. How would you determine whether physical problems contribute to symptoms?

INTRODUCTION

The population of older people is growing in every nation. Improvements in health care, preventive medicine and overall longevity have increased the numbers of people living to older and older ages. Also, the population explosion that took place in many countries in the mid-20th century is visible in the sheer numbers of people entering the stage we call being an older person. Estimates for the world population are that by the year 2050 the numbers of people over 85 years of age will continue to increase dramatically, especially in North America, China and India, as well as in Australia.

With this booming section of the population, the term 'elderly' or even 'geriatric'—meaning those over the age of 65—is insufficient to discuss a group of people whose ages may span four decades. The descriptive terms used to specifically group older people into relevant age categories include *young-old* (65 to 74), *middle-old* (75 to 84), and *old-old* (85 and older).

The norm is that many older people live independently with healthy lifestyles and satisfying experiences for all of their lives. As a consequence of improved pharmacological and other treatments, individuals affected by dementia and mood disorders (once associated with decreased longevity) will experience a relatively normal lifespan. An unprecedented growth in the number of older people with chronic mental illness will have a significant impact on the need for quality mental health care.

It is important to examine the age distribution of the over-65 population carefully. Grouping older people into an aggregate of all persons over the age of 65 tends to blur important distinctions. The old-old group tends to have the greatest incidences of depression, delirium, dementia and other chronic disabling conditions (Mackenzie, Reynolds, Chou, Pagura & Sareen, 2011; Unverzagt et al., 2011). The frail older people who consume many health care resources and community care services constitute only 5 per cent of the over-65 population. A large proportion of healthy older people, particularly single older women (who outnumber single older men by 2.5 to 1), will benefit most from supportive psychosocial services, which are often provided by psychiatric–mental health nurses.

Anticipating the varied mental health needs of a growing population of ageing 'baby boomers' is important for program planning and funding allocation. In Australia, the population of people aged over 65 will increase 86 per cent from 2011 to 2031, representing 20 per cent of the population (Hugo, 2013). The data clearly underscore a need for an increased number of health professionals who recognise that older people have multiple needs. Nursing's role in the mental health of older people and in aged care is expanding as the needs and real numbers of older people increase (Berlau, Corrada, Peltz & Kawas, 2011; Brooks, 2011).

The aim of this chapter is to provide a comprehensive discussion of health promotion and advocacy for older people with mental health needs. Contemporary issues, including end-of-life care, restorative programs and community-based support, are also addressed. We do not discuss the nursing care of older people with cognitive disorders in this chapter. Refer to Chapter 12 for nursing care strategies for cognitively impaired older people. Only a small percentage of older people have physical or mental health issues. This chapter will focus on that small percentage of older people who have disabling or distressing mental health problems.

OBSTACLES TO MENTAL HEALTH SERVICES FOR OLDER PEOPLE

Older people are the most underserved population in need of supportive and tertiary mental health care. This discussion highlights four roadblocks to mental health care services—ageism, myths, stigma and health care financing—and examines the demographic realities that compel us to break through these disabling roadblocks through self-awareness, health promotion and client advocacy (see Figure 22.1 ■).

Ageism

A primary roadblock to adequate mental health services for older people is ageism—prejudice against people because they are old. In many contemporary Western cultures, ageing is often viewed with disdain, dislike and trepidation. Nunney, Raynor, Knapp and Closs (2011) found a paternalistic attitude among health care providers who assumed older people would not be able to understand and function as well as younger people. That type of ageism marginalises and dehumanises older people, and has the potential to undermine self-respect and a sense of identity. Ageism stems from the belief that older people present a financial and emotional drain on the family and society. Ageism results from our fears of facing our own ageing process and mortality. Ageist attitudes can be internalised by older people, causing decreased self-worth and self-esteem, whatever the source.

Before considering any study about the health care needs of older people, it is important to keep a broad perspective on healthy ageing. Undergraduate nursing studies in the past have led to students developing a perception that ageing is a negative process of inevitable decline and disability. This is understandable when courses concentrate solely on chronic health problems, loss of function and/or pain that may be age-related, but which do not contextualise ageing appropriately. It has been well documented that many students develop a dislike of caring for older people and practise avoidance and discrimination as a result of being bombarded with experience of sickness and disability only.

When caring for older people, your personal biases can influence your clinical assessment and your decisions about interventions. You can provide invaluable support, insight and feedback to colleagues who are working with older people. Consider using the Self-awareness feature on the next page as a discussion point. We know that older people are as responsive to mental health services as are members of any other age group (Lysack, Lichtenberg & Schneider, 2011). By modelling positive attitudes towards ageing, and by advocating quality of life and health care for older people in all settings and at all levels of function, you can help dispel ageist influences. See Figure 22.2 ■ for a photograph of an older person and the supportive, candid and loving comments her family made about her.

Myths

Mental health care professionals and older people themselves often equate growing old with growing sad, lonely, disengaged, inactive, socially isolated and dependent. Such myths all too often inhibit people from seeking treatment for feelings and behaviours that they believe are a normal part of ageing. Misled by these myths, health professionals can be less inclined to refer older people for mental health services. We know that advancing age does not condemn an individual to senility, social isolation, loneliness or dependence. Most older people live independently and contentedly well into late life, unless they can no longer drive and live alone, live in rural areas without transportation, or live in urban areas with limited access to health care resources.

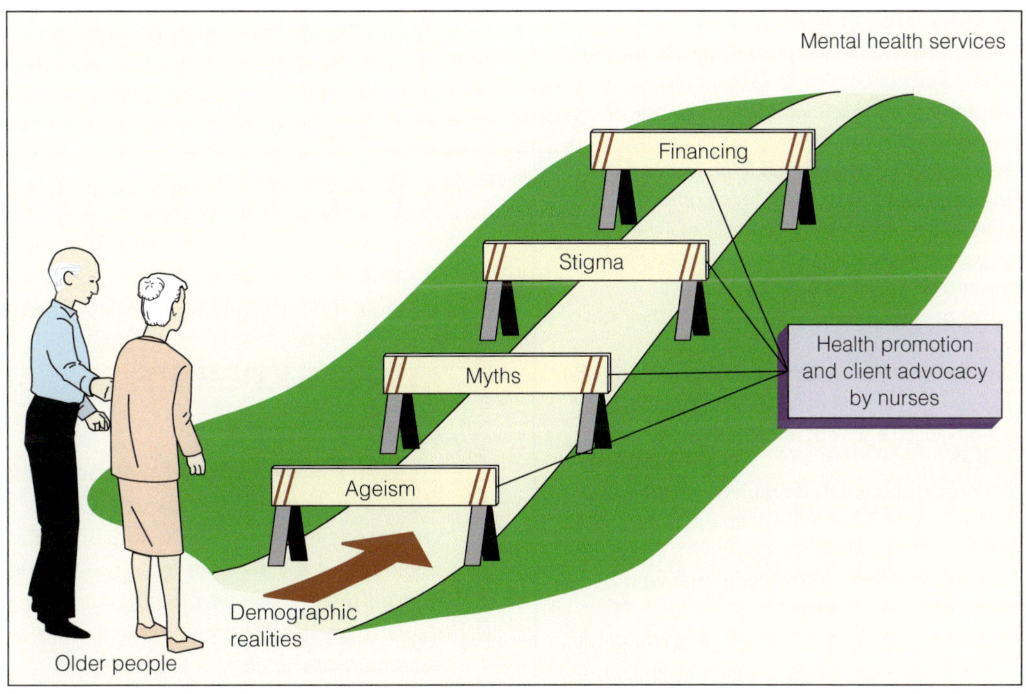

FIGURE 22.1 ■ Roadblocks to mental health services for older people.

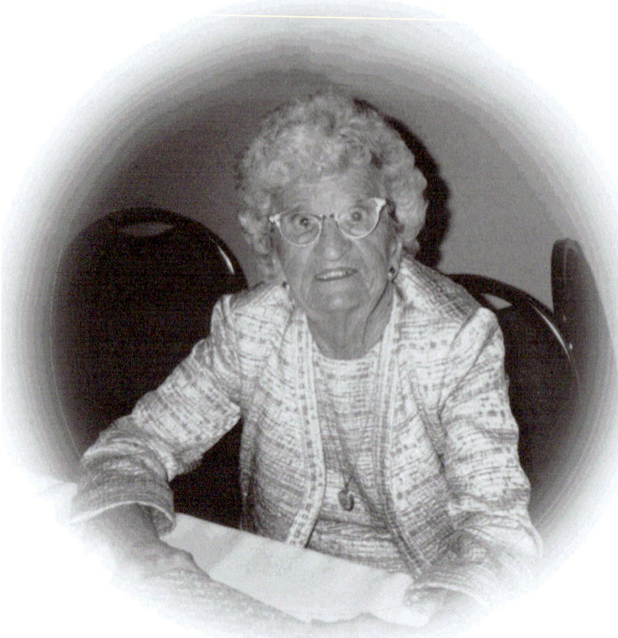

FIGURE 22.2 ■ In the eyes of her family and friends, this was a woman worthy of respect and admiration. She was 'strong-willed' and 'the epitome of ageing with style and grace'. 'She had a sense of humour, kept moving, spent 96 years living a full life rather than 50 years preparing to die, and enjoyed it to the last.' 'She was her own person, no matter what.'
Photo courtesy of © Dr Eileen Trigoboff.

SELF-AWARENESS
Attitudes towards ageing

A bias against older people because of their age can result in discrimination against them even by mental health professionals. Ask yourself the following questions, and discuss your responses with other students, faculty or colleagues.

1. Am I uncomfortable around people who are old, frail or confused?
2. Do I have positive role models for ageing with grace?
3. Do I dread growing old myself?
4. Should older people be encouraged to do as much as possible for themselves, or be cared for by others?
5. How do I feel about old people who are sexually active?
6. What are my specific ideas about how older people should look and act?
7. Do most older people become rigid and set in their ways once they age?
8. Am I well-informed about the differences between mental disorder in older people and the normal ageing process?
9. Do I equate advanced age with unattractiveness and incompetence?
10. Am I well-informed about the community resources and support systems available for older people and their family caregivers?
11. How do I feel when caring for an older person who appears demanding or dependent?

Reflecting on questions such as these can promote your awareness of attitudes that might interfere with providing quality care for older people.

Psychiatric–mental health nurses can serve as advocates by educating the public, other health care professionals, and older people and their families about the differences between normal ageing and changes associated with pathological conditions. Recognising that ageing itself is not depressing or a problem increases the likelihood that problems that do arise will be assessed and appropriately treated (Mezey & Mitty, 2011).

Stigma

Despite recent advances in mental health care, the stigma associated with mental illness remains very real to elderly people. Older people may not seek mental health services as readily as they should, and may hide their psychic pain for fear of being labelled 'crazy' or losing control and being institutionalised.

Nurses have the opportunity to educate the public about mental disorders and the state-of-the-art treatments that are available to all age groups. In so doing, we can help to decrease the stigma associated with psychiatric illness and treatment. Organisations such as beyondblue and the Black Dog Institute have made important advances in this direction by circulating information about the biological basis for many mental health disorders. You can refer older people who feel reluctant about

LIVED EXPERIENCE
Age discrimination

I suffered from age discrimination on two fronts. One was the age; and the other, ethnicity. In addition, they always resented having to allow more care time because of my diabetes and other ailments. In my experience, they hardly knew the difference between mental illness in older people and normal old age.

LIVED EXPERIENCE
Stigmatisation

I started suffering from stigmatisation a few days after I was admitted to hospital. One of my boys was attending a community function when he was asked about my absence from the function. Once he told them that I was in hospital because of depression, it has never been the same with some members of the community.

acknowledging a psychiatric problem to the www.beyondblue.org.au and www.blackdoginstitute.org.au websites. The Mental Illness Fellowship of Australia, at http://www.mifa.org.au, provides links to a range of other useful information sites.

As people learn more about research that confirms the brain mechanisms associated with psychiatric disorders, the traditional stigma associated with seeking mental health services is likely to decrease. At the present time, however, the primary care provider for many mentally ill older people is their family general practitioner.

Older people are seen by their general health care providers, surgeons, specialists for chronic illnesses such as arthritis or diabetes, and in clinics where they receive medications and have laboratory tests evaluated on a regular basis. Because of the likelihood that they will need specialised care, nurses specialising in a variety of settings need specific information about older people. What Every Nurse Should Know has information that is useful for nurses, especially those in rehabilitation services.

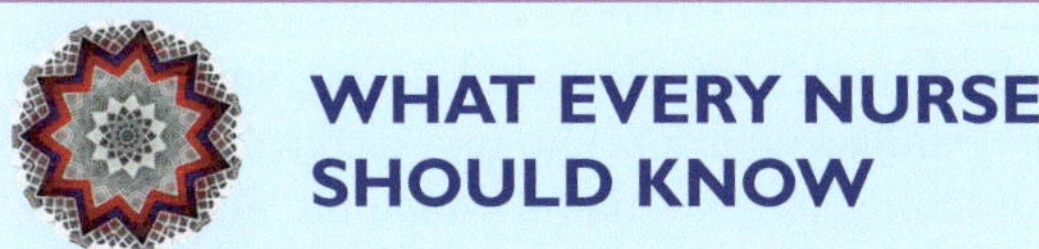

Psychological symptoms an older person may exhibit

Imagine you are a nurse in a medical/surgical unit. You need to be familiar with the likely symptoms that people over the age of 65 years may exhibit when spending time in an inpatient unit. The reason for the placement—post-stroke care, joint replacement, recovery from a fall—can direct you to anticipate what is likely to occur emotionally with the individual. Each of these events carries meaning for an older person that would not apply to someone younger. Stress, being in an unfamiliar environment, and struggling to adapt to body and emotional changes take a larger toll on older adults.

Symptoms may include (among many others) fear and anxiety, increased perception of pain, hallucinatory experiences, suspicion, irritability, disorientation, feelings of hopelessness or helplessness, worry about the future, poor concentration, lethargy and malaise. Behavioural changes may include withdrawal, crying, angry outbursts, poor cooperation with physical care and therapies, restlessness, wandering, intruding and accusations.

Nurses should be familiar with these symptoms, as each could be part of an emotional response requiring treatment, their presence can distort or mask symptoms of physical illnesses, and severe psychiatric distress can impair healing from medical and surgical procedures and injuries.

When an older person has symptoms that appear to be behavioural or psychiatric, be prepared and able to document, classify and report these symptoms correctly so that the person receives any necessary treatment. Knowing the proper interventions, pharmacological and nonpharmacological, can speed stabilisation and improve the quality of life that the people in your care experience.

Health care financing

Financial barriers, physical disability and transportation problems are some factors that limit access to services, especially for older people diagnosed with mental disorders. The financial barriers may be particularly serious. Australian primary care in general practice is supported by Medicare rebates. 'Bulk-billing', where the entire cost of a consultation is subsidised, is not universally available, and this may represent a barrier to accessing primary care on a regular basis. Public mental health community-based services, such as ongoing care coordination, are generally fee free, but inpatient admission often will incur a cost in the medium- to long-term. Access to private hospital mental health care is subsidised by private health insurance for those who are able to afford this insurance, but with restrictions to the length of hospitalisation. Many psychotropic medications are subsidised by the Pharmaceutical Benefits Scheme, but not all medications attract this subsidy for 'off-label' use. For example, some of the antipsychotic class of medications which are used to treat the severe agitation and psychosis in mid- to late-stage dementia disorders do not attract the subsidy.

Psychology services by referral from primary care are partially funded by Medicare, but have limits to the number of sessions. Some primary care networks provide access to psychology services, but subsidy and geographical availability are variable.

As baby boomers reach old age and require long-term care services, these gaps and lack of coverage may reach crisis levels unless service needs are addressed and resolved. For older people with a mental disorder, the crisis is even more acute, as long-term care facilities selectively admit/exclude clients with behavioural and psychological changes.

BIOPSYCHOSOCIAL THEORIES OF AGEING

Distinguishing between the changes associated with ageing and mental disorder in later life is a challenge. Many variables affect mental health as a person ages. Not all theories identified here have been fully confirmed through systematic research, and some—such as the disengagement theory—remain controversial.

Biological theories

Biological theories of ageing include genetic, wear-and-tear, immunology, nutritional and environmental theories.

Genetic theory

Throughout the Human Genome Project (initiated in 1990), which aimed to map and sequence the human genome in its entirety, definitions of health, illness and healthy ageing have been transformed by our increasing knowledge of genetics (Barzilai & Gabrieli, 2010). According to genetic theories, ageing is a process that operates over time to alter cellular structures. Harmful genes activate in late life to stop cell growth and division. This theory supports the idea that the lifespan is predetermined, and people's ageing experience is programmed by their genetic make-up.

Wear-and-tear theory

The wear-and-tear theory proposes that the accumulation of waste products from the metabolism damages DNA synthesis, leading eventually to organ malfunction. In short, cells wear out. Even though the theory allows for individual rates of cell decline that can be accelerated from abuse and slowed by care, the emphasis is one of loss and decline in later life.

Immunology theory

The immunology theory explains age-related decline in the immune system. As a person ages, their ability to defend against foreign organisms declines, with a corresponding increase in susceptibility to diseases, including cancer and serious infections.

Nutritional theory

Nutritional theory focuses on the idea that diet affects how one ages. The quality of one's diet (amounts of vitamin D, fresh fruits and vegetables especially) is as important as the quantity, because vitamin and nutrient deficiencies or excesses have an influence on disease processes.

Environmental theory

A number of environmental factors are known to threaten health, and may be associated with ageing. The ingestion of lead, arsenic, pesticides and other substances can seriously harm the body, as does smoking, exposure to second-hand smoke and air pollution. Environmental factors, such as crowded living conditions and high levels of noise, are known to be stressful and to drain a person's coping capacity (Volkers & Scherder, 2011). An older person's primary activities can also be an indication of health status or a threat to health; for example, sedentary TV-watching contributes to metabolic syndrome in older people. All of these factors can affect one's vulnerability or vigour while ageing.

Psychosocial theories

Psychosocial theories of ageing include the activity and disengagement theories, which contrast sharply with each other.

Activity theory

The activity theory proposes that the way to age successfully is to stay active and involved. Exercise and social interaction are believed to contribute to mental health and satisfaction in late life. Participation in regular exercise programs (both aerobic and strength-training) contributes to healthy ageing, and could play a role in preventing or reducing functional decline in older people (Lobo, Carvalho & Santos, 2011). Consequently, older people are encouraged to remain as active as possible for as long as possible. A number of consumer products, including computer and card-based activities, have been developed to encourage motor activity and mental activity contributing to successful ageing.

Disengagement theory

Disengagement theory is quite the opposite of activity theory. First proposed in the 1960s, the disengagement theory described what was considered an inevitable process in which older people willingly withdraw from social contact and responsibilities, relieved to turn matters over to the younger generation. This theory has become controversial, because many older adults continue to be engaged and responsible well into later life unless limited by immobility, which can lead to involuntary social isolation. Recent research discusses the negative impact of apathy on elder health and wellness (Adams, Roberts & Cole, 2011), and emphasises the need for continued mental activity in order to sustain health throughout the lifespan. See the section on restorative care later in this chapter.

Positive ageing theories

Changing patterns of illness in old age—with morbidity being compressed into fewer years, and effective interventions made to reduce disability in later life—make the goal of ageing successfully more realistic. Stability of personality traits into late life, high levels of integration in society, group heterogeneity and mature ego defence mechanisms appear to contradict the negative stereotypes of ageing. Successful ageing refers to the resilience in people who succeed in achieving a positive balance between gains and losses during ageing (Baltes & Baltes, 1990).

Biomedical models of successful ageing emphasise the absence or minimisation of chronic medical conditions, functional disability and psychiatric symptoms. Social models emphasise the importance of engagement with others. Psychological resources models emphasise self-efficacy, optimism, sense of purpose, playing a useful part, proactive coping, facing up to problems, resilience, self-confidence and self-worth.

Having positive attitudes to ageing may contribute to healthier mental and physical outcomes in older adults. Overcoming negative stereotypes of ageing through change at the societal and individual levels may help to promote more successful ageing (Bryant et al., 2012). See the Practice Example on the next page.

PSYCHIATRIC DISORDERS IN OLDER PEOPLE

Ageist attitudes in our culture account for some of the misconceptions about the prevalence of mental disorders among older people. Older people are believed to be more prone to mental illness than are young people. For several reasons, however, it is difficult to obtain exact incidence and prevalence rates for mental disorders in later life. Older people are often difficult to reach with community-wide surveys, some are reluctant to respond to personal questions that deal with emotional problems, and many either do not seek treatment for emotional problems or consult primary care providers rather than psychiatric professionals. Some epidemiological studies suggest very low rates of mental disorder among older people, but some of these may be fundamentally flawed and severely underestimate the unmet need among older people (Snowdon, Draper, Brodaty, Ames & Chiu, 2010).

When physical deterioration becomes a significant feature of an older person's life, the risk of comorbid psychiatric illness rises. Social isolation and financial burdens are additional

LIVED EXPERIENCE

Example of positive thinking and ageing

I have always had positive views on ageing, but during numerous stays in the hospital it was not possible to be positive about most things. In September 2011, I came home after a four-month stay, the longest ever. After a settling-in period of a few weeks, I decided to make some important decisions which would lead me to the path of long-term recovery.

The first thought that came to my mind was positive thinking. That did not require much effort; until 10 years ago, I was mostly a positive thinker, and in those days my husband's negative thinking used to annoy me.

The most useful thought that came to my mind was to get healthy and stay healthy. This was rather complicated, and required a substantial effort on many fronts, as staying well seemed the hardest part of it.

How should I manage my mental illness, I asked myself? I slept on that idea for a while, and finally a response to my question gave me so much relief. My mind told me that I had been a diabetic for 24 years and I had managed that very well, so why couldn't I manage my mental illness the same way? Since that day I have never had to look back. Life has been very kind to me; I steer my thinking according to my circumstances.

common difficulties older people experience. The sequelae of these social and physical pressures can evolve into symptoms of a psychiatric nature, to the extent that psychiatric diagnoses are not unusual. Results of lifetime prevalence indicate that psychiatric disorders and mental health problems, such as eating disorders, depressive symptoms and psychosocial stress, are public health concerns for this population.

Symptoms of mental illness in the older population often differ from those in other age groups. While the fifth edition of the *Diagnostic and statistical manual* (DSM-5; American Psychiatric Association [APA], 2013) has enhanced our ability to make valid and reliable diagnoses of mental disorders, there

Practice example

In the mid-1990s, Keith retired from a long and distinguished career as a professor at the university at the age of 60, although he continued to be energetic, motivated and productive in his work. He especially enjoyed researching and writing, but was happy to let go of teaching and the administrative aspects of his role in the faculty. Retirement gave him the time and opportunity to continue his academic research without other time pressures. He had resisted the impact of emerging technologies, preferring to make notes in a beautiful cursive script on quality paper, and to type manuscripts or formal correspondence on a manual typewriter. However, with the tradition of keeping an open and enquiring mind, he chose to learn the use of a personal computer in its early and most simple form, learning the functions of a basic operating system and word-processor.

Over the next decades, he continued to use these tools, which he believed were functional and efficient, producing large documents with adequate formatting, printing documents and envelopes, and keeping some household lists. Over this time, he did not see the need for internet search engines, multi-media integration, email communication or social media, but was genuinely impressed and openly interested in his grandchildren's mastery of 'smart' technologies. He chose to adopt only those technologies which he believed he needed.

EVIDENCE-BASED PRACTICE

Staying active and involved

Doris is 92 years old, lives in her own home and attends a seniors' day centre during the day. Her family is very close to her, and wants to make sure that she remains active enough to keep her mind and her body in the best possible form.

The program in which Doris is involved includes traditional activities as well as access to technological tools. Members of the centre are encouraged to use all of the technology to make their lives better through communication, education and physical activity. The staff are sensitive and realise that, while some older people are technologically sophisticated, others find technology frustrating and avoid it. Nursing staff are trained to be technologically competent and to educate others to become more technologically proficient. The following study noted that, importantly, techno-savvy older people can maintain and achieve health and wellbeing (associated with bodily comfort, social networks, self-efficacy and intellectual life) in and beyond their homes. You should base action on more than one study, but for this training program, the following research evidence was helpful:

Loe, M. (2010). Doing it my way: Old women, technology and wellbeing. *Sociology of Health and Illness, 32*(2), 319–334.

CRITICAL THINKING QUESTIONS

1. You have most probably used technology since you were a child. Older people have not. What are the implications of these generational differences?
2. What other evidence would you need to review before designing an intervention for Doris?

are few age-specific categories. Thus, despite the DSM's detailed descriptions of each category, clinicians and researchers continue to have difficulty applying the written descriptions of symptoms to older adults.

Dementia

Dementia is one of the more common psychiatric–mental health problems experienced by older people. It is an umbrella term covering the vast variety of neurocognitive impairments that interfere with memory and function. The most common is dementia of the Alzheimer's type (DAT); however, vascular dementia and dementia with Lewy bodies (DLB) are also quite common. Functional difficulties range from minor (such as not being able to do simple calculations) to extreme (such as the loss of ability to conduct basic hygiene). See Chapter 12 for details about cognitive disorders. A small percentage of people with dementia-related problems require some degree of mental health intervention for severe and persistent behavioural and psychological symptoms (Brodaty, Draper & Low, 2003).

Mood disorders

Mood disorders are primarily characterised by disturbed affect or emotional experience. When they occur in older people, they may present as:

- sustained elation and hyperactivity, such as in a manic episode
- changes from elation to depression, such as in bipolar disorder
- pervasive depressed mood (sometimes with agitation) such as in major depression.

Depression is the most preventable and most treatable mental disorder in later life.

Depression in older people

Depression among older people is widespread in general practice, and even higher in hospitals and nursing homes. Depression robs the person of later-life satisfaction, inhibits ego integrity, and may substantially decrease life expectancy. Older people, especially men, have the highest rate of suicide of any age group and a range of physical disturbances intensified by depression (Lapierre et al., 2011).

Although the signs and symptoms of depression are relatively consistent throughout the lifespan, certain characteristics of depression are particular to older people. It is crucial for clinicians to remember that depression in older adults that responds well to treatment may appear with cognitive changes similar to those that accompany other organically-based, irreversible disorders. Loss of executive function (often a diagnostic clue to dementia) includes disturbances in planning, sequencing, organising and abstracting. Such cognitive impairment can also be a sign of depression.

In addition to cognitive changes, another sign of depression in older adults is an excessive preoccupation with physical symptoms known as somatisation. Expressing discomfort through the body may be more familiar and comfortable than recognising and describing psychic pain. Such is the case in the following example.

Other possible somatic signs of depression to watch for include:

- chronic constipation
- muscular pain
- chest tightness
- headaches
- difficulty breathing
- chronic gastrointestinal upset.

LIVED EXPERIENCE

Seeking help

I first showed symptoms of depression when I was 54 years of age. I had lost my appetite, and even small, trivial tasks took a big effort to finish. Prior to that, my mother, who was overseas, had a third stroke, went into a coma and was on life-support for a year. That added a lot more anxiety to my existing fragile state, and all of a sudden life became very miserable. One night I was driving alone when I suddenly got frightened by the thought that I was alone and what if I had an accident? The next day I went to see my GP and told her what I was going through. She referred me to a psychiatrist.

I was prescribed an antidepressant and told that I would be fine in two weeks. When my mother died a few months later, I became totally withdrawn and did not want to see anyone other than my immediate family. Finally I left the city in a psychotic state, so had to be hospitalised on arrival in the new city.

LIVED EXPERIENCE

Depressive symptoms

I am a diabetic with high blood pressure and few other ailments. From my personal experience, the symptoms of depression always become exaggerated when my sugar levels are too high or too low.

I would get depressed all of a sudden without any known reason. Although this is still an ongoing problem, I have trained myself to monitor my moods at times like this and find an appropriate solution. As a result, my depression disappears in a short time. Sometimes I feel that I have been using CBT [cognitive behaviour therapy] without acknowledging it. For me it is a question of survival with a quality of life.

LIVED EXPERIENCE

Suicide among older people

Because of the religious influence—according to my religion, sanctity of life is very important and taking your own life is an unpardonable sin—I was dissuaded to even think about suicide. There were a couple of occasions (different times) when this thought did cross my mind, but it did not stay there for very long.

Strangely enough, I have no desire to kill myself or to do anything silly as I get old.

It is important to be persistent and perceptive in looking for signs of depression. Depressed, apathetic older people may believe that they are supposed to feel blue and 'down in the dumps' as they age. We need to support the view of depression as a pathological condition often caused by biochemical imbalances that can be corrected. Interventions for depression in older adults should be instituted as aggressively and comprehensively as they are with any other age group.

Depressive symptoms may also result from social and economic circumstances, such as social isolation and neglect. They may be the result of an acute or chronic medical condition, such as a stroke, Parkinson's disease or even a hip fracture. Consequently, it is imperative to include a comprehensive health assessment before beginning a treatment regimen. An older person's response to traumatic events may be tied to functional disability and require multiple areas of intervention.

Suicide among older people

Data from nearly all industrialised countries report that suicide rates rise progressively with age. People aged 65 and older have higher rates of suicide than other age groups (ABS, 2013). Compared with the general population, suicide attempts are more lethal and are approached with a greater degree of premeditation and planning when made by older people. Older adults who are at greater suicide risk include:

- men
- widowed or divorced people
- those of lower socioeconomic status
- those with chronic pain and terminal illness
- Indigenous people
- those with mental disorders/substance use
- those with neurological deficits due to stroke and brain injury
- those who fear becoming a burden.

Suicidal older people have been known to seek help from a general practitioner, often for a vague non-specific physical problem, prior to their self-destructive act. Accurate assessment of suicide potential requires active listening and direct questioning, and attending to anxious depression as a particular risk factor (Seo et al., 2011). Pay close attention to any of the following cues:

- verbal ('Life is not worth living'; 'I won't be around much longer'; 'I won't be here for the next holiday.')
- behavioural (completing a will, making funeral plans, giving away possessions, withdrawing, somatic complaints)
- situational (a recent move, loss of a loved one, the diagnosis of a terminal illness).

For detailed information on suicide and the assessment of suicide potential, including a lethality assessment, see Chapter 19.

Schizophrenia

The number and proportion of older people with schizophrenia will increase considerably with the movement of baby boomers into this population group over the next 30 years. This generation of people with chronic mental illness has not spent years in institutions as the mentally ill older people of past generations did. There is limited research on late-life schizophrenia, and less on its treatment. This population poses a particularly critical issue—85 per cent of older individuals with schizophrenia live in the community and are approaching the age when long-term care may become necessary.

An individual with *late-life schizophrenia* may have experienced psychosis lifelong and grown old, or may be a person who did not experience psychotic symptoms until late in life. People with late-onset schizophrenia are often women with less severe negative symptoms, better premorbid functioning in early adulthood, and less impairment in the areas of learning, abstraction and cognitive flexibility. They also require smaller doses of neuroleptic medication to manage their psychotic symptoms.

Adjustment disorders

Older people often experience dramatic life changes because of losses due to deaths, relocation, dependence, loss of autonomy, retirement, illness and financial stress. One or a combination of life changes and losses may contribute to the development of an *adjustment disorder*. The essential feature of adjustment disorders is a maladaptive reaction to an identifiable psychosocial stressor or stressors that occurs within three months after the onset of the stressor and has persisted for no longer than six months (APA, 2013). The following Mental Health in the Media discusses a movie about life changes within and between generations. People experiencing adjustment disorders may have a variety of psychiatric symptoms, including the following:

- anxious mood
- depressed mood
- mixed emotional features
- physical complaints
- withdrawal.

Psychotherapies can be enormously successful in the treatment of a person with an adjustment disorders.

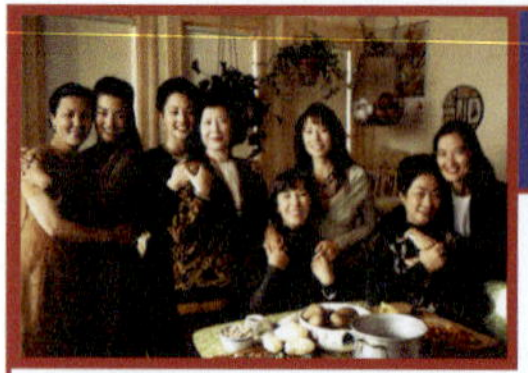

MENTAL HEALTH IN THE MEDIA

The Joy Luck Club

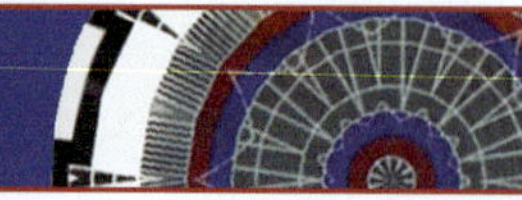

Every week, four older women, all Chinese immigrants, meet to tell stories, play mahjong and eat. The film reveals their hidden pasts—their brutal lives in feudal China. It is an exploration of the cultural conflict between the women and their daughters, how the mothers' experiences in pre-Revolutionary China continue to influence the lives of their American daughters, and the daughters' belief that they are very different from their mothers.

When one of the older women, Suyuan, dies, the three surviving members invite her daughter, June, to take her place. Catharsis and emotional fulfillment during the mahjong games come through the telling of the varied difficulties in the mother–daughter relationships. In America, the mothers find it difficult to understand the directions their daughters are taking. *The Joy Luck Club* reveals the importance of understanding culture and the differences between the generations. It illustrates how family roles and structures can be successfully negotiated when everyone gives a little.

Photo courtesy © Everett Collection.

Anxiety disorders

Anxiety is common across age groups, and increases in frequency with advancing age (Seo et al., 2011). Adjustments to physical, emotional and socioeconomic changes add to the variety of causes for anxiety. Anxiety reactions in the ageing individual may manifest themselves as somatic complaints, rigid thinking and behaviour, insomnia, fatigue, irritability, restlessness, confusion and increased dependence. Physiological indicators of anxiety include increased blood pressure, pulse, respirations, psychomotor restlessness and frequent voiding. Many of these manifestations are present in the following Practice Example.

Practice example

Mrs Pyun, age 82, was rushed to the emergency department by her bridge group with what they think might be a heart attack. She is short of breath and sweating, her pulse is rapid, her hands are shaking, and she cannot sit still during the assessment. She is tearful and cannot tell the triage nurse what is wrong. Mrs Pyun says, 'I don't know why I feel this way. I just know something bad is going to happen. I have to leave and get home. Why are you asking me all these questions? No, I don't have chest pain. I tried to tell them I was just nervous. I get this way sometimes.'

Unfortunately, anxiety disorders and panic attacks are often overlooked in older people, because, as with depression, a predominance of physical complaints mask the underlying disorder. In addition, anxiety in older people often co-occurs with depression. The anxiety is treated, but the depression persists, leading to a cycle of anxiety–depression and physical illness.

Delusional disorders

Delusions in older people are considered a cognitive mechanism for maintaining a sense of power and control. The delusions may be comforting ('I know I'm being guarded by an angel from God') or threatening ('The postman has reported me to the federal police because he thinks I am a terrorist'), but whatever the content, they customarily form a structure for understanding a situation that otherwise seems unmanageable. Delusions may also result from internalised ageist attitudes, sensory losses (particularly hearing impairment), and social isolation.

The delusions of older people are often associated with delirium, depression, dementia or anxiety disorders.

Persecutory delusions involve the belief that one is under investigation, being harassed, or at the mercy of some powerful force. Persecutory delusions may be a response to an older person's diminishing sense of self-mastery. Delusions involving suspiciousness and persecutory ideation are among the most unsettling for older people's caregivers and families. As older adults gradually give up important areas of function, such as financial management, driving, cooking and shopping, they may begin to develop delusions that people are robbing them or poisoning their food. They respond to these delusions by 'dismissing' or rejecting their caregivers in an effort to regain control over these areas of life.

With somatic delusions, the predominant theme is an imagined physical disorder or abnormality of appearance. Somatic delusions in older people are frequently characterised by extremely morbid content ('My blood is leaking into my skin and will poison anyone who touches me').

As a psychiatric–mental health nurse, you will find it crucial to establish trust and consistency with delusional older people. It is important to assess the situation to validate that any persecutory and somatic content is not based in reality. Social interaction with caring people and consistent reality-orientation are important needs. Relieving social isolation and correcting sensory losses may go far to solving some problems. Delusional processes associated with delirium often abate when the cause of the delirium is treated. Medication in small doses, geared towards relieving underlying anxiety or depressive disorder, may be helpful, although adherence is often a problem due to suspiciousness.

Substance-related disorders

A growing body of information suggests that substance use disorders, particularly alcoholism and prescription medication abuse, are more serious problems among older people than had been thought in the past (Arndt, Clayton & Schultz, 2011). Late-life losses and poor coping skills can lead to increased use of alcohol as a self-medication. Alcohol is both a psychological and physical depressant, thereby raising the risk for both depression and substance dependence. The multiplicity of prescription medications older people use can create problems with side-effects, cognitive impairments, drug–drug interactions, and metabolism. Prescribing practices can also inadvertently mask a substance abuse issue. The Practical Example that follows discusses an older person's benzodiazepine misuse.

LIVED EXPERIENCE

Medicines

I have only ever taken prescription medications most of my life. I have learnt a lot about prescription drugs and hard drugs. I do not drink alcohol, smoke or use any other substance. Most of my problems have been due to side-effects, drug–drug interactions and metabolic disorders. Some of the complications may be due to the long-term nature of my treatments for diabetes, high blood pressure and mental illness.

It is important for clinicians not to overlook making their patients aware of the side-effects and drug–drug interactions of most drugs used for depression. The most common side-effects I experienced include drowsiness, dizziness, insomnia and gastrointestinal symptoms. All antidepressants I have taken at different times caused too much elation and then more depression, even at very small doses. Some gave me excruciating tummy ache.

Practice example

Agnes Miller, a 78-year-old woman, has moved to an aged-care facility. Over the previous couple of years she has had increasing difficulty taking care of herself at home. The family reported the following problems prior to supporting her decision to move: leaving a stove turned on long after she had stopped cooking, putting household objects away in unusual places (the frying pan in the dryer, for example), and leaving the house dressed inappropriately for the weather. The family also noticed that her medication bottles were in a state of disarray, and she could not give them a coherent account of which medications she was taking or on what schedule.

Several days after Mrs Miller moved to the facility, staff members noticed that she was developing increasing symptoms of anxiety. These included physiological symptoms such as hyperventilation and diaphoresis, behavioural symptoms such as pacing and an inability to relax, and cognitive symptoms such as catastrophic thinking. However, she was not able to specify any cause for the anxiety. It appeared to be an adjustment disorder related to moving to the facility.

A psychiatric–mental health nurse interviewed Mrs Miller and, in the course of researching the problem, found that Mrs Miller's GP had been prescribing diazepam (Valium) for her for at least five years prior to admission. In gathering collateral information from family members, the nurse discovered that Mrs Miller appeared to have been inconsistently taking more diazepam on a daily basis than prescribed—six to eight pills a day, rather than the prescribed three. Since admission, the diazepam has been administered by the staff exactly as prescribed. Therefore the client's effective dose of diazepam has suddenly been reduced by 50 per cent to 75 per cent.

The upsurge in Mrs Miller's anxiety appeared to be a consequence of her previously undetected diazepam abuse, because she had difficulty tolerating the reduction in the dose. To address this problem, the mental health nurse worked with the other health care providers to reformulate the diazepam regimen so that Mrs Miller could be safely and slowly titrated off the diazepam and be prescribed a safer agent for the treatment of her anxiety.

It is important to note that older people are more vulnerable than younger people to the effects of alcohol and other substances, and that they consume more over-the-counter (OTC) preparations and prescribed medications than other population groups. Alcohol abuse and drug dependence among older people are serious problems. Alcohol abuse can predispose older people to accidents, nutritional deficiencies, and diseases that may lead to loss of autonomy. When older drinkers seek medical help for alcohol-related problems such as malnutrition, injuries from falls, and sleep problems, they rarely report alcoholism as their primary complaint. Unfortunately, the presenting problems may be treated and other symptoms mistakenly attributed to the ageing process.

Clinical manifestations of alcohol abuse in older people include:

- tolerance (requiring more of the substance for the same effect)
- alcohol-related physical health problems, such as gastritis, liver problems and pancreatitis
- physiological dependence on alcohol (the experience of withdrawal symptoms)
- unexpected reaction to prescription medications
- poor response to antipsychotic medications
- multiple social complications (problems with family relationships and social isolation)
- frequent behavioural problems, such as aggression, memory gaps, driving while impaired by alcohol, and traffic accidents
- self-care neglect, such as incontinence, malnutrition, dehydration, and poor hygiene and home maintenance.

Many people with late-onset problematic alcohol use are believed to have turned to drinking in response to stressful life events such as bereavement, illness, divorce, retirement, marital stress or depression. Assessment for drug and alcohol abuse in older people, especially socially isolated older people who have suffered recent losses, should be respectful and nonjudgmental. The risks of mixing medications with alcohol should be an important focus. Preventing drinking as a reaction to stress may be accomplished by providing social support and mental health services for older people at risk for social isolation and depression. Referral to resources such as Alcoholics Anonymous (http://www.alcoholics-anonymous.org) is a recommended intervention, especially when combined with other psychiatric supports. (See Chapter 13 for information about treating people with the dual diagnosis of mental illness and substance use.)

Disorders of arousal and sleep

Older people frequently experience sleep disruptions that may or may not meet the diagnostic criteria for a formal sleep disorder. For example, a lighter sleep phase pattern occurs with less deep sleep, as well as a common circadian rhythm sleep disorder called *advanced sleep-phase cycle* (*advanced* in terms of direction rather than severity; e.g. sleep and wake times are far earlier than desired). The result in older people is an inability to stay awake past 7pm, and then awakening—and being unable to return to sleep—at 3am (Gooneratne et al., 2011). This pattern can be mistakenly diagnosed as depression. Because older adults do have a disproportionately high incidence of depression, determining the presence of depression is also important.

The quantity and quality of sleep change with the ageing process. For example, the amount of REM sleep decreases with ageing. Older people experience more frequent awakenings during the night, spend an increased total time awake at night, and take longer to fall asleep. Changes in sleep architecture and resulting sleep patterns are believed to be related to changes in internal body rhythm, emotional stress, physical illness, and the effects of medications or drugs. Over one-third of people over 60 years of age complain of sleep disturbances (Gooneratne et al., 2011). Older people may nap more during the day and use a disproportionately high amount of OTC and prescription sleeping aids. Yet the chronic use of sedatives and hypnotics by older people has not been shown to improve the quality of sleep, and can lead to many undesirable and dangerous side-effects. Older people excrete these medications more slowly than the young, and thus are prone to developing toxic effects, including delirium, daytime drowsiness and loss of equilibrium. Respiration can be significantly disturbed with the use of sleeping medication.

Clinicians and clients alike must be cognisant of the risks associated with medications, especially when combined with alcohol or even herbal and other supplements. Frequently, sleep disturbances are treated with medications that treat the underlying cause of the sleep problem. Examples include mirtazapine (Avanza), an antidepressant that helps with the sleep and appetite problems of depression, and alprazolam (Xanax) if the sleep difficulty is associated with anxiety. The National Prescribing Service (NPS) hosts a Medicine Wise website www.nps.org.au which provides more detailed information to the public about specific medicines and more general topics.

Older people and their and health care providers should be more willing to try nonpharmacological therapies if indicated. Nonpharmacological guidelines that are recommended for improving sleep—sometimes called 'sleep hygiene'—for older people include the following:

- consistent daily physical activity
- a cool, well-ventilated room
- a light bedtime snack
- stress reduction to promote relaxation
- regular arousal time
- avoiding long naps during the day
- clean bed linens
- avoiding the consumption of caffeine, tobacco and alcohol.

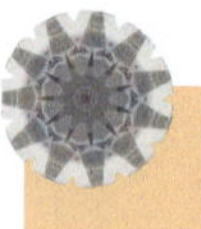

NURSING PROCESS
Older people

The following sections provide specific strategies for applying the nursing process when providing care to older people.

Assessment

Assessment includes an interview, a biological assessment, consideration of cognitive status, an assessment of psychological/emotional status, an assessment of strengths and coping strategies, an assessment of sexuality, an attempt to determine social and financial status, and a focused effort to be alert for any indicators of elder abuse.

The assessment interview

If feasible, a multi-disciplinary team approach is most effective in providing validation of assessment impressions, accurate diagnoses and appropriate intervention strategies. The interview is the initial step in the assessment process, and is important in differentiating between psychiatric disorders and the normal ageing process. Chapter 10 offers a comprehensive overview of the assessment procedures that should be adapted for older people. Insights on interviewing older people appear in Your Assessment Approach.

Interviewing requires skill and heightened sensitivity, and may take more time with older adults than with members of other age groups. Sensory loss, confusion, agitation, wandering, communication disorders, cultural influences, shame and the fear of stigmatisation may inhibit the expression of feelings in some older people. It is imperative to solicit

YOUR ASSESSMENT APPROACH
The key components of a biopsychosocial assessment

Guidelines for interviewing older people

1. Try to make the assessment interview as pleasant as possible by conveying a sense of respect and caring.
2. Be close to the person; use touch when appropriate.
3. Be clear in stating the purpose of the interview, and the length of time it will take.
4. Attend to verbal, non-verbal and environmental cues, as well as to the cognitive and behaviour status of the person.
5. Repeat the purpose and the timeframe of the interview if the older person forgets.

LIVED EXPERIENCE

Clinician's assessment approach

I would have felt most comfortable if somebody had explained the assessment process to me prior to the interview, and also what was to follow next after the interview, to relieve my mind of the symptoms of anxiety. I found questions about whether I was suicidal extreme and upsetting.

interpretations from family and other staff members to help fill in aspects of the clinical picture and validate information provided by the person in the individual interview, always with the consent of the person, when capable. Holistic assessment of older people should include objective and subjective information on: biological, cognitive, psychological function and strengths; coping strategies; and sexual, social and financial issues. In addition to the usual repertoire of screening tools, a variety of self-report screening tools have been designed for use specifically with older people. These require minimal special training to administer, and can help you obtain subjective assessment information. These tools may also be used as objective measures of the outcomes of interventions.

Biological assessment

Before a definitive psychiatric diagnosis can be made, all medically based illnesses with psychiatric symptoms (depression, cognitive deficits, restlessness and anxiety) must be ruled out. In addition, a complete medical and neurological examination is necessary to differentiate irreversible conditions from treatable conditions such as pseudodementia (discussed in Chapter 12). There are conditions, both chronic and systemic, that can predispose an older individual to changes in cognition. For older people, a urinary tract infection (UTI) is a common and debilitating problem that has accompanying pain and cognitive symptoms. Anaemia, infections, organ failure or cardiovascular disease can contribute to delirium. Many emergency department admissions for psychiatric problems in older adults prove to have an underlying biological aetiology, such as an infection, dehydration or adverse medication effects.

Objective assessment information includes laboratory results, a complete history, and physical examination, including weight, vital signs and a description of the physical appearance of the person. Standard diagnostic laboratory analyses appear in Figure 22.3 ■. Your medical/surgical nursing or general nursing texts offer specific biological assessment guides for older people.

Other procedures important for ruling out infections, space-occupying lesions, drug and medication toxicities, and cancers include chest radiography, drug toxicology screening, computed tomography (CT) scanning, positron-emission tomography (PET) scanning, electrocardiogram (ECG), electroencephalogram (EEG), and lumbar puncture.

Subjective assessment information includes the person's perceptions of their physical health, and a description of their chronic illnesses, symptoms, self-care activities, and any concerns and fears about their current situation.

Cognitive status

A thorough mental status examination is essential. Objective information includes the presence and extent of cognitive impairment. Include the family and other caregivers to determine the course of any changes. Ask: 'Did the changes happen gradually (dementia of the Alzheimer's type, drug/medication toxicity, metabolic imbalances), suddenly (depression, cerebrovascular accident, drug/medication toxicity), or in a graduated, stepwise fashion (vascular dementia)?' Family and other caregivers may have noticed changes at certain times of the day that could indicate specific problems (Gaugler, Roth, Haley & Mittelman, 2011). Ask: 'Have there

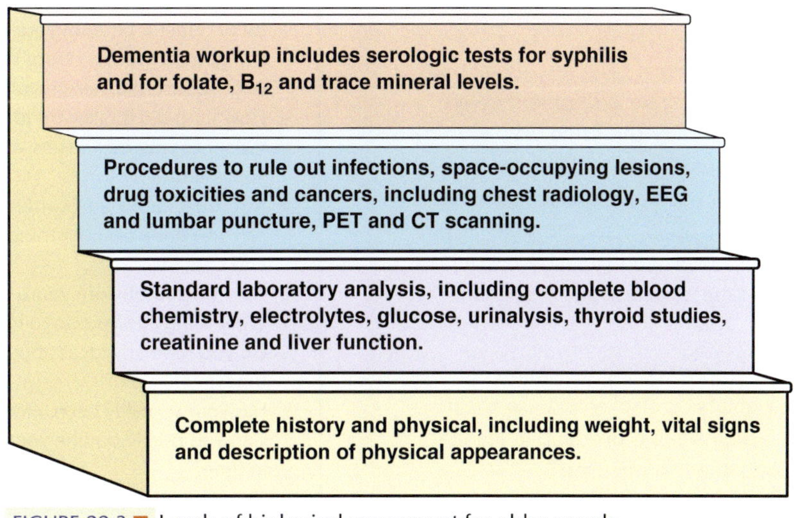

FIGURE 22.3 ■ Levels of biological assessment for older people.

been changes in mood, or has there been agitation in the late afternoon or early evening (sundowning)?' 'Have they been observed to have, or complained of having, trouble in making decisions or concentrating (depression)?'

There are some widely used cognitive screening tools, such as the Mini-Mental Status Examination (MMSE) or General Practitioner Assessment of Cognition (GPCOG). These are easy to administer and reasonably reliable screening tools, which can indicate the need for more robust evaluations, such as the Addenbrooke Cognitive Examination. Keep in mind, however, some important points when using standardised assessment tools with older people:

1. Older people are sensitive to fatigue, boredom, medications and environmental influences that can affect results on a mental status measurement tool.
2. Screening tools like the MMSE cannot distinguish delirium from dementia.
3. Assessment instruments designed for use with other age groups may not be accurate or complete for use with older people.
4. These tools may be less reliable for people with culturally diverse backgrounds.
5. Results may be misleading when used with people of very high or very low educational levels.

Subjective information regarding cognitive status includes the person's own perceptions of their mental status. Questions to ask include:

- How has your thinking been lately?
- Is your memory as good as it used to be?
- Have you been able to keep track of your medications? The days of the week? Mealtimes?

Psychological/emotional status

Objective data about the person's psychological and emotional status require synthesis of impressions from both the content and process of the assessment interview and the mental status examination. Avoid the overuse of psychiatric terminology, but rather strive for descriptions accompanied by examples of the person's behaviour and direct quotations. Be sure to include significant negative findings, such as the absence of delusional thoughts, suicidal ideation or hallucinations. Your assessment should include not only pathology and problems, but also health, adaptive strengths and personal assets.

Strengths and coping strategies

Ageing is a process punctuated by positive and negative stress-producing events. Older people (by definition) have lived for a longer time and may have developed resilience from coping with stressful life events. Information about coping strategies and strengths are as important as information about psychiatric symptoms. You can shift the conversation in this direction by making a statement such as: 'You certainly have lived a long, full life. Would you share with me some of your survival secrets?' Your Assessment Approach, below, provides sample questions to help you gather important information about strengths and coping strategies, such as spiritual practices, interests or reaching out to help others.

Spirituality can be a psychological support and a coping mechanism. Often, people who are facing novel stressors or significant threats to their security turn to religion or spirituality for the first time in their lives, or after an absence for a significant period of time. Is spirituality a recent focus for the person? If so, explore the concepts, meanings and emotions that spiritual expression offers them.

Sexuality

Sexuality is an important area which is often overlooked. Remember that sexual activity can and does continue into later life, and that sexuality is a broad, multi-dimensional component

LIVED EXPERIENCE

In my experience, the cognitive assessments were never conducted consistently the same way, even by the same person. Account needs to be taken of an individual's level of education or experiences in life, whether professional or otherwise, and their ethnic background, religious beliefs and language barriers, not to mention the type of illness and treatment-related factors.

It is very important to provide an environment conducive to their ability to display and use their cognitive skills in a positive and productive manner. This cannot be done in a few minutes.

YOUR ASSESSMENT APPROACH

Assessing psychological strengths

- Would you like to share with me some things about yourself?
- From memory, what were some of the upsetting, stressful or difficult times in your life?
- Did you ever recover from the traumatic experience of (e.g. spouse/partner's death?) If so, how?
- How long did it take you to accept that reality?
- What are your best assets when it comes to cheering yourself up?
- Are you a happy and content person by nature? If not, can you think of some things that might make you happy and content?
- How do you nurture yourself?
- What things do you do to have fun and relax?
- Do you have any ideas about how to get through rough times?
- Has your sexuality been affected over the years? If so, how?
- Can you briefly outline your major concerns at this point in time?
- Do you feel you need help? If so, what sort of help?

of personal identity. Films such as *Harold and Maude* and *Something's Gotta Give* portray richly, and with humour, sexual expression among older people. Sexual expression includes body image, affection, love, flirtation, social roles and interaction. Older people who do abstain from sexual expression often do so because they lack the opportunity, or perceive negative social pressure about sexuality in people their age.

Approach the topic of sexuality in a tactful, caring and nonjudgmental manner. An older person who does not wish to discuss sexual issues most likely will make that clear by stating it directly, not answering the question or changing the subject. People who were socialised in a different, more conservative era may not be comfortable discussing sex. Older adults who matured in the 1960s, however, may have entirely different attitudes towards their continuing sexuality.

Social and financial status

The quality and quantity of available social supports (past and present) are important for optimal functioning. A meaningful social network suggests that strong interpersonal skills can be mobilised to help negotiate stresses and losses in later life. Formation of a new social network when others have dissolved is easier for an older person with the personal resources of assertiveness, friendliness and warmth.

Older people who get by on a low, fixed income may be plagued by financial problems that affect their mental and physical health. Some communities offer services to help older people manage their finances. The removal of financial strain can dramatically improve the health of an ageing person. Sample questions for obtaining information about a client's social and financial status are listed in Your Assessment Approach, below.

Elder abuse

The mistreatment of older people is a serious, under-reported, under-detected phenomenon (Centers for Disease Control and Prevention, 2010). Mistreatment of older people may take many forms, including physical abuse, neglect, exploitation, abandonment and psychological abuse (see Your Assessment Approach on page 498). Older adults with fewer psychosocial resources or a number of psychosocial deficits seem to have an increased vulnerability to mistreatment. Mistreatment is particularly detrimental to psychological wellbeing (Luo & Waite, 2011). The term 'elder abuse' has been used to encompass a range of concerns, but some people believe that the term is unnecessary or disempowering. Abuse is abuse, no matter the ages of the perpetrator or survivor.

Older people who are at greatest risk for abuse and neglect are those who are dependent on others for care. The degree of dependence may overwhelm the caregiver, who may then harm the older person. Stressors related to caregiving can overwhelm any caregiver, but the caregiver of a frail person is often an adult child with additional family and work responsibilities or a spouse who is also ageing. (See Chapter 24 for more information on family stress and the burdens of caregiving.)

A growing number of states and territories provide legal alternatives such as guardianship. Long-term or respite care placement may be necessary. However, most older people react negatively to such placement and want to return to the potentially harmful home situation. In-home assistance is becoming available in most areas, and such home health services can decrease the strain on caregivers. Home visits made by a care coordinator or community health nurse can provide an opportunity to assess the possibility of abuse in any of its forms, or to prevent it by planning for services to meet the needs of older people and their family caregivers.

YOUR ASSESSMENT APPROACH
Guidelines for assessing social and financial status

Some examples may be:

- Does your social life involve sending and receiving emails and phone calls, or travelling to visit friends?
- How often do you need to travel for various purposes, e.g. shopping, visiting friends, meeting doctors' appointments, etc?
- Do you use public transport or are other means of transportation available to you?
- Are there times when you have to worry about your financial situation? Do you have someone like a partner, family members or close friend(s) whom you can rely on for extra financial and moral support?
- Do you enjoy your own company or feel lonely without others?
- Are you much happier in the presence of family and close friends? Are these the people you can rely on and confide in when in need?

Intervention

Once a comprehensive, multi-dimensional assessment is accomplished, problems, behaviours or issues are identified in a collaborative way. Specific issues likely to be associated with a diagnosed disorder are covered in earlier chapters. Chapters on anxiety (Chapter 8), cognition (Chapter 12), psychosis (Chapter 14), depression and mania (Chapter 15) and personality (Chapter 18) describe interventions for adults of all ages in great depth.

Planning and intervention

Mental health recovery is discussed in detail in Chapter 26 'Pathways to Care'. The **recovery** movement has developed into a dominant paradigm in mental health policy. The stories and experiences of people living with mental illness have driven changes in clinical practice and the expectations of mental health services. Recovery models evolved in response to adverse institutional experiences related to limited attention paid to the individual's psychosocial needs and their right to autonomy (Adams, 2010). Recovery-focused care actively seeks to maintain a person's integrity and autonomy, and resists the development of an illness-dominated identity, characterised by uselessness, worthlessness, hopelessness and sickness (Mancini, Hardiman & Lawson, 2005).

Little attention, though, has been given to what the concept of recovery means for older people living with a serious and

YOUR ASSESSMENT APPROACH **Forms of mistreatment of older people**

Determine whether the following have occurred:

Physical abuse	Neglect	Exploitation	Abandonment	Psychological abuse
■ Physical assault ■ Inflicting pain ■ Coercion (abrasions, bruises)	■ Withholding food/drink or medical attention	■ Taking social security or pension funds ■ Taking possessions ■ Removing excess funds from accounts when purchasing items	■ Dropping off at hospital or other health care facility ■ Leaving incapacitated person alone at home ■ Failing to provide basic services	■ Degrading comments ■ Threatening comments ■ Scare tactics (e.g. abandoning) when the person cannot provide for their own needs

persistent mental illness. The word 'recovery' is semantically difficult, as colloquially it suggests improvement or a return to a previous state. Using the word 'recovery' might cause confusion or create an expectation of the older person that might be hard to live up to. For some people, 'recovery' may seem an inappropriate term when the prognosis is irreversible decline, and misinterpretation may give people false hope (McKay, McDonald, Lie & McGowan, 2012).

An important reflection is that 'recovery' should be about what an older person is *recovering* in contrast to what the individual may be *recovering from* (e.g. illness or symptoms) (Collier, 2010). The older person may give priority to:

- maintaining a sense of *identity* from the past
- retaining *dignity* in the face of disability, and being respected by others
- exercising *control* over one's own lifestyle and goals
- perceiving a degree of *wellbeing*
- holding a sense of *hope* for the future.

This section describes some interventions which are not described elsewhere in the text, as well as commenting on some which are covered elsewhere but require some modification or comments regarding their use or adaptation with older people.

Reminiscence therapy and life review

Reminiscence therapy and life review are useful interventions for older people who are experiencing self-esteem disturbance, grief, hopelessness, powerlessness, altered role performance and social isolation. **Reminiscence therapy** uses the recall of past events, feelings and thoughts to facilitate pleasure, quality of life or adaptation to present circumstances. Although it can be used throughout the lifespan, it is of special significance when working with older people.

Reminiscing can and should be encouraged for older people, individually and in groups. Creative use of food, music, pets and special events can facilitate the process and make it fun. Materials such as photo albums, journals, cameras and video recorders provide ways for older people to establish a record of their lives, creating a legacy for those who follow. Storytelling, life review and reminiscence are discussed in the Practice Example.

Practice example

Listening to storytelling, life review and reminiscence

Encouraging the person to make an audiotape, dictate letters, create a photo album or scrapbook, or create other artistic expressions to depict the wholeness of their life can help establish a sense of satisfaction from a life well lived. Reminiscence and life review are identified as useful nursing interventions. Experts who teach about listening to stories suggest guidelines for nurses using this approach. One idea is developing a list of questions that encourage awareness of positive aspects of a life story, and reflection and enthusiasm on the part of the person telling the story. Questions might include: 'How would you like the rest of your story to be?' 'How has what has happened to you shaped who you are today?' 'What do you think are the major themes in your life story?'

Assisting with journal or diary writing

Keeping a journal offers a way to express inner thoughts. A journal can consist of narratives on topics such as 'What do I stand for?', 'What personal quality do I feel best about?' or 'What makes me feel joy?' However, a journal can also take the form of sketches, song lyrics, descriptions of dreams, poetry or prayers that can be original or collected from various sources.

Making and appreciating art as spiritual expression

Creating art and sharing it with others allows the person to leave a legacy, build a sense of community and make sense of experiences. You can encourage participation actively by drawing, painting or sculpting, or passively by collecting healing images such as mandalas, icons, or wilderness landscapes or photographs. Listening to music can help decrease anxiety, depression, agitation and aggressive behaviour, as well as improve relaxation and peace of mind.

The strategies for supporting and nurturing spirituality described here represent only a sample of the possibilities. They all require self-disclosure on the part of someone who may feel vulnerable. Extreme sensitivity is required to use them in practice. Some people prefer to discuss these topics with a member of the clergy or a spiritual advisor. These wishes must be respected.

Life review is a structured process involving the recall of past events in one's life in an effort to find meaning in those events. The process systematically reviews remote memories and addresses the expression of related feelings and the recognition of conflicts. A life review is a chance to re-examine one's life, solve old problems, make amends, establish perspective and restore harmony. As life review becomes an integral part of clinical care, it provides emotional and spiritual support. Approaching the second half of life with a positive perspective—a journey filled with new possibilities, and enriched by wisdom and learning from life experience—provides an opportunity to reflect on personal intentions, values, interpersonal relationships and a personal legacy (McSherry, 2011). Initiating and therapeutically directing the life review process requires your use of effective therapeutic listening skills (refer to Chapter 9) in order to enhance the psychological growth that can emerge as a result of this process.

Cognitive behaviour therapy

Cognitive and behavioural therapies (CBT) are formal structured therapies that share some basic principles:

- thoughts (cognitions) influence our behaviour and emotions
- thoughts can be monitored or altered
- behavioural or emotional change can be produced through changes in the way we think.

CBT is considered in great detail in Chapter 25. When considering any formal psychotherapy with an older person, there may be some special considerations. A key advantage of CBT is that treatment can be tailored to the specific situation and needs of the individual (Wilkinson, 2013). Some barriers that may arise in accessing therapy include mobility, transport and availability of skilled therapists. Depression in late life may be associated with deficits in executive function, working memory and processing speed, resulting in the need for modifications, such as increased structure in sessions and direct assistance with some techniques (Alexopoulos et al., 2008). Older people with more than mild impairment of verbal memory may struggle with both cognitive and behavioural strategies.

LIVED EXPERIENCE

Cognitive behavioural therapy (CBT) has helped me in the past four years while I have been well. My psychologist tells me that I have been using CBT all my life without knowing it.

During sick periods, the conceptual side of me must have been so bad that I found it difficult to grasp any depth of mindfulness, solution-based (being a scientist, still made sense) therapy and some home-grown versions of therapies which never made sense anyway.

Reality orientation

Reality orientation emphasises awareness of time, place, person and purpose. The approach provides consistency and a constant reminder to the person of where they are, why they are there and what is expected. The periodic use of reality orientation tests the older person's level of confusion and disorientation. The rationale for reality orientation is the need to use the part of the person's mind that remains intact.

Validation of emotions

Validation therapy is an emotion-oriented approach which guides skilled communication techniques for communicating with very old people who are diagnosed having Alzheimer's disease and related dementias. This approach classifies individuals with cognitive impairment as having one of four stages on a continuum of dementia: malorientation, time confusion, repetitive motion and vegetation. The benefits of validation therapy for patients are reported as restoration of self-worth, minimisation of the degree to which patients withdraw from the outside world, promotion of communication and interaction with other people, reduction of stress and anxiety, stimulation of dormant potential, help in resolving unfinished life tasks, and facilitation of independent living for as long as possible (Jones, 1997). The focus is on interpreting the emotions expressed, rather than the actual information, which is based on past realities rather than present reality. Errors in fact are given little focus, and the two-way communication between the disoriented person and the cognitively intact person is therefore not interrupted. The immediate and obvious benefits of stress reduction and conflict avoidance may theoretically lead to the resolution of emotions stemming from life review (Minardi & Hays, 2003).

Animal-assisted therapy

Animal-assisted therapy, or pet therapy, involves the purposeful use of animals to provide affection, attention, diversion and relaxation to people. The animals may be certified therapy animals and may be obtained from a variety of sources, such as the Delta Society (http://www.deltasociety.com.au/), or may live on the grounds of the facility. Animals that have physical contact with older people are trained to respond in a calm, non-threatening manner. Small animals can be held in an older person's lap, larger animals are trained to stand next to a chair and allow the person to stroke or pet them without having to hold them, and aviaries of birds provide sound, movement and interaction. Figure 22.4 ■ shows one such therapy animal.

Exercise and movement therapy

Exercise and movement therapy can help induce relaxation, maintain flexibility, restore balance and enhance joy in older people. Such interventions may include stretching and reaching activities, complex exercises such as T'ai Chi for those able to mirror the leader, or simple and concrete movements such as handholding for those who are physically or cognitively incapacitated.

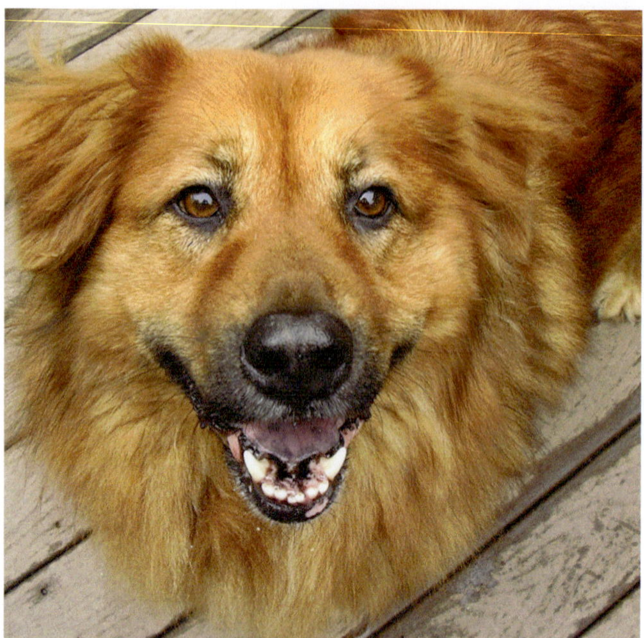

FIGURE 22.4 ■ Therapy animals like Bruno provide unconditional acceptance, and emotional, tactile and interactional opportunities for even significantly regressed or isolated older people.
Photo courtesy of Anne Garcia.

Support groups

Social support and group interventions are useful when working with people who experience dysfunctional or interrupted family processes, knowledge deficits, ineffective coping, dysfunctional grieving, social isolation and spiritual distress. The group situation or social environment provides emotional support as well as information for its members. Groups are the treatment of choice for many older people, especially those in long-term care facilities, because several people can benefit and transportation is not a problem.

Medication administration

Used judiciously, medications can be an effective adjunct to other interventions when working with people with mental disorders in later life. A key axiom to remember about medication dosing with older people is: 'Start low, go slow.' The high incidence of adverse medication reactions in older people underscores the need for careful monitoring and conservative dosages. Table 22.1 ■ summarises recommended dosages for categories of psychotropic medications used with older people. In general, information about dose adjustments and special considerations with older people are catalogued in medication references such as drug guides and medication manuals. (See also Chapter 7 of this text for in-depth information.)

It is important to recognise that older people are more prone to side-effects from psychiatric medications, and that nurses and older people should carefully observe or monitor for their occurrence. Among these side-effects are the following:

- extrapyramidal symptoms (dystonias, akathisia, tremor, pseudo-Parkinsonism)
- constipation
- anticholinergic effects (urinary retention, cognitive impairments, blurred vision, dry mouth, hallucinations, sexual dysfunction)
- cardiovascular effects (postural hypotension, arrhythmias)
- drug interactions resulting in delirium, confusion or disorientation
- over-sedation (drowsiness)
- paradoxical or idiosyncratic effects.

Medications within each psychotropic class vary widely in the intensity of side-effects. Complex interactions may require referral to an old-age psychiatrist who is knowledgeable about the complexities surrounding the appropriate doses and possible side-effects of these medications.

TABLE 22.1 ■ Dosage ranges of some commonly used psychotropic medications used with older people

Category	**Dosage range**
Antipsychotics: atypical	
olanzapine (Zyprexa)	5–10 mg/day
risperidone (Risperdal)	0.25–4 mg/day
quetiapine (Seroquel)	50–300 mg/day
Antipsychotics: conventional	
haloperidol	orally: 0.25–15 mg/day, intra muscularly: 2–5 mg four-hourly prescribe as needed
Anxiolytic agents (benzodiazepines)	
lorazepam	0.5–2.0 mg/day
oxazepam	10–30 mg/day
Mood stabilisers	
carbamazepine	200–800 mg/day
lithium	300 mg three times a day
valproate	250–1500 mg/day
lamotrigine	100–200 mg/day

(continued)

Table 22.1 ■ *(continued)*	
Sedative–hypnotic benzodiazepines	
temazepam	7.5–15 mg/bedtime
Atypical antidepressants	
mirtazapine	7.5–45 mg/bedtime
agomelatine	25–50 mg/bedtime
Selective serotonin reuptake inhibitors (SSRIs)	
citalopram (Cipramil)	10–20 mg/day
sertraline (Zoloft)	25–100 mg/day
escitalopram (Lexapro)	5–10 mg/day
Serotonin and noradrenaline reuptake inhibitors (SNRIs)	
venlafaxine (Effexor-XR)	150–225 mg/day
desvenlafaxine (Pristiq)	50 mg/day
duloxetine (Cymbalta)	20–60 mg/day
Tricyclic antidepressants	
nortriptyline (Allegron)	10–100 mg/day
Source: Jacobson, S. (2015). *Clinical manual of geriatric psychopharmacology* (2nd ed.). Washington, DC: American Psychiatric Publishing.	

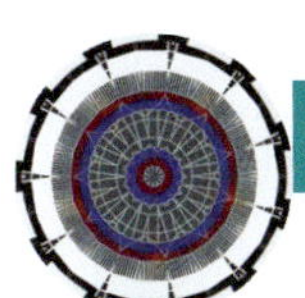

DEVELOPING CULTURAL COMPETENCE

Generational commonalities of older people

Cultural competence in mental health nursing with older people requires sensitivity to not only the ethnic, racial and cultural heritage of an older person, but also to their generational commonalities. Older people have their own history and a perspective in addition to their cultural identity. Even if an older person is of a majority culture, there is nothing routine or mainstream about the decades of experience the individual has accumulated.

Think about your culture and how you express it through religion, cooking, celebrations and traditions. Each culture may have a different definition of successful ageing, but their elders have all got similar wisdom based upon their life experiences.

What is defined as successful ageing in your generation within your culture? Do you think that your parents and grandparents defined successful ageing in the same way? Ageing well might include abstaining from drugs and alcohol, having a successful financial portfolio, demonstrating personal responsibility, or having wisdom based upon one's life experiences.

Older people who have lived with serious, lifelong and disabling mental health problems may have gone for years without the benefit of psychopharmacology (which was not developed until the late 1950s). Or they may have undergone unmodified electroconvulsive therapy (ECT) when muscle relaxants and anaesthesia were not used. They may have lived in under-served areas where mental health services were not available, or when the stigma was so palpable that no one went for treatment. Attitudes in our society towards mental health have undergone change, yet much more needs to change. Older people who have had lived with mental illness through the years will have experienced stigma and lack of services. This will inevitably have an influence on their attitudes towards mental health care. Cultural competence takes this perspective into account and increases our ability to establish and maintain therapeutic relationships together.

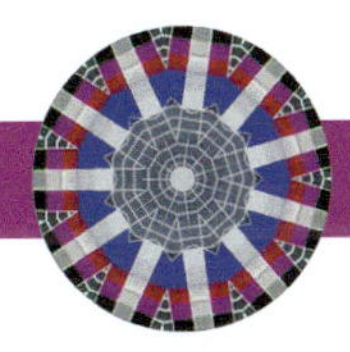

REFERENCES

Adams, K. B., Roberts, A. R., & Cole, M. B. (2011). Changes in activity and interest in the third and fourth age: Associations with health, functioning, and depressive symptoms. *Occupational Therapy International, 18*(1), 4–17.

Adams, T. (2010). The applicability of a recovery approach to nursing people with dementia. *International Journal of Nursing Studies, 47*, 626–634.

Alexopoulos, G. S., Raue, P. J., Kanellopoulos, D., Mackin, S., & Area, P. A. (2008). Problem solving therapy for the depression-executive dysfunction syndrome of late life. *International Journal of Geriatric Psychiatry, 23*, 782–788.

American Psychiatric Association (APA). (2013). *Diagnostic and statistical manual of mental disorders* (5th ed., Text Revision). Washington, DC: APA Publishing.

Arndt, S., Clayton, R., & Schultz, S. K. (2011). Trends in substance abuse treatment 1998–2008: Increasing older adult first-time admissions for illicit drugs. *American Journal of Geriatric Psychiatry, 19*(8), 704–711.

Australian Bureau of Statistics (ABS). (2013). *3303.0—Causes of death, Australia, 2011*. Retrieved from http://www.abs.gov.au/ausstats/abs@.nsf/mf/3303.0/

Baltes, P. B., & Baltes, M. M. (1990). Psychological perspectives on successful aging: The model of selective optimization with compensation. In P. B. Baltes & M. M. Baltes (Eds.), *Successful aging: Perspectives from the behavioral sciences* (pp. 1–34). New York, NY: Cambridge University Press.

Barzilai, N., & Gabrieli, I. (2010). Genetic studies reveal the role of the endocrine and metabolic systems in ageing. *Journal of Clinical Endocrinology and Metabolism, 95*(10), 4493–4500.

Berlau, D. J., Corrada, M. M., Peltz, C. B., & Kawas, C. H. (2011). Disability in the oldest-old: Incidence and risk factors in The 90+ Study. *American Journal of Geriatric Psychiatry, 20*(2), 159–168.

Brodaty, H., Draper, B. M., & Low, L. F. (2003). Behavioural and psychological symptoms of dementia: A seven-tiered model of service delivery. *Medical Journal of Australia, 178*(5), 231–234.

Brooks, C. L. (2011). Considering elderly competence when consenting to treatment. *Holistic Nursing Practice, 25*(3), 136–139.

Bryant, C., Bei, B., Gilson, K., Komiti, A., Jackson, H., & Judd, F. (2012). The relationship between attitudes to aging and physical and mental health in older adults. *International Psychogeriatrics, 24*(10), 1674–1683.

Centers for Disease Control and Prevention, National Center for Injury Prevention and Control, Division of Violence Prevention and Control. (2010). *Understanding elder maltreatment—fact sheet.* Retrieved from http://www.cdc.gov/violenceprevention/

Collier, E. (2010). Confusion of recovery: One solution. *International Journal of Mental Health Nursing, 19*, 16–21.

Gaugler, J. E., Roth, D. L., Haley, W. E., & Mittelman, M. S. (2011). Modeling trajectories and transitions: Results from the New York University caregiver intervention. *Nursing Research, 60*(Suppl.3), S28–S37.

Gooneratne, N. S., Tavaria, A, Patel, N., Madhusudan, L., Nadaraja, D., Onen, F., & Richards, K. C. (2011). Perceived effectiveness of diverse sleep treatments in older adults. *Journal of the American Geriatrics Society, 59*(2), 297–303.

Hugo, G. (2013). The changing demographics of Australia over the last 30 years. *Australian Journal on Ageing, 32*(Suppl.2), 18–27.

Jacobson, S. A. (2015). *Clinical manual of geriatric psychopharmacology* (2nd ed.). Washington, DC: American Psychiatric Publishing.

Jones, G. M. M. (1997). A review of Feil's validation method for communicating with and caring for dementia sufferers. *Current Opinion in Psychiatry, 10*(4), 326–332.

Lapierre, S., Erlangsen, A., Waern, M., De Leo, D., Oyama, H., Scocco, P., . . . Quinnett, P. (2011). A systematic review of elderly suicide prevention programs. *Crisis, 32*(2), 88–98. doi: 10.1027/0227-5910/a0000

Lobo, A., Carvalho, J., & Santos, P. (2011). Comparison of functional fitness in elderlies with reference values by Rikli and Jones and after one year of health intervention programs. *The Journal of Sports Medicine and Physical Fitness, 51*(1), 111–120.

Loe, M. (2010). Doing it my way: Old women, technology and well-being. *Sociology of Health and Illness, 32*(2), 319–334.

Luo, Y., & Waite, L. J. (2011). Mistreatment and psychological well-being among older adults: Exploring the role of psychosocial resources and deficits. *Journals of Gerontology, 66*(2), 217–229.

Lysack, C., Lichtenberg, P., & Schneider, B. (2011). Effect of a DVD intervention on therapists' mental health practices with older adults. *American Journal of Occupational Therapists, 65*, 297–305.

Mackenzie, C. S., Reynolds, K., Chou, K.-L., Pagura, J., & Sareen, J. (2011). Prevalence and correlates of generalized anxiety disorder in a national sample of older adults. *American Journal of Geriatric Psychiatry, 19*, 305–315.

Mancini, M. A., Hardiman, E. R., & Lawson, H. A. (2005). Making sense of it all: Consumer providers' theories about factors facilitating and impeding recovery from psychiatric disabilities. *Psychiatric Rehabilitation Journal, 29*(1), 48–55.

McKay, R., McDonald, R., Lie, D., & McGowan, H. (2012). Reclaiming the best of the biopsychosocial model of mental health care and 'recovery' for older people through a 'person-centred' approach. *Australasian Psychiatry, 20*(6), 492–495.

McSherry, C. B. (2011). The inner life at the end of life. *Journal of Hospice and Palliative Nursing, 13*(2), 112–120.

Mezey, M. D., & Mitty, E. (2011). A Bill of Rights for hospitalized older adults. *Journal of Nursing Administration, 41*(3), 115–121.

Minardi, H., & Hays, N. (2003). Nursing older adults with mental health problems. *Nursing Older People, 15*(7), 20–24.

Nunney, J., Raynor, D. K., Knapp, P., & Closs, S. J. (2011). How do the attitudes and beliefs of older people and healthcare professionals impact on the use of multi-compartment compliance aids? A qualitative study using grounded theory. *Drugs and Ageing, 28*(5), 403–414.

Seo, H. J., Jung, Y. E., Kim, T. S., Kim, J. B., Lee, M. S., Kim, J. M., . . . Jun, T. Y. (2011). Distinctive clinical characteristics and suicidal tendencies of patients with anxious depression. *Journal of Mental and Nervous Disease, 199*(1), 42–48. doi: 10.1097/NMD.0b013e3182043b60

Snowdon, J., Draper, B., Brodaty, H., Ames, D., & Chiu, E. (2010). Prevalence and treatment of late life depression. *Australian and New Zealand Journal of Psychiatry, 44*(11), 1054. doi: 10.3109/00048674.2010.514857

Unverzagt, F. W., Ogunniyi, A., Taler, V., Gao, S., Lane, K. A., Baiyewu, O., . . . Hall, K. S. (2011). Incidence and risk factors for cognitive impairment no dementia and mild cognitive impairment in African Americans. *Alzheimer Disease and Associated Disorders, 25*, 4–10. doi: 10.1097/WAD.0b013e3181f1c8b1

Volkers, K. M., & Scherder, E. D. (2011). Impoverished environment, cognition, ageing, and dementia. *Reviews in the Neurosciences, 22*(3), 259–266.

Wilkinson, Philip. (2013). Review: Cognitive behavioural therapy with older people *Maturitas, 76*(1), 5–9.

Therapeutic groups

23

CHRISTINE PALMER AND CAROLYN HYDE

LEARNING OUTCOMES

After completing this chapter, you will be able to:

1. Apply the general principles of the Johari Window to create opportunities for change and learning in small groups.
2. Encourage the assumption of appropriate task roles and maintenance roles among members of small groups.
3. Improve the dynamics of small groups by incorporating an understanding of the interpersonal needs of inclusion, control and affection.
4. Explain the purposes that therapeutic groups fulfil.
5. Design a therapeutic group based on the needs and personality characteristics of potential members.
6. Apply the process of here-and-now activation to a therapeutic group.
7. Develop process commentary appropriate to the level and purpose of the group.
8. Understand the importance of peer-led groups.

KEY TERMS

LIVED EXPERIENCE

Managing my borderline personality disorder

I was diagnosed with borderline personality disorder in 2009 aged 34 (along with depression, generalised anxiety disorder, social anxiety disorder and panic disorder). I have lived with anxiety since childhood, and at times I still feel self-conscious in social settings. I developed depression when I was 15 because I felt that I didn't belong in my family. I didn't know how to relate to them, and I felt alone, invisible and like an intruder.

From 2009 to 2013, I was developing self-awareness and learning how to manage symptoms through therapy. I started a peer support group for people with borderline personality disorder in Brisbane, Australia, after I learned that my mental health nurse was planning to leave. Thoughts of abandonment were triggered, but instead of becoming engulfed and trapped in feelings of anger, sadness, fearfulness and rejection, I became proactive, researching psychologists and support groups. I found the 'meetup.com' website. About 10 people had listed borderline personality disorder as an interest, but there was no active group. I decided to start a group, coming to this conclusion before my next appointment with my mental health nurse two weeks later. The decision was easy.

(continued)

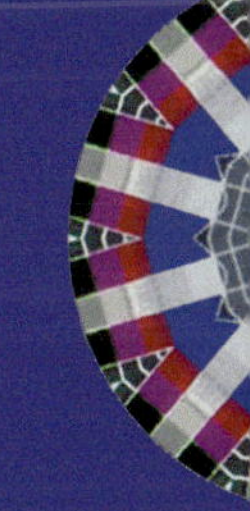

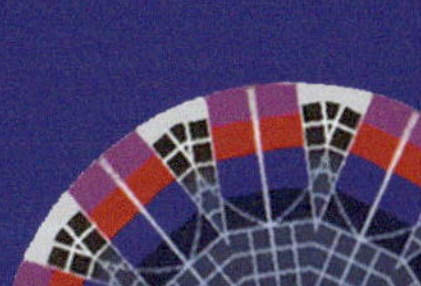

LIVED EXPERIENCE *(continued)*

The group was active on the website in 2013. I waited anxiously for people to join the group—however, I received requests to join the group the day after it was activated!

The benefits of being a member of the support group are: feeling less lonely and isolated; the ability to talk openly and honestly about your feelings without feeling judged; and being among people who understand what you are going through or have been through living with the disorder. We all get a better understanding of the disorder and also learn new coping skills.

INTRODUCTION

Why are groups important? Most people are born into a group—the family—and our survival from the moment of birth depends on relationships formed with other human beings. Our sense of self, of being, and of personal identity derives from the ways in which other members of the groups to which we belong perceive and respond to us. We interact with others at all stages of our lives in various groups—family groups, peer groups, work groups, play groups, worship groups. Many of the goals we set for ourselves cannot be achieved without our membership in groups. Through cooperation and coordination we can achieve objectives and reach goals that we could not through individual effort alone. In this way, groups help us to improve the quality of our lives.

Practice example

The staff members of a rehabilitation unit were required to provide two daily group sessions for all residents. The residents had varying psychiatric diagnoses—mainly bipolar affective disorder, schizophrenia, major depression, schizoaffective disorder and obsessive–compulsive disorder. The only area that could accommodate all of the residents (28–30 at any one time) was a large day room in which the chairs were set in a square. The nurses' station desk with telephones, and a locked door through which others entered and exited the unit, were located next to the day room.

1. Which elements of the environment might interfere with the smooth functioning of a group? Why?
2. How would the characteristics of the residents facilitate or hinder the group process?
3. What kinds of group activities would be appropriate, given the population of residents and the environmental circumstances?

LIVED EXPERIENCE

Belonging to a group is fantastic!

'I am just so chuffed to belong (at last!) to this group—we are special!!!!!! Thank you to everyone at group today, you are awesome!!!'

Much of our professional life is spent in groups—groups of people we work with as carers, and groups of colleagues with whom we plan and implement the delivery of health care services. Nurses have long been involved in working with people in small groups brought together for health teaching, psychoeducation or supportive purposes in inpatient facilities, and in community-based agencies as well. All nurses, regardless of their level of education, can lead therapeutic groups or psychoeducation groups, as long as they understand and apply group dynamics in their interventions. In fact, group interventions have become increasingly more important in this economy as a result of the need to provide treatments that are also cost-effective. However, the role of the psychiatric–mental health nurse as group psychotherapist is reserved for advanced practice registered nurses.

To use groups rationally and effectively, you must understand the forces that underlie small group interactional processes. Using group interventions, you can provide psychoeducation for the people you serve and their families. Therapeutic groups offer people the opportunity to seek validation, give and receive interpersonal feedback, and test new and different ways of being that may improve the quality of their lives. Mental health can be preserved, maintained and restored through interaction with others in productive groups.

SMALL GROUP DYNAMICS

Several forces modify and shape groups, influencing their effectiveness. These forces are discussed in the sections that follow.

Trust

Trust develops in relationships when people disclose more and more of their thoughts, perceptions, attitudes and reactions to one another, and find that their disclosures have been made in a safe environment among other people who respect their self-disclosures. The group member who makes a suggestion, discloses an attitude, feeling, experience or perception, gives feedback, or confronts another member, engages in trusting behaviour and assumes the risks inherent in trusting. Trusting and being trusted are intimately linked to risk-taking. The level of trust among the members of a group determines the extent of risk-taking behaviour in the group. Bear in mind, however, that the ways that people interact within the social microcosm of the group deeply reflects their usual interpersonal style (Goldberg & Hoyt, 2015). When trust exists, individual members will risk sharing more. Because trust takes some time to build, do not expect that trust will necessarily exist in short-term inpatient groups in which membership changes frequently in a brief period of time. It is the group leader's role to address safety and group cohesion when it is apparent that group members are having difficulty in openly expressing their views (Caruso et al., 2013).

Self-disclosure and self-awareness

There are many ways to think about self-awareness. Self-awareness is a complex, multi-dimensional phenomenon, often contradictory and partly undiscovered. The Johari Awareness Model, often called simply the **Johari Window**, is a theoretical tool used to represent self-awareness and self-disclosure in relation to other people.

Interpersonal interaction, in a group setting for example, is facilitated when people have sufficient knowledge about one another's attitudes, beliefs, actions and opinions to determine how safe it is to self-disclose. The Johari Window is a graphic representation of this self-awareness model. It is described here and illustrated in Figure 23.1 ■:

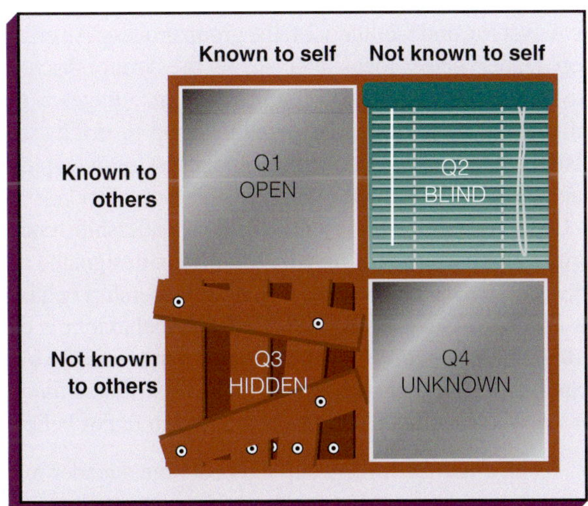

FIGURE 23.1 ■ Johari Window of self-disclosure.
Source: Adapted from Beebe, S. A., Beebe, S. J., & Redmond, M. V. (2011). *Interpersonal communication: Relating to others* (6th ed.). Boston, MA: Allyn & Bacon, p. 54.

- *Johari Window Quadrant 1:* Open activity (known to self and known to others). Quadrant 1 of the window represents aspects of the self that are known to you and are readily available and known to others as well. This is the part of the self that engages in daily social conversation. The more you reveal about yourself, the larger this quadrant will be.
- *Johari Window Quadrant 2:* Blind (not known to self but known to others). Quadrant 2 contains characteristics that are known to others but not to yourself. In this quadrant is information about how you affect others intentionally or unintentionally. It is an aspect of self about which you may get honest, genuine, uncensored feedback from others that may surprise you. In this case, the blind window gets smaller.
- *Johari Window Quadrant 3:* Hidden (known to self but not known to others). Quadrant 3 represents the private life space—knowledge you have about yourself that is not known to others. These are the secrets, the personal and private feelings, thoughts and fantasies that you have but that you do not want others to know.
- *Johari Window Quadrant 4:* Unknown (not known to self or others). Quadrant 4 contains knowledge about yourself that you do not know yet, and is also unknown to others. Eventually, some of this knowledge becomes known to you or to both you and others. This quadrant also represents unconscious processes that may be brought into awareness through psychotherapy.

Relations within the group

Major elements in this awareness model are its assumptions that humans respond to groups and that change or learning can follow opportunities for new interaction. The primary principle of change in relation to the Johari Window is that a change in one quadrant will affect all of the other quadrants. Certain other general principles of change that derive from the Johari Window are particularly suited to the understanding of small group behaviour. These principles are:

- A large open quadrant (Q1) facilitates working with others. Therefore, more of the resources and abilities of group members can be brought to bear on the group task when members have large Q1 areas.
- The open quadrant can be enlarged and awareness can be increased by learning about group processes as they are being experienced.
- The group's value system influences how a group confronts the unknown quadrant.

In a new and immature group, the open quadrant (Q1) is small, because free and spontaneous interaction does not immediately occur in new groups. As the group matures, the open quadrant expands and the private quadrant (Q3) shrinks accordingly. This means that members become freer to be themselves and to perceive others as they really are. An atmosphere of increasing trust, risk-taking and self-disclosure begins to form. An enlarged area of free activity means that the group uses more energy to work on the group task than to maintain or defend the hidden or avoided area of Q3. The blind quadrant (Q2) also diminishes as members learn more about themselves. Dealing with blind spots requires sensitivity, empathy and timing by the mental health nurse (Gans, 2011), and other group members might also develop some of these skills. The unknown quadrant (Q4) changes more slowly and to a lesser degree, because it represents an area in which unknown behaviours and motives reside. Figure 23.2 ■ compares the degrees of openness in immature and mature groups.

Cohesion

Cohesion can be defined as a spirit of common purpose. In groups that cohere (hang together), the members have a desire for mutual association. Cohesion is the primary factor keeping a group in existence and working effectively (Ellis, Peterson, Bufford & Benson, 2014; Norcross & Wampold, 2011).

A group is cohesive when its members are attracted to it. People are attracted to a therapeutic group for a wide variety of reasons. The group may meet their needs for affiliation, interpersonal security, self-knowledge or therapy. It may have members who not only are available for human interaction, but also have important shared attitudes, values, interests and beliefs. An attractive group has explicit, mutual and attainable group goals, with clear paths to goal attainment.

What indicates that the spirit of cohesion exists in a given group?

- Attendance is high.
- The members arrive on time.
- The members stay with the group.
- The members engage in an interdependence that is cooperative rather than competitive.
- The activities the group undertakes are satisfying and successful.
- There is a high degree of member participation.
- Communication networks are open, central and flexible in a warm and friendly atmosphere.
- 'We' is frequently heard in discussions.
- The members like and trust one another.
- The members enjoy interacting with one another.

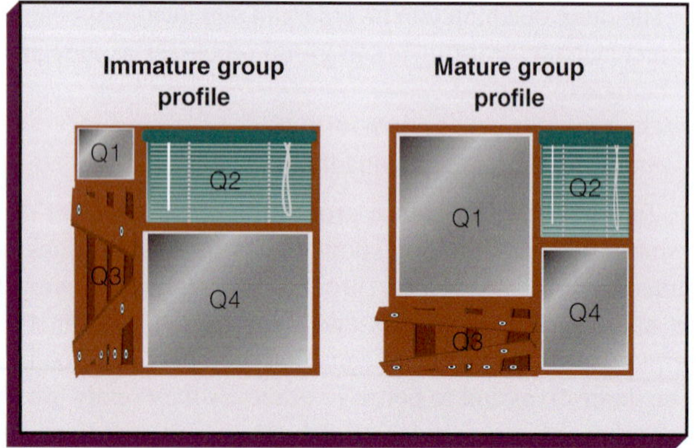

FIGURE 23.2 ■ Johari Window self-awareness configuration of the immature group versus the mature group.

LIVED EXPERIENCE

The value in sharing within a group

'Thank you Carolyn for dedicating your time and skills to ensure our meet-up. So wonderful to see so many new faces, and to share tales of each other's journey with such nonjudgment and compassion. I love this group; it truly brings a sense of belonging. Thank you to everyone for sharing and listening as you do—it's a huge honour. Sarah . . . thank you for volunteering your time, expertise and heart to us all yet again.'

Cohesive groups are not born—they are developed. Cohesion does not become evident until the group has come together long enough to have shared experiences that provide the basis for attraction. An outpatient group usually has an existence lengthy enough to provide time for cohesion to develop. Inpatient groups on acute care units are usually too brief to become cohesive.

How can a group's tendency to cohere be enhanced? Some methods include increasing the trusting and trustworthy behaviour of members through self-disclosure and through the acknowledgment of confidentiality, increasing the affection expressed among members, promoting inclusion and acceptance among members, and enhancing the influence that members have on one another. Another method for building cohesion is structuring cooperative relationships among the group members.

Group roles and leadership

Leadership is a process of influence. Group roles centre on the influence relationships that exist within the group. The primary influence relationship is leadership. An effective group leader is the catalyst for, and facilitator of, the group process. An effective group leader helps focus and shape the group discussion, motivates group members to participate, encourages a group to remain on track, and empowers the group to make creative decisions. In general, a good leader is successful in helping the group accomplish its goals (Harris & Sherblom, 2011).

Group dynamics theory tells us that leadership functions within a group can be fulfilled by the person designated as the leader, and by members who engage in leadership behaviour. This approach to understanding leadership behaviour is called the *distributed functions approach*, and stems from the classic research of Benne and Sheats (1948). The distributed functions approach to group leadership is based on two major beliefs:

1. any member of a group may become a leader by taking actions that serve group purposes
2. different members may perform various roles in a group.

Each member may play more than one role during a meeting of the group, and a wide range of roles in successive group sessions. Any member may play any or all of the roles. The various functional roles may be grouped into two categories:

1. **Task roles** are related to the task of the group. The job of people assuming these roles is to facilitate and coordinate group efforts in the selection, definition and solution of a group problem.
2. **Maintenance roles** are oriented towards building group-centred attitudes among the members and maintaining and perpetuating group-centred behaviour.

Sometimes members of a group satisfy their own individual needs that are irrelevant to the group task, and may also be negatively oriented to group maintenance functions. These are called **self-serving roles**. If a group is to function effectively, it must perform a self-diagnosis to determine what the needs of the group are and how they can be met, so that the self-serving roles no longer present obstacles to effective functioning. Task, maintenance and self-serving roles are described in Table 23.1 ■.

Distributing leadership functions among group members is important, because it teaches people the diagnostic skills and behaviours needed to accomplish the group's goals and maintain good interpersonal relationships. Of course, in psychotherapy groups, some functions or activities may be largely, or even solely, the province of the therapist. In psychotherapy groups, the quality of the therapeutic alliance with the group therapist has been found to be a consistent predictor of short-term group therapy outcome (Fasulo, Ball, Jurkovic & Miller, 2015).

Power and influence

It is impossible to discuss group dynamics without discussing power, because it is impossible to interact without influencing, and being influenced by, others. This process constantly occurs within groups, forcing members to adjust to one another and modify their behaviour and, sometimes, their attitudes and beliefs. *Power* is defined as the ability to do or act, to have possession of command or control over others, or to achieve the desired result. The terms 'power' and 'influence' are used interchangeably in this chapter.

Power and influence are not negative forces. Do not confuse the judicious use of power in building effective groups with the use of power to control, manage and manipulate others. Become aware of how you can employ power and influence in serving those in your care and your profession. Advocating for people, as well as conscious awareness of power imbalances in therapeutic relationships, are examples of this.

A group in which certain members have much power and others have little power is likely to be a group in trouble. The unequal distribution of power affects both the task and the maintenance functions of a group. Members who believe they have little influence within the group are unlikely to feel committed to group goals and to the implementation of group decisions. Their dissatisfaction with the group decreases its

TABLE 23.1 ■ Group roles and functions

Role	Function
Task roles	
Coordinator	Identifies the relationships among the group suggestions and ideas
Elaborator	Fleshes out ideas and suggestions (arranging seating; distributing handouts)
Information-giver	Offers facts, ideas and own experiences
Information-seeker	Asks for information that would clarify issues
Opinion-giver	States beliefs about group function and group values
Opinion-seeker	Asks for beliefs that would clarify group values
Maintenance roles	
Compromiser	Minimises conflict by seeking alternatives
Encourager	Moves the group in a positive direction by encouraging and praising the contributions of others
Follower	Goes along with the group
Group observer	Keeps the group records; interprets data
Harmoniser	Keeps the peace; smoothes over conflict
Standard-setter	Reminds the group of the standards to be achieved
Self-serving roles	
Aggressor	Attacks group members, ideas or values
Blocker	Disagrees, opposes and resists
Dominator	Manipulates others, seeks control through excessive talking; interrupts others
Playboy	Fails to become involved in group process
Recognition-seeker	Boasts, brags about accomplishments, calls attention to self
Self-confessor	Expresses personal and self-oriented, rather than group-oriented, insights and feelings

Source: Adapted from Harris, T. E., & Sherblom, J. C. (2011). *Small group and team communication* (5th ed.). Boston, MA: Allyn & Bacon, pp. 46–47.

attractiveness and reduces its cohesion, and ultimately group members will refuse to participate or they will leave the group.

Group developmental phases

Group development is not always orderly. Not all groups proceed through the stages in the order discussed here, although the following stages describe common experiences. As you will see, conflict is a normal and necessary part of the development of group cohesiveness. The stages of group development were first introduced by Tuckman (1965), when the first four stages were outlined at that time. Later, Tuckman and Jensen (1977) added the final stage.

Forming

In this beginning stage, the members are beginning to know one another, the purpose of the group, and their place or role in the group. Because the group has not yet established its norms (rules), unease, tension and awkwardness are normal (Harris & Sherblom, 2011). Gradually, people begin to relax and devote themselves to the task. Members are reluctant to self-disclose until issues of confidentiality are understood. Only then can members begin to build interpersonal trust. Getting to know other members of the group helps, but does not remove all anxiety. Concerns about other group members and their intentions, one's own role in the group, and the process, purpose and goals of the group remain. These concerns lead to the second group stage—storming.

Storming

In this phase, conflict inevitably erupts, usually over such issues as power, authority and competition within the group. In this stage, the politeness that characterised the first phase (forming) is replaced by more forthright opinions that are not based on keeping things 'nice'. In other words, the communication among members is more open and authentic. Successfully resolving this stage of conflict allows the group to move towards cohesion, as members become more interdependent upon one another. However, groups that avoid or suppress conflicts may create a continuing tension that stifles the development of cohesion, decision-making and problem-solving abilities. The secret to moving on and becoming an effective group is based on the ability of the group to air their conflicts and work through them.

Norming

Once differences are expressed and conflicts have subsided, the group begins to become more cohesive. The relationships among members are more open and trusting, and cooperation among the members has increased. The storming phase has given members the opportunity to test one another's reactions. However, just because conflicts have subsided does not mean that they are totally resolved. It is normal for groups to move back and forth between stages. Norming is an important stage in the group's development. During this stage, the group settles on specific rules—how discussions take place, how decisions will be made, which issues of the storming phase need to be revisited, how the labour in the group is to be divided, and how goals, roles and expectations are negotiated.

Performing

Performing is the real work phase of the group (Harris & Sherblom, 2011). Members increase their focus on the task at hand. There is an open exchange of information and the giving and receiving of feedback. Social tensions decrease as the group moves towards solving the tasks of the group. The group identifies possible solutions, and looks at what impact the possible solutions can have. In other words, they engage in the problem-solving process. Group members share the facts and data they possess, and make sure that all members understand the facts and data. They treat all ideas as welcome, and find direction from one another's ideas. They look at the positive and negative aspects of each solution before devising a plan of action.

Adjourning

The final phase in the group process is the termination of the group. Ideally, groups experience termination because they have completed their task and stop meeting together. Adjourning may be experienced in earlier phases of the group if members leave the group for any reason. The ending of a group is not without its stresses, especially if the group is a long-standing one and its purpose is more interpersonal (psychotherapy, support, self-awareness) than one oriented towards solving a specific problem (determining the unit rules on a psychiatric inpatient unit). Adjourning is an opportunity for members to say goodbye. Some groups mark the end of the group with a special event to experience a sense of closure.

Practice example

Adjourning stage

Eight third-year nursing students were ending their 10-week clinical experience on a community-based rehabilitation unit. They planned a special event for their last day—a combination psychoeducation experience with a special treat for the residents. The nursing students had developed a program for the residents that focused on the benefits to brain function and cognition of certain vitamins and minerals found in fruits. After a poster presentation and a show-and-tell of pineapples, papayas, mango, oranges, cantaloupe, strawberries and kiwifruit, the residents were given a bowl of these fruits which were not routinely available to them.

The activity allowed students and residents to finish on a positive note. The students delivered an educational experience, surprised the residents with an unusual treat, and provided an opportunity for residents and students to say their goodbyes to one another.

GROUP DEVELOPMENT THEORY

It is generally accepted that groups develop structure over time in a predictable way (MacKenzie, 1997). The interpersonal needs approach discussed in this section can be used to understand the development, dynamics and functioning of small groups, from mutual-help or self-help groups to psychoeducation groups to psychotherapy groups. The interpersonal needs approach helps us to understand how groups develop, and the factors that determine how effective they are.

The basic assumption of the interpersonal needs approach known as FIRO (Fundamental Interpersonal Relations Orientation), a classic group dynamics theory (Schutz, 1958b), is that people need people. In addition, people need to establish some equilibrium between themselves and the others in their environment. This equilibrium is determined by the interaction of three basic interpersonal needs, and it appears to be synonymous with interpersonal compatibility, or the extent to which people are able to get on with each other (Schutz, 1958b).

Three basic interpersonal needs

An interpersonal need is one that can be satisfied only through relationships with people. Schutz (1958b) reasoned that every individual has three interpersonal needs: inclusion, control and affection. It is the matching of these interpersonal needs between people that will help to build trust and to develop respectful relationships.

Inclusion

The interpersonal need for inclusion is the need to establish and maintain relationships with others that offer interactions and associations satisfying to you. In other words, the **inclusion need** consists of the ability to take an interest in others to a satisfactory degree, and the ability to allow other people to take an interest in you that is satisfying to yourself. This need determines whether a person is outgoing or prefers privacy. Compare the inclusion needs illustrated in Figure 23.3 ■.

Control

The interpersonal need for control is the need to establish and maintain a satisfactory relationship between yourself and other people with regard to power and influence. The **control need** consists of the ability to take charge to a satisfactory degree, and the ability to feel respect for the competence of others and their capacity to take responsibility. Compare the control needs illustrated in Figure 23.4 ■.

Affection

The interpersonal need for affection is the need to establish and maintain a satisfactory relationship between yourself and other people with regard to love, admiration and affection. The **affection need** consists of being able to love and admire other people or to be close and intimate to a satisfactory degree, and having others love you or be close and intimate with you to a satisfactory degree. Compare the affection needs illustrated in Figure 23.5 ■.

Interpersonal group phases

According to this approach, any group, given enough time, moves through three interpersonal phases—inclusion, control and affection, in that order—that correspond to the three basic interpersonal needs.

Inclusion phase

The first, or inclusion, phase is concerned with belonging. People attempt to find their place in the group, and are concerned with learning whether they will be acknowledged as individuals or left behind and ignored. Because these concerns give rise to

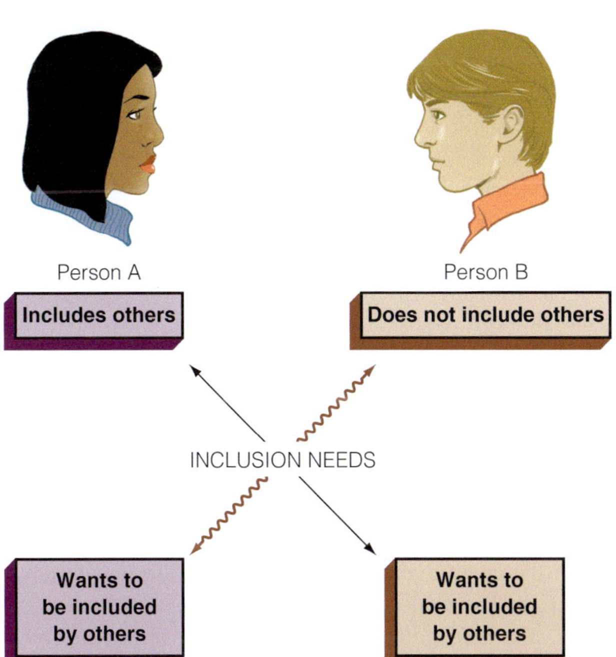

FIGURE 23.3 ■ Inclusion needs. While both people want to be included by others, only one (Person A) includes others. Therefore, Person B's needs for inclusion are met. However, Person A will feel frustrated because her need to be included is not being met.

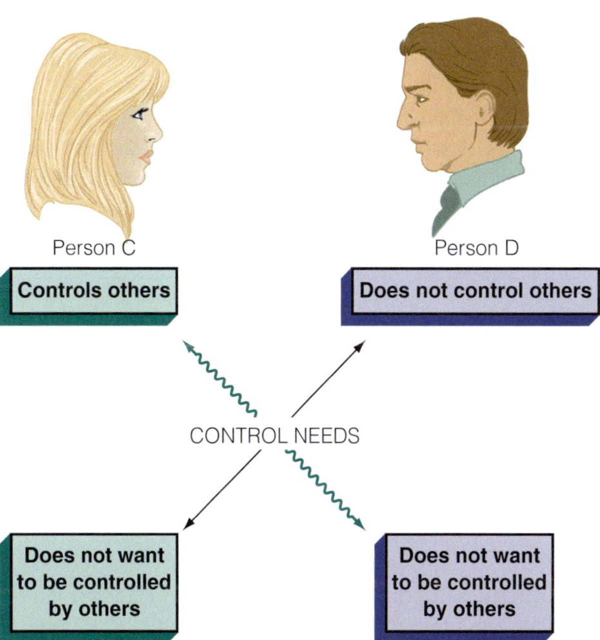

FIGURE 23.4 ■ Control needs. This situation has the potential for great conflict. Person D, who is happiest in a laid-back atmosphere, will resent, and perhaps sabotage, Person C's efforts to control him. Person C is likely to intensify her control efforts in response.

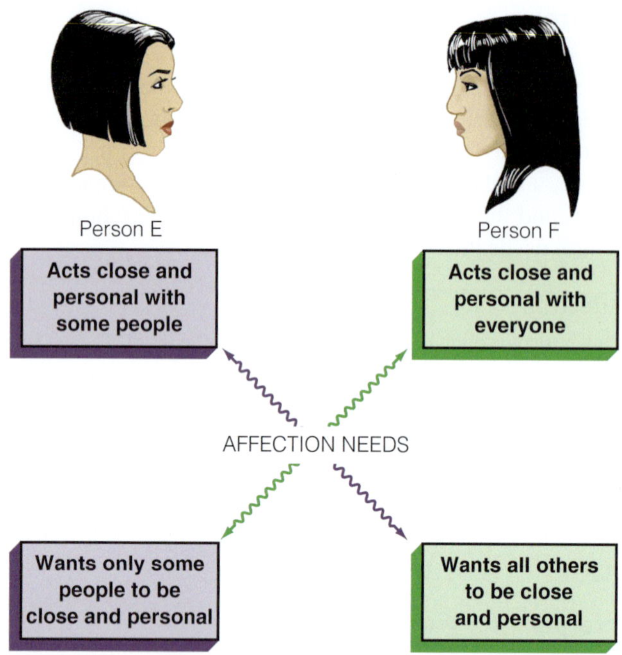

FIGURE 23.5 ■ Affection needs. Both people in this situation are getting some of their affection needs met if Person F is one of the people with whom Person E wishes to be close and personal. If not, Person E could back away emotionally if she views Person F as intrusive. Backing away would likely cause frustration for Person F.

anxiety, this phase is dominated by behaviour centred on the self. Over-talking, withdrawal, exhibitionism and sharing other group experiences and biographies are some examples.

Frequently, what Schutz (1958a) calls **goblet issues** predominate. These are issues of minor importance to the group that help the members get to know one another better and to test each other out. Goblet issues are a vehicle for sizing people up. Goblet issues may revolve around the weather, sports, rules of procedure and so on. If goblet issues continue to a significant extent beyond this initial phase of the group, they will impede group progress.

Control phase

The second, or control, phase is concerned with who has the power, and this becomes central after problems of inclusion have been resolved. Concern about decision-making procedures predominates. The problems that emerge in this phase centre on the following two concerns:

1. how responsibility is shared
2. how power and influence are distributed.

There are struggles for leadership and about the structure, rules of procedure, and methods of decision-making. Members attempt to establish comfortable positions for themselves in terms of responsibility and influence.

Affection phase

The third, or affection, phase is concerned with emotional proximity, and it follows satisfactory resolution of the preceding two phases. Individual members are now faced with the problem of becoming emotionally involved with one another. Concerns about not being liked by, being too close to, or not being close enough to others become relevant. The behaviour in this phase is generally characterised by high emotion—positive feelings, jealousy, hostility and pairing are some examples. Schutz (1958a) describes this phase as one in which, like porcupines, people attempt to get close enough to receive warmth, yet avoid the pain that sharp quills can inflict.

Interweaving of phases

None of these phases is distinct, because all three problem areas—inclusion, control and affection—are present at all times, even though only one predominates. Schutz (1958a) uses a tyre-changing analogy, what he calls tightening the bolts, to describe the sequence of the phases. Changing a tyre is best done by tightening the bolts just enough to hold the wheel in place. Then each bolt is tightened further until it is secured. The leader helps the group work on all three interpersonal need areas in similar fashion, returning to and working over each area to a more satisfactory level than was reached the last time. The interpersonal needs approach of Schutz is based on the belief that the way to attack problems within groups is by investigating what is going on among the individuals in the group and attempting to improve their interpersonal relations. You will discover a parallel between this group development theory and Yalom's group therapy theory, discussed in the next section.

GROUP THERAPY THEORY

There is great diversity and flux in the field of group therapy. Many types of groups are found in mental health care settings or in communities at large. Certain common principles seem to apply to all therapeutic groups, although specific methods and techniques may vary according to the purpose of the group or the skills and theoretical orientation of the therapist or group leader.

Irvin Yalom (2005) uses the term *interactional group therapy* to describe a process of group therapy in which member interaction plays a crucial role. In **group therapy**, six to eight members come together to learn about themselves and their relationships with others as a means of improving their mental health. (See Advantages of Group Therapy in the next section for a complete discussion of the purposes and the common principles that apply to interactional group therapy.)

The mental health nurse, even if not an advanced-practice nurse qualified as a group psychotherapist, can incorporate many of these principles of group therapy into the leadership role in therapeutic groups, as well as in informal groups in the milieu. The principles will have a sense of familiarity—Yalom, like Hildegard Peplau, was greatly influenced by the interpersonal theory of Harry Stack Sullivan. You will need to modify the principles for use in short-term groups, such as those on most inpatient units. Modifications for short-term inpatient groups are discussed throughout this section. Essential differences between inpatient and outpatient groups are identified in Table 23.2 ■.

TABLE 23.2 ■ Differences between inpatient and outpatient groups

Inpatient groups	Outpatient groups
The composition of the group changes depending on who has been admitted and who has been discharged.	The composition of the group is stable, usually over its life.
Members may be selected because they happen to be on a particular unit or assigned to a particular therapist.	Selection criteria play a major role in designing the group.
Attendance is compulsory and people are often wary of, or ambivalent about, attending the group.	Individuals usually choose whether to join a group. Those who choose to join are motivated.
Membership length is determined by the length of hospitalisation. When the individual is discharged, membership in the group ends.	The group continues for a predetermined length of time identified in the group contract—often one year or more.
The goal is relief of symptoms, possibly some degree of self-awareness, support and/or psychoeducation.	The goal is insight-oriented.
Sessions are usually 30–45 minutes long, daily or several times a week, and are based on the members' tolerance level.	Most outpatient groups are approximately 1½ hours in length, once a week.
Because of the continually changing membership, inpatient groups on acute care units rarely become cohesive.	Group cohesion can be expected to develop over time.
Group members have 24-hour exposure to one another; therefore, what goes on in the milieu outside of the group influences what goes on inside the group.	Members in outpatient groups don't usually have relationships with other members outside of the meetings.
The inpatient therapist provides a greater degree of structure and takes on a more active role because of the members' needs.	The outpatient therapist is less active and waits for the structure and the process to unfold.
Because the therapist has limited ability to select who will be in the group, the group tends to be heterogeneous in terms of vulnerability or ego strength, as well as personality characteristics.	Outpatient therapists usually design their groups to balance the behaviour and characteristics the members bring to the group. The members are more likely to be homogenous in terms of their ego strength.

Advantages of group therapy

The advantages of group therapy stem from one major factor: the presence of many people who participate in the therapeutic experience, rather than working with a solitary therapist. Specifically, group therapy provides the following:

- stimuli from multiple sources, revealing distortions in interpersonal relationships so that they can be examined and resolved
- multiple sources of feedback
- an interpersonal testing ground that allows members to try out old and new ways of being in an environment specifically structured for that purpose.

The curative factors

Yalom (2005) contends that 11 interdependent curative factors or mechanisms of change in group therapy help people. These factors constitute a rational basis for the therapist's choices of tactics and strategies, and are identified and defined in Table 23.3 ■. Yalom recommends group therapy as a means for achieving genuine encounters with other members and the group therapist (Yalom, 2009).

Types of group leadership

Groups can be led by a therapist working alone or by co-therapists working together in a variety of ways.

Single therapist approach

Groups led by a single therapist are common. They have an economic advantage in that only one therapist needs to be involved. A disadvantage is that the therapist cannot compare analyses of the group process with a co-therapist or get instant feedback or validation from a peer. Therapists working alone, however, do not have to direct their energies towards creating and maintaining a relationship with a colleague.

LIVED EXPERIENCE

Belonging and sharing improve my mood

'I always feel so good after these meet-ups. Thank you all for sharing your experiences and allowing me to share mine. It is great to no longer feel alone with this illness, and I am learning so much more from everybody.'

Co-therapy approach

Groups led by two therapists, who share responsibility for leadership of the group to varying degrees, are gaining in popularity. The two models seen most often are the junior–senior and the egalitarian styles of co-therapy.

Junior–senior co-therapy In the junior–senior approach, the therapists have unequal responsibilities towards the group. The senior member of the team is usually the more experienced or educated. Besides having major responsibility for the success

TABLE 23.3 ■ Curative factors of group therapy

Factor	Definition
Instilling hope	■ Establishing a sense of optimism for change and the success of the group therapy experience ■ Calling attention to the improvement that group members have made
Universality	■ Confirming that others experience similar pain and struggles ■ Disconfirming that the client is alone or unique in misery or hurt to provide a powerful sense of relief
Imparting information	■ Sharing didactic information or advice about recovery, strategies, resources and coping behaviours ■ Providing psychoeducation
Altruism	■ Finding that the members can be of importance to others and have something of value to give ■ Gaining from the act of giving
Corrective recapitulation of the primary family group	■ Reviewing and correctively reliving early familial conflicts and growth-inhibiting relationships in a more supportive environment ■ Challenging and exploring fixed roles ■ Working through unfinished business
Development of socialising techniques	■ Acquiring basic social skills; e.g. preparing for discharge, approaching a prospective employer, asking someone out on a date ■ Acquiring sophisticated social skills; e.g. resolving conflicts, being attuned to process, being facilitative towards others
Imitative behaviour	■ Trying out bits and pieces of the behaviour of the therapist and the members, and experimenting with those that fit well ■ Benefiting by observing the therapy of another member
Interpersonal learning	■ Learning that one constructs one's own interpersonal world, and therefore one has the power to change it ■ Comparing one's interpersonal evaluations with those of others, and altering distortions (consensual validation) ■ Learning how to adapt and to take on perspectives other than one's own
Group cohesiveness	■ Being attracted to the group and the other members with a sense of 'we'-ness rather than 'I'-ness ■ Being included, accepted and involved meaningfully with the other members
Catharsis	■ Being able to express feeling as a way of acquiring skills for the future ■ Feeling a sense of liberation by being able to get relief by expressing emotion in a supportive group
Existential factors	■ Being able to 'be' with others, to be a part of a group ■ Taking ultimate responsibility ■ Self-realisation

Source: Yalom, I. D. (2005). *The theory and practice of group psychotherapy* (5th ed.). New York, NY: Basic Books.

of the group, the senior therapist is responsible for training the junior member of the team.

This approach is commonly used in public mental health service settings, because it provides in-service training of new personnel and non-professionals under the guidance and watchful eye of an experienced group leader. However, the members of the group may be unclear about the subordinate/superordinate roles and unsure of how to deal with, and respond to, leaders of unequal abilities and responsibilities.

Egalitarian co-therapy In the egalitarian approach to co-therapy, two therapists of relatively equal ability and status share equally in responsibility for the group. Two nurses considering an egalitarian co-therapy relationship with each other need to engage in preliminary work to determine whether such a relationship is feasible for them. Exploration should include the following:

- discussing each therapist's theoretical approaches, intervention styles, past experiences with groups, sociocultural background and personality characteristics
- considering and resolving such issues as how and when feedback is to be given, how disagreements between them are to be handled in the session, and the general conditions under which they will work together
- agreeing that decisions on member selection, the length and number of sessions, the time and place are made together, and that decisions of an emergency nature made by one therapist in the absence of the other are based on mutually agreed-upon procedures for just such situations.

Obviously, egalitarian co-therapists must establish and maintain clear channels of communication. Not only must they expend a great deal of time and energy in preparation for the group experience, they must also plan for pre-session and post-session meetings, joint analysis of data, and joint supervision or consultation.

Creating the group

The effectiveness of a group depends greatly on the conditions under which it is created. Much as architects design buildings, therapists design groups with certain functions and characteristics in mind. Groups are often created for people who have similar health conditions. For example, people with early dementia have been found to benefit greatly from participating in music therapy groups (Sarkamo et al., 2014). The act or reminiscing within a group has also been found to be very therapeutic for people with dementia (Blake, 2013). Adults who have experienced childhood trauma benefit from art therapy groups (Schouten, de Niet, Knipscheer, Kleber & Hutschemaekers, 2015), as do people struggling to overcome eating disorders (Sporild & Bonsaken, 2014). An interesting example of a group of severely ill clients who manage to achieve their goals is described in Mental Health in the Media.

Selecting members

People may be admitted to an inpatient group on the basis of being hospitalised on a particular unit that mandates group therapy for all clients, being assigned to a particular therapist, or because group therapy has been determined to be the most appropriate form of treatment. Group therapists or leaders of therapeutic groups in inpatient units may have little leeway about including specific individuals in the group. Therefore, inpatient groups tend to have a more heterogeneous composition; that is, the members may vary significantly in terms of their personality characteristics, their vulnerabilities or their ego strengths. They also tend to be more ambivalent about group therapy. Nevertheless, it is possible to focus on the common human struggle of living with mental illness so that heterogeneous groups take on a homogeneous goal (Cook, Arechiga, Dobson & Boyd, 2014).

Group rules

The group rules identify the shared rights and responsibilities of therapists and members. It is a negotiated set of rules or arrangements for the structure and functioning of the group. They may be written or verbal, and should cover the following elements.

Practice example

I once held a joint academic and clinical leadership position. I had noticed that nurses were no longer running group activities in acute psychiatric inpatient units, so I arranged to go into the local unit and deliver a group once each month. I named the group the 'Pre-Discharge Planning Group' to ensure interest among the people in the ward. I would always have a group of people attending, as they were very keen to plan their exit from the ward! I insisted that a registered nurse from the ward also attended the group to demystify the process of group therapy and to provide an opportunity for observational learning (imitative behaviour, according to Yalom). The group also gave the staff an opportunity to see people interacting with each other, and enabled them to conduct ongoing assessments of mental state. For some time after I left the role I heard that the nurses were continuing to organise groups in that inpatient unit.

Goals and purposes The purpose of the group must be clear to all involved. In interactive group psychotherapy, the purpose is to bring about enduring behavioural and character change. The interactive group psychotherapy experience takes place largely in the present, in the here-and-now.

Goals may be long-term or short-term, and are both group-oriented and individualised. Some goals may be identified early, and others may be added as they emerge during the life of the group. You may alter goals as appropriate.

Time, length and frequency of meetings The time, length and frequency of meetings should be determined by the therapists after consideration of the clients' needs. Most outpatients find one 80- to 90-minute session per week useful. Shorter periods may not allow adequate time for discussion. Longer periods generally tax the endurance and alertness of both members and therapists. Inpatient groups generally meet several times per week, or even daily for about 30 to 45 minutes, although sessions may be longer or

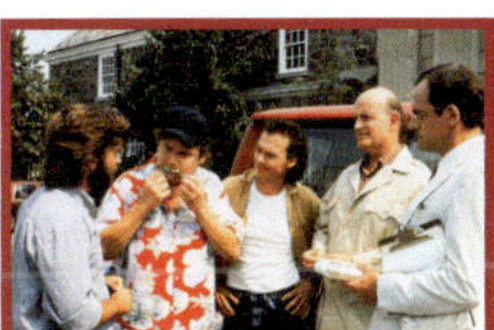

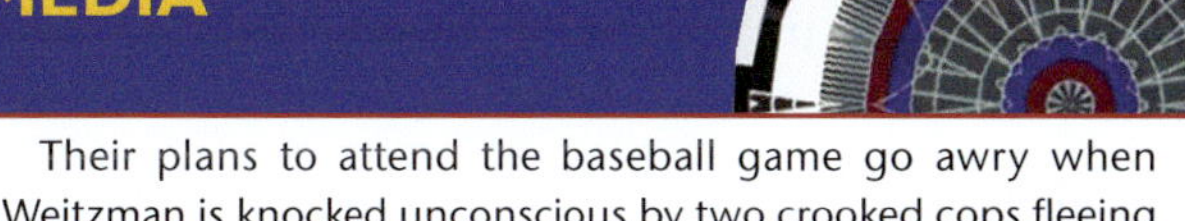

MENTAL HEALTH IN THE MEDIA

The Dream Team

Convinced that his four clients at a New Jersey mental hospital—Billy, Henry, Jack and Albert—need fresh air and time away from the hospital, Dr Jeff Weitzman (Dennis Boutsikaris) convinces the administration to allow him to take the group of four to see a baseball game at Yankee Stadium. Billy (Michael Keaton), an easy-to-anger, unpredictable pathological liar with delusions of grandeur, becomes the 'leader' of this group of four. Henry (Christopher Lloyd) is delusional—he believes he is a doctor at the hospital. Jack (Peter Boyle), also delusional, believes that he is Jesus Christ. Albert (Stephen Furst) is a simple and childlike man who needs direction to perform even everyday tasks. (Note that it is unlikely in real life that one staff member alone would independently take four people with severe psychotic symptoms for such an outing.)

Their plans to attend the baseball game go awry when Dr Weitzman is knocked unconscious by two crooked cops fleeing the scene of a crime. Stranded, and on their own in New York City without money or a phone, the group is forced to pull together and work in concert in order to cope with their circumstances.

The stereotyping of the people and their often outlandish, but humorous, behaviour are stigmatising elements of the film. However, the film's saving grace is its portrayal of the ability of four people to overcome their delusions and disorders in order to work together as a group to save Dr Weitzman. This positive message overshadows the over-the-top stereotypic portrayals of people with mental disorders.

Photo courtesy of KPA/Heritage Image/Glow Images.

shorter depending on the anxiety and tolerance levels of the particular group members.

Place of meetings The physical environment is important and influences the interaction among members. It is best to choose a pleasant room with comfortable chairs, preferably placed in a circle. The room should be private and free from external distractions.

Starting and ending dates If the group has a predetermined lifespan and the inclusive dates are known, inform the members of the dates. Groups without fixed termination dates usually plan termination individually, as each member is ready to move away from the group. Starting and ending dates are determined in inpatient groups by the length of the person's hospitalisation.

Addition of new members Open groups accept members after the first session; closed groups begin with a certain number of members and do not add new members. Open groups maintain their size by replacing members who leave the group. They may continue indefinitely or have a predetermined lifespan. Open groups are more common in short-term inpatient units where there is rapid turnover. Once the client leaves the inpatient setting, membership in the group ends. This means that because most hospitalisations in acute care settings are of one to three weeks' duration, there is little time for cohesion to develop. Cohesion develops in outpatient groups and in long-term inpatient units because of their length.

Closed groups are more common in settings where the stability of membership is likely. Such settings include private practice settings, residential facilities of various types and prisons. A major problem with the closed group is that it runs the risk of extinction as members leave the group for various reasons.

Attendance It is important that members make a commitment to attend every session. Absences hinder the establishment of cohesion and have a demoralising effect, especially when perceived as evidence that a member lacks interest or that the group is not attractive and valuable to its members. Stability of membership and high attendance are critical factors in the successful outcome of group therapy (Yalom, 2005).

Confidentiality Establish some rules regarding confidentiality, and explore the group members' concerns about who will have access to information about them. Many therapists like to use tape recorders so that their work can be evaluated by supervisors. They must first obtain consent before using a tape recorder.

The group leaders' employing agency may determine rules about confidentiality and access. In some instances, leaders may be required to make regular notes concerning each member's participation. Group leaders may also wish to establish with group members guidelines on confidentiality that allow the leaders to share content with professionals who provide clinical supervision to the therapist, or when members are dangerous to themselves or others. A good rule of thumb is: promise only what you can safely deliver. You should also hold members accountable for maintaining the confidentiality of the group.

Member interaction outside of the group Members in outpatient groups are discouraged from having relationships with other members outside of the meetings. Relationships outside of the group are likely to interfere with the group dynamics because of the formation of social coalitions or dyads. Limiting relationships is impossible in inpatient groups because the members may have 24-hour exposure to one another on the hospital unit or in a residential setting, and may also interact with the group therapist while the therapist is functioning in other roles. In fact, interaction with one another is encouraged in inpatient settings.

Participation of members and group leaders Members and leaders should reach an understanding about the responsibilities of participants. Group members should be fully informed participants in the therapeutic process. Participants should share their expectations about the behaviour and functions of members and therapists, and should clearly understand the modes of participation. Interaction patterns should form pathways between all members and the group leader(s), as illustrated in Figure 23.6 ■.

It is important for the inpatient group therapist to provide significantly more structure for the group and to take on a more active role than would be necessary in an outpatient group. Hospitalised inpatients are likely to be in crisis and to be more distressed and disorganised than outpatients. Passivity on the therapist's part would be destructive to the group and could increase a person's distress. Yalom (1998) suggests a protocol for structuring an inpatient group that is listed in the following Your Intervention Strategies.

Stages in therapy group development

There is comfort in being able to predict, to some extent, the behaviour of members at specific points in the group's life. Therapists organise predictions around stages or phases in the therapeutic experience, hoping to be prepared for expressions of behaviour. You must bear in mind, however, that human experiences are dynamic and fluid, and do not always progress as neatly as predicted.

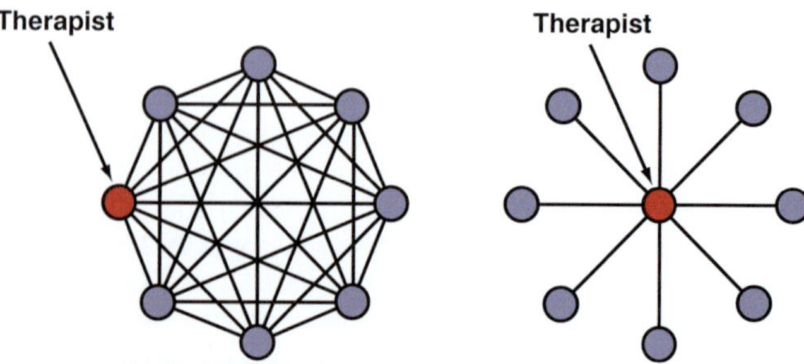

FIGURE 23.6 ■ Comparison of positive and negative interaction patterns in group therapy. The desirable interaction pattern is on the left. The diagram on the right, in which communication is primarily to or through the therapist, is undesirable.

YOUR INTERVENTION STRATEGIES
Structuring an inpatient group

1. 3–5 minutes of orientation, warm-up or preparation.
2. 20–30 minutes for an agenda go-around in which each member may share personal concerns or problems.
3. 20–30 minutes in which the therapist attempts to fit the members' agendas together by finding commonalities or threads to work on.
4. 3–5 minutes to review the work of the group and to identify the issues or concerns that remain unresolved.

The Schutz framework, presented earlier, gives clear indications of how group life develops in terms of meeting inclusion, control and affection needs, and the stages of group development discussed on pages 509–510 describe the common experiences of group members. This section focuses on the characteristics of member behaviour and therapist interventions in the orientation phase (where inclusion needs are more salient), the working phase (where control needs are more salient), and the termination phase (where affection needs are more salient) of interactional group therapy. As members' problems in living are revealed, group life becomes richer and more complex. Therefore, there is no 'recipe' that a therapist can follow to respond to every situation. Your Intervention Strategies, below, is simply a guide for identifying some common member behaviours and therapist interventions at various points in the life of the group.

Interactional group therapy

The core of interactional group therapy is the here-and-now. According to Yalom (2005), the here-and-now work of the interactional group therapist occurs on the following two levels:

1. focusing attention on each member's feelings toward other group members, the therapists and the group

YOUR INTERVENTION STRATEGIES
Characteristic member behaviours and nursing interventions in phases of group therapy

Member behaviour	Nursing interventions
Orientation phase	
Anxiety is high.	Recognise anxiety; avoid making demands until group anxiety has abated.
Members are unsure of what to do or say; need to be included.	Be active, and provide some structure and direction; suggest members introduce themselves; work to sustain the therapeutic role rather than the social role; include all members and encourage sharing but limit monopolising.
Members are unclear about the rules.	Clarify the rules; give information to dispel confusion or misunderstandings.
Members test therapists and other members in terms of trustworthiness, value stances, etc., often through goblet issues.	Capitalise on an opportunity to prove trustworthiness, and by being open to and accepting of the values of others.
Beginning attempts at self-disclosure and problem identification are made.	Focus on related themes; begin exploration; begin to focus on here-and-now experiences in session.
Members have sense of 'I'-ness, little sense of 'we'-ness.	Encourage involvement with others through curative factor of *universality*.
Working phase	
Sense of 'I'-ness is replaced by 'we'-ness.	Encourage cohesion; provide opportunity for expression of warm feelings.
Self-disclosure increases.	Encourage exploration, and move to problem-solving.
Members are more aware of interpersonal interactions in the here-and-now.	Encourage members to participate in observing and commenting on the here-and-now.
Additions and losses of members evoke strong reactions.	Prepare members for additions and losses where possible; provide an opportunity to talk about addition and loss experiences.
Ability to maintain focus on one topic increases.	Encourage exploration of the topic area in depth.
Termination phase	
Feelings about separation may extend from anger to joy.	Provide adequate time in as many sessions as necessary to work through affective responses; be sure members know the termination date in advance; help members leave with positive feelings by identifying positive changes that have occurred in individual members and in the group.
Members may feel lost and rudderless.	Explore the support systems available to individual members; bridge the gap where possible (to another agency, another therapist, etc.); keep in focus the task of resolving the loss.

2. illuminating the process (the relationship implications of interpersonal transactions).

Thus, group members need to become aware of the here-and-now events (what happened) and then reflect back on them (why it happened). Yalom (2005) calls this the **self-reflective loop** (see Figure 23.7 ■).

Steering the group into the here-and-now

The first task of the therapist is to steer the group into the here-and-now. Yalom calls this process **here-and-now activation**. As the group progresses and becomes comfortable with awareness of the here-and-now, much of the work is taken on by the members. Initially, however, a primary task of the therapist is to actively steer the group discourse towards here-and-now work. In other words, events in the session (the here-and-now) take precedence over those that occur outside or have occurred outside and in the past (the there-and-then).

Illuminating the process

If the group is to engage in interpersonal learning, the therapist must illuminate the process. This is the second task of prime importance. The group must move beyond a focus on content towards a focus on process—the how and the why of an interaction. The process can be considered from any number of perspectives. Choose the perspective based on the mood and needs of the group at that particular time. The members must recognise, examine and understand the process and be willing to self-disclose (review the discussion of self-disclosure earlier in this chapter). The task of illuminating the process belongs mainly to the therapist, as in the following Practice Example.

Process commentary is anxiety-producing for new or inexperienced therapists and group members, because there are so many injunctions against it in social situations. For example, commenting on someone's nervousness at a party is generally taboo. It not only makes the nervous person uncomfortable, but also puts the process commentator in a high-risk social situation. The comment may well be taken as criticism or viewed as inappropriate to the social context, and the commentator is vulnerable to retaliation from others. Be aware that process commentary may be difficult for you if you do not understand the differences between social and professional relationships. It is essential to educate group members about these differences and to prepare them to hear, respond to and eventually initiate process commentary themselves (Ulman, 2011). You will be unable to do so if you have not incorporated this understanding into your professional mental health nursing practice.

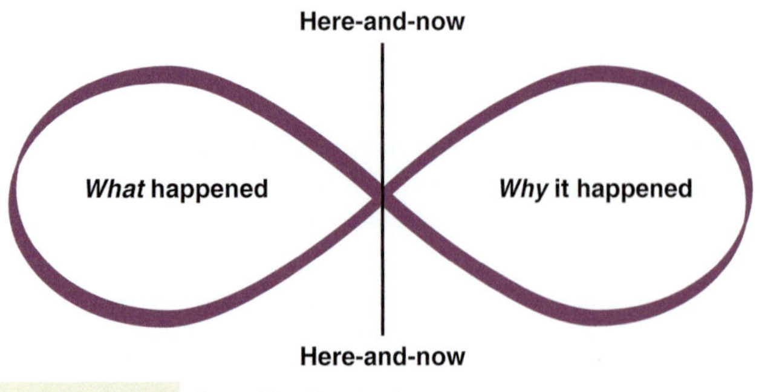

FIGURE 23.7 ■ The self-reflective loop.

Practice example

Every time Jim makes a comment in group, Al either sneers or smirks. As soon as Jim finishes speaking, Al contradicts whatever Jim has said. The group members focus on the content of the disagreements between Jim and Al. Margaret, the clinical nurse specialist who is the group therapist, steers the group in the direction of analysing the dynamics of the relationship between these members and the possible purposes their disagreements can serve for the group (e.g. controlling the direction of the group's efforts, meeting Al's control needs, or keeping the group anxiety down by keeping the focus away from other, more anxious members).

The process of focusing on the here-and-now is akin to the process that is called 'clearing the air' (making covert interpersonal difficulties overt) in Schutz's (1958b) framework. Clearing the air is a major step in the interpersonal needs approach. Although this step is initially uncomfortable, the final result is rewarding. The following are common interpersonal difficulties that occur in therapy groups that need to be made overt:

- withdrawal or silence by members
- inactivity or overactivity by members
- unintegrated behaviour by members
- destructive behaviour by members
- power struggles between members
- battles for attention among members
- dissatisfaction with the leader
- dissatisfaction with the amount of recognition a member receives for contributions
- dissatisfaction with the amount of affection and warmth demonstrated in the group.

In concert with Yalom's principles, Schutz's interpersonal needs approach is based on the belief that the way to attack problems within groups is by investigating what is going on interpersonally between the individuals in the group, and attempting to improve their interpersonal relations.

Focusing on the here-and-now experience differentiates interactive group psychotherapy from many other group therapies or therapeutic groups, such as those discussed in the next section.

THERAPEUTIC GROUPS

Nurses at all levels have long been involved in working with people and their families in small groups brought together for health teaching, psychoeducation or supportive purposes. This section discusses several different types of therapeutic groups that do not require the nurse to be an advanced-practice registered nurse.

Peer-led support groups

The major operating principle in mutual-help groups (also known as self-help groups) is that the help given to members comes from the members themselves. A mental health professional is viewed as unnecessary. In fact, many of these groups developed because of the failure of programs planned and implemented by professionals.

The role of the nurse in mutual-help groups is that of a resource person. You need to be informed about such groups so that you can refer potential members to groups appropriate to their needs, or provide consultation when invited to do so. Appropriate referral is important. When dually diagnosed clients (substance abuse and mental illness) were referred to a 12-step mutual-help group, they did better than those not in a mutual-help group (Hagler et al., 2015). In most mutual-help groups, leaders are former members. Alcoholics Anonymous is a well-known example of this principle.

There is a wide variety of mutual-help groups, for example:

- Mental Illness Fellowship Australia, support services for people with a mental illness (http://www.mifa.org.au/index.php/en/)
- The Black Dog Institute is a not-for-profit organisation and world leader in the diagnosis, treatment and prevention of mood disorders (http://www.blackdoginstitute.org.au/); Black Dog Institute also has clinician led groups such as Reach (http://www.blackdoginstitute.org.au/public/gettinghelp/blackdogsupportgroups.cfm)
- Al-Anon and Alateen, concerned with the families of people who abuse alcohol/substances (http://www.al-anon.alateen.org/australia/)
- GROW, free peer-led support groups regardless of diagnosis (http://www.grow.org.au/)
- Gamblers Anonymous, concerned with people who gamble compulsively (http://gaaustralia.org.au/)
- Gam-Anon, concerned with the families and friends of people who gamble compulsively (http://www.gam-anon.org/)
- Mental Health Carers ARAFMI Australia, a collective of organisations whose members are mental health carers (http://www.arafmiaustralia.asn.au/).

Psychoeducation groups

Psychoeducation groups led by nurses have the sharing of mental health care information as a primary goal. They also have the secondary benefit of facilitating the discussion of feelings such as isolation, helplessness, sadness, stigmatisation and/or anger, and possible strategies for dealing with these feelings. Psychoeducation groups may be specifically designed for family members. Even a brief psychoeducation group can be helpful in reducing the psychosocial burdens that relatives of people with depression face (Katsuki et al., 2011), the burdens that partners of veterans with post-traumatic stress disorder have to manage (Sones, Madsen, Jakupcak & Thorp, 2015), or that caregivers of people with dementia face (Haberstroh, Neumeyer, Krause, Franzman & Pantel, 2011).

LIVED EXPERIENCE

Groups help me to feel comfortable around others

For me, being a part of the group means that I am no longer alone living with this disorder. I have a sense of belonging and connection, and of being supported as well as being supportive. I learn from others' experiences, and I'm also listened to and not being judged. It has assisted me in my personal growth by continuing the development of self-awareness and insight, and I have grown in confidence (to the extent that I successfully completed a Diploma in Community Services Work in 2015). It has also helped me in managing the fear I sometimes feel when meeting new people, and to accept my awkwardness in social settings.

Medication education groups

Non-adherence to psychopharmacological prescription medication is the leading cause of relapse or recurrence of psychotic illness (Chan et al., 2015). Many studies have shown that the causes of medication non-adherence are related to a lack of insight and understanding by the person or their families of their illness and of their medication treatment (Chan et al., 2015), as well as the shame associated with self-stigma (Uhlmann et al., 2014). However, medication side-effects, such as dry mouth, blurred vision, impotence, sedation, weight gain and akathisia, can be difficult to tolerate, and it is understandable that people wish to make informed decisions about the medications they take, how long they take them for and under what circumstances.

Medication education groups provide an opportunity for psychiatric–mental health nurses to provide information about medications and their side-effects, and balance these against the positive effect that medications can have on their lives. Research has shown that increased adherence to treatment and insight often result from medication teaching groups (Bond & Anderson, 2015; Tay, 2007), and that they are as effective as individual cognitive behavioural therapy, while being significantly cheaper to deliver (Parikh et al., 2012).

It is also now known that people who are lifetime-compliant with antipsychotic medication can have worse physical and mental health outcomes than those who only use these medications in relapse, or those who have stopped their medication altogether. These new understandings provide opportunities for mental health professionals to have honest and open conversations about the usefulness of medications for people in their care, the risks associated with medications, and the balancing of the reduction of symptoms with the short- and long-term deleterious effects of many antipsychotics.

Social skills training groups

Groups can effectively provide social skills training for people, as well as for their family members. Small groups provide structure and support, while members are coached in simple yet essential social interactions. It is best to form groups of people who function at similar levels. Provide structure by clearly setting the time for group meetings, beginning and ending each session with a statement of goals, and recapping what the group has accomplished. The combination of social skills training with cognitive behavioural therapy (CBT) or dialectical behaviour therapy appears to be powerful (Granholm, Holden, Link & McQuaid, 2014).

Social skills training continues to be found useful for varying populations. Through cognitive behavioural training in a social skills depression-prevention program, adolescents increased their perception of social support by friends (Stice, Rohde, Gau & Wade, 2010). Perception of social support by others is inversely related to depressive symptoms—the greater the social support, the fewer the depressive symptoms. The positive effects were maintained through one- and two-year follow-up (Stice, Rohde, Gau & Ochner, 2011). After a 24-session social skills training group, psychiatric outpatients showed an improvement in social cognition (Horan et al., 2011). A decrease in positive, depressive and anxiety symptoms in first-episode psychosis participants, as well as improved quality of life, and improvement in negative symptoms, was found by another group of researchers who also combined CBT with social skills training (Gaynor, Dooley, Lawlor, Lawoyin & O'Callaghan, 2011). People with severe and persistent schizophrenia can learn and maintain new skills, and report improved functioning after cognitive behavioural social skills training (Granholm et al., 2014). Social skills training groups that focus on communication skills can reduce relationship risk factors for couples by teaching conflict resolution and communication skills.

Groups of medically ill people and their families

Groups composed of medically ill people are increasingly common, as psychiatric–mental health nurses move into general health care settings, offering liaison and consultation services to ill people and staff. Group work is useful for chronically ill or disabled people, preoperative and postoperative individuals, people with regulative medical problems (such as diabetes, cardiac disease or kidney disease), those who are dying or elderly, and those who have medical conditions with associated psychological factors (see Chapter 8), among others. Such groups generally focus on the stress associated with illness, and have as their goal the reduction of stress. While groups may not prolong life, they may improve the quality of life, including protection against depression, by enhancing coping skills in, for example, breast cancer survivors (Carlson et al., 2015). The therapeutic group has also been found helpful in teaching primary prevention strategies to people with metabolic syndrome at high risk for cardiovascular disease and type-2 diabetes (Dunkley et al., 2011). Groups may be composed of individuals alone, family members alone, or a combination.

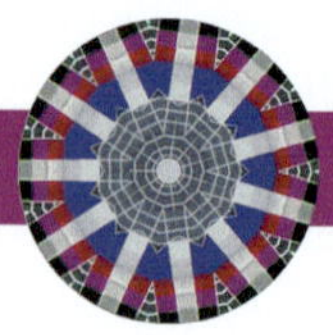

REFERENCES

Beebe, S. A., Beebe, S. J., & Redmond, M. V. (2011). *Interpersonal communication: Relating to others*. Boston, MA: Allyn & Bacon.

Benne, K. D., & Sheats, P. (1948). Functional roles of group members. *Journal of Social Issues, 4*, 41–49.

Blake, M. (2013). Group reminiscence therapy for adults with dementia: A review. *British Journal of Community Nursing, 18*(5), 228–233.

Bond, K., & Anderson, I. M. (2015). Psychoeducation for relapse prevention in bipolar disorder: A systematic review of efficacy in randomized controlled trials. *Bipolar Disorders, 17*(4), 349–362.

Carlson, L. E., Beattie, T. L., Giese-Davis, J., Faris, P., Tamagawa, R., Fick, L. J., . . . Speca, M. (2015). Mindfulness-based cancer recovery and supportive-expressive therapy maintain telomere length relative to controls in distressed breast cancer survivors. *Cancer, 121*(3), 476–484.

Caruso, R., Grassi, L., Biancosino, B., Marmai, L., Bonatti, L., Moscara, M., . . . Priebe, S. (2013). Exploration of experiences in therapeutic groups for patients with severe mental illness: Development of the Ferrara group experiences scale (FE-GES). *BMC Psychiatry, 13*, 242–250.

Chan, K. W., Wong, M. H., Hui, C. L., Lee, E. H., Chang, W. C., & Chen, E. Y. (2015). Perceived risk of relapse and role of medication: Comparison between patients with psychosis and their caregivers. *Social Psychiatry and Psychiatric Epidemiology, 50*(2), 307–315.

Cook, W. G., Arechiga, A., Dobson, L. A. V., & Boyd, K. (2014). Brief heterogeneous inpatient psychotherapy groups: A process-oriented psychoeducational (POP) model. *International Journal of Group Psychotherapy, 64*(2), 180–206.

Dunkley, A. J., Davies, M. J., Stone, M. A., Taub, N. A., Troughton, J., Yates, T., & Krunte, K. (2011). The reversal intervention for metabolic syndrome (TRIMS) study: Rationale, design, and baseline data. *Trials, 12*(1), 107.

Ellis, C. C., Peterson, M., Bufford, R., & Benson, J. (2014). The importance of group cohesion in inpatient treatment of combat-related PTSD. *International Journal of Group Psychotherapy, 64*(2), 208–226.

Fasulo, S. J., Ball, J. M., Jurkovic, G. J., & Miller, A. L. (2015). Towards the development of an effective working alliance: The application of DBT validation and stylistic strategies in the adaptation of a manualised complex trauma group treatment program for adolescents in long-term detention. *American Journal of Psychotherapy, 62*(2), 219–239.

Gans, J. S. (2011). Unwitting self-disclosures in psychodynamic psychotherapy: Deciphering their meaning and accessing the pain within. *International Journal of Group Psychotherapy, 61*(2), 218–237.

Gaynor, K., Dooley, B., Lawlor, E., Lawoyin, R., & O'Callaghan, E. (2011). Group cognitive behavioral therapy as a treatment for negative symptoms in first-episode psychosis. *Early Interventional Psychiatry*, 5(2), 168–173.

Goldberg, S. B., & Hoyt, W. T. (2015). Group as social microcosm: Within-group interpersonal style is congruent with outside group relational tendencies. *Psychotherapy, 52*(2), 195–204.

Granholm, E., Holden, J., Link, P. C., & McQuaid, J. R. (2014). Randomized clinical trial of cognitive behavioural social skills training for schizophrenia: Improvement in functioning and experiential negative symptoms. *Journal of Consulting and Clinical Psychology, 82*(6), 1173–1185.

Haberstroh, J., Neumeyer, K., Krause, K., Franzmann, J., & Pantel, J. (2011). TANDEM: Community training for informal caregivers of people with dementia. *Aging and Mental Health, 15*(3), 405–413.

Hagler, K. J., Rice, S. L., Munoz, R. E., Salvador, J. G., Forcehimes, A. A., & Bogenschutz, M. P. (2015). 'It might actually work this time': Benefits and barriers to adapted 12-step facilitation therapy and mutual-help group attendance from the perspective of dually diagnosed individuals. *Journal of Addictions Nursing, 26*(3), 120–128.

Harris, T. E., & Sherblom, J. C. (2011). *Small group and team communication* (5th ed.). Boston, MA: Allyn & Bacon.

Horan, W. P., Kern, R. S., Tripp, C., Hellemann, G., Wynn, J. K., Bell, M., . . . Green, M. F. (2011). Efficacy and specificity of social cognitive skills training for outpatients with psychiatric disorders. *Journal of Psychiatric Research, 45*(8), 1113–1122.

Katsuki, F., Takeuchi, H., Konishi, M., Sasaki, M., Murase, Y., Naito, A., . . . Furukawa, T. A. (2011). Pre-post changes in psychosocial functioning among relatives of patients with depressive disorders after brief multifamily psychoeducation: A pilot study. *BMC Psychiatry, 11, 56*. doi: 10.1186/1471-244X-11-56

MacKenzie, R. (1997). Clinical application of group development ideas. *Group Dynamics: Theory, Research and Practice, 1*(4), 275–287.

Norcross, J. C., & Wampold, B. E. (2011). Evidence-based therapy relationships: Research conclusions and clinical practices. *Psychotherapy, 48*(1), 98–102.

Parikh, S. V., Zaretsky, A., Beaulieu, S., Yatham, L. N., Young, L. T., Patelis-Siotis, I., . . . Streiner, D. L. (2012). A randomized controlled trial of psychoeducation or cognitive behavioural therapy in bipolar disorder: A Canadian network for mood and anxiety treatments. *Journal of Clinical Psychiatry, 73*(6), 803–810.

Sarkamo, T., Tervaniemi, M., Laitinen, S., Numminen, A., Kurki, M., . . . Rantanen, P. (2014). Cognitive, emotional, and social benefits of regular music activities in early dementia: Randomised controlled study. *The Gerontologist, 54*(4), 634–650.

Schouten, K. A., de Niet, G. J., Knipscheer, J. W., Kleber, R. J., & Hutschemaekers, G. J. M. (2015). The effectiveness of art therapy in the treatment of traumatized adults: A systematic review on art therapy and trauma. *Trauma, Violence, and Abuse. 16*(2), 220–228.

Schutz, W. C. (1958a). Interpersonal underworld. *Harvard Business Review, 36*, 123–135.

Schutz, W. C. (1958b). *The interpersonal underworld: FIRO*. Palo Alto, CA: Science and Behavior Books.

Sones, H. M., Madsen, J., Jakupcak, M., & Thorp, S. R. (2015). Evaluation of an educational group therapy program for female partners of veterans diagnosed with PTSD: A pilot study. *Couple and Family Psychology: Research and Practice, 4*(3), 150–160.

Sporild, I. A., & Bonsaken, T. (2014). Therapeutic factors in expressive art therapy for persons with eating disorders. *Groupwork: An Interdisciplinary Journal for Working with Groups, 24*(3), 46–60.

Stice, E., Rohde, P., Gau, J., & Ochner, C. (2011). Relationship of depression to perceived social support: Results from a randomized adolescent depression prevention trial. *Behavioral Research and Therapy, 49*(5), 361–366. doi: 10.1016/j.brat.2011.02.009

Stice, E., Rohde, P., Gau, J. M., & Wade, E. (2010). Efficacy trial of a brief cognitive-behavioral depression prevention program for high-risk adolescents: Effects at 1- and 2-year follow-up. *Journal of Consulting and Clinical Psychology, 78*(6), 856–867.

Tay, S. E. (2007). Compliance therapy: An intervention to improve inpatients' attitudes toward treatment. *Journal of Psychosocial Nursing and Mental Health Services, 45*(6), 29–37.

Tuckman, B. (1965). Developmental sequence in small groups. *Psychological Bulletin, 63*(6), 384–399.

Tuckman, B., & Jensen, M. (1977). Stages of small group development. *Group and Organisational Studies, 2*, 419–427.

Uhlmann, C., Kaehler, J., Harris, M. S., Unser, J., Arolt, V., & Lencer, R. (2014). Negative impact of self-stigmatization on attitude toward medication adherence in patients with psychosis. *Journal of Psychiatric Practice, 20*(5), 405–410.

Ulman, K. H. (2011). The present moment and implicit communication in group psychotherapy. *International Journal of Group Psychotherapy, 61*(2), 275–284.

Yalom, I. D. (1983). *Inpatient group psychotherapy*. New York, NY: Basic Books.

Yalom, I. D. (1998). *The Yalom reader*. New York, NY: Basic Books.

Yalom, I. D. (2005). *The theory and practice of group psychotherapy* (5th ed.). New York, NY: Basic Books.

Yalom, I. D. (2009). *The gift of therapy: An open letter to a new generation of therapists and their patients*. New York, NY: HarperCollins.

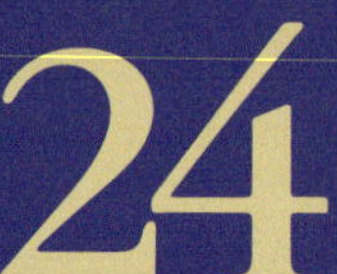

24 Family-focused interventions

DEB O'KANE AND TIM HEFFERNAN

KEY TERMS

diffuse boundary 524
disengaged families 526
enmeshed families 526
family burden 528
family system 524
family therapy 532
genogram 529
life script 525
pseudo-hostility 527
pseudo-mutuality 527
rigid boundaries 524
schismatic families 525
self-fulfilling prophecy 525
skewed families 526

LEARNING OUTCOMES

After completing this chapter, you will be able to:

1. Reflect on your own values and beliefs of family life, including your own experiences, and discuss the possible implications of these when working with carers and those in your care.
2. Describe families and their dynamics in terms of structure, relationships, boundaries and connections.
3. Differentiate between schism, skew, enmeshment, disengagement, pseudo-mutuality and pseudo-hostility as concepts of intimacy and control in families.
4. Develop a family assessment, incorporating the data obtained from the family into a care plan for the individual.
5. Partner with the individual and their families in implementing family interventions or family therapy, as appropriate, to improve recovery.

LIVED EXPERIENCE

Staying connected

Mental health is always a family issue—no member of a family is untouched when someone develops depression, anxiety or psychosis. The trouble is we tend to disconnect people from their families when they become unwell. Traditional acute care, especially involuntary care, takes people from their home into a medicalised clinical mental health unit where mobile phones and computers are banned, visiting hours are limited, and recovery begins with a ward full of strangers. Sometimes the wards are far away from home, especially if you come from the country.

We know that connectedness is a key to our recovery, and that connections frayed during an episode of illness often need more than the work of the individual to repair. It is difficult for your mother, father or your partner to seek help when you will not seek it yourself. It is difficult for families to be told that with this diagnosis comes a life diminished. Families need to recover, too, so it is always essential to promote hope, and to expect that people will regain their lives and their dreams.

A new way of responding to psychosis is called *Open Dialogue*. First developed in Western Lapland, where levels of diagnosed schizophrenia had become concerning, it is an intervention that is family-focused and centred on finding the meaning in each individual's experience.

(*continued*)

LIVED EXPERIENCE *(continued)*

This approach aims to support the individual's network of family and friends, as well as respect the decision-making of the individual. Working with families and social networks, as much as possible in their own homes, Open Dialogue teams work to help those involved in a crisis situation to be together and to engage in dialogue. It has been their experience that if the family/team can bear the extreme emotion in a crisis situation, and tolerate the uncertainty, in time, shared meaning usually emerges and healing is possible. Open Dialogue teams can include doctors and nurses, and in the United Kingdom Peer-supported Open Dialogue teams include peer workers.

It is about keeping families together, not treating the individual in isolation.

INTRODUCTION

We encounter families in many areas of our practice—in the emergency department, the intensive care unit, the school, the community health setting, and the mental health care setting, among others. It is for this reason that the knowledge you gain by reading this chapter will apply no matter what your practice setting will be. This chapter specifically discusses family dynamics, family assessment, family interventions such as psychoeducation and family therapy. They are recognised as important components of treatment for a person's recovery.

The family is the context in which most people, including nurses, develop their first relationships with other people. Our view of the larger social world outside our own unique family is moulded by the events that happen within our families and influence our development. Preventive approaches to family mental health, assessment of families in crisis, and intervention on their behalf must be based on an understanding of how families grow and interact, and how family coping patterns develop.

Box 24.1 Critical thinking questions

You are present at a multi-disciplinary discharge planning meeting. Mark James, a 22-year-old in your care, is being discharged from his first mental health hospital admission to the home he shares with his father and two sisters. Mark has been alienated from his mother since his parents' divorce when he was 17 years old. Mark's mother has failed to show up for the discharge meeting. The mental health team has recommended family-focused work to the James family. You perceive what you think is annoyance on Mr James's face, and one of Mark's sisters appears embarrassed. Although you would not be the person working with the family, you recognise how important Mark's family can be to his progress.

1. What might be some of the family's unspoken concerns and needs?
2. What actions can you take to address the family's unspoken needs and concerns?
3. Why would family-focused work be appropriate, rather than individual therapy?

NURSING SELF-AWARENESS

Assessing and intervening with the families of those in your care is an essential role. Family work should be seen as part of core, comprehensive, integrated mental health care to achieve the best outcomes for all involved.

Unfortunately, some mental health care professionals still have a bias against family involvement. This bias is a remnant of now-discredited theories that poor parenting and dysfunctional family interaction patterns give rise to mental illness. A related bias is the belief by some that if families 'cause' schizophrenia, then the family's contact with the person should be limited for the person's sake. Besides violating family rights, this bias prevents social interaction with family members that might serve as a normalising force on the person's journey to recovery. That is, circumstances within a family may not be ideal, but they are real and require coping skills. Here is a question you can use to check whether you have a bias against the family's rights: 'Am I responding to this family any differently than I would to the family of a person with a non-mental medical condition?'

SELF-AWARENESS
The influences of your own family experiences

It is helpful when working with families to first come to an understanding of the experiences you bring with you from your own family. Complete the following statements to facilitate your self-understanding and recognition of the biases you bring to your work with families.

1. When someone in my family talks too much, I usually . . .
2. When one of my family members is silent, I usually . . .
3. When someone in my family cries, I usually . . .
4. When my family members are excessively polite and unwilling to confront each other, I usually . . .
5. When there is conflict in my family, I usually . . .
6. When one individual in my family is verbally attacked, I usually . . .
7. If there is physical violence in my family, I usually . . .
8. My typical intervention 'rhythm' is (fast/slow) . . .
9. My style is characteristically more (nurturing/confronting) . . .
10. The things that make me most uncomfortable in my family are . . .

In addition, your experiences in your own family influence how you perceive and react to the families of those in your care. Truthfully answering the self-assessment questions in the above Self-awareness feature will help you to determine how your own family experiences might influence your behaviour with your clients' families.

FAMILY DYNAMICS

While there are common factors and mechanisms of change that underpin most forms of successful interventions, there are several unique dynamics that take place in families and influence both family and individual functioning. A selection of relevant theories that help to explain family dynamics and family treatment are discussed next. The section on family therapy will help you to understand and explain family therapy to those in your care, and support them and their families during the therapeutic experience. It does not prepare you to be a family therapist. As you will learn later in the chapter, the nurse family therapist role is an advanced-practice role.

Family structures

Defining 'family' within Australia is complex. The traditional family in Western society is a two-parent, two-generation family consisting of a married couple and their children by birth. In today's society, fewer than one in five children have grown up in this traditional family structure. In fact, relying on physical connections alone to define family means the reality of many families in contemporary society is not reflected. Contemporary families may look like any one of the following:

- a mother, a father and two children (traditional nuclear family)
- a couple with five children—two of hers, two of his, and one of theirs (blended family)
- a 32-year-old single man and his three foster children
- a divorced woman and her two teenagers
- a widowed man, his child and his parents
- a grandmother raising her three grandchildren
- two lesbian mothers and their child
- two gay fathers and their child
- a lesbian couple and a gay couple co-parenting their shared child
- three single women friends sharing an apartment as none could afford alone
- an elderly 'aunty' with various members of kin staying with her at various times.

Consideration must be given to the concept of family within other cultures. For instance, in Aboriginal communities, 'family' often refers to a kinship systems rather than blood ties, and can fluctuate in their composition (Australian Institute of Health and Welfare [AIHW], 2011). As Australian family forms continue to change, the task of defining the family is a difficult one (Qu & Weston, 2013), and for that reason, sensitive mental health nurses are required to adapt their clinical practice to the wide variety of family constellations that exists in contemporary society.

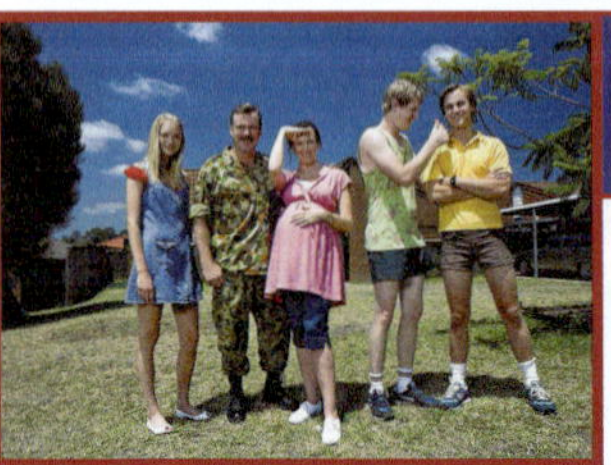

MENTAL HEALTH IN THE MEDIA
The Black Balloon

Themes of family dynamics, family responsibilities and roles, and family coping consistently run through the Australian movie *The Black Balloon*, especially the relationship between two of the main characters, Thomas and his older brother, Charlie.

Thomas is a 15-year-old boy who lives at home with his parents and his 17-year-old brother, Charlie. Charlie is autistic and can exhibit some challenging behaviour on occasion. Charlie is mainly cared for by his mother. However, within the film the mother requires hospital care due to some pregnancy complications, leaving the father and Thomas with the role of caring for Charlie on a daily basis. This causes many confronting and embarrassing situations for Thomas, at a time when he is struggling to 'fit in' within a new neighbourhood, peer group and school, after recently moving to the area due to his father's job in the army.

The film follows Thomas and the many emotions he faces in his teenage years, as well as attempting to adjust to the changes in family responsibility. Issues the film explores are his attraction to a young girl at his school, his role changes within the family, and having to contend with people seeing his brother as an object of disdain alongside the stigma of disability.

The film is both heart-warming and heart-breaking as you see Thomas attempting to find his place as a son, brother, carer and independent young teenager.

Family life cycle

The notion of universal family stages has attracted criticism over several decades. Critics of family development theory point to it as a limiting way of thinking about ethnically and racially diverse populations, gender and families without children (Anderson & Sabatelli, 2011). They propose that the notion of families moving through rigid, predetermined stages is a less productive method of understanding the dynamics that take place in families. Many family therapists believe that it is not necessary to understand a family's past in order to help them (Nichols, 2010). It is also important to recognise that the universality of family life-cycle stages and tasks have not been empirically validated through research. Despite these criticisms, the notion of a family life cycle helps us to understand the family's organisation in the present. Understanding families requires consideration of the challenges they face in each stage, how well they resolve the challenges, and how well they transition to the next stage.

Theories to explain family development were originally proposed by Duvall in 1957, and expanded upon by Duvall and Miller (Duvall & Miller, 1985). Duvall's formulations focused on the patterns and changes in family development as families move through stages. Duvalls' framework was enriched by McGoldrick, Preto and Carter (2015), whose multi-generational point of view, discussed in Table 24.1 ■, expanded the framework to include divorce, remarriage and culturally diverse patterns. The family life cycle is the period of time in which the structure and interactions of role relationships are noticeably distinct from other periods. The stages are inferred from events spurred on by a change in family membership.

Family characteristics and dynamics

Whether they are functional or dysfunctional, families have certain characteristics and dynamics. In a family, each person's behaviour is contingent on, and affects the behaviour of, the others. This creates some interesting and complex turns in family relationships.

Family roles

Members of a family must determine how to accomplish family tasks. They do so by establishing roles—patterns of behaviour sanctioned by the culture. Jackson (1968) believes that families set roles by operating as a rule-governed system, an ordered format designed so that members may be aware of their positions in relation to one another. Families decide which roles will exist within the system, socialise members into the roles, and then expend energy maintaining members within their roles.

When members are unable or unwilling to perform assigned roles, the family experiences stress. For the health of

TABLE 24.1 ■ Family developmental tasks

Stage of the family life cycle	Family developmental tasks
Leaving home as single young adults	■ Accepting emotional responsibility for self ■ Differentiating self from family of origin ■ Developing intimate peer relationships ■ Establishing self in respect to work and financial independence
Becoming a new couple through marriage	■ Forming a marital system ■ Committing to the new system ■ Realigning relationships with extended family and friends to include spouse
Making space for children	■ Adjusting the marital system to include children ■ Joining in childrearing, financial and household tasks ■ Realigning relationships with extended family to include parenting and grandparenting roles
Increasing flexibility of family boundaries	■ Increasing flexibility of parent–child relationships to support adolescent's independence ■ Increasing flexibility of family boundaries to support grandparents' frailties and caring for older generation ■ Refocusing on midlife marital and career issues
Accepting exits from and entries into the family system	■ Launching children and moving on ■ Renegotiating marital system as a dyad ■ Realigning relationships to include in-laws and grandchildren ■ Dealing with disabilities and deaths of parents (grandparents)
Accepting shifting generational roles in later life	■ Facing physiological decline while maintaining own and/or couple functioning and interests ■ Exploring new familial and social options ■ Supporting a more central role for the middle generation ■ Making room for the wisdom and experience of elders ■ Dealing with losses—of spouse, siblings and other peers—and preparing for death

Source: Nichols, M. P. (2010). *Family therapy: Concepts and methods* (9th ed.). Reprinted by permission of Pearson Education, Inc. Upper Saddle River, NJ.

the **family system**—which includes not only family members, but also their relationships, their communication with one another, and their interactions with the environment—roles must often be negotiated in other than stereotyped ways. When the roles are not negotiated satisfactorily, family disequilibrium results.

It is worth taking the time to consider the importance of roles within a family, and how these may change and fluctuate when living with a person experiencing mental illness. For instance, a person may enter into a relationship expecting to be a lifelong partner with equal responsibilities, yet find themselves in the role of caring for their partner, something they had never expected. Similarly, roles may change over the duration of the illness and the person's journey of recovery. Since recovery is different for each person, the implications of resuming their past role in the family may have substantially changed and need renegotiating.

Family boundaries

Families have boundaries which define who participates in the family, the amount or intensity of emotional investment in the family, the amount and kind of experiences available outside the family, and particular ways to evaluate experiences in terms of the family. Clear, stable and healthy boundaries allow for personal and meaningful relationships with others. A person with healthy boundaries has a solid sense of self. There are feelings of belongingness to the family as well as to others outside the family.

Boundaries may be clear or conflicting, rigid or diffuse. **Rigid boundaries**—those in which rules and roles are maintained under all conditions—keep members from having meaningful relationships with one another, and understanding one another. People with rigid boundaries can become isolated or withdrawn. The isolation extends to the outside community as a whole, and the family is cut off from others.

A **diffuse boundary** is the opposite of a rigid boundary—a person with diffuse boundaries has no clear, definable boundaries with others. In families, diffuse boundaries are characterised by family over-involvement in the lives of its members, leading to the loss of independence by one or all family members. Parents and children become increasingly dependent on one another at the expense of relationships outside the family. Diffuse boundaries increase the family's dependence on one another. Families that struggle with boundaries tend to raise children who struggle with boundaries.

Power structure

Most families have a hierarchical power structure in which the adults wield the power. The power structure is often developed in this way because it creates a safe environment in which young children can grow and develop, and because it is easy to operate. However, stress develops when disagreements exist about who holds the power.

In the Practice Example, once the adults in the Manson family were able to acknowledge their internal power struggle and come to an agreement on what rules were to be set and by whom, the family system was subject to less stress.

Practice example

Tom, the 18-year-old son in the Manson family, often used the family car without permission. Although some serious arguments ensued between Tom and his father, no restrictions were placed on Tom's behaviour, and the car keys continued to hang on a key rack in the front hall. Tom's paternal grandfather, who lived with the Manson family, took Tom's side in his arguments with his father. The grandfather took the stance that 'boys will be boys'.

One evening when the family car was at the garage for some minor work, Tom 'borrowed' his grandfather's new car. He was involved in a collision about an hour later. Although no one was injured, his grandfather's car was extensively damaged and had to be towed away. Later that night, the adults of the Manson family managed to come together to agree on a stance they could mutually support concerning Tom's use of the family cars.

When children mature and become capable of assuming greater responsibility for their own functioning, power is often diffused among the members of a family system in a more democratic fashion. Certain families, however, do not allow power to be redistributed, thus hindering the individual development of the members with less power. In some dysfunctional families, there is ongoing discord about power.

Relationship strains or conflicts

Relationship strains or conflicts can occur in the family or among various parts of the family, or outside of it. This commonly occurs when a previously and unanimously held family view is challenged by one or more members. A strain can exist between the individual members of a family—for instance, between two siblings with differing views on an issue. Conflict or strain can also occur between a member of the family and the rest of the family, or between a minority of family members and the other members.

Practice example

Charlene lives in the Coffs Harbour near the New South Wales–Queensland border. Her brother lives in Perth, one sister lives in North Queensland, and an estranged sister lives in Tasmania. Their 94-year-old mother, who lives in Byron Bay and needs increasing amounts of care, refuses to consider moving into a nursing home or an assisted-living facility. The burden of driving three hours to her mother's home every few weeks to check on her has fallen to Charlene because she lives the closest. Her sisters have begun to pressure Charlene to move to Byron Bay so that she can take care of their mother. However, Charlene is reluctant to do so. Her friends, church and job are in the community in which she lives. Currently, the two sisters are pitted against Charlene and her brother.

Strain can also exist between a family and the community when the family view differs from that of the community at large.

Relationship and communication intricacies in families

Some of the relationship complexities described next exist in all families, but dysfunctional families handle them differently than do functional families. Functional families allow for individuation and growth-producing experiences.

Self-fulfilling prophecy and life scripts

A **self-fulfilling prophecy** is an idea or expectation that is acted out, largely unconsciously, thus 'proving' itself. In families, self-fulfilling prophecies are often seen in the guise of family life scripts. A **life script** is a plan decided not by the fates, but by experiences early in life. People with life scripts are following forced, premature, early childhood decisions. Most people live a scripted life, at least to some extent.

There is an endless variety among life scripts. The Norm Smith Medal script is decided for the five-year-old boy whose parents enrol him in the community Junior Australian Football League and who attend weekly training. There are also scripts such as 'my son the doctor', 'my father the hero', 'my grandmother the matriarch'. A person with a script, whether 'good' or 'bad', is terribly disadvantaged in terms of autonomy or life potential. According to self-fulfilling prophecy, unless people recognise what the script is and take steps to change it, they are prevented from living to their potential.

Family scripts are similar, in that they are an unconscious process in which family members play out a role within the family according to past experiences. These are often repetitive unless the individual recognises the pattern and attempts to alter their script by 'correcting' what has occurred in the past (Rasheed, Rasheed & Marley, 2011). You will often hear parents say they will never make the same mistakes their own parents made with them, only to find themselves going to an extreme opposite, or occasionally replicating the things they said they never wanted to do.

Family myths and themes

Family myths and themes help families maintain balance by permitting them to resist change. *Family myths* are well-integrated beliefs, shared by all family members, about each other and their positions in family life. The beliefs are unchallenged, even though family members may have to resort to distortions to maintain the myth. The family myth is related to the family's inner image—how the family appears to its members.

Practice example

A myth in the Harpin family was that the father had the ability to make wise decisions. Individual members in this family participated to maintain the myth of the father as a wise man by gearing interactions with him in such a way that he appeared to make high-level family decisions single-handedly.

The *family theme* is the family's perception of its development and history. Family themes are important, because they shape the fates of individual members and determine the pressures with which each person must contend.

Practice example

The Weber family had a theme constructed around second-generation grandparents of Austrian descent, who were able to provide their oldest son with a law-school education through their hard work. This family conceived of people on welfare as 'lazy', thus reaffirming its view of the value of working hard and becoming educated.

Energy in the family is directed towards upholding particular images of the family—as the most hardworking, religious, popular, talented, financially successful, nonconformist or whatever—in order to maintain the front the family strives to present to others.

Family coalitions

Of all the forms of communicative exchange, dyadic communication is the most common. In fact, many families begin with a couple, a dyad. The presence of a third person always has an effect on an existing dyad. When the couple gives birth to or adopts a child, or a third person enters the family, the relationship becomes triadic. A triad is not a stable social situation, because it actually consists of a dyad plus one. Shifting alliances characterise triads or triangles in families. For example, adult partners may unite to discipline the child, mother and child may unite to argue for a family vacation, or father and child may join forces to go fishing together. Triangles are dysfunctional when issues are solved by shifting the intimacy among members rather than by working the actual issue through, or when interaction among family members is determined by fixed triangles. Fixed and rigid triangles are an effort to reduce stress and restore balance in a dysfunctional family. In actuality, fixed and rigid triangles perpetuate problems in families. Such coalitions always result in someone feeling 'left out' (Nichols, 2010). A problematic family triangle is illustrated in Figure 24.1 ■.

Coalitions arise basically to affect the distribution of power. By joining forces, two people can increase their influence over a third. Parents frequently pair up in order to discipline their child in a consistent manner. However, the child may also attempt to pair up with one parent to avoid discipline. In families with a number of children, typical coalitions involve the children closest in age or children of the same sex.

Deviations in the adult partners' coalition

In some families, problems develop from the couple's inability to form a satisfying coalition in terms of intimacy and control. Several common deviations within the family are examined in the sections that follow.

Schism Families in which the children are forced to join one or other camp of two warring spouses or adult caretakers are called **schismatic families**. The constant fighting in these families is most likely a defence against intimacy or closeness.

In schismatic families, the adult partners devalue and undercut each other. This makes it difficult for the children to want to be like either of them.

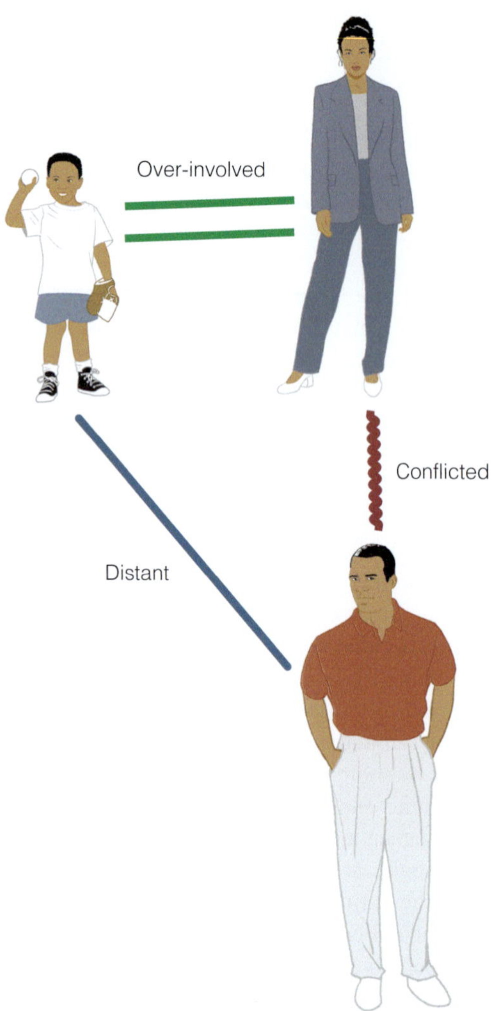

FIGURE 24.1 ■ A family triangle. In this family, the relationship between husband and wife is conflicted. Mother and son are over-involved. Father and son have a distant relationship.

Practice example

Patty and Krista joined their father in 'teasing' their mother whenever she was unclear about the latest news event, historical or geographical fact, movie or music. Their teasing gradually became increasingly derogatory and public. Patty, Krista and their father made it clear that they viewed her as incompetent and not very bright.

Skew Families in which one mate is severely dysfunctional are called **skewed families**. The other mate, who is usually aware of the dysfunction of the partner, assumes a passive, peace-making, submissive stance to preserve the relationship.

Practice example

Mick and Cindy loved to join their friends at elegant restaurants known for fine food. Cindy, who suffered with anorexia, usually ordered as her one and only entrée 'a small house salad, lemon only, please; no dressing'. At home, Cindy often ate only raw carrots. Dinner for her family was likely to be a scoop of mashed potatoes in a bowl of clear chicken broth. Mick did not acknowledge Cindy's unusual food preferences, her interest in recipes and restaurants, or her anorexia.

The passive partner is caught between effectively responding to the dysfunctional partner's view of 'reality' of the outside world and giving up this view within the home, thereby accepting the dysfunctional mate's view. On the surface, a skewed couple may appear to be complementary. However, their relationship is actually lopsided, and is unsuited to many basic family tasks.

Enmeshment A fast tempo of interpersonal exchange is characteristic of **enmeshed families**. Interactions within the family are of high intensity and are directed more towards issues of power than towards issues of affection.

Practice example

Gina is a university student and a single mother with a one-year-old daughter, who lives with her parents, second-generation Australians, in an enmeshed family. Gina has failed to maintain the life script expected of her—Little Miss Innocent—a chaste and innocent young woman who lives at home with her parents while she does her best to be the first in the family to graduate from university, thus improving her own and her family's circumstances. Gina's mother is especially embarrassed by the presence of Gina's young daughter, actually forcing Gina to hide her daughter away when relatives and friends come to visit. Gina and her father have no idea how to deal with her powerful and controlling mother. She feels stymied—unable to move out because of financial reasons, and reluctant to do so because of her own dependency needs—and torn, because she recognises that the family situation is not the best for her daughter.

In enmeshed families, one adult is often over-controlling and becomes anxious over the possibility of losing control over the children. Enmeshed families have diffuse boundaries. As you saw in this Practice Example, none of these categories are discrete. A family characterised as enmeshed may also be dealing with dysfunctional coalitions among the members, as well as life scripts that prevent them from living to their potential.

Disengagement Abandonment—at the other extreme from enmeshment—is characteristic of **disengaged families**. Family members seem oblivious to the effects of their actions on one another. They are unresponsive and unconnected to each other. Structure, order or authority in the family may be weak or non-existent. The responsibility of controlling and guiding increases the anxiety of the parent, who may feel overwhelmed and depressed. In these families, a child often assumes the parental role.

Practice example

Tony and Mary have eight children. Tony is seldom home, and works two full-time jobs in order to support his family financially. The little spare time he does have is spent with his friends at the local social club. Mary is tired, sleeps a lot and is probably clinically depressed. Rita, the oldest child, takes care of her seven younger siblings. She can't wait until she is old enough to get married and leave home.

Pseudo-mutuality and pseudo-hostility

In the 1950s, L. C. Wynne worked with families where a family member had a diagnosis of schizophrenia. He developed the concepts of **pseudo-mutuality** and **pseudo-hostility** as a way of describing both the positive and the negative emotions in dealing with family life (Goldenberg & Goldenberg, 2013).

A family with *pseudo-mutuality* functions as if it were a close, happy family. This pattern of relating has the following characteristics:

- persistent sameness in the structuring of roles
- insistence on the desirability and appropriateness of the role structures within the family, despite evidence to the contrary
- intense concern over deviations from the role structure or emerging autonomy
- marked absence of spontaneity, enthusiasm and humour in participating together.

In these families, the members do not form intimate bonds with one another as individuals. Instead, an inordinate amount of energy is expended in maintaining ritualised and stereotyped ways of behaving and relating. Such a family requires its members to give up their sense of personal identity.

Pseudo-hostility exists in families characterised by chronic conflict, alienation, tension and inappropriate remoteness. As in pseudo-mutuality, family members deny the problems in an attempt to negate the hostility. Family members view their differences as only minor ones. Both pseudo-mutual and pseudo-hostile family environments are stifling milieus.

Practice example

Jim and Ingrid had three children, only one of whom, a daughter, keeps in regular contact with them. Their children play out with them the relationships Jim and Ingrid had in their own families of origin. Jim has a brother, Fred, and Ingrid has several brothers and sisters in Finland. Jim is unconcerned about the fact that he has no idea where his brother is, or even whether his brother is still alive. Ingrid left her large family's home in Finland for Australia when she was 16 years old—they do not correspond, nor do they visit. This remoteness and lack of connectedness is mirrored in Jim and Ingrid's own family. When they are not ignoring one another, they and their children are in chronic conflict. The spouses of their two sons encourage their husbands to maintain contact with Jim and Ingrid, despite knowing that Ingrid undermines them at every opportunity. Occasions when they are together are marred by tension.

FAMILY ASSESSMENT

The family who has cared for the person with a lived experience of mental illness is most likely to have an in-depth understanding of the individual's illness, history and ability to function in the community. Including the family's insights in the assessment phase, and in the planning of care, is an important part of the recovery process. Family members want to be involved at an early stage, and to have their opinions heard and their experience with the ill family member respected (Nordby, Kjonsberg & Hummelvoll, 2010; Department of Health, 2013).

Family assessment involves gathering data in several different areas, and can be done both formally and informally. Do not overlook natural opportunities to assess families and their needs. During visits, join the family for a few minutes to learn about their understanding of the illness, available treatments and interventions, their concerns, and their questions. More formal assessments, using interview guides or strategies such as a family genealogy or timeline (discussed later in this chapter), are also available. Whichever methods you use, remember that a trusting relationship with key members of the person's family is essential for establishing a flow of information and planning care. Remember, however, to secure the person's permission before releasing information to their families, and encourage them to involve their families in their treatment. The individual rights of the person in your care and the carer in relation to the sharing of information is discussed in Chapter 11.

Demographic information

Obtain data pertaining to gender, age, occupation, religion and ethnicity. In addition to gathering discrete bits of information (the father is a 39-year-old Italian, laboratory assistant, and a member of St Ann's Roman Catholic parish), it is important to gather more detailed information that will give insight into family functioning:

- How actively does the family pursue religious/spiritual activities?
- What is the link of religion/spirituality to the family's value system, norms and practices?
- What is the family's racial, cultural and ethnic identification in relation to sense of identity and belonging?
- Who in the family is employed? What are their attitudes about employment?

Medical and mental health history

Here, you should also gather substantive information. You want to know about past medical and mental health treatment, including experiences with psychotropic medications, past and present illnesses, and pertinent health facts in the family of origin, in the extended family and in the family history.

Gather information about the developmental stage of the family.

- What were (are) the problems in transition from one developmental level to another?
- How has the family solved problems at earlier stages?
- What shifts in role responsibility have occurred over time?

Gaps in the collection of medical and mental health history were important in the unfortunate escalation of the situation summarised in the following Mental Health in the Media.

Family interactional data

This is probably the most complex data to obtain. For example, you want to gather information about family rules.

- What family rules foster stability in the family?
- What rules foster maladaptation?
- How are rules modified?

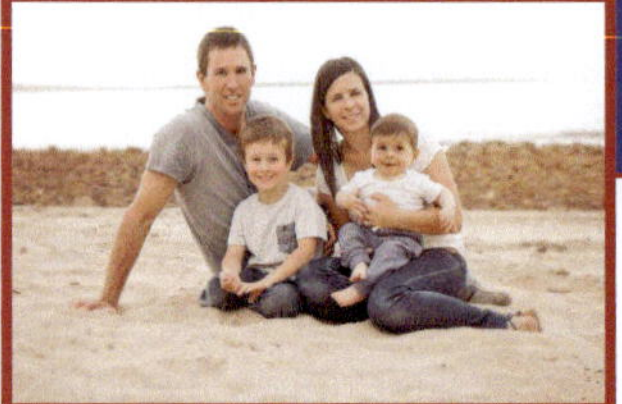

MENTAL HEALTH IN THE MEDIA

The Damien Little case

One of the most recent tragedies highlighting the importance of engaging with mental health services is the case of Damien Little, a father from Port Lincoln who killed his two sons (nine months and four years old) by shooting them, before taking his own life by driving his car off the end of a local wharf with both boys as passengers. Gunshot wounds were also found on the body of Damien. Media reports at the time indicate several issues, such as separation from his wife, possible financial difficulties and an ongoing three-year battle with mental illness that Damien refused to seek treatment for, despite requests from family and friends. Local community members and his wife publicly spoke out about Damien's struggle with depression, and that Damien should not be condemned for his actions. While no one can fully understand why familicide occurs, this case highlights the consequences of untreated mental illness and the lack of therapeutic family interventions.

Source: Based on Andrew Hough. (2016, January 9). Port Lincoln murder-suicide: Damien Little shot himself and his two sons befor he drove them off the wharf. *The Advertiser*. Retrieved from http://www.adelaidenow.com.au/news/south-australia/damien-little-shot-himself-and-his-two-children-before-he-drove-off-port-lincoln-wharf-in-murdersuicide/news-story/e63e4227442d8ddb970ccebf7db06cd1

- What happens when all members do not agree about the family rules?

You also need to determine the roles of family members.

- What are the formal roles for each member?
- What are the informal roles (scapegoat [scapegoating is explained in Chapter 21], controller, decision-maker and so on)?
- Do the roles seem to have a good fit in the family?

Most important, gather information on how family members communicate.

- What are the channels of communication—who speaks to whom?
- Are the messages clear?
- What is the extent of unclear or ambiguous messages, mixed messages or missed messages?
- Do members 'hear' one another?

Assess levels of cohesion by noting who accompanies the person and who visits if they are hospitalised. Visits from family are a rich source of information.

- Does the person come in alone?
- Who visits, how often, and for how long?
- Is it the whole family, or just one member?
- How do family visitors behave with the person experiencing mental illness?
- Do the members spend time interacting and sharing activities? Do they sit quietly together, or do they maintain physical and emotional distance from one another?

Document these patterns of family interactions, and monitor the effect of family visits on the person.

Family burden

More than 15 per cent of the Australian population are carers for a person with a lived experience of mental illness (Pirkis et al., 2010). Some families of those individuals experiencing mental illness report that caring for the ill member is a very important, largely underappreciated, stigmatised and frequently expensive, all-consuming task. **Family burden** is a term that refers to the difficulties and responsibilities of family members who assume a caretaking function for relatives with psychiatric disability, but comprises much more than the issues arising from providing practical care for a person. It involves subjective emotional difficulties and personal challenges faced by family members as a direct consequence of a person's illness. For some, the role of caregiver may be part of their family role, hence not perceived as a burden, whereas for others, new tasks or responsibilities they undertake may be unfamiliar and are identified as impacting on their life. While some family members may perceive the role to be a burden or a negative experience, many describe their role as rewarding, fulfilling and gratifying, having brought them closer in their relationship with the person in their care (Ennis & Bunting, 2013).

The burden of care can involve shame, embarrassment and feelings of guilt and self-blame (Lefley & Wasow, 2013), especially when the burden becomes great. This is the time when families may need the greatest level of support and understanding from professional staff.

You may ask the question: 'Do all families and all members in a family experience the family burden in the same way?' Studies that have examined the role of gender have found that relatives of males with schizophrenia frequently experience more social dysfunction than those of female clients (Awad & Voruganti, 2008). In addition, the more severe the symptoms the person has, the greater the family burden, although there is no agreement on which cluster of symptoms increases the family burden the most.

The family burdens reported most often are financial strain, violence in the household, reductions in the physical and mental health of family caregivers, disruption of family routines, worry about the future, the impact of stigma, the mental health system itself as a stressor, and feeling overwhelmed or unable to cope. Families also report having the following needs:

- information about the disorder itself
- information about how to manage day-to-day problems due to the ill family member's symptoms
- information and access to resources about medications and their side-effects

- strategies for helping the seriously mentally ill family member accept treatment
- support in their role as caregiver.

Gathering information about the family burden will help you to determine what kind of support would be most helpful to this family. A family s+upport group? Referral for their own mental health needs? Respite care to give the family a break from their caregiving role? Family therapy?

Remember, also, that many people experiencing mental illness are parents. With Reupert and colleagues (2012) reporting between 21 and 23 per cent of Australian children having one or more parents living with a mental illness, it is an area that must also be addressed when providing care for the person and their family. Unfortunately, children's voices are rarely heard, despite the fact that a parent's mental illness can have a significant psychosocial influence on the development of the children, particularly if other elements, such as social support, genetic disposition, the age of the child and the severity of the parent's mental illness are influencing the child's own mental health state (Reupert et al., 2012). It is good practice to remember that family burden is shared by everyone in the family, including children; therefore they, too, should be included in the support given to the family—being family-focused by involving all members of the family, delivering psychoeducation recovery-based interventions, and assessing family functioning supports strategies for early intervention and prevention of potential future problems.

What families want from mental health professionals

What better way to find out what families need from us than to ask them directly? When family members and people with schizophrenia were asked what elements were most important to them when in remission, consumers indicated that good, subjective wellbeing was the most important (Karow, Naber, Lambert & Moritz, 2011). Family members believed that symptom reduction, combined with good subjective well-being, was most important. In another study, Nordby and associates (2010) asked family members in focus-group interviews what they wanted from mental health professionals. Family members revealed that they wanted the following:

- an explicit invitation from mental health staff to participate
- the opportunity to get involved at an early stage
- staff members to treat their ill family member as a person and not a disease
- to be treated as resource people; to have their opinions and experiences respected and taken into consideration
- expressions of hopefulness from staff members and nurturance of hope, no matter the prognosis
- psychoeducation to help them learn what to say and how to behave towards their family member
- individual counselling and support.

These family members' requests will guide you in developing a therapeutic alliance (McGhee & Atkinson, 2010) with the person's family, and help you to diminish the social isolation and alienation from professional caregivers that family members often feel (Ewertzon, Lutzen, Svensson & Andershed, 2010).

Family system information

Determine how the family interacts with the outside world.

- How permeable or rigid are its boundaries?
- What is the extent to which the family fits into the larger culture of which it is a part?
- To what degree could the family be considered unusual or different from the larger culture?

Within the family, determine the family alliances.

- Who supports whom?
- Which members are in conflict with one another, or with the family as a whole?
- Are there extended-family supports?
- What other social supports are available to the family?

Needs, goals, values and aspirations

Determine whether essential needs are met.

- Are physical needs met?
- At what level does the family meet the social and emotional needs of its members?
- What are the individual needs of family members, and how do they fit with the family needs?
- Is the family willing or able to meet the individual needs of its members?

Determine the extent to which individual family members' goals, values and aspirations are articulated and understood by the other family members.

- Are the goals, values and aspirations shared by all?
- Do some members compromise?
- Do other members simply give up and give in?
- Does the family as a whole allow individual members to pursue individual goals and values?

Family genogram

From the study of families in detail, it becomes apparent that patterns are spread over generations. The timeline, or **genogram**, is highly effective as a visual representation of family patterns from one generation to the next. By drawing it on a long, narrow piece of paper and taping it to the wall during a family conference or family sessions, the treatment team or therapist can use it repeatedly as therapy progresses. Coloured lines can differentiate individual family members. Coloured flags, pins or stickers can identify and call attention to significant events in the family history. Note births, deaths, marriages and separations. You can use any of several family tree or genealogic tracing formats for the family timeline. One example is illustrated in Figure 24.2 ■. You can develop other genograms to explore specific issues.

Spiritual family genogram

A spiritual genogram—a multi-generational map of family members' religious and spiritual affiliations, events and conflicts—enables the person with a mental illness to make

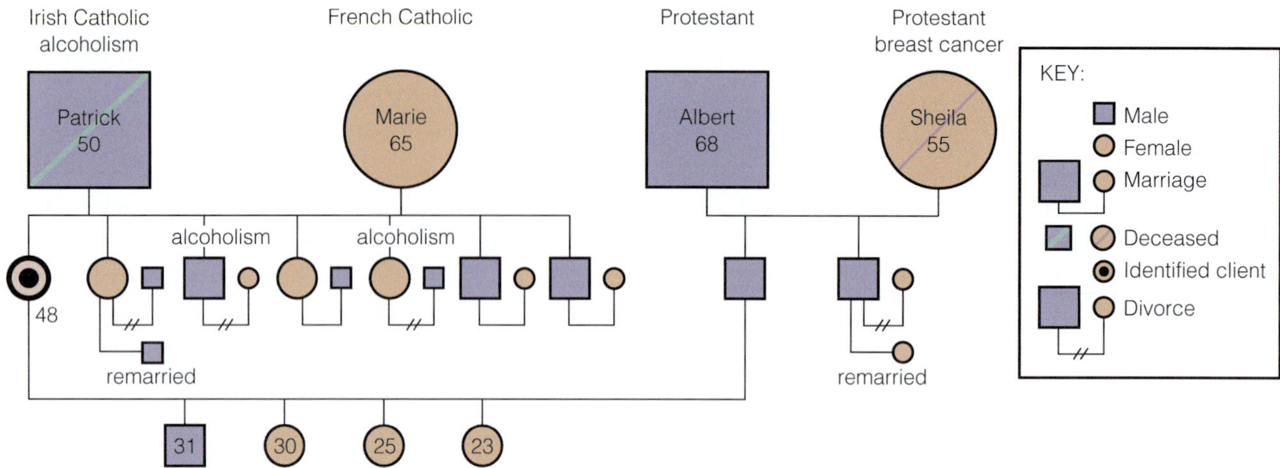

FIGURE 24.2 ■ One example of a family genogram.

sense of their family's religious/spiritual heritage. It also helps them to explore the ways in which their experiences with spirituality affect issues between the couple or family issues.

Cultural family genogram

A cultural family genogram is a useful tool for working with culturally diverse families. You can use a cultural family genogram to become more aware of the cultural differences between yourself and the family, and between the family and other families, to assess a family's strengths, and to point to areas where intervention may be useful. A cultural family genogram might include the elements discussed in Developing Cultural Competence.

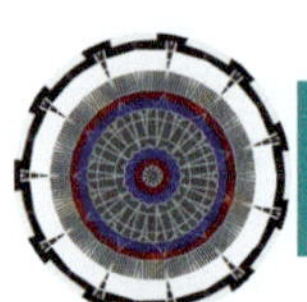

DEVELOPING CULTURAL COMPETENCE

The cultural family genogram

Identifying the following elements will help in developing a useful cultural family genogram:

- What language is spoken at home, and in the community?
- What significance does race, skin and hair colour play within the group?
- What role does religion and spirituality play within the everyday lives of the family members?
- What prejudices or stereotypes does this family have about themselves and other members of their cultural group?
- What prejudices or stereotypes does this family have about other cultural groups?
- What are the health beliefs in this family's culture?
- How does this culture view mental health professionals?
- What values does this family have about family, education and work?
- What are the pride/shame issues of this cultural group? How are they manifested in this family?

CRITICAL THINKING QUESTIONS

1. What benefit is there in knowing the role that religion and spirituality play in this family?
2. How could you use knowledge about how this family views mental health professionals?
3. How might the pride/shame issues of this family's cultural group affect the care plan?

Forensic family genogram

A forensic family genogram is a useful tool for forensic nurses for both assessment and intervention purposes. A two- or three-generational map can help offenders see the patterns in their lives as a way to begin to understand their personal circumstances. As part of the legal chart, it provides the courts with information about the events and factors in the individual lives of offenders in the form of a graphic database.

FAMILY INTERVENTIONS

More recently, with the abundance of information from contemporary research and government reports, the message to include families in all aspects of a person's care, from assessment to treatment, has been a clear directive to enhance a person's recovery. Three main goals for involving family members in an individual's treatment plan are:

1. enlisting the family as an ally in promoting and bringing about therapeutic progress and reducing relapse
2. improving the family environment
3. supporting family caregivers.

The main forms of family intervention in current use are: family psychoeducation, including knowledge and information about the illness, services, coping strategies and support; early identification and intervention; relapse prevention; management of complex needs; family therapy; and flexible respite options with support for all members of the family. Also important are availability of crisis management, and well-informed advocacy.

Services directed towards supporting the family caregivers of persons with serious and enduring mental illness may have the potential to improve outcomes for both the caregivers and the person they are caring for (Pahlavanzadeh, Heideri, Maghsudi, Glazavi & Semendari, 2010). Although there seems to be a consensus about the need for coordinated family-based services, they are not always implemented. According to the Mental Health Council of Australia, it is estimated that three-quarters of all those living with a complex mental illness are still living with their families (Mental Health Council of Australia [MHCA], 2012), yet a significant number of carers report they were rarely seen or never considered as a part of the team caring for the person with the lived experience of mental illness (National Mental Health Commission, 2012).

Family interventions are not always implemented into service delivery, despite Australian policy encouraging this as sound practice. Rarely are families integrated in care plans and seen as experts in the care package alongside the consumer. This could be for a variety of reasons, such as the service being frequently underfunded, the historical relationship between 'patient and medics', the misuse or misunderstanding of aspects of confidentiality and information-sharing, or the risk-averse nature of health services today (Bland & Foster, 2012). Often this is an area for active advocacy by the mental health nurse.

Family psychoeducation

Family members can benefit from psychoeducation groups designed specifically to help them cope with their loved one's illness. In studies of family caregivers of people with dementia, psychoeducation provided immediate help to reduce the family burden (Pahlavanzadeh et al., 2010), as well as support and information (Wilhelmson et al., 2011). Family psycho-education programs have emerged as a strongly supported evidence-based practice in the treatment of schizophrenia (Karow et al., 2011) and, when combined with the use of antipsychotics by people who are schizophrenic, is found to be cost-effective (Phanthunane, Vos, Whiteford & Bertram, 2011). Family psychoeducation has also been found to reduce relapse and rehospitalisation (Karow et al., 2011), and to improve the ill person's recovery and their family's wellbeing. Suggestions for elements to include in a family psychoeducation program are given in Collaborative Care.

Family psychoeducation educates family members about the specific mental illness, including its signs and symptoms, the medications being taken, the signs and stages of relapse, the treatment plan, and the fluctuating course of mental illness. They also learn about life events that cause stress for the person with mental illness, how to prevent relapse, and how to manage behaviour that may challenge others. Family psychoeducation should also address all of the family members' emotion regulation and interpersonal skills, particularly the strengths and resources they may not have realised already exist.

Some local areas facilitate family psychoeducation groups. These serve a supportive function in an accepting environment. Family members are informed about local and national groups and organisations that provide educational and counselling services and respite care.

COLLABORATIVE CARE

Psychoeducation for families

To assist families, you need to evaluate the family's current responses to living with, and caring for, a family member with a mental illness. The following suggestions apply to the time period shortly after a first hospital admission or first contact with mental health services, where the person in question has been recently diagnosed.

Suggestions	Rationale
Discuss the basic nature of the illness—for instance, the pathology of the illness—like any other biological disease.	Families misunderstand mental illness to be a personal failing, and so are at times comforted by the fact that it can have a biological basis.
Help families identify their responses to the early ambiguous signs of the illness, and notice how their responses have changed now that the diagnosis has been made.	Families often misinterpret early signs of the illness as acting out or developmentally inappropriate behaviour. On learning that these signs are part of the illness, they feel guilty for not seeking help sooner.
Reinforce the importance of families in supporting the ill family member to seek treatment.	Stigma about mental illness persists, and families need support for taking action and engaging with treatment systems.
Refer families to structured educational or psychoeducational programs in which they can learn about the illness, its treatment and recovery, as well as receive support.	Mental illness is extremely complex, and treatment is multi-faceted. Families can benefit from structured time to sit and discuss their concerns, issues and queries. Programs that offer support to families in addition to education have proven effective in improving the illness course for the ill member.
Inform families about how to reach the local support networks and resources. Hand out information that provides telephone numbers and people to contact.	Local and national organisations, such as SANE, COPMI, Life Without Barriers and Carers Australia, often provide peer support, education and advocacy for those with a lived experience of mental illness and their families/carers.
Provide families with access to appropriate, accurate and up-to-date information in books and manuals or articles. Referring them to their local library is a good starting point.	It is often useful for family members to have a quick-reference book available for help in managing symptoms and their own distress.

EVIDENCE-BASED PRACTICE

Decreasing family burden through psychoeducation

The program development committee at the mental health outreach clinic where you work has challenged you to provide a convincing rationale for your recent proposal. You believe that family psychoeducation helps to reduce family burden. However, in order to commit resources such as staff and funding, the committee has asked you to review the research to determine on what basis the agency can support your proposal.

Your review of the research found significant support for your proposal. Family psychoeducation groups for families with a family member with schizophrenia show a significant improvement in the person's social relationships, interest in obtaining a job and management of social conflicts. Family burden significantly improved, as did relatives' social contacts and perception of professional support. Family distress decreased as the confidence and skills of the family members increased. Similar results are found with studies of bipolar disorder, depression, suicide, borderline personality disorder and dementia of the Alzheimer's type.

You should base action on more than one study, but the following research was helpful in developing this proposal:

Karow, A., Naber, D., Lambert M., & Moritz, S. (2012). Remission as perceived by people with schizophrenia, family members and psychiatrists. *European Psychiatry, 27*(6), 426–431.

CRITICAL THINKING QUESTIONS

1. What are the purposes of reviewing the evidence before designing an intervention?
2. What specific areas of research should you review other than studies of family psychoeducation?
3. What might a structured family psychoeducation program look like?

Unfortunately, the use of family psychoeducation in routine clinical practice is limited. Family members are most likely to receive information about diagnosis and medications, and least likely to receive information about the treatment plan. However, nurses can be influential in persuading their agencies to develop family psychoeducation programs, as discussed in Evidence-based Practice, above.

Psychosocial interventions (PSI) are an integral part of recovery-orientated mental health service delivery, especially so with those people with enduring mental health issues. Psychosocial interventions have been around for many years, and are based on a collaboration between the consumer and carer(s). It includes interventions such as family work, psychoeducation, cognitive behavioural therapy, concordance therapy in medication management, self-management, coping strategy enhancement, strength-based assessment, solution-focused interventions and relapse prevention. It has been found to be effective in engaging and maintaining positive therapeutic relationships with both the person with mental illness and their family, as well as leading to better health care outcomes (Butler, Begley, Parahoo & Finn, 2014).

Family therapy

In general, family therapists believe that the emotional symptoms or problems of an individual are an expression of the emotional symptoms or problems in a family. Therefore, family therapists view the family system as a unit of treatment. Their concerns are basically with the relationships between the family members, not with the intrapsychic functioning of individual family members, and therapy is directed at changing the organisation of the family (Nichols, 2010). The discussion of **family therapy** in this chapter is designed to provide you with the information you need to know in order to formulate a referral for family therapy, and to educate and support individuals and their family members.

Forms of family therapy

There are two basic forms of family therapy—insight-oriented family therapy and behavioural-oriented family therapy—into which all schools of family therapy fit on some level. Some examples of insight-oriented family therapy approaches are as follows:

- *Psychodynamic:* Problems are believed to arise because of developmental delays, or current interactions or stresses.
- *Family of origin therapy:* The goal is to foster differentiation among the members and decrease emotional reactivity and triangulation (Bowen, 1992).

Some examples of behavioural-oriented family therapy and the theorists who developed them are:

- *Structural:* The focus is on systems, subsystems, boundaries and schismatic, skewed, enmeshed or disengaged families (Minuchin & Fishman, 1981; Navarre, 1998).
- *Strategic:* Problems arise because of inequality of power, flawed communication, and repetitive and maladaptive family interaction patterns (Haley, 1996; Satir, 1983).
- *Cognitive behavioural:* The focus is on changing thinking and behaviour, problem-solving, and the development of skills (see Chapter 25 for a complete discussion of cognitive behavioural strategies).

These lists are general, not exhaustive. Discussion of these theories and their specific interventions is beyond the scope of this book.

Qualifications of family therapists

Being a family therapist requires a firm and clear understanding of all of the dynamics and forces that influence families. Family therapists should be specially educated in the practice of family therapy, and strongly committed to a belief in the importance of the family. Nurse family therapists should be clinical specialists or advanced practitioners prepared in graduate programs that provide both theory and supervised clinical practice in this specialised area. It may be there is someone who takes on this role as part of the multi-disciplinary team. Families can receive help in finding a therapist on the website of the Australian Association of Family Therapy (www.aaft.asn.au/).

The family as a unit

Most family therapists recommend that all people in the family constellation participate in the assessment phase of family therapy. Not all agree on which people comprise the family constellation or the treatment unit. Some include all members of the nuclear family; others include members of the extended family; and still others, large numbers of people in the family's social network. Different coalitions may be seen together at different times to accomplish specific goals.

Children four years of age and younger are often not included in ongoing family therapy sessions. They may misinterpret, or be frightened by, the dialogue. In addition, small children tend to be disruptive. Some therapists, however, make it a point to bring all of the children into some family therapy sessions to see how the family as a whole operates.

Contract or goal negotiation

The negotiation phase of family therapy is begun by identifying what each member would like changed in the family. When each family member and the therapist have identified important goals, they begin negotiating a set of attainable goals that everyone is willing to work on. Compromise is needed to achieve a working goal. At this time, the family therapist, along with the family, may also identify the means—tasks, strategies and so on—that will be used to reach the negotiated goals.

Intervention

Therapy for a family system involves understanding and use of the here-and-now, and of the basic processes that occur in the system. Guidelines for common interventions employed by family therapists are listed in Your Intervention Strategies.

Terminating family therapy

Family therapists use various criteria to determine when termination is appropriate. Family therapy is often terminated when family members can do the following:

- see how they appear to others
- give feedback to others, telling them how they appear
- share their hopes, fears and expectations with one another
- openly discuss problems with one another
- openly disagree with one another when appropriate
- give clear messages
- check meanings with one another
- ask for clarification
- support one another
- achieve the family's goals.

Termination in family therapy occurs in a flexible way, helping families achieve realistic goals, thus ending therapy with a feeling of accomplishment.

YOUR INTERVENTION STRATEGIES

The role of the family therapist

- Creating a safe setting in which family members can risk looking at themselves and their actions
- Teaching family members how to share their observations with one another
- Asking for and giving information in a matter-of-fact, nonjudgmental, congruent way
- Responding as a role model whose meaning or intent can be queried without fear
- Setting rules for interaction to ensure that all family members participate; interruptions, acting-out, or making it impossible to converse are not tolerated; no one speaks for anyone else
- Clarifying the content and relationship aspects of messages
- Pointing out significant discrepancies, incongruities or double-level messages
- Helping everyone speak out clearly, so that each can be heard
- Viewing the family as a system, and not taking sides
- Validating that anger, pain and the 'forbidden' are safe to examine
- Re-educating family members to be accountable
- Delineating family roles and functions, and teaching explicitly about role responses and role choices

LIVED EXPERIENCE

Most families are resilient, even those we might consider dysfunctional. We need to build the capacity of families to nurture those in need, and we need to ensure that they have the appropriate resources with which to do so. For too many families the mental health system is impossible to navigate—it seems to them that the system's dysfunction makes their own recovery work so much harder. It is vital that nurses do not work in silos, but that they know the services available in a community. It seems a waste to spend most of our mental health budget on acute hospital care, while the pathways to the real world are littered with potholes, dead-end streets and collapsing bridges.

A mental health crisis should be reframed as an opportunity. For many of us an episode is cathartic, and it opens doors rather than closes them. Families need to hear about the strengths and ambitions of the person, not the problems and incapacity of the patient. It is important for nurses to be able to direct families to healthy, recovery-focused places when it comes time to hand over care.

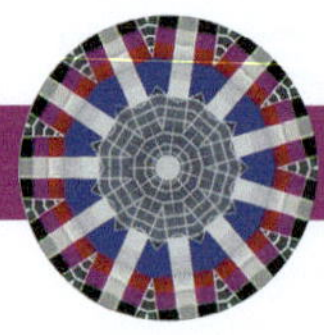

REFERENCES

Anderson, S. A., & Sabatelli, R. M. (2011). *Family interaction: A multigenerational developmental perspective* (5th ed.). Boston, MA: Allyn & Bacon.

Australian Institute of Health and Welfare (AIHW). (2011). *The health and welfare of Australia's Aboriginal and Torres Strait Islander people: An overview 2011*. Cat. No. IHW 42. Canberra, Australia: AIHW.

Awad, A. G., & Voruganti, L. I. (2008). The burden of schizophrenia on caregivers: A review. *Pharmacoeconomics, 26*(2), 149–162.

Bland, R., & Foster, M. (2012). Families and mental illness: Contested perspectives and implications for practice and policy. *Australian Social Work, 65*(4), 517–534.

Bowen, M. (1992). *Family therapy in clinical practice*. Northvale, NJ: Jason Aronson.

Butler, M., Begley, M., Parahoo, K., & Finn, S. (2014). Getting psychosocial interventions into mental health nursing practice: A survey of skill use and perceived benefits to service users. *Journal of Advanced Nursing, 70*(4), 866–877.

Department of Health. (2013). A national framework for recovery-oriented mental health services: Guide for practitioners and providers. Canberra, Australia: Commonwealth of Australia.

Duvall, E. M., & Miller, B. C. (1985). *Marriage and family development*. New York, NY: Harper & Row.

Ennis E., & Bunting B. (2013). Family burden, family health and personal mental health. *BMC Public Health, 13*(1), 255.

Ewertzon, M., Lutzen, K., Svensson, E., & Andershed, B. (2010). Family members' involvement in psychiatric care: Experiences of the healthcare professionals' approach and feeling of alienation. *Journal of Psychiatric and Mental Health Nursing, 17*(5), 422–432.

Goldenberg, H., & Goldenberg, I. (2013). *Family therapy: An overview* (8th ed.). Belmont. CA: Cengage Learning.

Haley, J. (1996). *Learning and teaching therapy*. New York, NY: Guilford Press.

Jackson, D. D. (1968). *Communication, family, and marriage*. Palo Alto, CA: Science and Behavior Books.

Karow, A., Naber, D., Lambert, M., & Moritz, S. (2012). Remission as perceived by people with schizophrenia, family members and psychiatrists. *European Psychiatry, 27*(6), 426–431.

Lefley, H. P., & Wasow, M. (2013). *Chronic mental illness, vol. 2: Helping families cope with mental illness*. Chur, Switzerland: Harwood Academic Publishers.

Maybery, D., & Reupert, A. (2009). Parental mental illness: A review of barriers and issues for working with families and children. *Journal of Psychiatric and Mental Health Nursing, 16*(9), 784–791.

McGhee, G., & Atkinson, J. (2010). The carer/key worker relationship cycle: A theory of the reciprocal process. *Journal of Psychiatric and Mental Health Nursing, 17*(4), 312–318.

McGoldrick, M., Garcia Preto, N., & Carter, B. (2015). *The expanded family life cycle: Individual, family and social perspectives* (5th ed.). Boston, MA: Pearson.

Mental Health Council of Australia (MHCA). (2012). *Recognition and respect: Mental health carers report*. Canberra, Australia: MHCA.

Minuchin, S., & Fishman, H. (1981). *Family therapy techniques*. Cambridge, MA: Harvard University Press.

National Mental Health Commission (NMHC). (2012). *A contributing life: The 2012 national report card on mental health and suicide prevention*. Canberra, Australia: NMHC, p. 36. Retrieved from http://www.mentalhealthcommission.gov.au/our-2013-report-card/2012-report-card.aspx (Accessed 2015, December 4.)

Navarre, S. (1998). Salvador Minuchin's structural family therapy and its application to multicultural family systems. *Issues in Mental Health Nursing, 19*, 557–565.

Nichols, M. (2010). *Family therapy: Concepts and methods* (9th ed). Boston, MA: Pearson.

Nordby, K., Kjonsberg, K., & Hummelvoll, J. R. (2010). Relatives of persons with recently discovered serious mental illness: In need of support to become resource persons in treatment and recovery. *Journal of Psychiatric and Mental Health Nursing, 17*(4), 304–311.

Pahlavanzadeh, S., Heideri, F. G., Maghsudi, J., Glazavi, A., & Semendari, S. (2010). The effects of family education programs on the caregiver burden of families of elderly with dementia disorders. *Iranian Journal of Nurse Midwifery and Research, 15*(3), 102–108.

Phanthunane, P., Vos, T., Whiteford, H., & Bertram, M. (2011). Cost-effectiveness of pharmacological and psychosocial interventions for schizophrenia. *Cost Effectiveness and Resource Allocation, 9*(1), 6.

Pirkis, J., Burgess, P., Hardy, J., Harris, M., Slade, T., & Johnston, A. (2010). Who cares? A profile of people who care for relatives with a mental disorder. *Australian and New Zealand Journal of Psychiatry, 44*(10), 929–937.

Qu, L., & Weston, R. (2013). *Australian households and families*. Australian Family Trends No. 4. Melbourne, Australia: Australian Institute of Family Studies.

Rasheed, J., Rasheed, M., & Marley, J. (2011). *Family therapy*. Los Angeles, CA: Sage Publications.

Reupert, A., Cuff, R., Drost, L., Foster, K., van Doesum K., & van Santvoort, F. (2012). Intervention programs for children whose parents have a mental illness: A review. *MJA Open, 1*(Suppl 1), 18–22. Retrieved from http://www.copmi.net.au/intervention-program (Accessed 2015, December 4.)

Satir, V. (1983). *Conjoint family therapy*. Palo Alto, CA: Science and Behavior Books.

Wilhelmson, K., Duner, A., Eklund, K., Gosman-Hedstrom, G., Blomberg, S., Hasson, H., . . . Dahlin-Ivanoff, S. (2011). Continuum of care for frail elderly people: Design of a randomized controlled study of a multi-professional and multidimensional intervention targeting frail elderly people. *BMC Geriatrics, 11*(1), 24.

Cognitive and behavioural interventions

25

CHRISTINE PALMER AND SHARON LAWN

LEARNING OUTCOMES

After completing this chapter, you will be able to:

1. Explain the central features of cognitive and behavioural interventions.
2. Relate conditioning to the process of human learning.
3. Analyse the effectiveness of a behavioural contract to promote a change in health-related behaviours.
4. Discuss how humans express themselves in cognitive and behavioural ways.
5. Describe how cognitive behavioural therapy (CBT) leads to changes in behaviour.
6. Explain how dialectical behavioural therapy (DBT) and acceptance and commitment therapy (ACT) differ from cognitive behavioural therapy.
7. Appraise strategies for community and family involvement in cognitive and behavioural therapies.

LIVED EXPERIENCE

CBT helped me to overcome my gambling addiction

I had a big problem with playing the pokies on the weekends at the local hotel. I had separated from my husband a few months before, and had become quite lonely and lost a lot of confidence. Initially, playing the poker machines got me out and made me feel better. The staff were friendly, the place was bright, and I could 'blend in', even when I was feeling down. But then I started having trouble paying my bills, and began to notice that I had trouble staying away from the local hotel. If I walked past on my way to the shops in the morning, I would be pulled to going inside to play the machines. Cognitive behaviour therapy (CBT) helped me to cope with the urge to gamble by helping me see my erroneous cognitions about winning, and be more aware of my rising excitement, blood pressure and breathing when I felt the urges.

KEY TERMS

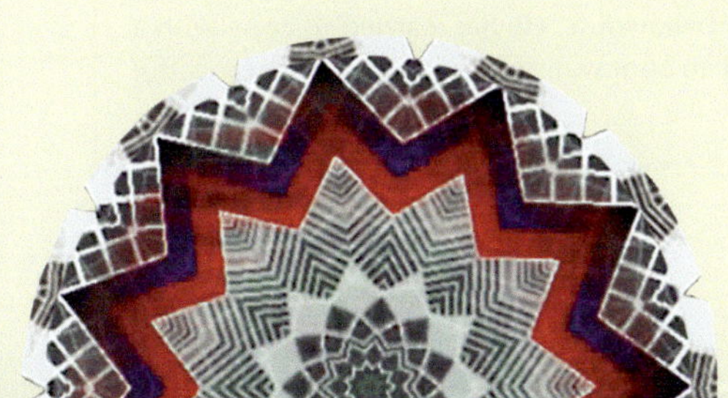

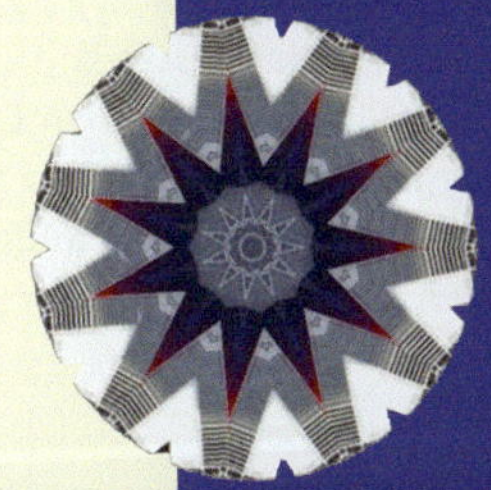

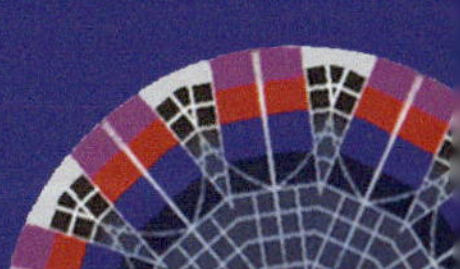

Practice example

Steven is a full-time university student. He has been depressed for some time, and has not made significant progress in long-term psychotherapy specifically focused on his childhood and developmental issues. You have discussed his treatment responses with other members of the treatment team during his recent hospitalisation for an exacerbation of his depression. Steven has expressed frustration at his inability to 'get better and leave the depression behind'. His depression and his routine ways of thinking and behaving continue in an unchanged, habitual manner.

The team believes a cognitive behavioural approach would give Steven a better chance at recovery from depression. Changing his thoughts and behaviours could change his feelings and diminish depressive thinking. Once changes begin to occur, Steven would have the opportunity to start feeling more hopeful, competent and successful, a distinct difference from his current view of himself.

1. How do you explain the notion that a change in thoughts and behaviours results in a change in feelings?
2. What should Steven know about this therapeutic method?
3. What differences would you expect to see in Steven's behaviour if the cognitive behavioural approach is effective?

INTRODUCTION

Amanda, a person who is most comfortable with structure and routine in her daily life, has finally decided to seek help to overcome her fear of flying. Her friends have invited Amanda to travel with them to Bali, a place she has always wanted to visit. Amanda always has several reasons why she cannot travel with them. Most of the time, she says that she needs to stay at home to care for her mother, who has a severe case of arthritis.

How might therapists with a variety of orientations approach Amanda's problem? A biologically-oriented therapist would first focus on diagnosing Amanda's problem as a specific phobia—fear of flying—once the presence of other anxiety disorders, specifically panic disorder with agoraphobia, have been ruled out. The biologically-oriented therapist would investigate Amanda's family history for the presence of phobias among first-degree biological relatives, and prescribe an antianxiety medication to alter her brain chemistry.

In contrast, a psychodynamic therapist would focus on Amanda's defensive style of avoidance. This therapist would identify Amanda's pattern of needing to have structure and control as a way of keeping anxiety in check. Treatment would be a talk therapy in which the therapist provides only minimal direction in the exploration of Amanda's past, her feelings and her frustrations. The therapeutic goal would be for Amanda to gain insight into her intrapsychic conflicts, interpersonal difficulties and defences.

A cognitive behavioural therapist would be aware of the issues in Amanda's life, but would approach therapy quite differently. A believer in the axiom that 'actions speak louder than words', the cognitive behavioural therapist looks for treatments that work, based on research evidence drawn from real-world trials. The therapist would focus on changing behaviour in the present, rather than focusing on gaining insight into the past. This change-oriented approach would pair relaxation training and systematic desensitisation (discussed later in this chapter) in Amanda's case.

In this chapter, you will learn that cognitive (thought) and behavioural (action) interventions have their base in human learning theory, and are comprised of diverse treatments based on empirical evidence. While not the only effective treatment—medications and other forms of talk therapy can also be effective—cognitive and behavioural strategies lend themselves to integration within a plan of care for people who may be receiving diverse, but effective, treatments for mental disorders. Frequently, cognitive behavioural therapy (CBT) is recommended for anger management. Mental Health in the Media describes the media's depiction of an 'appropriate' anger management program.

MENTAL HEALTH IN THE MEDIA

Anger Management

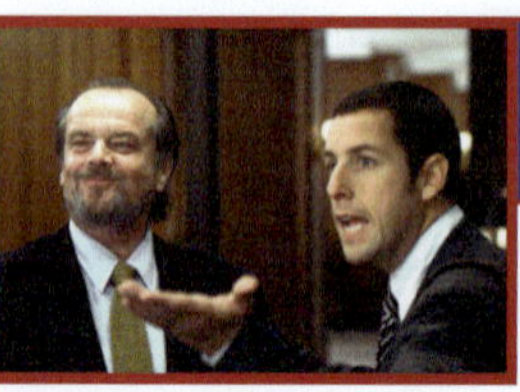

Sometimes media, such as movies, are not accurate primers for conducting cognitive behavioural interventions. In the movie *Anger Management*, the therapeutic process is bizarre and slapstick. However, it makes the point that we think and behave in ways that can be changed for the better.

After a small misunderstanding aboard an aeroplane escalates out of control, timid businessman Dave Buznik (Adam Sandler) is ordered by the court to undergo anger management therapy at the hands of specialist Dr Buddy Rydell (Jack Nicholson). Dave reluctantly accepts anger management counselling, but after another mishap Dr Rydell steps up his aggressive and unorthodox treatments by moving in with Dave. As Dr Rydell wreaks havoc with every aspect of Dave's life, Dave must decide whether to crawl back into his shell or finally stand up for himself. By the end of the movie, Dave's unrealistic and irrational thinking gives way to healthier behaviours. He has learned to cope with a disrespectful boss and an aggravating acquaintance by respectful assertiveness.

Photo courtesy © Photos 12/Alamy.

Historically, **behaviour therapy** was developed in the 1950s, and was considered the first wave of behaviour therapies. An emphasis on cognition during the 1970s led to the second wave of behavioural therapies, culminating in cognitive behavioural therapy (CBT) in the 1980s. The so-called third wave emerged in the late 1980s with the introduction of acceptance and commitment therapy (ACT), and later dialectical behavioural therapy (DBT) in the 1990s (Hayes, 2004). This chapter introduces concepts related to behaviour therapy and then cognitive therapy, before providing an overview of cognitive behavioural therapy. In more recent times, the term 'cognitive behavioural therapy' has largely replaced the terms 'behaviour therapy' and 'cognitive therapy' as a way of describing these therapeutic techniques. CBT focuses on changing thinking and behaviour, and improves problem-solving and the development of coping skills. Cognitive and behavioural interventions make use of the principles of cognitive functioning and behaviour listed in Box 25.1. Interventions are tailored to the individual's needs, and may be applied as single therapeutic entities or in combination. You can access the empirical evidence for cognitive behavioural therapy through the US National Library of Medicine National Institutes of Health (http://www.ncbi.nlm.nih.gov/pmc/?term=cognitive+behaviour+therapy).

This chapter also provides an introduction to ACT and DBT. These approaches to treatment have developed out of cognitive and behavioural therapies, and are therapeutic approaches of the so-called third wave of behavioural therapies, so reflect aspects of cognition and behaviour in their frameworks. Other third-wave behavioural therapies have continued to develop in the 21st century. According to Ost (2008), the third-wave therapies have some common characteristics, particularly mindfulness, values clarification and a focus on the therapeutic relationship. Regardless of the therapeutic approach we might use, it is always important to consider the person's cultural beliefs and practices, as culture informs our view of the world, and therefore how we view mental health and illness.

Box 25.1 Principles of cognitive functioning and behaviour

Principles of cognitive functioning

1. What people think affects how they feel.
2. What people think is often based on thinking habits.
3. If we change our thinking, we can effect a change in our feelings.

Principles of behaviour

People do things:	When they are rewarded in a way that is meaningful for them When something they don't like is removed
People don't do things:	When they get punished When something they like is taken away from them

BEHAVIOUR THERAPY

Behaviour has an impact on feelings and thoughts, as the following Practice Example demonstrates.

Practice example

An older woman with a hearing deficit is living with her daughter and son-in-law. She wears a hearing aid, but, to save on battery power, she removes it and turns it off immediately after dinner every night. When they try to talk to her, she cannot hear. She complains to others that her daughter and son-in-law are not interested in talking or interacting with her in the evening. Her behaviour isolates her, but she does not see the connection between her attempts at thriftiness and her feelings of loneliness.

The ways in which particular types of **behavioural therapy** can affect a variety of conditions are discussed next.

Classical conditioning

Generally, behaviour therapy reduces the occurrence of problematic behaviours. Behavioural therapy is very effective when used with a current problem that is relevant to the person's life (Keijsers, Maas, Opdorp & Minnen, 2016). It focuses on behavioural learning processes, including classical conditioning. The principles of **classical conditioning** are as follows:

- people learn to associate a particular feeling state with a particular circumstance that then becomes a conditioned stimulus for the feeling
- over time, the association between the circumstance and the feeling is strengthened through repetition and rehearsal.

The therapist's goal in behaviour therapy is to decrease or eliminate the association of a particular circumstance (the conditioned stimulus) with a particular feeling. See Figure 25.1 ■ for an example of a behaviour (gambling) that responds well to conditioning and intermittent reinforcement (occasional wins).

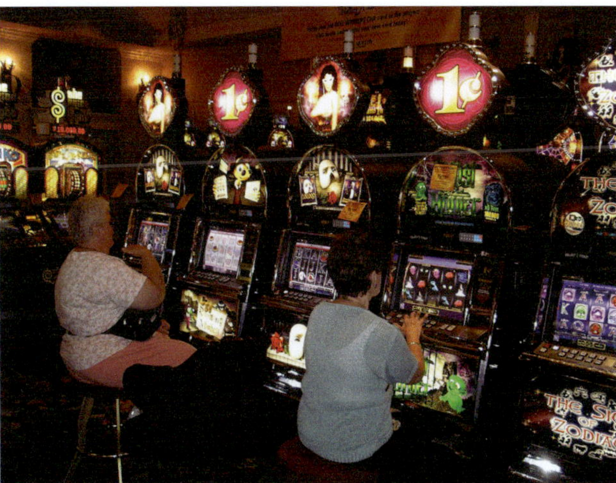

FIGURE 25.1 ■ Intermittent reinforcement. Operant conditioning involves an association between a stimulus and a response.
Photo courtesy of Greg Ward/DK Images.

Operant conditioning

Operant conditioning is another behavioural learning process, and is based on the following concepts:

- people are positively reinforced for certain behaviours
- people learn to seek further positive reinforcement (an environmental event that rewards, and thus increases the probability of, a behavioural response) by increasing that behaviour
- positive reinforcement results from either obtaining something desirable or avoiding something unpleasant.

The therapist's goal in operant conditioning is to help the individual increase positive reinforcement through more adaptive and effective behaviour. The effort to change health-related behaviour can be facilitated with a behavioural contract.

The behavioural contract

An effective **behavioural contract** must be tailored for the individual, and a comprehensive behavioural assessment is necessary to design such a contract and form practical, measurable and feasible objectives and goals.

Forming practical and measurable objectives and goals Formulating practical and measurable objectives and goals is the next step in developing a behavioural contract. Objectives are small steps leading to goal attainment; goals represent the overall desired outcomes. Prioritising the behavioural objectives involves the following four main features:

1. The goal should contribute directly to the desired result. In other words, how will tracking every cigarette a person smokes, and under what circumstances, help the person stop smoking? (It will sensitise the person and you to factors that contribute to smoking behaviour, and exactly how much and when the person smokes.)
2. The goal can be objectively monitored. (You know the objective is reached when the person completes the tracking mechanism.)
3. The goal is easily understood by the individual and all supportive significant others. (The person knows how to fill out the tracking mechanism, and knows why they are tracking the behaviour.)
4. The goal can be accomplished in the available time. (The person can fill out the form daily for one week.)

Behavioural goals should be objectively verifiable as contributing to positive treatment outcomes. The change is necessary and relevant, not outlandish. (It is relevant to track how often one smokes through keeping a daily journal; it is outlandish to set a goal of never having another craving to smoke.) The person, all significant others and the treatment team agree to and understand the goal. Also, the goal is not likely to negatively affect other important aspects of the person's health or psychosocial, interpersonal or intrapersonal functioning. Remember with whom you are formulating this contract—for example, you will not be asking a lifelong introvert to engage in sensitive self-disclosure in an intense psychotherapy group.

An obtainable goal could be for a person to develop better social skills. The combination of social skills training with CBT or DBT appears to be powerful. Social skills training is discussed in Chapter 23.

Negotiating a behavioural contract The basic rules for negotiating a behavioural contract include engaging the person and their family as colleagues, avoiding complex terminology or coercive formats, and making sure everyone completely understands, agrees to and, to the extent possible, feels comfortable with the contract. Your Intervention Strategies summarises the behavioural contracting process.

Potential problems can have a minimal impact if they are detected early in the process. If you anticipate and address them, people do not have to experience failure simply because the contract was poorly designed. Possible problems include a lack of understanding, a lack of commitment, a lack of adequate follow-up monitoring, and a lack of a defined format or contingency plan for unforeseen

YOUR INTERVENTION STRATEGIES Developing a behavioural contract

Step	Purpose	Action	Strategy
1	Comprehensive behavioural assessment	Interviewing	Collecting data on which the contract will be based
2	Formulating practical and measurable objectives and goals	Prioritising	Evaluating abilities
3	Negotiating a behavioural contract	Setting basic rules Identifying potential problems	Making adjustments Evaluating the relevance and usefulness of the behavioural contract
4	Optimising the person's ability to adhere to a behavioural contract	Determining barriers: ▪ intellectual ▪ emotional ▪ motivational ▪ physiological	Including constructive catalysts: ▪ psychotherapy ▪ relaxation training ▪ biofeedback ▪ family involvement

problems. A contract is poorly designed when it is in conflict with important and unchangeable aspects of the person's psychosocial functioning.

Continuing assessment, regular evaluations and trouble-shooting meetings will determine whether adjustments to the contract are necessary. Designing a contract which a person feels comfortable to follow will maximise the chance of success. Contracts can be adjusted in many ways, including providing formal supports, prioritisation of various objectives and appropriate revisions of goals. Creativity is an essential component in negotiating an effective behavioural contract.

Data on how well the person adheres to the contract can be collected through self-monitoring, self-reports at regular meetings, discussions in counselling sessions, and natural or scheduled observations. Further information can be collected from relatives, friends, colleagues and other treatment providers.

Careful determination and assessment of any potential barriers will help achieve success with behavioural contracting. Check for overall intellectual functioning as well as cognitive style (Hufford, Williams, Malec & Cravotta, 2012). Emotional perspectives can influence performance and outcome. Does the person manifest depression, irritability or anxiety that would interfere with contract adherence? It is important to design supports that will address these problems and promote success (Stice, Rohde, Gau & Ochner, 2011). Motivation can also play a large part in outcome. Did the person lack some motivation to begin with? What was done to address this problem? If design features to address motivation were implemented, check to see how they are working. Is there a decline in motivation? If so, why (psychiatric, social, economic or medical causation)? Address all underlying causative factors.

Physiology can affect outcome. Are medication side-effects a problem, or is the main effect of a medication (such as mood stabilisation for symptoms of mania) bothering the person? If this behavioural change is perceived as threatening to an established lifestyle and interaction pattern, or if the person becomes uncomfortable with the independence or responsibilities expected of them following the behavioural change, this could also sabotage adherence.

Provide constructive catalysts—those tools that will enhance the process without interference. Some psychotherapeutic interventions are useful with most clients undergoing stress. These include general stress management, preparing for the likely emotional consequences and adjustment difficulties that changes in health behaviours can cause, providing the opportunity to ventilate and disclose feelings, and setting up support services. More specialised treatment and techniques include relaxation training and biofeedback. Family involvement is a powerful and useful catalyst for promoting and maintaining behavioural change. Significant others, particularly those with whom the person resides or will reside, are likely to provide important input about the level of contract adherence. It is therefore important to involve them as much as appropriate in formulating and implementing the behavioural contract. If the details of the contract do not work for the involved family, they will not work for anyone.

Figure 25.2 ■ is a sample behavioural contract format and gives an overview of how the process of combining medications and behavioural change can be documented. Sections may be expanded or eliminated depending on the targeted behaviour and individual needs. Imagine a health behaviour of your own that you could change (such as doing more exercise or reducing sugar consumption), and walk yourself through this contract. If you can develop a plan to change your behaviour, you may very well be successful in helping others to change theirs.

In general, outcomes for behavioural change are easily identified. Behaviours are objective criteria by which progress can be tracked. They can be compared to previous behaviours for similarities or differences. If problematic behaviours occur less frequently, they may be considered to have a positive outcome. The following Practice Example illustrates positive outcomes with a person experiencing anxiety.

LIVED EXPERIENCE

Behavioural activation

I used to have trouble knowing how to keep my unit tidy. It would all just seem overwhelming and too hard, and I wouldn't do anything. I'd sit there and watch the dishes pile up. My nurse from the community mental health service worked with me to plan out some clear steps to manage my anxiety. Now I start with a set routine and keep on top of the dishes and mess in my kitchen.

Practice example

Kim, a 29-year-old man with a diagnosis of obsessive–compulsive disorder, worried obsessively that electrical appliances would cause fires. Kim's nurse taught him relaxation exercises and thought-stopping techniques to use when he found himself becoming anxious. The expected outcomes in Kim's situation are: he uses coping strategies to reduce anxiety, and reports decreased physical manifestations of anxiety. With practice, Kim found that within one week he was less anxious when in the kitchen or near other electrical appliances. Although his thoughts about appliance fires and his anxiety had not completely abated, they were definitely more manageable.

Behaviour modification

Behaviour modification frequently focuses on a target behaviour that is problematic for the individual (e.g., over-eating) or for the community (e.g., loud verbal outbursts). The behaviour is observed and tracked in objective and measurable terms, then addressed with a behaviour modification plan.

Sample behavioural contract

Client name ______________________________ Date ____________

Problem behaviour: ______________________________

Problem behaviour components

Behavioural	Affective
Cognitive	Physiological

Interview findings

Depression	Anxiety	Substance or alcohol use/abuse
Irritability	Psychotic symptomatology	Addictive/compulsive behaviour

Psychosocial variables

Present employment	Social/romantic functioning	Typical daily routines
Marital/family status	Avocational pursuits	Eating/sleeping/exercise habits
The client's expectations of how this behaviour change might alter any of the above		

Collateral information ______________________________

Cognitive style ______________________________

Which of the following apply for this contract?

- ☐ Psychotherapy for any current psychological problems
- ☐ Relaxation training/biofeedback
- ☐ General stress management
- ☐ Preparation for likely emotional consequences and adjustment difficulties
- ☐ The opportunity to ventilate and disclose feelings
- ☐ Support

Contract objectives and goals

This goal is agreed upon and understood by the client, all significant others, and the treatment team.

Signature ______________________________

Signature ______________________________

Signature ______________________________

Signature ______________________________

FIGURE 25.2 ■ Sample behavioural contract.

Both nonpharmacological and pharmacological interventions may be used to assist in the modification of behavioural disturbances. Nonpharmacological behavioural modification interventions are discussed here.

A behaviour modification program begins with the identification of a specific behaviour that requires change. It is important to monitor the target behaviour and develop a detailed database about it. The problem behaviour is carefully observed for the following:

- antecedents (what came before)
- precipitants (what appeared to cause or provoke the behaviour)
- how the behaviour is expressed
- timing
- frequency
- duration
- personal strengths to be capitalised on in designing the plan.

To enable a person to modify behaviour that is undesirable or unhealthy, giving support and involving that person in the plan of action are required (Kim, Park & Park, 2014; Morgan, Cousins, Middleton, Warriner-Gallyer & Ridsdale, 2016). One strategy organises the person's problem behaviour into a hierarchy. In this hierarchy, the least distressing changes are at the lowest level, and the most distressing are at the highest. For example, scores are assigned to levels of distress, ranging from zero, or none, to 100, the highest level of difficulty the person can imagine. Someone who overeats may feel only slight distress, or a score of 15, when thinking about not eating at a movie or a sporting event. A much higher distress level, with a score of 85, might occur when the same person considers being in an unfamiliar or uncomfortable social environment and not being able to eat.

Response prevention

Guiding an individual through imagining a situation at the lowest level of distress initially, and developing and rehearsing adaptive responses to the distress, establishes a new pattern that supplants the older, unhelpful response. This is called **response prevention**, meaning the automatic responses that have not been helpful are modified and replaced with more helpful or adaptive behaviours. Gradually, the person advances through their hierarchy of distress, learning to develop skills in responding competently at every step.

Systematic desensitisation

Systematic desensitisation, another behavioural modification treatment strategy, also uses a hierarchy to arrange treatment. Behaviours are identified and ordered according to the level of distress experienced by the person. The person then imagines being in certain situations at various levels of distress and learns to cope before moving on to the next level of distress. Deep breathing and relaxation are activities that are often used to help the person to manage the anxiety that is inevitably aroused as they work through the hierarchy. Your Intervention Strategies, above, provides a desensitisation hierarchy for a phobic fear of heights.

> **YOUR INTERVENTION STRATEGIES**
> **Desensitisation hierarchy for a phobic fear of heights**
>
> 1. Develop 10 to 12 scenes of increasing levels of fear.
>   *Example:* Ask the person to imagine the scene with the lowest level of fear:
>   'You are going up a kitchen stepladder. Step to the third rung, and look around.'
>   'Now you are going up to the top rung. You are at the top. Look around at the cupboards. Look at the floor.'
>   'Now you are on the second floor of an office building. Walk toward the window and look out.'
> 2. Continue in this manner, increasing the level of fear attached to the scene each time the person is able to visualise without undue anxiety:
>   'Now you go to the top of the Sydney Tower. Go over to the guardrail and look straight down.'
> 3. The final steps of the desensitisation process include encouraging the person to try some of these behaviours in real life, after successfully coping with the imagined scenes.

Assignments for graded exposures and response prevention are usually completed as homework, accompanied by self-monitoring (through diaries and/or graphs) and clinical assessment of progress through behavioural programming. The behaviour modification plan requires a realistic appraisal of the difficulties facing the person who wants to make a change, and includes a plan for handling those difficulties. Even someone with significant symptoms can make changes in this manner (Horan et al., 2011). A sample plan for someone who wants to quit smoking, for example, must include the following three steps:

1. understanding the mechanisms that trigger the urge to smoke
2. substituting other activities for the habit of smoking
3. recognising supports that will promote success in unlearning the rituals of smoking behaviour.

For a person trying to quit smoking, the environment should be smoke-free, and all smoking materials and accoutrements disposed of, in order to minimise relapses. Psychopharmacological supports are available to help with smoking cessation. The following Your Intervention Strategies lists behaviour modification tips for smoking cessation.

Rational emotive behavioural therapy

Rational emotive therapy (RET) was developed by Albert Ellis in 1975, and emphasises the cognitive causes of emotional problems, along with the importance of taking personal responsibility for maintaining health-damaging thought habits and irrational beliefs (Ellis, 2011). An irrational belief is a belief that lacks reason and sound judgment. Box 25.2 provides a list of some common irrational thoughts

YOUR INTERVENTION STRATEGIES

Smoking cessation behaviour modification guidance

Use the guidelines below to help a smoker quit:

- Set up a timeline of the typical smoking schedule.
- Develop a tracking mechanism for where the individual smokes (couch, corner bar, car).
- Use checklists for situations and interactions with others in which smoking is involved.
- Suggest a set of behaviours to substitute for smoking (e.g. replace the cigarette with a pen or go for a walk).
- Provide self-help literature.
- Encourage those in the environment to also quit smoking.
- Provide motivational material related to the person's current health status.
- Identify stressors.
- Enhance skills for coping with stressors.
- Emphasise the positive benefits of smoking cessation.
- Provide individual support.
- Reinforce short-term success.
- Provide support through group therapy.

that, when incorporated into an individual's belief system, are known to create unhealthy thoughts and feelings. The clinician who is skilled in RET helps identify irrational thought structures with the person seeking change, and then helps develop a plan to substitute more rational personal life philosophies and attitudes based on accurately perceived realities (Hyland & Boduszek, 2012). Healthy emotional consequences occur when rational thinking drives adequate functional behaviours.

Rational emotive behaviour therapy (REBT), as it is now known, identifies and corrects irrational beliefs. Rational and irrational beliefs, defined by REBT, form the basis of inferences (conclusions based on reasoning) derived to explain life experiences. Those inferences can be more or less functional, depending on the beliefs behind them. People who hold rational beliefs form inferences that are significantly more functional than those formed by people who hold irrational beliefs. The following Practice Example illustrates how firmly-held irrational beliefs can inhibit functioning.

The Socratic question-and-answer format is an important aspect of REBT. This method, illustrated in Box 25.3, allows the person to explore how a particular line of reasoning was allowed to develop and how it continues to function. It focuses on a logical perspective, which is an appealing and manageable therapeutic style to which many adults can relate. As with all therapeutic styles, however, there must be a fit between the person and the therapeutic intervention. Not all therapies will be useful, or even therapeutic, with everyone in all situations.

Box 25.2 Irrational thoughts

Rational therapy holds that certain core irrational ideas, which have been clinically observed, are at the root of most mental health disturbances. They are as follows:

- The idea that it is a dire necessity for adults to be loved by significant others for almost everything they do—*instead of their concentrating on their own self-respect, on winning approval for practical purposes, and on loving rather than on being loved.*
- The idea that certain acts are awful or wicked, and that people who perform such acts should be severely damned—*instead of the idea that certain acts are self-defeating or antisocial, and that people who perform such acts are behaving stupidly, ignorantly or neurotically, and would be better helped to change. People's poor behaviours do not make them rotten individuals.*
- The idea that it is horrible when things are not the way we like them to be—*instead of the idea that it is too bad, that we would be better to try to change or control bad conditions so that they become more satisfactory, and, if that is not possible, we had better temporarily accept and gracefully lump their existence.*
- The idea that human misery is invariably externally caused and is forced on us by outside people and events—*instead of the idea that misery is largely caused by the view that we take of unfortunate conditions.*
- The idea that if something is or may be dangerous or fearsome, we should be terribly upset and endlessly obsess about it—*instead of the idea that one would better frankly face it and render it non-dangerous or, when that is not possible, accept the inevitable.*
- The idea that it is easier to avoid than to face life difficulties and self-responsibilities—*instead of the idea that the so-called easy way is usually much harder in the long run.*
- The idea that we absolutely need something other or stronger or greater than ourselves on which to rely—*instead of the idea that it is better to take the risks of thinking and acting less dependently.*
- The idea that we should be thoroughly competent, intelligent and achieving in all possible respects—*instead of the idea that it would be better for us to simply do, rather than always need to do well, and accept ourselves as a quite imperfect creature, who has general human limitations and specific fallibilities.*
- The idea that because something once strongly affected our life, it should indefinitely affect it—*instead of the idea that we can learn from our past experiences, but not be overly attached to or prejudiced by them.*
- The idea that we must have certain and perfect control over things—*instead of the idea that the world is full of probability and chance, and that we can still enjoy life despite this.*
- The idea that human happiness can be achieved by inertia and inaction—*instead of the idea that we tend to be happiest when we are vitally absorbed in creative pursuits, or when we are devoting ourselves to people or projects outside ourselves.*
- The idea that we have virtually no control over our emotions, and that we cannot help feeling disturbed about things—*instead of the idea that we have real control over our destructive emotions if we choose to work at changing the belief that all of our needs and expectations must be met.*

Adapted from: Ellis, A. (2011). The essence of rational emotive behaviour therapy: A comprehensive approach to treatment. Retrieved from http://www.rebt.ws/albert_ellis_the_essence_of_rebt.htm

Practice example

Matt, a 38-year-old forklift operator, was injured on the job four years ago. His back injuries were treated, and all tests indicate a complete recovery; however, his ability to function at work is impaired, and he continues to complain of back pain. Matt has been referred to a specialist in psychotherapy for chronic pain.

In an REBT session, he describes an early experience of observing his father's lengthy struggle with cancer, during which his father was largely sedentary and his mother reacted hysterically whenever his father tried to be more active. In therapy it emerged that Matt had acquired an irrational core belief that problems or fears are best handled with rest, withdrawal and being sedentary. Matt's past pain symptoms were uncomfortable enough to trigger this response, consistent with his core belief. As he became more sedentary and less functional, his back became increasingly weak and prone to pain. The greater the pain, the less active he became, until he was caught in a vicious cycle of increasing pain and withdrawal.

REBT helped Matt learn to identify his irrational belief. This was accomplished through a Socratic question-and-answer format, so Matt recognised that withdrawal and inactivity led to more rather than fewer problems. The sources for Matt's irrational belief were clarified as well. The belief was reframed in a more rational direction—that many problems respond best to constructive and productive activity. Specifically, Matt's chronic pain was likely to improve with exercise, physical therapy and daily productive activity. Assignments were given between sessions to help Matt develop his repertoire in these areas. As he successfully proceeded to do so, his pain symptoms diminished and his self-esteem increased.

Box 25.3 The Socratic question-and-answer format

Matt:	'I spent the day in bed yesterday because my back hurt.'
Therapist:	'What did you hope that would accomplish?'
Matt:	'That my back would feel better.'
Therapist:	'Did it?'
Matt:	'No.'
Therapist:	'Can you ever remember a time when inactivity made your back feel better?'
Matt:	'No, it just gets worse.'
Therapist:	'So where and how did you come to believe that inactivity would make your back feel better?'
Matt:	'In my family we always rested when we were hurt.'
Therapist:	'Did that help your family?'
Matt:	'Come to think of it, not that I ever saw.'
Therapist:	'Maybe too much resting doesn't help?'
Matt:	'I never thought of it that way.'
Therapist:	'If too much resting doesn't help, what else might?'
Matt:	'Once when my back hurt, I went to a chiropractor and did some exercises. I remember that helped.'
Therapist:	'What does that tell you about resting too much?'
Matt:	'Maybe it's not such a good idea.'

COGNITIVE THERAPY

We know that our thoughts (cognitions) affect our feelings. **Cognitive therapy** is based on making cognitive changes, which, in turn, alters feelings. This is particularly useful for people who experience emotional problems, who are 'often trapped by a particularly negative or unhelpful way of looking at their situation and can only see this way of interpreting it' (Salkovskis, 1996, p. 49). Consider the routine and habitual thinking of most depressed persons: 'I'm no good at anything. I'm a failure in life.' With enough repetition, the depressed person comes to accept this particular self-evaluation as accurate.

The goal in cognitive therapy is to alter these thoughts to: 'There are things that I can do well, and there are things that I need to work on.' This type of thinking is more realistic and avoids adhering to an unhealthy perspective. Over time, a change in thinking allows the depressed person to replace disturbing and negative thoughts with neutral and positive thoughts; a cognitive change can influence an emotional change for the better. It will change the way they interpret situations (feelings/emotions), and lead to changes in behaviour. This process is the basis for cognitive therapy (Skinner, 1974, 1989). Aaron Beck's ideas have underpinned our understanding of cognitive therapy processes for several decades (Beck, 1995). Likewise, Albert Ellis's ABC model (Ellis & Harper, 1975) has helped to explain how and why the way we think affects the way we feel and behave. In this model, an activating event (A), followed by a particular belief or reaction to the event (B), is followed by emotional consequences (C).

Basic concepts

Three basic concepts are central to an understanding of cognitive therapy—attributions, modelling and self-efficacy.

Attributions

As humans, we constantly ascribe causes to the events in our lives. By labelling or assigning meaning to a circumstance or a set of circumstances, we make *attributions* ('I only got a grade of C. I'm no good at anything. Sarah and James got As. They can do anything'). Think of attributions as perceived causes that may or may not be objectively accurate. Depressed people often attribute failure to themselves and success to others; that is, they internalise responsibility for negative events rather than seeing them as having a range of potential causes beyond themselves. Then they attribute associated features or characteristics to that circumstance or set of circumstances (such as being a poor student or not knowing the material). Next, they expect a certain outcome from that circumstance, and they behave consistently with the expectation that they will not succeed. Finally, they have feelings that match, or are congruent with, the experience. The basic idea is that thoughts and behaviours lead to feelings. The concern is that this pattern can create a cycle that becomes self-fulfilling, which then maintains the person's depressed mood and hampers their recovery efforts and the efforts of those attempting to support them.

Modelling

Modelling involves imitating another (or others) in the expectation that one will receive rewards such as the rewards other people seem to be receiving. See Figure 25.3 ■ for an example of how people learn through modelling the behaviours of others. You have likely experienced modelling throughout your education, especially once you selected nursing as your career. You have doubtless observed nurses who are competent and effective, and you strive for that level of skill in order to receive the same rewards.

Self-efficacy

Human learning also occurs through self-efficacy. Self-efficacy involves believing that one's own actions are effective. People learn and adapt when they find themselves in circumstances demanding new or different skills. Under those circumstances, people who tend to believe that they can cope successfully with life and problems in living through acquiring skills, practising them, and observing successful outcomes will gain confidence and a sense of self-efficacy.

Over time, consistently making attributions, modelling behaviour and experiencing self-efficacy set a pattern of thinking in place. The pattern explains events while shaping expectations about interactions and other behaviours. The patterns can be shaped in adaptive or maladaptive ways, depending on the circumstances and the multiple variables that come into play. Unrealistic thought patterns are maladaptive, in that they make demands on the individual that cannot be met or cannot be resolved. For example, a 70-year-old woman who was adopted as a child may have believed for decades she has no worth because her birth mother gave her away. In her case, it is unrealistic to assume that the reason her mother gave her up for adoption was a malevolent one, and, because her birth mother is not likely to be found or identified in order to explain the circumstances of the adoption, this negative perception will continue to have negative impacts on her life.

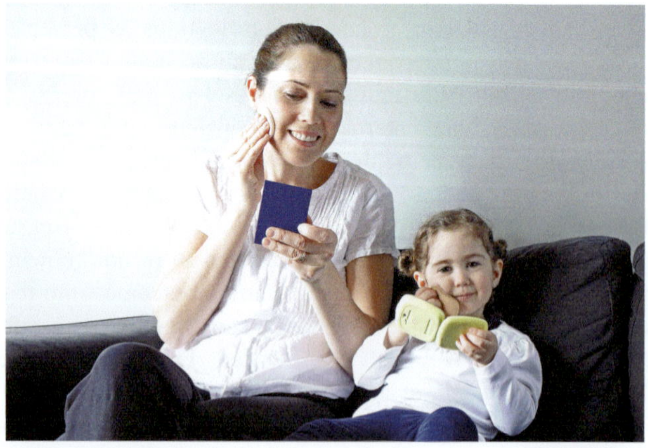

FIGURE 25.3 ■ Modelling. Imitative learning is a form of complex learning.
Photo courtesy of Elizabeth Crews Photography.

Cognitive therapy techniques

The purpose of cognitive therapy is first to identify thoughts that are unrealistic, negative or otherwise problematic. Once these thoughts are identified, they are examined for their impact on the individual. Nurses are instrumental in helping a person see how a particular set of thoughts can create a problem. When this connection is made, substituting neutral or positive thoughts for problematic thinking takes place over time. Correcting automatic problematic thinking is a retraining experience. The individual must unlearn their maladaptive cognitive style, and then learn adaptive cognitions (Hertenstein, Johann, Baglioni, Spiegelhalder & Reimann, 2016). The following Practice Example describes why cognitive changes are important to mental health.

Practice example

George is a 45-year-old man being treated for schizophrenia. His symptoms are coming under reasonable control with medications and therapy; however, he has been having difficulty lately with his mother. Whenever she cannot visit him at his home, he becomes depressed and agitated. The outpatient clinic nurse spoke with him about his current problems, and together they identified an irrational thought George has about his mother. He believes that if she doesn't visit him every seven days, regardless of whether she has to work overtime, that means she does not love him. George thought he would never be able to be 'a man' without his mother's love.

Once George identified his irrational conclusions about the meaning of her visits, he was able to talk to her about his feelings for her. George had to concentrate and work to replace his automatic and irrational thoughts with more realistic ones; his mother's love does not need to be renewed—it is always there. George came to recognise that the visiting schedule and their interpersonal relationship were not connected. He prepared a number of neutral and positive statements that he could repeat to himself whenever the old irrational thoughts appeared. Eventually, George was able to tolerate changes in the frequency of his mother's visits.

Positive imagery

Positive imagery consists of thinking in a positive way about how an event or experience will unfold, rather than anticipating disastrous results. This tends to promote the likelihood of a positive outcome.

Positive imagery can also be applied to past events. It is a reframing of actions taken. For example, a woman is attacked at her parked car and blames herself for being weak, unprepared and frightened. Positive imagery reframes the woman's actions as perfectly understandable under the circumstances, and walks her through the events with this different perspective. It gives her permission to react to frightening events with fear.

When directed towards an upcoming event, positive imagery can be a cognitive rehearsal. That is, thinking positively in advance about how a set of behaviours or an event occurs helps the individual perform more competently in a variety of situations and with a wider array of skills.

Mastery imagery

Mastery imagery shapes the individual's thoughts about being in control or having mastery over a particular situation. The point of this technique is to practise imagined successful behaviour change. An example of mastery imagery is imagining interacting competently and in an adult manner with someone who abused you in childhood. In the Practice Example that follows, Christine is achieving mastery over her work situation.

Practice example

Christine imagines and rehearses interacting with her usually demanding, critical and agitated supervisor. In the past, she would typically respond haphazardly and with agitation, which resulted in making errors and feeling ineffective. Christine's mastery imagery establishes a new routine that consists of interacting with her supervisor in a consistently calm and organised manner.

Negative imagery

Another useful cognitive therapy tool to help change unhelpful behaviours is *negative imagery*, or envisioning negative events and outcomes for those unhelpful behaviours. Envisioning the negative outcome of unhelpful behaviour can serve as a powerful educator. The scenario is played out in the person's thoughts, and can assist in predicting what is likely to happen unless changes are made.

It is possible to teach someone to identify the imagery invoked (the thoughts) when beginning an unhelpful behaviour, such as substance use. It may be something like: 'My favourite drug will be fun' or 'I am so much more relaxed and able to interact better when I use this stuff.' This is positive imagery. In this case, positive imagery promotes use of the substance even though that behaviour will interfere with and damage important relationships with others. The real impact of the behaviour is understood only when denial is dispensed with and consequences are recognised. Then substituting with negative imagery can begin.

For example, if a person uses alcohol, the positive imagery may be that it will make them feel good. Negatively envisioning alcohol use would consist of the person learning to say and think, 'If I drink alcohol, I will lose control of my thoughts and feelings. It will cost a lot of money, which I don't have, and will put a bigger emotional and physical gap between me and my wife.' Replacing positive imagery with negative imagery may reduce the automatic positive associations over time and reduce the urge to use the drug.

Attribution restructuring

The heart of cognitive therapy lies in recognising how we think and behave, and in identifying problematic learning. Learning involves schemas which comprise our beliefs and theories about other people, oneself and the world in general (Blackburn & Davidson, 1990, p. 26). These schemas serve as filters for ongoing experience and allow us to come to conclusions about events automatically. People develop patterns of thinking over time, often automatically, without active or conscious effort. Automatic thoughts can develop into specific (and frequently solidly crystallised) sets of automatic thinking. For example, a person who takes the same mental steps over and over comes to the same problematic conclusion. It is important to realise that unhelpful automatic thoughts and attributions require detection prior to intervention. That is, you can't make change unless you first recognise your negative automatic thoughts.

If a person has had a number of depressive episodes, the resulting *cognitive map* or *schema* (thinking in a particular path) must be factored into treatment. Each depressive episode generates negative cognitive maps that are likely to be reactivated the next time the person experiences even a mild dysphoric state, so that current experiences are interpreted more negatively. Each successive negative experience breeds another.

Attribution restructuring or retraining involves abandoning intuitive strategies in order to change the meanings associated with people, places and things. Once unhelpful cognitions (thoughts) are detected, evidence-based cognitive interventions can help to alter and restructure thinking. Schema-focused therapy, which was developed by Dr Jeff Young (Young, Klosko & Weishaar, 2006), who originally worked closely with Dr Aaron Beck, is one type of cognitive therapy used more recently, particularly with people who have experienced abuse or people with personality disorder (David & Freeman, 2015).

COGNITIVE BEHAVIOURAL THERAPY

The goal in **cognitive behavioural treatment** (CBT) is to develop healthier thinking that leads to more desirable feelings and a greater feeling of self-efficacy. CBT approaches examine underlying beliefs about illness, treatment and recovery. They aim to promote recovery, reduce distressing symptoms, help the person manage or prevent illness relapse and help the person improve their overall functioning. CBT is important because, in spite of advances in medication management of emotional problems, a considerable number of people with diagnosed mental health concerns experience persistent symptoms that they must learn to manage in order to improve their quality of life. Many people also experience unpleasant side-effects from medication, so adherence can be difficult.

Beck (1976; Beck & Freeman, 1990) indicates that behavioural problems arise in childhood when people learn core beliefs and make associations between what they believe and what they expect to happen. Beck's theories are accessible at the website for the Beck Institute for Cognitive Therapy and Research (http://www.beckinstitute.org/).

Building on what we learn in childhood, our labels and expectations influence the strategies we select to compensate and cope. Jeremy copes with the following situation according to the particular pattern that he has developed over time.

Practice example

Jeremy is a marketing consultant who must drive long distances to meet with his clients. One day, during a meeting with a client, he experienced a panic attack. His symptoms included shortness of breath, rapid heartbeat and thoughts of wanting to escape the situation. Afterward he was very tired. He decided to leave work early and drive home. When he got home he felt more relaxed and relieved. He hoped the panic attack was an isolated event that would not happen again.

However, Jeremy had more panic attacks. He longed to be at home when they occurred, because he experienced relief and greater comfort there. He soon began to cut back on face-to-face client meetings and conducted meetings online or by telephone instead. The more he stayed at home, the more anxious he became when he needed to leave. Eventually he became almost completely unable to leave home, whether for business, social or any other purpose (such as an emergency with a friend). The mere thought of stepping outside the house precipitated a panic attack. Jeremy had developed diagnosable panic disorder with agoraphobia.

Cognitive and behavioural treatment consists of identifying and recognising unhelpful thinking styles, and working towards the acquisition of new skills for managing stressors. Features of treatment include teaching, interpreting, reframing, and learning and practising new behaviours, and are extremely beneficial for people with mild to moderate depression and anxiety, and post-traumatic stress disorder (Cohen, Mannarino & Iyengar, 2011; Goodkind et al., 2016; Høifødet, Strøm, Kolstrup, Eisemann & Waterloo, 2011). Significant improvements have also been found in the treatment of suicidal behaviours (Mewton & Andrews, 2016) and binge eating (McIntosh et al., 2016). Once thoughts and behaviours are realistically and rationally framed and implemented, emotional reactions will be consistent with them. That is, once we are able to change our thinking so that we can live our lives according to our hopes and values, we will feel better about our place in the world.

See Evidence-based Practice for a description of how these treatment strategies are incorporated into a group setting for the treatment of panic disorder.

The cognitive behavioural approach is important in the contemporary treatment of substance dependence. There is sufficient research evidence supporting both drug-free outpatient treatment programs and treatment methods involving medications such as naltrexone (Revia) and buprenorphine (Subutex). These programs, combined with psychosocial treatment or behavioural techniques, provide additional promise for outpatient-based drug abuse treatment. CBT can be used to teach new coping skills to people with substance problems as long as the interventions are tailored to the individual's cognitive functioning (Kiluk, Nich & Carroll, 2011).

People who have psychotic symptoms also benefit from CBT (Thomas, Rossell, Farhall, Shawyer & Castle, 2011). The presence of auditory hallucinations or a lack of insight into illness does not interfere with CBT, nor does it interfere with the reduction of negative symptoms of schizophrenia

EVIDENCE-BASED PRACTICE

Treating panic attacks

Adam, aged 45 years, experienced panic attacks for six years. He tried to control the attacks on his own, but after two years finally went for treatment. Adam took medications with only moderate success for four years, and was ready to try something different to address his problem. He agreed to participate in your cognitive behavioural therapy group in an outpatient clinic.

It was noted by Adam's general practitioner and reported to you that Adam had a number of automatic responses to his panic attacks. He would think and feel a particular way whenever he became anxious, was exposed to a stressor, or had a panic attack. His defence mechanism was usually avoidance, which meant that his life had become very contained.

Over four months, Adam and several other individuals attended 12 group sessions based on a cognitive behavioural curriculum. Muscle relaxation, diaphragmatic breathing skills, cognitive restructuring, and homework assignments formed the cognitive behavioural aspects of the therapy. There was also a component to the group where the therapist guided participants through exposure to each person's problematic trigger. At the end of the treatment period, Adam was able to respond to stressors in a more mature, satisfactory manner. His panic attacks and other symptoms were also reduced. Even one year after the group concluded, Adam was still benefiting from the cognitive behavioural therapy he received.

Base your actions on more than one study, but these interventions were developed using cognitive behavioural principles in conjunction with the following research:

Gloster, A. T., Wittchen, H. U., Einsle, F., Lang, T., Helbig-Lang, E., Fydrich, T., . . . Arolt, V. (2011). Psychological treatment for panic disorder with agoraphobia: A randomised controlled trial to examine the role of therapist-guided exposure in situ in CBT. *Journal of Consulting and Clinical Psychology, 79*(3), 406–420.

CRITICAL THINKING QUESTIONS

1. What elements would you take into consideration when planning to introduce behavioural change?
2. How can Adam and his family benefit from psychoeducation?
3. What exercises and rehearsals would be considered priorities for Adam?

(see Chapter 14). Early intervention with CBT when someone first begins having psychotic symptoms has also been supported in the literature (Gaynor, Dooley, Lawlor, Lawoyin & O'Callaghan, 2011; Stafford, Jackson, Mayo-Wilson, Morrison & Kendall, 2013).

Thought stopping

Thought stopping is an example of a cognitive behavioural psychotherapeutic technique that can help someone change thinking processes. Changing the thinking process is important, because feelings can be strongly influenced by the pattern and process of thoughts. We all sometimes have difficulty with repetitive, maladaptive thinking. For example, one person might worry incessantly about things she cannot control; another repeatedly has inaccurate, negative thoughts about himself. For these individuals, the cognitive behavioural therapist might implement the procedure known as *thought stopping*. We can learn to stop negative or maladaptive thinking by visualising or imagining a specific image, sensation or circumstance. Examples of thought stopping include the following:

- visualising a traffic stop sign
- imagining hearing the word 'stop' said loudly
- imagining the tactile sensation of leaning against a closed door
- visualising pushing the problematic thoughts out of one's room.

Thought stopping is done whenever the identified negative or maladaptive thought occurs. Over time, the individual learns to stop such thoughts in an almost reflexive manner. This technique is typically used as part of a larger set of techniques that might also include developing alternative thoughts and mastering behavioural skills to alter outcomes in various problematic circumstances.

> **LIVED EXPERIENCE**
>
> **I can challenge my voices**
>
> I have lots of stress at the moment. My mum has been unwell and needs to go into hospital for an operation. My mental health worker has been helping me manage my symptoms, especially the voices that tell me to harm myself. We sat down and wrote what I heard the voices say (take a knife and cut my arms), how I feel and what I do at the time (feel scared and start pacing around the house), and what I am thinking at the time (I am being punished; I have no control over what the voice says). We have been practising telling the voices to just STOP, and I've been learning to recognise that I am just worried for my mum, too.

Techniques used in CBT such as thought stopping are defined and explained on the website of the Australian Association for Cognitive and Behavioural Therapists (http://www.aacbt.org/viewStory/WHAT+IS+CBT%3F).

CARE COORDINATION, COMMUNITY-BASED CARE AND HOME CARE

In addition to family members and friends who might be present in a person's everyday environment, you also need to consider other service providers who are part of the person's support network in the community. As part of your CBT work with a person, it is important to focus on maintaining the routines and schedules of cognitive behavioural interventions once a plan of care has been established. Homework assignments and practising more competent responses will ensure that the person retains the skills developed in therapy. The care coordinator (historically referred to as a 'case manager') can be helpful in sustaining that structure. The variety of interventions, such as group or individual therapy, behavioural activation, goal-setting and achievement, graded exposure, and self-study, can all be promoted and supported through care coordination. You may be the provider of CBT or you may be the care coordinator providing ongoing support, for which it will be important to have good communication with the person and the CBT therapist in order to support the goals of therapy and the gains made during therapy.

Each of the problems addressed with cognitive behavioural interventions benefits from maintaining those interventions in the person's natural setting. Counselling, psychotherapy and other treatments discussed in this chapter are frequently conducted in the community. The behavioural contract can be designed to address inpatient issues and community living, and to enhance the transition from inpatient treatment to an outpatient setting. This is also the case where an intensive period of formal therapy occurs in the community, in the context of specialist referral and ongoing community care and comprehensive care planning that involves a range of support providers. Additional supports can be built into the contract to ensure a person's success after the transition. These interventions in the community maximise both quality of life and management of symptoms.

ACCEPTANCE AND COMMITMENT THERAPY (ACT)

Acceptance and commitment therapy, or ACT (pronounced as the word 'act' and not as initials), is a therapeutic technique created in 1986 by Steve Hayes. ACT developed out of cognitive behavioural therapy but has a specific focus on mindfulness, the Eastern practice of focusing on the present. ACT is based in six core principles or domains, with therapeutic activities designed to improve psychological flexibility through activities directed at each of these domains. The domains are: cognitive defusion, acceptance, contact with the present moment, the observing self, values, and committed action (Harris, 2006). The first four of these are mindfulness skills designed to increase awareness

COLLABORATIVE CARE

Promoting the effectiveness of CBT with families of people with schizophrenia

An important adjunct to your work with people and the success of CBT may be how you and the person with whom you are working enlist the support of their family. Families can be important in promoting the effectiveness of CBT, because they are often more constant in the person's life than health care providers. They can support the person's motivation and problem-solving efforts, and are a source of encouragement to the person to engage with services and to persist with treatments. Involving families can also help family members to understand symptoms and minimise their own stress responses to the person's symptoms or behaviours; this in turn can help the person in their recovery. Family psychoeducation can be an integral feature of community-based care and home care. Teaching about symptoms and how to address them with the planned interventions is supportive and reassuring. Involving significant others increases the likelihood that the plan of care is implemented, and that frustrations and misunderstandings are minimised.

This list can give you some quick pointers about the best ways families can promote the effectiveness of cognitive behavioural therapy (CBT) with people who have schizophrenia.

- Explain how what we think (cognition) and what we do (behaviour) form the basis of CBT.
- Explain the difference between a thought and a feeling.
- During family contacts with someone who has schizophrenia:
- Talk about thoughts and behaviours with the person with schizophrenia.
- Describe practical issues.
- Use words that do not create emotional responses (neutral words such as 'unusual' instead of 'odd', 'unexpected' instead of 'frightening').
- Reinforce functional behaviour.
- Recognise that some behaviour may be the result of misread or misinterpreted social cues.

Talking about thoughts and behaviours, instead of feelings, is not intended to lessen problematic behaviours, but may provide individuals and family members with a structure for conversations when the person is symptomatic.

of our thoughts and feelings, and the bodily sensations that accompany these, as well as being more conscious of the surrounding environment. Mindfulness involves really noticing the environment, using all of our senses. Acceptance, part of mindfulness, allows us to acknowledge our thoughts and feelings without judging them. Mindfulness allows us to tune into the present moment rather than being caught up in and struggling with the past, or worrying about the future.

Thoughts (cognitions) can overwhelm us, until they cause us to experience sensations that might be categorised as symptomatic of illnesses, like anxiety or depression or substance abuse/dependence. Learning how to acknowledge distressing thoughts as 'just thoughts' is central to ACT. However, the aim of ACT is not to eliminate symptoms, but to learn how to transform the way we interpret and respond to difficult and painful thoughts so that we can live our lives according to what is deeply important to us (i.e. our values). Therapeutic activities are directed at helping us to change the way we view our thoughts, so that those thoughts no longer hold the power over us that they have had in the past. While some therapeutic approaches provide a workbook approach to treatment, ACT uses 'an eclectic mix of metaphor, paradox, and mindfulness skills, along with a wide range of experiential exercises and values-guided behavioural interventions' (Harris, 2006, p. 2).

In ACT, what the person feels, thinks, remembers or experiences is not pinpointed as the problem to be changed. ACT views the behaviour as 'an opportunity to work on how powerful events in the here and now can become barriers to growth' (Hayes, 2004, p. 652). Human psychological problems are problems of psychological inflexibility due to cognitive fusion and experiential avoidance. Psychological flexibility has been defined by Hayes et al. (2006, p. 7) as 'the ability to contact the present moment more fully as a conscious human being, and to change or persist in behaviour when doing so serves valued ends'. It is clear from this definition that the combination of mindfulness processes with values-based committed action enables greater psychological flexibility enabling movement towards a life worth living.

ACT has been shown to be beneficial in the treatment of a wide range of conditions, including: chronic pain management (Baranoff, Hanrahan, Burke & Connor, 2015); binge eating disorder (Hill, Masyda, Melcher & Morgan, 2015); alcohol use disorder in people with co-occurring depression or bipolar disorder (Thekiso et al., 2015); smoking cessation (Kelly et al., 2015; Heffner, McClure, Mull, Anthenelli & Bricker, 2015); negative symptoms and depression in people following psychosis (White at al., 2011); and aggressive behaviour (Zarling, Lawrence & Marchman, 2015).

ACT has also been found to be applicable in the treatment of people with neurodevelopmental disorders (Leoni, Corti & Cavagnola, 2015), as well as being useful in supporting clinical psychology students through their study and practice supervision by working to enhance their self-care to moderate their stress (Pakenham, 2015). An Australian study (Pinto et al., 2015) found significant improvement in a range of psychological and behavioural dimensions for people with many different diagnoses attending a 10-week ACT group therapy program. They concluded that ACT encourages people to live their lives with meaning and purpose.

DIALECTICAL BEHAVIOUR THERAPY

Linehan and associates (1999) specifically developed *dialectical behaviour therapy* (DBT) for the outpatient treatment of people with borderline personality disorder who engaged in suicidal or self-harming behaviours. DBT is a specialised subset of the cognitive behavioural treatment modalities. The person with borderline personality disorder tends to be crisis-prone, with intense relational crisis episodes (Smoski et al., 2011). In other words, interactions with others have the potential to disrupt the person powerfully.

DBT is a biosocial behavioural model of treatment that assumes there is a disorder in how a person regulates emotions and tolerates stress (Grogan & Murphy, 2011). The numerous dysfunctional patterns of behaviour common in the diagnosis of borderline personality disorder (see Chapter 18), such as self-destructive behaviour, the inability to govern impulses, or severe dissociative phenomena, are regarded within the DBT framework as the person's attempts to problem-solve. DBT has also been used successfully in treating the adolescent who is at highest risk for suicidal behaviour and self-injury.

DBT is a psychosocial treatment program that focuses on teaching people the following four skills:

1. mindfulness (attention to one's experience)
2. interpersonal effectiveness
3. emotional regulation
4. distress tolerance.

Dialectical behaviour therapy focuses on the continuing balance between the necessity of accepting unhelpful and sometimes destructive behaviour patterns (a cognitive feature) in both an intrapsychic and interactional context, while still working to change them (the behavioural feature). This is the nature of dialectics; recognising that there is a simultaneous acknowledgment of the self as 'good enough', while also recognising the need to make some changes. DBT is a clearly structured therapy and integrates a wide choice of therapeutic strategies. It is a promising psychosocial intervention for improving interpersonal functioning among people with borderline personality disorder.

Cultural aspects of cognitive and behavioural interventions

Cultural considerations involve more than an individual's race or ethnicity. Culture is a concept that includes, among other characteristics, religion, spirituality, gender, sexual orientation and expression, social status and age. To be a competent provider of cognitive behavioural interventions, you must, at a minimum, understand these variables, be self-aware, and be comfortable working with those from a culture that differs from your own. The Self-awareness feature, below, will help sensitise you to the forces of a dominant culture. This is particularly important because, as a nurse, you provide care to diverse populations. This section will briefly describe how to implement this consciousness within a cognitive behavioural intervention framework.

The emphasis is on the individual in cognitive behavioural interventions (what the individual thinks, feels, interprets, assigns meanings to, etc.); therefore, it can be the ideal venue in which to address cultural diversity in treatment.

There is a further benefit to blending an understanding of cognitive and behavioural interventions and cultural diversity. The following Developing Cultural Competence indicates some of these.

LIVED EXPERIENCE

Developing understanding through DBT

I had always felt like the nurses and doctors didn't understand me until I started the DBT program. They seemed to think I was putting it on and I just needed to get a grip on myself. DBT is hard work and difficult sometimes, because I have to look at my behaviours and how they affect other people, but the therapist is always conscious of what I need and helps me to see the good parts of me, too. I get to learn how to manage my feelings; feelings that have been so uncomfortable to be with in the past. I have made a couple of good friends in the group. We understand each other.

SELF-AWARENESS

Influence of the dominant culture on cognitive behavioural interventions

What you think (cognition) and how you act (behaviour) are influenced by your culture. Being a member of the dominant cultural group shapes who you are. On the other hand, not being a member of the dominant cultural group also has the power to shape your identity. Determine whether there is a difference between you, the person for whom you are providing care, and the dominant culture on the major cultural characteristics in the following list. Be alert to the effect these differences will have on your cognitive behavioural interventions.

- religion
- spirituality
- gender
- ability/disability
- sexual orientation and expression
- social status
- age
- race
- ethnicity.

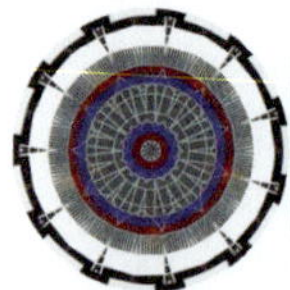

DEVELOPING CULTURAL COMPETENCE

Culture and cognitive behavioural interventions

Consider what it may be like to have someone discuss the following situation with you. Rachel is upset about being spoken to in a harsh and loud manner by her male supervisor at work. She feels demoralised after every interaction with him. Rachel is willing to make several changes in her thinking and behaviour in order to feel and function better, and agrees to work with you within a cognitive behavioural framework. She may require cognitive restructuring, mastery imagery, and assertiveness and communication assignments.

You examine each feature of Rachel's situation and Rachel's characteristics to determine whether there are any cultural contributions to the overall problem, and identify the following factors. Rachel is young, and therefore may not have a lot of experience with supervisors. She has an untreated 20 per cent hearing loss that may prompt people to speak louder to her than normal to ensure she hears all of what is being said. Because Rachel is Egyptian-Australian, it is important to assess Rachel's comfort level when speaking with males, her expectations when she interacts with males, and whether her heritage could contribute to the difficulties she is having with her supervisor. When you take cultural considerations into account, you may change the overall structure of her plan (or not), but you would certainly shape your interventions around these issues.

CRITICAL THINKING QUESTIONS

1. What cognitive behavioural changes would you recommend for Rachel?
2. What recommendations would you make for homework or rehearsals that Rachel could practise?

HOW I WILL USE MY MENTAL HEALTH SKILLS IN PRACTICE

Samantha's story: My best friend started therapy last year because she was depressed. I was so proud of Lynne for doing something none of us ever thought of doing—going to therapy—and she got a lot out of it. Her therapist, a psychiatric–mental health nurse, taught her that what you think and what you do affect how you feel. During my clinical rotations at psychiatric–mental health sites, I heard about cognitive behavioural counselling and psychotherapy, but wasn't able to see how well it worked until Lynne's experience. One example helped me plan my specialty area in nursing: Lynne learned that she had some unrealistic expectations of herself, and when she couldn't possibly achieve those goals she became sad, ashamed and depressed. In counselling, Lynne talked about these goals and gradually came to realise she could think and do things differently. The change in her is remarkable, and she is a healthier woman now. I hope that I, too, will develop the skills to help people to challenge their negative automatic thinking and improve their lives.

Providing physiological support with medications

Often, people feel anxious when faced with making behavioural changes. This anxiety is best handled through supportive and instructive interactions. However, some individuals require physiological support to prevent their anxiety from reaching panic levels. Anxiolytics, or antianxiety medications, could be administered in sufficient quantities to reduce the problematic feeling state, yet leave the person with enough motivation to learn behavioural techniques for anxiety management where appropriate. Recall from Chapter 8 that some anxiety is necessary for learning to take place. Therefore, levels of anxiolytics that completely eliminate anxiety are counter-therapeutic.

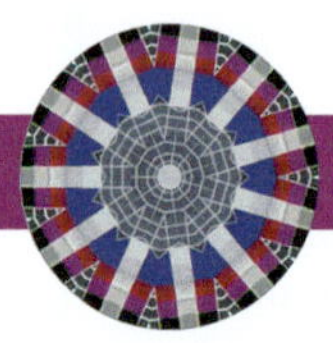

REFERENCES

Baranoff, J. A., Hanrahan, S. J., Burke, A. L. J., & Connor, J. P. (2015). Changes in acceptance in a low-intensity, group-based acceptance and commitment therapy (ACT) chronic pain intervention. *International Journal of Behavioral Medicine 23*(1), 30–38. doi:10.1007/s12529-015-9496-9 (Accessed 2015, December 16.)

Beck, A. T. (1976). *Cognitive therapy and the emotional disorders*. New York, NY: International Universities Press.

Beck, A. T., & Freeman, A. (1990). *Cognitive therapy of personality disorders*. New York, NY: Guilford Press.

Beck, J. S. (1995). *Cognitive therapy: Basics and beyond.* New York, NY: Guilford Press.

Blackburn, I., & Davidson, K. (1990). *Cognitive therapy for depression and anxiety: A practitioner's guide.* Oxford, England: Blackwell.

Cohen, J. A., Mannarino, A. P., & Iyengar, S. (2011). Community treatment of posttraumatic stress disorder for children exposed to intimate partner violence: A randomized controlled trial. *Archives of Pediatrics and Adolescent Medicine, 165*(1), 16–21.

David, D. O, & Freeman, A. (2015). Overview of cognitive-behavioral therapy of personality disorder. In A. T. Beck, D. D. Davis & A. Freeman (Eds.), *Cognitive therapy of personality disorders* (3rd ed.) (pp. 3–18). New York, NY: Guilford Press.

Ellis, A. (2011). The essence of rational emotive behavior therapy: A comprehensive approach to treatment. Retrieved from http://www.rebt.ws/albert_ellis_the_essence_ of_rebt.htm

Ellis, A., & Harper, R. (1975). *A new guide to rational living*. Chatworth, CA: Wilshire Book Co.

Gaynor, K., Dooley, B., Lawlor, E., Lawoyin, R., & O'Callaghan, E. (2011). Group cognitive behavioral therapy as a treatment for negative symptoms in first-episode psychosis. *Early Interventional Psychiatry, 5*(2), 168–173.

Gloster, A. T., Wittchen, H. U., Einsle, F., Lang, T., Helbig-Lang, E., Fydrich, T., . . . Arolt, V. (2011). Psychological treatment for panic disorder with agoraphobia: A randomized controlled trial to examine the role of therapist-guided exposure in situ in CBT. *Journal of Consulting and Clinical Psychology, 79*(3), 406–420. doi: 10.1037/a0023584

Goodkind, M. S., Gallagher-Thompson, D., Thompson, L. W., Kesler, S. R., Anker, L., Flournoy, J., . . . O'Hara, R. M. (2016). The impact of executive function on response to cognitive behavioral therapy in late-life depression. *International Journal of Geriatric Psychiatry, 31*(4), 334–339.

Grogan, S., & Murphy, K. P. (2011). Anticipatory stress response in PTSD: Extreme stress in children. *Journal of Child and Adolescent Psychiatric Nursing, 24*(1), 58–71.

Harris, R. (2006). Embracing your demons: An overview of acceptance and commitment therapy. *Psychotherapy in Australia, 12*(4), 2–8.

Hayes, S. C. (2004). Acceptance and commitment therapy, relational frame theory, and the third wave of behavioural and cognitive therapies. *Behavior Therapy, 35*(4), 639–665.

Hayes, S. C., Luoma, J. B., Bond, F. W., Masuda, A., & Lillis, J. (2006). Acceptance and commitment therapy: Model, processes, and outcomes. *Behaviour Research and Therapy, 44*, 1–25.

Heffner, J. L., McClure, J. B., Mull, K. E., Anthenelli, R. M., & Bricker, J. B. (2015). Acceptance and commitment therapy and nicotine patch for smokers with bipolar disorder: Preliminary evaluation of in-person and telephone-delivered treatment. *Bipolar Disorders, 17*(5), 560–566.

Hertenstein, E., Johann, A., Baglioni, C., Spiegelhalder, K., & Riemann, D. (2016). Treatment of insomnia: A preventive strategy for cardiovascular and mental disorders. *Mental Health and Prevention, 4*(2), 96–103.

Hill, M. L., Masuda, A., Melcher, H., & Morgan, J. R. (2015). Acceptance and commitment therapy for women diagnosed with binge eating disorder: A case-series study. *Cognitive and Behavioral Practice, 22*(3), 367–378.

Høifødet, R. S., Strøm, C., Kolstrup, N., Eisemann, M., & Waterloo, K. (2011). Effectiveness of cognitive behavioural therapy in primary health care: A review. *Family Practice, 28*(5), 489–504. doi: 10.1093/fampra/cmr017

Horan, W. P., Kern, R. S., Tripp, C., Hellemann, G., Wynn, J. K., Bell, M., . . . Green, M. F. (2011). Efficacy and specificity of social cognitive skills training for outpatients with psychiatric disorders. *Journal of Psychiatric Research, 45*(8), 1113–1122.

Hufford, B. J., Williams, M. K., Malec, J. F., & Cravotta, D. (2012). Use of behavioural contracting to increase adherence with rehabilitation treatments on an inpatient brain injury unit: A case report. *Brain Injury, 26*(13–14), 1743–1749.

Hyland, P., & Boduszek, D. (2012). Resolving a difference between cognitive therapy and rational emotive behaviour therapy: Towards the development of an integrated CBT model of psychopathology. *Mental Health Review Journal, 17*(2), 104–116.

Keijsers, G. P. J., Maas, J., Opdorp, A., & Minnen, A. (2016). Addressing self-control cognitions in the treatment of trichotillomania: A randomized controlled trial comparing cognitive therapy to behaviour therapy, *Cognitive Therapy and Research, 40*, 522–531.

Kelly, M. M., Sido, H., Forsyth, J. P., Ziedonis, D. M. Kalman, D., & Cooney, J. L. (2015). Acceptance and commitment therapy smoking cessation treatment for veterans with posttraumatic stress disorder: A pilot study. *Journal of Dual Diagnosis, 11*(1), 50–55.

Kiluk, B. D., Nich, C., & Carroll, K. M. (2011). Relationship of cognitive function and the acquisition of coping skills in computer assisted treatment for substance use disorders. *Drug and Alcohol Dependence, 114*(2–3), 169–176.

Kim, C.-J., Park, J.-W., & Park, H.-R. (2014). Effects of a community-based intervention on cardio-metabolic risk and self-care behaviour in older adults with metabolic syndrome. *International Journal of Nursing Practice, 20*(2), 212–220.

Leoni, M., Corti, S., & Cavagnola, R. (2015). Third generation behavioural therapy for neurodevelopmental disorders: Review and trajectories. *Advances in Mental Health and Intellectual Disabilities, 9*(5), 265–274.

Linehan, M. M., Schmidt III, H., Dimeff, L. A., Craft, J. C., Kanter, J., & Comtois, K. A. (1999). Dialectical behavior therapy for patients with borderline personality disorder and drug-dependence. *American Journal on Addictions, 8*, 279–292.

McIntosh, V. V. W., Jordan, J., Carter, J. D., Frampton, C. M. A., McKenzie, J. M., Latner, J. D., & Joyce, P. R. (2016). Psychotherapy for transdiagnostic binge eating: A randomized controlled trial of cognitive-behavioural therapy, appetite-focused cognitive-behavioural therapy, and schema therapy. *Psychiatry Research, 240*, 412–420.

Mewton, L., & Andrews, G. (2016). Cognitive behavioural therapy for suicidal behaviours: Improving patient outcomes. *Psychology Research and Behaviour Management, 9*, 21–29.

Morgan, M., Cousins, S., Middleton, L., Warriner-Gallyer, G., & Ridsdale, L. (2016). Patients' experiences of a behavioural intervention for migraine headache: A qualitative study. *The Journal of Headache and Pain, 17*, ArtID 16.

Ost, L-G. (2008). Efficacy of the third wave of behaviour therapies: A systematic review and meta-analysis. *Behavior Research and Therapy, 46*(3), 296–321.

Pakenham, K. I. (2015). Investigation of the utility of the acceptance and commitment therapy (ACT) framework for fostering self-care in clinical psychology trainees. *Training and Education in Professional Psychology, 9*(2), 144–152.

Pinto, R. A., Kienhuis, M., Slevison, M., Chester, A., Sloss, A., & Yap, K. (2015). The effectiveness of an outpatient acceptance and commitment therapy group programme for a transdiagnostic population. *Clinical Psychologist*. doi:10.1111/cp.12057 (Accessed 2015, December 16.)

Salkovskis, P. M. (1996). *Trends in cognitive behavioural therapies*. Chichester, England: Wiley.

Skinner, B. F. (1974). *About behaviorism*. New York, NY: Knopf.

Skinner, B. F. (1989). The origins of cognitive thought. *American Psychologist, 44*, 12–18.

Smoski, M. J., Salsman, N., Wang, L., Smith, V., Lynch, T. R., Dager, S. R., . . . Linehan, M. M. (2011). Functional imaging of emotional reactivity in opiate-dependent borderline personality disorder. *Personality Disorders: Theory, Research, and Treatment, 2*(3), 230–241. doi: 10.1037/a0022228

Stafford, M. R., Jackson, H., Mayo-Wilson, E., Morrison, A. P., & Kendall, T. (2013). Early interventions to prevent psychosis: systematic review and meta-analysis. *British Medical Journal, 346*, f185 www.bmj.com/content/346/bmj.f185

Stice, E., Rohde, P., Gau, J., & Ochner, C. (2011). Relationship of depression to perceived social support: Results from a randomized adolescent depression prevention trial. *Behavioral Research and Therapy, 49*(5), 361–366. doi: 10.1016/j.brat.2011.02.009

Thekiso, T. B., Murphy, P., Milnes, J., Lambe, K., Curtin, A., & Farren, C. F. (2015). Acceptance and commitment therapy in the treatment of alcohol use disorder and comorbid affective disorder: A pilot matched control trial. *Behavior Therapy, 46*(6), 717–728.

Thomas, N., Rossell, S., Farhall, J., Shawyer, F., & Castle, D. (2011). Cognitive behavioural therapy for auditory hallucinations: Effectiveness and predictors of outcome in a specialist clinic. *Behavioural and Cognitive Psychotherapy, 39*(2), 129–138.

White, R., Gumley, A., McTaggart, J., Rattrie, L., McConville, D., Cleare, S., & Mitchell, G. (2011). A feasibility study of Acceptance and Commitment Therapy for emotional dysfunction following psychosis. *Behavioral Research and Therapy, 49*(12), 901–907.

Young, J. E., Klosko, J. S., & Weishaar, M. E. (2006). *Schema therapy: A practitioner's guide*. New York, NY: Guilford Press.

Zarling, A., Lawrence, E., & Marchman, J. (2015). A randomized controlled trial of acceptance and commitment therapy for aggressive behavior. *Journal of Consulting and Clinical Psychology, 83*(1), 199–212.

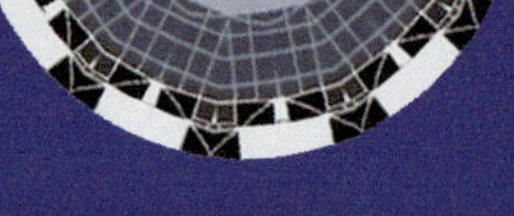

26 Pathways of care

CHRISTINE PALMER AND MATTHEW HALPIN

KEY TERMS

LEARNING OUTCOMES

After completing this chapter, you will be able to:

1. Explain the central concepts of recovery and psychiatric rehabilitation.
2. Understand the difference between personal recovery and clinical recovery.
3. Appreciate the conditions necessary to support a person towards recovery from mental illness.
4. Describe the types of maturational and situational crises a person can experience.
5. Analyse the sequence of a crisis, and determine its significance for the nursing care of a person in crisis.
6. Understand how to assess the risk factors and balancing factors integral to the experience of crisis.
7. Analyse the personal feelings and responses that may affect professionals when caring for people in crisis or people with mental illness.

LIVED EXPERIENCE

It takes time for people to accept their illness and work with clinicians

When I was diagnosed with mental illness, I thought my life was over. I questioned everything I knew about my life. I asked myself, what does this mean for me? Does this mean I will always be unwell? Does this mean I will spend a lot of my life in hospital? I also asked myself, what do I have to look forward to now? My understanding of mental illness was that my life was over. It meant I had to forget about goals and dreams. I had to forget about university, a good job, marriage, children and everything I had ever looked forward to. I thought a diagnosis of mental illness meant there was no hope for recovery, no future and that my life would be forever changed. I thought my life was now 'mental illness' and I was no longer the person I thought I was. I was now something else. I had a complete lack of understanding of mental illness. I had the same stigmatising ideas that society held, but, most of all, I had self-stigma. I had all of the negative ideas that others had about people with mental illness and I applied them to myself. This was because I knew nothing about mental illness other than what I had seen on TV and in the movies. I thought it meant my life was over.

INTRODUCTION

There is no single 'recipe' for the provision of psychiatric–mental health care. Indeed, you have likely read about pathways to care in a range of different settings with quite some variation in how we might work with a person with a mental illness. Nevertheless, there are some key strategies and philosophies that underpin our approach to nursing care. The concept of personal recovery can be difficult to understand, perhaps because it is not a biological concept. Because it is so important, it is elaborated in quite some detail in this chapter. Psychiatric rehabilitation is a separate concept from recovery, although rehabilitation services usually adopt a recovery philosophy to guide processes and practices. Rehabilitation is designed to support the development of skills and capacities in people who have lost these as a result of living with a serious mental illness.

Crisis intervention is a quite different pathway to care from that described in recovery and rehabilitation. Crisis work is short-term, and is designed to restore balance in the lives of people who have experienced a critical life event, as well as to attempt to avert the development of mental illness.

Regardless of whether you find yourself working with people with a mental illness or with someone challenged by crisis, it is important to be aware of the impact of this work on your own mental wellbeing. Listening to the stories of others that contain traumatic events and memories can lead to health problems if you are not consciously processing them. The final section of this chapter points to some of the ways you can help to manage the effects of vicarious traumatisation.

SELF-AWARENESS

What does mental illness mean to you?
What has been your experience of knowing someone or working with someone with a mental illness?
Which preconceived ideas were maintained, and which were dispelled, as a result of your experience(s)?

RECOVERY

William Anthony (1993) wrote one of the first articles guiding mental health services to embrace a recovery-oriented philosophy. Anthony (1993, p. 527) defined **recovery** as:

> a deeply personal, unique process of changing one's attitudes, values, feelings, goals, skills and/or roles. It is a way of living a satisfying, hopeful, and contributing life even with limitations caused by the illness. Recovery involves the development of new meaning and purpose in one's life as one grows beyond the catastrophic effects of mental illness.

Despite more than two decades of seeking to achieve recovery-oriented mental health service systems, it is argued that there is still much to be achieved to reduce disparity and improve recovery outcomes for people with severe mental illness (Drake & Whitley, 2014). As a health professional, your understanding of recovery is important in changing attitudes and in the acceptance of a recovery-oriented philosophy of care (Feeney, Jordan & McCarron, 2013). Recovery-oriented service provision has been shown to positively impact on a range of outcomes (Malinovsky et al., 2013).

Recovery from mental illness shares some similarities with the concept of recovery in physical health care settings, but also has some important differences. Just as a person with a severe physical injury can recover, a person diagnosed with a mental illness is able to recover; however, their life might be significantly different (Anthony, 1993). Consider a person having a car accident and severing their spinal cord, for example. In this situation, even with significant treatment, the person may not be able to walk again, but will rather learn to adapt their life to being in a wheelchair. If a person is diagnosed with schizophrenia and they have a severe and disabling course to their illness, they can still engage in the process of recovery. We know that around two-thirds of people diagnosed with schizophrenia will have a complete recovery or a significant recovery with few ongoing difficulties (Lysaker & Buck, 2008). About a third will have a more disabling course to their illness, and experience periods of illness and wellness throughout their lives. Recovery from mental illness does not mean that the person will never get unwell again, but rather that if they do they will have more effective coping strategies to help minimise the relapse, they will know how to plan for this, and they will also know when to seek help when it is needed.

As part of this recovery journey, the person will need to make changes to their life, learn to understand their illness and symptoms, and learn ways to manage any side-effects from treatment (which sometimes can be significant). People diagnosed with mental illness may also experience stigma from the community, as well as their own self-stigma, which is an internalised form of societal stigma. Internalised stigma can be a powerfully negative force that ultimately impedes recovery (Boyd, Otilingam & DeForge, 2014). Some diagnostic labels, such as schizophrenia, attract more stigma than others (Bentall, 2013). To combat this, it will be important to help the other people in the person's life to get a better understanding of the illness (Corrigan, Kosyluk & Rusch, 2013).

They may also need to look at increasing their own understanding of mental illness. Talking to others who have similar experiences is an excellent strategy to achieve this (Conner, McKinnon, Ward, Reynolds & Brown, 2015). Many mental health services now employ peer workers, who are people who also live with a mental illness, and whose role it is to support others diagnosed with a mental illness through sharing what they have learned from their own experiences. People are able to learn, through the observation of others, that it is possible to live a satisfying and full life regardless of their diagnosis. It has also been determined that volunteer peer support workers have better outcomes through personal growth and increased hope for the future (Firmin, Luther, Lysaker & Sayers, 2015; Ha, 2016).

Some of the key components of recovery are:

- hope
- empowerment
- understanding
- identity
- personal responsibility.

Hope

One of the key components of recovery is **hope** (McCauley, McKenna, Keeney & McLaughlin, 2015). The role of hope in recovery has been an interest of health professionals for many years. What hope means in the mental health context is looking beyond the illness and being able to look forward to your future. Miller (1992), cited in Landeen et al. (1996, p. 459), defines hope as:

> a state characterised by an anticipation of a continued good state, an improved state, or a release from a perceived entrapment. The anticipation may or may not be founded on concrete, real-world evidence. Hope is an anticipation of a future which is good and is based upon: mutuality (relationships with others), a sense of personal competence, coping ability, psychological well-being, purpose and meaning in life, as well as a sense of 'the possible.'

Hope is about the person with mental illness being able to look forward to tomorrow and to the future. Often, people who experience mental illness can lose hope, and at times have suicidal thoughts based in the belief that they have nothing to live for. Hope is what drives us all, and is what helps us plan and achieve goals and look forward to the future. As students in nursing you undoubtedly hope to achieve the goal of becoming a nurse and having a satisfying and rewarding career in the future. You will most likely have many other goals in your life which are driven by hope. This may include having a family, meeting new people, owning your own house and travelling the world, for example.

Can you imagine if you had nothing to look forward to, no plans and no reason to get up in the morning? People experiencing depression and other mental illnesses often lose hope. As a health professional, the work you do can contribute to a person recapturing that hope and once again looking forward to tomorrow. It is important to understand that health professionals can promote hope or equally destroy optimism for the future (Bird et al., 2014; Eriksen, Arman, Davidson, Sundfor & Karlsson, 2014). Hope is an important part of everyone's life, and such an important part of any person's recovery journey as this provides the foundation for moving forward to achieve important life goals.

Hope is considered fundamental before a person can choose to embark on recovery. Jacobson and Curtis (2000, p. 335) refer to hope as the emotional aspect of recovery and that it holds 'a promise that things can and do change, that today is not the way it will always be'. Curtis (1997) identified a number of factors considered critical to recovery, as reported by consumers, and the top-ranked factor was 'just one person who believed in me'. Morse and Penrod (1999) have developed a process model for the development of hope following a critical life experience, such as being told that you have breast cancer or that you have a mental illness. This model was developed from qualitative enquiry, exploring emotional responses to the experience of illness (refer to Figure 26.1 ■).

The 'event' is the experience of illness and, for the purpose of this section, we will reflect on these processes in relation to being informed that you have a mental illness. *Enduring* is the initial response, and this involves suspending

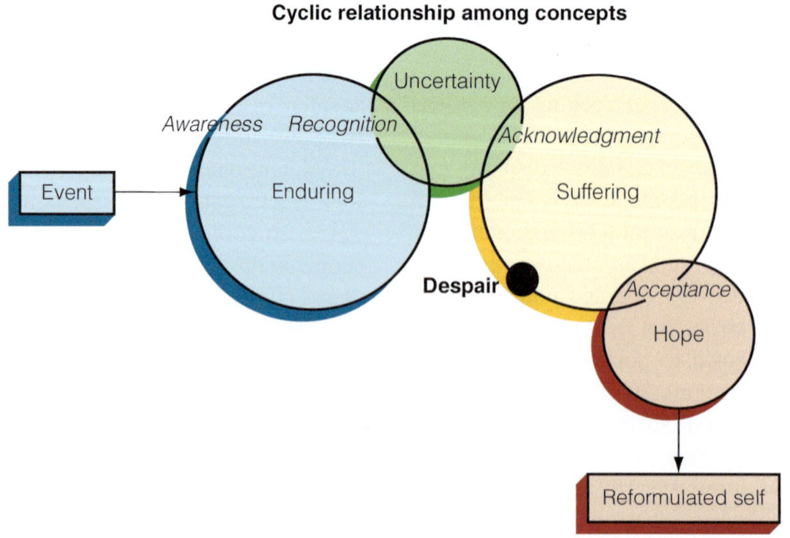

FIGURE 26.1 ■ Model for the development of hope.
Source: Morse, J. M., & Penrod, J. (1999). Linking concepts of enduring, uncertainty, suffering, and hope. *Image: Journal of Nursing Scholarship, 31*(2), 145–150, p. 149.

or suppressing emotions and remaining in control. We do this because we worry that we will 'lose it' or disintegrate. The level of knowing here is *awareness*.

Uncertainty is evident when we begin to recognise what has happened and know what our goals are for the future, but we are unable to choose a course of action from a range of options. Unfortunately, this state of uncertainty paralyses hope. At this time we simply exist in an emotional state, and suffer as a result of not being able to act. When we are in a state of uncertainty, we have no other choice but to tolerate the present, and this can be very difficult to do.

Suffering involves acknowledgment of what is happening to us. We begin to grasp the situation, and consequently suffer emotionally. Morse and Penrod (1999) point out that 'the depth of the state of suffering is despair, utter hopelessness' (p. 148). Out of this overwhelming emotional experience, we begin to piece reality together, and begin to develop a view of what the future might look like. 'This process of piecing together a new future begins in small incremental pieces, eventually building to . . . acceptance of the event and identification of both a goal and the means to attain it, which eventually leads to hope' (Morse and Penrod, 1999, p. 148). So, according to this model, suffering is viewed as integral to moving on and ultimately to repair.

Suffering leads to hope. The level of knowing is now *acceptance*, and we become future-oriented. With hope, we are now able to develop an action plan designed to achieve the desired goals for the future. Hope is bolstered by supportive relationships, and this can include relationships with health professionals. This leads to a new state. There is a sense of becoming a 'better person' for having suffered. This state has been labelled the '*reformulated self*', whereby the past is accepted and we also accept that the future has been irrevocably changed, and a choice is made to 'make the most of life'.

As a nurse, it is important that you understand where a person is in relation to the process of developing hope. This understanding will help you to know how to respond to a person during the phases of enduring, uncertainty and suffering. If these phases are acknowledged as normal or expected, nurses won't make the mistake of attempting to force people to have hope when they are unable to accept it. The trauma involved in dealing with a critical life experience, such as the diagnosis of mental illness, results in a range of responses. These responses are part of a process that is not linear. People move back and forth, and an understanding of this may also explain the delays for some in developing hope. These are normal responses, so should not be assessed as being part of an illness.

Empowerment

Empowerment is defined in different ways; however, most definitions of empowerment in mental health focus on the person who is ill and their carers feeling included and involved in decisions relating to them or the person they care for (Crane-Ross, Lutz & Roth, 2006) The essence of empowerment in mental health is about helping people feel in control of their life and their mental health (Patterson et al., 2016). This involves active collaboration in decision-making, leading to a sense of control over their health and illness. Empowerment is about the person being in the driver's seat and knowing that, regardless of the re-emergence of symptoms of their illness, they are living a life that they choose.

Recovery in mental illness, as discussed previously, does not mean that a person will never experience symptoms again or never get unwell again. It means that, despite the re-emergence of symptoms, they are still living a hopeful and contributing life (Whitley, Palmer & Gunn, 2015). However, there are often times when people might feel disempowered or not in control due to the symptoms they are experiencing. They may feel that they don't have a say in decisions relating to their treatment. This may be because they are told they must take medication or be in hospital when they think they don't need to be, and this may be enforced through legislation. Even in these situations, it is possible for nurses to include people in decisions, and to help provide choice, support and education so that they will feel like a partner in their care.

Knowledge/understanding

The first thing most people tend to do when they have been diagnosed with any sort of illness is to research and read about it to better understand what is happening and which treatments are likely to be helpful. The same applies for people who have been diagnosed with a mental illness. Developing an understanding of the illness, the treatment they are receiving and how this will benefit their mental health is an important part of a person's journey of recovery. Often, in the early stages of their illness, a person might not understand what is happening to them, why they are receiving treatment, how this treatment will help them, and even what a diagnosis may mean for them in the short- and long-term. The more understanding a person has about their illness, treatment and recovery, the greater the benefit will be to the person. As a health professional, it is part of your role to assist people (and their carers) to understand their mental illness, and the available self-management strategies and treatment options. By doing this, you assist them in commencing or continuing their recovery journey. A good way to guide what could help the person or their family is to consider what you would like to know if you had just been diagnosed with a serious physical or mental illness.

Identity

Having a sense of identity is important for everyone. Identity is about who you are, how you see yourself, what characterises you and how you are viewed by others. When someone is diagnosed with a mental illness, their sense of identity is often something that is questioned. Identity is often viewed negatively, particularly in the early stages. Often when people are diagnosed with a mental illness, they will question who they are and struggle to view themselves in the same way they did before. This internal questioning can lead to negative thoughts and further depression (Cruwys & Gunaseelan, 2016). They may have self-defeating thoughts, such as 'I can't do this because I have a mental illness' or 'They won't like me because I have a mental illness.' Having experienced mental

LIVED EXPERIENCE

Finding my identity

When I was diagnosed with bipolar affective disorder in my late teens, it was a shock that led me to question my identity and ask questions like 'Who am I now?', 'How can I be the person I was planning to be?' and 'What will this mean for my life?' At that stage of my life I was in Year 12 and was planning to go to university straight out of school and study in the area of health science or sports science. I was also training a lot in martial arts, and wanted it live in Japan and train full-time for three to six months with my Karate school's headquarters. This diagnosis led to me to believe that this was no longer an option and that my life was over. I had started to define myself by my illness based on stigma, and what I thought I knew about mental illness. I had already started to view my future negatively.

It took a number of years before I started to define my identity more positively and begin to look forward to the future. One of the major contributors to this change, which led me to recapture hope and redefine my identity, was the work of some health professionals seven years after I was diagnosed with mental illness. These health professionals, including nurses, helped me better understand my illness and treatment, and introduced me to my first understandings of what recovery meant.

One of the things they did was to challenge my negative beliefs, and this made me think differently. They asked me 'Why do you think you can't go to university?', 'Why do you think your life is over?' and 'Why can't you achieve what you want to achieve?' From these seeds of hope, my life began to change. Ten years on, I am married, living somewhere I love, I have almost finished a psychology degree, and I'm working in a managerial role in a mental health service setting. To get here took support, hard work and motivation, but those first steps were possible because health professionals helped me regain my personal identity and my path to recovery.

illness, people can experience a profound challenge to their identity, and part of their recovery may include redefining who they are (Bonney & Stickley, 2008).

Recovery often involves accepting, understanding and managing psychological experiences (Bonney & Stickley, 2008), and part of the recovery process may be to reconstruct a sense of self (Davidson & Strauss, 1992). Reconstructing a person's identity is not always a negative, and it can be an important part of the recovery journey, which can lead to a new-found sense of hope and sense of self (Bird et al., 2014).

Personal responsibility

Personal responsibility is a crucial component of recovery. Recovery from a mental illness doesn't happen in a vacuum. The health professional's role is to provide support, but a health professional can't make a person recover. Ultimately, it is up to the person with mental illness to embrace possibility and accept responsibility for making change. Health professionals can assist with the process by providing support, effective treatment and education. Mead and Copeland (2000, p. 5) note

> It's up to each individual to take responsibility for their own wellness. There is no one else who can do this for us. When our perspective changes from reaching out to be saved to one in which we work to heal ourselves and our relationships, the pace of our recovery increases dramatically

When symptoms are persistent and severe, taking responsibility can be hard, and at these times the assistance from health professionals can provide the support necessary to take even the smallest steps. This can significantly contribute to a person's recovery, as sometimes the small steps are just what is needed to get through a difficult and challenging period in one's journey (Mead & Copeland, 2000). Taking responsibility can mean a range of things in a person's life. It can mean taking responsibility for taking medication as prescribed, and working closely with doctors before making any change to this. It can also mean taking responsibility for things that may be having a negative impact on recovery, such as self-medicating with drugs and/or alcohol, which is quite common for people with a mental illness (Bolton, Robinson & Sareen, 2009).

The person who uses drugs and alcohol may believe the substances help calm them or reduce the symptoms, but it is well-known that self-medicating with drugs and alcohol actually increases and worsens symptoms and negatively impacts on psychological wellbeing (Margoles, Malchy, Negrete, Tempier & Gill, 2005). Other triggers that impact on a person's wellbeing include not getting enough sleep, taking on too much work, or putting themselves in situations that may be risky to their health. As a health professional, it can be useful for you to think about the sorts of things that have a negative effect on your own wellbeing, and this may give you some ideas of the triggers that might have a negative effect on the people you are working with. Many of the things that impact on wellbeing can have even worse ramifications when you have a mental illness.

When working with people about triggers and personal responsibility, pros and cons charts can be useful, as this helps the person to see the positives and negatives of something that is impacting on their mental wellbeing. This is a useful tool to help people see the impact for themselves, and to think more about how it affects their mental health. Peer support can also be useful

LIVED EXPERIENCE

Personal responsibility

Taking personal responsibility was a key step in my recovery, but it took many years for me to realise that I needed to take responsibility for my illness. For many years I lived in denial that I had a bipolar illness. On a daily basis I used drugs, believing they would make the symptoms go away, but I was really only self-medicating and trying to hide how I was feeling from the world and from myself. The drugs were doing the opposite, and every time I used them my symptoms would get worse. This resulted in frequent visits to the emergency department, often after trying to take my life. I also didn't take responsibility for my treatment, and would often not turn up to doctors' appointments and not take my medication. This even included taking on high-pressure jobs and continuing to push myself harder and harder. I was trying to win a battle against my illness. Each time I did this, my work colleagues noticed something was wrong, and after a period of time they tried to counsel me. When this happened, I denied that anything was wrong and I usually quit my job. The cycle would then repeat in the next job.

The first major event that led to change was after a longer admission in hospital, and with the assistance of the clinical team I started to take responsibility for my mental health. I started by giving up drugs and accepting counselling. This was followed by taking my medication as prescribed and engaging in treatment, and then working with my doctors and workers to learn more about my illness. This included doing a lot of individual work and really examining myself; looking at what was helping my recovery, and what was making things worse. This is still something that I do every day. Taking personal responsibility has been a crucial part of my recovery. It remains an ongoing journey, but each day I learn more about myself and get better at managing the 'ups and downs' of my illness.

when working with a person about taking responsibility, as these peer workers have lived through mental illness themselves, and can give first-hand examples and guide others through the steps needed to take responsibility for their recovery.

Is recovery different for different people?

For people living with a mental illness, recovery means being able to have a life they are happy with, regardless of the symptoms of mental illness. People living with mental illness want to be able to have a life that is not defined by their illness, but a life that is meaningful, where they have goals to look forward to, where they can plan for the future, have close relationships and are able to look forward to each day. People living with a mental illness often have similar aspirations and goals to anyone else. They want to be able to live a life that they are happy with, and this includes having somewhere to live, having good relationships with friends and family and meaningful activity, which might include work, or being engaged in hobbies, study or socialising with friends. Being part of the broader community is integral to having a life worth living.

Recovery can differ from person to person, just as individual goals differ. Recovery for one person may mean being out of hospital and living in supported accommodation. This person may need a high level of assistance with daily living, such as the provision of meals and assistance with medication, and they may need to be seen regularly by their health professional. This person may attend the local clubhouse or community centre and attend art classes. They might be happy to just be out of hospital, having somewhere to live, and having the support they need as well as hobbies they enjoy. Recovery for someone else might mean having their own home, working full-time, being in a relationship and needing minimal assistance from mental health services. Although these two examples of recovery may look completely different, they have one thing in common: each person has a life that they are happy with, and they are achieving their goals.

As a psychiatric–mental health nurse, you have an important role in supporting people in their recovery journey. To do this you will use a range of clinical skills, including supporting, questioning, coaching, assisting with an understanding of their illness and available treatments, challenging their beliefs about their illness, and encouraging them through the steps needed in their ongoing journey of recovery. One of the most important components of your role as a mental health professional will be to provide the hope for recovery when a person might be at the lowest point in their illness and at other points in their recovery. Holding hope for others until they can reclaim it for themselves is a powerful way of expressing your support and encouragement. Your clinical expertise and your understanding of recovery are essential in supporting people though their journey and helping them to achieve their goals.

Personal recovery and clinical recovery

Recovery has historically meant cure from illness or disease. *Clinical recovery* is recovery measured against clinical indicators, such as the presence of symptoms, time away from treatment, the level of symptoms experienced and the medication dosage required. Most health services are interested in measuring clinical recovery (Slade, 2009). According to the clinical recovery model, staying well is an indicator of recovery. The person-centred recovery model, as already indicated, is much more about living a good life even if the symptoms of the illness recur. *Personal recovery* is consumer- and strengths-based, and the focus is on the person's life, their capacity for happiness and wellbeing, and how people define themselves rather than being identified by their illness. Personal recovery has emerged from the lived experience of people with mental illness, and is quite different to clinical recovery (Slade & Longden, 2015).

People with mental illness also often confuse clinical and personal recovery, and so measure their own personal recovery according to the clinical recovery model. Health professionals need to clarify the difference between clinical recovery and personal recovery, not only for themselves, but for the people they serve. Personal recovery is values-based, and is geared more towards choice and empowerment than clinical recovery is. Personal recovery is about promoting wellbeing rather than purely treating an illness. Personal recovery is the philosophy that underpins mental health service system policies in Australia, and guides the provision of mental health service delivery (Leamy, Bird, Le Boutillier, Williams & Slade, 2011). Personal recovery is defined within the Australian national recovery framework (Commonwealth of Australia, 2013, p. 11) as 'being able to live and create a meaningful and contributing life in a community of choice with or without the presence of mental health issues'.

Readiness for recovery

Recovery is different for each person and everyone's journey of recovery is unique. Readiness for recovery also differs from person to person, and is a stage where the person is able to take steps, through support and personal responsibility, towards their own recovery. As a nurse, you have an important role in assisting people with their recovery. One of the key components to this is assisting the person you are working with to see hope for the future, to set goals, and to help them to take their first steps towards their personal recovery. These first steps may be somewhat small—like sleeping less, preparing a meal for themselves, engaging in treatment for the first time, or assisting with helping to improve interpersonal relationships.

Although some of these things may seem very small, these steps can be foundational to the change needed. For example, you might support someone to go out shopping, which may not be something they have done for a while or had the confidence to do. Symptoms like anxiety, depression, social phobia and auditory hallucinations can keep some people very socially isolated. By assisting the person to take these first steps, you might give them the confidence to continue and to achieve more. This step might be the first of many small goals that they achieve that helps them on their recovery journey.

Examples follow of rehabilitation goals, ranging from basic functioning to quality-of-life issues:

- washing their own clothes
- shopping for their own food
- maintaining healthy and appropriate nutrition
- remaining active in the community—regardless of their living setting
- seeking sufficient intellectual stimulation
- enhancing their quality of life
- continuing a relationship with mental health care providers
- collaborating with caregivers to monitor psychotropic medications
- participating in a plan to reduce or eliminate—when clinically safe to do so—psychotropic medications
- expressing feelings assertively
- coping with increases in symptoms and personal crises.

Different people you work with may be in different stages of their illness and recovery, so this means that some may be ready to take small steps while others might not. Encouragement and support should be still provided, as, even if the person isn't quite ready for recovery right now, the support might assist them to move towards readiness.

People are more likely to be able to strive for and achieve these goals when they acknowledge their own strengths and needs. As a nurse facilitating recovery, you are involved in every aspect of a person's psychological growth and development (O'Baire-Kark & Klevay, 2011). The likelihood that a person will have symptom reduction to the point of recovery seems to be affected by the person's coping style (Staring, van der Gaag & Mulder, 2011). In a 2011 study by Staring and associates, people who integrated important features—such as who they are, what their needs are, and what seems to help keep them stable and healthy—had significantly better odds for recovery. This study was conducted with people who have schizophrenia, and was remarkable, in that having insight and a therapeutic alliance did not contribute meaningfully to recovery. Recovery and remission seem to be more associated with putting the pieces together in a way that works for the individual, rather than insisting on a particular path or on understanding how and why a problem exists (LeBel, 2011).

Once people express a need for greater autonomy, planning for recovery can begin. All involved parties must be flexible to the changing circumstances of stress and illness, triggers and relapse, and the barriers to overcoming them. Recovery is an individualised state defined by each person. It cannot be imposed from without; recovery must be achieved from within.

People with mental illness who are working towards recovery may have discovered many ways to function effectively. However, the individual needs to evaluate, on an ongoing basis, the usefulness of a particular coping strategy or interaction style, and develop an array of responses to problems. What might be helpful for one person might not be at all helpful for another, so it is important that people try many different strategies until they find something that works well for them. Figure 26.2 ■ illustrates the steps to take to learn about what works and what needs to be changed so people can progress toward recovery.

Realistic and attainable expectations of change

What kind of supports do people need to begin the process of changing to recovery-focused behaviours? Expectations of change must be realistic and attainable, keeping in mind that they may need to be flexible depending on crises and depleted resources (emotional and financial). The 10 main components of mental health recovery have been determined by an expert

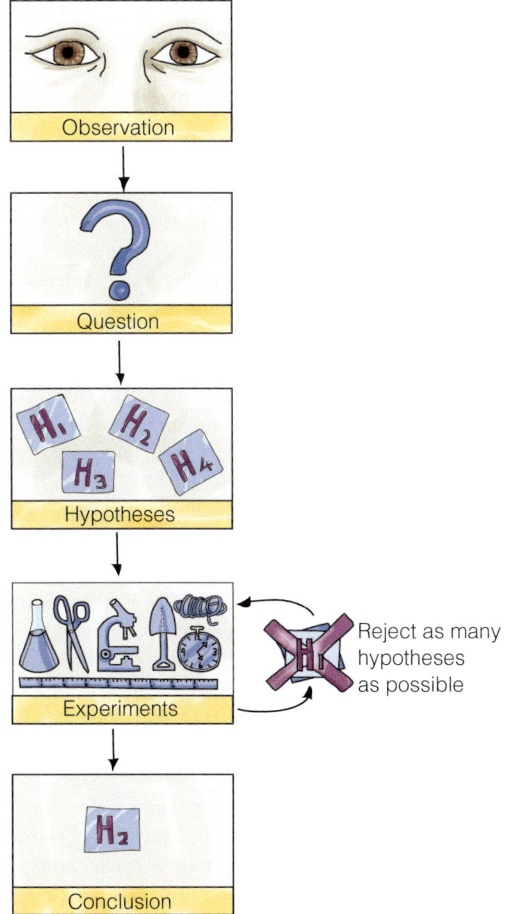

FIGURE 26.2 ■ Developing recovery skills that work for the individual.

panel on mental health (see Box 26.1). Change is not immediate, instantaneous or initially permanent. Every person trying to make a change in behaviour must go through transitional stages before, during and after the change is made.

Relapse

Relapse is a return of significant symptoms that are problematic for the person in a number of areas of functioning. There are degrees of relapse from mild to total and severe, although a severe level of relapse can often be avoided if early symptoms are detected and addressed. Identifying stressors and triggers for relapse, developing coping skills, and recognising each victory helps to make interactions effective and life meaningful. Relapse can be disheartening, and can lead to feelings of self-doubt and a further loss of confidence.

This can also be hard for you as a nurse, as you may have been working closely with a person who has achieved goals, made great progress and is feeling more in control of their illness. A few months later you might see the person back in hospital and back to how they were feeling before. Your role as a nurse and how you work with the person in this experience can make a great difference to how the person feels. You could be judgmental and not provide hope—for example, by asking what the person did wrong—which can make the person feel worse. On the other hand, you can provide hope by emphasising that this is only small setback, and advising them to view this relapse as a learning opportunity to better understand the illness and what may have triggered the return of symptoms. By providing this perspective you are able to support the person's confidence, acknowledge their strengths and help them to see the learning opportunity within, which may assist with their recovery in the future.

Onken, Dumont, Ridgway, Dornan and Ralph (2002) examined what hindered and helped people with their recovery. As a part of this study, they examined from a consumer's perspective what was helpful from mental health staff and what was unhelpful or hindered their recovery. Onken et al. (2002) found that staff who were parental, who didn't understand the person's experience, who had low expectations of the person's recovery, and who acted as superior and disrespectful, had a negative impact on a person's recovery journey. Conversely, people found that staff who were hopeful, had positive expectations and held the belief that recovery is possible had a positive impact on their journey.

Practice example

Michael is someone who has paranoid schizophrenia with frightening delusions. He was stabilised for several months, but then became uncomfortable when he thought his neighbours were deliberately shining their headlights into his living room window in order to bother him. His symptoms steadily worsened, and he stated at his clinic appointment, 'Why do I have to revisit this hell? I was there already and got out. Now I'm back in hell again.'

Peer support

Peer support is the employment (paid or voluntary) of a person with a lived experience of mental illness, either as a consumer or a carer, whose role is to support people and/or their carers in their recovery journey. Peer support workers use their personal lived experience to help people or carers to develop recovery skills, navigate the mental health service system and understand mental illness (Holmes, Molloy, Beckett, Field & Stratford, 2013). Peer support involves people who have a lived experience of mental illness and have made significant steps in their own recovery from a mental illness, who then provide support either individually or in a group to people who are experiencing mental illness and may be just starting their own recovery journey (Mead & MacNeil, 2006).

During the past 10 years, there has been a significant growth in the peer support workforce across Australia, the United States, New Zealand and the United Kingdom (Gallagher & Halpin, 2014), with many mental health services now employing peer workers in a range of settings, including acute inpatient units, community teams, day programs or psychosocial rehabilitation programs. Peer support workers are now an important part of multi-disciplinary teams across mental health services.

A South Australian study reviewing the role of peer support workers or lived-experience staff found that consumers and carers, as well as clinical staff, value the role of peer

Box 26.1 National Consensus Statement on Mental Health Recovery: the 10 fundamental components of recovery

The following are the fundamental components for recovery from a mental health condition:

- ***Self-direction.*** People with mental illness lead, control, exercise choice over, and determine their own path of recovery by optimising autonomy, independence and control of resources to achieve a self-determined life. By definition, the recovery process must be self-directed by the individual, who defines their own life goals, and designs a unique path toward those goals.
- ***Individualised and person-centred.*** There are multiple pathways to recovery based on an individual's unique strengths and resiliencies, as well as their needs, preferences, experiences (including past trauma), and cultural background in all of its diverse representations. Individuals also identify recovery as being an ongoing journey and an end result, as well as an overall paradigm for achieving wellness and optimal mental health.
- ***Empowerment.*** People have the authority to choose from a range of options and to participate in all decisions—including the allocation of resources—that will affect their lives, and are educated and supported in so doing. They have the ability to join with others to collectively and effectively speak for themselves about their needs, wants, desires and aspirations. Through empowerment, an individual gains control of their own destiny, and influences the organisational and societal structures in their life.
- ***Holistic.*** Recovery encompasses an individual's whole life, including mind, body, spirit and community. Recovery embraces all aspects of life, including housing, employment, education, mental health and healthcare treatment and services, complementary and naturalistic services, addictions treatment, spirituality, creativity, social networks, community participation, and family supports as determined by the person. Families, providers, organisations, systems, communities and society play crucial roles in creating and maintaining meaningful opportunities for the person's access to these supports.
- ***Non-linear.*** Recovery is not a straightforward step-by-step process; it is based on continual growth, occasional setbacks, and learning from experience. Recovery begins with an initial stage of awareness in which a person recognises that positive change is possible. This awareness enables the person to move on to fully engage in the work of recovery.
- ***Strengths-based.*** Recovery focuses on valuing and building on the multiple capacities, resiliencies, talents, coping abilities, and inherent worth of individuals. By building on these strengths, they leave unsuccessful life roles behind them and engage in new life roles (e.g., partner, caregiver, friend, student, employee). The process of recovery moves forward through interaction with others in supportive, trust-based relationships.
- ***Peer support.*** Mutual support—including the sharing of experiential knowledge and skills and social learning—plays an invaluable role in recovery. People with a lived experience of mental illness encourage and engage others in recovery, and provide each other with a sense of belonging, supportive relationships, valued roles, and community.
- ***Respect.*** Community, systems, and societal acceptance and appreciation of people with mental illness—including protecting their rights and eliminating discrimination and stigma—are crucial in achieving recovery. Self-acceptance and regaining belief in one's self are particularly vital. Respect ensures the inclusion and full participation of all people in all aspects of their lives.
- ***Responsibility.*** People with mental illness have a personal responsibility for their own self-care and journeys of recovery. Taking steps toward their goals may require great courage. People must strive to understand and give meaning to their experiences, and identify coping strategies and healing processes to promote their own wellness.
- ***Hope.*** Recovery provides the essential and motivating message of a better future—that people can and do overcome the barriers and obstacles that confront them. Hope is internalised, but can be fostered by peers, families, friends, providers and others. Hope is the catalyst of the recovery process.

Adapted from: The National Consensus Statement on Health Recovery, U.S. Department of Health and Human Services, Substance Abuse and Mental Health Services Administration (SAMHSA), Center for Mental Health Services. National Mental Health Information Center.

LIVED EXPERIENCE

Helping others through lived experience

When I started my journey of recovery, I soon found out I was not alone, and the more I spoke to friends and family, the more I realised many people had their own lived experience, and they, too, had been affected by mental illness. Soon I realised that what I learnt from my experience could help others, and I found that there were many other people out there who were already helping others through their own personal experiences. These people were working in peer support and using their lived experience in powerful ways. They talked about their recovery journey, helped people realise they were not alone, and they provided hope. By doing this, they empowered me to believe that I, too, could recover.

These peer workers could say: 'Mate, I know—I have been there, too, and it gets better, and you will get through this.' By sharing their lived experience, they helped me start my own journey of recovery. At that stage I realised I wanted to do this, too, and soon I began working as a peer support worker, and each day I was able to help another person realise that they could look forward to their future. I helped people to see that recovery was possible for everyone with a mental illness.

support workers within mental health services (Gallagher & Halpin, 2014). People with mental illness described peer support workers as providing hope for recovery, and that they assisted them in identifying positive coping strategies, and helped them to find ways to manage the symptoms of mental illness. Mental health service staff also saw the value of lived-experience staff in promoting recovery, and reported that they found that when peer workers shared their lived experience, this reduced people's distress. They also found that the peer worker role supported the work of other clinical staff (Gallagher & Halpin, 2014), while improving recovery outcomes for the peer workers themselves (Firmin et al., 2015).

Peer support workers can assist in providing a bridge in communication between the person and their carer and/or the clinical team. Peer support is a valued addition to many mental health services, and can assist the clinical team to further support consumer and carer recovery (Kidd, Kenny & McKinstry, 2015; Repper & Carter, 2011).

The Australian national recovery framework

The *National framework for recovery-oriented mental health services* provides the policies designed to underpin mental health services with a recovery philosophy (Commonwealth of Australia, 2013). This policy document brings together recovery approaches from across Australia, based on both Australian and international research, to form a consistent approach for recovery-based practices across mental health services in Australia. This framework complements professional standards and competency frameworks at a state and national level. Some of the core principles describing recovery, which are common across research and inform this policy frame work, are that recovery is:

- a non-linear journey
- a normal human process
- an ongoing journey, and not the same as a cure or having an endpoint
- often not done alone
- a unique and personal journey.

An overview of the Australian recovery framework is presented in Figure 26.3 ■.

Psychiatric disability

Some people with mental illness have a severe and persistent course to their illness that requires more intensive support. This is a clinically diverse population, with different diagnoses

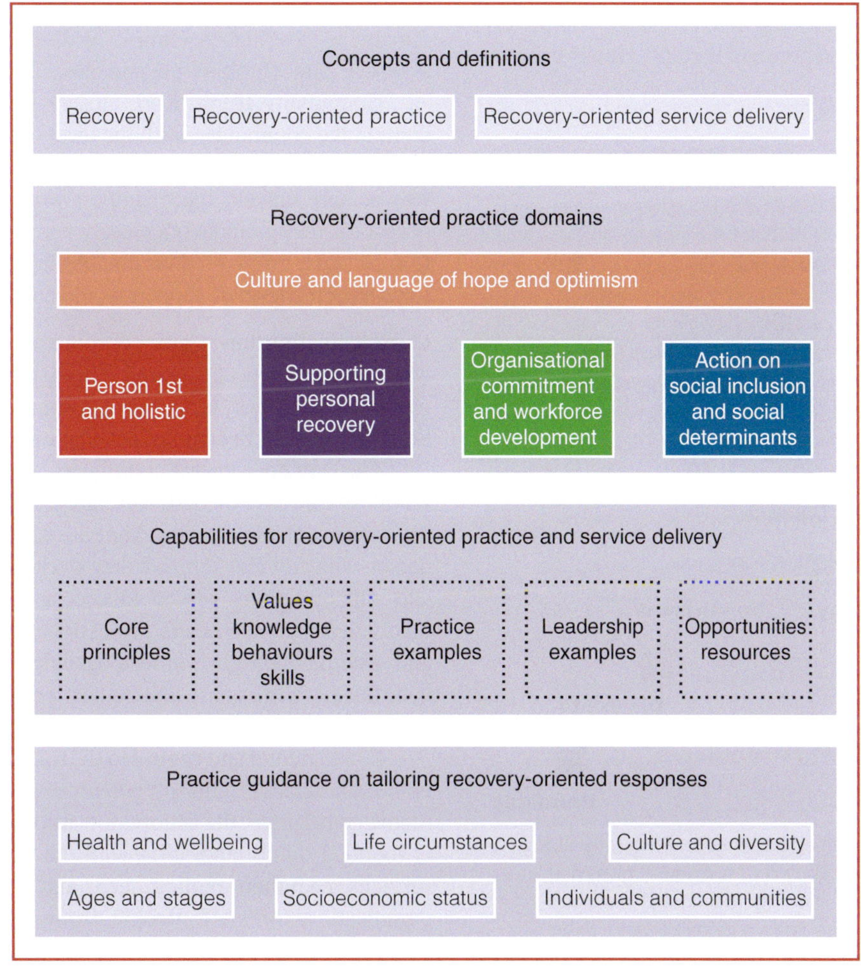

FIGURE 26.3 ■ The national framework for recovery-oriented mental health services: at a glance.
Commonwealth of Australia. (2013). *A national framework for recovery-oriented mental health services: Guide for practitioners and providers.* Canberra, Australia: Commonwealth of Australia.

and varied patterns of illness. There is considerable variation in symptom profile, pattern of relapse or acute exacerbations, and quality of life across a range of disorders. People with major depressive disorder (MDD), bipolar affective disorders, schizophrenia, anxiety disorders, and many of the personality disorders, for example, can all suffer enduring and disabling conditions resulting in disadvantage.

The core feature of a severe and persistent disorder is not diagnosis or prognosis, but the experience of ***psychiatric disability***. In 1980, the World Health Organization (WHO) developed and published a classification system (Figure 26.4 ■) for the phases of a long-term illness that also relates to mental illness or psychiatric disorders. Whether mild or severe, whether ongoing, recurring or remitting, these disorders require services that go beyond the limits of an acute disease model.

The profile that emerges of people with persistent and disabling mental illness is that of a highly vulnerable subgroup within the mental health care service systems. This subgroup accounts for the majority of people being treated within hospital-based systems and in many community programs. They are at risk for developing secondary or concurrent mental health concerns, and for problems associated with the social determinants of living. They account for a significant percentage of homeless people. These multiple, interacting problems require complex approaches to service provision.

Some disorders run their course and resolve completely, either spontaneously or in response to therapy. However, some disorders leave residual impairment or disability of short or long duration. While there is a substantial amount of disability associated with acute disorders, the extended disability resulting from enduring illnesses is distressing at individual, family and community levels.

Practice examples

Jacqui, aged 33 years, has long-standing mental health problems. Years of irregular adherence to treatment, and intermittent episodes of substantial substance abuse, have resulted in unacceptable behaviours. These unacceptable behaviours caused Jacqui to be evicted from her apartment. She is now homeless.

David stopped taking his medication for bipolar disorder after he became homeless. Months later, his symptom level began to interfere with every aspect of his functioning. David began critiquing the outfits of people he passed on the street, and then demanding consultation fees from them.

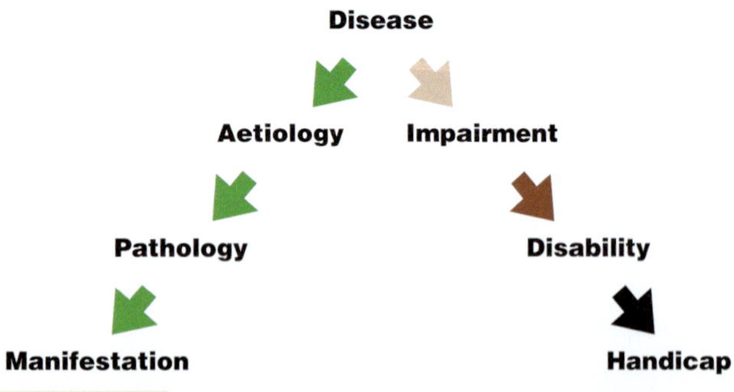

FIGURE 26.4 ■ The WHO parallel sequence for long-term illness. The aetiology of the disorder, known or unknown, gives rise to changes in structure or functioning, manifested as signs and symptoms, and collectively known as *impairment*. If the impairment alters functional performance or behaviour, it produces *disability*. When the impairment or disability places the person at a disadvantage within the community, a *handicap* occurs.

Community support programs

Community support programs offer a range of treatment and rehabilitation services, with a care coordination component to assess needs, coordinate care, monitor outcomes and assist the person to achieve recovery.

Community mental health support

Community mental health support is a vital component of care and the provision of clinical support to people with mental illness in the community. This support can range from short-term follow-up post-hospitalisation to assisting people in their recovery and re-engaging in their life, to longer-term support, depending on the needs of the person and the severity of their illness.

Community mental health care is provided through community mental health teams, which are comprised of a range of disciplines, including psychiatrists, nurses, occupational therapists, social workers and psychologists. Some teams also include peer workers. The community mental health teams provide an integrated approach to care, and this may include outpatient psychiatry clinics, walk-in services, acute and assertive clinical follow-up, and clinical rehabilitation services.

Community teams work closely with people, supporting them in the community, with the level of support catering to the individual needs of the person. This may mean that, if the person was acutely unwell, more support would be provided and, if necessary, they would work closely with the acute inpatient team to facilitate a hospital admission. As the person's mental health improved, the level of support would change to suit their needs.

Care coordination Care coordination is the linchpin for community support programs. This avoids the duplication and overlap of services. It also avoids shunting vulnerable people between services because of fluctuations in their clinical status.

The care coordinator coordinates a person's care to ensure seamless care is provided, and navigates their journey through the many available services. The care coordinator is not the only person who provides care, but they work as a guide, collaborating and supporting the person to access services. This includes involving a range of health professionals from within the team, and external non-government agencies as needed. The care coordinator is the consistent contact person and coordinator of care, regardless of where the person is in their recovery journey.

Fundamental and central to the role of the care coordinator is the relationship with the person requiring care. To be truly recovery-oriented, the negotiation and coordination of services is founded on collaboration with the person in need, so that services meet their explicit needs and not purely the needs of organisations or staff. People from high-risk groups, such as people with dual diagnoses, those who are homeless as well as mentally ill, and people who are frequently hospitalised may receive more intensive and clinically sophisticated forms of community-based care and specific care coordination to address their unique service requirements.

Residential services Recent reports continue to document the lack of affordable and decent housing options for many who are severely mentally ill, and their consequent concentration in what may be marginal or unsafe areas. Many people who are severely and persistently mentally ill live with families, but those who live alone frequently depend on residential hostels and boarding homes. It is difficult to generalise about the quality of these housing options, because they vary a great deal. For example, some boarding arrangements encourage autonomy and provide a warm, stable environment for residents. Other arrangements, however, fall far below standards that should be applied to living environments for people requiring intensive support, such as that described in the following Practice Example. While supported accommodation in hostels might offer some stability in housing and connection to others, research has also shown that people can experience hostel living arrangements as oppressive and gloomy, and this can cause a disconnect from their sense of identity (Bengtsson-Tops, Ericsson & Ehliasson, 2014).

Practice example

Lewis moved from one apartment to another in a different neighbourhood. During his clinic appointment, he told the nurse that the new apartment had a bug problem. There were huge numbers of cockroaches, spiders and moths in every room. The rental agency told Lewis to 'just handle it'.

The question of housing satisfaction can also be highly subjective. Some people prefer the privacy of a flat, despite what may be other negative features, such as location or limited living space. Other people prefer a more cozy, homelike environment. Programs with an active treatment component may be attractive to some people, but others appreciate a fairly calm and non-demanding environment, despite its monotony. For this reason, a community support system focuses not only on accessing some form of acceptable housing, but on evaluating the quality of that housing for the individual, working with the person to find a 'good fit'.

Medication use Medication regimens remain important aspects of treatment programs for the severely and persistently mentally ill. Research on the efficacy of medication, particularly neuroleptic regimens for schizophrenia, has historically demonstrated that these agents reduce rates of relapse and hospital re-admission. However, more recent research challenges this perception (Gotzsche, Young & Crace, 2015), and they are certainly not problem-free. Medication regimens demand adherence, tolerance of temporary and long-term side effects, and acceptance of the risk of long-term health problems, such as developing type 2 diabetes. Some secondary effects of medications can be uncomfortable and embarrassingly visible (e.g. obesity).

Medication can also come with a range of other problems, which are important to discuss with the person and develop effective plans to manage them. These side-effects can be managed, but take additional effort, and the person may need additional assistance. As mentioned above, a common side-effect is weight gain. Imagine how you would feel if you were a fit and healthy young person, and then you gained 20 kilos due to medication. This can have a very negative effect on the person's health and self-esteem, and can lead to a refusal to take medication. To manage this, the person needs support to have a healthy diet and regular exercise, and to work with the treating team to closely monitor the body's response, including blood screens for cholesterol and blood glucose. The impact of poor physical health is one of the biggest causes of reduced life expectancy in people with mental illness. Nonetheless, this can be managed, and a person can be fit and healthy, with support, education and commitment.

Medication services for the mentally ill should address the impact of medications on quality of life, and should promote collaboration with the person to develop a regimen that is tolerable and beneficial. *Depot medication therapy*, usually consisting of an injection every two to four weeks, forgoes the need to take medications several times a day, and is a valuable strategy for some people. Current advances in psychopharmacology have produced new classes of

HOW I WILL USE MY MENTAL-HEALTH SKILLS IN PRACTICE

Madison's story

I was 17 years old when I began working as a nurse's aide in a small long-term care facility. I was just starting university to become a nurse, and wanted experience working in the field. There were not very many people being cared for in the facility, because it was a private enterprise with the goal of making it as homelike as possible. I became close to all of the residents while learning to take care of them.

One woman, Louise, was extra special. She was only 50 years old, but had such debilitating and deforming arthritis that she could not care for herself and was no longer able to work as a psychiatric–mental health nurse. She was bright and personable, and I admired her strength of character in dealing with a chronic illness. Louise's roommate, Ida, was a bitter and negative woman, who rarely said anything neutral about her world or the people in it. A positive statement from Ida was unheard of. Ida's granddaughter came in to visit her, and she was so excited to show off her boyfriend's gift—a pretty pearl ring in a gold band. Ida's only comment was: 'Pearls mean sorrow.' Ida's granddaughter was devastated and left in tears. Ida's response to her roommate was: 'See? Pearls do mean sorrow.' Louise then reassured Ida that, even though her granddaughter was becoming close to her boyfriend, no one could take Ida's place. Ida, Louise told her, would always be Grandmother, and nothing could change that.

When I asked Louise later, in private, what was the connection between Ida being mean-spirited and Louise reassuring Ida, Louise's reply opened my eyes to the value of psychological sophistication. Louise said, 'When people feel threatened about being hurt by someone, they will put the energy into hurting that person first. Ida wasn't being mean, she was being hurt.' Being able to help someone cope with feelings, with what I now know are psychiatric–mental health nursing interactions, helped me choose the area for my nursing career.

medications that may prove less uncomfortable and socially limiting than standard treatments, and may help people who in the past have been resistant to medication, or non-adherent. The introduction of newer therapies makes the medication component of community care all the more important. At the same time, it is important to be aware of how disempowering it can be for people to be forcibly medicated when they question the benefits of those medications and/or when they experience very uncomfortable adverse effects.

Practice example

Ms Linnea is a 57-year-old widow who came into the medication clinic for her monthly injection, accompanied by her care coordinator. Ms Linnea has had a diagnosis of schizophrenia, paranoid type, for many years, but was maintained well with outpatient care and medications, requiring only brief crisis intervention and two short hospital stays by the time she was 50.

After her husband died, Ms Linnea had a severe decompensation, experiencing frightening hallucinations and delusions, and threatened her neighbours. The police were called, and she was hospitalised. Ms Linnea was stabilised on depot medications, and referred to a community-support program for assistance with both housing and rehabilitation. A care coordinator helped Ms Linnea apply for the Disability Support Pension (DSP), arranged for a shared apartment, facilitated medication and clinic appointments, visited her weekly, and encouraged regular participation in a social rehabilitation program. Ms Linnea has not required hospitalisation in six years. Although she still hears voices, she is able to monitor them and, whenever necessary, she seeks support to live with her voice-hearing experiences (Corstens, Longden, McCarthy-Jones, Waddington & Thomas, 2014).

Outpatient treatment Traditional outpatient psychotherapies that address *problems in living* may not meet the needs of all mentally ill persons, because some people require a broader range of support services to function well in the community. Many severely mentally ill individuals also require rehabilitation interventions that address their specific functional deficits and treatment goals, rather than insight-oriented therapies. These people need individual, family and group treatments that are sensitive to their particular problems and needs. Because the principles of rehabilitation for people with severe mental illness are followed in community treatment centres, they are an ideal option for this population.

Crisis stabilisation People with mental illness are at risk for acute exacerbations of their illness. This may be particularly true during times of stress or transition. But, in some cases, acute exacerbations are entirely unpredictable. In any case, this population requires access to acute assessment and treatment services as part of a package of community support, including 24-hour emergency and **crisis** units and outreach programs. Nursing expertise is extremely important in these emergency settings, because of the need for skilled and comprehensive assessment of acute problems. Crisis intervention can be disempowering and frightening. Boscarato et al. (2014) found that people prefer the involvement of known supports like family or friends, general practitioners, or mental health key workers. However, when this was not possible, research participants expressed a preference for the collaborative involvement of Crisis Assessment and Treatment (CAT) workers and police, rather than the police alone (Boscarato et al., 2014).

In addition to the need for crisis stabilisation because of acute exacerbation of psychiatric illness, people with severe mental illness are also frequent victims of violent crime. Up to one-third of people with severe mental illness are victims of violent crime, and the rate of being victimised is, in some circumstances, double that of the general population. When alcohol and drug use is involved, the rate of victimisation can be 140 times the rate of victimisation of the general population (Maniglio, 2009). Crisis stabilisation is often required in these situations, as well.

Mental Health in the Media discusses an individual who had ups and downs and subsequent homelessness as a result of substance abuse. He achieved sobriety, but relapsed when stressors affected his stability.

General health care People with severe mental illness are a medically under-served group in the community, with needs in the areas of primary health care, dental care and vision care. Health needs are most pronounced in subgroups such as those with co-occurring substance use problems and the elderly mentally ill, who have concurrent physical disorders. However, many people who are severely mentally ill are, to some extent, at risk from lifestyle factors (problematic housing or nutrition) or from the consequences of psychiatric treatment (problematic medication side-effects or medication interactions). Any person with a serious psychiatric diagnosis risks under-diagnosis of medical illness by both primary care and psychiatric providers.

In psychiatric services, clinicians may focus on mental disorders with inadequate attention to the total person. Only a small proportion of medical problems are diagnosed in physical assessments. Individuals most likely to be under-diagnosed are those who abuse substances, are elderly or are female. Community support and care coordination interventions can help those with severe mental illness obtain services, despite 'falling between the cracks' in systems that are poorly organised to meet the needs of people with multiple diagnoses.

Day programs Day treatment and partial hospitalisation programs provide continuity of care between the hospital and the outpatient sector in a less restrictive setting. These programs can also provide an alternative to hospital care for individuals who need complex treatment monitoring.

Day treatment programs offer groups and activities that provide for recreation and socialisation, and that help people function in the community. The role of leisure activities in improving recovery has been well established (Iwasaki et al., 2014). They may be used on a short-term basis for specific goals, or on a long-term basis for relapse prevention. Day programs are increasingly incorporating a recovery-oriented rehabilitation philosophy that maximises opportunities for meaningful activities in environments that are as 'normal' as possible, focusing on strengths rather than on pathology.

Family and network support Family support interventions are directed at reducing stress in the person's interpersonal environment and minimising the burden of care for family members. If people have little contact with families, interventions may target the people in their networks who provide them with support: friends, landlords, service providers.

With this emphasis on support to the supporters, interventions include the following:

- psychoeducational activities that increase knowledge about the disorder and reduce family stress
- practical assistance with information about homemaking or legal services
- respite services (short-term placements to relieve the family of the burden of care).

Such services have been widely recommended as a way to reduce the family's burden and enhance the quality of life of both client and family for the long-term (Spijker et al., 2011).

When you work with families of the severely and persistently mentally ill, becoming attuned to their concerns promotes recovery. Families may express ambivalence about caregiving. For example, they may want to promote the person's autonomy, yet feel discomfort or guilt about the type of living situation the person is able to maintain independently. Clear information and nonjudgmental attitudes from you and other providers can do much to alleviate a family's distress and assure them that there may not be a single ideal solution to their problems.

Advocacy Many of the difficulties people with severe mental illness experience in the community reflect a poor understanding of psychiatric illness among the general population, and inadequate resources for their needs. For example, access to housing is a function of resources and community acceptance. Attention to housing is futile if no residential resources exist, and vocational programs require access to employers. For this reason, one component of community support for people with severe and enduring mental illness is advocacy, or activities that increase access to resources. Advocacy can occur on an individual basis; for example, a care coordinator might intervene with a landlord to help a person obtain housing. Advocacy activities also occur at the level of the community, such as in programs for community education or outreach to employers.

When you provide rehabilitation services, you must have clear ideas of the person's rights as well as their responsibilities. Nurses often refer to these concepts in advocating for appropriate referrals and authorisations for treatment. A statement of rights helps focus our awareness on the most fundamental aspect of the nursing role, that of being an advocate. When you carry out your role in this framework, you bring to the multi-disciplinary team skills and knowledge that extend beyond biological or pathological aspects of care. You view the person through a holistic perspective. You piece together any fragmented pieces of the person's care to form a cohesive plan with the goal of recovery. This cannot be done in the isolation of an office or simply by telephone. It requires an active, on-site presence, interviews, meetings, attendance at treatment planning conferences, and appropriate documentation. The extent of your involvement is detailed in the Practice Example.

Practice example

Helen wanted to work in a nearby hotel food-service department. She was clear about her right to be hired without being discriminated against, but she was not clear about her responsibilities. Helen's care coordinator/nurse discussed the following responsibilities with her: behaving appropriately even if she is experiencing symptoms, interacting civilly even if she is angry, and telling her supervisor when she is having difficulty and needs help or support.

Families of people with more severe and disabling forms of mental illness have also assumed a much greater advocacy role than in the past. Family advocacy arose in response to

MENTAL HEALTH IN THE MEDIA

Ted Williams, the 'golden voice'

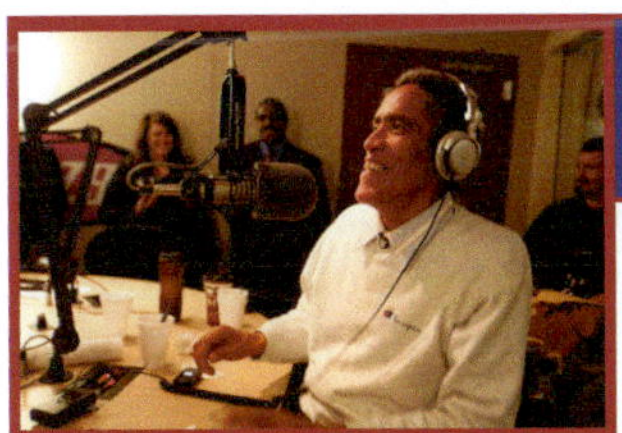

It all began with a cardboard sign held by a dishevelled homeless man standing on a wintry street. On the sign, the homeless man, Ted Williams, had written that he had a golden voice and would gladly accept donations. A journalist asked Ted Williams to demonstrate his voice, and Mr Williams, on the spot, recorded an accomplished radio promo. During the interview with the journalist, Mr Williams detailed how he had been a radio voice-over artist until his fortunes changed as a result of substance abuse (narcotics and alcohol), and he became homeless. The video was posted on YouTube and immediately went viral.

Mr Williams was subsequently interviewed on a number of television programs, where he discussed his life and his problems, and asserted that he had been clean and sober for two years and wanted a chance to prove himself to be a capable voice-over artist again. Subsequently, he received numerous job offers. He became the voice in advertisements for a food product, did network voice-over work, and hosted a television program. Reconciliations with many long-estranged family members accompanied the extensive media coverage.

Shortly thereafter, Mr Williams began drinking again when it became difficult for him to manage the stress of the media attention. During a television interview with a psychologist, Mr Williams agreed to enter a rehabilitation program. He was admitted, but checked himself out 12 days later. Within three months, Mr. Williams returned to a rehabilitation facility, and his job offers were withdrawn or put on hold indefinitely.

Ted Williams, the golden voice of radio, continues to pursue a successful course of recovery from substance abuse and a sober lifestyle. Along with many others in similar circumstances, he has encountered some difficulties and setbacks. However, his continued motivation and efforts are the necessary precursors to success.

Photo courtesy of Doral Chenoweth III/MCT/Newscom.

problems accompanying the deinstitutionalisation process that placed an enormous burden of care on families. It also developed in reaction to the stigmatisation of parents by the historical attribution of serious mental disorders to childrearing practices. The major family organisation for people with severe and persistent mental disorders is the Association of Relatives and Friends of the Mentally Ill (ARAFMI). The national and local chapters of ARAFMI have grown tremendously over the past 30 years, and have become a recognised force in mental health policy development.

PSYCHIATRIC REHABILITATION

Although the components of community support models provide the structure for services to people who are severely and persistently mentally ill, their effectiveness depends on the content of these component services. **Psychiatric rehabilitation** has an emphasis on the prevention or reduction of impairment or handicap (see Figure 26.4), as opposed to the treatment of disease, and serves as a guide for the content of practice at many levels of care. It includes an overall treatment philosophy, as well as specific interventions and programs.

Psychiatric rehabilitation philosophy

Psychiatric rehabilitation has its roots in theory about physical disabilities, and includes training and supportive interventions intended to increase functional status. Research in schizophrenia and related severe mental illness suggests that psychiatric rehabilitation facilitates social inclusion and functioning (Odes et al., 2011). Treatment addresses the disease process and its consequent symptoms. Rehabilitation approaches emphasise specific interventions to address targeted areas of functioning. Rehabilitation approaches are also strongly grounded in beliefs about empowerment, emphasising feelings of control and worth, particularly through the achievement of personal goals and wishes (Bitter, Roeg, van Nieuwenhuizen & van Weeghel, 2015).

Rehabilitation-oriented services begin with functional assessment and identification of highly individualised goals. A plan is developed to meet objectives by behavioural interventions that target specific functional deficits, or by environmental interventions that enable functioning with an existing deficit. From a rehabilitation perspective, it is important to extend support as long as possible. Support is not necessarily withdrawn because a person improves. For example, people doing well in supported employment programs would not be expected to necessarily 'graduate' to independent employment and thereby forfeit the support.

Rehabilitation philosophy is entirely consistent with the self-care and symptom management interventions developed by psychiatric–mental health nurses. In fact, rehabilitation theory and conceptual models in nursing share a common focus on functional adaptation in supportive environments.

Psychosocial rehabilitation centres/clubhouses

Although a rehabilitation philosophy can inform and enhance many treatment modalities, some specific rehabilitation programs make a unique contribution to service systems. One of the most important types of psychiatric rehabilitation programs is psychosocial rehabilitation. This particular model helps people reintegrate within their communities, improve their quality of life, and limit—or eliminate—frequent re-admission to hospital (Petersen, Lund & Stein, 2011; Svedberg, Svensson, Hansson & Jormfeldt, 2014; Wong, Stanton & Sands, 2014). Under a community support system structure, psychosocial rehabilitation modalities could be available at a day programming centre. Psychosocial services emphasise a collaborative relationship between staff and people seeking support, and provide experiences in a supportive but realistic milieu for the development of abilities for functioning in the real world, as in the Practice Example.

Practice example

Jackson has been attending a psychosocial rehabilitation centre, which functions as a clubhouse, regularly for a number of weeks. Playing pool and cards and taking classes in hip-hop provide him with opportunities to socialise with his peers. He can bring up his concerns informally with the professional staff, or in any one of a variety of planned group sessions.

The clubhouse model of psychosocial rehabilitation began in 1948 in New York, and was set up by a group of people recently discharged from a psychiatric hospital. There are now more than 300 clubhouses operating in 33 countries, including Australia and New Zealand. With a focus on strengths and abilities rather than deficits and symptoms, clubhouses welcome participants as 'members' rather than as clients or patients, and emphasise vocational achievement within the supported environment of the clubhouse. The supportive relationships developed between members change people's lives and help them to engage in the process of recovery (Raeburn, Halcomb, Walter & Cleary, 2013; Raeburn, Schmied, Hungerford & Cleary, 2014).

Supported employment

While all mental health programs have some emphasis on vocational rehabilitation, not all vocational programs conform to a psychiatric rehabilitation model. Supported employment models reflect a rehabilitation perspective because of their emphasis on adding support to the normal environment. This model delineates basic competencies that are necessary for employment, and offers classes that prepare people to set goals and choose a job focus. Once people are placed, they are supported by job coaches, who serve as role models, provide feedback and act as liaisons to employers.

Practice example

Mick was very good with numbers, organising and filing. His job coach found him a position in a shoe department of a large department store. His job was to take the shoes the customers tried on, return them to the proper box and file the box according to its number in the shoe storage area. Alicia, the job coach, accompanied Mick for the first several days in his new job. On his second day there was a shoe sale, and Mick became distressed and agitated because customers left so many shoes lying about. The job coach helped Mick calm down when he began yelling at the customers. Alicia ultimately had to find another placement for Mick, as an ability to manage stress turned out to be more important to his job success than his skill with numbers.

YOUR INTERVENTION STRATEGIES

Making something different happen: a scenario you can use to help people change

Making a change involves specific steps. This is a scenario you can use with people for whom you are caring: a person is walking down a particular street and falls into a huge hole. This happens over and over again: the person walks down the same street and falls into the same hole. Imagine the hole is a stressor or an interaction with someone that doesn't go well.

Making something different happen in your life will not be an automatic or instantaneous event. Change is a process and requires progressive steps of mental action.

Think of the following five steps to making a change:

1. At some point, you realise you are dissatisfied with a particular behaviour and you want it to change. 'I keep doing this, and I don't want to. I need to make a change.' *The idea that change is needed is an important first step.*
2. Now you walk down the street with the huge hole in it, and try to see the hole before you fall in it. *You may very well continue to perform the original, unsuccessful coping or interaction, but this step encourages you to recognise that you use it even though it does not work.*
3. Try to see the hole as soon as you walk down the street, then continue walking and fall in the hole. *The goal is to progress to anticipating earlier and earlier in the process your use of the unsuccessful coping or interaction.*
4. Walk down the street, see the hole as soon as you begin walking, and walk around the hole when you get to it. *This is an exciting step. You start coping or interacting. You recognise your tendency to use the original unsuccessful coping or interaction, and use the healthier and more competent step instead.*
5. Walk down a street that does not have a huge hole in it. *From now on you will use the effective coping or competent interaction. You have successfully made a change in your life.*

Social skills training

Social skills training methods are based on principles of social learning, and use behavioural techniques, such as role-playing, practising and reinforcement to promote the learning of instrumental role behaviour, as well as problem-solving abilities and interpersonal skills. Social skills training techniques may be incorporated into individual, group and family treatment modalities, where they may add measurable benefits. Your Intervention Strategies, above, suggests a useful analogy that you can use when encouraging people to change their behaviour.

Recognising and supporting people at risk

Subgroups of people with severe and enduring mental illness are at particularly high risk for poor outcomes, and are also extraordinarily difficult to serve in conventional programs. These subgroups include the following:

- people who have substance-related problems
- people who are homeless
- people with frequent re-admissions to acute care
- people who are frequently involved in the criminal justice system.

The interrelationships among these problems are complex, making it difficult to separate them or to distinguish root problems from their consequences. For example, substance use may exacerbate symptoms and lead to rehospitalisation. This in turn may disrupt stability of residence, increasing the possibility of arrest and reducing the likelihood of medication adherence. In other words, if individuals belong to one subgroup at risk, it is likely that they belong to several, thus increasing their overall vulnerability.

Concurrent substance-related disorders

Psychiatric illness greatly increases the odds of having a substance-related disorder. Alcohol has typically been the drug of choice with people who are severely mentally ill, perhaps because it is relatively inexpensive and easily accessible. Psychostimulant use has also increased among this population, a phenomenon partially attributed to the emergence of crack cocaine and methamphetamine as increasingly common drugs of abuse. Concurrent substance-related disorders are probably the most consistent predictor of re-admission to psychiatric hospitals.

Substance use contributes to a host of undesirable outcomes, which are thoroughly discussed in Chapter 13. It is highly correlated with homelessness and criminal justice system involvement (Maniglio, 2009). It is also a cause of concurrent medical morbidity, including exposure to HIV. Several of these risk-related behaviours are evident in the Practice Example.

Practice example

On her last admission to the inpatient unit for treatment of a manic episode, Emily had a persistent vaginal fungal infection that resisted treatment. Testing came back positive for the presence of HIV. Prior to this last admission, Emily had not taken her lithium for two months. As Emily's mania increased, so did her risk behaviour. When elated, Emily was disinhibited, so was willing to try anything, from alcohol to crack cocaine to unprotected sex with men she met at several bars she frequented. When her mood was elevated, Emily felt invulnerable.

For a variety of reasons involving different funding streams and different treatment philosophies, substance abuse services and psychiatric care are often poorly integrated. In mental health care systems, the dually-diagnosed person encounters little specific expertise related to drug or alcohol use. Severely mentally ill people sometimes do poorly in substance abuse programs that stress confrontation or demand sobriety as a precondition to treatment. Integrated programs for the dually-diagnosed mentally ill include inpatient and day treatment programs as well as group interventions.

Homelessness and mental illness

Homelessness is at an all-time high among people with mental illness (Paquin, 2011). The goal of providing acceptable and long-term housing remains elusive, particularly in urban centres. While the proportion of people with mental illness in the community who are permanently homeless is thought to be relatively small, a large and heterogeneous group experiences spells of residential instability (see Figure 26.5 ■). Although mental health service policy in Australia aims to ensure discharge from hospital into stable accommodation, it is not always possible (Williams & Stickley, 2011; Moore, Gerdtz, Hepworth & Manias, 2011).

Practice example

Rob, aged 29 years, was referred to an intensive care coordination team after his third hospital admission within a year. Rob has a diagnosis of schizoaffective disorder, but it is unclear whether his diagnosis accounts for his frequent acute episodes, or whether the episodes are precipitated by his use of stimulants and alcohol. Rob has no stable place of residence, and has stayed in shelters over the past few years. He describes himself as too preoccupied with his survival needs to seek treatment between emergency episodes. He claims that alcohol helps him manage his anxiety and his 'voices' when he is on the streets.

The homeless outreach team will first address Rob's need for safe housing. The team will then work with Rob to help him acknowledge that alcohol and drugs can increase his discomfort, and to support his use of psychotropic medication. When Rob is stabilised, he will work with the team and consider other treatment goals.

Whether these periods of homelessness involve movement between transient accommodations or actual street dwelling, they impose very harsh living conditions on people who are highly vulnerable. Homelessness interferes with the ability to use services, including the use of psychotropic medications. It increases the risk of trauma, substance abuse, infectious disease exposure and victimisation. Homelessness also makes conventional services unworkable, because the undomiciled can rarely store medication and use regular outpatient services. Those who are homeless and mentally ill are likely to experience several barriers to beginning, maintaining and completing treatment. Several practical matters—establishing a medication routine, having access to health care providers, having an actual address or telephone, and being supported by friends and family—are the usual barriers faced by homeless people. Living independently in the community is possible when there is a consistent set of circumstances, daily routines, privacy and a secure base in which to feel capable (Pati, 2011). In many geographical locations, a dominant 'treatment first' approach persists, whereby individuals must meet a hierarchy of program requirements before becoming eligible for an apartment of their own. This persists as a barrier.

Services to the homeless include supported housing models with care coordination components, shelter-based rehabilitation and substance abuse services, and mobile outreach teams to identify people needing support and link them with services. Care coordination services are particularly important to manoeuvre through the labyrinth of services and entitlements. While shelters and emergency programs serve a

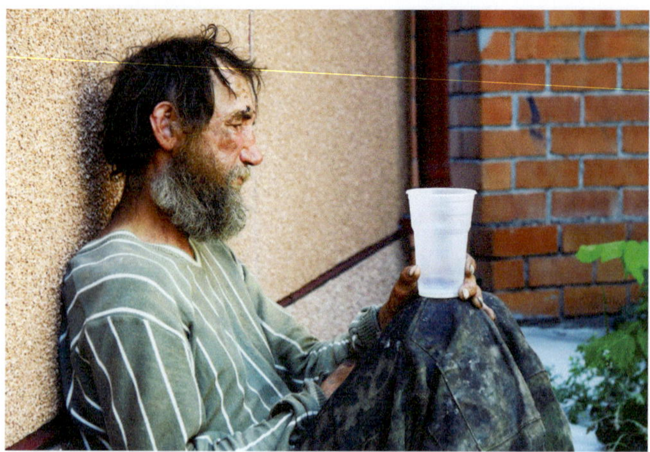

FIGURE 26.5 ■ Estimates of the extent of homelessness among the mentally ill range from 25 per cent to more than 50 per cent. Whichever number is more accurate, it is clear that the mentally ill constitute a prominent subgroup among the homeless.
Photo courtesy of Wrangler/Shutterstock.

critical short-term need, they also contribute to instability. It is preferable, by far, to develop permanent housing for people with psychiatric disabilities. In Australia, the national peak body for homelessness is Homelessness Australia (HA), which provides systemic advocacy for the homelessness sector. They work in collaboration with homelessness assistance services, state and national homelessness peak organisations, other peak organisations, government agencies and the broader community (http://www.homelessnessaustralia.org.au/).

HIV

The homeless mentally ill who live in urban areas, particularly those who live in municipal shelters, are at particular risk for HIV and other communicable diseases. The high incidence of injection drug use in this population, along with exchanging sex for drugs or money, makes them more vulnerable. The specific cognitive barriers that result from mental illness and HIV infection add to the difficulty of obtaining prophylactic or early treatment. Nevertheless, Australia has maintained a low rate of HIV infection and a high rate of treatment for those infected, compared with the rest of the world.

HIV disease is disproportionately prevalent among individuals already at the economic edge, and those who are targets of discrimination in housing and medical care: people of colour, homosexuals, injection drug users, and homeless and runaway youth. Fatigue, repeated hospitalisations and recurring illnesses all require time off from work, resulting first in the loss of employment, then in the loss of housing. Although most people with an impaired immune system can live independently, they require a safe environment that helps them avoid exposure to infectious diseases, and allows them to get adequate rest, meet their special nutritional needs, and have access to support services and home help when necessary.

People requiring frequent re-admission

Virtually all severe and persistent disorders will involve some kind of relapse at some time; more than one or two admissions

Box 26.2 Why frequent re-admissions are problematic

Frequent re-admission to acute psychiatric settings is a problem for several reasons, including:

1. it represents a considerable expense
2. it is a signal of relapse, indicating severe difficulties for the individual
3. it suggests a failure of the community system to link the individual between acute episodes with meaningful and accessible services, and to institute the type of treatment and monitoring that might manage symptomatic shifts without hospitalisation.

in 12 months exceed norms. Box 26.2 identifies why frequent admissions are unhealthy and problematic.

Individual-based factors that contribute to frequent re-admission include substance abuse, which may be the best predictor of re-admission. Cycling through emergency and acute care has been attributed to a 'chronic crisis' style among people in some diagnostic groups, particularly those with certain personality disorders. However, many younger people with schizophrenia and bipolar disorder use alcohol and drugs to combat boredom and medication side-effects, and to self-medicate or treat symptoms in what they consider a 'normal' way.

On a systems level, re-admission may reflect a failure to link the person with services that they consider meaningful and accessible. The system as a whole may respond best to people who 'fit' into programs and benefit from treatment alone. Those with more social needs or less acceptance of their illness may not consider ambulatory services relevant to their needs, and may instead require assertive outreach to link them with appropriate outpatient providers.

Frequent criminal justice system involvement

The prevalence rates of major psychiatric disorders in jails have increased gradually but continuously, at least in part because of deinstitutionalisation policies. Society has a low tolerance for disordered behaviour, and the lack of services for the severely and persistently mentally ill in the mental health care system leads to a funnelling into the criminal justice system. Almost half of prisoners (49 per cent) in Australia had been told by a professional that they had a mental illness (including substance abuse disorders) (Australian Institute of Health and Welfare [AIHW], 2015). This represented an overall increase of 29 per cent from 2012 data. Almost 27 per cent of prisoners were currently taking prescribed medication for a mental illness. The AIHW (2015) also reported that, of young Australian adults aged 20–30 years, nearly one-third (32 per cent) of those with a mental illness has been arrested across a 10-year period. Quite often the first arrest occurred before the person had been engaged with mental health services and diagnosed with an illness.

Unemployment, homelessness and substance abuse contribute to the profile of the severely mentally ill forensic person. Many forensic inpatient services are filled to capacity. Most mentally ill offenders end up in jails rather than in forensic mental hospitals; they rarely become connected with local mental health networks, and are frequently counted among the homeless because they have no fixed address. Psychiatric–mental health nurses provide valuable care coordination and advocacy services for this specific population, as well as for people with severe mental illness at high-risk in general.

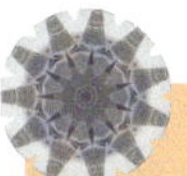

STEPS TO RECOVERY

Recovery is a process that has important components that have previously been discussed. However, keep in mind that changes in an individual person's circumstances and preferences require ongoing needs assessment and adjustment of the plan for achieving recovery.

Assessing needs

Nurses who work collaboratively with people with the goal of recovery interact with all members of the health care team to create, with the person, a recovery plan. Trust, mutual support and clear communication among team members are necessary. If the person is determined to need, and want, particular educational activities, your role as the nurse is to develop a plan in a collaborative manner to promote the successful acquisition of an educational experience. Similarly, stable living arrangements contribute significantly to the ability of a person to achieve recovery. Your involvement in person-centred care includes prioritising, so that people have the underpinnings that maximise the probability of success.

Planning for rehabilitation and recovery

In this phase of care, you can bring valuable information concerning benefits, limits, family resources, expectations and other pertinent data to the recovery planning table. For example, the Commonwealth Government has funded programs supporting people with serious mental illness to live, with support, in the community. Notable programs include the Personal Helpers and Mentors Scheme (PHaMS), Partners in Recovery (PIR) and the Mental Health Nurse Incentive Program (MHNIP). Using the formal and informal support systems, the treatment team is able to set mutually agreed-upon goals with desired outcomes, and can begin to plan action steps, using person-driven timeframes or critical pathways as a guide.

Spirituality

An important component of coping with a chronic illness, and having successful experiences, is having an outlet for spirituality. This portion of the recovery plan honours the person's preferences and needs. People who find a system of meaning within which to function tend to have more satisfying outcomes (Onyango et al., 2011). Spirituality can enhance and support a person's recovery through strengthening psychosocial wellbeing.

There is no need to have formal religiosity in order to be a spiritual person, although many people do prefer the structure of the rituals and religious practices. Being a member of a community seems to be the important feature. A spiritual person who has contact with other like-minded individuals, and feels accepted and appreciated, is unlikely to be or feel alone in the world.

Voluntary community activities

Having a structure and purpose to one's daily activities provides healing and a sense of accomplishment (Arbesman & Logsdon, 2011). Voluntary activity is a way to be involved with others in a variety of settings that do not place premature demands on the person. Volunteering also offers a way for people to master complex skills at their own pace while experiencing an activity level that can meet their individual needs.

Another benefit of volunteering comes from helping another person cope with a problem similar to one's own (Firmin et al., 2015). This is a feature of adult learning that reinforces learning. Most people find that teaching others is an excellent way to incorporate meaningful information. This, along with contributing to someone else's recovery, is a powerful message that the person has succeeded to a certain degree on the road to recovery and has something to offer the community.

Psychopharmacology and recovery

Combining maintenance antipsychotic medication therapy with psychosocial approaches has been found to be more effective than pharmacotherapy alone in delaying or preventing relapse, and promoting clinical recovery. When symptoms become less manageable or stressors increase, early intervention has been found to be effective in preventing relapse in people with a mental disorder. This could be accomplished through close personal, collaborative or family monitoring for the person's particular *early warning signs* (those symptoms that occur early in the relapse process for that person, such as a change in sleep pattern). Once identified, discussion about the need for intervention with antipsychotic medication needs to occur, as it might reduce the overall intensity of the relapse event (Emsley, Kilian & Phahladira, 2016).

Programs for relapse prevention typically combine standard doses of maintenance antipsychotic medication with psychosocial treatment, and result in lower relapse rates (Geddes & Miklowitz, 2013). Weekly group therapy is an opportunity to discuss early warning symptoms, as it is important that people learn to identify them for themselves so that they might seek help early. A multi-family group component might be helpful to support and educate the families, as well as provide peer contacts and here-and-now experiences.

Those who live more independently and experience relapses could benefit from a community contact, such as a regular follow-up with their general practitioner, or a mental health nurse providing services under the Medicare initiative known as the Mental Health Nurse Incentive Program (MHNIP) (Happell, Palmer & Tennent, 2011). Prevention is more effective when people and their families understand the likely relapse triggers, as outlined in Table 26.1 ■.

Other aspects of relapse prevention have been implemented clinically with good results. People with a psychosis not responsive

TABLE 26.1 ■ Relapse triggers in mental disorder

Physiological stressors		
Infection	Pain	Dehydration
Acute illness	Fatigue	Surgery
Chronic illness	Side-effects of medications	Injury
Failure to take prescribed medications	Appetite changes	Insomnia
Personal stressors		
Negative symptoms of schizophrenia	Financial difficulties Depression	Exacerbation/relapse of illness
Spiritual distress	An increase in responsibility	Pet loss/illness/ageing
Recreational activity	Maturational/developmental changes	Decreased access to resource choice
Interpersonal stressors		
Interpersonal conflict	Loss of job or status within a job	Conflict, anger
Relationship changes (family, intimate relationships, friendships)	Altered contact with another or others	Perceived rejection/abandonment
Community stressors		
Difficulties making living arrangements	Disruption of living situation	Roommate/family stressors
	Transportation	Community disruption

to pharmacotherapy may benefit from specific cognitive behavioural therapies (see Chapter 25), while people with persistent negative symptoms and limited social competence may find social skills training useful. Successful outcomes for individuals and their families occur with psychological support, behavioural treatments, social and cognitive rehabilitation, assistance in social and scholastic activities, enhancement of social skills, and family support (Masi & Liboni, 2011). In addition, new programs of supported employment may enable some people to maintain competitive employment.

Implementing the rehabilitation and recovery plan

The next phase of the recovery process is to ensure that the person obtains any needed care. You and the person will take the opportunity to look at the whole picture of their needs and abilities, and keep up-to-date on changes in the plan. As a care coordinator, you will contribute time and resources to monitor the quantity and quality of care delivered.

Keep in mind during the implementation phase that your role involves conflict resolution. The skills needed to work with a person and manage relationships within a large mental health provision system include:

- setting limits tactfully
- arbitrating differences
- maintaining the focus on successful outcomes for all.

LIVED EXPERIENCE

What recovery really means to me

Recovery is about capturing that hope again, finding who you are and who you want to be, and not letting your life be defined by your illness. For me, when I took those first steps towards recovery after many years of illness, I looked forward to my future. I had renewed confidence and thought to myself, 'Why can't I think about future plans instead of thinking that they're not possible just because I'm sick?' For me, recovery was realising that I had a life I could look forward to, and not the feeling that my life was over. I started to look at my goals, my hopes and my future, and started thinking about what I needed to do. Recovery also made me look at my illness in a different way. It made me ask questions about my diagnosis and treatment, and it made me realise that it's okay to ask for help, and with help I could still live the life I had hoped for.

In order to contribute positively to an outcome of rehabilitation and recovery, you need patience, maturity and experience. You may also be called upon to provide additional data or consumer/family education where a denial or extension of service is in question. As an advocate, you may identify gaps in care that require action in the community, in a treatment facility or within the nursing system. Your recovery focus makes you the best consultant to nursing departments for improving quality, because you view problems in the system from the person's perspective.

Evaluating the rehabilitation and recovery plan

Evaluating progress towards the recovery goal consists of continuous monitoring of intervention responses and progress towards desired outcomes. This may include discussions to discover and manage side-effects of psychotropic medications (see Chapter 7), medication monitoring for dosage and adherence, as well as monitoring individual responses to other therapies, such as counselling and activities. The evaluation is made together with the person, incorporating ancillary information when available. Perhaps the process is moving too slowly for the person, or the plan needs to be adjusted for more realistic shorter-term goals.

An important feature of any recovery plan is the active participation of the person. Flexibility and honest discussion help establish a workable document that is not static. Focus on proximal goals and make a point of acknowledging achievement at every stage. Every individual has the right to expect recovery; every nurse has the responsibility to contribute faithfully and energetically to that goal.

LIVED EXPERIENCE

Crisis is unmanageable

I usually manage my life quite well. I work and I have some good friends and family around me. There are also times when everything gets to be too much. I feel pressured at work, or something goes wrong and I feel like a failure. I start to feel very tense and anxious, and I feel like a dark cloud has moved in. Then I feel completely unable to cope . . . and that's when I cut myself.

CRISIS INTERVENTION

On 11 September 2001, hijackers crashed two airliners into New York City's World Trade Center, toppling its twin 110-story towers. This disaster was witnessed on television screens across the world as a third plane slammed into the Pentagon, and a fourth crashed outside Pittsburgh. The death toll, numbering almost 3000, included firefighters, police officers and medical personnel killed while attempting to rescue victims. The impact on New York City was horrific. Many people lost their jobs, because business premises were demolished and tourists stayed away. Even the usual winter holiday festivities, for which New York City is famous, were conducted with an air of great sadness. Consider your own experience of this event by working through the questions in Box 26.3. The impact on the rest of the country—survivors, citizens and visitors alike—and around the world was tremendous, as these Practice Examples illustrate.

Practice examples

Nguyen, a visitor from Malaysia, was walking across the Brooklyn Bridge, admiring the view of lower Manhattan, when he saw the plane hit the first tower. He stood on the bridge in horror, watching the fireball and then people jumping from the high-rise buildings. Although he has long since returned to Malaysia, he has nightmares in which he relives the experience over and over.

Two teenagers were at home in Arizona watching TV while getting ready for school when they saw the news. First they experienced sadness, then disbelief, confusion, anger and, finally, fear. One said, 'Now I know that terrorism isn't just something you see on the evening news that happens on the other side of the world. My life has been changed forever.'

Tadeusz works at an airport outside Warsaw, Poland. People were gathered around him, chatting about the disaster, crying and praying. Tadeusz left work sick that day. He told his supervisor that he felt nauseated and weak in the knees at the thought that airplanes at his airport could be targeted and that life was so fragile.

The research literature suggests that more people need treatment for mental health difficulties than for physical symptoms following an injury-causing agent or event. The mental health risks include not only post-traumatic stress

Box 26.3 Your experience of crisis

Do you remember how you felt on Tuesday, 11 September 2001 (12 September in Australia and New Zealand)? Did you feel helpless? Did you know what to do or say to others? Did you fear for someone you knew who was in the United States at the time? Did you call anyone? Did you talk about the event with others? Did you want it all to go away? If you answered 'yes' to any of these questions, you know what a crisis feels like. Chances are that you, your family and your community were in crisis, along with many other individuals, families and communities.

disorder (PTSD), but also acute stress disorder, depression, complicated bereavement reactions, substance use disorders, fear, anxiety, somatisation, anger control, and arrest or regression of childhood developmental progression (DelGaizo, Elhai & Weaver, 2011; Claassen, Kashner, Kashner, Xuan & Larkin, 2011). Communities exposed to a crisis, even communities distant from the threat or the disaster, face an acute 'mental health surge' that can overwhelm available community mental health resources. Recent developments in health care preparedness have addressed some of these needs; however, further investigation and investment are required (Raphael & Ma, 2011).

A crisis is an acute, time-limited state of disequilibrium resulting from situational, developmental or societal sources of stress. An individual can be said to be in crisis when they are in a situation in which their usual problem-solving or adaptive methods are inadequate to resolve a problem or conflict, causing a state of disequilibrium. People involved in these incidents may be unable to effectively manage stressful events or environmental changes. They may be unable to function and may feel paralysed and powerless. Some examples of key crises that are deeply etched into the memories of Australians include:

- the Eureka stockade riot and insurrection, which occurred at Ballarat, Victoria, on 3 December 1854, during which at least 27 people died
- the West Gate bridge collapse in Melbourne in 1970, which resulted in the deaths of 35 construction workers
- Cyclone Tracey, which decimated the city of Darwin on 24 December 1974 and 71 people died
- the Ash Wednesday fires across Victoria and South Australia in February 1983, resulting in the deaths of 75 people
- the Port Arthur massacre on 28 April 1996, which left 35 people dead
- the Thredbo landslide on 30 July 1997, resulting in 18 lives lost
- the Black Saturday bushfires in Victoria in February 2009, resulting in the deaths of 173 people
- the Queensland floods from December 2010 to January 2011, leaving 38 people dead with six missing, presumed dead.

Similar critical events affecting New Zealanders include:

- the eruption of Mount Tarawera on 10 June 1886, which destroyed the Pink and White Terraces, then the 8th Wonder of the World, with a significant loss of life
- the Napier earthquake on 3 February 1931, and its subsequent fires, which, combined, killed 256 and left thousands injured
- the Tangiwai disaster, when a lahar (a volcanic mudflow) at 10.21pm on Christmas Eve 1953 plunged an express train into a flooded river at Tangiwai, killing 151 people
- the sinking of the ferry *Wahine* in a storm on 10 April 1968, killing 53, witnessed by the people of Wellington
- the crashing of Air New Zealand Flight 901 into Mount Erebus, in Antarctica, during a white-out on 28 November 1979, killing all 257 passengers and crew
- the Canterbury earthquakes on 4 September 2010 and 22 February 2011, the second, at 6.3 on the Richter scale, killing 165 people, injuring 1500–2000, and leaving thousands more homeless
- the Pike River Mine disaster, a lethal gas explosion in a coal mine on 19 November 2010, which left 29 miners trapped underground, who were later believed to have died after a second explosion on 24 November.

It is likely that the New York terrorist attack in 2001 (and other large-scale crisis events) will continue to have effects such as PTSD far into the future (DiGrande, Neria, Brackbill, Pulliam & Galea, 2011; Raphael & Ma, 2011). Years after the event, mothers and adolescents—who were children when 9/11 occurred—had symptoms of depression and post-traumatic stress disorder (Gershoff, Aber, Ware & Kotler, 2010). Those who study what happens to the survivors of catastrophes—natural or manmade—find similar disruptions of psychosocial health of great concern (Berger, 2011). Adolescents who experienced or witnessed violence had different coping mechanisms regardless of gender (Reid-Quiñones et al., 2010). Aggressive and avoidant responses by victims as well as witnesses indicate that more attention should be given to how youth cope with violence. Other examples of situations that have caused a crisis are outlined in the following Practice Examples.

Practice examples

An ex-employee comes into an office building and shoots people; a tragic school bus accident claims five six-year-old children and their teacher; two teenagers from the same high school kill themselves in the same week; a 66-year-old man retires and feels useless and considers suicide; a 23-year-old woman finds out that she has a fatal illness; a premature baby is born; a 12-year-old child is kidnapped while walking home from school.

Nurses are intimately connected with crises. We often interact with people who are faced with new, frightening and troublesome situations. Because of who we are, where we work, and our accessibility to individuals and families, we are in a position to offer supportive and therapeutic interventions that can change people's lives. You can help if you understand how to effectively intervene; that is, if you understand how to implement crisis intervention skills. *Crisis intervention* is a conceptual framework for intervention that calls for short-term, action-oriented assistance focused on problem-solving, with a goal of restoring the individual's equilibrium. Effective crisis intervention will call for all the skills that a well-prepared nurse can muster (Yin, He, Arbon & Zhu, 2011).

Crisis intervention is not the specialty of any one professional group. People who intervene in crises come from the fields of nursing, medicine, psychology, social work and theology. Police officers, teachers, school guidance counsellors, rescue workers and bartenders, among others, are often on-the-spot crisis interveners.

Crisis as a turning point

The word 'crisis' stems from the Greek *krinein*, 'to decide'. In Chinese, two characters are used to write the word: one is the character for danger, and the other the character for opportunity. The interaction between danger and opportunity will become clearer as you read the rest of this chapter.

Crisis situations are turning points or junctures in a person's life that result in a new equilibrium. The new equilibrium may be close to that of the pre-crisis state, or it may be a more positive or more negative state. If the new equilibrium is more positive, the person experiences personal growth, increased competence, a better social network, new-found problem-solving abilities or an improved self-image. If the new equilibrium is more negative, the individual may lose skills, regress to an earlier developmental stage, develop socially unacceptable behaviours, or develop a mental disorder. Unsuccessful negotiation of a crisis leaves the person feeling anxious, threatened and ineffective. Individuals may also respond to a crisis event with disturbed personal coping or with frankly psychotic behaviour. This process is illustrated in Figure 26.6 ■.

Because a state of disequilibrium is so uncomfortable, a crisis is self-limiting. That is, even without intervention, a crisis will resolve itself with either a favourable or an unfavourable conclusion. Studies indicate that those who experience crisis with an unfavourable conclusion, and do not seek or are not involved in some form of mental health treatment, tend to be more vulnerable to mental health issues such as depression and PTSD. This is why crisis intervention is sometimes called 'primary prevention for PTSD'. The following Evidence-based Practice discusses the characteristics of those at risk for mental health problems following a crisis.

Common characteristics of crises

To understand the concept of crisis fully, and to appreciate the interaction of risk factors, we must differentiate among levels of distress to illustrate what a crisis is not. Stress is not crisis. Everyone feels stress at various times, in a variety of forms (see the discussion in Chapter 8). Stress is pressure and tension. Stressful situations may demand our attention and may be exhausting, but they are not crises. An emergency is a situation that often demands an immediate response to ensure the survival of an individual. Although neither stress nor an emergency are themselves a crisis, stress or an emergency can ultimately precipitate a crisis. A crisis is not a mental disorder. A crisis can happen to someone who has never had a mental disorder or to someone who is currently experiencing a mental disorder. Common characteristics of crises are discussed in Box 26.4.

Resilience, risk factors and balancing factors

Why do some people effectively manage disequilibrium while others go into crisis? This capacity is called resilience. *Resilience* is the ability not only to survive and bounce back from difficult and traumatic experiences, but also to continue to grow and develop emotionally and psychologically. The notion

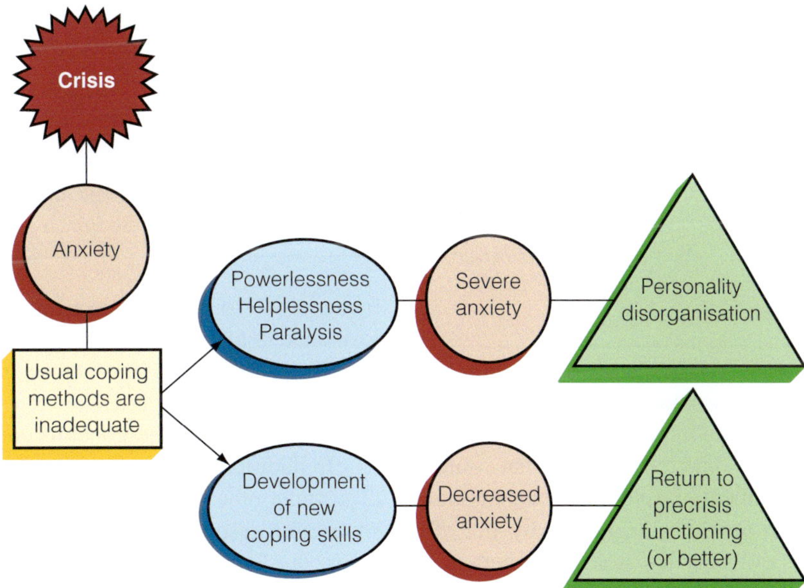

FIGURE 26.6 ■ The progression of a crisis to either successful or unsuccessful resolution depends on what people do when they discover that their usual coping mechanisms are ineffective.

EVIDENCE-BASED PRACTICE

Tangible support for a person in crisis

Crises occur when someone is personally attacked, has a dire set of circumstances or has their worldview disrupted. Nurses practise with people in these situations in a variety of settings. One of the main goals is to minimise the risk of psychological disorder, or a worsening of a disorder, for people experiencing the crisis. The set of common symptoms to assess and address would be depressive symptoms.

Mrs Taylor, a middle-aged Australian Aboriginal woman, has been referred for a crisis evaluation to the Crisis Assessment and Treatment team (CAT) in which you work. It has been several weeks since the death of her husband from a medical condition. In reviewing her records, you note that she has had several hospitalisations for crisis-type episodes, severe anxiety and depression over recent years.

She is tearful and anxious, and appears to be suffering from depression. She expresses sadness at the death of her husband. She has three adult children and many grandchildren, but has no siblings or surviving parents. It transpires that Mrs Taylor has recently met with a commissioner who interviewed her as part of the Royal Commission into Institutional Responses to Child Sexual Abuse. It seems that Mrs Taylor has been re-experiencing trauma from her childhood following the interview. She was taken into care by government authorities when she was only a few months old, and so she lost all connection with her family. She spent her childhood in institutional care, and suffered extreme verbal, physical, emotional and sexual abuse until she met and married her husband, who was also an Australian Aborigine. She describes their relationship as a 'pretty good' one, and says 'I don't know what I'll do without him.'

You know by your review of the literature that the risk of depression and other mental illnesses are significantly increased in Aboriginal people, particularly those who belong to what is now known as 'the Stolen Generations' (children who were forcibly removed from their families on the basis of their race—being Aboriginal—according to government policy in operation from 1905 until the 1970s). The subsequent loss of connection to family and culture continues to have severe effects on the mental health and wellbeing of Indigenous Australians today (Cunningham & Paradies, 2012; Li, D'Arcy & Meng, 2016). It is also known that racism continues to contribute to the incidence of depressive symptoms in Indigenous Australians (Paradies & Cunningham, 2012).

CRITICAL THINKING QUESTIONS

1. How would you support Mrs Taylor at this time?
2. How is it possible for Mrs Taylor to overcome the trauma and loss associated with her childhood experiences?

Source: Commonwealth of Australia. (1997). *Report of the National Inquiry into the Separation of Aboriginal and Torres Strait Islander Children From Their Families*. Canberra, Australia: Commonwealth of Australia.

Box 26.4 Common characteristics of crises

- Many situational crises are experienced as sudden. The person is usually not aware of a warning signal, whether or not others could 'see it coming'. The individual or family may feel that they have had little or no preparation for the event or trauma.
- The crisis may be experienced as ultimately life-threatening, whether this perception is realistic or not.
- Communication with significant others is often reduced or cut off.
- There may be perceived or real displacement from familiar surroundings or significant loved ones.
- All crises have an aspect of loss, whether actual or perceived. The losses can include an object, a person, a hope, a dream or any significant factor for that individual.

Box 26.5 Risk factors for crisis

- Intensity of exposure to the situation
- Pre-existing psychiatric symptoms and diagnosis
- Prior history of traumatic exposure
- Family history of psychiatric problems, anxiety and/or antisocial behaviour
- Early separation from parents
- Childhood abuse
- Poverty
- Cultural expectations that prohibit asking others for help
- Degree of threat to life (being on a plane that crashes versus watching a plane crash from a distance)

of resilience encompasses the biological and psychological characteristics intrinsic to an individual, such as personality style and the quality of interpersonal relationships that confer protection against the development of psychopathology (Bhui & Dinos, 2011). Resilience probably explains why not all people who are stressed and socially isolated experience mental health problems (Cacioppo, Reis & Zautra, 2011). Researchers and clinicians alike have been surprised by the prevalence of the capacity for resilience, and clinicians are beginning to focus on uncovering and energising pathways to resilience in their clients (Shpiegel, 2016).

There are several risk factors, in addition to the nature of the trauma or the experience itself, that place individuals at high risk for crisis. These factors are identified in Box 26.5.

In addition to these risk factors, the presence or absence of certain other events or situations are important to the successful resolution of disequilibrium. These are called *balancing factors*. For example, how do individuals perceive and understand the event/crisis in their lives? Are they being punished? Is this happening only to them and never to anyone else? How will the event affect their future? Do they see the situation realistically, or is it distorted? *Situational supports* are also important. Are there people in their lives who can help them solve the problem? Meaningful relationships with others give support and assistance during the crisis. Individuals with inadequate support are likely to experience a decrease in self-esteem. In turn, lowered self-esteem may make an event appear more threatening. An individual's *coping mechanisms* may add or detract from the successful resolution of disequilibrium caused by crisis.

All people use mechanisms to cope with anxiety and tension. Because the individual has used these coping mechanisms with success in the past, they become part of the coping repertoire. These tension-relieving mechanisms can be obvious or subtle; see the discussion in Chapter 8. If an individual has a realistic perception of the traumatic event or crisis, adequate situational support, and adequate coping mechanisms, the problem will be resolved and equilibrium will be regained, making it unlikely that a crisis will result. If, however, one or more of these important factors are absent, the problem is likely to be unresolved, disequilibrium is likely to continue, and a state of crisis will result (Aguilera, 1998).

Biopsychosocial theories of crisis

The recognition of crisis has a long history. It was not until the 20th century, however, that strategies for helping people to cope with crisis were developed. Theories of crisis and crisis intervention resulted from early research studies that are now classics, as well as more recent events in the field of mental health. Some of these are described in the following section.

The aetiology, psychobiology, epidemiology, comorbidity and treatment of crisis and its sequelae are complicated. Mental Health in the Media highlights one such complicated crisis. Some theories that attempt to explain what happens in a crisis, and how to intervene in a crisis, are described next.

Tyhurst's stages of disaster

Tyhurst (1957) identified three overlapping stages in response to a disaster. They are:

1. impact
2. recoil
3. post-trauma.

These stages are as relevant today as they were then, and they help mental health care workers understand the experiences of the victims of hurricanes, floods, fires, terrorist attacks and other disasters, as well as the people who experienced the disaster by watching it at home on their television sets.

Impact The first stage, impact, is stimulated by the catastrophe. Victims recognise what is happening to them, and are concerned mainly with the present. During this acute phase, the victim's major concern may be staying alive. According to Tyhurst, about 75 per cent of victims experience shock and confusion. Although they appear dazed, they also exhibit the physical signs of fear. Another group of people, up to 25 per cent, remain coherent. They logically and rationally assess the situation, and develop and implement a plan for dealing with the immediate problems brought on by the catastrophe. A third group, also up to 25 per cent, may panic or become immobilised with fear. They may behave hysterically, or they may be overlooked because they sit and silently stare into space, despite the possibility that remaining fixed to the spot might put them at further risk.

Recoil In recoil, the second stage, the initial stress of the disaster has passed, and victims may no longer find their lives in immediate danger, although injuries and other discomforts come to their awareness. Emergency shelter, food and clothing become available. The victims' behaviour is usually dependent—they want to be taken care of. Weeping is common as survivors begin to realise all that has happened to them.

Post-trauma The full impact of the losses the victims have experienced comes in the third, or post-trauma, period. Grief is a predominant response to the losses in their lives. Disturbed and psychotic responses may occur.

Caplan's stages of a crisis reaction

Caplan (1964) studied various developmental crises, such as reactions to premature births, infancy, childhood and adolescence, as well as accidental crises such as illness and death. Caplan built upon Tyhurst's work with disaster

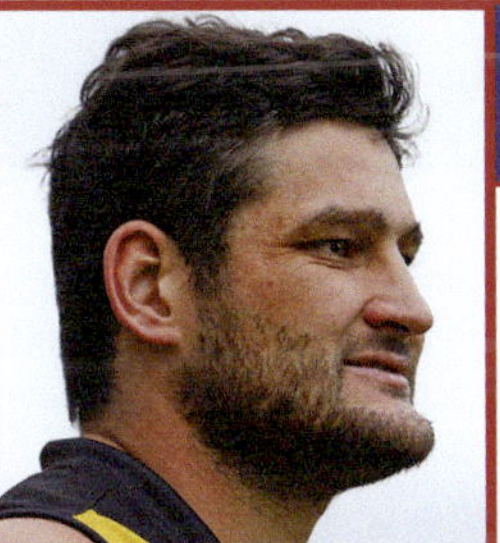

MENTAL HEALTH IN THE MEDIA

Brendan Fevola

Brendan Fevola, a celebrated Australian Rules football player, recently won the 2016 *I'm a celebrity, get me out of here* television show in Australia. However, his life has not always been so rosy. Brendan's parents separated when he was eight years old. His marriage had broken down following allegations of infidelity against Fevola, and he became addicted to gambling. This led to him ultimately declaring bankruptcy.

While considered a promising AFL player, his off-field bad behaviour caused problems for him in the League, leading to his sacking in 2011. During filming of *I'm a celebrity*, Fevola admitted that this episode in his life was the best thing that had happened to him. He admitted that he had suffered depression for some years and began to drink heavily, and that his gambling addiction was out of control. Following his sacking, he went to rehabilitation and began the journey back to good health and recovery. He and his wife have reunited, and the latest reports are that they are planning to have a fourth child.

victims. According to Caplan, the four stages of a crisis reaction are:

1. *Phase 1:* The individual experiences an initial increase in tension because of the emotionally hazardous crisis-precipitating event.
2. *Phase 2:* When the individual is unable to resolve the crisis quickly, tension and disruption of daily living increase.
3. *Phase 3:* If the individual attempts but fails to resolve the crisis by the usual problem-solving techniques, tension increases to such a level that the individual may become depressed.
4. *Phase 4:* At the final stage, the person may partly resolve the crisis by using new coping skills. Mental disruption or disorder may occur if the person does not develop new coping skills to manage the crisis.

Roberts's model of crisis intervention

Roberts's seven-stage model of crisis intervention (2005), shown in Figure 26.7 ■, has been used to help people in acute psychological crisis and acute situational crisis, persons in high-risk populations such as suicidal juvenile offenders (Roberts & Bender, 2006), and persons diagnosed with acute stress disorder. The seven stages are:

1. Plan and conduct a thorough assessment (including lethality assessment [refer to Chapter 10], assessment of dangerousness to self or others, and assessment of immediate psychosocial needs).
2. Make interpersonal contact, establish rapport, and rapidly establish the relationship (conveying genuine regard and respect for the person, acceptance, reassurance and a nonjudgmental attitude; refer to Chapter 2).
3. Examine the dimensions of the problem in order to define it (including the 'last straw' of the precipitating event).
4. Encourage an exploration of feelings and emotions through active listening (refer to Chapter 9).
5. Explore and assess past coping attempts, and generate and explore alternatives and previously untried coping methods or solutions.
6. Restore cognitive functioning through the implementation of an action plan based on cognitive mastery (refer to Chapter 25).
7. Follow up with the person and leave the door open for future contact, especially around the time of the anniversary of the event (exactly one month or one year after the victimisation).

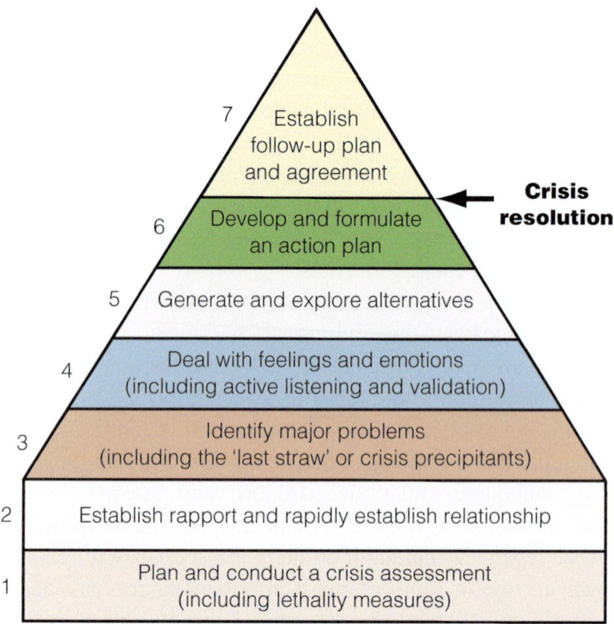

FIGURE 26.7 ■ Roberts's seven-stage model of crisis intervention.
Source: From Roberts, A. R. (2005). Bridging the past and present to the future of crisis intervention and crisis management. In A. R. Roberts (Ed.), *Crisis intervention handbook: Assessment, treatment, and research* (3rd ed.) (Figure 1-1, p. 20). New York, NY: Oxford University Press. Used by permission of Oxford University Press, Inc.

Types of crises

In the contemporary view, the origin of a crisis is as important as the type of crisis. Roberts (2005) points out that if we know how the crisis began, we have a better opportunity to intervene effectively. Two general categories of crisis origins are situational and maturational.

Situational crisis

A *situational crisis* can originate from three sources: material or environmental (fire, natural disaster, manmade biohazards, terrorist attacks); personal or physical (heart attack, diagnosis of fatal illness, bodily disfigurement); and interpersonal or social (death of a loved one or divorce). Often these life-changing events motivate people to take significant action in their close relationships that alter their life course.

Because the event leading to the situational crisis is usually unanticipated, one generally cannot do anything directly to prevent it. In a more indirect sense, an individual can attempt to keep healthy and focus on the most effective methods of interacting with others. However, the complexity of the experience influences the ability of the individual to resolve the trauma. For instance, a person coping with one traumatic incident is more likely to resolve the experience than someone faced with multiple traumas or factors (Melamed & Castro, 2011). An example of a situational crisis (in which the origin of the crisis is the husband's diagnosis of terminal cancer) follows in the Practice Example.

Practice example

Jessie, age 52, is a social worker at a local mental health clinic who is feeling increasingly less able to function since she learned that her husband has a terminal, inoperable form of cancer. Many arrangements need to be made, including finding adequate medical treatment and doing appropriate evaluations of her husband.

Jessie has been unable to work for two to three days, and now tells a psychiatric–mental health nurse that she can no longer function—she has been unable to make any of the required phone calls, despite knowing that she is the person who must coordinate everything. Jessie speaks of feeling overwhelmed, shakes her head, and says, 'Can you believe it? I do this all the time for others, but I can't do it now. Isn't that a joke?'

Maturational crisis

A *maturational crisis* involves life cycle changes or normal transitions of human development. These are the traditional stages of human development that include infancy, childhood, puberty, adolescence, adulthood, middle age and old age. During each stage, the individual is subject to unique stressors. Each stage of development is characterised by developmental tasks the individual must accomplish in order to progress to the next level. A failure at any one level compromises the next stage of development.

Maturational crises also include such changes as marriage, retirement and the transition from being a student to a worker. Crises associated with these states arise when the individual enters a new area of development or functioning and cannot adapt to functioning at that level. If the person experiences additional trauma or change, the risk for experiencing a crisis increases. Whenever people experience more than two life changes or traumatic events, their coping capacity may be strained, and the potential for crisis becomes greater.

An example of a maturational crisis, in which the origin of the crisis is a decision to divorce complicated by multiple stressors, follows in the Practice Example.

Practice example

Bernie, aged 62 years, has been hospitalised several times for paranoid schizophrenia over the past 40 years. Bernie's wife, Alice, moved out of their apartment and told Bernie that she has decided to seek a divorce. After Alice moved out, the apartment caught fire and burned. Bernie moved to a boarding house and became depressed and stopped taking his medication. He began to have auditory hallucinations. Bernie has come to the crisis centre accompanied by the police, who found him on the street crying, sobbing and mumbling incoherently.

Nursing self-awareness

It is important that you develop increased awareness of yourself, and are able to handle your feelings, so that you can intervene in a crisis situation. It will help to reflect on your answers to the questions posed in the Self-awareness feature, below.

SELF-AWARENESS
Am I ready for crisis work?

Thoughtfully consider and reflect on your answers to the following questions:

- Do I believe that people who are in crisis are helpless?
- Can I contain my own anxiety when I am working with someone who is severely anxious?
- How do I feel when I'm not in control in certain situations?
- How do I react to people who are frightened?
- How do I react to people who are angry?
- How do I react to people who threaten me?
- Do I have ideas that will hinder my ability to help others? For example, do I believe any of the following: women who are raped are asking for it; men should be strong and not show emotions; children should be seen and not heard?

To remain effective in crisis work, and to continue to grow personally and professionally, you should practise the following important behaviours:

- Respect and believe in a person's capacity to grow and change.
- Be aware of the impact on yourself of repeatedly listening to traumatic stories.
- Formulate your own outlets for stress, frustration and anger.
- Deal with your own fears about violence, and your own vulnerability to stress and conflict.
- Develop realistic expectations about what you can do for others.
- Respect each person's own unique timetable for crisis resolution.
- Collaborate with other crisis interveners and community groups.

You will become more skilled as you incorporate each of these behaviours into your professional repertoire. Do not underestimate the impact of vicarious trauma. When we hear the traumatic stories of others' experiences, we are sometimes emotionally harmed by those stories and the distress we can see in the person. Much has been written about the impact of vicarious trauma (Cieslak et al., 2014; Iqbal, 2015) and professional development clinical supervision is a very helpful strategy for processing these experiences (Abassary & Goodrich, 2014).

Some additional activities that you can undertake to take care of yourself and lessen the personal impacts of disaster and crises involve self-nurturance. Focus on what you did right every day, monitor your own reactions, keep a journal in which you write your personal thoughts and feelings, and practise the self-care tips in the following Self-awareness: Self-care Tips for Emergency and Disaster Response Workers. People in crisis will expect you to help them regain control of themselves, not to control them. Being self-assured and composed will help people to regain control.

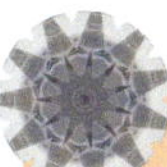

CARING FOR PEOPLE IN CRISIS

Crisis intervention as a therapeutic strategy is strongly humanistic. People are viewed as capable of personal growth, and as having the ability to influence and control their own lives. According to these concepts, the task of the intervener is to help the individual in crisis to understand the combination of events that led to the crisis, and to guide the individual, prior to a maladaptive response, towards a resolution that will meet the person's unique needs and foster future growth and strength. Especially during the acute phase, the goal of crisis intervention is to restore the person to the pre-trauma level of functioning as quickly as possible.

In addition to the interventions discussed in this section, other strategies that are employed with people in crisis can be found in other chapters. They are cognitive behavioral therapy interventions (Chapter 25), pharmacological interventions (Chapter 7), and stress management techniques (Chapter 10).

SELF-AWARENESS
Self-care tips for emergency and disaster response workers

Normal reactions to a disaster event

- No one who responds to a mass casualty event is untouched by it.
- Profound sadness, grief and anger are normal reactions to an abnormal event.
- You may not want to leave the scene until the work is finished.
- You will likely try to over-ride stress and fatigue with dedication and commitment.
- You may deny the need for rest and recovery time.

Signs that you may need stress management assistance

- Difficulty communicating thoughts
- Difficulty remembering instructions
- Difficulty maintaining balance
- Uncharacteristic argumentativeness
- Difficulty making decisions
- Limited attention span
- Unnecessary risk-taking
- Tremors/headaches/nausea
- Tunnel vision/muffled hearing
- Colds or flulike symptoms
- Disorientation or confusion
- Difficulty concentrating
- Loss of objectivity
- Greater tendency towards feeling easily frustrated
- Inability to engage in problem-solving
- Inability to disconnect from work when off-duty
- Refusal to follow orders
- Refusal to leave the scene
- Increased use of drugs/alcohol
- Unusual clumsiness

Ways to help manage your stress

- Limit on-duty work hours to no more than 12 hours per day.
- Make work rotations from high-stress to lower-stress functions.
- Make work rotations from the scene to routine assignments, as feasible.
- Use counselling assistance programs available through your agency.
- Practise deep breathing, yoga and/or mindfulness.
- Drink plenty of water and eat healthy snacks, like fresh fruit or dried fruit, nuts, trail mix, whole grain breads and other energy foods at the scene.
- Keep yourself hydrated with water, mineral water, decaffeinated coffee or tea, juice and electrolyte supplements.
- If you are able to, take calcium supplements, which can counteract the high levels of lactic acid produced by tension, and vitamin C, which may help you to maintain alertness.
- Take frequent, brief breaks from the scene, as feasible.
- Talk about your emotions, to process what you have seen and done.
- Stay in touch with your family and friends.
- Participate in memorials, rituals and the use of symbols as a way to express feelings.
- Pair up with another responder so that you can monitor one another's stress.

Source: Adapted from USDHHS Substance Abuse and Mental Health Services Administration. (2011). *Self-care tips for emergency and disaster response workers*. Retrieved from http://www.samhsa.gov

Providing psychoeducation for survivors of trauma helps them to better understand their own stress responses. Learning coping strategies provides a sense of control over these responses.

It is equally important that nurses are educated and prepared to respond to crises and disasters. Disaster preparedness plans are created by individual health care facilities, and most nurses undergo a program of continuing education training in their agency. However, it would be an effective primary prevention strategy to prepare nursing students for just such contingencies. For example, psychological crisis intervention has been identified as a core nursing skill for disaster response training (Yin et al., 2011).

Assessment

Assessment takes place on three levels: individual, family and sociocultural.

Individual assessment

Assessment of the individual is the first phase of crisis intervention. The nurse or helper must focus on assessing the following elements that relate to the person and the problem. Collect data about the following:

- the person's resilience
- the person's coping style
- the precipitating event
- the situational supports
- the person's perception of the crisis
- any guilt a disaster survivor may feel about having survived, or about actions taken in order to survive
- the person's ability to handle the problem.

The following Communication feature shows an example of assessing a person's coping style.

Assessment is an essential step of crisis intervention, and the basis for later decisions about how and when to intervene, and who to call (the first step of Roberts's model). Another feature of an individual assessment in the face of a crisis is how the person is managing spiritually. See Box 26.6, Crisis As a Test of Faith, as a tool to help clients use their faith to heal. Intellectual capabilities would also contribute to decisions about needed interventions (Lunsky & Elserafi, 2011).

It is also very important to assess and evaluate the person's suicide potential. (See Chapter 19 for lethality assessment.) During this time, an individual may need to be hospitalised to ensure their safety, and a referral to a therapist or an emergency department in a general hospital or a psychiatric emergency room may be necessary. Part of

COMMUNICATION

Person in crisis

FATHER: 'How will I ever be able to get my son back from foster care? I never seem to do anything right with him.'

NURSE RESPONSE 1: 'Jim, if you could rank yourself as a dad on a scale of 1 to 10, with 10 meaning always doing everything "right" and 1 meaning never doing anything "right", where would you rank yourself?'

RATIONALE: Using a scaling question will open the door to discussing with Jim the skills and competencies that are within his control and those that need to be worked on.

NURSE RESPONSE 2: 'Let's talk about what you have been doing with Jimmy that is "right".'

RATIONALE: This intervention has two goals: eliciting a behavioural description of the interaction between father and son, and helping Jimmy's father to identify his parenting strengths.

Box 26.6 Crisis as a test of faith

It may be that a psychiatric crisis has also brought forth a spiritual crisis. The person may, for the first time, be faced with looking at the three spiritual issues of life.

1. 'Of what value is my life? Why was I born, anyway? I have nothing to give.' These are the words of someone who is depressed or actively suicidal.
2. 'What do I hold to be sacred?' What things are important to the person, what things have meaning?
3. 'How do I know what's true?' The person with anxiety or psychosis has great difficulty sorting out what's real and what's not real, determining what's true and what's not true. Life as we know it has many dichotomies. The unanswerable becomes even more of a challenge when a psychiatric crisis emerges.

Recall what happened to your relationships with friends and family when you were in a personal crisis. Did the relationships change? Our cognitive sphere, our affective sphere and our relational sphere are all affected. We lose our centring of purpose, of sacredness, of reality. We lose our spirit and become disconnected. Do you think the relationships of the person in your care change when they are in a crisis?

the overall assessment is to determine what is necessary to return this person to a state of equilibrium; this may be different from what is necessary to solve the problem.

Family assessment

Family assessment is important when an individual has been traumatised, because trauma reverberates through an entire family as well as when a crisis involves all or several members within a family (de Jong & Schout, 2011). Meet with as many family members as possible, to assess family resilience, family resources, coping skills and interpersonal styles. Crises often accompany role changes in families, or increase stresses in families that do not have the resources to meet the challenge.

Some common family crises are the death of a family member, the terminal illness of a family member, single parenting, divorce, drug/alcohol dependence, family violence, infidelity, remarriage, mental illness, incest and the departure of children from home (empty-nest syndrome).

Sociocultural assessment

A critically important source of the meaning of an individual's response to stress or trauma is the broader sociocultural context in which the person lives. A person's culture influences the sources of distress a person experiences, as well as the person's symptomatology, interpretation of symptoms, and methods of coping.

How one is raised influences how one experiences distress, whether one seeks help, and whether one allows oneself to be disabled by a mental health problem. For example, in some cultures, anxiety is considered a problem of individual strength or moral code, as opposed to a mental health problem. In some cultures, it may be more acceptable to have a physical problem than an emotional problem.

Cultural competence requires knowledge about other cultures and sensitivity to the culture of others in order to select the interventions that will likely be most helpful. Cultural sensitivity involves much more than simply identifying a family's ethnic origins or health practices. Think about developing a cultural family genogram as an aid to assessing culturally diverse families. The cultural family genogram is discussed in Chapter 24 as it applies to family-based interventions. It is just as relevant a tool for working with culturally diverse families in crisis.

To be effective in sociocultural assessment, you must also become aware of the influences and beliefs from your own experiences. If you are not familiar with a person's cultural needs, ask respectful questions to help the person fully express their distress. For example, 'I want to understand how all of this might affect you. Tell me more about how you feel about this situation. Tell me how your neighbours (your friends/your family) might feel about it.'

Disaster assessment

Nurses as citizens are often at the scene of natural disasters, or may be called on to help. Nurses can be particularly helpful during the initial stage of a disaster, because, in addition to having the ability to provide care to the injured, they have the skills needed to perform physical assessments and assess psychological distress.

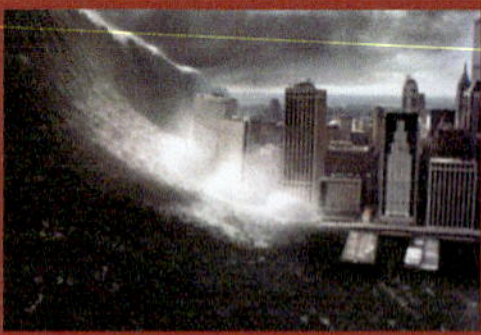

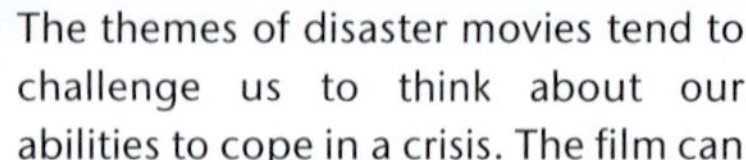

MENTAL HEALTH IN THE MEDIA

Disaster movies

The themes of disaster movies tend to challenge us to think about our abilities to cope in a crisis. The film can take the form of a special vacation trip we can all relate to being spoiled by volcanoes, asteroids or dinosaurs. Or a futuristic view of the world can spark our imaginations, and then introduce the element of intrusions by alien beings or dark mega-deities from the ninth dimension. While different scenarios are presented, the overarching question seems to be 'What would you do if faced with . . . ?'

The main themes of disaster movies can be categorised by our responses to the story. Generally, these themes, and our possible responses, are as follows:

Escapism—The movie takes you away from your everyday difficulties and can prompt you to say to yourself, 'At least my current problems are not as bad as that.'

Reinforcing our current skill level—Throughout the film, you could say to yourself, 'I can manage that situation better than the people in the movie are doing.'

Shock and awe—Being surprised or not having any idea what is coming can give you an adrenaline surge while you are sitting comfortably at the movies.

Challenging our coping—This movie theme can give us pause, where we consider, 'What could be done to deal with this set of circumstances?'

Despite the seemingly superficial manner with which disaster movies treat our psychological underpinnings, they do awaken our sensibilities to the human condition. Whether it is appreciating how people have the strength of character to perform under horrible conditions, or to be able to imagine yourself managing and coping, disaster movies can serve a purpose beyond pure entertainment.

Photo courtesy of Everett Collection Inc.

Supporting a person in crisis

Effective planning for crisis intervention must be:

- based on careful assessment and an understanding of human dependence needs
- developed in active collaboration with the person in crisis and the significant people in that person's life
- focused on immediate, concrete, contributing problems
- appropriate to the person's level of thinking, feeling and behaving
- consistent with the person's lifestyle and culture
- time-limited, concrete and realistic
- mutually negotiated and renegotiated
- organised to provide for follow-up.

Many of these principles form the basis for therapeutic communication strategies.

Effective intervention is based on the ability to implement the second step of Roberts's model—make interpersonal contact, establish rapport and rapidly establish the relationship (conveying genuine regard and respect for the person, acceptance, reassurance and a nonjudgmental attitude). One-to-one interventions that enable interpersonal contact, establish rapport and establish the relationship are important to an individual in crisis. However, nurses who work with people in crisis often need to use many non-traditional interventions, which can be as important as any verbal interventions. Working successfully with people in crisis is based on having a flexible, open view of what may be therapeutic with different individuals. You must have a full repertoire of skills and interventions that can be individualised to help all types of people in crisis, including the ability to assist with spiritual needs. Box 26.7, Helping People to Recuperate from Crisis, offers suggestions that will help a person in crisis integrate body, mind and spirit.

Several different types of crisis intervention are discussed next.

Box 26.7 Helping people to recuperate from crisis

It is important for people who have experienced a crisis or trauma to stay grounded. Suggest the following exercises to someone who is feeling confused, upset, in disbelief or hopeless.

1. Sit on a chair, feel your feet on the ground, press on your thighs, feel your behind on the seat and your back supported by the chair. Look around you and pick six objects that have red or blue in them. This should allow you to feel in the present, more grounded, and in your body. Notice how your breath gets deeper and calmer. You may want to go outdoors and find a peaceful place to sit on the grass. As you do, feel how your body is held and supported by the ground.
2. Gently pat the different parts of your body with your hand, with a loose wrist. Your body may feel more tingling, more alive, sharp, and you may feel more connected to your feelings.
3. Tense your muscles, each group at a time. Hold your shoulders with your arms across your chest, tighten your grip, and pat your arms up and down. Do the same with your legs, tighten them and hold them from the outside, patting through their length. Tighten your back, tighten your front, then gently release the tension. This may help you to feel more balanced.
4. If you believe in prayer or in a greater power, pray for the rest of the souls of the dead, for the healing of the wounded, and for the consolation of the grieving. Pray for peace, understanding, wisdom, and for the forces of good to prevail. Do not give up faith in the ultimate goodness of being, and keep your trust in humanity.

Take comfort in knowing that we humans are extremely resilient and have been able to recuperate from the most horrendous tragedies.

Source: Adapted from USDHHS Substance Abuse and Mental Health Services Administration. *After a disaster: Self-care tips for dealing with stress*. Retrieved from http://www.samhsa.gov.

Crisis counselling

Crisis counselling is a type of brief, solution-focused therapy. Unlike therapies that focus on bringing about major personality change, crisis counselling focuses on strengths and solving immediate problems. Focusing on strengths is a resilience-oriented approach (Honig, 2010).

Crisis counselling usually lasts for five or six sessions, and involves individuals, groups or families. The following techniques are used:

- listening actively and with concern (Your Intervention Strategies, below, discusses communication strategies specific to working with a person in crisis)
- exploring the dimension of the problem, including the 'last straw', in order to define it (Roberts's third step)
- encouraging the open expression of feelings (Roberts's fourth step)
- helping the person gradually accept reality
- assessing past coping attempts, and helping the person explore new ways of coping with problems (Roberts's fifth step)
- linking the person to a social network
- engaging in decision counselling or problem-solving with the person, thus restoring cognitive mastery (Roberts's sixth step)
- reinforcing newly learned coping devices
- following up on the person after resolution of the crisis and leaving the door open for future contact, especially around the time of the anniversary of the event (Roberts's seventh step).

Telephone counselling

Suicide prevention and crisis intervention centres rely heavily on telephone counselling by volunteers who have professional consultation available to them. Also known as 'hotlines' and often available around the clock, they allow callers to remain anonymous and test what it feels like to ask for assistance. No appointment, travel time, or money is necessary, and help is immediately available. The volunteers usually work within a protocol that indicates what information they need from the person to assess the crisis. Their goal is to plan steps to provide immediate relief and then long-term follow-up, if necessary.

The calls made to a hotline usually fall into one of four categories: crisis calls, ventilation calls (getting a problem 'off one's chest'), combinations of ventilation and information calls, or information-only calls. Calls that request information and ventilation are handled by supportive listening and giving information. Crisis calls need special techniques. Workers in crisis intervention centres generally follow a step-by-step agency protocol. For more information on suicide prevention hotlines, refer to Chapter 19.

Anticipatory guidance

Anticipatory guidance is providing assistance in anticipation of the potential for crisis, thus averting it. These are some examples of anticipatory guidance: discussing methods of contraception with adolescents or young adults; preparing a child and the family for a tonsillectomy; arranging for a volunteer from the Reach for Recovery Program to visit a woman who has had a mastectomy; and preparing a list of helpful phone numbers for a person who is being discharged from acute hospital care back to the community.

Helping develop social supports

Immediate and tangible social support is crucial for people in crisis. Many people who are at risk for major depressive episodes following a crisis perceive their social supports to be very low (Salguerro, Fernandez-Berrocal, Iruarrizaga, Cano-Vindel & Galea, 2011). Many people in crisis have limited social supports, and are not always sure about how to access supports or develop them. You can help a person develop tangible social supports by: introducing a woman whose husband is an alcoholic to Alcoholics Anonymous groups in her community, referring a family with a terminally ill member

YOUR INTERVENTION STRATEGIES Communication strategies in crisis work

- ***Use silence***—this gives the person time to reflect and become more aware of feelings. Silence can prompt elaboration. Simply being with the person is supportive.
- ***Use non-verbal communication***—maintaining eye contact, head nodding, caring facial expressions, and occasional 'uh-huhs' lets the person know that you are in tune.
- ***Paraphrase***—understanding, empathy and interest are conveyed by repeating portions of what the person has said. Paraphrasing also checks for accuracy, clarifies misunderstandings, and lets people know that they have been heard. You could say, 'So, you are saying that ...' or 'I have heard you say that ...'.
- ***Reflect feelings***—this helps the person identify and articulate emotions. You could say, 'You sound angry/scared/etc. Does that fit for you?'
- ***Allow the expression of emotions***—this is an important part of healing. Venting often helps the person work through feelings in order to better engage in constructive problem-solving.

Some things to say

- 'These are normal reactions to an abnormal situation.'
- 'It is understandable that you feel this way.'
- 'It wasn't your fault; you did the best you could.'
- 'I am sorry that this happened.'
- 'Things will get better, and you will feel better, although they may never be the same again.'
- 'You had a special relationship with your pet/car/house/child.'
- 'It is a good idea for you to talk about how you feel.'
- 'I care about how you feel.'
- 'You have the right to have these feelings.'

Source: Adapted from USDHHS Substance Abuse and Mental Health Services Administration. *Disaster counseling*. Retrieved from http://www.samhsa.gov.

to a local hospice, giving a rape victim the telephone number of the rape crisis hotline, or informing the newly discharged person and their family about the Association of Relatives and Friends of the Mentally Ill (ARAFMI) (www.arafmiaustralia.asn.au), the Mental Illness Fellowship (www.mifellowship.org.au), Mind Australia (www.mindaustralia.org.au) and a range of other government and non-government agencies.

Critical incident stress management

Critical incident stress management (CISM) is a comprehensive, integrative and multi-faceted approach to crisis intervention that spans the time sequence of a crisis. It is based on the notion that no single intervention alone is effective in crisis work (Pack, 2013). CISM consists of multiple components that can be applied to individuals, families, small groups, large groups, communities and organisations. It can be best understood as a strategic delivery platform for primary, secondary and tertiary prevention programs in the wake of large and small critical incidents (crises), rather than simply a crisis intervention treatment (Strand, Felices & Williams, 2010; Yin et al., 2011). Table 26.2 ■ describes the elements of CISM according to Everly and Mitchell (2008), and their intents.

The term 'CISM' replaces the term '*critical incident stress debriefing (CISD)*' to describe this approach. CISD was originally formulated in the 1980s by Mitchell and Everly (1996) in response to an air disaster in Washington, DC. The original approach, known as critical incident stress debriefing, was intended to include four major elements: on-scene crisis intervention; post-incident small-group discussion (known as *defusing*); a more formalised several-phase group discussion, which included debriefing; and follow-up support services. In practice, however, only one element, the group discussion (often to the exclusion of the others), became the focus of disaster mental health intervention. Its ease of use, and the perception that it prevented PTSD, led to its popularity. Although the small-group meeting has both psychological and psychoeducational elements, described later in this section, it should not by itself be considered psychotherapy. According to the criticisms voiced by its developers, Everly and Mitchell (2008), and evidence in recent research (Strand et al., 2010; Wei, Szumilas & Kutcher, 2010), CISM is not a singular stand-alone crisis intervention or an effective way to prevent PTSD. Its most effective use appears to be in mitigating (decreasing, but not preventing) PTSD in soldiers and emergency services personnel. CISM is a more contemporary and broader approach, and includes debriefing as one of its several components.

The debriefing process remains a valuable crisis intervention. The debriefing process offers an opportunity for individuals affected by a traumatic event to share their thoughts and feelings in a safe and controlled environment. Box 26.8 discusses the phases of the small-group debriefing process in detail.

The typical settings in which debriefing as a component of CISM is used are: with staff on an inpatient unit after a suicide; with inmates after a murder in a jail; with military medical teams; with crisis line volunteers; with first responders, such as police, fire and paramedical officers; and with rescue and health care workers after natural disasters or terrorist attacks (Everly & Mitchell, 2008; Honig, 2010; Strand, Felices & Williams, 2010).

TABLE 26.2 ■ Components of critical incident stress management (CISM)

Component	Intent
1. Pre-event planning and preparation	To provide anticipatory guidance and foster resilience
2. Assessment	To determine the need for intervention for those directly and indirectly exposed
3. Strategic planning	To improve the crisis response
4. Individual crisis intervention	To provide psychological first aid to individuals
5. Large-group crisis intervention	To provide large-group psychological first aid
6. Small-group crisis intervention	To provide small-group psychological first aid and powerful event group support
7. Family crisis intervention	To provide psychological first aid to families
8. Organisational and community intervention	To deliver services to organisations and communities, and to improve preparedness
9. Pastoral crisis intervention	To provide faith-based support
10. Follow-up and referral	To ensure continuity of care for those directly and indirectly exposed

VICARIOUS TRAUMATISATION

Disasters and traumatic experiences shake the foundations of our beliefs about how other people behave towards one another, and can shatter our assumption that the world is a safe place. In evaluating the after-effects of a disaster, remember that there may be an impact on those who are not direct victims, including helpers.

A disaster can affect the mental health of various groups—a condition known as **vicarious traumatisation**. Also known as *secondary trauma response*, vicarious traumatisation is a condition in which psychological after-effects are experienced by those who are not direct victims of the traumatic event. The groups most commonly at increased risk are identified in the following list. Those individuals who are most affected are listed first.

1. next-of-kin
2. injured survivors and their close ones
3. uninjured survivors
4. onlookers (the helpless helpers, who are at particularly high risk)
5. rescuers
6. body handlers
7. health personnel (many mass-injury situations may demand difficult prioritising)
8. people responsible for the disaster

Box 26.8 The small-group debriefing process

Introduction phase (setting the tone for the subsequent phases)

- Explain the purpose of the meeting.
- Explain and give an overview of the process.
- Motivate the participants.
- Assure the participants that information will be confidential.
- Explain the guidelines.
- Identify the team members.
- Answer questions or concerns.

Fact phase (imparting power to the participants through giving information)

- Assist the participants to discuss the facts of the incident.
- Ask the participants to introduce themselves.
- Ask the participants to talk about how they were involved in the incident.
- Ask the participants to talk about what happened from their perspective (tell their story).

Thought phase (transitioning between impersonal outside facts and that which is internal, close and personal)

- Ask each participant to discuss their first thoughts or most prominent thoughts about the traumatic event. Expect to hear emotional comments.

Reaction phase (ventilating with a potential for emotional abreaction)

- Most of the discussing is done by the participants.
- Discussion is freewheeling.
- Ask participants what the worst thing was about the situation, what they would choose to erase, and what aspect of the situation causes the most pain.

Symptom phase (normalising and attacking the myth of unique weakness or vulnerability)

- Move the group towards more cognitively-oriented material.
- Ask participants to describe any cognitive, physical, emotional or behavioural experiences they encountered at the scene of the incident.
- Ask about any symptoms that followed subsequently.

Teaching phase (moving further away from the emotional content of the reaction phase)

- Acknowledge the symptoms described in the symptom phase.
- Reaffirm that symptoms are normal, typical or predictable after what they have been through.
- Forewarn the group about possible symptoms they might experience in the future.
- Involve the participants in stress management activities.

Re-entry phase (identifying consistent themes that may be used to facilitate closure and provide a psychological uplift)

Participant roles

- Introduce any new material they wish to discuss.
- Review old material already discussed.
- Ask any questions.
- Discuss whatever would help them to bring closure to the debriefing.

Debriefing team roles

- Answer any questions.
- Inform and reassure.
- Provide appropriate handouts and other written material.
- Provide referral sources for assessment, therapy and so on.
- Summarise the debriefing experience with words of respect, encouragement, appreciation, support and direction.

9. coworkers in workplace disasters
10. evacuees.

Nurses and other crisis workers are routinely exposed to victim suffering and to the after-effects of crisis, trauma and inhumane acts. They are at risk for becoming what has been called 'wounded healers'. Awareness of the psychological risk can prevent the loss of necessary personnel (Walden, 2010). This Practice Example illustrates how vicarious traumatisation can affect rescue workers.

Practice example

Barbara was a mental health nurse at a hospital in Darwin, Australia, when Cyclone Tracey destroyed much of the city. She was also a volunteer who assisted survivors and first responders (firefighters, police officers, paramedics), and counselled them for several weeks. Barbara became preoccupied with the stories she heard. Her insomnia and angry outbursts at home prompted Barbara to seek counselling for herself.

Expect to be vulnerable to this condition if you work with people in the highly disorganised crisis period; with those who are victims of sexual assault, violence or disaster; or with those, such as sexual offenders, who traumatise others. Vicarious traumatisation can also affect your own physical health by inducing gastrointestinal problems (such as gastritis or peptic ulcer), hypertension and fatigue. In the home or in the workplace, you could experience the following:

- an increase in the number of sick days you take
- indecision or difficulty with problem-solving
- isolation or withdrawal
- behavioural outbursts.

Should this happen, seek additional support, supervision, and referral for professional assistance.

The opposite of vicarious traumatisation, *vicarious resilience*, is an emerging topic for study. Vicarious resilience, a new concept put forth by Hernandez, Gangsei and Engstrom (2007), addresses the question of how psychotherapists who work with survivors of political violence or kidnapping are affected by others' stories of resilience. Their study illustrates, yet again, that therapists are affected by hearing other people's stories (this time positively) and that stories of resilience and constructive coping with adversity can contribute to sustaining and empowering trauma therapists.

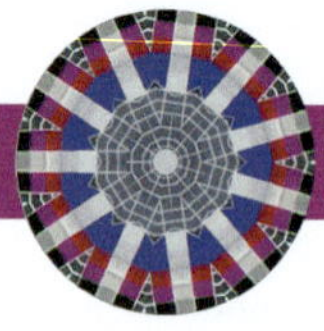

REFERENCES

Abassary, C., & Goodrich, K. M. (2014). Attending to crisis-based supervision for counselors: The CARE model of crisis-based supervision. *The Clinical Supervisor, 33*(1), 63–81.

Aguilera, D. C. (1998). *Crisis intervention: Theory and methodology* (8th ed.). St Louis, MO: Mosby.

Anthony, W. (1993). Recovery from mental illness: The guiding vision of the mental health service system in the 1990s. *Psychosocial Rehabilitation Journal, 16*(4), 11.

Arbesman, M., & Logsdon, D. W. (2011). Occupational therapy interventions for employment and education for adults with serious mental illness: A systematic review. *American Journal of Occupational Therapy, 65*, 238–246.

Australian Institute of Health and Welfare (AIHW). (2015). *The health of Australia's prisoners 2015*. Cat. No. PHE 207. Canberra, Australia: AIHW.

Bengtsson-Tops, A., Ericsson, U., & Ehliasson, K. (2014). Living in supportive housing for people with serious mental illness: A paradoxical everyday life, *International Journal of Mental Health Nursing, 23*(5), 409–418.

Bentall, R. P. (2013). Would a rose, by any other name, smell sweeter? *Psychological Medicine, 43*(7), 1560–1562.

Berger, J. T. (2011). Imagining the unthinkable: Illuminating the present. *Journal of Clinical Ethics, 22*(1), 17–19.

Bhui, K., & Dinos, S. (2011). Preventive psychiatry: A paradigm to improve population mental health and well-being. *British Journal of Psychiatry, 198*, 417–419.

Bird, V., Leamy, M., Tew, J., Le Boutillier, C., Williams, J., & Slade, M. (2014). Fit for purpose? Validation of a conceptual framework for personal recovery with current mental health consumers. *Australian and New Zealand Journal of Psychiatry, 48*(7), 644–653.

Bitter, N. A., Roeg, D. P. K., van Nieuwenhuizen, C., & van Weeghel, J. (2015). Effectiveness of the Comprehensive Approach to Rehabilitation (CARe) methodology: Design of a cluster randomized controlled trial. *BMC Psychiatry, 15*, 165–175. doi: 10.1186/s12888-015-0564-0

Bolton, J. M., Robinson, J., & Sareen, J. (2009). Self-medication of mood disorders with alcohol and drugs in the national epidemiologic survey on alcohol and related conditions. *Journal of Affective Disorders, 115*(3), 367–375.

Bonney, S., & Stickley, T. (2008). Recovery and mental health: A review of the British literature. *Journal of Psychiatric and Mental Health Nursing, 15*(2), 140–153.

Boscarato, K., Lee, S., Kroschel, J., Hollander, Y., Brennan, A., & Warren, N. (2014). Consumer experience of formal crisis-response services and preferred methods of crisis intervention. *International Journal of Mental Health Nursing, 23*(4), 287–295.

Boyd, J. E., Otilingam, P. G., & DeForge, B. R. (2014). Brief version of the Internalized Stigma of Mental Illness (ISMI) scale: Psychometric properties and relationship to depression, self esteem, recovery orientation, empowerment, and perceived devaluation and discrimination, *Psychiatric Rehabilitation Journal, 37*(1), 17–23.

Cacioppo, J. T., Reis, H. T., & Zautra, A. J. (2011). Social resilience: The value of social fitness with an application to the military. *American Psychologist, 66*(1), 43–51.

Caplan, G. (1964). *Principles of preventive psychiatry*. New York, NY: Basic Books.

Cieslak, R., Shoji, K., Douglas, A., Melville, E., Luszczynska, A., & Benight, C. C. (2014). A meta-analysis of the relationship between job burnout and secondary traumatic stress among workers with indirect exposure to trauma, *Psychological Services, 11*(1), 75–86.

Claassen, C., Kashner, T. M., Kashner, T. K., Xuan, L., & Larkin, G. L. (2011). Psychiatric emergency 'surge capacity' following acts of terrorism and mass violence with high media impact: What is required? *General Hospital Psychiatry, 33*(3), 287–293. doi: 35400018984980.0110

Commonwealth of Australia. (2013). *A national framework for recovery-oriented mental health services: Guide for practitioners and providers*. Canberra, Australia: Commonwealth of Australia.

Conner, K. O., McKinnon, S. A., Ward, C. J., Reynolds III, C. F., & Brown, C. (2015). Peer education as a strategy for reducing internalized stigma among depressed older adults. *Psychiatric Rehabilitation Journal, 38*(2), 186–193.

Corrigan, P. W., Kosyluk, K. A., & Rusch, N. (2013). Reducing self-stigma by coming out proud, *American Journal of Public Health, 103*(5), 794–800.

Corstens, D., Longden, E., McCarthy-Jones, S., Waddingham, R., & Thomas, N. (2014). Emerging perspectives from the hearing voices movement: Implications for research and practice. *Schizophrenia Bulletin, 40*(Suppl. 4), S285–S294.

Crane-Ross, D., Lutz, W. J., & Roth, D. (2006). Consumer and case manager perspectives of service empowerment: relationship to mental health recovery. *Journal of Behavioral Health Services and Research, 33*(2), 142–155.

Cruwys, T., & Gunaseelan, S. (2016). 'Depression is who I am': Mental illness identity, stigma and wellbeing. *Journal of Affective Disorders, 189*, 36–42.

Cunningham, J., & Paradies, Y. C. (2012). Socio-demographic factors and psychological distress in Indigenous and non-Indigenous Australian adults aged 18–64 years: Analysis of national survey data. *BMC Public Health, 12*, 95. doi: 10.1186/1471-2458-12-95

Curtis, L. (1997). *New directions: International overview of best practices in recovery and rehabilitation services for people with serious mental illness*. Wellington, New Zealand: The Mental Health Commission.

Davidson, L., & Strauss, J. S. (1992). Sense of self in recovery from severe mental illness. *British Journal of Medical Psychology, 65*(2), 131–145.

de Jong, G., & Schout, G. (2011). Family group conferences in public mental health care: An exploration of opportunities. *International Journal of Mental Health Nursing, 20*(1), 63–74.

DelGaizo, A. L., Elhai, J. D., & Weaver, T. L. (2011). Posttraumatic stress disorder, poor physical health and substance use behaviors in a national trauma-exposed sample. *Psychiatry Research, 188*(3), 390–395. doi: 10.1016/j.psychres.2011.03.016

DiGrande, L., Neria, Y., Brackbill, R. M., Pulliam, P., & Galea, S. (2011). Long-term posttraumatic stress symptoms among 3,271 civilian survivors of the September 11, 2001 terrorist attacks on the World Trade Center. *American Journal of Epidemiology, 173*(3), 271–281.

Drake, R. E., & Whitley, R. (2014). Recovery and severe mental illness: Description and analysis. *Canadian Journal of Psychiatry, 59*(5), 236–242.

Emsley R., Kilian S., & Phahladira L. (2016). How long should antipsychotic treatment be continued after a single episode of schizophrenia? *Current Opinion in Psychiatry, 29*(3), 224–229.

Eriksen, K. A., Arman, M., Davidson, L., Sundfor, B., & Karlsson, B. (2014). Challenges in relating to mental health professionals: Perspectives of persons with severe mental illness. *International Journal of Mental Health Nursing, 23*(2), 110–117.

Everly, G. S., & Mitchell, J. T. (2008). *Integrative crisis intervention and disaster mental health*. Ellicott City, MD: Chevron Publishing Corporation.

Feeney, L., Jordan, I., & McCarron, P. (2013). Teaching recovery to medical students, *Psychiatric Rehabilitation Journal, 36*(1), 35–41.

Firmin, R. L., Luther, L., Lysaker, P. H., & Salyers, M. P. (2015). Self-initiated helping behaviors and recovery in severe mental illness: Implications for work, volunteerism, and peer support. *Psychiatric Rehabilitation Journal, 38*(4), 336–341.

Gallagher, C., & Halpin, M. (2014). *Lived experience workforce in South Australian public mental health service, what we have learned, what we have achieved and future direction*. Adelaide, Australia: Central Adelaide Local Health Network Mental Health Directorate, SA Health.

Geddes, J. R., & Miklowitz, D. J. (2013). Treatment of bipolar disorder. *The Lancet, 381*(9878), 1672–1682.

Gershoff, E. T., Aber, J. L., Ware, A., & Kotler, J. A. (2010). Exposure to 9/11 among youth and their mothers in New York City: Enduring associations with mental health and sociopolitical attitudes. *Child Development, 81*(4), 1142–1160.

Gotzsche, P. C., Young, A. H., & Crace, J. (2015). Maudsley debate: Does long term use of psychiatric drugs cause more harm than good? *British Medical Journal, 350*, h2435.

Ha, K. (2016). The companion project: Recovery among volunteer peer support providers in South Korea. *Psychiatric Rehabilitation Journal, 39*(1), 71–73.

Happell, B., Palmer, C., & Tennent, R. (2011). The mental health nurse incentive program: Desirable knowledge, skills and attitudes from the perspective of nurses. *Journal of Clinical Nursing, 20*(5–6), 901–910.

Hernandez, P., Gangsei, D., & Engstrom, D. (2007). Vicarious resilience: A new concept in work with those who survive trauma. *Family Process, 46*(2), 229–241.

Holmes, D., Molloy, L., Beckett, P., Field, J., & Stratford, A. (2013). Peer support workers hold the key to opening up recovery-orientated service in inpatient units. *Australasian Psychiatry, 21*(3), 282–283.

Honig, A. L. (2010). War then and now: From surviving to thriving. *International Journal of Emergency Mental Health, 12*(3), 207–212.

Iqbal, A. (2015). The ethical considerations of counselling psychologists working with trauma: Is there a risk of vicarious traumatisation? *Counselling Psychology Review, 30*(1), 44–51.

Iwasaki, Y., Coyle, C., Shank, J., Messina, E., Porter, H., Salzer, M., . . . Koons, G. (2014). Role of leisure in recovery from mental illness. *American Journal of Psychiatric Rehabilitation, 17*(2), 147–165.

Jacobson, N., & Curtis, L. (2000). Recovery as policy in mental health services: Strategies emerging from the States. *Psychiatric Rehabilitation Journal, 23*(4), 333–341.

Kidd, S., Kenny, A., & McKinstry, C. (2015). Exploring the meaning of recovery-oriented care: An action-research study, *International Journal of Mental Health Nursing, 24*(1), 38–48.

Landeen, J., Kirkpatrick, H., Woodside, H., Byrne, C., Bernardo, A., & Pawlick, J. (1996). Factors influencing staff hopefulness in working with people with schizophrenia. *Issues in Mental Health Nursing, 17*, 457–467.

Leamy, M., Bird, V., Le Boutillier, C., Williams, J., & Slade, M. (2011). Conceptual framework for personal recovery in mental health: Systematic review and narrative synthesis. *British Journal of Psychiatry, 199*(6), 445–452.

LeBel, J. L. (2011). Coercion is not mental health care. *Psychiatric Services, 62*, 453.

Li, M., D'Arcy, C., & Meng, X. (2016). Maltreatment in childhood substantially increases the risk of adult depression and anxiety in prospective cohort studies: Systematic review, meta-analysis, and proportional attributable fractions. *Psychological Medicine, 46*(4), 717–730.

Lunsky, Y., & Elserafi, J. (2011). Life events and emergency department visits in response to crisis in individuals with intellectual disabilities. *Journal of Intellectual Disability, 55*(7), 714–718. doi: 10.1111/j.1365-2788.2011.01417.x

Lysaker, P. H., & Buck, K. D. (2008). Is recovery from schizophrenia possible? An overview of concepts, evidence and clinical implications. *Primary Psychiatry, 15*(6), 60–65.

Malinovsky, I., Lehrer, P., Silverstein, S. M., Shankman, S. A., O'Brien, W., . . . van Nostrand, G. (2013). An empirical evaluation of recovery transformation at a large community psychiatric rehabilitation organization. *Psychological Services, 10*(4), 428–441.

Maniglio, R. (2009). Severe mental illness and criminal victimization: A systematic review. *Acta Psychiatrica Scandinavia, 119*(3), 180–191.

Margolese, H. C., Malchy, L., Negrete, J. C., Tempier, R., & Gill, K. (2004). Drug and alcohol use among patients with schizophrenia and related psychoses: Levels and consequences. *Schizophrenia Research, 67*(2), 157–166.

Masi, G., & Liboni, F. (2011). Management of schizophrenia in children and adolescents: Focus on pharmacotherapy. *Drugs, 71*(2), 179–208.

McCauley, C. O., McKenna, H. P., Keeney, S., & McLaughlin, D. F. (2015). Concept analysis of recovery in mental illness in young adulthood. *Journal of Psychiatric and Mental Health Nursing, 22*(8), 579–589.

Mead, S., & Copeland, M. E. (2000). What recovery means to us: Consumers' perspectives. *Community Mental Health Journal, 36*(3), 315–328.

Mead, S., & MacNeil, C. (2006). Peer support: What makes it unique. *International Journal of Psychosocial Rehabilitation, 10*(2), 29–37.

Melamed, B. G., & Castro, C. (2011). Observations and insights about strengthening our soldiers (SOS). *Journal of Clinical Psychology in Medical Settings, 18*(2), 210–223. doi: 10.1007/s10880-011-9253-4

Mitchell, J. T., & Everly Jr, G. S. (1996). *Critical incident stress debriefing: An operations manual*. Ellicott City, MD: Chevron Publishing.

Moore, G., Gerdtz, M. F., Hepworth, G., & Manias, E. (2011). Homelessness: Patterns of emergency department use and risk factors for re-presentation. *Emergency Medicine Journal, 28*, 422–427.

Morse, J. M., & Penrod, J. (1999). Linking concepts of enduring, uncertainty, suffering, and hope. *Image: Journal of Nursing Scholarship, 31*(2), 145–150.

O'Baire-Kark, M., & Klevay, A. (2011). Another perspective on finger replantation surgery: Nursing support for the psychological levels of recovery. *Journal of Trauma Nursing, 18*(1), 34–42.

Odes, H., Katz, N., Noter, E., Shamir, Y., Weizman, A., & Valevski, A. (2011). Level of function at discharge as a predictor of readmission among inpatients with schizophrenia. *American Journal of Occupational Therapy, 65*, 314–319.

Onken, S. J., Dumont, J. M., Ridgway, P., Dornan, D. H., & Ralph, R. O. (2002). Mental health recovery: What helps and what hinders? A national research project for the development of recovery facilitating system performance indicators. Retrieved from http://akmhcweb.org/docs/RecoveryPIWebDescription.pdf (Accessed 2003, November 1.)

Onyango, G. R., Paratharayil, M., van den Berg, S., Reiffers, R., Snider, L., & Erikson, C. (2011). Spirituality and psychosocial work in emergencies: Four commentaries and a response. *Intervention, 9*(1), 61–73.

Pack, M. J. (2013). Critical incident stress management: A review of the literature with implications for social work. *International Social Work, 56*(5), 608–627.

Paquin, S. O. (2011). Social justice advocacy in nursing: What is it? How do we get there? *Creative Nursing, 17*(2), 63–67.

Paradies, Y. C. & Cunningham, J. (2012). The DRUID study: Racism and self-assessed health status in an indigenous population, *BMC Public Health, 12*, 131. doi: 10.1186/1471-2458-12-131

Pati, A. (2011). Brighter prospects. *Nursing Standard, 25*(20), 20–21.

Patterson, C., Moxham, L., Taylor, E., Sumskis, S., Perlman, D., Brighton, R., . . . Keough, E. (2016). Perceived control among people with severe mental illness: A comparative study. *Archives of Psychiatric Nursing, 30*(5), 563–567. doi: http://dx.doi.org/10.1016/j.apnu.2016.04.002

Petersen, I., Lund, C., & Stein, D. J. (2011). Optimizing mental health services in low-income and middle-income countries. *Current Opinion in Psychiatry, 24*, 318–323.

Raeburn, T., Halcomb, E., Walter, G., & Cleary, M. (2013). An overview of the clubhouse model of psychiatric rehabilitation. *Australasian Psychiatry, 21*(4), 376–378.

Raeburn, T., Schmied, V., Hungerford, C., & Cleary, M. (2014). Clubhouse model of psychiatric rehabilitation: How is recovery reflected in documentation? *International Journal of Mental Health Nursing, 23*(5), 389–397.

Raphael, B., & Ma, H. (2011). Mass catastrophe and disaster psychiatry. *Molecular Psychiatry, 16*(3), 247–251.

Reid-Quiñones, K., Kliewer, W., Shields, B. J., Goodman, K., Ray, M. H., & Wheat, E. (2010). Cognitive, affective, and behavioral responses to witnessed versus experienced violence. *American Journal of Orthopsychiatry, 814*(1), 51–60.

Repper, J., & Carter, T. (2011). A review of the literature on peer support in mental health services. *Journal of Mental Health, 20*(4), 392–411.

Roberts, A. R. (Ed.). (2005). *Crisis intervention handbook: Assessment, treatment, and research* (3rd ed.). New York, NY: Oxford University Press.

Roberts, A. R., & Bender, K. (2006). Juvenile offender suicide: Prevalence, risk factors, assessment, and crisis intervention protocols. *International Journal of Emergency Mental Health, 8*(4), 255–265.

Salguero, J. M., Fernandez-Berrocal, P., Iruarrizaga, I., Cano-Vindel, A., & Galea, S. (2011). Major depressive disorder following terrorist attacks: A systematic review of prevalence, course, and correlates. *BMC Psychiatry, 11*(1), 96. doi: 10.1186/1471-244X-11-96

Shpiegel, S. (2016). Resilience among older adolescents in foster care: The impact of risk and protective factors. *International Journal of Mental Health and Addiction, 14*(1), 6–22.

Slade, M. (2009). *Personal recovery and mental illness: A guide for mental health professionals*. Cambridge, England: Cambridge University Press.

Slade, M., & Longden, E. (2015). Empirical evidence about recovery and mental health. *BMC Psychiatry, 15*, 285–298.

Spijker, A., Wollersheim, H., Teerenstra, S., Graff, M., Adang, E., . . . Vernooij-Dassen, M. (2011). Systematic care for caregivers of patients with dementia: A multicenter, cluster-randomized, controlled study. *American Journal of Geriatric Psychiatry, 19*, 521–531.

Staring, A.B. P., van der Gaag, M., & Mulder, C. L. (2011). Recovery style predicts remission at one-year follow-up in outpatients with schizophrenia spectrum disorders. *Journal of Nervous and Mental Disease, 199*(5), 295–300.

Strand, R., Felices, K., & Williams, K. (2010). Critical incident stress management (CISM) in support of special agents and other first responders to the Fort Hood shooting: Summary and recommendations. *International Journal of Mental Health, 12*(3), 151–160.

Substance Abuse and Mental Health Services Administration (SAMHSA). (2006). *National consensus statement on mental health recovery*. Rockville, MD: Center of Mental Health Services, SAMHSA. Retrieved from http://store.samhsa.gov/product/National-Consensus-Statement-on-Mental-Health-Recovery/ SMA05-4129

Svedberg, P., Svensson, B., Hansson, L., & Jormfeldt, H. (2014). A 2-year follow-up study of people with severe mental illness involved in psychosocial rehabilitation. *Nordic Journal of Psychiatry, 68*(6), 401–408.

Tyhurst, J. S. (1957). The role of transition states—including disasters—in mental illness. In *Symposium on preventive and social psychiatry, 15–17 April 1957* (pp. 1–23). Washington, DC: Walter Reed Army Institute of Research.

Walden, P. (2010). Wounded healers: Nurses and depression. *Nursing Made Incredibly Easy! 8*(6), 6–7.

Wei, Y., Szumilas, M., & Kutcher, S. (2010). Effectiveness on mental health of psychological debriefing for crisis intervention in schools. *Educational Psychology Review, 22*(3), 339–347.

Whitley, R., Palmer, V., & Gunn, Jane. (2015). Recovery from severe mental illness. *Canadian Medical Association Journal, 187*(13), 951–952.

Williams, S., & Stickley, T. (2011). Stories from the streets: People's experiences of homelessness. *Journal of Psychiatric and Mental Health Nursing, 18*(5), 432–439.

Wong, Y.-L. I., Stanton, M. C., & Sands, R. G. (2014). Rethinking social inclusion: Experiences of persons in recovery from mental illness. *American Journal of Orthopsychiatry, 84*(6), 685–695.

Yin, H., He, H., Arbon, P., & Zhu, J. (2011). A survey of the practice of nurses' skills in Wenchuan earthquake disaster sites: Implications for disaster training. *Journal of Advanced Nursing, 67*(10), 2231–2238. doi: 10.1111/j.1365-2648.2011.05699.x

APPENDIX A

DSM-5 CLASSIFICATIONS

Each disorder is named and then coded firstly with the ICD-9-CM code, and then in parentheses the ICD-10-CM code as outlined in the DSM-5.

__._ (__._) Blank lines indicated that the code is not applicable.

Neurodevelopmental disorders

Intellectual disabilities (Intellectual development disorder)

__._ (__._) Intellectual disabilities (Intellectual development disorder)
Specify current severity:
317 (F70) Mild
318.0 (F71) Moderate
318.1 (F72) Severe
318.2 (F73) Profound
315.8 (F88) Global developmental delay
319 (F79) Unspecified intellectual disability (Intellectual developmental disorder)

Communication disorders

315.39 (F80.9) Language disorder
315.39 (F80.0) Speech sound disorder
315.35 (F80.81) Childhood-onset fluency disorder (Stuttering)
315.39 (F80.89) Social (Pragmatic) communication disorder
307.9 (F80.9) Unspecified communication disorder

Autism spectrum disorder

299.00 (F84.0) Autism spectrum disorder
Specify if: Associated with a known medical or genetic condition or environmental factor or associated with another neurodevelopmental, mental or behavioural disorder
Specify: Current severity requiring very substantial support, requiring substantial support, requiring support
Specify if: With or without accompanying intellectual or language impairment, with catatonia

Attention-deficit/hyperactivity disorder

__._ (__._) Attention-deficit/hyperactivity disorder
Specify whether:
314.01 (F90.2) Combined presentation
314.00 (F90.0) Predominantly in attentive presentation
314.01 (F90.1) Predominantly hyperactive/impulsive presentation
Specify if: In partial remission
Specify current severity: Mild, moderate, severe
314.01 (F90.8) Other specified attention-deficit/hyperactivity disorder
314.01 (F90.9) Unspecified attention-deficit/hyperactivity disorder

Specific learning disorder

__._ (__._) Specific learning disorder
Specified if:
315.00 (F81.0) With impairment in reading (*specify if:* with word reading accuracy, reading rate or fluency, reading comprehension)
315.2 (F81.81) With impairment in written expression (*specify if:* with spelling accuracy, grammar and punctuation accuracy, clarity or organisation of written expression)
315.1 (F81.2) With impairment in mathematics (*specify if:* with number sense, memorisation of arithmetic facts, accurate or fluent calculation, accurate maths reasoning)
Specify current severity: Mild, moderate, severe

Motor disorders

315.4 (F82) Developmental coordination disorder
307.3 (F98.4) Stereotypic movement disorder
Specify if: With self-injurious behaviour, without self-injurious behaviour
Specify if: Associated with a known medical or genetic condition, neurodevelopmental disorder, or environmental factor
Specify current severity: Mild, moderate, severe

Tic disorders

307.23 (F95.2) Tourette's disorder
307.22 (F95.1) Persistent (chronic) motor or vocal tic disorder
Specify if: With motor tics only, with vocal tics only
307.21 (F95.0) Provisional tic disorder
307.20 (F95.8) Other specific tic disorder
307.20 (F95.9) Unspecified tic disorder

Other neurodevelopmental disorders

315.8 (F88) Other specified neurodevelopment disorder
315.9 (F89) Unspecified neurodevelopment disorder

Schizophrenia spectrum and other psychotic disorders

Specify if: The following course specifiers are only to be used after one year duration of the disorder: first episode, currently in acute episode; first episode, currently in partial remission; first episode, currently in full remission; multiple episodes, currently in acute episode; multiple episodes, currently in partial remission; multiple episodes, currently in full remission; continuous; unspecified
Specify if: With catatonia

Specify if: Current severity of delusions, hallucinations, disorganised speech, abnormal psychomotor behaviour, negative symptoms, impaired cognition, depression and mania symptoms
301.22 (F21) Schizotypal (personality) disorder
297.1 (F22) Delusional disorder
Specify whether: Erotomanic type, grandiose type, jealous type, persecutory type, somatic type, mixed type, unspecified type
Specify if: With bizarre content
298.8 (F23) Brief psychotic disorder
Specify if: With marked stressor(s), without marked stressor(s), with postpartum onset
295.40 (F20.9) Schizophreniform disorder
Specify if: With good prognostic features, without good prognostic features
295.90 (F20.9) Schizophrenia
__._ (__._) Schizoaffective disorder
Specify whether:
295.70 (F25.0) Bipolar type
295.70 (F25.1) Depressive type
__._ (__._) Substance/medication-induced psychotic disorder
Specify if: With onset during intoxication, with onset during withdrawal
__._ (__._) Psychotic disorder due to another medical condition
Specify whether:
293.81 (F06.2) With delusions
293.82 (F06.0) With hallucinations
293.89 (F06.1) Catatonia associated with another medical disorder (Catatonia specifier)
293.89 (F06.1) Catatonia disorder due to another medical condition
293.89 (F06.1) Unspecified catatonia
298.8 (F28) Other specified schizophrenia spectrum and other psychotic disorder
298.9 (F29) Unspecified schizophrenia spectrum and other psychotic disorder

Bipolar and related disorders

Specify: With anxious distress (*specify:* current severity: mild, moderate, moderate–severe, severe); with mixed features; with rapid cycling; with melancholic features; with atypical features; with mood-congruent psychotic features; with mood-incongruent psychotic features; with catatonia; with peri-partum onset; with seasonal pattern
__._ (__._) Bipolar 1 disorder
__._ (__._) Current or most recent episode manic
296.41 (F31.11) Mild
296.42 (F31.12) Moderate
296.43 (F31.13) Severe
296.44 (F31.2) With psychotic features
296.45 (F31.73) In partial remission
296.46 (F31.74) In full remission
296.40 (F31.9) Unspecified
296.40 (F31.0) Current or most recent episode hypomanic
296.45 (F31.73) In partial remission
296.46 (F31.74) In full remission
296.40 (F31.9) Unspecified
__._ (__._) Current or most recent episode depressed
296.51 (F31.31) Mild
296.52 (F31.32) Moderate
296.53 (F31.4) Severe
296.54 (F31.5) With psychotic features
296.55 (F31.75) In partial remission
296.56 (F31.76) In full remission
296.50 (F31.9) Unspecified
296.7 (F31.9) Current or most recent episode unspecified
296.89 (F31.81) Bipolar II disorder
Specify: Current or most recent episode Hypomanic, Depressed
Specify course in full criteria for a mood episode are not currently met: In partial remission, in full remission
Specify severity if all criteria for a mood episode are not currently met: mild, moderate, severe
301.13 (F34.0) Cyclothymic disorder
Specify if: With anxious distress
__._ (__._) Substance/medication-induced bipolar and related disorder
Specify if: With onset during intoxication, with onset during withdrawal
293.83 (__._) Bipolar and related disorder due to another medical condition
Specify if:
293.83 (F06.33) With manic features
293.83 (F06.33) With manic or hypomanic-like episode
293.83 (F06.34) With mixed features
296.89 (F31.89) Other specified bipolar and related disorder
296.80 (F31.9) Unspecified bipolar and related disorder

Depressive disorders

Specify if: With anxious distress (*specify current severity:* mild, moderate, moderate–severe, severe); with mixed features; with melancholic features; with atypical features; with mood-congruent psychotic features; with mood-incongruent psychotic features; with catatonia; with peri-partum onset; with seasonal pattern
296.99 (F34.8) Disruptive mood dysregulation disorder
__._ (__._) Major depressive disorder
__._ (__._) Single episode
296.21 (F32.0) Mild
296.22 (F32.1) Moderate
296.23 (F32.2) Severe
296.24 (F32.3) With psychotic features
296.25 (F32.4) In partial remission
296.26 (F32.5) In full remission
296.20 (F32.9) Unspecified
__._ (__._) Recurrent episode
296.31 (F33.0) Mild
296.32 (F33.1) Moderate
296.33 (F33.2) Severe
296.34 (F33.3) With psychotic features
296.35 (F33.41) In partial remission
296.36 (F33.42) In full remission
296.30 (F33.9) Unspecified
300.4 (F34.1) Persistent depressive disorder (Dysthymia)
Specify if: In partial remission, in full remission

Specify if: Early-onset, late-onset
Specify if: With pure dysthymic syndrome; with persistent major depressive episode; with intermittent major depressive episode; with current episode; with intermittent major depressive episode; without current episode
Specify if: Current severity mild, moderate, severe
625.4 (N94.3) Premenstrual dysphoria disorder
__._ (__._) Substance/medication-induced depressive disorder
Specify if: With onset during intoxication, with onset during withdrawal
293.83 (__._) Depressive disorder due to another medical condition
Specify if:
293.83 (F06.31) With depressive features
293.83 (F06.32) With major depressive like episode
293.83 (F06.34) With mixed features
311 (F32.8) Other specified depressive disorder
311 (F32.9) Unspecified depressive disorder

Anxiety disorders

309.21 (F93.0) Separation anxiety disorder
312.23 (F94.0) Selective mutism
300.29 (__._) Specify phobia
Specify if:
(F40.218) Animal
(F40.228) Natural environment
__._ (__._) Blood-injection injury
(F40.230) Fear of blood
(F40.231) Fear of injections and transfusion
(F40.232) Fear of other medical care
(F40.233) Fear of injury
(F40.248) Situational
(F40.298) Other
300.23 (F40.10) Social anxiety disorder social phobia
Specify if: Performance only
300.01 (F41.0) Panic disorder
__._ (__._) Panic attack specify
300.22 (F40.00) Agoraphobia
300.02 (F41.1) Generalised anxiety disorder
__._ (__._) Substance/medication-induced anxiety disorder
Specify if: With onset during intoxication, with onset during withdrawal, with onset during medication use
293.84 (F06.4) Anxiety disorder due to another medical condition
300.09 (F41.8) Other specified anxiety disorder
300.00 (F41.9) Unspecified anxiety disorder

Obsessive–compulsive and related disorders

Specify if: With good or fair insight, with poor insight, with absent insight/delusional beliefs
300.3 (F42) Obsessional compulsive disorder
Specify if: Tic-related
300.7 (F45.22) Body dysmorphic disorder
Specify if: With muscle dysmorphic
300.3 (F42) Hoarding disorder
Specify if: With excessive acquisition
312.39 (F63.3) Trichotillomania (Hair-pulling disorder)
698.4 (L98.1) Excoriation (Skin-picking disorder)
_._ (_._) Substance/medication-induced obsessive–compulsive and related disorder
Specify if: With onset during intoxication, with onset during withdrawal, with onset after medication use
294.8 (F06.8) Obsessive–compulsive and related disorder due to another medical condition
Specify if: With obsessive–compulsive disorder-like symptoms, with appearance preoccupations, with hoarding symptoms, with hair-pulling symptoms, with skin-picking symptoms
300.3 (F42) Other specified obsessive–compulsive and related disorder
300.3 (F42) Unspecified obsessive–compulsive and related disorder

Trauma- and stressor-related disorders

313.89 (F94.1) Reactive attachment disorder
Specify if: Persistent
Specify current severity: Severe
313.89 (F94.2) Disinhibited social engagement disorder
Specify if: Persistent
Specify current severity: Severe
309.81 (F43.10) Post-traumatic stress disorder includes post-traumatic stress disorder for children six years and younger
Specify whether: With dissociative symptoms
Specify if: With delayed expression
308.3 (F43.0) Acute stress disorder
_._ (_._) Adjustment disorders
Specify whether:
309.0 (F43.21) With depressed mood
309.24 (F43.22) With anxiety
309.28 (F43.23) With mixed anxiety and depressed mood
309.3 (F43.24) With disturbance of conduct
309.4 (F43.25) With mixed disturbance of emotions and conduct
309.9 (F43.20) Unspecified
309.89 (F43.8) Other specified trauma- and stressor-related disorder
309.9 (F43.9) Unspecified trauma- and stressor-related disorder

Dissociative disorders

300.14 (F44.81) Dissociative identity disorder
300.12 (F44.0) Dissociative amnesia
Specify if:
300.13 (F44.1) With associative fugue
300.6 (F48.1) Depersonalisation/derealisation disorder
300.15 (F44.89) Other specified dissociative disorder
300.15 (F44.9) Unspecified dissociative disorder

Somatic symptom and related disorders

300.82 (F45.1) Somatic symptom disorder
Specify if: With predominant pain
Specify if: Persistent
Specify current severity: Mild, moderate, severe
300.7 (F45.21) Illness anxiety disorder
Specify whether: Care seeking type, care avoidant type
300.11 (__._) Conversion disorder (Functional neurological symptom disorder)

Specify symptom type:
(F44.4) With weakness or paralysis
(F44.4) With abnormal movement
(F44.4) With swallowing symptoms
(F44.4) With speech symptoms
(F44.5) With attacks or seizures
(F44.6) With amnesia all sensory loss
(F44.6) With special sensory symptom
(F44.7) With mixed symptoms
Specify if: Acute episode, persistent
Specify if: With psychological distress (specify stressor), without psychological stressor
316 (F54) Psychological factors affecting other medical condition
Specify current severity: Mild, moderate, severe, extreme
300.19 (F68.10) Factitious disorder (includes factitious disorder imposed on self, factitious disorder imposed on another)
Specify: Single episode, recurrent episodes
300.89 (F45.8) Other specified somatic symptom and related disorder
300.82 (F45.9) Unspecified somatic symptom and related disorder

Feeding and eating disorders

Specify if: In remission
Specify if: In partial remission, in full remission
Specify current severity: Mild, moderate, severe, extreme
307.52 (__._) Pica
(F98.3) In children
(F50.8) In adults
307.53 (F98.21) Rumination disorder
307.59 (F50.8) Avoidant/restrictive food intake disorder
307.1 (__._) Anorexia nervosa
Specify whether:
(F50.01) Restricting type
(F50.02) Binge-eating/purging type
307.51 (F50.2) Bulimia nervosa
307.51 (F50.8) Binge-eating disorder
307.59 (F50.8) Other specified food or eating disorder
307.50 (F50.9) Unspecified feeding or eating disorder

Elimination disorders

307.6 (F98.0) Enuresis
Specify whether: Nocturnal only, diurnal only, nocturnal and diurnal
307.7 (F98.1) Enocopresis
Specify whether: With constipation and overflow incontinence, without constipation and overflow incontinence
__._ (__._) Other specified elimination disorder
788.39 (N39.498) With urinary symptoms
787.60 (R15.9) With faecal symptoms
__._ (__._) Unspecified elimination disorder
788.30 (R32) With urinary symptoms
787.60 (R15.9) With faecal symptoms

Sleep–wake disorders

Specify if: Episodic, persistent, recurrent
Specify if: Acute, subacute, persistent
Specify current severity: Mild, moderate, severe
780.52 (G47.00) Insomnia disorder
Specify if: With non-sleep disorder mental comorbidity, with other medical comorbidity, with other sleep disorder
780.54 (G47.10) Hypersomnolence disorder
Specify if: With mental disorder, with medical condition, with another sleep disorder
__._ (__._) Narcolepsy
Specify whether:
347.00 (G47.419) Narcolepsy without cataplexy but with hypocretin deficiency
347.01 (G47.411) Narcolepsy with cataplexy but without hypocretin deficiency
347.00 (G47.419) Autosomal dominant cerebella ataxia, deafness and narcolepsy
347.00 (G47.419) Autosomal dominant narcolepsy, obesity and type 2 diabetes
347.10 (G47.429) Narcolepsy secondary to another medical condition

Breathing-related sleep disorders

327.23 (G47.33) Obstructive sleep apnoea hypopnea
__._ (__._) Central sleep apnoea
Specify whether:
327.21 (G47.31) Idiopathic central sleep apnoea
786.06 (R06.3) Cheyne–Stokes breathing
780.57 (G47.37) Central sleep apnoea comorbid with opioid use
Specify current severity:
__._ (__._) Sleep-related hypoventilation
Specify whether:
327.24 (G47.34) Idiopathic hypoventilation
327.25 (G47.35) Congenital central alveolar hypoventilation
327.26 (G47.36) Comorbid sleep-related hypoventilation
Specify current severity:
__._ (__._) Circadian rhythm sleep–wake disorders
Specify whether:
307.45 (G47.21) Delayed sleep phase type
Specify if: Familial, overlapping with non-24-hour sleep–wake type
307.45 (G47.22) Advanced sleep phase type
Specify if: Familial
307.45 (G47.23) Irregular sleep–wake type
307.45 (G47.24) Non-24 hour sleep–wake type
307.45 (G47.26) Shiftwork type
307.45 (G47.20) Unspecified type

Parasomnias

__._ (__._) Non-rapid eye movement sleep arousal disorders
Specify whether:
307.45 (G51.3) Sleepwalking type
Specify if: With sleep-related eating, with sleep-related sexual behaviour (sexsomnia)
307.46 (G51.4) Sleep terror type
307.47 (G51.5) Nightmare disorder
Specify if: During sleep onset

Specify if: With associated non-sleep disorder, with associated other medical condition, with associated other sleep disorder
327.42 (G47.52) Rapid-eye-movement sleep behaviour disorder
333.94 (G25.81) Restless legs syndrome
__._ (__._) Substance/medication-induced sleep disorder
Specify whether: Insomnia type, daytime sleepiness type, parasomnias type, mixed type
Specify if: With onset during intoxication, with onset during discontinuation/withdrawal
780.52 (G47.09) Other specified insomnia disorder
780.52 (G47.00) Unspecified insomnia disorder
780.54 (G47.19) Other specified hypersomnolence disorder
780.54 (G47.10) Unspecified hypersomnolence disorder
780.59 (G47.8) Other specified sleep–wake disorder
780.59 (G47.9) Unspecified sleep–wake disorder

Sexual dysfunctions

Specify whether: Lifelong, acquired
Specify whether: Generalised, situational
Specify current severity: Mild, moderate, severe
302.74 (F52.32) Delayed ejaculation
302.72 (F52.21) Erectile disorder
302.73 (F52.21) Female orgasmic disorder
Specify if: Never experienced an orgasm under any situation
302.72 (F52.22) Female sexual interest/arousal disorder
302.76 (F52.6) Genito-pelvic pain/penetration disorder
302.71 (F52.0) Male hypoactive sexual desire disorder
302.75 (F52.4) Premature (early) ejaculation
__._ (__._) Substance/medication-induced sexual dysfunction
Specify if: With onset during intoxication, with onset during withdrawal, with onset after medication use
302.79 (F52.8) Other specific sexual dysfunction
302.70 (F52.9) Unspecified sexual dysfunction

Gender dysphoria

__._ (__._) Gender dysphoria
302.6 (F64.2) Gender dysphoria in children
Specify if: With a disorder of sexual development
302.85 (F64.1) Gender dysphoria in adolescents and adults
Specify if: With a disorder of sexual development
Specify if: Post-transition
302.6 (F64.8) Other specified gender dysphoria
302.6 (F64.9) Unspecified gender dysphoria

Disruptive, impulse-control and conduct disorders

313.81 (F91.3) Oppositional defiant disorder
Specify current severity: Mild, moderate, severe
312.34 (F63.81) Intermittent explosive disorder
__._ (__._) Conduct disorder
Specify whether:
312.81 (F91.1) Childhood-onset type
312.82 (F91.2) Adolescent-onset type
312.89 (F91.9) Unspecified onset
Specify if: With limited prosocial emotions
Specify current severity: Mild, moderate, severe
301.7 (F60.9) Antisocial personality disorder
312.33 (F63.1) Pyromania
312.32 (F63.2) Kleptomania
312.89 (F91.8) Other specified disruptive, impulsive-control and conduct disorder
312.9 (F91.9) Unspecified disruptive, impulsive-control and conductive disorder

Substance-related and addictive disorders

Specify if: In early remission, in sustained remission
Specify if: In a controlled environment
Specify if: With perceptual disturbances

Substance-related disorders

Alcohol-related disorders

__._ (__._) Alcohol use disorder
Specify current severity:
305.00 (F10.10) Mild
303.90 (F10.20) Moderate
303.90 (F10.20) Severe
303.00 (__._) Alcohol intoxication
(F10.129) With use disorder, mild
(F10.229) With use disorder, moderate or severe
(F10.929) Without use disorder
291.81 (__._) Alcohol withdrawal
(F10.239) Without perceptual disturbances
(F10.232) Other alcohol-induced disorders
291.9 (F10.99) Unspecified alcohol-related disorder

Caffeine-related disorders

305.90 (F15.929) Caffeine intoxication
292.0 (F15.93) Caffeine withdrawal
__._ (__._) Other caffeine-induced disorders
292.9 (F15.99) Unspecified caffeine-related disorder

Cannabis-related disorders

__._ (__._) Cannabis use disorder
Specify current severity:
305.20 (F12.10) Mild
304.30 (F12.20) Moderate
304.30 (F12.20) Severe
292.89 (__._) Cannabis intoxication
Without perceptual disturbances
(F12.129) With use disorder, mild
(F12.229) With use disorder, moderate or severe
(F12.929) Without use disorder
With perceptual disturbances
(F12.122) With use disorder, mild
(F12.222) With use disorder, moderate or severe
(F12.922) Without use disorder
292.0 (F12.288) Cannabis withdrawal
__._ (__._) Other cannabis-induced disorders
292.9 (F12.99) Unspecified cannabis-related disorder

Hallucinogen-related disorders

__._ (__._) Phencyclidine use disorder
Specify current severity:
305.90 (F16.10) Mild
304.60 (F16.20) Moderate
304.60 (F16.20) Severe
__._ (__._) Other hallucinogen use disorder
Specify: The particular hallucinogen
Specify current severity:
305.30 (F16.10) Mild
304.50 (F16.20) Moderate
304.50 (F16.20) Severe
292.89 (__._) Phencyclidine intoxication
(F16.129) With use disorder, mild
(F16.229) With use disorder, moderate or severe
(F16.929) Without use disorder
292.89 (__._) Other hallucinogen intoxication
(F16.129) With use disorder, mild
(F16.229) With use disorder, moderate or severe
(F16.929) Without use disorder
292.89 (F16.983) Hallucinogen persisting perception disorder
__._ (__._) Other phencyclidine-induced disorders
__._ (__._) Other hallucinogen-induced disorders
292.9 (F16.99) Unspecified phencyclidine-related disorder
292.9 (F16.99) Unspecified hallucinogen-related disorder

Inhalant-related disorders

__._ (__._) Inhalant use disorder
Specify: the particular inhalant
Specify current severity:
305.90 (F18.10) Mild
304.60 (F18.20) Moderate
304.60 (F18.20) Severe
292.89 (__._) Inhalant intoxication
(F18.129) Use with disorder, mild
(F18.229) Use with disorder, moderate or severe
(F18.929) Without use disorder
__._ (__._) Other inhalant-induced disorders
292.9 (F18.99) Unspecified inhalant-related disorder

Opioid-related disorders

__._ (__._) Opioid use disorder
Specify if: On maintenance therapy, in a controlled environment
Specify current severity:
305.50 (F11.10) Mild
304.00 (F11.20) Moderate
304.00 (F11.20) Severe
292.89 (__._) Opioid intoxication
Without perceptual disturbances
(F11.129) With use disorder, mild
(F11.229) With use disorder, moderate or severe
(F11.929) Without use disorder
With perceptual disturbances
(F11.122) With use disorder, mild
(F11.222) With use disorder, moderate or severe
(F11.922) Without use disorder
292.0 (F11.23) Opioid withdrawal
__._ (__._) Other opioid-induced disorders
292.9 (F11.99) Unspecified opioid-related disorder

Sedative, hypnotic or anxiolytic-related disorders

__._ (__._) Sedative, hypnotic or anxiolytic use disorder
Specify current severity:
305.40 (F13.10) Mild
304.10 (F13.20) Moderate
304.10 (F13.20) Severe
292.89 (__._) Sedative, hypnotic or anxiolytic intoxication
(F13.129) With use disorder, mild
(F13.229) With use disorder, moderate or severe
(F13.929) Without use disorder
292.0 (__._) Sedative, hypnotic or anxiolytic withdrawal
(F13.239) Without perceptual disturbances
(F13.232) With perceptual disturbance
__._ (__._) Other sedative, hypnotic or anxiolytic-induced disorders
292.9 (F13.99) Unspecified sedative, hypnotic or anxiolytic-induced disorders

Stimulant-related disorders

__._ (__._) Stimulant use disorders
Specify current severity:
__._ (__._) Mild
305.70 (F15.10) Amphetamine-type substance
305.60 (F14.10) Cocaine
305.70 (F15.10) Other or unspecified stimulant
__._ (__._) Moderate
304.40 (F15.20) Amphetamine-type substance
304.20 (F14.20) Cocaine
304.40 (F15.20) Other or unspecified stimulant
__._ (__._) Severe
304.40 (F15.20) Amphetamine-type substance
304.20 (F14.20) Cocaine
304.40 (F15.20) Other or unspecified stimulant
292.89 Stimulant intoxication
Specify: The specify intoxicant
292.89 (__._) Amphetamine or other stimulant, without perceptual disturbances
(F15.129) With use disorder, mild
(F15.229) With use disorder, moderate or severe
(F15.929) Without use disorder
292.89 (__._) Cocaine, without perceptual disturbances
(F14.129) With use disorder, mild
(F14.229) With use disorder, moderate or severe
(F14.929) Without use disorder
292.89 (__._) Amphetamine or other stimulant, with perceptual disturbances
(F15.122) With use disorder, mild
(F15.222) With use disorder, moderate or severe
(F15.922) Without use disorder
292.89 (__._) Cocaine, with perceptual disturbances
(F14.122) With use disorder, mild
(F14.222) With use disorder, moderate or severe
(F14.922) Without use disorder

292.0 (__._) Stimulant withdrawal
Specify: The specific substance causing the withdrawal syndrome
(F15.23) Amphetamine or other stimulant
(F14.23) Cocaine
__._ (__._) Other stimulant-induced disorder
292.9 (__._) Unspecified stimulant-related disorder
(F15.99) Amphetamine or other stimulant
(F14.99) Cocaine

Tobacco-related disorders

__._ (__._) Tobacco use disorder
Specify if: On maintenance therapy, in a controlled environment
Specify current severity:
305.1 (Z72.0) Mild
305.1 (F17.200) Moderate
305.1 (F17.200) Severe
292.0 (F17.203) Tobacco withdrawal
__._ (__._) Other tobacco-induced disorders
292.9 (F17.209) Unspecified tobacco-induced disorder
__._ (__._) Other (or unknown) substance use disorder
Specify current severity:
305.90 (F19.10) Mild
304.90 (F19.20) Moderate
304.90 (F19.20) Severe
292.89 (__._) Other (or unknown) substance intoxication
(F19.129) With use disorder, mild
(F19.229) With use disorder, moderate or severe
(F19.929) Without use disorder
292.0 (F19.239) Other (or unknown) substance withdrawal
__._ (__._) Other (or unknown) substance-related disorder
292.9 (F19.99) Unspecified other (or unknown) substance-related disorder

Non-substance-related disorder

312.31 (F63.0) Gambling disorder
Specify if: Episodic, persistent
Specify current severity: mild, moderate, severe

Neurocognitive disorders

__._ (__._) Delirium
Specify whether:
__._ (__._) Substance intoxication delirium
__._ (__._) Substance withdrawal delirium
292.81 (__._) Medication induced delirium
293.0 (F05) Delirium due to another medical condition
293.0 (F05) Delirium due to multiple aetiologies
Specify if: Acute, persistent
Specify if: Hyperactive, hypoactive, mixed level of activity
780.09 (R41.0) Other specified delirium
780.09 (R41.0) Unspecified delirium

Major and minor neurocognitive disorders

Specify whether: Due to Alzheimer's disease, fronto-temporal lobar degeneration, Lewy body disease, vascular disease, traumatic brain injury, substance/medication use, HIV infection, prion disease, Parkinson's disease, Huntington's disease, another medical condition, multiple aetiologies, unspecified
Specify: Without behavioural disturbance, with behavioural disturbance
Specify current severity: Mild, moderate, severe

Major or mild neurocognitive disorder due to Alzheimer's disease

__._ (__._) Probable major neurocognitive disorder due to Alzheimer's disease
294.11 (F02.81) With behavioural disturbance
294.10 (F02.80) Without behavioural disturbance
331.9 (G31.9) Possible major neurocognitive disorder due to Alzheimer's disease
331.83 (G31.84) Mild neurocognitive disorder due to Alzheimer's disease

Major or minor fronto-temporal neurocognitive disorder

__._ (__._) Probable major neurocognitive disorder due to fronto-temporal lobar degeneration
294.11 (F02.81) With behavioural disturbance
294.10 (F02.80) Without behavioural disturbance
331.9 (G31.9) Possible major neurocognitive disorder due to fronto-temporal lobar degeneration
331.83 (G31.84) Mild neurocognitive disorder due to fronto-temporal lobar degeneration

Major or mild neurocognitive disorder with Lewy bodies

__._ (__._) Probable major neurocognitive disorder with Lewy bodies
294.11 (F02.81) With behavioural disturbance
294.10 (F02.80) Without behavioural disturbance
331.9 (G31.9) Possible major neurocognitive disorder with Lewy bodies
331.83 (G31.84) Mild neurocognitive disorder with Lewy bodies

Major or mild vascular neurocognitive disorder

__._ (__._) Probable major vascular neurocognitive disorder
290.40 (F01.51) With behavioural disturbance
290.40 (F01.50) Without behavioural disturbance
331.9 (G31.9) Possible major vascular neurocognitive disorder
331.83 (G31.84) Mild vascular neurocognitive disorder

Major or mild neurocognitive disorders due to traumatic brain injury

__._ (__._) Major neurocognitive disorder due to traumatic brain injury
294.11 (F02.81) Without behavioural disturbance
294.10 (F02.80) Without behavioural disturbance
331.83 (G31.84) Mild neurocognitive disorder due to traumatic brain injury

Substance/medication-induced major or mild neurocognitive disorder

Specify if: Persistent

Major or mild neurocognitive disorder due to HIV

__._ (__._) Major neurocognitive disorder due to HIV infection
294.11 (F02.81) With behavioural disturbance
294.10 (F02.80) Without behavioural disturbance
331.83 (G31.84) Mild neurocognitive disorder due to HIV infection

Major or mild neurocognitive disorder due to prion disease

__._ (__._) Major neurocognitive disorder due to prion disease
294.11 (F02.81) With behavioural disturbance
294.10 (F02.80) Without behavioural disturbance
331.83 (G31.84) Mild neurocognitive disorder due to prion disease

Major or mild neurocognitive disorders due to Parkinson's disease

__._ (__._) Major neurocognitive disorder probably due to Parkinson's disease
294.11 (F02.81) With behavioural disturbance
294.10 (F02.80) Without behavioural disturbance
331.9 (G31.9) Major neurocognitive disorder possibly due to Parkinson's disease
331.83 (G31.84) Mild neurocognitive disorder due to Parkinson's disease

Major or mild neurocognitive disorder due to Huntington's disease

__._ (__._) Major neurocognitive disorder due to Huntington's disease
294.11 (F02.81) With behavioural disturbance
294.10 (F02.80) Without behavioural disturbance
331.83 (G31.84) Mild neurocognitive disorder possibly due to Huntington's disease

Major or mild neurocognitive disorder due to another medical condition

__._ (__._) Major neurocognitive disorder due to another medical condition
294.11 (F02.81) With behavioural disturbance
294.10 (F02.80) Without behavioural disturbance
331.83 (G31.84) Mild neurocognitive disorder due to another medical condition

Major or mild neurocognitive disorder due to multiple aetiologies

__._ (__._) Major neurocognitive disorder due to multiple aetiologies
294.11 (F02.81) With behavioural disturbance
294.10 (F02.80) Without behavioural disturbance
331.83 (G31.84) Mild neurocognitive disorder due to multiple aetiologies

Unspecified neurocognitive disorder

799.59 (R41.9) Unspecified neurocognitive disorder

Personality disorders

Cluster A personality disorders

301.0 (F60.0) Paranoid personality disorder
301.20 (F60.1) Schizoid personality disorder
301.22 (F21) Schizotypal personality disorder

Cluster B personality disorders

301.7 (F60.2) Antisocial personality disorder
301.83 (F60.3) Borderline personality disorder
301.50 (F60.4) Histrionic personality disorder
301.81 (F60.81) Narcissistic personality disorder

Cluster C personality disorders

301.82 (F60.6) Avoidant personality disorder
301.6 (F60.7) Dependent personality disorder
301.4 (F60.5) Obsessive–compulsive personality disorder

Other personality disorders

301.1 (F07.0) Personality change due to another medical condition
Specify whether: Labile type, disinhibited type, aggressive type, apathetic type, paranoid type, other type, combined type, unspecified type
301.89 (F60.89) Other specified personality disorder
301.9 (F60.9) Unspecified personality disorder

Paraphilic disorders

Specify if: In a controlled environment, in full remission
302.82 (F65.3) Voyeuristic disorder
302.4 (F65.2) Exhibitionist disorder
Specify whether: Sexually aroused by exposing genitals to pre-pubertal children, sexually aroused by exposing genitals to physically mature individuals, sexually aroused by exposing genitals to pre-pubertal children and to physically mature individuals
302.89 (F65.81) Frotteuristic disorder
302.83 (F65.51) Sexual masochism disorder
Specify if: With asphyxiophilia
302.84 (F65.52) Sexual sadism disorder
302.2 (F65.4) Paedophilic disorder
Specify whether: Exclusive type, non-exclusive type
Specify if: Sexually attracted to males, sexually attracted to females, sexually attracted to both
Specify if: Limited to incest
302.81 (F65.0) Fetishistic disorder
Specify if: Body part(s), non-living object(s), other
302.3 (F65.1) Transvestic disorder
Specify if: With fetishism, with autogynephilia
302.89 (F65.89) Other specific paraphilic disorder
302.9 (F65.9) Unspecified paraphilic disorder

Other mental disorders

294.8 (F06.8) Other specified mental disorder due to another medical condition

294.9 (F09) Unspecified medical disorder due to another medical condition
300.9 (F99) Other specified mental disorder
300.9 (F99) Unspecified mental disorder

Medication-induced movement disorders and other adverse effects of medication

332.1 (G21.11) Neuroleptic-induced Parkinsonism
332.1 (G21.19) Other medical-induced Parkinsonism
333.92 (G21.0) Neuroleptic malignant syndrome
333.72 (G24.02) Medication-induced acute dystonia
333.99 (G25.71) Medication-induced acute akathisia
333.85 (G24.01) Tardive dyskinesia
333.72 (G24.09) Tardive dystonia
333.99 (G25.71) Tardive akathisia
333.1 (G25.1) Medication-induced postural tremor
333.99 (G25.79) Other medication-induced movement disorder
__._ (__._) Antidepressant discontinuation syndrome
995.29 (T43.205A) Initial encounter
995.29 (T43.205D) Subsequent encounter
995.29 (T43.205S) Sequelae
__._ (__._) Other adverse effect of medication
995.20 (T50.905A) Initial encounter
995.20 (T50.905D) Subsequent encounter
995.20 (T50.905S) Sequelae

Other conditions that may be a focus of clinical attention

Relational Problems

Problems related to family upbringing

V61.20 (Z62.820) Parent–child relational problem
V61.8 (Z62.891) Sibling relational problem
V61.8 (Z62.29) Upbringing away from parents
V61.29 (Z62.898) Child affected by parental relationship distress

Other problems related to primary support group

V61.10 (Z63.0) Relationship distress with spouse or intimate partner
V61.03 (Z63.5) Disruption of family by separation or divorce
V61.8 (Z63.8) High expressed emotion level within family
V62.82 (Z63.4) Uncomplicated bereavement

Abuse and Neglect

Child maltreatment and neglect problems

Child physical abuse

Child physical abuse, confirmed
995.54 (T74.12XA) Initial encounter
995.54 (T74.12XD) Subsequent encounter
Child physical abuse, suspected
995.54 (T76.12XA) Initial encounter
995.54 (T76.12XD) Subsequent encounter
Other circumstances related to child physical abuse
V61.21 (Z69.010) Encounter for mental health services for victim of child abuse by parent
V61.21 (Z69.020) Encounter for mental health services for victim of non-parental child abuse
V15.41 (Z62.810) Personal history (past history) of physical abuse in childhood
V61.22 (Z69.011) Encounter for mental health services for perpetrator of parental child abuse
V62.83 (Z69.021) Encounter for mental health services for perpetrator of non-parental child abuse

Child sexual abuse

Child sexual abuse, confirmed
995.53 (T74.22XA) Initial encounter
995.53 (T74.22XD) Subsequent encounter
Child sexual abuse, suspected
995.53 (T76.22XA) Initial encounter
995.53 (T76.22XD) Subsequent encounter
Other circumstances related to child sexual abuse
V61.21 (Z69.010) Encounter for mental health services for victim of child sexual abuse by parent
V61.21 (Z69.020) Encounter for mental health services for victim of non-parental child sexual abuse
V15.41 (Z62.810) Personal history (past history) of sexual abuse in childhood
V61.22 (Z69.011) Encounter for mental health services for perpetrator of parental child sexual abuse
V62.83 (Z69.021) Encounter for mental health services for perpetrator of non-parental child sexual abuse

Child neglect

Child neglect, confirmed
995.52 (T74.02XA) Initial encounter
995.52 (T74.02XD) Subsequent encounter
Child neglect, suspected
995.52 (T76.02XA) Initial encounter
995.52 (T76.02XD) Subsequent encounter
Other circumstances related to child neglect
V61.21 (Z69.010) Encounter for mental health services for victim of child neglect by parent
V61.21 (Z69.020) Encounter for mental health services for victim of non-parental child neglect
V15.42 (Z69.812) Personal history (past history) of neglect in childhood
V61.22 (Z69.011) Encounter for mental health services for perpetrator of parental child neglect
V62.83 (Z69.021) Encounter for mental health services for perpetrator of non-parental child neglect

Child psychological abuse

Child psychological abuse, confirmed
995.51 (T74.32XA) Initial encounter
995.51 (T74.32XD) Subsequent encounter
Child psychological abuse, suspected
995.51 (T76.32XA) Initial encounter
995.51 (T76.32XD) Subsequent encounter

Other circumstances related to child psychological abuse
V61.21 (Z69.010) Encounter for mental health services for victim of child psychological abuse by parent
V61.21 (Z69.020) Encounter for mental health services for victim of non-parental child psychological abuse
V15.42 (Z62.811) Personal history (past history) of psychological abuse in childhood
V61.22 (Z69.011) Encounter for mental health services for perpetrator of parental child psychological abuse
V62.83 (Z69.021) Encounter for mental health services for perpetrator of non-parental child psychological abuse

Adult maltreatment and neglect problems

Spouse or partner violence, physical

Spouse or partner violence, physical, confirmed
995.81 (T74.11XA) Initial encounter
995.81 (T74.11XD) Subsequent encounter
Spouse or partner violence, physical, suspected
995.81 (T76.11XA) Initial encounter
995.81 (T76.11 XD) Subsequent encounter
Other circumstances related to spouse or partner violence, physical
V61.11 (Z69.11) Encounter for mental health services for victim of spouse or partner violence, physical
D15.41 (Z91.410) Personal history (past history) of spouse or partner violence, physical
V61.12 (Z69.12) Encounter for mental health services for perpetrator of spouse or partner violence, physical

Spouse or partner violence, sexual

Spouse or partner violence, sexual, confirmed
995.83 (T74.21XA) Initial encounter
995.83 (T74.21XD) Subsequent encounter
Spouse or partner violence, sexual, suspected
995.83 (T76.21XA) Initial encounter
995.83 (T76.21XD) Subsequent encounter
Other circumstances related to spouse or partner violence, sexual
V61.11 (Z69.81) Encounter for mental health services for victim of spouse or partner violence, sexual
V15.41 (Z91.410) Personal history (past history) of spouse or partner violence, sexual
V61.12 (Z69.12) Encounter for mental health services for perpetrator of sexual or partner violence, sexual

Spouse or partner, neglect

Spouse or partner in neglect, confirmed
995.85 (T74.01XA) Initial encounter
995.85 (T74.01XD) Subsequent encounter
Spouse or partner neglect, suspected
995.85 (T76.01XA) Initial encounter
995.85 (T76.01XD) Subsequent encounter
Other circumstances related to spouse or partner neglect
V61.11 (Z69.11) Encounter for mental health services for victim of spouse or partner neglect
V15.42 (Z91.412) Personal history (past history) of spouse or partner neglect
V61.12 (Z69.12) Encounter for mental health services for perpetrator of spouse or partner neglect

Spouse or partner abuse, psychological

Spouse or partner abuse, psychological, confirmed
995.82 (T74.31XA) Initial encounter
995.82 (T74.31XVD) Subsequent encounter
Spouse or partner abuse, psychological, suspected
995.82 (T76.31XA) Initial encounter
995.82 (T76.31XD) Subsequent encounter
Other circumstances related to spouse or partner abuse, psychological
V61.11 (Z69.11) Encounter for mental health services for victim of spouse or partner psychological abuse
V15.42 (Z91.411) Personal history (past history) of spouse or partner psychological abuse
V61.12 (Z69.12) Encounter for mental health services for perpetrator of spouse or partner psychological abuse

Adult abuse by non-spouse or non-partner

Adult physical abuse by non-spouse or non-partner, confirmed
995.81 (T74.11XA) Initial encounter
995.81 (T74.11XD) Subsequent encounter
Adult physical abuse by non-spouse or non-partner, suspected
995.81 (T76.11XA) Initial encounter
995.81 (T76.11XD) Subsequent encounter
Adult sexual abuse by non-spouse or non-partner, confirmed
995.83 (T74.21XA) Initial encounter
995.83 (T74.21XD) Subsequent encounter
Adult sexual abuse by non-spouse or non-partner, suspected
995.83 (T76.21XA) Initial encounter
995.83 (T76.21XD) Subsequent encounter
Adult psychological abuse by non-spouse or non-partner, confirmed
995.82 (T74.31XA) Initial encounter
995.82 (T74.31XD) Subsequent encounter
Adult psychological abuse by non-spouse or non-partner, suspected
995.82 (T76.31 XA) Initial encounter
995.82 (T76.31XD) Subsequent encounter
Other circumstances related to adult abuse by non-spouse or non-partner
V65.49 (Z69.81) Encounter for mental health services for victim of non-spousal adult abuse
V62.83 (Z69.82) Encounter for mental health services for perpetrator of non-spousal adult abuse

EDUCATIONAL AND OCCUPATIONAL PROBLEMS

Educational problems
V62.3 (Z55.9) Academic or educational problem

Occupational problems
V62.21 (Z56.82) Problem related to current military deployment status
V62.29 (Z56.9) Other problem related to employment

HOUSING AND ECONOMIC PROBLEMS

Housing problems

V60.0 (Z59.0) Homelessness
V60.1 (Z59.1) Inadequate housing
V60.89 (Z59.2) Discord with neighbour, lodger or landlord
V60.6 (Z59.3) Problem related to living in a residential institution

Economic problems
V60.2 (Z59.4) Lack of adequate food or safe drinking water
V60.2 (Z59.5) Extreme poverty
V60.2 (Z59.6) Low income
V60.2 (Z59.7) Insufficient social insurance or welfare support
V60.9 (Z59.9) Unspecified housing or economic problem

Other Problems Related to The Social Environment

V62.89 (Z60.0) Phase of life problem
V60.3 (Z60.2) Problem related to living alone
V62.4 (Z60.3) Acculturation difficulty
V62.4 (Z60.4) Social exclusion or rejection
V62.4 (Z60.5) Target of (perceived) adverse discrimination or persecution
V62.9 (Z60.9) Unspecified problem related to social environment

Problems Related to Crime or Interaction with The Legal System

V62.89 (Z65.4) Victim of crime
V62.5 (Z65.0) Conviction in civil or criminal proceedings without imprisonment
V62.5 (Z65.1) Imprisonment or other incarceration
V62.5 (Z65.2) Problems related to release from prison
V62.5 (Z65.3) Problems related to other legal circumstances

Other Health Service Encounters for Counselling and Medical Advice

V65.49 (Z70.9) Sexual counselling
V65.40 (Z71.9) Other counselling or consultation

Problems Relates to Other Psychosocial, Personal and Environmental Circumstances

V62.89 (Z65.8) Religious or spiritual problem
V61.7 (Z64.0) Problems related to unwanted pregnancy
V61.5 (Z64.1) Problems related to multiparity
V62.89 (Z64.4) Discord with social service provider, including probation officer, case manager or social services worker
V62.89 (Z65.4) Victim of terrorism or torture
V62.22 (Z65.5) Exposure to disaster, war or other hostilities
V62.89 (Z65.8) Other problem related to psychosocial circumstances
V62.9 (Z65.9) Unspecified problem related to unspecified psychosocial circumstances

Other Circumstances of Personal History

V15.49 (Z91.49) Other personal history of psychological trauma
V15.59 (Z91.5) Personal history of self-harm
V62.21 (Z91.82) Personal history of military deployment
V15.89 (Z91.89) Other personal risk factors
V69.9 (Z72.9) Personal problem related to lifestyle
V71.01 (Z72.811) Adult antisocial behaviour
V71.02 (Z72.810) Child or adolescent antisocial behaviour
Problems related to access to medical or other healthcare
V63.9 (Z75.3) Unavailability or inaccessibility of healthcare facilities
V63.8 (Z75.4) Unavailability or inaccessibility or of other helping agencies
Non-adherence to medical treatment
V15.81 (Z91.19) Non-adherence to medical treatment
278.00 (E66.9) Overweight or obesity
V65.2 (Z76.5) Malingering
V40.31 (Z91.83) Wandering associated with a mental disorder
V62.89 (R41.83) Borderline intellectual functioning

Source: Kneisl, C. R. & Trigoboff, E. (2013). *DSM-5 Transition Guide for Contemporary Psychiatric–Mental Health Nursing* (3rd ed.). ©2013 Pearson Inc, ISBN13: 9780133597301.

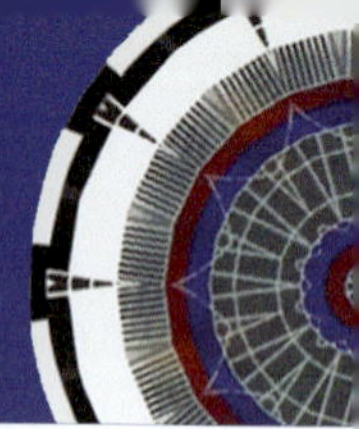

APPENDIX B

ICD-10 CLASSIFICATIONS

❖ This symbol denotes an Australian addition to the World Health Organization's ICD-10

NOS = not otherwise specified
NEC = not elsewhere classified

Mental and behavioural disorders

F00–F09 Organic, including symptomatic, mental disorders

F00 Dementia in Alzheimer's disease

F00.0 Dementia in Alzheimer's disease with early onset
F00.1 Dementia in Alzheimer's disease with late onset
F00.2 Dementia in Alzheimer's disease, atypical or mixed-type
F00.9 Dementia in Alzheimer's disease, unspecified

F01 Vascular dementia

F01.0 Vascular dementia of acute onset
F01.1 Multi-infarct dementia
F01.2 Subcortical vascular dementia
F01.3 Mixed cortical and subcortical vascular dementia
F01.8 Other vascular dementia
F01.9 Vascular dementia, unspecified

F02 Dementia in other diseases classified elsewhere

F02.0 Dementia in Pick's disease
F02.1 Dementia in Creutzfeldt–Jakob disease
F02.2 Dementia in Huntington's disease
F02.3 Dementia in Parkinson's disease
F02.4 Dementia in human immunodeficiency virus (HIV) disease
F02.8 Dementia in other specified diseases classified elsewhere

F03 Unspecified dementia

F04 Organic amnesia syndrome, not induced by alcohol and other psychoactive substances

F04.0 Post-traumatic amnesia
- ❖ F04.00 Post-traumatic amnesia, unspecified
- ❖ F04.01 Post-traumatic amnesia, duration < 24 hours
- ❖ F04.02 Post-traumatic amnesia, duration > 24 hours and < 14 days
- ❖ F04.03 Post-traumatic amnesia, duration > 14 days

F04.9 Amnesic syndrome, unspecified

F05 Delirium, not induced by alcohol and other psychoactive substances

F05.0 Delirium not superimposed on dementia, so described
F05.1 Delirium superimposed on dementia
F05.8 Other delirium
F05.9 Delirium, unspecified

F06 Other mental disorders due to brain damage and dysfunctional and to physical disease

F06.0 Organic hallucinosis
F06.1 Organic catatonic disorder
F06.2 Organic delusional (schizophrenia-like) disorder
F06.3 Organic mood (affective) disorders
F06.4 Organic anxiety disorder
F06.5 Organic dissociative disorder
F06.6 Organic emotionally labile (asthenic) disorder
F06.7 Mild cognitive disorder
F06.8 Other specified mental disorders due to brain damage and dysfunctional and to physical disease
F06.9 Unspecified mental disorder due to brain damage and dysfunctional and to physical disease

F07 Personality and behavioural disorders due to brain damage, damage and dysfunction

F07.0 Organic personality disorder
F07.1 Post-encephalitic syndrome
F07.2 Post-concussional syndrome
F07.8 Other organic personality and behavioural disorders due to brain damage, damage and dysfunction
F07.9 Unspecified organic personality and behavioural disorder due to brain damage, damage and dysfunction

F09 Unspecified organic or symptomatic mental disorder

F10–F19 Mental and behavioural disorders due to psychoactive substance use

Categories for F10–F19
.0 Acute intoxication
.1 Harmful use
.2 Dependence syndrome
.3 Withdrawal state
.4 Withdrawal state with delirium
.5 Psychotic disorder
.6 Amnesic syndrome
.7 Residual and late-onset psychotic disorder
.8 Other mental and behavioural disorder
.9 Unspecified mental and behavioural disorder

F10 Mental and behavioural disorders due to use of alcohol

F11 Mental and behavioural disorders due to use of opioids

F12 Mental and behavioural disorders due to use of cannabinoids

F13 Mental and behavioural disorders due to use of sedatives or hypnotics

F14 Mental and behavioural disorders due to use of cocaine

F15 Mental and behavioural disorders due to of other stimulants, including caffeine

F16 Mental and behavioural disorders due to use of hallucinogens

F17 Mental and behavioural disorders due to use of tobacco

F18 Mental and behavioural disorders due to use of volatile solvents

F19 Mental and behavioural disorders due to multiple drug use and use of other psychoactive substances

F20–F29 Schizophrenia, schizotypal and delusional disorders

F20 Schizophrenia

F20.0 Paranoid schizophrenia
F20.1 Hebephrenic schizophrenia
F20.2 Catatonic schizophrenia
F20.3 Undifferentiated schizophrenia
F20.4 Post-schizophrenic depression
F20.5 Residual schizophrenia
F20.6 Simple schizophrenia
F20.8 Other schizophrenia
F20.9 Schizophrenia, unspecified

F21 Schizotypal disorder

F22 Persistent delusional disorders

F22.0 Delusional disorder
F22.8 Other persistent delusional disorders
F22.9 Persistent delusional disorder, unspecified

F23 Acute and transient psychotic disorders

F23.0 Acute polymorphic psychotic disorder without symptoms of schizophrenia
F23.1 Acute polymorphic psychotic disorder with symptoms of schizophrenia
F23.2 Acute schizophrenia-like psychotic disorder
F23.3 Other acute predominantly delusional psychotic disorders
F23.8 Other acute and transient psychotic disorders
F23.9 Acute and transient psychotic disorder, unspecified

F24 Induced delusional disorder

F25 Schizoaffective disorders

F25.0 Schizoaffective disorder, manic type
F25.1 Schizoaffective disorder, depressive type
F25.2 Schizoaffective disorder, mixed type
F25.8 Other schizoaffective disorders
F25.9 Schizoaffective disorder, unspecified

F28 Other non-organic psychotic disorders

F29 Unspecified non-organic psychosis

F30–F39 Mood (affective) disorders

F30 Manic episode

F30.0 Hypomania
F30.1 Mania without psychotic symptoms
F30.2 Mania with psychotic symptoms
F30.8 Other manic episodes
F30.9 Manic episode, unspecified

F31 Bipolar affective disorder

F31.0 Bipolar affective disorder, current episode hypomanic
F31.1 Bipolar affective disorder, current episode manic without psychotic symptoms
F31.2 Bipolar affective disorder, current episode manic with psychotic symptoms
F31.3 Bipolar affective disorder, current episode mild or moderate depression
F31.4 Bipolar affective disorder, current episode severe depression without psychotic symptoms
F31.5 Bipolar affective disorder, current episode severe depression with psychotic symptoms
F31.6 Bipolar affective disorder, current episode mixed
F31.7 Bipolar affective disorder, currently in remission
F31.8 Other bipolar affective disorders
F31.9 Bipolar affective disorder, unspecified

F32 Depressive episode

- 0 not specified as arising in the postnatal period
- 1 arising in the postnatal period

F32.0 Mild depressive episode
F32.1 Moderate depressive episode
F32.2 Severe depressive episode without psychotic symptoms
F32.3 Severe depressive episode with psychotic symptoms
F32.8 Other depressive episodes
F32.9 Depressive episode, unspecified

F33 Recurrent depressive disorder

F33.0 Recurrent depressive disorder, current episode mild
F33.1 Recurrent depressive disorder, current episode moderate
F33.2 Recurrent depressive disorder, current episode severe without psychotic symptoms
F33.3 Recurrent depressive disorder, current episode severe with psychotic symptoms
F33.4 Recurrent depressive disorder, currently in remission
F33.8 Other recurrent depressive disorders
F33.9 Recurrent depressive disorder, unspecified

F34 Persistent mood (affective) disorder

F34.0 Cyclothymia
F34.1 Dysthymia
F34.8 Other persistent mood (affective) disorders
F34.9 Persistent mood (affective) disorder, unspecified

F38 Other mood (affective) disorders

F38.0 Other single mood (affective) disorders
F38.1 Other recurrent mood (affective) disorders

F38.8 Other specified mood (affective) disorders

F39 Unspecified mood (affective) disorder

F40–F48 Neurotic, stress-related and somatoform disorders

F40 Phobic anxiety disorders

F40.0 Agoraphobia
- ❖ F40.00 Agoraphobia without mention of panic disorder
- ❖ F40.01 Agoraphobia with panic disorder

F40.1 Social phobias
F40.2 Specific (isolated) phobias
F40.8 Other phobic anxiety disorders
F40.9 Phobic anxiety disorder, unspecified

F41 Other anxiety disorders

F41.0 Panic disorder (episodic paroxysmal anxiety)
F41.1 Generalised anxiety disorder
F41.2 Mixed anxiety and depressive disorder
F41.3 Other mixed anxiety disorders
F41.8 Other specified anxiety disorders
Anxiety hysteria
F41.9 Anxiety disorder, unspecified
Anxiety NOS

F42 Obsessive–compulsive disorder

F42.0 Predominantly obsessional thoughts or ruminations
F42.1 Predominantly compulsive acts (obsessional rituals)
F42.2 Mixed obsessional thoughts and acts
F42.8 Other obsessive–compulsive disorders
F42.9 Obsessive–compulsive disorder, unspecified

F43 Reaction to severe stress, and adjustment disorders

F43.0 Acute stress reaction
F43.1 Post-traumatic stress disorder
F43.2 Adjustment disorders
F43.8 Other reactions to severe stress
F43.9 Reaction to severe stress, unspecified

F44 Dissociative (conversion) disorders

F44.0 Dissociative amnesia
F44.1 Dissociative fugue
F44.2 Dissociative stupor
F44.3 Trance and possession disorders
Dissociative disorders of movement and sensation
F44.4 Dissociative motor disorders
F44.5 Dissociative convulsions
F44.6 Dissociative anaesthesia and sensory loss
F44.7 Mixed dissociative (conversion) disorders
F44.8 Other dissociative (conversion) disorders
- ❖ F44.80 Ganser's syndrome
- ❖ F44.81 Multiple personality disorder
- ❖ F44.82 Transient dissociative (conversion) disorders occurring in childhood and adolescence
- ❖ F44.88 Other specified dissociative (conversion) disorders

F44.9 Dissociative (conversion) disorder, unspecified

F45 Somatoform disorders

F45.0 Somatisation disorder
F45.1 Undifferentiated somatoform disorder
F45.2 Hypochondriacal disorder
F45.3 Somatoform autonomic dysfunction
- ❖ F45.30 Somatoform autonomic dysfunction, unspecified organ or system
- ❖ F45.31 Somatoform autonomic dysfunction, heart and cardiovascular system
- ❖ F45.32 Somatoform autonomic dysfunction, upper gastrointestinal tract
- ❖ F45.33 Somatoform autonomic dysfunction, lower gastrointestinal tract
- ❖ F45.34 Somatoform autonomic dysfunction, respiratory system
- ❖ F45.35 Somatoform autonomic dysfunction, genito-urinary system
- ❖ F45.38 Somatoform autonomic dysfunction, other organ or system
- ❖ F45.39 Somatoform autonomic dysfunction, multiple organs or systems

F45.4 Persistent somatoform pain disorder
F45.8 Other somatoform disorders
F45.9 Somatoform disorder, unspecified

F48 Other neurotic disorders

F48.0 Neurasthenia
F48.1 Depersonalisation–derealisation syndrome
F48.8 Other specified neurotic disorders
F48.9 Neurotic disorder, unspecified

F50–F59 Behavioural syndromes associated with psychological disturbances and physical factors

F50 Eating disorders

F50.0 Anorexia nervosa
F50.1 Atypical anorexia nervosa
F50.2 Bulimia nervosa
F50.3 Atypical bulimia nervosa
F50.4 Overeating associated with other psychological disturbances
F50.5 Vomiting associated with other psychological disturbances
F50.8 Other eating disorders
F50.9 Eating disorder, unspecified

F51 Non-organic sleep disorders

F51.0 Non-organic insomnia
F51.1 Non-organic hypersomnia
F51.2 Non-organic disorder of the sleep–wake schedule
F50.3 Sleepwalking (somnambulism)
F50.4 Sleep terrors (night terrors)
F51.5 Nightmares
F51.8 Other non-organic sleep disorders
F51.9 Non-organic sleep disorder, unspecified

F52 Sexual dysfunction, not caused by organic disorder or disease

F52.0 Lack or loss of sexual desire
F52.1 Sexual aversion and lack of sexual enjoyment
F52.2 Failure of genital response
F52.3 Organismic dysfunction
F52.4 Premature ejaculation
F52.5 Non-organic vaginismus
F52.6 Non-organic dyspareunia
F52.7 Excessive sexual drive
F52.8 Other sexual dysfunction, not caused by organic disorder or disease
F52.9 Unspecified sexual dysfunction, not caused by organic disorder or disease

F53 Mental and behavioural disorders associated with the puerperium, not elsewhere classified

F53.0 Mild mental and behavioural disorders associated with the puerperium, not elsewhere classified
Depression: post-natal NOS, postpartum NOS
F53.1 Severe mental and behavioural disorders associated with the puerperium, not elsewhere classified
Puerperal psychosis NOS
F53.8 Other mental and behavioural disorders associated with the puerperium, not elsewhere classified
Post-partum: blues NOS, dysphoria NOS, mood disturbance NOS, sadness NOS
F53.9 Puerperal mental disorder, unspecified

P54 Psychological and behavioural factors associated with disorders or diseases classified elsewhere

F55 Harmful use of non-dependence-producing substances

- F55.0 Antidepressants
- F55.1 Laxatives
- F55.2 Analgesics
- F55.3 Antacids
- F55.4 Vitamins
- F55.5 Steroids or hormones
- F55.6 Specific herbal or folk remedies
- F55.8 Other substances that do not produce dependence
- F55.9 Unspecified

F59 Unspecified behavioural syndromes associated with physiological disturbances and physical factors

F60–F69 Disorders of adult personality and behaviour

F60 Specific personality disorders

F60.0 Paranoid personality disorder
F60.1 Schizoid personality disorder
F60.2 Dissocial personality disorder
F60.3 Emotionally unstable personality disorder

- F60.30 Impulsive type
- F60.31 Borderline type

F60.4 Histrionic personality disorder
F60.5 Anankastic personality disorder
F60.6 Anxious (avoidant) personality disorder
F60.7 Dependent personality disorder
F60.8 Other specific personality disorders
F60.9 Personality disorder, unspecified

F61 Mixed and other personality disorders

F62 Enduring personality changes, not attributable to brain damage and disease

F62.0 Enduring personality change after catastrophic experience
F62.1 Enduring personality change after psychiatric illness
F62.8 Other enduring personality changes
F62.9 Enduring personality change, unspecified

F63 Habit and impulse disorders

F63.0 Pathological gambling
F63.1 Pathological fire-setting (pyromania)
F63.2 Pathological stealing (kleptomania)
F63.3 Trichotillomania
F63.8 Other habits and impulse disorders
F63.9 Habit and impulse disorder, unspecified

F64 Gender identity disorders

F64.0 Transsexualism
F64.1 Dual-role transvestism
F64.2 Gender identity disorder of childhood
F64.8 Other gender identity disorders
F64.9 Gender identity disorder, unspecified

F65 Disorders of sexual preference

F65.0 Fetishism
F65.1 Fetishistic transvestism
F65.2 Exhibitionism
F65.3 Voyeurism
F65.4 Paedophilia
F65.5 Sadomasochism
F65.6 Multiple disorders of sexual preference
F65.8 Other disorders of sexual preference
F65.9 Disorder of sexual preference, unspecified

F66 Psychological and behavioural disorders associated with sexual development and orientation

F66.0 Sexual maturation disorder
F66.1 Egodystonic sexual orientation
F66.2 Sexual relationship disorder
F66.8 Other psychosexual development disorders
F66.9 Psychosexual development disorder, unspecified

F68 Other disorders of adult personality and behaviour

F68.0 Elaboration of physical symptoms for psychological reasons

F68.1 Intentional production of feigning of symptoms or disabilities, either physical or psychological (factitious disorder)
F68.8 Other specified disorders of adult personality and behaviour

F69 Unspecified disorder of adult personality and behaviour

F70–F79 Mental retardation

.0 With the statement of no, or minimal, impairment of behaviour
.1 Significant impairment of behaviour requiring attention or treatment
.8 Other impairments of behaviour
.9 Without mention of impairment of behaviour

F70 Mild mental retardation

F71 Moderate mental retardation

F72 Severe mental retardation

F73 Profound mental retardation

F78 Other mental retardation

F79 Unspecified mental retardation

F80–F89 Disorders of psychological development

F80 Specific development disorders of speech and language

F80.0 Specific speech articulation disorder
F80.1 Expressive language disorder
F80.2 Receptive language disorder
F80.3 Acquired aphasia with epilepsy (Landau–Kleffner)
F80.8 Other developmental disorders of speech and language
F80.9 Developmental disorder of speech and language, unspecified

F81 Specific developmental disorders of scholastic skills

F81.0 Specific reading disorder
F81.1 Specific spelling disorder
F81.2 Specific disorder of arithmetical skills
F81.3 Mixed disorder of scholastic skills
F81.8 Other developmental disorders of scholastic skills
F81.9 Developmental disorder of scholastic skills, unspecified

F82 Specific development disorder of motor function

F83 Mixed specific development disorders

F84 Pervasive development disorders

F84.0 Childhood autism
F84.1 Atypical autism
F84.2 Rett's syndrome
F84.3 Other childhood disintegrative disorder
F84.4 Overactive disorder associated with mental retardation and stereotyped movements
F84.5 Asperger's syndrome
F84.8 Other pervasive development disorders
F84.9 Pervasive development disorder, unspecified

F88 Other disorders of psychological development

F89 Unspecified disorder of psychological development

F90–F98 Behavioural and emotional disorders with onset usually occurring in childhood and adolescence

F90 Hyperkinetic disorders

F90.0 Disturbance of activity and attention
F90.1 Hyperkinetic conduct disorder
F90.8 Other hyperkinetic disorders
F90.9 Hyperkinetic disorder, unspecified

F91 Conduct disorders

F91.0 Conduct disorder confined to the family context
F91.1 Unsocialised conduct disorder
F91.2 Socialised conduct disorder
F91.3 Oppositional defiant disorder
F91.8 Other conduct disorders
F91.9 Conduct disorder, unspecified

F92 Mixed disorders of conduct and emotion

F92.0 Depressive conduct disorder
F92.8 Other mixed disorders of conduct and emotions
F92.9 Mixed disorder of conduct and emotions, unspecified

F93 Emotional disorders with onset specific to childhood

F93.0 Separation anxiety disorder of childhood
F93.1 Phobic anxiety disorder of childhood
F93.2 Social anxiety disorder of childhood
F93.3 Sibling rivalry disorder
F93.8 Other childhood emotional disorders
F93.9 Childhood emotional disorder, unspecified

F94 Disorders of social functioning with onset specific to childhood and adolescence

F94.0 Elective mutism
F94.1 Reactive attachment disorder of childhood
F94.2 Disinhibited attachment disorder of childhood
F94.8 Other childhood disorders of social functioning
F94.9 Childhood disorder of social functioning, unspecified

F95 Tic disorders

F95.0 Transient tic disorder
F95.1 Chronic motor or vocal tic disorder
F95.2 Combined vocal and multiple motor tic disorder (de la Tourette)
F95.8 Other tic disorders
F95.9 Tic disorder, unspecified

F98 Other behavioural and emotional disorders with onset usually occurring in childhood and adolescence

F98.0 Non-organic enuresis
F98.1 Nonorganic encopresis
F98.2 Feeding disorder of infancy and childhood
F98.3 Pica of infancy and childhood
F98.4 Stereotyped movement disorders
F98.5 Stuttering (stammering)
F98.6 Cluttering
F98.8 Other specified behavioural and emotional disorders with onset usually occurring in childhood and adolescence
F98.9 Unspecified behavioural and emotional disorders with onset usually occurring in childhood and adolescence

F99 Unspecified mental disorder

F99 Mental disorder, not otherwise specified

Sources: Pain Ladder from ICD-10 Version 2016, reprinted from the World Health Organization 2016; ICD-10 Category classification from ICD-10 Version 2016, World Health Organization.

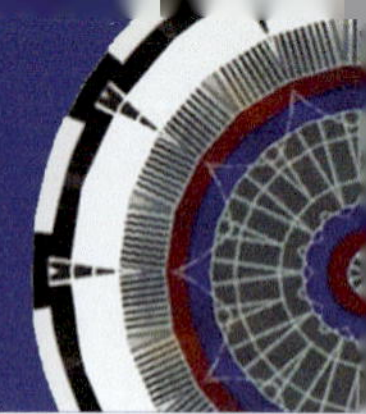

MAPPING TO THE NMBA REGISTERED NURSE STANDARDS FOR PRACTICE (JUNE 2016)

Chapter number	Standard	Criteria (sub-standard)	Evidence-based examples (including page no.)
1	1. Thinks critically and analyses nursing practice	1.1 Accesses, analyses, and uses the best available evidence, that includes research findings, for safe and competent nursing practice	Access to Australian epidemiological data sets through the website www.aihw.gov/mental-health-information-sources, in Mental Illness as a Global Problem, p. 5
		1.2 Develops practice through reflection on experiences, knowledge, actions, feelings and beliefs to identify how these shape and impact practice	Examines the history of psychiatric nursing and mental illness and the approaches to care in Important Dates in the Shifting Approaches to Mental Disorder, pp. 10–11, 14–15; Figure 1–2, pp. 12–13
		1.3 Respects and values all cultures and experiences, which includes responding to the role of carers and community that underpin the health of Aboriginal and Torres Strait Islander peoples and people of other cultures	Understand the stigmatisation associated with mental illness in Box 1.3: Stigmatising beliefs about mental illness, p. 15; Figure 1.7: The effect of stigma on personal recovery from mental illness, p. 16
	2. Engages in therapeutic and professional relationships	2.2 Communicates effectively, and is respectful of a person's dignity, culture, values, beliefs and rights	Respects individuals seeking mental health interventions in People, Not Patients, p. 4
		2.4 Provides support and directs people to resources to optimise health-related decisions and health-seeking behaviours	Identifies individuals vulnerable to mental illness in Table 1.2: Sociocultural dislocation, violence and mental illness, p. 9
		2.5 Advocates on behalf of people in a manner that respects the person's autonomy and capacity	Advocates for individuals seeking mental health interventions in People, Not Patients, p. 4
	3. Maintains the capability for practice	3.2 Provides the information and education required to enhance people's control over health	Identifies characteristics of individuals who are mentally healthy in Box 1.1: Characteristics of people considered to be mentally healthy, p. 4
	4. Comprehensively conducts assessments	4.1 Conducts assessments that are holistic as well as culturally appropriate	Assesses individuals from immigrant and refugee backgrounds in Box 1.2: Questions for assessing people from refugee and immigrant backgrounds, p. 10
		4.3 Works in partnership to determine factors that affect, or potentially affect, the health and wellbeing of people and populations to determine priorities for action and/or for referral	Actively seeks to prevent stigmatisation in Self-awareness: Respectful language to combat stigma, p. 17
	5. Develops a plan for nursing practice	5.2 Collaboratively constructs nursing practice plans until contingencies, options priorities, goals, actions, outcomes and timeframes are agreed with the relevant persons	Refers individuals to appropriate mental health organisations in Table 1.1: Mental health support organisations, p. 8

Chapter number	Standard	Criteria (sub-standard)	Evidence-based examples (including page no.)
2	2. Engages in therapeutic and professional relationships	2.1 Establishes, sustains and concludes relationships in a way that differentiates the boundaries between professional and personal relationships	Practices according to appropriate type of relationship in Table 2.1: Differences between professional and social relationships, p. 23; Table 2.2: Similarities and differences in informal and formal one-to-one relationships, p. 24 Establishes the therapeutic relationship according to identified phases: Orientation, pp. 30–36; Your Intervention: Strategies goals, tasks and interventions of the orientation phase, p. 35 Working phase, pp. 36–40; Your Intervention Strategies: Goals, tasks and interventions of the working phase, p. 37; Your Intervention Strategies: Problem-solving strategies, p. 39 Termination phase, pp. 40–43; Your Assessment Approach: Termination readiness, p. 40; Your Intervention Strategies: Goals, tasks and interventions of the termination phase, p. 42
		2.2 Communicates effectively, and is respectful of a person's dignity, culture, values, beliefs and rights	Engages in the therapeutic relationship in Figure 2.1: Nurse and consumer characteristics that enhance the one-to-one therapeutic relationship, p. 20; The Initial Contract, p. 30
	3. Maintains the capability for practice	3.1 Considers and responds in a timely manner to the health and wellbeing of self and others in relation to the capability for practice	Practices self-awareness when engaging in a therapeutic relationship in Self-awareness: Common concerns of nursing students and new graduate nurses, p. 22
		3.3 Uses a lifelong learning approach for continuing professional development of self and others	Recognises and implements strategies to support transference and countertransference, pp. 27–28; Self-awareness: Countertransference, p. 28
		3.4 Accepts accountability for decisions, actions, behaviours and responsibilities inherent in their role, and for the actions of others to whom they have delegated responsibilities	Engages in self-disclosure when appropriate in Self-awareness: Self-disclosure, p. 30
	4. Comprehensively conducts assessments	4.1 Conducts comprehensive assessments that are holistic as well as culturally appropriate	Conducts comprehensive assessment during the orientation phase of the therapeutic relationship, pp. 31–32

Chapter number	Standard	Criteria (sub-standard)	Evidence-based examples (including page no.)
			Conducts comprehensive assessment during the working phase of the therapeutic relationship, pp. 36–37 Conducts comprehensive assessment during the termination phase of the therapeutic relationship, pp. 40–41
	5. Develops a plan for nursing practice	5.1 Uses assessment data and best available evidence to develop a collaborative plan	Plans care with the consumer during the orientation phase of the therapeutic relationship, pp. 32–36 Plans care with the consumer during the working phase of the therapeutic relationship, pp. 37–39 Plans care with the consumer during the termination phase of the therapeutic relationship, pp. 41–42
	7. Evaluates outcomes to inform nursing practice	7.1 Evaluates and monitors progress toward the expected goals and outcomes	Evaluates achievement of expectations with the consumer at the conclusion of the orientation phase of the therapeutic relationship, p. 36 Evaluates achievement of expectations with the consumer at the conclusion of the working phase of the therapeutic relationship, pp. 39–40 Evaluates achievement of expectations with the consumer of the termination phase of the therapeutic relationship, p. 43
3	1. Thinks critically and analyses nursing practice	1.4 Complies with legislation, regulations, policies, guidelines and other standards or requirements relevant to the context of practice when making decisions	Adheres to the Australian College of Mental Health Nurses Standards of Practice for Australian Mental Health in What is Mental Health Nursing, pp. 46–47; Standards of Practice for Australian Mental Health Nurses, pp. 52–54
		1.7 Contributes to quality improvement and relevant research	Utilises nursing theory to promote mental health practice in Nursing's Theoretical Heritage, pp. 55–58
	2. Engages in therapeutic and professional relationships	2.8 Participates in and/or leads collaborative practice	Engages in collaborative practice relationships in Partnership and Collaboration, pp. 54–55; Your Intervention Strategies: Lessons on collaboration, p. 55
	3. Maintains the capability for practice	3.3 Uses a lifelong learning approach for continuing professional development of self and others	Remains current in the practice of mental health nursing in the New Millennium, pp. 50–51; The Education of Mental Health Nurses, pp. 51–52

Chapter number	Standard	Criteria (sub-standard)	Evidence-based examples (including page no.)
		3.7 Identifies and promotes the integral role of nursing practice and the profession in influencing better health outcomes for people	Applies the caring process when delivering mental health care in Box 3.1: Watson's clinical caritas processes, p. 57
	6. Provides safe, appropriate and responsive quality nursing practice	6.2 Practises within their scope of practice	Adheres to the Australian College of Mental Health Nurses Standards of Practice for Australian Mental Health in What is Mental Health Nursing, pp. 46–47; Standards of Practice for Australian Mental Health Nurses, pp. 52–54
		6.5 Practises in accordance with relevant policies, guidelines, standards, regulations and legislation	Adheres to the Australian College of Mental Health Nurses Standards of Practice for Australian Mental Health in What is Mental Health Nursing, pp. 46–47; Standards of Practice for Australian Mental Health Nurses, pp. 52–54
4	1. Thinks critically and analyses nursing practice	1.2 Develops practice through reflection on experiences, knowledge, actions, feelings and beliefs to identify how these shape practice	Examines beliefs about mental illness in Box 4.1: Blind and irrational beliefs about mental illness, p. 63
	2. Engages in therapeutic and professional relationships	2.1 Establishes, sustains and concludes relationships in a way that differentiates the boundaries between professional and personal relationships	Participates in activities to improve therapeutic relationships in Qualities That Enhance Therapeutic Relationships, pp. 68–72
		2.2 Communicates effectively, and is respectful of a person's dignity, culture, values, beliefs and rights	Acknowledges and addresses spiritual needs in Box 4.2: Spirituality: helping others rediscover their spiritual path, p. 71
	3. Maintains the capability for practice	3.1 Considers and responds in a timely manner to the health and wellbeing of self and others in relation to the capability for practice	Engages in self-analysis of feelings in Figure 4.1 Self-awareness of feelings, p. 62; Personal Integration, pp. 61–65
		3.3 Uses a lifelong learning approach for continuing professional development of self and others	Practices self-awareness in Self-awareness: Influence of sociocultural heritage, p. 65; Taking Care of the Self, pp. 65–67; Self-awareness: Comparing your own passive, aggressive and assertive behaviours, p. 69
5	1. Thinks critically and analyses nursing practice	1.1 Accesses, analyses, and uses the best available evidence, that includes research findings, for safe, quality practice	Identifies appropriate theoretical base when planning practice approaches in Humanistic Interactionism and Psychobiology: The Mind–Body–Spirit Connection, pp. 76–79
	2. Engages in therapeutic and professional relationships	2.8 Participates in and/or leads collaborative practice	Engages in interdisciplinary mental health practice in Theories for Interdisciplinary Mental Health care, pp. 79–88; Table 5.1: Comparison of major features of traditional psychiatric theories, p. 79

Chapter number	Standard	Criteria (sub-standard)	Evidence-based examples (including page no.)
	6. Provides safe, appropriate and responsive quality nursing practice	6.1 Provides comprehensive safe, quality practice to achieve agreed goals and outcomes that are responsive to the nursing needs of people	Implements theoretical-supported approaches when applying mental health nursing care Box 5.5: Fundamental principles of cognitive behavioural therapy, p. 83
		6.2 Practises within their scope of practice	Adheres to actions with the scope of practice in Scope of Psychiatric–Mental Health Nursing Practice pp. 75–76
6	1. Thinks critically and analyses nursing practice	1.1 Accesses, analyses, and uses the best available evidence, which includes research findings, for safe, quality practice	Understands brain function and the role of brain structures to support mental health in Brain, Mind and Behaviour, pp. 91–93, 95–99 Utilises information about the role of neurotransmitters for mental health function in Neurons, synapses, receptors and neurotransmission, pp. 100–101, 103–105; Table 6.1: The major known neurotransmitters, p. 102
	3. Maintains the capability for practice	3.2 Provides the information and education required to enhance people's control over health	Informs individuals impacted by mental illness in Collaborative Care: Teaching about genetics and schizophrenia, p. 107
	4. Comprehensively conducts assessments	4.3 Works in partnership to determine factors that affect, or potentially affect, the health and wellbeing of people and populations to determine priorities for action and/or for referral	Accesses information about individual mental illness to support assessment findings in Biological Basis of Mental Illness, pp. 105–109
7	1. Thinks critically and analyses nursing practice	1.3 Respects all cultures and experiences, which includes responding to the role of family and community that underpin the health of Aboriginal and Torres Strait Islander peoples and people of other cultures	Employs approaches to enhance medication adherence with Indigenous cultures in Box 7.1: Recommendations for working with Aboriginal and Torres Strait Islander peoples, p. 116
	2. Engages in therapeutic and professional relationships	2.2 Communicates effectively, and is respectful of a person's dignity, culture, values, beliefs and rights	Engages in conversation about herbal medications in Communication: Communicating with a person about herbal medicines, p. 139
		2.7 Actively fosters a culture of safety and learning that includes engaging with health professionals and others, to share knowledge and practice that supports person-centred care	Examines the use of complementary/alternative therapies in the treatment of mental illness, in Herbal Medicines, pp. 139–140
	3. Maintains the capability for practice	3.2 Provides the information and education required to enhance people's control over health	Implements teaching plans to support person-centred care in Collaborative Care features: Teaching about antipsychotic medications, p. 122; Teaching about a low-tyramine diet, p. 128; Teaching about antidepressants, p. 131–132
			Facilitates education on strategies to enhance medication adherence in Your Intervention Strategies: Lithium maintenance considerations, p. 135

Chapter number	Standard	Criteria (sub-standard)	Evidence-based examples (including page no.)
	4. Comprehensively conducts assessments	4.2 Uses a range of assessment techniques to systematically collect relevant and accurate information and data to inform practice	Assesses and evaluates medications for potential interactions in Your Assessment Approach: Antipsychotic medication interactions, p. 122 Assesses for medication adverse effects in Your Assessment Approach: Extrapyramidal side-effects (EPSEs), p. 124 Assesses for medication interactions in Your Assessment Approach: Antidepressant medication interactions, p. 129 Assesses for manifestations when medications are not taken as prescribed in Your Assessment Approach: SSRI discontinuation syndrome, p. 131 Assesses for medication interactions in Your Assessment Approach: Mood stabiliser medication interactions, p. 133 Assesses for medication interactions in Your Assessment Approach: Anxiolytic medication interactions, p. 136
		4.4 Assesses the resources available to inform planning	Accesses information about the effects of medications on sleep in What Every Nurse Should Know: Medications that affect sleep, p. 138
	5. Develops a collaborative plan for nursing practice	5.1 Uses assessment data and best available evidence to develop a collaborative plan	Accesses information to support collaborative medication planning in Box 7.2: Recommendations on the medication management of schizophrenia and related disorders and mood disorders, p. 117
	6. Provides safe, appropriate and responsive quality nursing practice	6.1 Provides comprehensive safe, quality practice to achieve agreed goals and outcomes that are responsive to the nursing needs of individuals	Implements strategies to enhance medication adherence in Your Intervention Strategies: Enhancing adherence to medication, p. 113
8	1. Thinks critically and analyses nursing practice	1.1 Accesses, analyses, and uses the best available evidence, that includes research findings, for safe, quality practice	Reviews current theory on anxiety in Anxiety, pp. 149–151; Box 8.1: General causes of anxiety, p. 149
		1.5 Uses ethical frameworks when making decisions	Examines theories of stress prior to planning care for a person with this health issue in Biopsychosocial Theories of Stress, pp. 145–149 Analyses theories that can cause anxiety in Biopsychosocial Theories, pp. 158–160

Chapter number	Standard	Criteria (sub-standard)	Evidence-based examples (including page no.)
	2. Engages in therapeutic and professional relationships	2.2 Communicates effectively, and is respectful of a person's dignity, culture, values, beliefs and rights	Engages in a therapeutic conversation in Communication: Person with a social anxiety disorder, p. 167
	3. Maintains the capability for practice	3.2 Provides the information and education required to enhance people's control over health	Implements strategies to reduce life stressors in Collaborative Care: Teaching about life changes, p. 147 Instructs on approaches to reduce anxiety in Your Intervention Strategies: Activities that promote relaxation, p. 165 Encourage medication adherence through teaching provided in Collaborative Care: Teaching about medications for anxiety disorder, p. 166 Utilises approaches to enhance sleep in Collaborative Care: Teaching about improving sleep quality, p. 168
	4. Comprehensively conducts assessments	4.2 Uses a range of assessment techniques to systematically collect relevant and accurate information and data to inform practice	Assesses for sources of anxiety in Assessing Anxiety, pp. 151–152 Recognises anxiety-related illnesses in Anxiety-Related Disorders, pp. 154–158; Table 8.2: Common obsessions and compulsions, p. 157 Conducts an assessment for an anxiety disorder, pp. 160–163; Your Assessment Approach: Person with an anxiety disorder, p. 160
		4.3 Works in partnership to determine factors that affect, or potentially affect, the health and wellbeing of people and populations to determine priorities for action and/or for referral	Determines coping mechanisms used prior to planning care in Coping with Stress and Anxiety, p. 152; Table 8.1: Common defence mechanisms, pp. 153–154
	5. Develops a plan for nursing practice	5.1 Uses assessment data and best available evidence to develop a plan	Creates a collaborative plan of care to address an anxiety disorder in Planning and Implementation, p. 163
	6. Provides safe, appropriate and responsive quality nursing practice	6.1 Provides comprehensive safe, quality practice to achieve agreed goals and outcomes that are responsive to the nursing needs of people	Implements strategies to reduce anxiety in Your Intervention Strategies: Person experiencing panic, p. 164; Your Intervention Strategies: Person with anxiety, p. 164 Utilises therapeutic techniques as required in Box 8.2: Therapeutic techniques for people with anxiety, trauma and stressor-related disorders, p. 166; Table 8.4: Cognitive behavioural techniques for treating phobias, p. 167

Chapter number	Standard	Criteria (sub-standard)	Evidence-based examples (including page no.)
	7. Evaluates outcomes to inform nursing practice	7.1 Evaluates and monitors progress towards the expected goals and outcomes	Evaluates care provided as identified in Evaluation, p. 168
9	1. Thinks critically and analyses nursing practice	1.3 Respects all cultures and experiences, which includes responding to the role of family and community that underpin the health of Aboriginal and Torres Strait Islander peoples and people of other cultures	Engages in culturally appropriate communication techniques in Developing Cultural Competence: Role of culture, p. 175
		1.5 Uses ethical frameworks when making decisions	Recognises the appropriate theory to explain method of communication in Biopsychosocial Theories and Models of Human Communication, pp. 179–184
	2. Engages in therapeutic and professional relationships	2.2 Communicates effectively, and is respectful of a person's dignity, culture, values, beliefs and rights	Reviews mechanism of communication prior to engaging in conversations, in The Process of Human Communication, pp. 173–179 Utilises appropriate communication approaches in Your Assessment Approach: Preferred predicates, p. 184; Facilitating Communication and Building a Relationship, pp. 184–186
	3. Maintains the capability for practice	3.3 Uses a lifelong learning approach for continuing professional development of self and others	Employs strategies to improve communication skills in Self-awareness: Guidelines for improving non-verbal communication, p. 185; Therapeutic Communication Skills, pp. 186–191
10	2. Engages in therapeutic and professional relationships	2.2 Communicates effectively, and is respectful of a person's dignity, culture, values, beliefs and rights	Utilises effective communication techniques in Communication: Assessing the person, p. 199
	3. Maintains the capability for practice	3.3 Uses a lifelong learning approach for continuing professional development of self and others	Engages in active self-evaluation of assessment skills in Self-awareness: Evaluating your own assessment skills, p. 204
	4. Comprehensively conducts assessments	4.1 Conducts assessments that are holistic as well as culturally appropriate	Completes an assessment in an emergency situation in What Every Nurse Should Know: Assessing a person experiencing mental distress in an emergency department, p. 196
		4.2 Uses a range of assessment techniques to systematically collect relevant and accurate information and data to inform practice	Conducts data collection through the use of a variety of assessment tools in Mental State Assessment, pp. 195–200 Determines when to use the Mini-Mental State Exam, pp. 200–201 Incorporates the assessment of physiological (pp. 201–202), neurological (pp. 202–203), psychological (p. 203, and Box 10.2: Common psychological tests), and psychosocial (pp. 206–207) statuses as appropriate

Chapter number	Standard	Criteria (sub-standard)	Evidence-based examples (including page no.)
	5. Develops a plan for nursing practice	5.1 Uses assessment data and best available evidence to develop a plan	Plans collaborative care according to appropriate taxonomies in Psychiatric Diagnostic Practice According to the DSM: The Problem With Taxonomies, pp. 203–206
11	1. Thinks critically and analyses nursing practice	1.4 Complies with legislation, regulations, policies, guidelines and other standards or requirements relevant to the context of practice when making decisions	Implements appropriate laws when addressing mental health issues, in Law, Mental Health and Involuntary Treatment Issues, pp. 216–219; Table 11.1: Mental health care law: 10 basic principles, p. 219
		1.5 Uses ethical frameworks when making decisions	Implements appropriate ethical principles when providing mental health care in Principles of Bioethics, and Ethical Guidelines for Psychiatric–Mental Health Nurses, p. 212
	2. Engages in therapeutic and professional relationships	2.2 Communicates effectively, and is respectful of a person's dignity, culture, values, beliefs and rights	Recognises ethical dilemmas in Ethical Dilemmas in Psychiatric–Mental Health Nursing, p. 213; Neuroethics: An Emerging Field, pp. 213–215
		2.5 Advocates on behalf of people in a manner that respects the person's autonomy and legal capacity	Ensures that the rights of individuals with mental health issues are protected in The Rights of People with a Mental Illness, pp. 222–223; Your Intervention Strategies: The rights of people with mental illness, p. 223; Your Intervention Strategies: When the right to privacy can be breached, p. 223; Mental Health Advance Directives, p. 224
	6. Provides safe, appropriate and responsive quality nursing practice	6.5 Practises in accordance with relevant policies, guidelines, standards, regulations and legislation	Provides mental health interventions according to legal guidelines, in Psychiatry and Criminal Law, pp. 219–221; Forensic Mental Health Nursing, pp. 221–222
12	1. Thinks critically and analyses nursing practice	1.1 Accesses, analyses, and uses the best available evidence, that includes research findings, for safe, quality practice	Applies the most current theory on cognitive disorders when caring for consumers with these disorders in Delirium, pp. 228–229; Dementia, pp. 229–230, 232–237; Table 12.1: Comparing delirium, dementia and depression, pp. 230–231
		1.5 Uses ethical frameworks when making decisions	Reviews theories of cognitive alterations in Biopsychosocial Theories, pp. 237–238
	2. Engages in therapeutic and professional relationships	2.2 Communicates effectively, and is respectful of a person's dignity, culture, values, beliefs and rights	Engages in meaningful conversation in Communication: Person with dementia, p. 243; Person with dementia at risk for self-harm, p. 243; Communication: Person with dementia and hallucinations, p. 244

Chapter number	Standard	Criteria (sub-standard)	Evidence-based examples (including page no.)
	3. Maintains the capability for practice	3.2 Provides the information and education required to enhance people's control over health	Engages in caregiving teaching to enhance care of the consumer with a cognitive disorder in Collaborative Care: Family strategies, p. 244; Your Intervention Strategies: Strategies for working with the person who wanders, p. 245; Your Intervention Strategies: Strategies for supporting memory function, p. 246, and Collaborative Care: Nutrition and feeding, p. 248
	4. Comprehensively conducts assessments	4.1 Conducts assessments that are holistic as well as culturally appropriate	Assesses for different levels of Alzheimer's disease in Box 12.1: Behavioural changes of dementia of the Alzheimer's type (DAT), p. 234
		4.2 Uses a range of assessment techniques to systematically collect relevant and accurate information and data to inform practice	Conducts an assessment of a consumer with a cognitive disorder in Nursing Process: People with cognitive disorders, pp. 238–242
	5. Develops a plan for nursing practice	5.1 Uses assessment data and best available evidence to develop a plan	Identifies care issues based upon assessment findings in Nursing Care pp. 242–244
		5.2 Collaboratively constructs nursing practice plans until contingencies, options priorities, goals, actions, outcomes and timeframes are agreed with the relevant persons	Creates a plan of care based upon assessment findings, in Planning and Implementation, pp. 244–247
		5.5 Coordinates resources effectively and efficiently for planned actions	Actively engages with caregivers to monitor and evaluate care needs in Care Coordination, p. 247
	6. Provides safe, appropriate and responsive quality nursing practice	6.1 Provides comprehensive, safe, quality practice to achieve agreed goals and outcomes that are responsive to the nursing needs of people	Implements strategies to support cognitive function in Self-awareness: Triggering semantic memory, p. 246
	7. Evaluates outcomes to inform nursing practice	7.1 Evaluates and monitors progress towards the expected goals and outcomes	Reviews the plan of care in collaboration with caregivers to determine achievement of expected outcomes, p. 247
13	1. Thinks critically and analyses nursing practice	1.1 Accesses, analyses, and uses the best available evidence, that includes research findings, for safe, quality practice	Reviews the DSM classifications for substance use disorders, in Diagnostic Feature: DSM-5 criteria, pp. 252–253 Applies various theories to enhance comprehension of substance use disorders in Theories Related to the Development of Substance Use Disorders, pp. 254–258
		1.3 Respects all cultures and experiences, which includes responding to the role of family and community that underpin the health of Aboriginal and Torres Strait Islander peoples and people of other cultures	Analyses substance abuse in different cultures in Developing Cultural Competence: Substance use in specific cultures, p. 257

Chapter number	Standard	Criteria (sub-standard)	Evidence-based examples (including page no.)
	2. Engages in therapeutic and professional relationships	2.2 Communicates effectively, and is respectful of a person's dignity, culture, values, beliefs and rights	Engages in meaningful conversation in Communication: Person intoxicated with alcohol, p. 282; Communication: Person with a history of substance use but not currently using them, p. 285
		2.9 Reports notifiable conduct of health professionals, health workers and others	Recognises signs of substance abuse in health care professionals, in Your Assessment Approach: Warning signs of health care providers with substance use disorders, p. 279
	3. Maintains the capability for practice	3.2 Provides the information and education required to enhance people's control over health	Provides teaching to assist persons and families to understand enabling behaviour in Box 13.1: How significant others enable, p. 258; in Collaborative Care: Teaching about relapse, p. 285
		3.3 Uses a lifelong learning approach for continuing professional development of self and others	Maintains personal health when caring for persons with substance use disorders in Self-awareness, p. 259; Self-awareness: Maintaining therapeutic optimism, p. 273; Self-awareness: Your stress response and susceptibility to substance use, p. 280
	4. Comprehensively conducts assessments	4.1 Conducts assessments that are holistic as well as culturally appropriate	Applies assessment techniques according to abused substance, in Your Assessment Approach: Stages of alcohol withdrawal, p. 262; What Every Nurse Should Know: People with substance use disorders, p. 264; in Assessment pp. 280–282; Your Assessment Approach: Interview questions for substance use, p. 281
		4.2 Uses a range of assessment techniques to systematically collect relevant and accurate information and data to inform practice	Examines populations at risk and implements appropriate assessment techniques in Alcohol Withdrawal Syndrome, pp. 260–262; What Every Nurse Should Know: Pain medication use, p. 265; Groups at Risk for Substance use disorders, pp. 276–280 Applies information about commonly occurring symptoms in the assessment of individuals misusing substances in Substance Use Disorders, pp. 252–254; Diagnostic Feature: Substance use disorders, intoxication, tolerance and withdrawal, p. 253; Table 13.1: Alcohol and effects on behaviour, p. 259; Table 13.2: 'How much in a standard drink?', p. 259; Table 13.3: Main signs and symptoms of alcohol withdrawal, p. 261; Table 13.4: Symptoms and signs of opioid withdrawal, p. 266; Table 13.5: Effects of psychostimulants, p. 268

Chapter number	Standard	Criteria (sub-standard)	Evidence-based examples (including page no.)
		4.3 Works in partnership to determine factors that affect, or potentially affect, the health and wellbeing of people and populations to determine priorities for action and/or for referral	Analyses concurrent use of substances with a mental illness, in Box 13.2: Consequences of using substances when living with a mental illness, p. 277
	5. Develops a plan for nursing practice	5.1 Uses assessment data and best available evidence to develop a plan	Creates a collaborative plan of care to address substance use, in Planning and implementation, pp. 282–286
	6. Provides safe, appropriate and responsive quality nursing practice	6.1 Provides comprehensive safe, quality practice to achieve agreed goals and outcomes that are responsive to the nursing needs of people	Implements the plan of care to address substance misuse, in Box 13.3: The 12 steps of Alcoholics Anonymous, p. 284
	7. Evaluates outcomes to inform nursing practice	7.1 Evaluates and monitors progress towards the expected goals and outcomes	Evaluates effectiveness of interventions in Evaluation, p. 286
14	1. Thinks critically and analyses nursing practice	1.1 Accesses, analyses, and uses the best available evidence, that includes research findings, for safe, quality practice	Reviews the DSM Essential Features in Schizophrenia, p. 291 Applies various theories to enhance comprehension of schizophrenia in Biopsychosocial Theories, pp. 298–302
		1.3 Respects all cultures and experiences, which includes responding to the role of family and community that underpin the health of Aboriginal and Torres Strait Islander peoples and people of other cultures	Addresses issues associated with culture, religion and schizophrenia in Developing Cultural Competence: Culture, religion and schizophrenia, p. 313
	2. Engages in therapeutic and professional relationships	2.2 Communicates effectively, and is respectful of a person's dignity, culture, values, beliefs and rights	Engages in meaningful conversation in Communication: A person with clang associations, p. 297; and Communication: Unfocused person, p. 300
	3. Maintains the capability for practice	3.2 Provides the information and education required to enhance people's control over health	Provides teaching to families in Collaborative Care: People living with schizophrenia and their families: teaching about the negative symptoms of schizophrenia, p. 308; and Your Intervention Strategies: Increasing medication adherence for people living with schizophrenia, p. 312
		3.3 Uses a lifelong learning approach for continuing professional development of self and others	Maintains self-awareness when caring for persons with schizophrenia in Self-awareness: Working with people living with schizophrenia, p. 310
	4. Comprehensively conducts assessments	4.1 Conducts assessments that are holistic as well as culturally appropriate	Completes comprehensive assessments of the individual with schizophrenia in Assessment, pp. 303–309; Your Assessment Approach: The person who is hallucinating, p. 303; Box 14.1: Neurological soft and hard signs, p. 304; Box 14.2: Problematic communication patterns common in schizophrenia, p. 305; and What Every Nurse Should Know: Primary symptoms of schizophrenia, p. 307

Chapter number	Standard	Criteria (sub-standard)	Evidence-based examples (including page no.)
		4.2 Uses a range of assessment techniques to systematically collect relevant and accurate information and data to inform practice	Applies information about commonly occurring symptoms in the assessment of individuals with schizophrenia in Symptoms of Schizophrenia, pp. 291–296; Table 14.1: Types of hallucinations, p. 292; Table 14.2: Types of delusions, p. 292; Table 14.3: Positive symptoms, pp. 293–294; Table 14.4: Negative symptoms, p. 294; and Other Psychotic Disorders, pp. 297–298
	5. Develops a plan for nursing practice	5.1 Uses assessment data and best available evidence to develop a plan	Plans care to address the needs of the person with schizophrenia in Objective data, pp. 303–309; and Box 14.3: Important issues for the person living with schizophrenia, p. 309
	6. Provides safe, appropriate and responsive quality nursing practice	6.1 Provides comprehensive, safe, quality practice to achieve agreed goals and outcomes that are responsive to the nursing needs of people	Implements the plan of care to address schizophrenia in Planning and implementation, pp. 309–316; Box 14.4: Challenges to adherence, p. 311; Your Intervention Strategies: Helping a person manage hallucinations, p. 314; and Your Intervention Strategies: Helping a person living with schizophrenia manage delusions, p. 315
	7. Evaluates outcomes to inform nursing practice	7.1 Evaluates and monitors progress towards the expected goals and outcomes	Evaluates effectiveness of interventions in Evaluation, pp. 316–317
15	1. Thinks critically and analyses nursing practice	1.1 Accesses, analyses and uses the best available evidence, that includes research findings, for safe, quality practice	Reviews the Diagnostic Features for Bipolar disorders, p. 323 Understands and applies various theories to enhance comprehension of major depressive disorders in Biopsychosocial Theories, pp. 326–329
	2. Engages in therapeutic and professional relationships	2.2 Communicates effectively, and is respectful of a person's dignity, culture, values, beliefs and rights	Implements communication techniques to assist the person with a depressive disorder in Box 15.2: A sample process-recording with a person who is depressed, p. 331; Communication: Client experiencing major depressive episode, p. 334; and Communication: The person with bipolar disorder, p. 341
	3. Maintains the capability for practice	3.2 Provides the information and education required to enhance people's control over health	Provides teaching to persons and families in Collaborative Care: Teaching about aggressive, passive, and assertive behaviours, p. 333
		3.3 Uses a lifelong learning approach for continuing professional development of self and others	Maintains self-awareness when caring for persons with a depressive disorder in Minimising maladaptive dependence, p. 333 Maintains self-awareness when caring for persons with a bipolar disorder in Self-awareness: Potential reactions to working with people who have mania, p. 339

Chapter number	Standard	Criteria (sub-standard)	Evidence-based examples (including page no.)
	4. Comprehensively conducts assessments	4.1 Conducts assessments that are holistic as well as culturally appropriate	Completes comprehensive assessments of the individual with a major depressive disorders in Your Assessment Approach: Abnormal biological findings in affective disorders, p. 327; and Assessment, pp. 329–330 Completes comprehensive assessments of persons with bipolar disorders, pp. 337–338; and Box 15.3: Mania symptoms: DIGFAST, p. 337
		4.2 Uses a range of assessment techniques to systematically collect relevant and accurate information and data to inform practice	Applies information about commonly occurring symptoms in the assessment of individuals with a major depressive disorder in Major Depressive Disorder, pp. 321–323; Box 15.1: Key facts about major depression, p. 321; Persistent Depressive Disorder (Dysthymia), p. 323; Bipolar and Related Disorders, pp. 323–325; and Affective Disorders Due to Another Medical Condition, pp. 325–326; What Every Nurse Should Know: Physical complaints and depression, p. 330; and What Every Nurse Should Know: Grief and depression, p. 337
	5. Develops a plan for nursing practice	5.1 Uses assessment data and best available evidence to develop a plan	Plans care to address issues related to individuals experiencing a depressive disorder, pp. 330–331 Plans care to address issues related to persons with an elevated mood and mania pp. 338–339
	6. Provides safe, appropriate and responsive quality nursing practice	6.1 Provides comprehensive, safe, quality practice to achieve agreed goals and outcomes that are responsive to the nursing needs of people	Implements the plan of care to address major depressive disorders in Care planning and implementation, pp. 331–335; Your Intervention Strategies: Preventing inpatient suicide and promoting safety, p. 332; Your Intervention Strategies: Working with people receiving ECT p. 335 Implements the plan of care to address bipolar disorders in Care planning, pp. 339–342; and Your Intervention Strategies: Setting and enforcing limits, p. 340
		6.5 Practises in accordance with relevant policies, guidelines, standards, regulations and legislation	Participates in care coordination and community-based care in the ongoing care of the person with a depressive disorder, pp. 336–337 Participates in care coordination and community-based care for the person with a bipolar disorder p. 343

Chapter number	Standard	Criteria (sub-standard)	Evidence-based examples (including page no.)
	7. Evaluates outcomes to inform nursing practice	7.1 Evaluates and monitors progress towards the expected goals and outcomes	Evaluates effectiveness of interventions for a major depressive disorder in Evaluation, pp. 335–336 Evaluates effectiveness of interventions for bipolar disorder in Evaluation, pp. 342–343
16	1. Thinks critically and analyses nursing practice	1.1 Accesses, analyses and uses the best available evidence, that includes research findings, for safe, quality practice	Reviews the Diagnostic Features: Dissociative disorders, p. 349; Diagnostic Features: Somatoform symptom and related disorders, p. 357 Applies various theories to enhance comprehension of somatoform disorders in Biopsychosocial Theories, pp. 351–352; somatic symptom disorders in Biopsychosocial Theories, pp. 360–361
		1.3 Respects all cultures and experiences, which includes responding to the role of family and community that underpin the health of Aboriginal and Torres Strait Islander peoples and people of other cultures	Analyses Developing Cultural Competence: Culture-bound syndromes that can be misdiagnosed as dissociative disorders, p. 352; Developing Cultural Competence: Culture-bound syndromes that can be misdiagnosed as somatic symptom disorders, p. 361
	2. Engages in therapeutic and professional relationships	2.2 Communicates effectively, and is respectful of a person's dignity, culture, values, beliefs and rights	Utilises therapeutic communication techniques in Communication: The person with depersonalisation/derealisation disorder, p. 355; Communication: The person with somatic symptom disorder, p. 364
	3. Maintains the capability for practice	3.2 Provides the information and education required to enhance people's control over health	Provides teaching to persons and families in Collaborative Care: Teaching about somatic symptom disorders, p. 364
		3.3 Uses a lifelong learning approach for continuing professional development of self and others	Participates in self-awareness activities when caring for the person with somatic symptom and related disorders, p. 361
	4. Comprehensively conducts assessments	4.1 Conducts assessments that are holistic as well as culturally appropriate	Completes comprehensive assessments of the individual with a dissociative disorder in Assessment, pp. 352–354; Your Assessment Approach: Individual with depersonalisation/derealisation disorder, p. 353; Your Assessment Approach: Person with dissociative identity disorder, p. 353 Completes comprehensive assessments of the individual with somatic symptom and related disorders in Assessment, pp. 361–362; Your Assessment Approach: The person with somatic symptom disorder, p. 362; and What Every Nurse Should Know: Somatic symptom and related disorders, p. 362

Chapter number	Standard	Criteria (sub-standard)	Evidence-based examples (including page no.)
		4.2 Uses a range of assessment techniques to systematically collect relevant and accurate information and data to inform practice	Applies information about commonly occurring symptoms in the assessment of individuals with Dissociative Disorders, pp. 349–351 Applies information about commonly occurring symptoms in the assessment of the person with Somatic Symptom and Related Disorders, pp. 356–358, Malingering, p. 358; Factitious disorders, pp. 358–359; What Every Nurse Should Know: Factitious disorder imposed on another and child abuse, pp. 359–360
	5. Develops a plan for nursing practice	5.1 Uses assessment data and best available evidence to develop a plan	Plans collaborative care to address issues common to people with dissociative disorders, in Nursing Practice, p. 354 Plans collaborative care for people with somatic symptoms and related disorders in Nursing Practice, p. 363
	6. Provides safe, appropriate and responsive quality nursing practice	6.1 Provides comprehensive, safe, quality practice to achieve agreed goals and outcomes that are responsive to the nursing needs of people	Implements the plan of care for the person with dissociative disorders, in Care planning and implementation, pp. 354–355 Implements the plan of care to address somatic symptoms and related disorders in Care planning and implementation, pp. 363–364; and Your Intervention Strategies: The person with somatic symptom disorder, p. 363
		6.5 Practises in accordance with relevant policies, guidelines, standards, regulations and legislation	Participates in care coordination and community care for the person with a dissociative disorder, p. 356 Participates in care coordination and community care for the individual with somatic symptom disorder, p. 365
	7. Evaluates outcomes to inform nursing practice	7.1 Evaluates and monitors progress towards the expected goals and outcomes	Evaluates effectiveness of interventions for dissociative disorder in Evaluation, pp. 355–356 Evaluates effectiveness of interventions for somatic symptom disorder in Evaluation, pp. 364–365
17	1. Thinks critically and analyses nursing practice	1.1 Accesses, analyses and uses the best available evidence, that includes research findings, for safe, quality practice	Reviews Diagnostic Features: Eating disorders, p. 371 Applies various theories to enhance comprehension of eating disorders in Biopsychosocial Theories, pp. 372–375

Chapter number	**Standard**	**Criteria (sub-standard)**	**Evidence-based examples (including page no.)**
		1.3 Respects all cultures and experiences, which includes responding to the role of family and community that underpin the health of Aboriginal and Torres Strait Islander peoples and people of other cultures	Analyses the cultural effects of eating disorders in Developing Cultural Competence: When thin is in, p. 375
	2. Engages in therapeutic and professional relationships	2.2 Communicates effectively, and is respectful of a person's dignity, culture, values, beliefs and rights	Utilises therapeutic communication techniques in Communication: Woman with anorexia nervosa, p. 381; Communication: Person with Bulimia Nervosa, p. 386
	3. Maintains the capability for practice	3.2 Provides the information and education required to enhance people's control over health	Provides teaching to individuals and families in Collaborative Care: Family-based therapies, pp. 379–380
		3.3 Uses a lifelong learning approach for continuing professional development of self and others	Participates in self-awareness activities in Self-awareness: Possible reactions to working with people with eating disorders, p. 376
	4. Comprehensively conducts assessments	4.1 Conducts assessments that are holistic as well as culturally appropriate	Completes comprehensive assessments of the person with anorexia nervosa in Assessment, pp. 376–377 Completes comprehensive assessments of the person with bulimia nervosa in Assessment, pp. 383–384
		4.2 Uses a range of assessment techniques to systematically collect relevant and accurate information and data to inform practice	Critiques and applies information about commonly occurring identifying factors for anorexia nervosa, p. 371, and bulimia nervosa, p. 372
	5. Develops a plan for nursing practice	5.1 Uses assessment data and best available evidence to develop a plan	Collaboratively plans care to address the needs of the person with anorexia nervosa in Nursing implications, pp. 377–378 Plans care to address the needs of the person with bulimia nervosa in Nursing implications, p. 384
	6. Provides safe, appropriate and responsive quality nursing practice	6.1 Provides comprehensive, safe, quality practice to achieve agreed goals and outcomes that are responsive to the nursing needs of people	Implements the plan of care for the person with anorexia nervosa, in Planning and implementation, pp. 378–382; Your Intervention Strategies: Guidelines for graded nutritional therapy, p. 378; Box 17.1: Criteria for inpatient admission, p. 378 Implements the plan of care for the person with bulimia nervosa, in Planning and implementation, pp. 384–386; and Box 17.2: Affirmations for those who compulsively overeat, p. 385
		6.5 Practises in accordance with relevant policies, guidelines, standards, regulations and legislation	Participates in care coordination and community-based care in the ongoing care of a person with anorexia nervosa, p. 383 Participates in care coordination and community-based care in the ongoing care of a person with bulimia nervosa, p. 387

Chapter number	Standard	Criteria (sub-standard)	Evidence-based examples (including page no.)
	7. Evaluates outcomes to inform nursing practice	7.1 Evaluates and monitors progress towards the expected goals and outcomes	Evaluates effectiveness of interventions for the person with anorexia nervosa in Evaluation, p. 382 Evaluates effectiveness of interventions for bulimia nervosa in Evaluation, p. 386–387
18	1. Thinks critically and analyses nursing practice	1.1 Accesses, analyses and uses the best available evidence, that includes research findings, for safe, quality practice	Reviews the approaches for classification in Classification and Diagnosis, pp. 395–396; Personality Disorder Classification, pp. 396–400; Table 18.1: DSM Essential features—Cluster A personality disorders: odd–eccentric, p. 396; Box 18.2: Criteria for diagnosis of personality disorder, p. 396; Table 18.2: Essential features—Cluster B personality disorders: dramatic–emotional, p. 398; Table 18.3: Essential features—Cluster C personality disorders: anxious–fearful, p. 399; Recovery and Self-discovery, pp. 400–402 Applies various theories to enhance comprehension of personality disorders in Theories of Personality, pp. 391–392; Theories of Disorder, p. 392; and Theories of Causation, pp. 392–395
		1.3 Respects all cultures and experiences, which includes responding to the role of family and community that underpin the health of Aboriginal and Torres Strait Islander peoples and people of other cultures	Analyses the impact of culture in Developing Cultural Competence: Assessing people with schizoid and schizotypal personalities, p. 397
	2. Engages in therapeutic and professional relationships	2.2 Communicates effectively, and is respectful of a person's dignity, culture, values, beliefs and rights	Utilises therapeutic communication techniques in Communication: Person with paranoid personality disorder, p. 406
	3. Maintains the capability for practice	3.2 Provides the information and education required to enhance people's control over health	Provides teaching to individuals and carers in Collaborative Care: Teaching about personality disorders, p. 408
		3.3 Uses a lifelong learning approach for continuing professional development of self and others	Participates in self-awareness activities in Self-awareness: Explore your thoughts and feelings toward people with personality disorder, p. 404; Box 18.3: Key principles for working with people with personality disorders, p. 405; Self-awareness: Working with traumatised people, p. 409
	4. Comprehensively conducts assessments	4.1 Conducts assessments that are holistic as well as culturally appropriate	Completes comprehensive assessments of the person with a personality disorder in Assessment, pp. 405, 407; Your Assessment Approach: People with dramatic–emotional personality disorders and their families, p. 406

Chapter number	Standard	Criteria (sub-standard)	Evidence-based examples (including page no.)
		4.2 Uses a range of assessment techniques to systematically collect relevant and accurate information and data to inform practice	Applies information about commonly occurring identifying factors for personality disorders in What Every Nurse Should Know: Person with borderline personality disorder, p. 397; What Every Nurse Should Know: Person with dependent personality disorder, p. 399; Box 18.5: The role of self-harm, p. 407; Box 18.7: Trauma triggers, p. 409; Box 18.8: What helps and what hurts, p. 409
		4.3 Works in partnership to determine factors that affect, or potentially affect, the health and wellbeing of people and populations to determine priorities for action and/or for referral	Participates in the care and treatment of individuals with personality disorders in Treatment, pp. 402–403; Table 18.4: Personality disorder psychological therapies, p. 402
	6. Provides safe, appropriate and responsive quality nursing practice	6.1 Provides comprehensive, safe, quality practice to achieve agreed goals and outcomes that are responsive to the nursing needs of people	Implements the plan of care for the individual with a personality disorder in Box 18.4: Intervention strategies for responding to a person in crisis, p. 405; Your Intervention Strategies: Guidelines for people with paranoid personality disorder, p. 406; and Box 18.6: Intervention strategies for people who use self-harm, p. 407
19	1. Thinks critically and analyses nursing practice	1.1 Accesses, analyses and uses the best available evidence, that includes research findings, for safe, quality practice	Applies various theories to enhance comprehension of self-destructive behaviour in Biopsychosocial Theories, pp. 416–419; Box 19.3: Suicide myths versus suicide facts, p. 417
	2. Engages in therapeutic and professional relationships	2.2 Communicates effectively, and is respectful of a person's dignity, culture, values, beliefs and rights	Utilises therapeutic communication techniques in Communication: A person who attempts suicide, p. 416
		2.7 Actively fosters a culture of safety and learning that includes engaging with health professionals and others, to share knowledge and practice that supports person-centred care	Reviews and implements suicide prevention actions in Suicide Prevention, pp. 419–420; Box 19.5: Risk factors and protective factors for suicide, p. 420 Support counselling efforts for survivors, in Survivors of Suicide, pp. 429–431
	3. Maintains the capability for practice	3.2 Provides the information and education required to enhance people's control over health	Provides teaching to people, and families in Collaborative Care: Helping families prevent suicide, p. 428; Collaborative Care: Helping an individual develop a family suicide crisis plan, p. 429
		3.3 Uses a lifelong learning approach for continuing professional development of self and others	Participates in self-awareness activities about destructive behaviour in Nursing Self-awareness, p. 420; Self-awareness: An attitude inventory for working with people who are suicidal, p. 421

Chapter number	Standard	Criteria (sub-standard)	Evidence-based examples (including page no.)
	4. Comprehensively conducts assessments	4.1 Conducts assessments that are holistic as well as culturally appropriate	Completes comprehensive assessments of The person who is suicidal or self-harming in Assessment, pp. 421–424; Box 19.6: Lethality of suicide methods, p. 423; and Your Assessment Approach: Suicide risk assessment, p. 423
		4.2 Uses a range of assessment techniques to systematically collect relevant and accurate information and data to inform practice	Applies information about commonly occurring identifying factors for Self-Harming Behaviour, pp. 414–416; Box 19.1: Suicide facts, p. 414; Box 19.2: Continuum of suicidal behaviour, p. 415; What Every Nurse Should Know: Suicidal ideation in primary care, p. 415; Box 19.4: Characteristics most closely associated with suicide, p. 418
	5. Develops a plan for nursing practice	5.1 Uses assessment data and best available evidence to develop a plan	Creates a plan of care appropriate for a person at risk for suicide in Planning and implementation, pp. 424–428
		5.3 Documents, evaluates and modifies plans accordingly to facilitate the agreed outcomes	Identifies realistic outcomes for a person with suicidal or self-destructive behaviour, in Identification of outcomes, p. 424
	6. Provides safe, appropriate and responsive quality nursing practice	6.1 Provides comprehensive safe, quality practice to achieve agreed goals and outcomes that are responsive to the nursing needs of people	Implements the plan of care for people with suicidal or self-destructive behaviour in Planning and implementation, pp. 424–428; Your Intervention Strategies: How to develop no-self-harm/no-suicide contracts, p. 425; Your Intervention Strategies: Sample protocols for suicide precautions, p. 426
		6.5 Practises in accordance with relevant policies, guidelines, standards, regulations and legislation	Participates in care coordination, community-based, or home care in the ongoing care of a person with self-destructive or suicidal behaviour, pp. 428–429
	7. Evaluates outcomes to inform nursing practice	7.1 Evaluates and monitors progress towards the expected goals and outcomes	Evaluates effectiveness of interventions for individuals who are suicidal or have self-harming behaviour in Evaluation, p. 428
20	1. Thinks critically and analyses nursing practice	1.1 Accesses, analyses and uses the best available evidence, that includes research findings, for safe, quality practice	Applies various theories to enhance comprehension of Family Violence: Physical Abuse in Biopsychosocial Theories, pp. 439–440 Applies various theories to enhance comprehension of Family Violence: Sexual Abuse in Biopsychosocial Theories, pp. 447–448
	3. Maintains the capability for practice	3.2 Provides the information and education required to enhance people's control over health	Provides teaching to the person and families in Collaborative Care: Teaching about family violence, p. 442
		3.3 Uses a lifelong learning approach for continuing professional development of self and others	Participates in self-awareness activities in Self-awareness: Working with survivors of family violence, p. 441; Self-awareness: Working with survivors of child sexual abuse, p. 445

Chapter number	Standard	Criteria (sub-standard)	Evidence-based examples (including page no.)
	4. Comprehensively conducts assessments	4.1 Conducts assessments that are holistic as well as culturally appropriate	Completes comprehensive assessments of the person with family physical abuse, in Assessment, p. 440; Your Assessment Approach: Nursing history tool for assessing survivors of family violence, p. 441 Completes comprehensive assessments of the person who has experienced family sexual abuse, in Assessment, p. 448; Your Assessment Approach: Nursing history tool for the assessment of individuals and families for family sexual abuse, p. 449; Your Assessment Approach: Physical assessment of the sexual abuse victim, p. 450
		4.2 Uses a range of assessment techniques to systematically collect relevant and accurate information and data to inform practice	Applies information about commonly occurring identifying factors for Family Violence: Physical Abuse, pp. 433–439; What Every Nurse Should Know: Assessing for emotional and physical abuse during pregnancy, p. 437; and Box 20.2: Why do they stay? Why do they go back?, p. 439 Applies information about commonly occurring identifying factors for Family Violence: Sexual Abuse, pp. 444–447; Box 20.3: Typical threatening statements by sexual abusers, p. 446
	5. Develops a plan for nursing practice	5.1 Uses assessment data and best available evidence to develop a plan	Identifies problems to address family violence in Problem identification, pp. 440–441 Identifies problems to address family sexual abuse in Problem identification, p. 448 Determines appropriate outcomes of care for the person who has experienced family sexual abuse in Outcomes of intervention, pp. 449–450
		5.2 Collaboratively constructs nursing practice plans until contingencies, options priorities, goals, actions, outcomes and timeframes are agreed with the relevant persons	Creates a collaborative plan of care to address family violence in Planning and implementation, pp. 441–443
			Creates a plan of care to address family sexual abuse in Planning and implementation, pp. 450–451
	6. Provides safe, appropriate and responsive quality nursing practice	6.1 Provides comprehensive, safe, quality practice to achieve agreed goals and outcomes that are responsive to the nursing needs of people	Implements a plan of care to address family violence in Planning and implementation, pp. 441–443

Chapter number	Standard	Criteria (sub-standard)	Evidence-based examples (including page no.)
			Implements a plan of care to address family sexual abuse in Planning and implementation, pp. 450–451
		6.5 Practises in accordance with relevant policies, guidelines, standards, regulations and legislation	Participates in care coordination community-based, or home care in the ongoing care of the person who has experienced family violence, p. 444 Participates in care coordination community-based, or home care in the ongoing care of the person who has experienced family sexual abuse, pp. 451–452
	7. Evaluates outcomes to inform nursing practice	7.1 Evaluates and monitors progress towards the expected goals and outcomes	Evaluates effectiveness of interventions for the person who has experienced family violence in Evaluation, p. 443 Evaluates effectiveness of interventions for the person who has experienced family sexual abuse in Evaluation, p. 451
21	1. Thinks critically and analyses nursing practice	1.1 Accesses, analyses and uses the best available evidence, that includes research findings, for safe, quality practice	Reviews the Diagnostic Features: Adolescent depression, p. 472 Applies various theories to enhance comprehension of young people and mental illness in Biopsychosocial Theories, pp. 457–460
		1.3 Respects all cultures and experiences, which includes responding to the role of family and community that underpin the health of Aboriginal and Torres Strait Islander peoples and people of other cultures	Advocates for young people with mental illness in Box 21.2: The health and wellbeing of young Australians, p. 461; Developing Cultural Competence: Preventing and dealing with cyberbullying, p. 477; Developing Cultural Competence: Cultural and societal obstacles to displaced and disenfranchised youth, p. 481
	2. Engages in therapeutic and professional relationships	2.2 Communicates effectively, and is respectful of a person's dignity, culture, values, beliefs and rights	Utilises therapeutic communication techniques in Communication: The person using swearing or obscenities, p. 468; Communication: The young person with sexual acting-out behaviour, p. 471
		2.6 Uses delegation, supervision, coordination, consultation and referrals in professional relationships to achieve improved health outcomes	Advocates for young people experiencing mental illness in The Role of the Nurse, pp. 460–465; Box 21.1: Student problems in the school setting that call for early intervention, p. 461
	3. Maintains the capability for practice	3.2 Provides the information and education required to enhance people's control over health	Facilitates the learning of parents and caregivers with young people with mental illnesses in Your Intervention Strategies: Encouraging more effective parenting behaviours, p. 464; Collaborative Care: Preventing and dealing with cyberbullying, pp. 477–478

Chapter number	Standard	Criteria (sub-standard)	Evidence-based examples (including page no.)
		3.3 Uses a lifelong learning approach for continuing professional development of self and others	Participates in self-awareness activities with Self-awareness: A self-awareness inventory for working with young people, p. 469
	4. Comprehensively conducts assessments	4.1 Conducts assessments that are holistic as well as culturally appropriate	Completes comprehensive assessments for young people in Assessment pp. 465–473; What Every Nurse Should Know: Working with young people who are upset, p. 465; Your Assessment Approach: Behavioural changes associated with teenage drug abuse, p. 473
		4.2 Uses a range of assessment techniques to systematically collect relevant and accurate information and data to inform practice	Applies information about young people and mental illness, pp. 456–457; What Every Nurse Should Know: Allaying the stress of parents and family members of young people, p. 457; What Every Nurse Should Know: Helping young people cope with the stress of a cancer diagnosis, p. 458; Your Assessment Approach: Exploring the meaning of a young person's identified problem or behaviour, p. 459; What Every Nurse Should Know: Teen pregnancy, p. 461
	5. Develops a plan for nursing practice	5.1 Uses assessment data and best available evidence to develop a plan	Focuses on the needs of the young adult in Responding to the needs of a young person living with mental illness, pp. 473–474 Develops a collaborative plan of care for the young person with a mental illness in Planning and implementation, pp. 474–479
		5.2 Collaboratively constructs nursing practice plans until contingencies, options priorities, goals, actions, outcomes and timeframes are agreed with the relevant persons	Select outcomes appropriate for the young person with a mental illness in Identifying Outcomes, p. 474
	6. Provides safe, appropriate and responsive quality nursing practice	6.1 Provides comprehensive safe, quality practice to achieve agreed goals and outcomes that are responsive to the nursing needs of people	Implements a plan of care for the young person with a mental illness in Planning and implementation, pp. 474–479
		6.5 Practises in accordance with relevant policies, guidelines, standards, regulations and legislation	Participates in care coordination, community-based, primary care in the ongoing care for young person with a mental illness, p. 480
	7. Evaluates outcomes to inform nursing practice	7.1 Evaluates and monitors progress towards the expected goals and outcomes	Evaluates effectiveness of interventions to address young people with mental illness in Evaluation, pp. 479–480
22	1. Thinks critically and analyses nursing practice	1.1 Accesses, analyses and uses the best available evidence, that includes research findings, for safe, quality practice	Applies various theories to enhance comprehension of ageing and mental illness in Biopsychosocial Theories, pp. 487–488
		1.3 Respects all cultures and experiences, which includes responding to the role of family and community that underpin the health of Aboriginal and Torres Strait Islander peoples and people of other cultures	Applies cultural principles with Developing Cultural Competence: Generational commonalities of older people, p. 501

Chapter number	Standard	Criteria (sub-standard)	Evidence-based examples (including page no.)
	3. Maintains the capability for practice	3.3 Uses a lifelong learning approach for continuing professional development of self and others	Engages in self-awareness in Self-awareness: Attitudes toward ageing, p. 486
	4. Comprehensively conducts assessments	4.1 Conducts assessments that are holistic as well as culturally appropriate	Completes comprehensive assessments of older people in Assessment, pp. 494–497; Your Assessment Approach: The key components of a biopsychosocial assessment: guidelines for interviewing older people, p. 494; Assessing psychological strengths, p. 496; Your Assessment Approach: Guidelines for assessing social and financial status, p. 497; Your Assessment Approach: Forms of mistreatment of older people, p. 498
		4.2 Uses a range of assessment techniques to systematically collect relevant and accurate information and data to inform practice	Applies information about Obstacles to Mental Health Services for Older people, pp. 485–487; What Every Nurse Should Know: Psychological symptoms an older person may exhibit, p. 487; and Psychiatric Disorders in Older People, pp. 488–494
	5. Develops a plan for nursing practice	5.1 Uses assessment data and best available evidence to develop a plan	Develops a plan of care for an older person with a mental illness pp. 497–500
	6. Provides safe, appropriate and responsive quality nursing practice	6.1 Provides comprehensive, safe, quality practice to achieve agreed goals and outcomes that are responsive to the nursing needs of people	Implements a plan of care for an older person with a mental illness pp. 497–500
23	1. Thinks critically and analyses nursing practice	1.1 Accesses, analyses and uses the best available evidence, that includes research findings, for safe, quality practice	Applies various theories to support therapeutic groups in Group Development Theory, pp. 508–510; and Group Therapy Theory, pp. 510–516
	2. Engages in therapeutic and professional relationships	2.1 Establishes, sustains and concludes relationships in a way that differentiates the boundaries between professional and personal relationships	Participates in group development and group work in Small Group Dynamics, pp. 504–508; Table 23.1: Group roles and functions, p. 507
		2.8 Participates in and/or leads collaborative practice	Participates in the creation of groups in Creating groups, pp. 512–514; and Therapeutic Groups, pp. 516–518
	4. Comprehensively conducts assessments	4.2 Uses a range of assessment techniques to systematically collect relevant and accurate information and data to inform practice	Applies information about types of groups in Table 23.2: Differences between inpatient and outpatient groups, p. 511; and Table 23.3: Curative factors of group therapy, p. 512
	6. Provides safe, appropriate and responsive quality nursing practice	6.1 Provides comprehensive safe, quality practice to achieve agreed goals and outcomes that are responsive to the nursing needs of people	Engage in therapy group development in Stages in therapy group development, pp. 514–516; Your Intervention Strategies: Structuring an inpatient group, p. 515; and Characteristic member behaviours and nursing interventions in phases of group therapy, p. 515
24	1. Thinks critically and analyses nursing practice	1.3 Respects all cultures and experiences, which includes responding to the role of family and community that underpin the health of Aboriginal and Torres Strait Islander peoples and people of other cultures	Applies cultural principles in family dynamics in Developing Cultural Competence: The cultural family genogram, p. 530

Chapter number	Standard	Criteria (sub-standard)	Evidence-based examples (including page no.)
	2. Engages in therapeutic and professional relationships	2.1 Establishes, sustains and concludes relationships in a way that differentiates the boundaries between professional and personal relationships	Recognises actions that support positive family dynamics in Family Dynamics, pp. 522–527; Table 24.1: Family developmental tasks, p. 523
	3. Maintains the capability for practice	3.2 Provides the information and education required to enhance people's control over health	Provides teaching to support with Collaborative Care: Psychoeducation for families, p. 531; Your Intervention Strategies: The role of the family therapist, p. 533
		3.3 Uses a lifelong learning approach for continuing professional development of self and others	Participates in self-awareness activities in Nursing Self-awareness, pp. 521–522; Self-awareness: The influences of your own family experiences, p. 522
	4. Comprehensively conducts assessments	4.2 Uses a range of assessment techniques to systematically collect relevant and accurate information and data to inform practice	Engages in techniques in conducting a Family Assessment, pp. 527–530
	6. Provides safe, appropriate and responsive quality nursing practice	6.1 Provides comprehensive, safe, quality practice to achieve agreed goals and outcomes that are responsive to the nursing needs of people	Implement interventions to support the family in Family Interventions, pp. 530–533
25		1.3 Respects all cultures and experiences, which includes responding to the role of family and community that underpin the health of Aboriginal and Torres Strait Islander peoples and people of other cultures	Applies cultural principles in Developing Cultural Competence: Culture and cognitive behavioural interventions, p. 550
	2. Engages in therapeutic and professional relationships	2.8 Participates in and/or leads collaborative practice	Utilises information about cognitive and behavioural interventions in Behavioural Therapy, pp. 537–543; Box 25.2: Irrational thoughts, p. 542; Cognitive Therapy, pp. 543–545; Cognitive Behavioural Therapy, p. 545; Acceptance And Commitment Therapy (ACT), pp. 547–549; and Dialectical Behavioural Therapy, pp. 549–550
	3. Maintains the capability for practice	3.1 Considers and responds in a timely manner to the health and wellbeing of self and others in relation to the capability for practice	Employs a variety of techniques when using cognitive and behavioural interventions in Box 25.1: Principles of cognitive functioning and behaviour, p. 537; Box 25.3: The Socratic question-and-answer format, p. 543
		3.2 Provides the information and education required to enhance people's control over health	Provides teaching to the person and families with Collaborative Care: Promoting the effectiveness of CBT with families of people with schizophrenia, p. 548
		3.3 Uses a lifelong learning approach for continuing professional development of self and others	Participates in self-awareness activities about cognitive and behavioural interventions in Self-awareness: Influence of the dominant culture on cognitive behavioural interventions, p. 549

Chapter number	Standard	Criteria (sub-standard)	Evidence-based examples (including page no.)
	6. Provides safe, appropriate and responsive quality nursing practice	6.1 Provides comprehensive, safe, quality practice to achieve agreed goals and outcomes that are responsive to the nursing needs of people	Implement strategies to cognitive and behavioural interventions in Your Intervention Strategies: Developing a behavioural contract, p. 538; Your Intervention Strategies: Desensitisation hierarchy for a phobic fear of heights, p. 541; Your Intervention Strategies: Smoking cessation behaviour modification guidance, p. 542
		6.5 Practises in accordance with relevant policies, guidelines, standards, regulations and legislation	Participates in care coordination, community-based care and home care, p. 547
26	1. Thinks critically and analyses nursing practice	1.1 Accesses, analyses and uses the best available evidence, that includes research findings, for safe, quality practice	Applies appropriate theories of crisis in Biopsychosocial theories of crisis, pp. 575–577
		1.4 Complies with legislation, regulations, policies, guidelines and other standards or requirements relevant to the context of practice when making decisions	Adheres to the National framework for recovery-oriented mental health services, p. 561
	2. Engages in therapeutic and professional relationships	2.2 Communicates effectively, and is respectful of a person's dignity, culture, values, beliefs and rights	Utilises therapeutic communication techniques in Communication: Person in crisis, p. 579; Your Intervention Strategies: Communication strategies in crisis work, p. 581
		2.4 Provides support and directs people to resources to optimise health-related decisions	Employs actions to support individuals experiencing vicarious trauma in Box 26.8 The small-group debriefing process, p. 583
		2.6 Uses delegation, supervision, coordination, consultation and referrals in professional relationships to achieve improved health outcomes	Refers to the components for personal recovery from a mental health condition in Box 26.1: National Consensus Statement on Mental Health Recovery: the 10 fundamental components of recovery, p. 560
	3. Maintains the capability for practice	3.2 Provides the information and education required to enhance people's control over health	Supports families and others who have experienced a traumatic event in Vicarious Traumatisation, pp. 582–583
		3.3 Uses a lifelong learning approach for continuing professional development of self and others	Participates in self-awareness activities as described in Box 26.3: Your experience of crisis, p. 572; Nursing self-awareness, p. 577; Self-awareness: Self-care tips for emergency and disaster response workers, p. 578
	4. Comprehensively conducts assessments	4.1 Conducts assessments that are holistic as well as culturally appropriate	Completes comprehensive assessments of persons with mental illness during their personal recovery, in Assessing needs, p. 569 Completes a comprehensive assessment of the person in crisis, in Assessment, pp. 578–579; Box 26.6: Crisis as a test of faith, p. 579

Chapter number	Standard	Criteria (sub-standard)	Evidence-based examples (including page no.)
		4.2 Uses a range of assessment techniques to systematically collect relevant and accurate information and data to inform practice	Utilises information about the recovery process to aid persons experiencing mental illness in Recovery, pp. 553–560, 561–562 Utilises information about crisis intervention in Crisis intervention, pp. 571–575; Box 26.4: Common characteristics of crises, p. 574; Box 26.5: Risk factors for crisis, p. 574
		4.3 Works in partnership to determine factors that affect, or potentially affect, the health and wellbeing of people and populations to determine priorities for action and/or for referral	Analyses the impact of hospital readmissions in Box 26.2: Why frequent re-admissions are problematic, p. 569
	5. Develops a plan for nursing practice	5.1 Uses assessment data and best available evidence to develop a plan	Creates a comprehensive plan of care for the individual during their personal recovery journey in Planning for rehabilitation and recovery, pp. 569–570 Designs a plan of care to address all aspects of the person experiencing a crisis in Supporting a person in crisis, pp. 580–582
		5.5 Coordinates resources effectively and efficiently for planned actions.	Refers individuals with mental illnesses to community programs, in Psychiatric disability, pp. 561–566
	6. Provides safe, appropriate and responsive quality nursing practice	6.1 Provides comprehensive, safe, quality practice to achieve agreed goals and outcomes that are responsive to the nursing needs of people	Encourages the use of health prevention in the care of people with mental illnesses in Psychiatric Rehabilitation, pp. 566–569; Your Intervention Strategies: Making something different happen: a scenario you can use to help people change, p. 567 Implements the plan of care of persons recovering from a mental illness in Implementing the rehabilitation and recovery plan, pp. 570–571; Table 26.1: Relapse triggers in mental disorder, p. 570 Implements a plan of care to support the person experiencing a crisis in Supporting a person in crisis, pp. 580–582; Box 26.7: Helping people to recuperate from crisis, p. 580; Table 26.2: Components of critical incident stress management (CISM), p. 582
	7. Evaluates outcomes to inform nursing practice	7.1 Evaluates and monitors progress towards the expected goals and outcomes	Evaluates the success of the psychiatric rehabilitation plan in Evaluating the rehabilitation and recovery plan, p. 571

INDEX

Page numbers followed by *f* indicate figures, and those followed by *t* indicate tables, boxes or special features. Page numbers in **bold** refer to a definition of a key term.

A

G

H

M

N

T

U

V